COMPLETE GUIDE TO PRESCRIPTION & NONPRESCRIPTION

DRUGS

By H. WINTER GRIFFITH, M.D.

Revised and Updated by Stephen W. Moore, M.D.

Technical Consultants:
Kevin Boesen, Pharm.D.
Cindy Boesen, Pharm.D.

Over 6000 Brand Names
Over 1000 Generic Names

A Perigee Book

A PERIGEE BOOK
Published by the Penguin Group
Penguin Group (USA) Inc.
375 Hudson Street, New York, New York 10014, USA

USA | Canada | UK | Ireland | Australia | New Zealand | India | South Africa | China

Penguin Books Ltd., Registered Offices: 80 Strand, London WC2R 0RL, England
For more information about the Penguin Group, visit penguin.com.

COMPLETE GUIDE TO PRESCRIPTION AND NONPRESCRIPTION DRUGS

PUBLISHING HISTORY
2014 Perigee trade paperback edition / November 2013

ISBN: 978-1-59463-197-9
ISSN: 1082-2585

PRINTED IN THE UNITED STATES OF AMERICA

10 9 8 7 6 5 4 3 2 1

Neither the publisher nor the author is engaged in rendering professional advice or services to the individual reader. The ideas, procedures, and suggestions contained in this book are not intended as a substitute for consulting with your physician. All matters regarding your health require medical supervision. Neither the author nor the publisher shall be liable or responsible for any loss or damage allegedly arising from any information or suggestion in this book.

While the author has made every effort to provide accurate telephone numbers, Internet addresses, and other contact information at the time of publication, neither the publisher nor the author assumes any responsibility for errors, or for changes that occur after publication. Further, the publisher does not have any control over and does not assume any responsibility for author or third-party websites or their content.

Most Perigee books are available at special quantity discounts for bulk purchases for sales promotions, premiums, fund-raising, or educational use. Special books, or book excerpts, can also be created to fit specific needs. For details, write: Special.Markets@us.penguingroup.com.

Contents

Drugs and You....................iv
Guide to Drug Charts....................vi
Checklist for Safer Drug Use....................xiii
Compliance with Doctors' Instructions....................xv
Cough and Cold Medicines....................xvi
Pregnancy Risk Category Information....................xviii
Buying Prescription Drugs Online....................xix
Information about Substances of Abuse....................xx
Medical Conditions and Their Commonly Used Drugs....................xxii
Drug Charts
(Alphabetized by drug generic name or drug class name)....................1
Generic and Brand Name Directory....................862
Additional Drug Interactions....................898
Glossary....................931
Index
(Generic names, brand names and class names)....................957
Emergency Guide for Overdose Victims....................1088
Emergency Guide for Anaphylaxis Victims....................1090

About the Author

H. Winter Griffith, M.D., authored 25 medical books, including the *Complete Guide to Symptoms, Illness & Surgery* and *Complete Guide to Sports Injuries*, each published by The Body Press/Perigee Books. Others include *Instructions for Patients; Drug Information for Patients; Instructions for Dental Patients; Information and Instructions for Pediatric Patients; Vitamins, Minerals and Supplements;* and *Complete Guide to Medical Tests*. Dr. Griffith received his medical degree from Emory University in Atlanta, Georgia. After 20 years in private practice, he established and was the first director of a basic medical science program at Florida State University. He then became an associate professor of Family and Community Medicine at the University of Arizona College of Medicine. Until his death in 1993, Dr. Griffith lived in Tucson, Arizona.

Editor

Stephen Moore, M.D.
Family physician, Tucson, Arizona

Technical Consultants

Kevin Boesen, Pharm.D.
Clinical Assistant Professor, College of Pharmacy, University of Arizona

Cindy Boesen, Pharm.D.
Clinical Instructor, College of Pharmacy, University of Arizona

Technical Editor

Jo A. Griffith

Drugs and You

What is in This Book

The purpose of this book is to give you information about the most widely used drugs (prescription and nonprescription). The information is derived from many authoritative sources and represents the consensus of many experts. Every effort has been made to ensure accuracy and completeness. However, because drug information is constantly changing, you should always talk to your doctor or pharmacist if you have any questions or concerns.

The information applies to generic drugs in both the United States and Canada. Generic names do not vary in these countries, but brand names do. Each year, new drug charts are added and existing charts are updated when appropriate. For the most part, drugs that are injected by a medical professional, used mainly in a hospital (or medical clinic) or have rare usage are not included.

A drug cannot "cure." It aids the body's natural defenses to promote recovery. Likewise, a manufacturer or doctor cannot guarantee a drug will help every person. The complexity of the human body, individual responses in different people and in the same person under different circumstances, past and present health, age and gender impact how well a drug works.

All effective drugs produce desirable changes in the body, but can also cause undesirable adverse reactions or side effects. Before you decide whether to take a drug, you or your doctor must decide, "Will the benefits outweigh the risks?"

In the United States, it is the responsibility of the Food and Drug Administration (FDA) to ensure that drugs are safe and effective. For more information, you may contact the FDA at 1-888-INFO-FDA or visit the website: www.fda.gov.

Your Role

Learn the generic names and brand names of all your medicines. For example, acetaminophen is the generic name for the brand Tylenol. Write them down to help you remember. If a drug is a combination, learn the names of its generic ingredients.

Filling a Prescription

Once a prescription is written you may purchase the medication from various sources. Pharmacies are usually located in a drug or grocery store. You may need to consider your options: Does your health insurance limit where prescriptions can be filled? Is the location convenient? Does the pharmacy maintain patient records and are the employees helpful and willing to answer drug related questions?

Insurance companies or an HMO (Health Maintenance Organization) may specify certain pharmacies. Some insurance companies have chosen a mail-order pharmacy. Normally a prescription is sent to the mail-order pharmacy or phoned in by the physician. Mail order is best used for maintenance (long-term medications). Short-term medications such as antibiotics should be purchased at a local pharmacy.

Once a pharmacy has been chosen it is best to stay with that one so an accurate drug history can be maintained. The pharmacist can more easily check for drug interactions that may be potentially harmful to the patient or decrease the efficacy of one or more of the medications.

You can phone the pharmacy for a refill. Provide the prescription number, name of medication, and name of the patient.

Taking A Drug

Read the instructions provided with the drug and follow all directions for taking or using it.

Never take medicine in the dark! Recheck the label before each use. You could be taking the wrong drug!

Tell your doctor about any unexpected new symptoms you have while taking or using a drug. You may need to change drugs or have a dose adjustment.

Storage

Keep all medicines out of children's reach and in childproof containers. Store drugs in a cool, dry place, such as a kitchen cabinet or bedroom. Avoid medicine cabinets in bathrooms. They get too moist and warm at times.

Keep medicine in its original container, tightly closed. Don't remove the label! If directions call for refrigeration, keep the medicine cool, but don't freeze it.

Discarding

Don't save leftover medicine to use later. Discard it on or before the expiration date shown on the container. Dispose safely to protect children and pets. See page xiv.

Alertness

Many of the medicines used to treat disorders may alter your alertness. If you drive, work around machinery, or must avoid sedation, discuss the problem with your doctor; usually there are ways (e.g., the time of day you take the medicine) to manage the problem.

Alcohol & Medications

Alcohol and drugs of abuse defeat the purpose of many medications. For example, alcohol causes depression; if you drink and are depressed, antidepressants will not relieve the depression. If you have a problem with drinking or drugs, discuss it with your doctor. There are ways to help.

Learn About Drugs

Study the information in this book's charts regarding your medications. Read each chart completely. Because of space limitations, most information that fits more than one category appears only once. Any time you are prescribed a new medication, read the information on the chart for that drug, then take the time to review the charts on other medications you already take. Read any instruction sheets or printed warnings provided by your doctor or pharmacist.

Drug Advertising

Ads can cause confusion. Be sure and get sufficient information about any drug you think may help you. Ask your doctor or pharmacist.

Be Safe! Tell Your Doctor

Some suggestions for wise drug use apply to all drugs. Always give your doctor, dentist, or healthcare provider complete information about the drugs and supplements you take, including your medical history, your medical plans and your progress while under medication.

Medical History

Tell the important facts of your medical history including illness and previous experience with drugs. Include allergic or adverse reactions you have had to any medicine or other substance in the past. Describe the allergic symptoms you have, such as hay fever, asthma, eye watering and itching, throat irritation and reactions to food. People who have allergies to common substances are more likely to develop drug allergies.

List all drugs you take. Don't forget vitamin and mineral supplements; skin, rectal or vaginal medicines; eyedrops and eardrops; antacids; antihistamines; cold and cough remedies; inhalants and nasal sprays; aspirin, aspirin combinations or other pain relievers; motion sickness remedies; weight-loss aids; salt and sugar substitutes; caffeine; oral contraceptives; sleeping pills; laxatives; "tonics" or herbal preparations.

Future Medical Plans

Discuss plans for elective surgery (including dental surgery), pregnancy and breast-feeding. These conditions may require discontinuing or modifying the dosages of medicines you may be taking.

Questions

Don't hesitate to ask questions about a drug. Your doctor or pharmacist will be able to provide helpful information if they are familiar with you and your medical history.

Guide to Drug Charts

The drug information in this book is organized in condensed, easy-to-read charts. Each drug is described in a two-page format, as shown in the sample chart below and opposite. Charts are arranged alphabetically by drug generic names, such as ACETAMINOPHEN or by drug class name, such as ANTIHISTAMINES.

A generic name is the official chemical name for a drug. A brand name is a drug manufacturer's registered trademark for a generic drug. Brand names listed on the charts include those from the United States

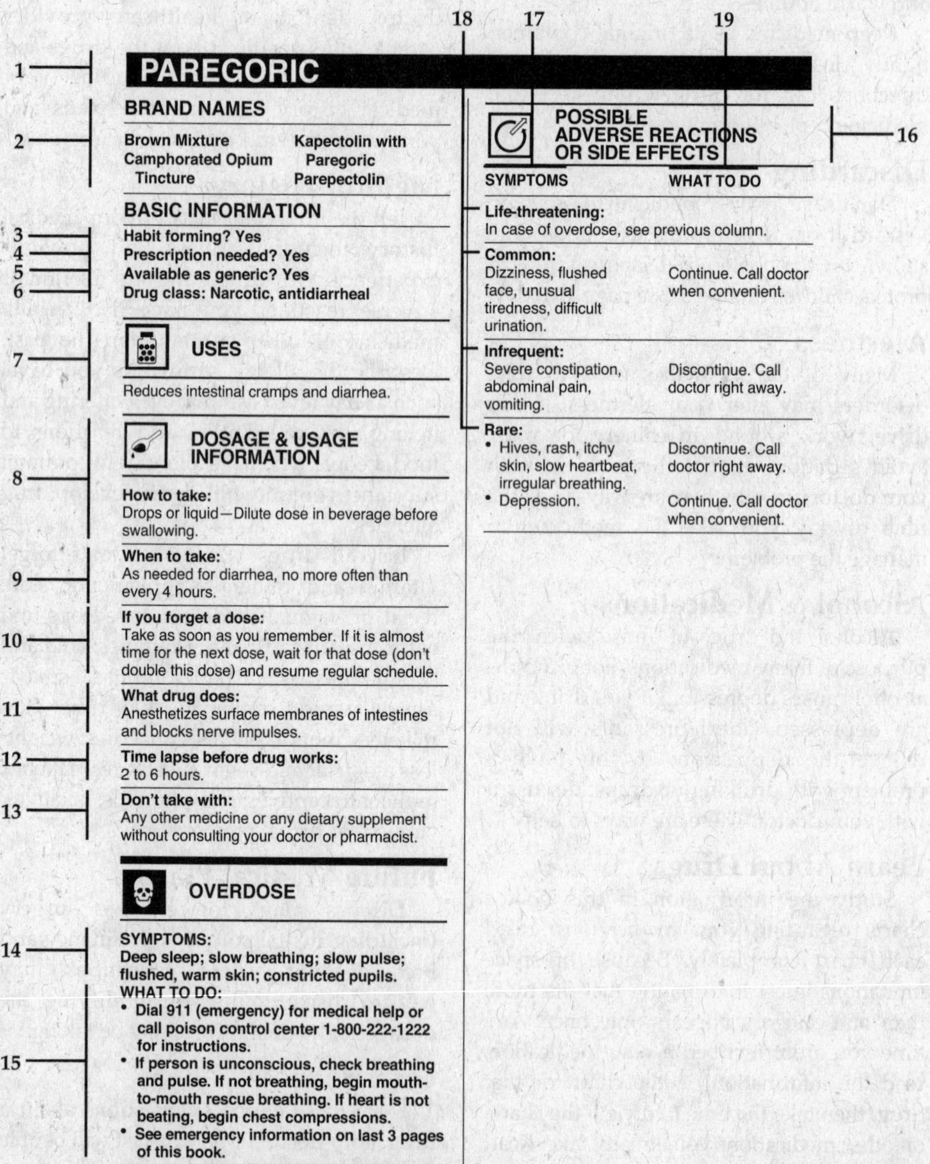

and Canada. A generic drug may have one, a few, or many brand names.

To find information about a generic drug, look it up in the index. To learn about a brand name, check the index, where each brand name is followed by the name(s) of its generic ingredients and their chart page number(s).

The chart design is the same for every drug. When you are familiar with the chart, you can quickly find information you want to know about a drug.

On the next few pages, each of the numbered chart sections below is explained. This information will guide you in reading and understanding the charts that begin on page 2.

PAREGORIC

20 **WARNINGS & PRECAUTIONS**

21 **Don't take if:**
You are allergic to any narcotic.*

22 **Before you start, consult your doctor if:**
You have impaired liver or kidney function.

23 **Over age 60:**
More likely to be drowsy, dizzy, unsteady or constipated.

24 **Pregnancy:**
Risk factor varies with length of pregnancy. See category list on page xviii and consult doctor.

25 **Breast-feeding:**
Drug filters into milk. May depress infant. Avoid.

26 **Infants & children:**
Use only under medical supervision.

27 **Prolonged use:**
Causes psychological and physical dependence.

28 **Skin & sunlight:**
No problems expected.

29 **Driving, piloting or hazardous work:**
Don't drive or pilot aircraft until you learn how medicine affects you. Don't work around dangerous machinery. Don't climb ladders or work in high places. Danger increases if you drink alcohol or take medicine affecting alertness and reflexes, such as antihistamines, tranquilizers, sedatives, pain medicine, narcotics and mind-altering drugs.

30 **Discontinuing:**
May be unnecessary to finish medicine. Follow doctor's instructions.

31 **Others:**
Great potential for abuse.

POSSIBLE INTERACTION WITH OTHER DRUGS 32

GENERIC NAME OR DRUG CLASS	COMBINED EFFECT
Analgesics*	Increased analgesic effect.
Anticholinergics*	Increased risk of constipation.
Antidepressants*	Increased sedation.
Antidiarrheal preparations*	Increased sedative effect. Avoid.
Antihistamines*	Increased sedation.
Central nervous system (CNS) depressants*	Increased central nerve system depression.
Naloxone	Decreased paregoric effect.
Naltrexone	Decreased paregoric effect.
Narcotics,* other	Increased narcotic effect.

POSSIBLE INTERACTION WITH OTHER SUBSTANCES 33

INTERACTS WITH	COMBINED EFFECT
Alcohol:	Increases alcohol's intoxicating effect. Avoid.
Beverages:	None expected.
Cocaine:	None expected.
Foods:	None expected.
Marijuana:	Impairs physical and mental performance.
Tobacco:	None expected.

1—Generic or Class Name

Each drug chart is titled by generic name or by the name of the drug class, such as DIGITALIS PREPARATIONS.

All drugs have a generic name. These generic names are the same worldwide. Sometimes a drug is known by more than one generic name. The chart is titled by the most common one. Less common generic names appear in parentheses. For example, vitamin C is also known as ascorbic acid. Its chart title is VITAMIN C (Ascorbic Acid). The index will include both names.

Your drug container may show a generic name, a brand name or both. If you have only a brand name, use the index to find the drug's generic name(s) and chart page number(s).

If your drug container shows no name, ask your doctor or pharmacist for the name and write it on the container.

2—Brand Names

A brand name is usually shorter and easier to remember than the generic name. The brand name is selected by the drug manufacturer

The brand names listed for each generic drug in this book do not include all brands available in the United States and Canada. The more common names are listed. New brands appear on the market, and brands are sometimes removed from the market. No list can reflect every change. In the instances in which the drug chart is titled with a drug class name instead of a generic name, the generic and brand names all appear under the heading GENERIC AND BRAND NAMES. The GENERIC NAMES are in capital letters and the BRAND NAMES are in lower-case letters.

Inclusion of a brand name does not imply recommendation or endorsement. Exclusion does not imply that a missing brand name is less effective or less safe than the ones listed. Some drug charts have too many generic and brand names to list on the page. A complete list is on the page indicated on the chart.

Lists of brand names don't differentiate between prescription and nonprescription drugs. The active ingredients are the same.

If you buy a nonprescription drug, look for generic names of the active ingredients on the container. Common nonprescription drugs are described in this book under their generic components. Many are also listed in the index by brand name.

Most drugs contain inert, or inactive, ingredients that are fillers, dyes or solvents for the active ingredients. Manufacturers choose inert ingredients that preserve the drug without interfering with the action of the active ingredients.

Inert substances are listed on labels of nonprescription drugs. They do not appear on prescription drugs. Your pharmacist can tell you all active and inert ingredients in a prescription drug.

Occasionally, a tablet, capsule or liquid may contain small amounts of sodium, sugar or potassium. If you are on a diet that severely restricts any of these, ask your pharmacist or doctor to suggest another form.

Some liquid medications contain alcohol. Avoid them if you are susceptible to the adverse effects of alcohol consumption.

BASIC INFORMATION

3—Habit Forming?

Yes—means the drug is capable of leading to physical and/or psychological dependence.

Physical dependence includes tolerance (requiring larger dosages or repeated use) and withdrawal symptoms (mental and physical) when it is stopped.

Psychological dependence involves repeated use of a drug to bring about effects that are pleasurable or satisfying, or it reduces undesirable feelings.

4—Prescription Needed?

Yes—means a doctor must prescribe the drug for you. "No" means you can buy the drug without prescription. Sometimes low strengths of a drug are available without prescription, while higher strengths require prescription.

The information about the drug applies whether it requires prescription or not. If the generic ingredients are the same, nonprescription drugs have the same dangers, warnings, precautions and interactions as prescription drugs. A nonprescription (over-the-counter) drug has dosing and other instructions printed on the container label. Always read them carefully before you take the drug. The information and warnings on containers for nonprescription drugs may not be as complete as the information in this book. Check both sources.

5—Available as Generic?

Some drugs have patent restrictions that protect the manufacturer or distributor of that drug. These drugs may be purchased only by a specific brand name.

Drugs purchased by generic name are usually less expensive than brand names. Once the patent expires, other drug companies can sell that particular drug. They will choose their own brand name.

Some states allow pharmacists to fill a prescription by brand name or generic name (if one is available). This allows patients to buy the least expensive form of a drug.

A doctor may specify a brand name because he or she trusts a known source more than an unknown manufacturer of generic drugs. You and your doctor should decide together whether you should buy a medicine by generic name or brand name.

Generic drugs manufactured in other countries are not subject to regulation by the U.S. Food and Drug Administration. All drugs manufactured in the United States are subject to regulation.

6—Drug Class

Drugs that possess similar chemical structures or similar therapeutic effects are grouped into classes. Most drugs within a class produce similar benefits, side effects, adverse reactions and interactions with other drugs and substances. For example, all the generic drugs in the narcotic drug class will have similar effects on the body.

Some information on the charts applies to all drugs in a class. The index lists the classes (such as narcotics) and lists the drug charts in that class.

Names for classes of drugs are not standardized; class names listed in other references may vary from the class names in this book.

7— Uses

This section lists the disease or disorder for which a drug is prescribed.

Most uses listed are approved by the U.S. Food and Drug Administration. Some uses are listed if experiments and clinical trials indicate effectiveness and safety. Still, other uses are included that may not be officially sanctioned, but for which doctors may prescribe the drug.

The use for which your doctor prescribes the drug may not appear. You and your doctor should discuss the reason for any prescription medicine you take. You alone will probably decide whether to take a nonprescription drug. This section may help you make a wise decision.

DOSAGE & USAGE INFORMATION

8—How To Take

Drugs are available in forms of tablets, capsules, chewables, liquids, powders, thin film, specialty tablets, suppositories, injections, transdermal patches (used on the skin), aerosol inhalants and topical forms such as drops, sprays, creams, gels, ointments and lotions. This section gives brief instructions for taking or using each form.

The information here supplements the drug label information. If your doctor's instructions differ from these suggestions, follow your doctor's instructions.

Instructions are left out for how much to take. Dose amounts can't be generalized. Dosages of prescription drugs must be individualized for you by your doctor. Be sure the dosage instructions are on the label. Advice to "take as directed" is not helpful if you forget the doctor's instructions or didn't understand them. Nonprescription drugs have instructions on the labels regarding how much to take.

9—When To Take

Dose schedules vary for medicines and for patients.

Drugs prescribed on a schedule should usually be taken at approximately the same times each day. Some must be taken at regular intervals to maintain a steady level of the drug in the body. If the schedule interferes with your sleep, consult your doctor.

Instructions to take on an empty stomach mean the drug is absorbed best in your body this way. Other drugs must be taken with liquid or food because they irritate the stomach.

Instructions for other dose schedules are usually on the label. Variations in standard dose schedules may apply because some medicines interact with others if you take them at the same time.

10—If You Forget a Dose

Suggestions in this section vary from drug to drug. Most tell you when to resume taking the medicine if you forget a scheduled dose.

Establish good habits so you won't forget doses. Forgotten doses decrease a drug's therapeutic effect.

11—What Drug Does

This is a simple description of the drug's action in the body. The wording is generalized and may not be a complete explanation of the complex chemical process that takes place. For some drugs, the method of action is unknown.

12—Time Lapse Before Drug Works

The times given are approximations. Times vary a great deal from person to person, and from time to time in the same person. The figures give you some idea of when to expect improvement or side effects.

13—Don't Take With

Some drugs create problems when taken in combination with other substances. Most problems are detailed in the Interaction section of each chart.

Occasionally, an interaction is singled out if the combination is particularly harmful.

OVERDOSE

14—Symptoms

The symptoms listed are most likely to develop with accidental or purposeful overdose. Overdosage may not cause all symptoms listed. Sometimes symptoms are identical to ones listed as side effects. The difference is intensity and severity. You will have to judge. Consult a doctor or poison control center if you have any doubt.

15—What To Do

If you suspect an overdose, whether symptoms are apparent or not, get medical help or advice, and if needed, follow instructions in this section. Additional instructions for emergency treatment for overdose are at the end of the book.

16—Possible Adverse Reactions or Side Effects

Adverse reactions or side effects are symptoms that may occur when you take a drug. They are effects on the body other than the desired therapeutic effect.

The term side effects implies expected and usually unavoidable effects of a drug. Side effects have nothing to do with the drug's intended use.

For example, the generic drug paregoric reduces intestinal cramps and vomiting. It also often causes a flushed face. The flushing is a side effect that is harmless and does not affect the drug's therapeutic potential. Many side effects disappear in a short time without treatment.

The term adverse reaction is more significant. For example, paregoric can cause a serious adverse allergic reaction in some people. This reaction can include hives, rash and severe itch.

Some adverse reactions can be prevented, which is one reason this information is included in the book. Most adverse reactions are minor and last only a short time. With many drugs, adverse reactions that might occur will frequently diminish in intensity as your body adjusts to the medicine.

The majority of drugs, used properly for valid reasons, offer benefits that outweigh potential hazards.

17—Symptoms

Symptoms of commonly known side effects and adverse reactions are listed. Other drug responses may be listed under "Prolonged Use," "Skin & Sunlight" or "Others." You may experience a symptom that is not listed. It may be a side effect or adverse reaction to the drug, or it may be an additional symptom of the illness. If you are unsure, call your doctor.

18—Frequency

This is an estimation of how often symptoms occur in persons who take the drug. The four most common categories of frequency can be found under the SYMPTOMS heading and are as follows: Life-threatening means exactly what it says; seek emergency treatment immediately. Common means these symptoms are expected and sometimes inevitable. Infrequent means the symptoms occur in approximately 1% to 10% of patients. Rare means symptoms occur in fewer than 1%.

19—What To Do

Follow the guidelines provided opposite the symptoms that apply to you. These are general instructions. If you are concerned or confused, always call your doctor.

20— Warnings & Precautions

Read these entries to determine special information that applies to you.

21—Don't Take If

This section lists circumstances when drug use is not safe. On some drug labels and in formal medical literature, these circumstances are called contraindications.

22—Before You Start, Consult Your Doctor If

This section lists conditions, especially disease conditions, under which a drug should be used only with caution and medical supervision.

23—Over Age 60

As a person ages, physical changes occur that require special considerations. Liver and kidney functions decrease, metabolism slows and the prostate gland enlarges in men.

Most drugs are metabolized or excreted at a rate dependent on kidney and liver functions. Smaller doses or longer intervals between doses may be necessary to prevent unhealthy concentration of a drug. Toxic effects and adverse reactions occur more frequently and cause more serious problems in older people.

24—Pregnancy

The best rule to follow during pregnancy is to avoid all drugs, including tobacco and alcohol. Any medicine—prescription or nonprescription—requires medical advice and supervision.

This section will alert you if there is evidence that a drug harms the unborn child. Lack of evidence does not guarantee a drug's safety.

The definitions of the pregnancy risk categories of drugs used by the Food and Drug Administration (FDA) are listed on page xviii.

25—Breast-feeding

Many drugs filter into a mother's milk. Some drugs have dangerous or unwanted effects on the nursing infant. This section suggests ways to minimize harm to the child.

26—Infants & Children

Many drugs carry special warnings and precautions for children because of a child's size and immaturity. In medical terminology, newborns are babies up to 2 weeks old, infants are 2 weeks to 1 year, and children are 1 to 12 years.

27—Prolonged Use

With the exception of immediate allergic reactions, most drugs produce no ill effects during short periods of treatment. However, relatively safe drugs taken for long periods may produce unwanted effects. These are listed. Drugs should be taken in the smallest doses and for the shortest time possible. Nevertheless, some diseases and conditions require a prolonged or even lifelong period of treatment. Therefore, follow-up medical examinations and laboratory tests recommended when a drug is used for long periods are listed. Your doctor may want to change drugs occasionally or alter your treatment regimen to minimize problems.

The words "functional dependence" sometimes appear in this section. This does not mean physical or psychological addiction. Sometimes a body function ceases to work naturally because it has been replaced or interfered with by the drug. The body then becomes dependent on the drug to continue the function.

28—Skin & Sunlight

Many drugs cause photosensitivity, which means increased skin sensitivity to ultraviolet rays from sunlight or artificial rays from a sunlamp. This section will alert you to this potential problem.

29—Driving, Piloting or Hazardous Work

Any drug that alters moods or that decreases alertness, muscular coordination or reflexes may make these activities particularly hazardous. The effects may not appear in all people, or they may disappear after a short exposure to the drug. If this section contains a warning, use caution until you determine how a new drug affects you.

30—Discontinuing

This section gives special warnings about discontinuing a drug.

Some patients stop taking a drug when symptoms begin to go away, although complete recovery may require longer treatment.

Other patients continue taking a drug when it is no longer needed.

Some drugs cause symptoms days or weeks after they have been discontinued.

31—Others

Warnings and precautions appear here if they don't fit into the other categories. This section includes special instructions, reminders, storage instructions, warnings to persons with chronic illness and other information.

32—Possible Interaction With Other Drugs

People often must take two or more drugs at the same time. Many of these drug combinations have the potential to interact adversely. Fortunately, this adverse reaction occurs in only a small proportion of people who take the interacting combinations. Drugs interact in your body with other drugs, whether prescription or nonprescription. Interactions affect absorption, metabolism, elimination or distribution of either drug. Other factors that can influence drug interactions are the patient's age, state of health and the way the drugs are administered: Time taken, how taken, dosage, dosage forms and duration of treatment. The chart lists interactions by generic name, drug class or drug-induced effect. An asterisk (*) in this column reminds you to "See Glossary" in the back of the book, where that entry is further explained.

If a drug class appears, the drug you are looking up may interact with any drug in that class. Drugs in each class that are included in the book are listed in the index. Occasionally drugs that are not included in this book appear in the Interaction column.

Interactions are sometimes beneficial. You may not be able to determine from the chart which interactions are good and which are bad. Don't guess. Consult your doctor or pharmacist if you take drugs that interact. Some combinations can be fatal.

Some drugs have too many interactions to list on one chart. The additional interactions appear on the continuation page indicated at the bottom of the list.

Testing has not been done on all possible drug combinations. It is important to let your doctor or pharmacist know about any drugs you take, both prescription and nonprescription.

33— Possible Interaction With Other Substances

The substances listed here are repeated on every drug chart. All people eat food and drink beverages. Many adults consume alcohol. Some people use cocaine and/or smoke tobacco or marijuana. This section shows possible interactions between these substances and each drug.

Checklist for Safer Drug Use

- Tell your doctor about any drug you take (even aspirin, allergy pills, cough and cold preparations, antacids, laxatives, herbal preparations, vitamins, etc.) before you take any new drug.
- Learn all you can about drugs you may take *before* you take them. Information sources are your doctor, your nurse, your pharmacist, this book, other books in your public library and the Internet.
- Keep an up-to-date list of all the medicines you take in a wallet or purse. Include name, dose and frequency.
- Don't take drugs prescribed for someone else—even if your symptoms are the same.
- Keep your prescription drugs to yourself. Your drugs may be harmful to someone else.
- Tell your doctor about any symptoms you believe are caused by a drug—prescription or nonprescription—that you take.
- Take only medicines that are *necessary*. Avoid taking nonprescription drugs while taking prescription drugs for a medical problem.
- Before your doctor prescribes for you, tell him about your previous experiences with any drug—beneficial results, side effects, adverse reactions or allergies.
- Take medicine in good light after you have identified it. If you wear glasses to read, put them on to check drug labels. It is easy to take the wrong drug or take a drug at the wrong time.
- Don't keep any drugs that change mood, alertness or judgment—such as sedatives, narcotics or tranquilizers—by your

bedside. These can cause accidental deaths. You may unknowingly repeat a dose when you are half asleep or confused.

- Know the names of your medicines. These include the generic name, the brand name and the generic names of all ingredients in a combination drug. Your doctor, nurse or pharmacist can give you this information.
- Study the labels on all nonprescription drugs. If the information is incomplete or if you have questions, ask the pharmacist for more details.
- If you must deviate from your prescribed dose schedule, tell your doctor.
- Shake liquid medicines before taking (if directed).
- Store all medicines away from moisture and heat. Bathroom medicine cabinets are usually unsuitable.
- If a drug needs refrigeration, don't freeze.
- Obtain a standard measuring spoon from your pharmacy for liquid medicines. Kitchen teaspoons and tablespoons are not accurate enough.
- Follow diet instructions when you take medicines. Some work better on a full stomach, others on an empty stomach. Some drugs are more useful with special diets. For example, medicine for high blood pressure may be more effective if accompanied by a sodium-restricted diet.
- Tell your doctor about any allergies you have to any substance (e.g., food) or adverse reactions to medicines you've had in the past. A previous allergy to a drug may make it dangerous to prescribe again. People with other allergies, such as eczema, hay fever, asthma, bronchitis and food allergies, are more likely to be allergic to drugs.
- Prior to surgery, tell your doctor, anesthesiologist or dentist about any drug you have taken in the past few weeks. Advise them of any cortisone drugs you have taken within two years.
- If you become pregnant while taking any medicine, including birth control pills, tell your doctor immediately.
- Avoid *all* drugs while you are pregnant, if possible. If you must take drugs during pregnancy, record names, amounts, dates and reasons.
- If you see more than one doctor, tell each one about drugs others have prescribed.
- When you use nonprescription drugs, report it so the information is on your medical record.
- Store all drugs away from the reach of children.
- Note the expiration date on each drug label. Discard outdated ones safely. If no expiration date appears and it has been at least one year since taking the medication, it may be best to discard it. Follow any specific disposal instructions on the drug label or patient information that came with the medication. Do not flush prescription drugs down the toilet unless this information specifically instructs you to do so. If no instructions are given, throw the drugs in the household trash, but first: Take them out of their original containers and mix them with an undesirable substance, such as used coffee grounds or kitty litter. Alternatively, check if local household hazardous-waste collection programs—where you're supposed to take motor oil and batteries—accept expired medicines.
- Pay attention to the information in the drug charts about safety while driving, piloting or working in dangerous places.
- Alcohol, cocaine, marijuana or other mood-altering drugs, as well as tobacco—mixed with some drugs—can cause a life-threatening interaction, prevent your medicine from being effective or delay your return to health. Be sure that you avoid them during illness.
- Some medications are subject to theft. For example, a repair person in your home who is abusing drugs may ask to use your bathroom, and while there "check

out" your medicine cabinet. Sedatives, stimulants and analgesics are especially likely to be stolen, but almost any medication is subject to theft.

- If possible, use the same pharmacy for all your medications. Every pharmacy keeps a "drug profile," and if it is complete, the pharmacist may stop medications that are likely to cause serious interactions. Also, having a record of all your medications in one place helps your doctor or an emergency room doctor get a complete picture in case of an emergency.

- If you have a complicated medical history or a condition that might render you unable to communicate (e.g., diabetes or epilepsy), wear some type of medical identification (small tag, bracelet, neck chain or other) to identify your condition. (The MedicAlert Corporation provides this type of product. Call 888-633-4298 or go online www.medicalert.org for information.) Some people carry a wallet card with the information. A newer type of medical alert ID is the USB tag. It is basically a USB flash drive that contains a person's medical emergency information and can store much more information if desired. Emergency medical people can access the information using any available computer.

- If you are giving medicine to children, read all instructions carefully. Use the specific dosing device (dropper, cup, etc.) that comes with the product. Don't exceed recommended dose. It does not help and can cause health risks.

- Ask your pharmacist if they will provide an extra, prescription-labeled small bottle or container to use for one or two doses of your medication. It can be used when going out for a meal, during short trips or for a student in school. This avoids carrying all your medications with you.

Compliance with Doctors' Instructions

For medical purposes, compliance is defined as the extent to which a patient follows the instructions of a doctor and includes taking medications on schedule, keeping appointments and following directions for changes in lifestyle, such as changing one's diet or exercise.

Although the cost of obtaining medical advice and medication is one of the largest items in a family budget, many people defeat the health-care process by departing from the doctor's recommendations. This failure to carry out the doctor's instructions is the single most common cause of treatment failure. Perhaps the instructions were not presented clearly, or you may not have understood them or realized their importance and benefits.

Factors That Can Cause Problems With Compliance:

- Treatment recommendations that combine two or more actions (such as instructions to take medication, see a therapist and join a support group).
- Recommendations that require lifestyle changes (such as dieting).
- Recommendations that involve long-term treatment (such as taking a medication for life).
- Recommendations for very young patients or for the elderly (when another person has to be responsible for following the instructions).
- Other factors include traveling and time changes, busy work schedules and lack of organization.

Examples of Noncompliance:

- Medications are forgotten or discontinued too soon. Forgetting to take a medication is the most common of all shortcomings, especially if a medication must be taken more than once a day. If you need to take a medication several times a day, set out a week's supply in an inexpensive pill box that you can carry with you.

- Side effects of medications are a common problem. Almost all medications have some unpleasant side effects. Often these disappear after a few days, but if they don't, let your doctor know right away. Side effects can often be controlled by changing dosage, switching to a similar medication or by adding medications that control the side effects.
- Not taking a drug because it is unpleasant (e.g., bad tasting). Ask your doctor about options.
- Cost is another reason why there are treatment failures. Because of a tight budget, a person may take a medication less frequently than prescribed or just not purchase it. If you can't afford a medication, perhaps a less costly one can be prescribed or your doctor can find other ways to provide it.
- Laboratory tests, x-rays or other recommended medical studies are not obtained, perhaps due to concerns about costs or fear of the tests themselves.
- Recommendations about behavioral changes such as diet or exercise are ignored (old habits are difficult for anyone to change).
- Suggested immunizations are not obtained, sometimes due to fear of needles.
- Follow-up visits to the doctor are not made, or appointments are canceled, perhaps due to problems finding transportation or long waiting times in the doctor's office.

Communicating With Your Doctor:

- If you don't understand something, ask.
- If there are reasons why you cannot follow a recommendation, speak up.
- If you have reservations or fears about treatment, discuss them.

Remember, it is your health and your money that are at issue. You and your doctor are—or should be—working together to make you well and keep you healthy.

Cough and Cold Medicines

There are hundreds of nonprescription (over-the-counter or OTC) drugs available to treat symptoms of the common cold and other minor respiratory illnesses.

Some of these drugs contain a single active ingredient that relieves one specific symptom (such as a cough). Other drugs contain combinations of two or more ingredients intended to relieve a number of different symptoms (such as a cough, stuffy nose and pain).

Each of the active ingredients in a drug has a generic (or chemical) name. Generics are names such as acetaminophen, ibuprofen, aspirin, pseudoephedrine, guaifenesin, diphenhydramine and others.

Cough and cold drugs can be sorted into five categories (or classes). They include:

Antihistamines dry up secretions of the respiratory tract and help control allergy symptoms. Antihistamines may cause drowsiness, slow reflexes and decrease ability to concentrate. Therefore, don't drive vehicles or pilot aircraft until you learn how this medicine affects you. Don't work around dangerous machinery. Don't climb ladders or work in high places. The danger increases if you drink alcohol or take other medicines that affect alertness and reflexes. Antihistamines can cause other side effects or adverse reactions.

Decongestants relieve symptoms of nasal or bronchial congestion. Decongestants may cause nervousness, irregular heartbeats in some people, dizziness, confusion and other side effects. Conduct your daily activities with these effects in mind.

Antitussives (Cough suppressants) reduce the frequency and severity of a cough. These may be either narcotic (e.g., codeine and hydrocodone) or non-narcotic (e.g., dextromethorphan or carbetapentane). Narcotic cough suppressants are habit-forming and may cause some of the same mental changes that can take place with antihistamines. The most common non-narcotic antitussive medicine, dextromethorphan, is not habit-forming but has other side effects. Carbetapentane is similar (but not covered in this book).

Expectorants loosen secretions to make them easier to cough up. The most common expectorant is guaifenesin, which has very few side effects.

Analgesics relieve aches, pains and fever. Common analgesics in cough and cold medicines are aspirin, acetaminophen and ibuprofen.

These nonprescription drugs are generally recognized as safe, but they do have side effects, possible interactions with other drugs, and need to be used with caution in certain individuals.

There is no drug that will cure a cold (including antibiotics). If you decide to take a drug for specific symptoms, a single ingredient one is usually a better choice, unless each of the drug's ingredients is necessary to relieve your particular symptoms. Before taking a drug, read the label and follow all the directions. Also, read the information in this book about the drug's generic ingredients. To find information about a drug:

- Look on the label for the generic ingredients that are in the drug product.
- Consult the index for each generic name and find the page number for its drug chart. Then look up each drug chart. Read all the information, especially regarding the adverse reactions and side effects, precautions, and interactions with other drugs you may be taking.

Always consult a doctor if any cold symptoms cause you concern.

Practice prevention—wash your hands often and keep your hands away from your face.

Nonprescription cough and cold drugs in children

- Read the label to be sure it is approved for your child's age. Labels advise you not to use these medicines in children under age 4. Do not give children medications labeled only for adults.

- Choose nonprescription cough and cold medicines with child-resistant safety caps, when available. After using, make sure to close the cap tightly and store the medicine out of the sight and reach of children.

- Check the "active ingredients" section of the DRUG FACTS label of the medicines that you choose. This will help you know what symptoms the "active ingredients" in the medicine are intended to treat.

- Be careful about giving more than one medicine to a child. If you do, make sure they do not have the same type of "active ingredients." If you use two medicines that have the same or similar active ingredients, a child could get too much of an ingredient and that may hurt your child.

- Carefully follow the directions for how to use the medicine in the DRUG FACTS part of the label. The directions tell you how much medicine to give and how often you can give it. If you have a question about how to use the medicine, ask your pharmacist or doctor. Overuse or misuse of these products can lead to serious and potentially life threatening side effects.

- Only use measuring devices that come with the medicine or those specially made for measuring drugs.. Do not use common household spoons to measure medicines for children because household spoons come in different sizes and are not meant for measuring medicines.

- Understand that using nonprescription cough and cold medicines does not cure the cold or cough. These medicines only treat the symptom(s) such as runny nose, congestion, fever and aches. They do not shorten the length of time your child is sick.

Pregnancy Risk Category Information

The pregnancy risk category assigned to a medication identifies the potential risk for that particular drug to cause birth defects or death to an unborn child (fetus). These categories are assigned by applying the definitions of the Food and Drug Administration (FDA) to the available clinical information about the drug. Most drugs are tested only on animals and not on humans for safety during pregnancy, because such testing would subject unborn children to unnecessary risks.

It is best to avoid all drugs during pregnancy, but this rating system can help you and your doctor to assess the risk-to-benefit ratio should drug treatment become necessary. You and your doctor should discuss these benefits and risks carefully before any drug treatment is initiated. You should not take any medications (including nonprescription drugs such as laxatives or cold remedies) without your doctor's approval.

A brief explanation and the definitions of the drug categories, labeled A, B, C, D, and X, are listed below:

- A: *No evidence of risk exists.* Adequate and well-controlled studies in pregnant women have not shown an increased risk of fetal abnormalities.
- B: *The risk of fetal harm is possible but remote.* Animal studies have revealed no evidence of harm to the fetus; however, there are no adequate and well-controlled studies in pregnant women, or animal studies have shown an adverse effect, but adequate and well-controlled studies in pregnant women have failed to demonstrate a risk to the fetus.
- C: *Fetal risk can't be ruled out.* Animal studies have shown an adverse effect, and there are no adequate and well-controlled studies in pregnant women, or no animal studies have been conducted, and there are no adequate and well-controlled studies in pregnant women.
- D: *Positive evidence of fetal risk exists, but, potential benefits from the drug may outweigh the risk. For example, the drug may be acceptable in a life-threatening situation or serious disease if safer drugs can't be used or are ineffective.* Adequate well-controlled or observational studies in pregnant women have demonstrated a risk to the fetus.
- X: *Contraindicated during pregnancy.* Adequate well-controlled or observational studies in animals or pregnant women have demonstrated positive evidence of fetal abnormalities. The use of the product is contraindicated in women who are or who may become pregnant.
- NR: Not rated.

Buying Prescription Drugs Online

The Food and Drug Administration (FDA) offers these suggestions. When it comes to buying medicine online, it is important to be very careful. Some websites sell medicine that may not be safe to use and could put your health at risk.

• Some websites that sell medicine:

1. Aren't U.S. state-licensed pharmacies or aren't pharmacies at all.
2. May give a diagnosis that is not correct and sell medicine that is not right for you or your condition.
3. Won't protect your personal information.

• Some medicines sold online:

1. Are fake (counterfeit or "copycat" medicines).
2. Are too strong or too weak.
3. Have dangerous ingredients.
4. Have expired (are out-of-date).
5. Aren't FDA-approved (haven't been checked for safety and effectiveness).
6. Aren't made using safe standards.
7. Aren't safe to use with other medicine or products you use.
8. Aren't labeled, stored, or shipped correctly.

What you should do:

1. Talk with your doctor and have a physical exam before you get any new medicine for the first time.
2. Use only medicine that has been prescribed by your doctor or another trusted professional who is licensed in the U.S. to write prescriptions for medicine.
3. Ask your doctor if there are any special steps you need to take to fill your prescription.

These tips will help protect you if you buy medicines online:

• Know your source to make sure it's safe.

• Make sure a website is a state-licensed pharmacy that is located in the United States. Pharmacies and pharmacists in the United States are licensed by a state's board of pharmacy. Your state board of pharmacy can tell you if a website is a state-licensed pharmacy, is in good standing, and is located in the United States. Find a list of state boards of pharmacy on the National Association of Boards of Pharmacy (NABP) website at www.nabp.info.

• The NABP has a program to help you find some of the pharmacies that are licensed to sell medicine online. Internet websites that display the seal of this program have been checked to make sure they meet state and federal rules. For more on this program and a list of pharmacies that display the Verified Internet Pharmacy Practice Sites™ Seal, (VIPPS® Seal), go to www.vipps.info.

• Look for websites with practices that protect you. A safe website should:

1. Be located in the United States and licensed by the state board of pharmacy where the website is operating.
2. Have a licensed pharmacist to answer your questions.
3. Require a prescription from your doctor or other health care professional who is licensed in the United States to write prescriptions for medicine.
4. Have a way for you to talk to a person if you have problems.

• Be sure your privacy is protected.

1. Look for privacy and security policies that are easy-to-find and easy-to-understand.
2. Don't give any personal information (such as social security number, credit card, or medical or health history), unless you are sure the website will keep your information safe and private.
3. Make sure that the site will not sell your information, unless you agree.

Report websites you are not sure of, or if you have complaints about a site.

Go to www.fda.gov/buyonline and click on "Your Guide to Reporting Problems to FDA."

Information about Substances of Abuse

Each of the drug charts list the interactions of alcohol, marijuana and cocaine. These three drugs are singled out because of their wide use and abuse.

Drugs of abuse include those that are addictive and harmful.

Common drugs of abuse:

Tobacco (nicotine)

What it does: Tobacco smoke contains noxious, addictive and cancer-producing ingredients. They include nicotine, carbon monoxide, ammonia and tars. Carcinogens probably come from the tars. Tars are present in chewing tobacco, snuff, cigarettes, cigars and pipes.
Short-term effects of average amount: Relaxation of mood if you are a steady smoker. Constriction of blood vessels.
Short-term effects of large amount inhaled: Headache, appetite loss, nausea.
Long-term effects: Risk of lung cancer and other cancers. Breathing problems and chronic lung disease, heart and blood vessel disease, risk of abortion and reduced birth weight of baby born to women who smoke during pregnancy.

Alcohol

What it does:

• *Central Nervous System*
It depresses normal mental activity and normal muscle function. Alcoholism is associated with accidents of all types. Marital, family, work, legal and social problems also occur. Abuse of alcohol may result in nerve damage and cause various types of brain disorders.

• *Gastrointestinal System*
Increases stomach acid, poisons liver function. Chronic alcoholism frequently leads to permanent damage to the liver.

• *Heart and Blood Vessels*
Decreased normal function, leading to heart diseases such as cardiomyopathy and disorders of the blood vessels and kidney, such as high blood pressure. Bleeding from the esophagus and stomach frequently accompany liver disease.

• *Unborn Fetus (teratogenicity)*
Alcohol abuse in the mother carrying a fetus causes *fetal alcohol spectrum disorder (FASD). It* includes mental deficiency, facial abnormalities, slow growth and other major and minor problems in a newborn.

Signs of Use:
Early signs: Smell of alcohol on the breath, behavior changes (aggressive; passive; lack of sexual inhibition; poor judgment; uncontrolled emotion, such as rage).
Intoxication signs: Unsteady gait, slurred speech, poor performance of any brain or muscle function, stupor or coma in *severe* alcoholic intoxication.

Long-term effects:
Addiction: Compulsive alcohol use. Persons addicted to alcohol have severe withdrawal symptoms if alcohol is unavailable.
Liver disease: Usually cirrhosis.
Loss of sexual function: Impotence, erectile dysfunction, loss of libido.
Increased incidence of cancer: Lung and other types. Interferes with medications.

Marijuana (cannabis, hashish)

What it does: Heightens perception, causes mood swings, relaxes mind and body.
Signs of use: Red eyes, lethargy, uncoordinated body movements.
Long-term effects: Decreased motivation. Possible brain, heart, lung and reproductive system damage, schizophrenia.

Amphetamines (including ecstasy)

What they do: Speed up physical and mental processes to cause a false sense of energy and excitement. The moods are temporary and unreal.
Signs of use: Dilated pupils, insomnia, trembling.
Long-term effects or overdose: Violent behavior, paranoia, inflammation of blood

vessels, renal failure, possible death from overdose.

Anabolic Steroids

What they do: Enhance strength, increase muscle mass.
Signs of use: Significant mood swings, aggressiveness.
Long-term effects or overdose: Possible heart problems, paranoia and mania, liver damage, male infertility and impotence, male characteristics in females.

Barbiturates

What they do: Produce drowsiness and lethargy.
Signs of use: Confused speech, lack of coordination and balance.
Long-term effects or overdose: Disrupt normal sleep pattern. Possible death from overdose, especially with alcohol abuse.

Sedative-hypnotics (benzodiazepines, "party drugs" that include gammahydroxybutyrate and rohypnol)

What they do: Produce drowsiness and lethargy.
Signs of use: Slow breathing, low blood pressure, vomiting, delirium, amnesia, possible coma.
Long-term effects or overdose: Disrupt normal sleep pattern. Possible death from overdose, especially in combination with alcohol.

Cocaine

What it does: Stimulates the nervous system, heightens sensations and may produce hallucinations.
Signs of use: Trembling, intoxication, dilated pupils, constant sniffling.
Long-term effects or overdose: Soreness of nasal passages. Itching all over body, some with open sores. Possible brain damage or heart rhythm disturbance. Possible death from overdose.

Crystal Methamphetamine

What it does: Stimulates the nervous system, heightens sensations and has long-lasting euphoric effects.
Signs of use: Obsessively picking at the face or body, hallucinations, teeth grinding, extreme energy and no sleep for 2-3 days, major loss of weight.
Long-term effects or overdose: Rapid heart rate, high blood pressure, damaged blood vessels in the brain, fever, convulsions and death.

Opiates (codeine, heroin, morphine, methadone, opium)

What they do: Relieve pain, create temporary and false sense of well-being.
Signs of use: Small pupils, mood swings, slurred speech, sore eyes, lethargy, weight loss, sweating.
Long-term effects or overdose: Loss of appetite, infections, need to increase drug amount to produce same effects, death.

Phencyclidine (PCP, angeldust)

What they do: Produce euphoria along with a feeling of numbness.
Signs of use: Violent behavior, dizziness, loss of motor skills, disorientation.
Long-term effects or overdose: Seizures, high or low blood pressure, rigid muscles. Possible death from overdose.

Psychedelic Drugs (LSD, mescaline)

What they do: Produce hallucinations, either pleasant or frightening.
Signs of use: Dilated pupils, sweating, trembling, fever, chills.
Long-term effects or overdose: Lack of motivation, unpredictable behavior, hallucinations, death from overdose.

Volatile Substances (glue, solvents, nitrous oxide, other volatile compounds)

What they do: Produce hallucinations, false sense of well-being, loss of consciousness.
Signs of use: Dilated pupils, flushed face, confusion, respiratory failure, coma.
Long-term effects or overdose: Permanent brain, liver, kidney damage; death.

Medical Conditions and Their Commonly Used Drugs

This list contains the names of many medical problems and the names of drugs that may be used for their treatment. The drugs are listed either as a generic name (e.g., Acetaminophen) or class name (e.g., Antihistamines). Specific brand or trade names of drugs are not shown. This list of drugs is intended only as a guide and is not meant to be 100% complete. Use it for a general reference.

The inclusion of a drug name does not mean it is necessarily an appropriate treatment for you. Also, your doctor may prescribe a drug for you that is not listed, but is quite appropriate for treatment. Your doctor knows your medical history and can prescribe the drug that should work best for you.

You can find information about the drugs listed by looking up the name in the General Index and referring to the page listed. Do not be concerned if the drug chart does not list your specific illness in the USES section. For example, that section may state that a drug is used for bacterial infections and not list specific bacterial disorders (such as a vaginal infection or urinary tract infection).

Acid Indigestion & Upset Stomach
- Antacids
- Bismuth Salts
- Histamine H_2 Receptor Antagonists
- Hyoscyamine
- Proton Pump Inhibitors
- Simethicone
- Sodium Bicarbonate

Acne
- Antiacne Cleansing (Topical)
- Antibacterials for Acne (Topical)
- Azelaic Acid
- Benzoyl Peroxide
- Erythromycins
- Isotretinoin
- Keratolytics
- Nitroimidazoles
- Retinoids (Topical)
- Tetracyclines

Actinic Keratoses
- Fluorouracil (Topical)
- Masoprocol

Acute Myocardial Infarction
- Angiotensin-Converting Enzyme (ACE) Inhibitors

Addison's Disease
- Adrenocorticoids (Systemic)

Aging
- Dehydroepiandrosterone (DHEA)

AIDS – See HIV Infection

Alcohol Withdrawal
- Acamprosate
- Benzodiazepines
- Beta-Adrenergic Blocking Agents
- Carbamazepine
- Disulfiram
- Hydroxyzine
- Lithium
- Naltrexone
- Thiamine

Allergies & Allergic Reactions
- Adrenocorticoids (Nasal Inhalation)
- Adrenocorticoids (Oral Inhalation)
- Adrenocorticoids (Systemic)
- Antihistamines
- Antihistamines (Nasal)
- Antihistamines, Nonsedating
- Antihistamines, Phenothiazine-Derivative
- Cromolyn
- Decongestants (Ophthalmic)
- Ephedrine
- Hydroxyzine
- Leukotriene Modifiers

Alopecia
- 5-Alpha Reductase Inhibitors
- Minoxidil

Altitude Illness
- Carbonic Anhydrase Inhibitors

Alzheimer's Disease
- Cholinesterase Inhibitors
- Memantine

Amebiasis
- Chloroquine
- Iodoquinol
- Nitroimidazoles

Amenorrhea
- Bromocriptine
- Progestins

Amyotrophic Lateral Sclerosis (ALS)
- Riluzole

Anemia
- Adrenocorticoids (Systemic)
- Androgens
- Cyclosporine
- Folic Acid
- Iron Supplements
- Leucovorin
- Vitamin B-12

Angina
- Antithyroid Drugs
- Beta-Adrenergic Blocking Agents
- Calcium Channel Blockers
- Dipyridamole
- Nitrates
- Ranolazine

Ankylosing Spondylitis
- Adrenocorticoids (Systemic)
- Anti-inflammatory Drugs, Nonsteroidal (NSAIDs)
- Anti-inflammatory Drugs, Nonsteroidal (NSAIDs) COX-2 inhibitors
- Aspirin
- Methotrexate
- Sulfasalazine

Tumor Necrosis Factor Blockers

Anorexia
Antidepressants, Tricyclic
Progestins
Selective Serotonin Reuptake Inhibitors (SSRIs)

Anxiety
Antidepressants, Tricyclic
Barbiturates
Benzodiazepines
Beta-Adrenergic Blocking Agents
Buspirone
Haloperidol
Hydroxyzine
Loxapine
Meprobamate
Phenothiazines
Selective Serotonin Reuptake Inhibitors (SSRIs)
Serotonin & Norepinephrine Reuptake Inhibitors (SNRIs)
Thiothixene

Appetite Stimulant
Antihistamines
Dronabinol

Appetite Suppressant
Appetite Suppressants

Arrhythmias – See Heart Rhythm Disorders

Arthritis
Acetaminophen
Adrenocorticoids (Systemic)
Anakinra
Anti-Inflammatory Drugs, Nonsteroidal (NSAIDs)
Anti-Inflammatory Drugs, Nonsteroidal (NSAIDs) COX-2 Inhibitors
Aspirin
Azathioprine
Capsaicin
Chloroquine
Cyclosporine
Diclofenac (Topical)
Gold Compounds
Hydroxychloroquine
Leflunomide
Meloxicam
Methotrexate
Salicylates
Tofacitinib
Tumor Necrosis Factor Blockers

Asthma
Adrenocorticoids (Nasal Inhalation)
Adrenocorticoids (Oral Inhalation)
Adrenocorticoids (Systemic)
Bronchodilators, Adrenergic
Bronchodilators, Xanthine
Cromolyn
Ephedrine
Ipratropium
Leukotriene Modifiers

Athlete's Foot
Antibacterials, Antifungals (Topical)
Antifungals (Topical)

Attention Deficit Hyperactivity Disorder (ADHD) & ADD
Amphetamines
Atomoxetine
Central Alpha Agonists
Stimulant Medications
Stimulants, Amphetamine-Related

Autism
Aripiprazole
Haloperidol
Olanzapine
Quetiapine
Selective Serotonin Reuptake Inhibitors (SSRIs)
Serotonin-Dopamine Antagonists
Stimulant Medications

Bacterial Infections
Acetohydroxamic Acid (AHA)
Cephalosporins
Chloramphenicol
Clindamycin
Erythromycins
Fluoroquinolones
Kanamycin
Lincomycin
Linezolid
Macrolide Antibiotics
Neomycin (Oral)
Nitrofurantoin
Nitroimidazoles
Penicillins
Penicillins & Beta-Lactamase Inhibitors
Rifamycins
Sulfonamides
Telithromycin
Tetracyclines
Trimethoprim
Vancomycin

Baldness – See Hair Loss

Bedwetting (Enuresis)
Antidepressants, Tricyclic
Desmopressin

Bipolar Disorder
Aripiprazole
Asenapine
Carbamazepine
Lithium
Divalproex
Quetiapine
Serotonin-Dopamine Antagonists
Valproic Acid
Ziprasidone

Birth Control – See Contraception

Bites & Stings
Adrenocorticoids (Topical)
Anesthetics (Topical)

Bladder Infection – See Cystitis

Bladder, Overactive – See Overactive Bladder

Bladder Spasms
Clidinium
Propantheline

Bleeding
Antifibrinolytic Agents
Vitamin K

Blood Circulation
Cyclandelate
Intermittent Claudication Agents
Isoxsuprine
Vitamin E

Blood Clots
Anticoagulants (Oral)
Dabigatran
Dipyridamole
Factor Xa Inhibitors
Platelet Inhibitors
Ticagrelor

Bronchial Spasms
Anticholinergics
Bronchodilators, Adrenergic

Bronchitis
Bronchodilators, Anticholinergic
Bronchodilators, Xanthine
Cephalosporins
Dextromethorphan
Fluoroquinolones
Ipratropium
Macrolide Antibiotics
Sulfonamides
Tetracyclines

Bulimia
Antidepressants, Tricyclic
Lithium

Selective Serotonin Reuptake Inhibitors (SSRIs)

Burns
Anesthetics (Topical)
Zinc Supplements

Bursitis
Adrenocorticoids (Systemic)
Anti-Inflammatory Drugs, Nonsteroidal (NSAIDs)
Aspirin
Salicylates

Cancer
Adrenocorticoids (Systemic)
Aminoglutethimide
Androgens
Antiandrogens, Nonsteroidal
Antifungals, Azoles
Busulfan
Capecitabine
Chlorambucil
Cyclophosphamide
Estramustine
Estrogens
Etoposide
Hydroxyurea
Imatinib
Levamisole
Lomustine
Melphalan
Mercaptopurine
Methotrexate
Paclitaxel
Procarbazine
Progestins
Raloxifene
Tamoxifen
Thioguanine
Thyroid Hormones
Toremifene

Cancer of the Skin
Fluorouracil (Topical)
Masoprocol
Mechlorethamine (Topical)

Canker Sores
Amlexanox
Anesthetics (Mucosal-Local)

Chickenpox
Acetaminophen
Antihistamines
Antivirals for Herpes Virus

Cholesterol, High
Cholestyramine
Colestipol
Ezetimibe
Gemfibrozil
HMG-CoA Reductase Inhibitors
Neomycin (Oral)
Niacin
Raloxifene

Chronic Obstructive Pulmonary Disease (COPD)
Adrenocorticoids (Systemic)
Bronchodilators, Adrenergic
Bronchodilators, Anticholinergic
Bronchodilators, Xanthine
Ipratropium
Roflumilast

Cirrhosis
Colchicine
Cyclosporine
Thiamine (Vitamin B-1)

Colds & Cough
Acetaminophen
Anticholinergics
Antihistamines
Antihistamines, Nonsedating
Anti-Inflammatory Drugs, Nonsteroidal (NSAIDs)
Aspirin
Dextromethorphan
Ephedrine
Guaifenesin
Oxymetazoline
Phenylephrine
Phenylephrine (Ophthalmic)
Pseudoephedrine

Colic
Hyoscyamine
Simethicone

Colitis – See Inflammatory Bowel Disease

Congestion, Chest
Bronchodilators, Adrenergic
Ephedrine
Oxymetazoline
Phenylephrine
Pseudoephedrine
Xylometazoline

Congestive Heart Failure
Angiotensin-Converting Enzyme (ACE) Inhibitors
Beta-Adrenergic Blocking Agents
Beta-Adrenergic Blocking Agents & Thiazide Diuretics
Digitalis Preparations
Diuretics, Loop
Diuretics, Potassium-Sparing
Diuretics, Potassium-Sparing & Hydrochlorothiazide
Diuretics, Thiazide
Nitrates

Conjunctivitis (Pink Eye)
Antibacterials (Ophthalmic)
Antivirals (Ophthalmic)

Conjunctivitis, Seasonal Allergic
Anti-Inflammatory Drugs, Nonsteroidal (Ophthalmic)
Antiallergic Agents (Ophthalmic)

Constipation
Laxatives, Bulk-Forming
Laxatives, Osmotic
Laxatives, Softener/Lubricant
Laxatives, Stimulant
Linaclotide
Lubiprostone
Tegaserod

Contraception
Contraceptives, Oral & Skin
Contraceptives, Vaginal
Selective Progesterone Receptor Modulators

Convulsions (Epilepsy; Seizures)
Anticonvulsants, Hydantoin
Anticonvulsants, Succinimide
Barbiturates
Benzodiazepines
Carbamazepine
Divalproex
Felbamate
Gabapentin
Lacosamide
Lamotrigine
Levetiracetam
Oxcarbazepine
Primidone
Tiagabine
Topiramate
Valproic Acid
Zonisamide

Corneal Ulcers
Antibacterials (Ophthalmic)

Crohn's Disease – See Inflammatory Bowel Disease

Cushing's Disease
Adrenocorticoids (Systemic)
Aminoglutethimide
Antifungals, Azoles
Metyrapone
Trilostane

Cystitis
Phenazopyridine
Sulfonamides & Phenazopyridine
See also – Bacterial Infections

Dandruff
Antifungals (Topical)
Antiseborrheics (Topical)
Coal Tar

Deep Vein Thrombosis – See Blood Clots

Dementia
Buspirone
Cholinesterase Inhibitors
Ergoloid Mesylates
Haloperidol

Depression
Antidepressants, Tricyclic
Aripiprazole
Bupropion
Ergoloid Mesylates
Loxapine
Maprotiline
Mirtazapine
Monoamine Oxidase (MAO) Inhibitors
Monoamine Oxidase Type B (MAO-B) Inhibitors
Nefazodone
Selective Serotonin Reuptake Inhibitors (SSRIs)
Serotonin & Norepinephrine Reuptake Inhibitors (SNRIs)
Stimulant Medications
Trazodone
Vilazodone

Dermatitis
Adrenocorticoids (Systemic)
Adrenocorticoids (Topical)
Anesthetics (Topical)
Antiseborrheics (Topical)
Coal Tar
Colchicine
Dapsone
Keratolytics

Dermatomyositis
Adrenocorticoids (Systemic)
Methotrexate

Diabetes
Acarbose
Bromocriptine
Colesevelam
DPP-4 Inhibitors
GLP-1 Receptor Agonists
Insulin
Insulin Analogs
Meglitinides
Metformin
Miglitol
Pramlintide
Sulfonylureas
Thiazolidinediones

Diarrhea
Attapulgite
Bismuth Salts
Charcoal, Activated
Difenoxin & Atropine
Diphenoxylate & Atropine
Kaolin & Pectin
Loperamide
Nitazoxanide
Paregoric
Rifaximin

Dietary Supplement
Calcium Supplements
Iron Supplements
Niacin
Vitamin A
Vitamin B-12 (Cyanocobalamin)
Vitamin C (Ascorbic Acid)
Vitamin D
Vitamin E
Vitamin K
Zinc Supplements

Digestive Spasms
Clidinium
Dicyclomine
Difenoxin & Atropine
Hyoscyamine
Propantheline

Diverticulitis
Cephalosporins
Clindamycin
Fluoroquinolones
Nitroimidazoles
Penicillins

Drowsiness
Caffeine
Orphenadrine, Aspirin & Caffeine

Dry Eyes
Protectant (Ophthalmic)

Dry Mouth
Pilocarpine (Oral)

Dysmenorrhea – See Menstrual Cramps

Ear Infections or Problems
Antibacterials (Otic)
Anti-Inflammatory Drugs, Steroidal (Otic)
Antipyrine & Benzocaine (Otic)
Phenylephrine
See also – Bacterial Infections

Ear Wax
Antipyrine & Benzocaine (Otic)

Eczema
Adrenocorticoids (Topical)
Antibacterials, Antifungals (Topical)
Coal Tar
Doxepin (Topical)
Keratolytics

Edema – See Fluid Retention

Emphysema
Adrenocorticoids (Systemic)
Bronchodilators, Adrenergic
Bronchodilators, Anticholinergic
Bronchodilators, Xanthine
Ipratropium

Endometriosis
Danazol
Nafarelin

Epilepsy – See Convulsions

Erectile Dysfunction
Alprostadil
Erectile Dysfunction Agents
Papaverine

Esophagitis
Histamine H_2 Receptor Antagonists
Metoclopramide
Proton Pump Inhibitors

Estrogen Deficiency
Estrogens

Eye Allergies
Antiallergic Agents (Ophthalmic)

Eye Conditions
Antibacterials (Ophthalmic)
Cromolyn
Cycloplegic, Mydriatic (Ophthalmic)
Cyclopentolate (Ophthalmic)
Decongestants (Ophthalmic)
Natamycin (Ophthalmic)
Phenylephrine (Ophthalmic)

Fatigue
Caffeine

Fever
Acetaminophen
Anti-Inflammatory Drugs, Nonsteroidal (NSAIDs)
Aspirin
Barbiturates, Aspirin & Codeine
Narcotic Analgesics & Aspirin
Salicylates

Fibrocystic Breast Disease
Danazol
Vitamin E

Fibromyalgia
Pregabalin

Flu – See Influenza

Fluid Retention
Angiotensin-Converting Enzyme (ACE) Inhibitors & Hydrochlorothiazide
Carbonic Anhydrase Inhibitors
Diuretics, Loop
Diuretics, Potassium-Sparing
Diuretics, Thiazide
Guanethidine & Hydrochlorothiazide
Hydralazine & Hydrochlorothiazide
Indapamide
Reserpine, Hydralazine & Hydrochlorothiazide

Fungal Infections
Antifungals, Azoles
Antifungals (Topical)
Antifungals (Vaginal)
Griseofulvin
Nystatin
Terbinafine (Oral)

Gallstones
Ursodiol

Gastroesophageal Reflux
Histamine H_2 Receptor Antagonists
Proton Pump Inhibitors
Sucralfate

Genital Warts
Condyloma Acuminatum Agents

Giardiasis
Furazolidone
Nitroimidazoles
Quinacrine

Gingivitis & Gum Disease
Chlorhexidine
Erythromycins
Penicillins
Tetracyclines

Glaucoma
Antiglaucoma, Adrenergic Agonists
Antiglaucoma, Anticholinesterases
Antiglaucoma, Beta Blockers
Antiglaucoma, Carbonic Anhydrase Inhibitors
Antiglaucoma, Cholinergic Agonists
Antiglaucoma, Prostaglandins
Carbonic Anhydrase Inhibitors

Gonorrhea
Cephalosporins
Erythromycins
Fluoroquinolones
Macrolide Antibiotics
Penicillins
Tetracyclines

Gout
Adrenocorticoids (Systemic)
Antigout Drugs
Anti-Inflammatory Drugs, Nonsteroidal (NSAIDs)
Colchicine
Meloxicam
Probenecid
Sulfinpyrazone

Hair, Excess Facial
Eflornithine

Hair Loss
5-Alpha Reductase Inhibitors
Anthralin (Topical)
Minoxidil (Topical)

Hay Fever
Antiallergic Agents (Ophthalmic)
Antihistamines
Antihistamines, Nonsedating
Antihistamines, Phenothiazine-Derivative
Antihistamines, Piperazine
Ephedrine
Guaifenesin
Hydroxyzine
Orphenadrine
Phenylephrine (Ophthalmic)

Headache (Cluster, Migraine, Sinus, Tension, Vascular)
Acetaminophen
Antidepressants, Tricyclic
Antihistamines
Anti-Inflammatory Drugs, Nonsteroidal (NSAIDs)
Aspirin
Barbiturates, Aspirin & Codeine
Beta-Adrenergic Blocking Agents
Buspirone
Butorphanol
Caffeine
Calcium Channel Blockers
Central Alpha Agonists
Divalproex
Ergot Derivatives
Lithium
Monoamine Oxidase Inhibitors
Topiramate
Triptans

Heart Rhythm Disorders
Antiarrhythmics, Benzofuran-Type
Beta-Adrenergic Blocking Agents
Calcium Channel Blockers
Digitalis Preparations
Disopyramide
Dofetilide
Flecainide Acetate
Mexiletine
Propafenone
Quinidine

Heartburn
Antacids
Histamine H_2 Receptor Antagonists
Proton Pump Inhibitors
Sodium Bicarbonate

Hemorrhoids
Adrenocorticoids (Topical)
Anesthetics (Rectal)
Hydrocortisone (Rectal)

Herpes
Antivirals (Topical)
Antivirals for Herpes Virus

Hepatitis B
Nucleotide Reverse Transcriptase Inhibitors

High Blood Pressure – See Hypertension

HIV Infection
Fusion Inhibitors
Integrase Inhibitors
Maraviroc
Non-Nucleoside Reverse Transcriptase Inhibitors
Nucleoside Reverse Transcriptase Inhibitors
Nucleotide Reverse Transcriptase Inhibitors
Protease Inhibitors

Hives (Urticaria)
Antihistamines
Antihistamines, Nonsedating
Antihistamines, Phenothiazine-Derivative
Hydroxyzine

Huntington's
Haloperidol

Hypercalcemia
Colesevelam
Colestipol
Dextrothyroxine
HMG-CoA Reductase Inhibitors

Hypertension
Alpha Adrenergic Receptor Blockers
Angiotensin II Receptor Antagonists
Angiotensin-Converting Enzyme (ACE) Inhibitors

Angiotensin-Converting Enzyme (ACE) Inhibitors & Hydrochlorothiazide
Beta-Adrenergic Blocking Agents
Beta-Adrenergic Blocking Agents & Thiazide Diuretics
Calcium Channel Blockers
Central Alpha Agonists
Diuretics, Loop
Diuretics, Potassium-Sparing
Diuretics, Potassium-Sparing & Hydrochlorothiazide
Diuretics, Thiazide
Eplerenone
Guanadrel
Guanethidine
Guanethidine & Hydrochlorothiazide
Hydralazine
Hydralazine & Hydrochlorothiazide
Indapamide
Minoxidil
Rauwolfia Alkaloids
Reserpine, Hydralazine & Hydrochlorothiazide

Hyperthyroidism
Antithyroid Drugs

Hypertriglyceridemia
Fibrates
Gemfibrozil
HMG-CoA Reductase Inhibitors
Omega-3-acid Ethyl Esters

Hypoglycemia
Glucagon

Hypothyroidism
Thyroid Hormones

Impotence - See Erectile Dysfunction

Incontinence
Antidepressants, Tricyclic
Estrogens
Flavoxate
Muscarinic Receptor Antagonists

Indigestion – See Heartburn

Infertility
Bromocriptine
Clomiphene
Danazol
Progestins

Inflammation
Anti-Inflammatory Drugs, Nonsteroidal (NSAIDs)
Anti-Inflammatory Drugs, Nonsteroidal (NSAIDs) COX-2 Inhibitors
Aspirin
Mesalamine
Narcotic Analgesics & Aspirin
Salicylates

Inflammatory Bowel Disease
Adrenocorticoids (Systemic)
Cyclosporine
Infliximab
Mesalamine
Nitroimidazoles
Olsalazine

Influenza
Antivirals for Influenza
Antivirals for Influenza, Neuraminidase Inhibitors
Ribavirin

Insomnia
Barbiturates
Belladonna Alkaloids & Barbiturates
Benzodiazepines
Eszopiclone
Melatonin
Meprobamate
Ramelteon
Trazodone
Triazolam
Zaleplon
Zolpidem

Intermittent Claudication
Intermittent Claudication Agents
Pentoxifylline

Irregular Heartbeat – See Heart Rhythm Disorders

Irritable Bowel Syndrome
Linaclotide
Tegaserod

Itching
Adrenocorticoids (Topical)
Doxepin (Topical)

Jet Lag
Melatonin

Jock Itch
Antifungals (Topical)

Joint Pain
Anti-Inflammatory Drugs, Nonsteroidal (NSAIDs)
Anti-Inflammatory Drugs, Nonsteroidal (NSAIDs) COX-2 Inhibitors
Aspirin

Kidney Stones
Antigout Drugs
Citrates
Diuretics, Thiazide
Penicillamine
Sodium Bicarbonate
Tiopronin

Labyrinthitis
Antihistamines, Phenothiazine-Derivative
Antihistamines, Piperazine
Benzodiazepines

Leg Pain or Cramps
Cyclandelate
Intermittent Claudication Agents
Orphenadrine
Pentoxifylline
Quinine

Leukemia
Imatinib
Thioguanine

Lice
Pediculicides

Lupus (Skin & Systemic)
Adrenocorticoids (Systemic)
Adrenocorticoids (Topical)
Anti-Inflammatory Drugs, Nonsteroidal (NSAIDs)
Anti-Inflammatory Drugs, Nonsteroidal (NSAIDs) COX-2 Inhibitors
Hydroxychloroquine
Methotrexate
Quinacrine

Lyme Disease
Cephalosporins
Erythromycins
Macrolide Antibiotics
Penicillins
Tetracyclines

Malabsorption
Quinacrine
Vitamin K

Malaria
Antimalarial
Atovaquone
Chloroquine
Hydroxychloroquine
Primaquine
Proguanil
Quinidine
Quinine
Sulfadoxine & Pyrimethamine
Tetracyclines

Male Hormone Deficiency
Androgens

Melanoma
- Hydroxyurea
- Levamisole
- Melphalan

Meniere's Disease
- Antihistamines
- Antihistamines, Piperazine
- Benzodiazepines
- Scopolamine (Hyoscine)

Menopause
- Estrogens
- Progestins

Menorrhagia – See Menstruation, Excessive

Menstrual Cramps
- Anti-Inflammatory Drugs, Nonsteroidal (NSAIDs)
- Anti-Inflammatory Drugs, Nonsteroidal (NSAIDs) COX-2 Inhibitors
- Contraceptives, Oral & Skin

Menstruation, Excessive (Menorrhagia)
- Antifibrinolytic Agents
- Contraceptives, Oral & Skin
- Danazol
- Estrogens
- Progestins

Mental & Emotional Disturbances
- Loxapine
- Rauwolfia Alkaloids
- Serotonin-Dopamine Antagonists

Motion Sickness
- Antihistamines
- Antihistamines, Nonsedating
- Antihistamines, Phenothiazine-Derivative
- Antihistamines, Piperazine
- Clotrimazole
- Diphenidol
- Scopolamine

Multiple Sclerosis
- Adrenocorticoids (Systemic)
- Baclofen
- Tizanidine

Muscle Cramp, Spasm, Strain
- Baclofen
- Cyclobenzaprine
- Dantrolene
- Muscle Relaxants, Skeletal
- Orphenadrine
- Orphenadrine, Aspirin & Caffeine
- Quinine
- Tizanidine

Myasthenia Gravis
- Adrenocorticoids (Systemic)
- Antimyasthenics
- Azathioprine
- Cyclosporine

Narcolepsy
- Amphetamines
- Pemoline
- Stimulant Medications
- Stimulants, Amphetamine-Related

Narcotic Withdrawal
- Buprenorphine & Naloxone
- Central Alpha Agonists
- Naltrexone

Nasal Allergy
- Adrenocorticoids (Nasal Inhalation)
- Antihistamines (Nasal)

Nausea & Vomiting
- Antihistamines, Phenothiazine-Derivative
- Bismuth Salts
- Diphenidol
- Dronabinol
- Hydroxyzine
- Metoclopramide
- Nabilone
- Phenothiazines
- Scopolamine
- Trimethobenzamide

Nerve Disorders
- Pregabalin

Neural Tube Defects (prevention)
- Folic Acid

Obesity
- Appetite Suppressants
- Lorcaserin
- Orlistat
- Selective Serotonin Reuptake Inhibitors (SSRIs)

Obsessive Compulsive Disorder
- Antidepressants, Tricyclic
- Selective Serotonin Reuptake Inhibitors (SSRIs)

Ocular Hypertension
- Antiglaucoma, Carbonic Anhydrase Inhibitors
- Beta-Adrenergic Blocking Agents (Ophthalmic)

Osteoarthritis – See Arthritis

Osteoporosis
- Bisphosphonates
- Bone Formation Agents
- Calcitonin
- Calcium Supplements
- Estrogens
- Raloxifene
- Sodium Fluoride
- Vitamin D

Otitis Media – See Ear Infection

Overactive Bladder
- Mirabegron
- Muscarinic Receptor Antagonists

Paget's Disease
- Bisphosphonates
- Colchicine

Pain
- Acetaminophen
- Anti-Inflammatory Drugs, Nonsteroidal (NSAIDs)
- Anti-Inflammatory Drugs, Nonsteroidal (NSAIDs) COX-2 Inhibitors
- Aspirin
- Barbiturates, Aspirin & Codeine
- Butorphanol
- Carbamazepine
- Narcotic Analgesics
- Narcotic Analgesics & Acetaminophen
- Narcotic Analgesics & Aspirin
- Orphenadrine, Aspirin & Caffeine
- Salicylates
- Tapentadol
- Tramadol
- Trazodone

Pain In Mouth
- Anesthetics (Mucosal-Local)

Panic Disorder
- Antidepressants, Tricyclic
- Benzodiazepines
- Monoamine Oxidase Inhibitors

Parasites
- Anthelmintics
- Pentamidine

Parkinson's Disease
- Antidyskinetics
- Antihistamines
- Antivirals for Influenza
- Bromocriptine
- Carbidopa & Levodopa
- COMT Inhibitors
- Dopamine Agonists, Nonergot
- Levodopa
- Monoamine Oxidase Type B (MAO-B) Inhibitors

Orphenadrine

Parkinson's Tremors
Antihistamines
Niacin

Peripheral Neuropathy
Serotonin & Norepinephrine Reuptake Inhibitors (SNRIs)

Peyronie's Disease
Aminobenzoate Potassium

Pneumocystis Jiroveci
Atovaquone
Dapsone
Primaquine
Trimethoprim

Pneumonia
Fluoroquinolones
Ribavirin
Sulfonamides

Pneumonia, Community Acquired
Telithromycin

Poisoning
Charcoal, Activated

Potassium Deficiency
Potassium Supplements

Premature Labor
Isoxsuprine

Premenstrual Syndrome (PMS)
Antidepressants, Tricyclic
Anti-Inflammatory Drugs, Nonsteroidal (NSAIDs)
Buspirone
Calcium Supplements
Contraceptives, Oral & Skin
Danazol
Pyridoxine (Vitamin B-6)
Selective Serotonin Reuptake Inhibitors (SSRIs)
Vitamin E

Pressure Sores
Benzoyl Peroxide

Prostate Hyperplasia, Benign
5-Alpha Reductase Inhibitors
Alpha Adrenergic Receptor Blockers

Psoriasis
Adrenocorticoids (Topical)
Anthralin (Topical)
Biologics for Psoriasis
Coal Tar
Cyclosporine
Keratolytics
Methotrexate
Psoralens
Retinoids (Oral)
Retinoids (Topical)
Tumor Necrosis Factor Blockers
Vitamin D (Topical)

Psychotic Disorders
Aripiprazole
Asenapine
Carbamazepine
Clozapine
Haloperidol
Loxapine
Lurasidone
Olanzapine
Phenothiazines
Quetiapine
Serotonin-Dopamine Antagonists
Thiothixene
Ziprasidone

Pulmonary Arterial Hypertension (PAH)
Endothelin Receptor Antagonists

Rashes – See Skin Disorders

Rectal Fissures
Anesthetics (Rectal)

Respiratory Syncytial Virus (RSV)
Ribavirin

Restless Legs Syndrome
Antidyskinetics
Benzodiazepines
Carbidopa & Levodopa
Dopamine Agonists, Nonergot
Narcotic Analgesics

Rheumatoid Arthritis – See Arthritis

Rickets
Vitamin D

Ringworm – See Fungal Infections

Rosacea
Antibacterials (Topical)
Antibacterials for Acne (Topical)
Azelaic Acid
Benzoyl Peroxide
Nitroimidazoles
Tetracyclines

Scabies
Pediculicides

Schizophrenia
Aripiprazole
Carbamazepine
Clozapine
Haloperidol
Olanzapine
Phenothiazines
Quetiapine
Serotonin-Dopamine Antagonists

Scleroderma
Aminobenzoate Potassium

Seasonal Affective Disorder (SAD)
Bupropion
Selective Serotonin Reuptake Inhibitors (SSRIs)

Seizures – See Convulsions

Shingles
Antivirals (Topical)
Antivirals for Herpes Virus
Capsaicin

Sickle Cell Disease
Hydroxyurea

Sinusitis
Cephalosporins
Erythromycins
Macrolide Antibiotics
Penicillins
Penicillins & Beta-Lactamase Inhibitors
Sulfonamides
Tetracyclines
Trimethoprim
Xylometazoline

Skin Cancer – See Cancer of the Skin

Skin Disorders
Anesthetics (Topical)
Antibacterials (Topical)
Antibacterials, Antifungals (Topical)
Cyclophosphamide
Condyloma Acuminatum Agents
Fluorouracil (Topical)
Isotretinoin
Neomycin (Topical)
Retinoids (Topical)

Skin Lines & Wrinkles
Botulinum Toxin Type A

Smoking Cessation
Bupropion
Central Alpha Agonists
Nicotine
Varenicline

Sore Throat
Anesthetics (Mucosal-Local)
See also – Bacterial Infections

Stroke Prevention
Platelet Inhibitors

Sunburn
Adrenocorticoids (Topical)
Anesthetics (Topical)

Swelling – See Fluid Retention

Thyroid Disorders – See Hyperthyroidism; Hypothyroidism

Tonsillitis
Cephalosporins
Macrolide Antibiotics

Tourette's Syndrome
Antidyskinetics
Haloperidol

Toxoplasmosis
Atovaquone

Transplantation, Organ (Antirejection)
Azathioprine
Cyclosporine
Immunosuppressive Agents

Tremors
Benzodiazepines
Beta-Adrenergic Blocking Agents

Trichomoniasis
Nitroimidazoles

Trigeminal Neuralgia
Baclofen
Carbamazepine

Tuberculosis
Cycloserine
Ethionamide
Isoniazid
Nitroimidazoles
Rifamycins

Ulcers
Antacids
Anticholinergics
Bismuth Salts
Glycopyrrolate
Histamine H_2 Receptor Antagonists
Nitroimidazoles
Proton Pump Inhibitors
Sodium Bicarbonate
Sucralfate
Tetracyclines

Ulcers, Skin
Becaplermin

Ulcerative Colitis
Olsalazine
Sulfasalazine

Urethra Spasms
Clidinium
Propantheline

Urethritis
Erythromycins
Fluoroquinolones
Macrolide Antibiotics
Phenazopyridine
Sulfonamides & Phenazopyridine
Tetracyclines

Urinary Frequency
Muscarinic Receptor Antagonists

Urinary Retention
Antimyasthenics
Bethanechol

Urinary Tract Infection
Acetohydroxamic Acid (AHA)
Atropine, Hyoscyamine, Methenamine
Cephalosporins
Cinoxacin
Cycloserine
Flavoxate
Fluoroquinolones
Methenamine
Penicillins
Penicillins & Beta-Lactamase Inhibitors
Phenazopyridine
Sulfonamides
Tetracyclines
Trimethoprim

Urine Acidity
Citrates
Vitamin C

Uveitis
Anti-Inflammatory Drugs, Steroidal (Ophthalmic)

Vaginal Infections or Irritation
Clindamycin
Estrogens
Nitroimidazoles
Progestins

Vaginal Yeast Infections
Antifungals (Vaginal)

Vertigo
Antihistamines, Piperazine
Niacin

Virus Infections of the Eye
Antivirals (Ophthalmic)

Vitamin Deficiency
Pantothenic Acid
Riboflavin
Vitamin A
Vitamin B-12
Vitamin C
Vitamin D
Vitamin E
Vitamin K

Vitiligo
Psoralens

Vomiting – See Nausea & Vomiting

Warts
Keratolytics
Retinoids (Topical)

Wilson's Disease
Penicillamine
Zinc Supplements

Worms
Anthelmintics

Zinc Deficiency
Zinc Supplements

Drug Charts

5-ALPHA REDUCTASE INHIBITORS

GENERIC AND BRAND NAMES

DUTASTERIDE
- **Avodart**
- **Duagen**
- **Jalyn**
- **Neulasta**

FINASTERIDE
- **Propecia**
- **Proscar**

BASIC INFORMATION

Habit forming? No
Prescription needed? Yes
Available as generic? Yes, for some
Drug class: Dihydrotestosterone inhibitor

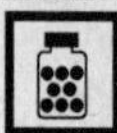

USES

- Treats noncancerous enlargement of the prostate gland in men (benign prostatic hypertrophy or BPH).
- Theoretically, may prevent the development of prostate cancer. Studies are ongoing.
- Treatment of male pattern hair loss in men.

DOSAGE & USAGE INFORMATION

How to take:
Tablet or capsule—Swallow with liquid. If you can't swallow whole, crumble tablet and take with liquid or food.

When to take:
Once a day or as directed, with or without meals.

If you forget a dose:
Take as soon as you remember. If it is almost time for the next dose, wait for the next scheduled dose (don't double this dose).

What drug does:
Inhibits the enzyme needed for the conversion of testosterone to dihydrotestosterone. Dihydrotestosterone is required for the development of benign prostatic hypertrophy.

Time lapse before drug works:
- May require up to 6 months for full therapeutic effect for BPH.
- For treatment of hair loss, may not see any benefit for 3 months or more.

Don't take with:
Any other medicine or dietary supplement without consulting your doctor or pharmacist, especially nonprescription decongestants.

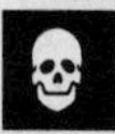

OVERDOSE

SYMPTOMS:
Effects unknown.
WHAT TO DO:
Overdose unlikely to threaten life. If person uses much larger amount than prescribed or if accidentally swallowed, call doctor or poison control center 1-800-222-1222 for help.

POSSIBLE ADVERSE REACTIONS OR SIDE EFFECTS

SYMPTOMS	WHAT TO DO
Life-threatening: None expected.	
Common: None expected.	
Infrequent: Decreased volume of ejaculation, back or stomach pain, headache.	Continue. Call doctor when convenient.
Rare:	
• Impotence, decreased libido, breast enlargement and tenderness.	Continue. Call doctor when convenient.
• Allergic reaction (skin rash, swelling of lips).	Discontinue. Call doctor right away.

WARNINGS & PRECAUTIONS

Don't take if:
- You are allergic to dutasteride or finasteride.
- You are a female, are pregnant or a child.

Before you start, consult your doctor if:
- You have not had a blood test to check for prostate cancer.
- Your sexual partner is pregnant or may become pregnant.
- You have a liver disorder.
- You have reduced urinary flow.
- You have large residual urinary volume.

Over age 60:
No special problems expected.

Pregnancy:
- Not recommended for women.
- Pregnant women should not handle the crushed tablets.
- Ask your doctor if you should avoid exposure to mate's semen if he takes these drugs.
- Risk category X (see page xviii).

Breast-feeding:
These drugs are not recommended for women.

Infants & children:
Not recommended.

Prolonged use:
Talk to your doctor about the need for follow-up medical examinations or laboratory studies to check the effectiveness of the treatment.

Skin & sunlight:
No special problems expected.

Driving, piloting or hazardous work:
No special problems expected.

Discontinuing:
Don't discontinue without medical advice.

Others:
- Advise any doctor or dentist whom you consult that you take this medicine.
- May affect results of some medical tests (especially prostate specific antigen [PSA] which is a test for prostate cancer).
- For those who respond well, the drug must be continued indefinitely.
- Some adverse effects of finasteride may continue after drug is stopped. For Propecia brand, these include libido, ejaculation and orgasm disorders. For Proscar brand, this includes decreased libido.
- Reports show that finasteride use may lead to male infertility and/or poor semen quality. Once drug is stopped, these effects improve or return to normal.

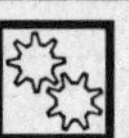

POSSIBLE INTERACTION WITH OTHER DRUGS

GENERIC NAME OR DRUG CLASS	COMBINED EFFECT
None expected.	

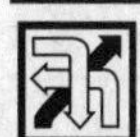

POSSIBLE INTERACTION WITH OTHER SUBSTANCES

INTERACTS WITH	COMBINED EFFECT
Alcohol:	No proven problems.
Beverages:	Grapefruit juice may increase effect of finasteride.
Cocaine:	No proven problems.
Foods:	No proven problems.
Marijuana:	No proven problems.
Tobacco:	No proven problems.

ACAMPROSATE

BRAND NAMES

Campral

BASIC INFORMATION

Habit forming? No
Prescription needed? Yes
Available as generic? No
Drug class: Alcohol-abuse deterrent

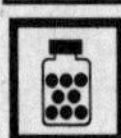

USES

Treatment for alcohol dependence. It is used after alcohol withdrawal to help maintain abstinence by reducing cravings. The drug should be part of a complete treatment plan (e.g., counseling, behavior therapy and support of family and friends). The drug does not diminish or eliminate withdrawal symptoms.

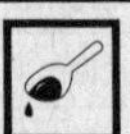

DOSAGE & USAGE INFORMATION

How to take:
Tablet—Swallow whole with liquid. May be taken with or without food.

When to take:
Usually three times a day at the same time each day (such as at mealtimes).

If you forget a dose:
Take as soon as you remember. If it is almost time for the next dose, wait for that dose (don't double this dose) and resume regular schedule.

What drug does:
Action is not fully understood. It appears to affect chemicals (called neurotransmitters) in the brain and reduces the craving for alcohol.

Time lapse before drug works:
About one week.

Don't take with:
Any other medicine or any dietary supplement without consulting your doctor or pharmacist.

OVERDOSE

SYMPTOMS:
Diarrhea and possibly other symptoms.
WHAT TO DO:
Overdose unlikely to threaten life. If person uses much larger amount than prescribed or if accidentally swallowed, call doctor or poison control center 1-800-222-1222 for help.

POSSIBLE ADVERSE REACTIONS OR SIDE EFFECTS

SYMPTOMS	WHAT TO DO
Life-threatening: None expected.	
Common: Diarrhea, dizziness, itching, nausea, gas, bloating, vomiting, abdominal pain, headache, insomnia.	Continue. Call doctor when convenient.
Infrequent: Depression, anxiety, increase or decrease in sexual desire, rash or other skin reaction, heart palpitations, fainting, muscle pain, swelling (face, feet or ankles).	Continue. Call doctor when convenient.
Rare:	
• Thoughts of suicide or patient talks of suicide.	Discontinue. Get emergency help.
• Low blood pressure, increased heart rate, other symptoms that may occur (can be due to the drug or are a result of alcohol abuse or alcohol withdrawal symptoms).	Continue. Call doctor when convenient.

WARNINGS & PRECAUTIONS

Don't take if:
You are allergic to acamprosate.

Before you start, consult your doctor if:
- You have kidney (renal) disease or severe kidney impairment.
- You suffer from depression or have thoughts about suicide.

Over age 60:
No special problems expected.

Pregnancy:
Decide with your doctor if drug benefits justify risk to unborn child. Risk category C. (See page xviii).

Breast-feeding:
It is unknown if drug passes into milk. Avoid drug or discontinue nursing until you finish medicine. Consult doctor for advice on maintaining milk supply.

Infants & children:
Safety and effectiveness of use in children under age 18 not established.

Prolonged use:
Talk to your doctor about the need for follow-up medical examinations or laboratory studies to determine drug's effectiveness and to monitor for symptoms and suicidal thoughts.

Skin & sunlight:
No problems expected.

Driving, piloting or hazardous work:
- Avoid if the drug makes you feel dizzy, otherwise no problems expected.
- If you start drinking alcohol again, avoid driving, piloting or hazardous work.

Discontinuing:
Do not stop taking acamprosate without talking to your doctor. Continue taking acamprosate even if you start drinking alcohol again.

Others:
- Advise any doctor or dentist whom you consult that you take this medicine.
- Drug may affect the accuracy of some medical tests.
- Contact your doctor if you develop symptoms of depression, have suicidal thoughts or start drinking alcohol again.

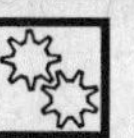

POSSIBLE INTERACTION WITH OTHER DRUGS

GENERIC NAME OR DRUG CLASS	COMBINED EFFECT
None expected.	

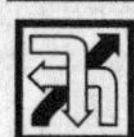

POSSIBLE INTERACTION WITH OTHER DRUGS

INTERACTS WITH	COMBINED EFFECT
Alcohol:	None expected, but all alcohol should be avoided.
Beverages:	None expected.
Cocaine:	Effects unknown. Avoid.
Foods:	None expected. Avoid foods that contain alcohol.
Marijuana:	Effects unknown. Avoid.
Tobacco:	None expected.

ACARBOSE

BRAND NAMES

Precose

BASIC INFORMATION

Habit forming? No
Prescription needed? Yes
Available as generic? Yes
Drug class: Antihyperglycemic, antidiabetic

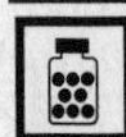

USES

Treatment for hyperglycemia (excess sugar in the blood) that cannot be controlled by diet alone in patients with type 2 diabetes. It may be used alone or in combination with other antidiabetic drugs.

DOSAGE & USAGE INFORMATION

How to take:
Tablet—Swallow with liquid. Take at the very beginning of a meal.

When to take:
Usually 3 times a day or as directed by doctor. Dosage may be increased at 4- to 8-week intervals until maximum benefits are achieved.

Continued next column

OVERDOSE

SYMPTOMS:

- **Symptoms of lactic acidosis (acid in the blood)—chills, diarrhea, severe muscle pain, sleepiness, slow heartbeat, breathing difficulty, unusual weakness.**
- **Symptoms of hypoglycemia (not a problem with acarbose used alone)—stomach pain, anxious feeling, cold sweats, chills, confusion, convulsions, cool pale skin, excessive hunger, nausea or vomiting, rapid heartbeat, nervousness, shakiness, unsteady walk, unusual weakness or tiredness, vision changes, unconsciousness.**

WHAT TO DO:

- **For mild low blood sugar symptoms, drink or eat something containing sugar right away.**
- **For more severe symptoms, dial 911 (emergency) for medical help or call doctor or poison control center 1-800-222-1222 for instructions.**
- **See emergency information on last 3 pages of this book.**

If you forget a dose:
Take as soon as you remember. If it is almost time for the next dose, then skip the missed dose and wait for your next scheduled dose (don't double this dose).

What drug does:
Impedes the digestion and absorption of carbohydrates and their subsequent conversion into glucose, improving control of blood glucose, and may reduce the complications of diabetes. However, acarbose does not cure diabetes.

Time lapse before drug works:
May take several weeks for full effectiveness.

Don't take with:
Any other medicine or any dietary supplement without consulting your doctor or pharmacist.

POSSIBLE ADVERSE REACTIONS OR SIDE EFFECTS

SYMPTOMS	WHAT TO DO
Life-threatening:	
In case of overdose or low blood sugar, see previous column.	
Common:	
Diarrhea, stomach cramps, gas, bloating, feeling of fullness in stomach, nausea.	Continue. Call doctor when convenient.
Infrequent:	
None expected.	
Rare:	
Lactic acidosis or severe low blood sugar (see symptoms under Overdose).	Discontinue. Call doctor right away or seek emergency help.

WARNINGS & PRECAUTIONS

Don't take if:
You are allergic to acarbose.

Before you start, consult your doctor if:
- You have any kidney or liver disease or any heart or blood vessel disorder.
- You have any chronic health problem.
- You have an infection, illness or any condition that can cause low blood sugar.
- You have a history of acid in the blood (metabolic acidosis or ketoacidosis).
- You have inflammatory bowel disease or any other intestinal disorder.
- You are allergic to any medication, food or other substance.

Over age 60:
No special problems expected. A lower starting dosage may be recommended by your doctor.

Pregnancy:
Decide with your doctor if drug benefits justify risks to unborn child. Risk category B (see page xviii).

Breast-feeding:
It is unknown if drug passes into milk. Avoid drug or discontinue nursing until you finish medicine. Consult doctor for advice on maintaining milk supply.

Infants & children:
Safety and efficacy have not been established. Use only under close medical supervision.

Prolonged use:
- Schedule regular doctor visits to determine if the drug is continuing to be effective in controlling the diabetes and to check for any problems in kidney function.
- You will most likely require an antidiabetic medicine for the rest of your life.
- You will need to test your blood glucose levels several times a day; or for some, once to several times a week.
- Acarbose may reduce absorption of iron, causing anemia. Discuss with your doctor.

Skin & sunlight:
No special problems expected.

Driving, piloting or hazardous work:
No special problems expected.

Discontinuing:
Don't discontinue without consulting your doctor even if you feel well. You can have diabetes without feeling any symptoms. Untreated diabetes can cause serious problems.

Others:
- Advise any doctor or dentist whom you consult that you take this medicine. Drug may interfere with the accuracy of some medical tests.
- Follow any special diet your doctor may prescribe. It can help control diabetes.
- Consult doctor if you become ill with vomiting or diarrhea.
- Use caution when exercising. Ask your doctor about an appropriate exercise program.
- Wear medical identification stating that you have diabetes and take this medication.
- Learn to recognize the symptoms of low blood sugar. You and your family need to know what to do if these symptoms occur.
- Have a glucagon kit and syringe in the event severe low blood sugar occurs.
- High blood sugar (hyperglycemia) may occur with diabetes. Ask your doctor about symptoms to watch for and treatment steps to take.
- Educate yourself about diabetes.

POSSIBLE INTERACTION WITH OTHER DRUGS

GENERIC NAME OR DRUG CLASS	COMBINED EFFECT
Amylase (Pancreatic enzyme)	Decreased acarbose effect.
Charcoal, activated	Decreased acarbose effect.
Hyperglycemia-causing medications*	Increased risk of hyperglycemia.
Metformin	Decreased acarbose effect. Increased risk of side effects.
Pancreatin (Pancreatic enzyme)	Decreased acarbose effect.
Pramlintide	Decreased absorption of nutrients.

POSSIBLE INTERACTION WITH OTHER SUBSTANCES

INTERACTS WITH	COMBINED EFFECT
Alcohol:	May increase effect of acarbose. Avoid excessive amounts.
Beverages:	No special problems.
Cocaine:	No special problems.
Foods:	No special problems.
Marijuana:	No special problems.
Tobacco:	No special problems.

*See Glossary

ACETAMINOPHEN

BRAND NAMES

See full list of brand names in the *Generic and Brand Name Directory*, page 862.

BASIC INFORMATION

Habit forming? No
Prescription needed? No
Available as generic? Yes
Drug class: Analgesic, fever reducer

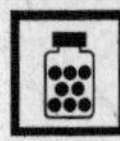

USES

Treatment of mild to moderate pain and fever. Acetaminophen does not relieve redness, stiffness or swelling of joints or tissue inflammation. Use other drugs for inflammation.

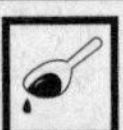

DOSAGE & USAGE INFORMATION

How to take:

- Note—Acetaminophen comes in several dosage forms and is also an ingredient in many cold, cough and flu remedies. Read labels carefully. Do not use, or give, more than the dosage recommended for adults or children. Too much acetaminophen can result in liver or kidney damage.
- Tablet or capsule—Swallow with liquid. Do not open, crush or chew tablet or capsule.
- Chewable tablet—Chew and swallow.
- Liquid drops—Follow package instructions.
- Liquid—Follow instructions on label.
- Powder—Mix as instructed with water or other liquid and swallow. May be mixed with small amount of food and eaten.
- Granules—Mix with a small amount of applesauce, ice cream or jam and eat.
- Dissolving tablet—Place tablet on tongue and let dissolve (or chew) before swallowing.
- Rectal suppository—Remove wrapper and moisten suppository with water. Gently insert into rectum. Push well into rectum with finger.

When to take:
As needed, depending on the dosage. May range from 3-8 hours between dosages.

If you forget a dose:
Take as soon as you remember. Wait 3-8 hours for next dose (depending on dosage used).

What drug does:
Exact mechanism is not fully known. Blocks pain impulses in central nervous system. Reduces fever by acting on the hypothalamic heat regulating center.

Time lapse before drug works:
15 to 30 minutes. May last 4 or more hours.

Don't take with:

- Other drugs that contain acetaminophen. An overdose may occur.
- Any other medicine or any dietary supplement without consulting your doctor or pharmacist.

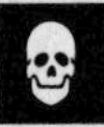

OVERDOSE

SYMPTOMS:
May take up to 12 hours after an overdose for symptoms to occur. Sweating, diarrhea, nausea, vomiting, stomach upset and cramping or pain, irritability, loss of appetite, yellow skin or eyes, seizures, coma.

WHAT TO DO:

- **If you suspect overdose, even if not sure, call doctor or poison control center 1-800-222-1222 for help. Symptoms may not appear until damage has occurred.**
- **Dial 911 (emergency) if symptoms occur.**
- **See emergency information on last 3 pages of this book.**

POSSIBLE ADVERSE REACTIONS OR SIDE EFFECTS

SYMPTOMS	WHAT TO DO
Life-threatening:	
Rare allergic reaction (hives, itching, rash, trouble breathing, tightness in chest, swelling of lips or tongue or face).	Seek emergency treatment immediately.
Common:	
None expected.	
Infrequent:	
None expected.	
Rare:	
Extreme fatigue, skin rash or itch or hives, sore throat and fever, unexplained bleeding or bruising, blood in urine, painful or decreased or frequent urination, yellow skin or eyes, black or tarry stools, illness symptoms not present before taking drug (sore throat, pain, fever).	Discontinue. Call doctor right away.

WARNINGS & PRECAUTIONS

Don't take if:
You are allergic to acetaminophen or aspirin.

Before you start, consult your doctor if:
- You have kidney or liver disease.
- You drink 3 or more alcoholic drinks a day.

Over age 60:
No problems expected as long as proper dosage is taken.

Pregnancy:
No proven harm to unborn child. Avoid if possible. Consult doctor. Risk category B (see page xviii).

Breast-feeding:
Small amounts of drug may pass into breast milk. There is no proven harm to nursing infant, but consult your doctor before taking drug.

Infants & children:
Read the label on the product to see if it is approved for your child's age. Always follow the directions on product's label about how to use. If unsure, ask your doctor or pharmacist.

Prolonged use:
- Don't take drug for a long period of time without medical approval.
- Talk to your doctor about the need for follow-up medical exams or lab studies to check liver and kidney functions.

Skin & sunlight:
No problems expected.

Driving, piloting or hazardous work:
Avoid if you feel drowsy. Otherwise, no problems expected.

Discontinuing:
Discontinue in 3-10 days if symptoms don't improve.

Others:
- May interfere with the accuracy of some medical tests.
- Advise any doctor or dentist whom you consult that you take this medicine (if you take it regularly).
- Diabetic patients may get false blood glucose results while taking this drug. Check with the doctor if any changes occur.
- There is a risk for severe liver injury if person takes more than recommended dose, takes high doses on regular basis or takes with other drug containing acetaminophen.
- If the sore throat or fever symptoms don't improve after 2 to 3 days use or if pain symptoms continue more than 5 to 10 days, call your doctor.

POSSIBLE INTERACTION WITH OTHER DRUGS

GENERIC NAME OR DRUG CLASS	COMBINED EFFECT
Acetaminophen-containing drugs	May increase risk of liver injury.
Anticoagulants, oral*	May increase anticoagulant effect. Consult doctor.
Anti-inflammatory drugs, nonsteroidal (NSAIDs)	Increased risk of adverse effects of both drugs.
Aspirin and other salicylates*	Increased risk of adverse effects of both drugs.
Caffeine-containing products	May increase stimulant effect. Take 8-12 hours apart.
Enzyme inducers*	Increased risk of liver damage.
Hepatotoxic medications*	Increased risk of liver damage.

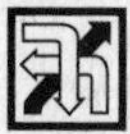

POSSIBLE INTERACTION WITH OTHER SUBSTANCES

INTERACTS WITH	COMBINED EFFECT
Alcohol:	Can cause liver damage. Avoid.
Beverages:	None expected.
Cocaine:	None expected. However, cocaine may slow body's recovery. Avoid.
Foods:	None expected.
Marijuana:	Increased pain relief. However, marijuana may slow body's recovery. Avoid.
Tobacco:	None expected.

*See Glossary

ACETOHYDROXAMIC ACID (AHA)

BRAND NAMES

Lithostat

BASIC INFORMATION

Habit forming? No
Prescription needed? Yes
Available as generic? No
Drug class: Antibacterial (antibiotic), antiurolithic

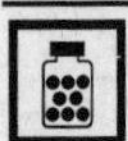

USES

- Treatment for chronic urinary tract infections.
- Prevents formation of urinary tract stones. Will not dissolve stones already present.

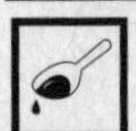

DOSAGE & USAGE INFORMATION

How to take:
Tablet—Swallow with liquid. If you can't swallow whole, crumble tablet and take with liquid or food.

When to take:
At the same time each day, according to instructions on prescription label.

If you forget a dose:
Take as soon as you remember. If it is almost time for the next dose, wait for the next scheduled dose (don't double this dose).

What drug does:
Stops enzyme action that makes urine too alkaline. Alkaline urine favors bacterial growth and stone formation and growth.

Time lapse before drug works:
1 to 3 weeks.

Don't take with:
- Alcohol or iron supplement.
- Any other medicine or any dietary supplement without consulting your doctor or pharmacist.

OVERDOSE

SYMPTOMS:
Loss of appetite, tremor, nausea, vomiting.
WHAT TO DO:
Overdose unlikely to threaten life. If person uses much larger amount than prescribed or if accidentally swallowed, call doctor or poison control center 1-800-222-1222 for help.

POSSIBLE ADVERSE REACTIONS OR SIDE EFFECTS

SYMPTOMS	WHAT TO DO
Life-threatening: In case of overdose, see previous column.	
Common: Appetite loss, nausea, vomiting, anxiety, depression, mild headache, unusual tiredness.	Continue. Call doctor when convenient.
Infrequent:	
• Loss of coordination, slurred speech, severe headache, sudden change in vision, shortness of breath, clot or pain over a blood vessel, sudden chest pain, leg pain in calf (deep vein blood clot).	Discontinue. Seek emergency treatment.
• Rash on arms and face.	Continue. Call doctor when convenient.
Rare:	
• Sore throat, fever, unusual bleeding, bruising.	Discontinue. Call doctor right away.
• Hair loss.	Continue. Call doctor when convenient.

WARNINGS & PRECAUTIONS

Don't take if:
You have severe chronic kidney disease.

Before you start, consult your doctor if:
- You are anemic.
- You have or have had phlebitis or thrombophlebitis.

Over age 60:
Adverse reactions and side effects may be more frequent and severe than in younger persons.

Pregnancy:
Studies inconclusive on harm to unborn child. Animal studies show fetal abnormalities. Don't use. Risk category X (see page xviii).

Breast-feeding:
Studies inconclusive. May have a potential for adverse reactions in nursing children. Avoid drug or discontinue nursing until you finish medicine. Consult doctor on maintaining milk supply.

Infants & children:
Not recommended. Safety and dosage have not been established.

Prolonged use:
Talk to your doctor about the need for follow-up medical examinations or laboratory studies to check blood pressure, liver function, kidney function, urinary pH.

Skin & sunlight:
No problems expected.

Driving, piloting or hazardous work:
Don't drive or pilot aircraft until you learn how medicine affects you. Don't work around dangerous machinery. Don't climb ladders or work in high places. Danger increases if you drink alcohol or take medicine affecting alertness and reflexes, such as antihistamines, tranquilizers, sedatives, pain medicines, narcotics and mind-altering drugs.

Discontinuing:
Don't discontinue without consulting doctor. Dose may require gradual reduction if you have taken drug for a long time. Doses of other drugs may also require adjustment.

Others:
Advise any doctor or dentist whom you consult that you take this medicine.

POSSIBLE INTERACTION WITH OTHER DRUGS

GENERIC NAME OR DRUG CLASS	COMBINED EFFECT
Iron	Decreased effects of both drugs.

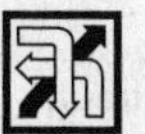

POSSIBLE INTERACTION WITH OTHER SUBSTANCES

INTERACTS WITH	COMBINED EFFECT
Alcohol:	Severe skin rash common in many patients within 30 to 45 minutes after drinking alcohol.
Beverages:	None expected.
Cocaine:	None expected.
Foods:	None expected.
Marijuana:	None expected.
Tobacco:	None expected.

ADRENOCORTICOIDS (Nasal Inhalation)

GENERIC AND BRAND NAMES

BECLOMETHASONE (nasal)
- Beconase
- Beconase AQ
- Qnasl
- Vancenase
- Vancenase AQ

BUDESONIDE (nasal)
- Rhinocort Aqua
- Rhinocort Nasal Inhaler
- Rhinocort Turbuhaler

CICLESONIDE (nasal)
- Omnaris
- Zetonna

DEXAMETHASONE (nasal)
- Dexacort Turbinaire

FLUTICASONE (nasal)
- Dymista
- Flonase
- Veramyst

MOMETASONE (nasal)
- Asmanex
- Nasonex
- Nasonex Aqueous Nasal Spray

TRIAMCINOLONE (nasal)
- AllerNaze
- Nasacort AQ
- Nasacort HFA
- Tri-Nasal

BASIC INFORMATION

Habit forming? No
Prescription needed? Yes
Available as generic? Yes, for some
Drug class: Adrenocorticoid (nasal); anti-inflammatory (steroidal), nasal

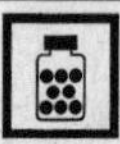

USES

- Treats allergic conditions such as hay fever (seasonal rhinitis).
- Treats nasal polyps and noninfectious-inflammatory nasal conditions.

OVERDOSE

SYMPTOMS:
None expected.
WHAT TO DO:
Overdose unlikely to threaten life. If person uses much larger amount than prescribed or if accidentally swallowed, call doctor or poison control center 1-800-222-1222 for help.

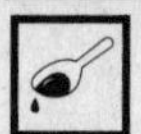

DOSAGE & USAGE INFORMATION

How to take:
Spray—Read patient instruction sheet supplied with your prescription. Usually 1 or 2 sprays into each nostril every 12 hours. Save container for possible refills.

When to take:
At the same time each day, according to instructions on prescription label.

If you forget a dose:
Use as soon as you remember up to an hour late. If you remember more than an hour late, skip this dose. Don't double the next dose.

What drug does:
- Subdues inflammation by decreasing secretion of prostaglandins in cells of the lining of the nose and by inhibiting release of histamine.
- Very little, if any, of the nasal adrenocorticoid gets absorbed into the bloodstream.

Time lapse before drug works:
Usually 5 to 7 days, but may be as long as 2 to 3 weeks.

Don't take with:
Any other medicine or any dietary supplement without consulting your doctor or pharmacist.

POSSIBLE ADVERSE REACTIONS OR SIDE EFFECTS

SYMPTOMS	WHAT TO DO
Life-threatening: None expected.	
Common: Burning or dryness of nose, sneezing.	Continue. Call doctor when convenient.
Infrequent: Crusting inside the nose, nosebleed, sore throat, ulcers in nose, cough, dizziness, headache, hoarseness, nausea, runny nose, bloody mucus.	Discontinue. Call doctor right away.
Rare:	
• White patches in nose or throat.	Discontinue. Call doctor right away.
• Eye pain, wheezing respiration.	Discontinue. Seek emergency treatment.

WARNINGS & PRECAUTIONS

Don't take if:
You are allergic to cortisone or any cortisone-like medication.

Before you start, consult your doctor if:
- You are allergic to any of the propellants in the spray. These include benzalkonium chloride, disodium acetate, phenylethanol, fluorocarbons and propylene glycol.
- You have sores in the nose, have had recent surgery or injury involving the nose.
- You have amebiasis, asthma, type 2 diabetes, glaucoma, herpes eye infection, liver disease, tuberculosis, underactive thyroid, any heart condition or any infection.

Over age 60:
No special problems expected.

Pregnancy:
Risk factors vary for drugs in this group. See category list on page xviii and consult doctor.

Breast-feeding:
Drug may pass into milk. Avoid drug or discontinue nursing until you finish medicine. Consult doctor on maintaining milk supply.

Infants & children:
- Approval for use in children varies for these drugs (ranging from ages over 2, 4 and 6).
- Adrenocorticoids taken by mouth may slow or decrease growth rate or cause reduced adrenal gland function. The nasal form is generally considered safer than the oral form. Be sure you and your child's doctor discuss all benefits and risks of the drug.

Prolonged use:
Not recommended.

Skin & sunlight:
No special problems expected.

Driving, piloting or hazardous work:
Don't drive or pilot aircraft until you learn how medicine affects you. Don't work around dangerous machinery. Don't climb ladders or work in high places. Danger increases if you drink alcohol or take medicine affecting alertness and reflexes.

Discontinuing:
No special problems expected.

Others:
Advise any doctor or dentist whom you consult that you use this medicine.

POSSIBLE INTERACTION WITH OTHER DRUGS

GENERIC NAME OR DRUG CLASS	COMBINED EFFECT
Ephedrine	Decreased effect of nasal adrenocorticoid.
Phenobarbital	Decreased effect of nasal adrenocorticoid.
Rifampin	Decreased effect of nasal adrenocorticoid.
Ritonavir	Increased effect of fluticasone.

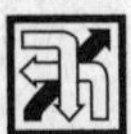

POSSIBLE INTERACTION WITH OTHER SUBSTANCES

INTERACTS WITH	COMBINED EFFECT
Alcohol:	None expected.
Beverages:	None expected.
Cocaine:	None expected.
Foods:	None expected.
Marijuana:	None expected.
Tobacco:	None expected.

ADRENOCORTICOIDS (Oral Inhalation)

GENERIC AND BRAND NAMES

BECLOMETHASONE (oral inhalation)
- Beclodisk
- Becloforte
- Qvar
- Vanceril

BUDESONIDE (oral inhalation)
- Pulmicort Flexhaler
- Pulmicort Respules
- Symbicort

CICLESONIDE (oral inhalation)
- Alvesco Inhalation

DEXAMETHASONE (oral inhalation)
- Decadron Respihaler

FLUTICASONE (oral inhalation)
- Advair Diskus
- Advair HFA
- Flovent
- Flovent HFA

MOMETASONE (oral inhalation)
- Dulera

TRIAMCINOLONE (oral inhalation)
- Azmacort

BASIC INFORMATION

Habit forming? No
Prescription needed? Yes
Available as generic? Yes, for some
Drug class: Anti-inflammatory (inhalation), antiasthmatic

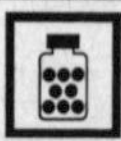

USES

Treatment for prevention of symptoms in patients with chronic bronchial asthma. Does not relieve the symptoms of an acute asthma attack.

DOSAGE & USAGE INFORMATION

How to take:
Oral inhaler—Follow instructions that come with your prescription or from your doctor. If you don't understand the instructions or have any questions, consult your doctor or pharmacist. Most effective if taken regularly. More effective if taken with a spacer.

Continued next column

When to take:
Your doctor will determine the dosage amount and schedule that will help control the asthma symptoms and lessen risks of side effects. Usually 1 to 2 inhaled puffs 3 to 4 times a day is sufficient.

If you forget a dose:
Take as soon as you remember. Then spread out the remaining doses for that day at regularly spaced intervals.

What drug does:
Helps prevent inflammation in the lungs and breathing passages. May decrease progression of severe disease.

Time lapse before drug works:
1 to 4 weeks for the initial response and up to several months for full benefits.

Don't take with:
Any other medicine or any dietary supplement without consulting your doctor or pharmacist.

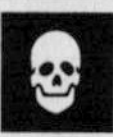

OVERDOSE

SYMPTOMS:
None expected.
WHAT TO DO:
Overdose unlikely to threaten life. If person uses much larger amount than prescribed or if accidentally swallowed, call doctor or poison control center 1-800-222-1222 for help.

POSSIBLE ADVERSE REACTIONS OR SIDE EFFECTS

SYMPTOMS	WHAT TO DO
Life-threatening: None expected.	
Common: Dry mouth, cough, throat irritation, hoarseness or other voice changes.	Continue. Call doctor when convenient.
Infrequent: Dry throat, headache, nausea, skin bruising, unpleasant taste, white curd-like patches in mouth or throat, pain when eating or swallowing (thrush).	Continue. Call doctor when convenient.
Rare: Increased wheezing; difficulty in breathing; pain, tightness or burning in chest; behavior changes (restlessness, nervousness, depression) with budesonide.	Continue, but call doctor right away.

WARNINGS & PRECAUTIONS

Don't use if:
You are allergic to any corticosteroids.*

Before you start, consult your doctor if:
- You have osteoporosis.
- You have or have had tuberculosis.
- You are taking oral corticosteroid drugs.

Over age 60:
No special problems expected.

Pregnancy:
Risk factors may vary for drugs in this group. See category list on page xviii and consult doctor.

Breast-feeding:
Unknown effect. Decide with your doctor if you should continue breast-feeding while using this drug.

Infants & children:
- Should be safe with regular low-dosage regimen. These drugs may slow or decrease growth rate or cause reduced adrenal gland function. Be sure you and your child's doctor discuss all benefits and risks of the drug.
- Children using large doses of this drug are more susceptible to infectious disease (chicken pox, measles). Avoid exposure to infected people and keep all immunizations up to date.

Prolonged use:
- Talk to your doctor about the need for follow-up medical examinations or laboratory studies to check adrenal function, growth and development in children, pulmonary function and inhalation technique.
- The drug may lose its effectiveness. If this occurs, consult your doctor.

Skin & sunlight:
No special problems expected.

Driving, piloting or hazardous work:
No special problems expected.

Discontinuing:
Don't discontinue this drug after prolonged use without consulting doctor. Dosage may require a gradual reduction before stopping to avoid any withdrawal symptoms.

Others:
- Advise any doctor or dentist whom you consult that you use this medicine.
- Carry or wear identification to state that you use this medicine.
- Call your doctor if you have any injury, infection or other stress to your body.
- Take medicine only as directed. Do not increase or reduce dosage without doctor's approval.

POSSIBLE INTERACTION WITH OTHER DRUGS

GENERIC NAME OR DRUG CLASS	COMBINED EFFECT
None significant.	

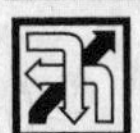

POSSIBLE INTERACTION WITH OTHER SUBSTANCES

INTERACTS WITH	COMBINED EFFECT
Alcohol:	None expected.
Beverages:	None expected.
Cocaine:	Effects not known. Best to avoid.
Foods:	None expected.
Marijuana:	Effects not known. Best to avoid.
Tobacco:	Asthma patients should avoid.

*See Glossary

ADRENOCORTICOIDS (Systemic)

GENERIC AND BRAND NAMES

See full list of generic and brand names in the *Generic and Brand Name Directory*, page 864.

BASIC INFORMATION

Habit forming? No
Prescription needed? Yes
Available as generic? Yes, for most
Drug class: Anti-inflammatory (steroidal), corticosteroid, immunosuppressant

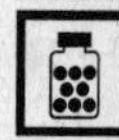

USES

- Used for their anti-inflammatory and immunosuppressive effect in the treatment of many medical disorders,
- Treats allergies, asthma, arthritis, Addison's disease, skin problems, ulcerative colitis, some cancers and numerous other conditions.

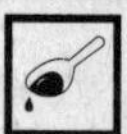

DOSAGE & USAGE INFORMATION

How to take:

- Tablet or capsule—Swallow with liquid. Take with food to lessen stomach irritation. If you have trouble swallowing drug, ask doctor or pharmacist for advice.
- Extended-release tablet or extended-release capsule—Swallow whole with liquid. Take with food to lessen stomach irritation.
- Oral disintegrating tablet—Let tablet dissolve in mouth. Do not chew or swallow tablet.
- Oral suspension, syrup or enema—Follow instructions on label.

When to take:
At the same time(s) each day. Take once-a-day or once-every-other-day doses in mornings.

If you forget a dose:
Take as soon as you remember. If it is almost time for the next dose, wait for the next scheduled dose (don't double this dose).

Continued next column

OVERDOSE

SYMPTOMS:
May have psychological changes, heart rhythm problems or allergic symptoms (e.g., shortness of breath).
WHAT TO DO:

- **Dial 911 (emergency) for medical help or call poison control center 1-800-222-1222 for instructions.**
- **See emergency information on last 3 pages of this book.**

What drug does:
Decreases inflammatory responses. Suppresses immune response. Stimulates bone marrow.

Time lapse before drug works:
Starts working within hours, but may take days to weeks for full benefit.

Don't take with:
Any other medicine or any dietary supplement without consulting your doctor or pharmacist.

POSSIBLE ADVERSE REACTIONS OR SIDE EFFECTS

SYMPTOMS	WHAT TO DO
Life-threatening:	
Hives, rash, intense itching, faintness, swelling soon after a dose (anaphylaxis).	Seek emergency treatment immediately.
Common:	
Increased appetite, indigestion, stomach irritation, insomnia, mood changes, feeling nervous or restless; with long term use—high blood pressure or puffy face or weak bones or fractures.	Continue. Call doctor when convenient.
Infrequent:	
• Infections, blurred or decreased vision, frequent urination, increased thirst, unusual mental or emotional changes.	Continue. Call doctor right away.
• Feeling dizzy or lightheaded, changes in skin color, flushing, hiccups, sweating, spinning sensation, acne, hair loss.	Continue. Call doctor when convenient.
Rare:	
Long term use or high doses—pain (stomach, bone, joint, other), black or tarry stools, eye pain or redness or sensitive to light, muscle cramps, menstrual problems, headaches, irregular heartbeat, stretch marks or thin skin, nausea or vomiting, child's growth stunted, sleep problems, unusual hair growth or bruising, tiredness or weakness, rapid weight gain, slow wound healing, feet or ankle swelling.	Continue. Call doctor when convenient.

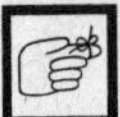

WARNINGS & PRECAUTIONS

Don't take if:
- You are allergic to any cortisone* drug.
- You have an active case of tuberculosis, systemic fungal infection, herpes infection of eyes or peptic ulcer disease.

Before you start, consult your doctor if:
You have, or have had, heart disease, congestive heart failure, diabetes, AIDS, HIV infection, glaucoma, underactive or overactive thyroid, high blood pressure, myasthenia gravis, blood clots in legs or lungs, peptic ulcer disease, tuberculosis, recent or current chickenpox or measles, kidney or liver disease, esophagitis, cold sores, osteoporosis, systemic lupus erythematosus or hyperlipidemia.

Over age 60:
With long term use, the adverse reactions and side effects may be more frequent or severe; may have increased risk of osteoporosis, eye problems or high blood pressure.

Pregnancy:
Risk category varies for drugs in this group. See category list on page xviii and consult doctor.

Breast-feeding:
Drug passes into milk. Avoid drug or discontinue nursing until you finish medicine. Consult doctor for advice on maintaining milk supply.

Infants & children:
- Use only under close medical supervision. These drugs may slow or decrease growth rate or cause reduced adrenal gland function. Be sure you and your child's doctor discuss all benefits and risks of the drug.
- Children using large doses of this drug are more susceptible to infectious disease.

Prolonged use:
- Greatly increases the risk of adverse effects.
- Talk to your doctor about the need for follow-up medical exams or laboratory studies.

Skin & sunlight:
No problems expected.

Driving, piloting or hazardous work:
No problems expected (unless you feel dizzy).

Discontinuing:
- Don't discontinue without doctor's advice until you complete prescribed dose, even though symptoms diminish or disappear.
- Don't stop drug suddenly. Drug dose usually needs to be gradually reduced (tapered). Consult doctor if withdrawal symptoms occur (e.g., fatigue, weakness, stomach pain, nausea or vomiting, diarrhea or low blood pressure).
- Drug can affect your response to surgery, illness, injury or stress for 2 years after discontinuing. Tell anyone who takes medical care of you within 2 years about use of this drug.

Others:
- Consult your doctor before receiving any type of vaccination. Some vaccines may be less effective in persons taking this drug.
- Resistance to infection is less while taking this medicine. Consult doctor if infection occurs.
- Call doctor about swelling or rapid weight gain.
- Advise any doctor or dentist whom you consult that you take this medicine.
- May cause recurrence of tuberculosis.
- Can interfere with the accuracy of some medical tests.
- Wear or carry medical identification that indicates use of this drug (if using long term).

POSSIBLE INTERACTION WITH OTHER DRUGS

GENERIC NAME OR DRUG CLASS	COMBINED EFFECT
Antacids*	May decrease effect of adrenocorticoid.
Anticholinergics*	Risk of glaucoma.
Anticoagulants,* oral	May increase or decrease anti-coagulant effect.
Antidepressants, tricyclic*	Increased risk of side effects.
Antidiabetics,* oral	Decreased anti-diabetic effect.
Antifungals, azole	Increased effect of adrenocorticoid.
Anti-inflammatory drugs, nonsteroidal (NSAIDs)*	Increased risk of side effects.

Continued on page 898

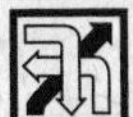

POSSIBLE INTERACTION WITH OTHER SUBSTANCES

INTERACTS WITH	COMBINED EFFECT
Alcohol:	Stomach ulcer risk.
Beverages: Grapefruit juice.	Ask your doctor or pharmacist.
Cocaine:	Unknown. Avoid.
Foods: Grapefruit.	Ask your doctor or pharmacist.
Marijuana:	Unknown. Avoid.
Tobacco:	May decrease adrenocorticoid effect.

***See Glossary**

ADRENOCORTICOIDS (Topical)

GENERIC AND BRAND NAMES

See full list of generic and brand names in the *Generic and Brand Name Directory*, page 864.

BASIC INFORMATION

Habit forming? No
Prescription needed? Yes, for some
Available as generic? Yes
Drug class: Adrenocorticoid (topical)

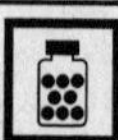

USES

Relieves redness, swelling, itching, skin discomfort of hemorrhoids; insect bites; poison ivy, oak, sumac; soaps, cosmetics; jewelry; burns; sunburn; numerous skin rashes; eczema; discoid lupus erythematosus; swimmer's ear; sun poisoning; hair loss; scars; pemphigus; psoriasis; pityriasis rosea.

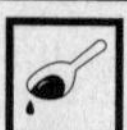

DOSAGE & USAGE INFORMATION

How to use:

- Cream, lotion, ointment, gel—Apply small amount and rub in gently.
- Foam—Follow directions on container. Don't breathe vapors.
- Other forms—Follow directions on container.

When to use:
When needed or as directed. Don't use more often than directions allow.

If you forget an application:
Use as soon as you remember.

What drug does:
Reduces inflammation by affecting enzymes that produce inflammation.

Time lapse before drug works:
15 to 20 minutes.

Don't use with:
Any other topical medicine without consulting your doctor or pharmacist.

OVERDOSE

SYMPTOMS:
None expected.
WHAT TO DO:
If person swallows or inhales drug, call doctor or poison control center 1-800-222-1222 for help.

POSSIBLE ADVERSE REACTIONS OR SIDE EFFECTS

SYMPTOMS	WHAT TO DO
Life-threatening: None expected.	
Common: None expected.	
Infrequent: Infection on skin with pain, redness, blisters, pus; skin irritation with burning, itching, blistering or peeling; acne-like skin eruptions.	Continue. Call doctor when convenient.
Rare: None expected.	

Note: Side effects are unlikely if topical adrenocorticoids are used in low doses for short periods of time. High doses for long periods can possibly cause the adverse reactions of cortisone, listed under ADRENOCORTICOIDS (Systemic).

WARNINGS & PRECAUTIONS

Don't take if:
You are allergic to any topical adrenocorticoid (cortisone) preparation.

Before you start, consult your doctor if:
- You plan pregnancy within medication period.
- You have diabetes.
- You have infection at treatment site.
- You have stomach ulcer.
- You have tuberculosis.

Over age 60:
Adverse reactions and side effects may be more frequent and severe than in younger persons, especially thinning of the skin.

Pregnancy:
Decide with your doctor whether drug benefits justify risk to unborn child. Risk category C (see page xviii).

Breast-feeding:
No problems expected.

Infants & children:
- Use only under medical supervision. Too much for too long can be absorbed into blood stream through skin and retard growth.
- For infants in diapers, avoid plastic pants or tight diapers.

Prolonged use:
- Increases chance of absorption into blood stream to cause side effects of oral cortisone drugs.
- May thin skin where used.
- Talk to your doctor about the need for follow-up medical examinations or laboratory studies to check complete blood counts (white blood cell count, platelet count, red blood cell count, hemoglobin, hematocrit), adrenal function.

Skin & sunlight:
Desoximetasone may cause rash or intensify sunburn in areas exposed to sun or ultraviolet light (photosensitivity reaction). Avoid over-exposure. Notify doctor if reaction occurs.

Driving, piloting or hazardous work:
No problems expected.

Discontinuing:
May be unnecessary to finish medicine. Follow doctor's instructions.

Others:
- Don't use a plastic dressing longer than 2 weeks.
- Aerosol spray—Store in cool place. Don't use near heat or open flame or while smoking. Don't puncture, break or burn container.
- Don't use for acne or gingivitis.

POSSIBLE INTERACTION WITH OTHER DRUGS

GENERIC NAME OR DRUG CLASS	COMBINED EFFECT
Antibacterials* (topical)	Decreased antibiotic effect.
Antifungals* (topical)	Decreased antifungal effect.

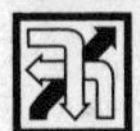

POSSIBLE INTERACTION WITH OTHER SUBSTANCES

INTERACTS WITH	COMBINED EFFECT
Alcohol:	None expected.
Beverages:	None expected.
Cocaine:	None expected.
Foods:	None expected.
Marijuana:	None expected.
Tobacco:	None expected.

***See Glossary**

ALPHA ADRENERGIC RECEPTOR BLOCKERS

GENERIC AND BRAND NAMES

ALFUZOSIN
UroXatral
DOXAZOSIN
Cardura
Cardura XL
PRAZOSIN
Minipress
Minizide
SILODOSIN
Rapaflo
TAMSULOSIN
Flomax
Jalyn
TERAZOSIN
Hytrin

BASIC INFORMATION

Habit forming? No
Prescription needed? Yes
Available as generic? Yes, for some
Drug class: Antihypertensive

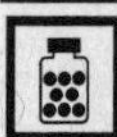

USES

- Treatment for high blood pressure.
- May improve congestive heart failure.
- Treatment for Raynaud's disease.
- Treatment for benign prostatic hyperplasia.

DOSAGE & USAGE INFORMATION

How to take:
- Tablet (doxazosin)—Swallow with liquid. If you can't swallow whole, crush or crumble tablet and take with liquid or food.
- Tablet or capsule or extended-release tablet—Swallow whole with liquid. Do not crumble or crush or chew tablet or open capsule.

Continued next column

OVERDOSE

SYMPTOMS:
Extreme weakness; rapid or irregular heartbeat; loss of consciousness; cold, sweaty skin; weak, rapid pulse; coma.
WHAT TO DO:
- **Dial 911 (emergency) for medical help or call poison control center 1-800-222-1222 for instructions.**
- **If person is unconscious, check breathing and pulse. If not breathing, begin mouth-to-mouth rescue breathing. If heart is not beating, begin chest compressions.**
- **See emergency information on last 3 pages of this book.**

When to take:
At the same times each day.

If you forget a dose:
Take as soon as you remember. If it is almost time for the next dose, wait for the next scheduled dose (don't double this dose).

What drug does:
Expands and relaxes blood vessel walls to lower blood pressure.

Time lapse before drug works:
30 minutes; may take days or weeks for full effect.

Don't take with:
Any other medicine or any dietary supplement without consulting your doctor or pharmacist.

POSSIBLE ADVERSE REACTIONS OR SIDE EFFECTS

SYMPTOMS	WHAT TO DO
Life-threatening:	
In case of overdose, see previous column.	
Common:	
Headache, dizziness.	Continue. Call doctor when convenient.
Infrequent:	
• Rash or itchy skin, blurred vision, shortness of breath, difficulty breathing, chest pain, rapid heartbeat.	Discontinue. Call doctor right away.
• Appetite loss, constipation or diarrhea, abdominal pain, nausea, vomiting, fluid retention, joint or muscle aches, tiredness, weakness and faintness when arising from bed or chair, little or no semen when ejaculating.	Continue. Call doctor when convenient.
• Headache, irritability, depression, dry mouth, stuffy nose, increased urination, drowsiness.	Continue. Tell doctor at next visit.
Rare:	
Decreased sexual function, numbness or tingling in hands or feet.	Continue. Call doctor when convenient.

ALPHA ADRENERGIC RECEPTOR BLOCKERS

WARNINGS & PRECAUTIONS

Don't take if:
You are allergic to alpha adrenergic receptor blockers.

Before you start, consult your doctor if:
- You experience lightheadedness or fainting with other antihypertensive drugs.
- You are easily depressed.
- You have impaired brain circulation or have had a stroke.
- You will have surgery within 2 months, including dental surgery, requiring general or spinal anesthesia.
- You have coronary heart disease (with or without angina).
- You have kidney disease or impaired liver function.

Over age 60:
Begin with no more than 1 mg. per day for first 3 days. Increases should be gradual and supervised by your doctor. Don't stand while taking. Sudden changes in position may cause falls. Sit or lie down promptly if you feel dizzy. If you have impaired brain circulation or coronary heart disease, excessive lowering of blood pressure should be avoided. Report problems to your doctor immediately.

Pregnancy:
Risk category varies for drugs in this group. See category list on page xviii and consult doctor.

Breast-feeding:
It is unknown if drug passes into milk. Avoid drug or discontinue nursing until you finish medicine. Consult doctor for advice on maintaining milk supply.

Infants & children:
Not recommended.

Prolonged use:
Talk to your doctor about the need for follow-up medical examinations or laboratory studies.

Skin & sunlight:
No problems expected.

Driving, piloting or hazardous work:
Don't drive or pilot aircraft until you learn how medicine affects you. Don't work around dangerous machinery. Don't climb ladders or work in high places.

Discontinuing:
Don't discontinue without doctor's advice until you complete prescribed dose, even though symptoms diminish or disappear.

Others:
- First dose likely to cause dizziness or lightheadedness. Take drug at night and get out of bed slowly next morning.
- Advise any doctor or dentist whom you consult that you take this medicine.
- May affect the results in some medical tests.

POSSIBLE INTERACTION WITH OTHER DRUGS

GENERIC NAME OR DRUG CLASS	COMBINED EFFECT
Amphetamines*	Decreased alpha adrenergic blocker effect.
Antihypertensives, other*	Increased antihypertensive effect. Dosages may require adjustments.
Anti-inflammatory drugs, nonsteroidal (NSAIDs)*	Decreased effect of alpha adrenergic blocker.
Enzyme inhibitors*	Increased effect of alpha adrenergic blocker.
Estrogen	Decreased effect of alpha adrenergic blocker.
Ritonavir	Increased effect of alfuzosin.
Sympathomimetics*	Decreased effect of alpha adrenergic blocker.

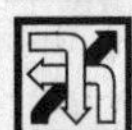

POSSIBLE INTERACTION WITH OTHER SUBSTANCES

INTERACTS WITH	COMBINED EFFECT
Alcohol:	Excessive blood pressure drop.
Beverages:	Grapefruit juice may increase effect of one or more of these drugs.
Cocaine:	Increased risk of heart block and high blood pressure.
Foods:	None expected.
Marijuana:	Fainting. Avoid.
Tobacco:	Possible spasm of coronary arteries. Avoid.

*See Glossary

ALPROSTADIL

BRAND NAMES

Caverject
Edex
Muse

BASIC INFORMATION

Habit forming? No
Prescription needed? Yes
Available as generic? No
Drug class: Impotence therapy

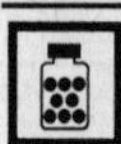

USES

Treatment for impotence in some men who have erectile dysfunction due to neurologic, vascular, psychological or mixed causes.

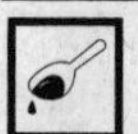

DOSAGE & USAGE INFORMATION

How to use:

- Injection—The first injection will be given in the doctor's office to determine proper dosage and to train you in preparing and self-injecting the drug. When using it at home, follow the instructions provided with the prescription or use as directed by your doctor to inject drug into the penis.
- Intraurethral—Use as a single dose suppository 10 to 30 minutes prior to intercourse.

When to take:
Usually 10 to 30 minutes prior to sexual intercourse. Do not use injection more than 3 times in one week and do not use more than once in a 24-hour period. Do not use more than 2 suppositories in one 24-hour period.

If you forget a dose:
Not used on a scheduled basis.

What drug does:
Increases the blood flow into the penis and decreases the blood flow from the penis. The change in blood flow causes the penis to swell and elongate.

Continued next column

Time lapse before drug works:
5 to 20 minutes. Erections may last up to 60 minutes.

Don't take with:
Any other medicine or any dietary supplement without consulting your doctor or pharmacist.

OVERDOSE

SYMPTOMS:
Prolonged penile erection.
WHAT TO DO:
Overdose unlikely to threaten life. If person uses much larger amount than prescribed or if accidentally swallowed, call doctor or poison control center 1-800-222-1222 for help.

POSSIBLE ADVERSE REACTIONS OR SIDE EFFECTS

SYMPTOMS	WHAT TO DO
Life-threatening: None expected.	
Common:	
• Pain at site of injection, aching or burning pain during erection.	Discontinue. Call doctor when convenient.
• Pinching sensation at injection site.	Continue. Tell doctor at next visit.
Infrequent: None expected.	
Rare:	
• Erection lasting more than 4 hours is not priapism; (priapism is defined as an erection lasting more than 6 hours). Could cause permanent damage to the penis.	Call doctor right away or seek emergency care.
• Bruising or bleeding at site of injection; redness, swelling, tenderness, lumpiness, itching, rash, irritation, strange feeling, numbness or curving of the erect penis; slight bleeding from urethra, swelling of leg veins, dizziness, fainting, rapid pulse. Female partners may have mild vaginal itching or burning.	Discontinue. Call doctor when convenient.

WARNINGS & PRECAUTIONS

Don't use if:
You are allergic to alprostadil or you have been advised not to have sex.

Before you start, consult your doctor if:
- You have liver disease.
- You have sickle cell anemia or trait.
- You have multiple myeloma or leukemia.
- You have a penile implant or any type of penile malformation.
- You are allergic to any other medications.
- You have a history of priapism (prolonged penile erection).

Over age 60:
Effects on this age group are variable. Consult doctor.

Pregnancy:
Not used by females. Men should not use the product to have sexual intercourse with a pregnant woman unless the couple uses a condom barrier.

Breast-feeding:
Not used by females.

Infants & children:
Not used in this age group.

Prolonged use:
Have regular checkups with your doctor while using this drug to determine the effectiveness of the treatment and to check for any penile problems.

Skin & sunlight:
No special problems expected.

Driving, piloting or hazardous work:
No special problems expected.

Discontinuing:
No special problems expected.

Others:
- Don't increase dosage or frequency of use without your doctor's approval.
- Follow label instructions and dispose of all needles properly after use. Do not reuse or share needles.
- The injection of this drug provides no protection from sexually transmitted diseases. Other protective measures, such as condoms, should be used when necessary to prevent the spread of sexually transmitted diseases.
- Slight bleeding may occur at injection site. Apply pressure if this occurs. If bleeding persists, consult doctor.

POSSIBLE INTERACTION WITH OTHER DRUGS

GENERIC NAME OR DRUG CLASS	COMBINED EFFECT
None significant.	

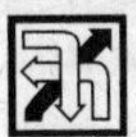

POSSIBLE INTERACTION WITH OTHER SUBSTANCES

INTERACTS WITH	COMBINED EFFECT
Alcohol:	No special problems expected.
Beverages:	No special problems expected.
Cocaine:	No special problems expected.
Foods:	No special problems expected.
Marijuana:	No special problems expected.
Tobacco:	No special problems expected.

*See Glossary

AMINOGLUTETHIMIDE

BRAND NAMES

Cytadren

BASIC INFORMATION

Habit forming? No
Prescription needed? Yes
Available as generic? No
Drug class: Antiadrenal, antineoplastic

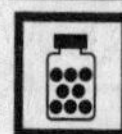

USES

- Treats Cushing's syndrome.
- Treats breast and prostate cancer.

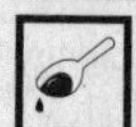

DOSAGE & USAGE INFORMATION

How to take:
Tablet—Swallow with liquid. If you can't swallow whole, crumble tablet and take with liquid or food. Instructions to take on empty stomach mean 1 hour before or 2 hours after eating.

When to take:
Follow doctor's instructions exactly.

If you forget a dose:
Take as soon as you remember. If it is almost time for the next dose, wait for the next scheduled dose (don't double this dose).

What drug does:
Suppresses adrenal cortex.

Time lapse before drug works:
1 to 2 hours.

Don't take with:
Any other medicines (including over-the-counter drugs such as cough and cold medicines, laxatives, antacids, diet pills, caffeine, nose drops, vitamins or other diet supplements) without consulting your doctor or pharmacist.

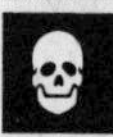

OVERDOSE

SYMPTOMS:
None expected.
WHAT TO DO:
Overdose unlikely to threaten life. If person uses much larger amount than prescribed or if accidentally swallowed, call doctor or poison control center 1-800-222-1222 for help.

POSSIBLE ADVERSE REACTIONS OR SIDE EFFECTS

SYMPTOMS	WHAT TO DO
Life-threatening: None expected.	
Common:	
• Skin rash on face and hands, feeling drowsy.	Continue, but call doctor right away.
• Nausea, loss of appetite.	Continue. Call doctor when convenient.
Infrequent:	
Dizziness, clumsiness, unusual tiredness or weakness, unusual eye movements, depression, fast heartbeat, feeling shaky, slurred speech.	Continue, but call doctor right away.
Rare:	
• Unusual bleeding or bruising, black or tarry stools, fever and chills along with cough or low back pain or painful urination, shortness of breath, pinpoint spots on skin, blood in urine.	Discontinue. Call doctor right away.
• Tenderness or swelling of the neck, headache, vomiting, menstrual changes, hair growth or deeper voice in females, muscle pain.	Continue. Call doctor when convenient.

WARNINGS & PRECAUTIONS

Don't take if:
You are allergic to aminoglutethimide or glutethimide,

Before you start, consult your doctor if:
- You have recently been exposed to chicken pox.
- You have shingles (herpes zoster).
- You have decreased thyroid function (hypothyroidism).
- You have any liver or kidney disorder.
- You have any form of infection.

Over age 60:
Adverse reactions and side effects may be more frequent and severe than in younger persons. You may need smaller doses for shorter periods of time.

Pregnancy:
Risk category D (see page xviii).

Breast-feeding:
Unknown effect. Decide with your doctor if you should continue breast-feeding while using this drug.

Infants & children:
Effect not documented. Consult your doctor.

Prolonged use:
Talk to your doctor about the need for follow-up medical examinations or laboratory studies to check thyroid function, liver function, serum electrolytes (sodium, potassium, chloride) and blood pressure.

Skin & sunlight:
No problems expected.

Driving, piloting or hazardous work:
No problems expected.

Discontinuing:
No special problems expected.

Others:
- Advise any doctor or dentist whom you consult that you take this medicine.
- May affect results in some medical tests.
- May cause decreased thyroid function.

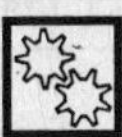

POSSIBLE INTERACTION WITH OTHER DRUGS

GENERIC NAME OR DRUG CLASS	COMBINED EFFECT
Anticoagulants*	Decreased anticoagulant effect.
Central nervous system (CNS) depressants*	Increased risk of drowsiness.
Cortisone-like drugs*	Decreased cortisone effects.
Dexamethasone	Decreased dexamethasone effect.

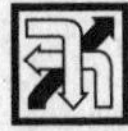

POSSIBLE INTERACTION WITH OTHER SUBSTANCES

INTERACTS WITH	COMBINED EFFECT
Alcohol:	Increased stomach irritation.
Beverages: Coffee, tea, cocoa.	Increased stomach irritation.
Cocaine:	No proven problems.
Foods:	No proven problems.
Marijuana:	No proven problems.
Tobacco:	No proven problems.

*See Glossary

AMLEXANOX

BRAND NAMES

Aphthasol | OraDisc

BASIC INFORMATION

Habit forming? No
Prescription needed? Yes
Available as generic? No
Drug class: Antiaphthous ulcer agent

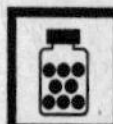

USES

Treatment for severe canker sores (aphthous ulcers) in the mouth.

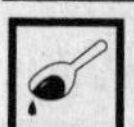

DOSAGE & USAGE INFORMATION

How to use:

- Oral paste—Use fingertips to apply paste directly to each canker sore following oral hygiene.
- Patch—Apply to affected area in the mouth. The drug will dissolve slowly.

When to use:
Use as soon as symptoms of a canker sore appear. Apply four times a day—after meals and before bedtime. Wash hands after application.

If you forget a dose:
Use as soon as you remember. If it is almost time for the next dose, wait for the next dose (don't double this dose).

What drug does:
Exact healing mechanism is unknown. Appears to stop the inflammatory process and hypersensitivity reaction.

Time lapse before drug works:
Pain relief may occur within hours or up to 24 hours. Complete healing time will take several days.

Don't use with:
Any other medicine for mouth ulcers without consulting your doctor or pharmacist.

OVERDOSE

SYMPTOMS:
None expected.
WHAT TO DO:
If person accidentally swallows drug, call doctor or poison control center 1-800-222-1222 for help.

POSSIBLE ADVERSE REACTIONS OR SIDE EFFECTS

SYMPTOMS	WHAT TO DO
Life-threatening:	
None expected.	
Common:	
None expected.	
Infrequent:	
Slight pain, stinging or burning at site of application.	No action necessary.
Rare:	
Diarrhea, nausea, rash.	Discontinue. Call doctor when convenient.

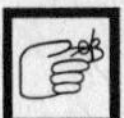

WARNINGS & PRECAUTIONS

Don't take if:
You are allergic to amlexanox.

Before you start, consult your doctor if:
- You are allergic to any medication, food or other substance.
- You have a weak immune system due to drugs or illness.

Over age 60:
No problems expected.

Pregnancy:
Decide with your doctor if drug benefits outweigh risks to unborn child. Risk category B (see page xviii).

Breast-feeding:
It is unknown if drug passes into milk. Absorption into the body has occurred with this drug. Avoid drug or discontinue nursing until you finish medicine. Consult doctor for advice on maintaining milk supply.

Infants & children:
Safety and efficacy have not been established. Use only under close medical supervision.

Prolonged use:
Normally only used for up to 10 days of treatment.

Skin & sunlight:
No problems expected.

Driving, piloting or hazardous work:
No problems expected.

Discontinuing:
May be unnecessary to finish medicine. Discontinue when canker sores heal.

Others:
- If canker sores do not heal after 10 days, consult your dentist or health care provider.
- Advise any doctor or dentist whom you consult that you take this medicine.

POSSIBLE INTERACTION WITH OTHER DRUGS

GENERIC NAME OR DRUG CLASS	COMBINED EFFECT
None expected.	

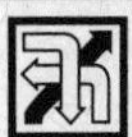

POSSIBLE INTERACTION WITH OTHER SUBSTANCES

INTERACTS WITH	COMBINED EFFECT
Alcohol:	None expected.
Beverages:	None expected.
Cocaine:	None expected.
Foods:	None expected.
Marijuana:	None expected.
Tobacco:	None expected.

AMPHETAMINES

GENERIC AND BRAND NAMES

AMPHETAMINE & DEXTRO-AMPHETAMINE
- Adderall
- Adderall XR

DEXTROAMPHETAMINE
- Dexedrine
- Dexedrine Spansule
- Liquadd
- Oxydess
- Spancap

LISDEXAMFETAMINE
- Vyvanse

METHAMPHETAMINE
- Desoxyn
- Desoxyn Gradumet

BASIC INFORMATION

Habit forming? Yes
Prescription needed? Yes
Available as generic? Yes
Drug class: Central nervous system stimulant

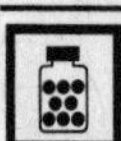

USES

- Treats narcolepsy (sleep attacks).
- Treats attention deficit hyperactivity disorder in adults, adolescents and children.

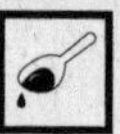

DOSAGE & USAGE INFORMATION

How to take:
- Tablet—Swallow with liquid.
- Extended-release capsule or tablet—Swallow each dose whole with liquid; do not crush.
- Solution—Follow instructions on prescription.

When to take:
- Short-acting form—Don't take later than 6 hours before bedtime.
- Long-acting form—Take on awakening.

If you forget a dose:
Take as soon as you remember. If it is almost time for the next dose, wait for that dose (don't double this dose) and resume regular schedule.

Continued next column

OVERDOSE

SYMPTOMS:
Rapid heartbeat, hyperactivity, high fever, hallucinations, suicidal or homicidal feelings, convulsions, coma.

WHAT TO DO:
- **Dial 911 (emergency) for medical help or call poison control center 1-800-222-1222 for instructions.**
- **See emergency information on last 3 pages of this book.**

What drug does:
- Hyperactivity—Decreases motor restlessness and increases ability to pay attention.
- Narcolepsy—Increases motor activity and mental alertness; diminishes drowsiness.

Time lapse before drug works:
Takes several weeks to see if drug is effective.

Don't take with:
Any other medicine or any diet supplement without consulting your doctor or pharmacist.

POSSIBLE ADVERSE REACTIONS OR SIDE EFFECTS

SYMPTOMS	WHAT TO DO
Life-threatening:	
In case of overdose, see previous column.	
Common:	
• Irritability, nervousness, insomnia, euphoria. signs of addiction.*	Continue. Call doctor when convenient.
• Dry mouth.	Continue. Tell doctor at next visit.
• Fast, pounding heartbeat.	Discontinue. Call doctor right away.
Infrequent:	
• Dizziness, reduced alertness, blurred vision, unusual sweating.	Discontinue. Call doctor right away.
• Headache, diarrhea or constipation, appetite loss, stomach pain, nausea, vomiting, weight loss, diminished sex drive, impotence.	Continue. Call doctor when convenient.
Rare:	
• Rash, hives, chest pain, irregular heartbeat, trouble breathing, fainting, hallucinations, becoming suspicious, manic behavior, uncontrollable movements (head, neck, arms, legs).	Discontinue. Call doctor right away.
• Mood changes, swollen breasts.	Continue. Call doctor when convenient.

WARNINGS & PRECAUTIONS

Don't take if:
You are allergic to any amphetamine.

Before you start, consult your doctor if:
- You plan to become pregnant.
- You have glaucoma.
- You have diabetes, overactive thyroid, anxiety or tension.

- You have a history of substance abuse.
- You will have surgery within 2 months, requiring general or spinal anesthesia.
- Adult or child patient has a mental illness.

Over age 60:
Adverse reactions and side effects may be more frequent and severe than in younger persons.

Pregnancy:
Decide with your doctor if drug benefits justify risk to unborn child. Consult doctor. Risk category C (see page xviii).

Breast-feeding:
Drugs pass into breast milk. Consult your doctor.

Infants & children:
- Amphetamine-dextroamphetamine is used to treat attention deficit disorder in children age 3 and older. Do not use this drug in children under the age of 12 years for weight loss.
- Reports of sudden unexplained death (SUD) in children has been associated with amphetamine abuse and reported in children with underlying heart defects taking amphetamines. A very small number of cases of SUD have been reported in children without heart defects taking amphetamines. Talk to your child's doctor about this risk.

Prolonged use:
- Drug can be habit forming. Ask your doctor about the risks involved.
- Talk to your doctor about the need for follow-up medical examinations or laboratory studies to check blood pressure, growth charts in children and need for continued treatment.

Skin & sunlight:
No problems expected.

Driving, piloting or hazardous work:
Don't drive or pilot aircraft until you learn how medicine affects you. Don't work around dangerous machinery. Don't climb ladders or work in high places. Danger increases if you drink alcohol or take medicine affecting alertness and reflexes.

Discontinuing:
May be unnecessary to finish medicine, but don't suddenly stop. Follow doctor's instructions.

Others:
- Use of this drug must be closely supervised. Don't use for appetite control or depression.
- Advise any doctor or dentist whom you consult that you take this medicine.
- During a withdrawal phase, may cause prolonged sleep of several days.
- Don't use for fatigue or to replace rest.
- Drug may cause serious heart and psychiatric (mental) problems, including sudden death. Read warning information provided with prescription. Call doctor right away if symptoms develop (e.g., chest pain, shortness of breath, fainting or hallucinations).

POSSIBLE INTERACTION WITH OTHER DRUGS

GENERIC NAME OR DRUG CLASS	COMBINED EFFECT
Antidepressants, tricyclic*	Decreased amphetamine effect.
Antihypertensives*	Decreased anti-hypertensive effect.
Beta-adrenergic blocking agents*	High blood pressure, slow heartbeat.
Carbonic anhydrase inhibitors*	Increased amphetamine effect.
Central nervous system (CNS) stimulants,* other	Excessive CNS stimulation.
Doxazosin	Decreased doxazosin effect.
Furazolidone	Sudden and severe high blood pressure.
Haloperidol	Decreased amphetamine effect.
Monoamine oxidase (MAO) inhibitors*	Severe increase in blood pressure.
Phenothiazines*	Decreased amphetamine effect.
Prazosin	Decreased prazosin effect.
Sodium bicarbonate	Increased amphetamine effect.

Continued on page 898

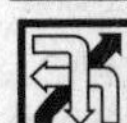

POSSIBLE INTERACTION WITH OTHER SUBSTANCES

INTERACTS WITH	COMBINED EFFECT
Alcohol:	Decreased amphetamine effect. Avoid.
Beverages: Caffeine drinks.	Overstimulation. Avoid.
Cocaine:	Dangerous risk to body's nervous system. Avoid.
Foods:	None expected.
Marijuana:	Frequent use—Severely impaired mental function.
Tobacco:	None expected.

***See Glossary**

ANAGRELIDE

BRAND NAMES

Agrylin

BASIC INFORMATION

Habit forming? No
Prescription needed? Yes
Available as generic? Yes
Drug class: Platelet count-reducing agent; antithrombocythemia

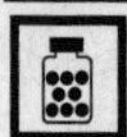

USES

Reduces elevated platelet counts and the risk of thrombosis (formation of a blood clot); also makes symptoms more tolerable in patients with essential thrombocythemia.

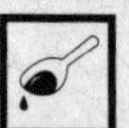

DOSAGE & USAGE INFORMATION

How to take:
Capsule—Swallow with liquid. Take with or without food.

When to take:
At the same time each day. Dose may be adjusted to maintain proper platelet count.

If you forget a dose:
Take as soon as you remember. If it is almost time for the next dose, then skip the missed dose and wait for your next scheduled dose (don't double this dose).

What drug does:
Exact mechanism is unknown.

Time lapse before drug works:
One to two weeks.

Don't take with:
Any other medicine or any dietary supplement without consulting your doctor or pharmacist.

OVERDOSE

SYMPTOMS:
None expected immediately. May lower platelet count, leading to increased bleeding.
WHAT TO DO:
Overdose unlikely to threaten life. If person uses much larger amount than prescribed or if accidentally swallowed, call doctor or poison control center 1-800-222-1222 for help.

POSSIBLE ADVERSE REACTIONS OR SIDE EFFECTS

SYMPTOMS	WHAT TO DO
Life-threatening:	
Severe headache or weakness; pain or pressure in chest, jaw, neck, back or arms; swelling of feet or legs; severe tiredness or weakness; increased heart rate; difficulty breathing or shortness of breath.	Seek emergency treatment immediately.
Common:	
• Abdominal pain, weakness, dizziness palpitations, shortness of breath.	Continue, but call doctor right away.
• Diarrhea, heartburn, gas, bloating, headache, loss of appetite, general feeling of discomfort or illness, nausea, pain.	Continue. Call doctor if symptoms persist.
Infrequent:	
• Blurred or double vision, painful or difficult urination, blood in urine, tingling in hands or feet, unusual bruising or bleeding, flushing, faintness.	Discontinue. Call doctor right away.
• Canker sore, joint pain, back pain, confusion, fever or chills, insomnia, constipation, leg cramps, runny nose, depression, nervousness, ringing in ears, skin rash, sensitivity to light, itching, sleepiness, vomiting.	Continue. Call doctor if symptoms persist.
Rare:	
Hair loss.	Continue. Tell doctor at next visit.

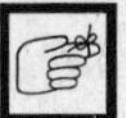

WARNINGS & PRECAUTIONS

Don't take if:
You are allergic to anagrelide.

Before you start, consult your doctor if:
- You have any kidney or liver disease or any heart or blood vessel disorder.
- You have any chronic health problem.
- You are pregnant or nursing.

Over age 60:
No problems expected.

Pregnancy:
Decide with your doctor if drug benefits justify risk to unborn child. Risk category C (see page xviii).

Breast-feeding:
It is unknown if drug passes into milk. Avoid drug or discontinue nursing until you finish medicine. Consult doctor for advice on maintaining milk supply.

Infants & children:
Safety and efficacy have not been established in patients under 16. Use only under close medical supervision.

Prolonged use:
Schedule regular visits with your doctor for laboratory examinations to monitor the continued effectiveness of the medication.

Skin & sunlight:
No problems expected.

Driving, piloting or hazardous work:
No problems expected.

Discontinuing:
Don't discontinue without consulting your doctor even if you feel well.

Others:
- Close medical supervision, including frequent platelet counts, required at start of therapy with this drug.
- Advise any doctor or dentist whom you consult that you are using this medicine.

POSSIBLE INTERACTION WITH OTHER DRUGS

GENERIC NAME OR DRUG CLASS	COMBINED EFFECT
Sucralfate	May interfere with anagrelide absorption. Don't take at the same time.

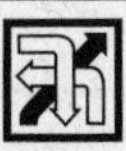

POSSIBLE INTERACTION WITH OTHER SUBSTANCES

INTERACTS WITH	COMBINED EFFECT
Alcohol:	None expected.
Beverages:	None expected.
Cocaine:	Effects unknown. Avoid.
Foods:	None expected.
Marijuana:	Effects unknown. Avoid.
Tobacco:	None expected.

ANAKINRA

BRAND NAMES

Kineret

BASIC INFORMATION

Habit forming? No
Prescription needed? Yes
Available as generic? No
Drug class: Antirheumatic; biological response modifier

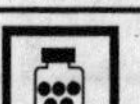

USES

Treatment of moderately to severely active rheumatoid arthritis. Used for patients who have not responded to one or more disease modifying antirheumatic drugs (DMARDs). May be used alone or in combination with certain other arthritis drugs.

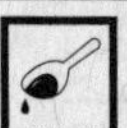

DOSAGE & USAGE INFORMATION

How to take:
Injection—The drug is self-injected under the skin (subcutaneously). Follow your doctor's instructions and the directions provided with the prescription on how and where to inject. Do not use the medication unless you are sure about the proper method for injection. Store medication in the refrigerator (do not freeze) until you plan to use it. After each use, throw away the syringe and any medicine left in it (ask your pharmacist about disposal methods). Never reuse the needle or syringe.

When to take:
Inject every day at the same time each day.

If you forget a dose:
Inject as soon as possible. If it is almost time for your next dose, skip the missed dose and go back to your regular dosing schedule. Do not double doses.

What drug does:
Reduces the actions of chemicals in the body that cause inflammatory and immune responses. It helps prevent progressive joint destruction.

Continued next column

Time lapse before drug works:
It will take several weeks before full benefits of the drug are noticeable.

Don't use with:
Any other medicine or any dietary supplement without consulting your doctor or pharmacist.

OVERDOSE

SYMPTOMS:
None expected.
WHAT TO DO:
If an overdose is suspected, call doctor or poison control center 1-800-222-1222 for help.

POSSIBLE ADVERSE REACTIONS OR SIDE EFFECTS

SYMPTOMS	WHAT TO DO
Life-threatening: None expected.	
Common: Diarrhea, headache, nausea, mild stomach pain.	Continue. Call doctor when convenient.
Infrequent: Reaction at injection site (pain, purple discoloration, inflammation), pain in bones or joints, fever or chills, chest pain, skin symptoms (itching, redness, swelling, hot), cold or flu symptoms (sneezing, cough, sore throat, muscle aches, runny or stuffy nose), trouble with breathing, insomnia, unusual tiredness, vomiting, other signs or symptoms of an infection.	Discontinue. Call doctor right away.
Rare: Allergic reaction (itching, rash, hives, swelling of face or lips, wheezing).	Discontinue. Call doctor right away.

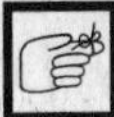

WARNINGS & PRECAUTIONS

Don't take if:
You are allergic to anakinra or the components of the drug (including proteins made from bacterial cells such as *E coli*).

Before you start, consult your doctor if:
- You have a chronic disorder or infection or are immunosuppressed.
- You have asthma (increases risk of infections).
- You have a kidney disorder.
- You have an active infection.
- You are allergic or sensitive to latex.

Over age 60:
Used with caution in elderly patients, since infections are more common in this age group.

Pregnancy:
Usually safe, but decide with your doctor if drug benefits justify any possible risk to unborn child. Risk category B (see page xviii).

Breast-feeding:
It is unknown if drug passes into milk. Consult doctor for advice on breast-feeding if you use this medication.

Infants & children:
Not recommended for children under age 18.

Prolonged use:
- No specific problems expected, but medical studies are ongoing.
- Talk to your doctor about the need for follow-up medical examinations or laboratory studies to check effectiveness of the drug and to monitor for infections.

Skin & sunlight:
No problems expected.

Driving, piloting or hazardous work:
No problems expected.

Discontinuing:
No problems expected. Consult doctor.

Others:
- Advise any doctor or dentist whom you consult that you take this medicine.
- Using this drug increases the risk of infections. Consult your doctor if any signs or symptoms of infection occur.
- Avoid immunizations unless approved by your doctor.

POSSIBLE INTERACTION WITH OTHER DRUGS

GENERIC NAME OR DRUG CLASS	COMBINED EFFECT
Tumor necrosis factor blockers	Increased risk of infections. Use only with close medical supervision.
Vaccines, live	Vaccines may not be effective.

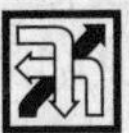

POSSIBLE INTERACTION WITH OTHER SUBSTANCES

INTERACTS WITH	COMBINED EFFECT
Alcohol:	None expected.
Beverages:	None expected.
Cocaine:	None expected. However, cocaine may slow body's recovery. Avoid.
Foods:	None expected.
Marijuana:	None expected. However, marijuana may slow body's recovery. Avoid.
Tobacco:	None expected.

ANDROGENS

GENERIC AND BRAND NAMES

See full list of generic and brand names in the *Generic and Brand Name Directory*, page 866.

BASIC INFORMATION

Habit forming? No
Prescription needed? Yes
Available as generic? Yes, for some
Drug class: Androgen

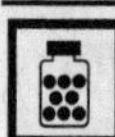

USES

- Corrects male hormone deficiency. Reduces "male menopause" symptoms (loss of sex drive, depression, anxiety).
- Decreases calcium loss of osteoporosis (softened bones).
- Blocks breast cancer cell growth in women.
- Stimulates beginning of puberty in certain boys.
- Augments treatment of aplastic anemia.
- Stimulates weight gain after illness, injury or for chronically underweight persons.
- Stimulates growth in treatment of dwarfism.

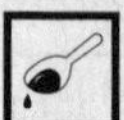

DOSAGE & USAGE INFORMATION

How to take:

- Tablet or capsule—Take with food to lessen stomach irritation.
- Gel, cream, buccal system, transdermal (skin patch), topical solution—Follow instructions provided with prescription or by your doctor.
- Injection—Given as needed for the condition by medical professional. May be self-injected as prescribed by your doctor.

When to take:
Follow directions provided with your prescription.

If you forget a dose:
Take or use as soon as you remember. If it is almost time for the next dose, wait for the next scheduled dose (don't double this dose). For gel or patch, usually wait for next scheduled time.

Continued next column

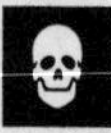

OVERDOSE

SYMPTOMS:
None expected.
WHAT TO DO:
Overdose unlikely to threaten life. If person uses much larger amount than prescribed or if accidentally swallowed, call doctor or poison control center 1-800-222-1222 for help.

What drug does:

- Stimulates cells that produce male sex characteristics.
- Replaces hormone deficiencies.
- Stimulates red-blood-cell production.
- Suppresses production of estrogen (female sex hormone).

Time lapse before drug works:
Varies with problems treated. May require 2 or 3 months of regular use for desired effects.

Don't take with:
Any other medicine or any dietary supplement without consulting your doctor or pharmacist.

POSSIBLE ADVERSE REACTIONS OR SIDE EFFECTS

SYMPTOMS	WHAT TO DO
Life-threatening:	
Intense itching, weakness, loss of consciousness.	Seek emergency treatment immediately.
Common:	
Acne or oily skin, deep voice, enlarged clitoris in females; frequent or continuing erections, sore or swollen breasts in men, pain or sores under patch.	Discontinue. Call doctor right away.
Infrequent:	
• Yellow skin or eyes, depression or confusion, other changes in moods, flushed face, rash or itch, nausea, vomiting, diarrhea, swollen feet or legs, headache, rapid weight gain, difficult or frequent urination, unusual bleeding, scrotum pain.	Discontinue. Call doctor right away.
• Sore mouth, higher or lower sex drive, decreased testicle size, impotence in men, mild redness or itching at site of patch, hair loss, pubic hair growth.	Continue. Call doctor when convenient
Rare:	
Black stools, ongoing symptoms at patch, site, vomiting blood, fever, chills, hives or spots on body.	Discontinue. Call doctor right away.

WARNINGS & PRECAUTIONS

Don't take if:
You are allergic to any male hormone.

Before you start, consult your doctor if:
- You might be pregnant.
- You have cancer of- or enlarged prostate.
- You have heart disease or arteriosclerosis.
- You have kidney or liver disease.
- You have breast cancer (male or female).
- You have high blood pressure.
- You have diabetes (drug can affect blood sugar).

Over age 60:
- May stimulate sexual activity.
- In males, can enlarge prostate, worsen prostate cancer and cause urinary retention. Have a prostate exam before starting this medication.

Pregnancy:
Risk to unborn child outweighs drug benefits. Don't use. Risk category X (see page xviii).

Breast-feeding:
Drug passes into milk. Avoid drug or discontinue nursing until you finish medicine. Consult doctor for advice on maintaining milk supply.

Infants & children:
Use with children only under close medical supervision.

Prolonged use:
- May cause liver cancer, possible kidney stones. In women may cause unnatural hair growth and deep voice.
- Talk to your doctor about the need for follow-up medical examinations or laboratory studies to check effectiveness or unwanted effects of the drug.

Skin & sunlight:
No problems expected.

Driving, piloting or hazardous work:
No problems expected.

Discontinuing:
No problems expected.

Others:
- Reduces sperm count and volume of semen. This effect is usually temporary.
- With patch or gel, drug can pass to sexual partner. Consult doctor if partner starts getting any of the side effects listed.
- Wash hands carefully after applying gel and cover area where gel applied.
- Children and women need to avoid contact with areas of skin where men have applied the gel. It can cause serious side effects, especially in children. Consult doctor if symptoms occur.
- Will not increase strength in athletes.
- Advise any doctor or dentist whom you consult that you take this medicine.
- In women, may cause changes such as deepened voice, increased hair growth, enlarged clitoris. Some changes may not go away after drug is discontinued.

POSSIBLE INTERACTION WITH OTHER DRUGS

GENERIC NAME OR DRUG CLASS	COMBINED EFFECT
Anticoagulants*	Increased anticoagulant effect.
Antidiabetic agents*	Increased antidiabetic effect.
Chlorzoxazone	Decreased androgen effect.
Cyclosporine	Increased cyclosporine effect.
Hepatotoxic drugs* (other)	Increased liver toxicity.
Insulin	Increased antidiabetic effect.
Oxyphenbutazone	Decreased androgen effect.
Phenobarbital	Decreased androgen effect.
Phenylbutazone	Decreased androgen effect.

POSSIBLE INTERACTION WITH OTHER SUBSTANCES

INTERACTS WITH	COMBINED EFFECT
Alcohol:	None expected.
Beverages:	None expected.
Cocaine:	No proven problems.
Foods:	
Salt.	Excessive fluid retention (edema). Decrease salt intake while taking male hormones.
Marijuana:	Decreased blood levels of androgens.
Tobacco:	No proven problems.

***See Glossary**

ANESTHETICS (Mucosal-Local)

GENERIC AND BRAND NAMES

BENZOCAINE
- Anbesol Baby Gel
- Anbesol Maximum Strength Gel
- Anbesol Maximum Strength Liquid
- Baby Anbesol
- Baby Orabase
- Baby Oragel
- Baby Oragel Nighttime Formula
- Benzodent
- Children's Chloraseptic Lozenges
- Dentapaine
- Dentocaine
- Dent-Zel-Ite
- Hurricaine
- Numzident
- Num-Zit Gel
- Num-Zit Lotion
- Orabase-B with Benzocaine
- Orajel Extra Strength
- Orajel Liquid
- Orajel Maximum Strength
- Oratect Gel
- Rid-A-Pain
- SensoGARD Canker Sore Relief
- Spec-T Sore Throat Anesthetic
- Topicaine

BENZOCAINE & MENTHOL
- Chloraseptic Lozenges Cherry Flavor

BENZOCAINE & PHENOL
- Anbesol Gel
- Anbesol Liquid
- Anbesol Regular Strength Gel
- Anbesol Regular Strength Liquid

DYCLONINE
- Children's Sucrets
- Sucrets Maximum Strength
- Sucrets Regular Strength

LIDOCAINE
- Xylocaine
- Xylocaine Viscous
- Zilactin-L

TETRACAINE
- Supracaine

BASIC INFORMATION

Habit forming? No
Prescription needed? Yes, for some
Available as generic? Yes, for some
Drug class: Anesthetic (mucosal-local)

OVERDOSE

SYMPTOMS:
Overabsorption by body—Dizziness, blurred vision, seizures, drowsiness.
WHAT TO DO:
- **Dial 911 (emergency) for medical help or call poison control center 1-800-222-1222 for instructions.**
- **Not for internal use. If child accidentally swallows, call numbers above.**
- **See emergency information on last 3 pages of this book.**

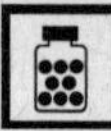

USES

Relieves pain or irritation in mouth caused by toothache, teething, mouth sores, dentures, braces, dental appliances. Also relieves pain of sore throat for short periods of time.

DOSAGE & USAGE INFORMATION

How to use:
- For mouth problems—Apply to sore places with cotton-tipped applicator. Don't swallow.
- For throat—Gargle, but don't swallow.
- For aerosol spray—Don't inhale.

When to use:
As directed by physician or label on package.

If you forget a dose:
Use as soon as you remember.

What drug does:
Blocks pain impulses to the brain.

Time lapse before drug works:
Immediately.

Don't use with:
Any other medicine for your mouth without consulting your doctor or pharmacist.

POSSIBLE ADVERSE REACTIONS OR SIDE EFFECTS

SYMPTOMS	WHAT TO DO
Life-threatening:	
Unusual anxiety, excitement, nervousness, irregular or slow heartbeat.	Discontinue. Seek emergency treatment.
Common:	
None expected.	
Infrequent:	
Redness, irritation, sores not present before treatment, rash, itchy skin, hives.	Discontinue. Call doctor right away.
Rare:	
None expected.	

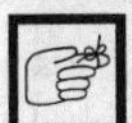

WARNINGS & PRECAUTIONS

Don't take if:
You are allergic to any of the products listed.

Before you start, consult your doctor if:
- You are allergic to anything.
- You have infection, canker sores or other sores in your mouth.
- You take medicine for myasthenia gravis, eye drops for glaucoma or any sulfa medicine.

Over age 60:
Adverse reactions and side effects may be more frequent and severe than in younger persons. Ask doctor about smaller doses.

Pregnancy:
Risk factors vary for drugs in this group. See category list on page xviii and consult doctor.

Breast-feeding:
No problems expected, but check with doctor.

Infants & children:
No problems expected, but check with doctor.

Prolonged use:
Not intended for prolonged use.

Skin & sunlight:
No problems expected.

Driving, piloting or hazardous work:
Wait to see if causes dizziness, sweating, drowsiness or blurred vision. If not, no problems expected.

Discontinuing:
No problems expected.

Others:
- Keep cool, but don't freeze.
- Don't puncture, break or burn aerosol containers.
- Don't eat, drink or chew gum for 1 hour after use.
- Heat and moisture in bathroom medicine cabinet can cause breakdown of medicine. Store someplace else.
- Before anesthesia, tell dentist about any medicines you take or use.

POSSIBLE INTERACTION WITH OTHER DRUGS

GENERIC NAME OR DRUG CLASS	COMBINED EFFECT
None expected.	

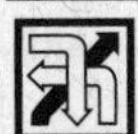

POSSIBLE INTERACTION WITH OTHER SUBSTANCES

INTERACTS WITH	COMBINED EFFECT
Alcohol:	Adverse reactions more common.
Beverages:	None expected.
Cocaine:	May cause too much nervousness and trembling. Avoid.
Foods:	None expected.
Marijuana:	None expected.
Tobacco:	Avoid. Tobacco makes mouth problems worse.

ANESTHETICS (Rectal)

GENERIC AND BRAND NAMES

BENZOCAINE
Americaine Hemorrhoidal
Ethyl Aminobenzoate
DIBUCAINE
Nupercainal
LIDOCAINE
Anamantle HC Cream Kit
Peranex HC Cream
Recticare Anorectal
Xyralid RC
PRAMOXINE
Fleet Relief
ProCort
Proctofoam
Tronolane
Tronothane
TETRACAINE
Pontocaine Cream
TETRACAINE & MENTHOL
Pontocaine Ointment

BASIC INFORMATION

Habit forming? No
Prescription needed? Yes, for some
Available as generic? Yes
Drug class: Anesthetic (rectal)

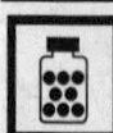

USES

- Relieves pain, itching and swelling of hemorrhoids (piles).
- Relieves pain of rectal fissures (breaks in lining membrane of the anus).

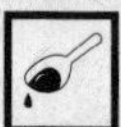

DOSAGE & USAGE INFORMATION

How to use:
- Rectal cream or ointment—Apply to surface of rectum with fingers. Insert applicator into rectum no farther than 1/2 and apply inside. Wash applicator carefully or discard.
- Aerosol foam—Read patient instructions. Don't insert into rectum. Use the special applicator and wash carefully after using.
- Suppository—Remove wrapper and moisten with water. Lie on side. Push blunt end of suppository into rectum with finger. If suppository is too soft, run cold water over wrapper or put in refrigerator for 15 to 45 minutes before using.

Continued next column

OVERDOSE

SYMPTOMS:
None expected.
WHAT TO DO:
Not intended for internal use. If child accidentally swallows, call doctor or poison control center 1-800-222-1222 for help.

- Pads—For external use only. Follow instructions on label. Do not use for more than 1 week without doctor's approval.

When to use:
As directed on the product's label.

If you forget a dose:
Use as soon as you remember.

What drug does:
Deadens nerve endings to pain and touch.

Time lapse before drug works:
5 to 15 minutes.

Don't use with:
Any other topical rectal medicine without consulting your doctor or pharmacist.

POSSIBLE ADVERSE REACTIONS OR SIDE EFFECTS

SYMPTOMS	WHAT TO DO
Life-threatening:	
None expected.	
Common:	
None expected.	
Infrequent:	
• Nervousness, trembling, hives, rash, itch, inflammation or tenderness not present before application, slow heartbeat.	Discontinue. Call doctor right away.
• Dizziness, blurred vision, swollen feet.	Continue. Call doctor when convenient.
Rare:	
• Blood in urine.	Discontinue. Call doctor right away.
• Increased or painful urination.	Continue. Call doctor when convenient.

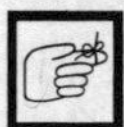

WARNINGS & PRECAUTIONS

Don't use if:
You are allergic to any topical anesthetic.

Before you start, consult your doctor if:
- You have skin infection at site of treatment.
- You have had severe or extensive skin disorders such as eczema or psoriasis.
- You have bleeding hemorrhoids.

Over age 60:
Adverse reactions and side effects may be more frequent and severe than in younger persons.

Pregnancy:
Risk factors vary for drugs in this group. See category list on page xviii and consult doctor.

Breast-feeding:
No problems expected. Consult doctor.

Infants & children:
Use caution. More likely to be absorbed through skin and cause adverse reactions.

Prolonged use:
Possible excess absorption. Don't use longer than 3 days for any one problem.

Skin & sunlight:
No problems expected.

Driving, piloting or hazardous work:
No problems expected.

Discontinuing:
May be unnecessary to finish medicine. Follow doctor's instructions.

Others:
- Report any rectal bleeding to your doctor.
- Keep cool, but don't freeze.

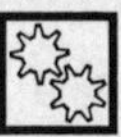

POSSIBLE INTERACTION WITH OTHER DRUGS

GENERIC NAME OR DRUG CLASS	COMBINED EFFECT
Sulfa drugs*	Decreased anti-infective effect of sulfa drugs.

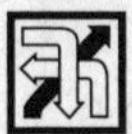

POSSIBLE INTERACTION WITH OTHER SUBSTANCES

INTERACTS WITH	COMBINED EFFECT
Alcohol:	None expected.
Beverages:	None expected.
Cocaine:	Possible nervous system toxicity. Avoid.
Foods:	None expected.
Marijuana:	None expected.
Tobacco:	None expected.

*See Glossary

ANESTHETICS (Topical)

GENERIC AND BRAND NAMES

See full list of generic and brand names in the *Generic and Brand Name Directory*, page 866.

BASIC INFORMATION

Habit forming? No
Prescription needed?
High strength: Yes
Low strength: No
Available as generic? Yes
Drug class: Anesthetic (topical)

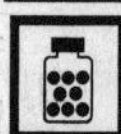

USES

Relieves pain and itch of sunburn, insect bites, scratches and other minor skin irritations.

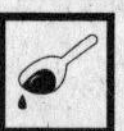

DOSAGE & USAGE INFORMATION

How to use:
All forms—Use only enough to cover irritated area. Follow instructions on label or use as directed by doctor. Avoid using on large areas of skin.

When to use:
When needed for discomfort, no more often than every hour.

If you forget an application:
Use as needed.

What drug does:
Blocks pain impulses from skin to brain.

Time lapse before drug works:
3 to 15 minutes.

Don't take with:
Any other topical medicine without consulting your doctor or pharmacist.

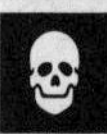

OVERDOSE

SYMPTOMS:
If swallowed or inhaled—Dizziness, nervousness, trembling, seizures.
WHAT TO DO:
- **Dial 911 (emergency) for medical help or call poison control center 1-800-222-1222 for instructions.**
- **See emergency information on last 3 pages of this book.**

POSSIBLE ADVERSE REACTIONS OR SIDE EFFECTS

SYMPTOMS	WHAT TO DO
Life-threatening: None expected.	
Common: None expected.	
Infrequent: Hive-like swellings on skin or in mouth or throat, skin problems not present before treatment (rash, burning, stinging, tenderness, redness).	Discontinue. Call doctor right away.
Rare: If too much of drug absorbed into body (very rare)—Nervousness, slow heartbeat, dizziness, blurred or double vision, confusion, convulsions, noises in ears, feeling hot or cold, numbness, trembling, anxiety, paleness, tiredness or weakness.	Discontinue. Call doctor right away.

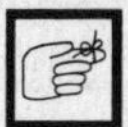

WARNINGS & PRECAUTIONS

Don't use if:
You are allergic to any topical anesthetic.

Before you start, consult your doctor if:
- You have skin infection at site of treatment.
- You have had severe or extensive skin disorders such as eczema or psoriasis.
- You have bleeding hemorrhoids.

Over age 60:
Adverse reactions and side effects may be more frequent and severe than in younger persons.

Pregnancy:
Risk factors vary for drugs in this group. See category list on page xviii and consult doctor.

Breast-feeding:
No problems expected. Consult doctor.

Infants & children:
Use caution. More likely to be absorbed through skin and cause adverse reactions.

Prolonged use:
Possible excess absorption.

Skin & sunlight:
May cause rash or intensify sunburn in areas exposed to sun or ultraviolet light (photosensitivity reaction). Avoid overexposure. Notify doctor if reaction occurs.

Driving, piloting or hazardous work:
No problems expected.

Discontinuing:
May be unnecessary to finish medicine. Follow doctor's instructions.

Others:
- Contact doctor if condition being treated doesn't improve within a week. Call sooner if new symptoms develop or pain worsens.
- Wash hands carefully after use.

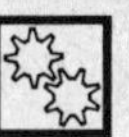

POSSIBLE INTERACTION WITH OTHER DRUGS

GENERIC NAME OR DRUG CLASS	COMBINED EFFECT
Sulfa drugs*	Decreased effect of sulfa drugs for infection.

POSSIBLE INTERACTION WITH OTHER SUBSTANCES

INTERACTS WITH	COMBINED EFFECT
Alcohol:	None expected.
Beverages:	None expected.
Cocaine:	Possible nervous system toxicity. Avoid.
Foods:	None expected.
Marijuana:	None expected.
Tobacco:	None expected.

***See Glossary**

ANGIOTENSIN II RECEPTOR ANTAGONISTS

GENERIC AND BRAND NAMES

AZILSARTAN
- Edarbi
- Edarbyclor

CANDESARTAN
- Atacand
- Atacand Plus

EPROSARTAN
- Teveten
- Teveten HCT

IRBESARTAN
- Avalide
- Avapro

LOSARTAN
- Cozaar
- Hyzaar

OLMESARTAN
- Azor
- Benicar
- Benicar HCT
- Tribenzor

TELMISARTAN
- Micardis
- Micardis HCT
- Micardis Plus
- Twynsta

VALSARTAN
- Diovan
- Diovan HCT
- Diovan Oral
- Exforge
- Exforge HCT
- Valturna

BASIC INFORMATION

Habit forming? No
Prescription needed? Yes
Available as generic? Yes, for some
Drug class: Antihypertensive, angiotensin II receptor antagonist

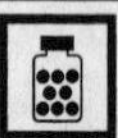

USES

- Treatment for hypertension (high blood pressure) and heart failure. May be used alone or in combination with other anti-hypertensive medications.
- Reduces risk of heart attack or stroke in certain patients.

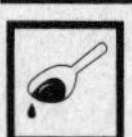

DOSAGE & USAGE INFORMATION

How to take:
Tablet—Swallow with liquid. May be taken with or without food.

Continued next column

OVERDOSE

SYMPTOMS:
Slow or irregular heartbeat, faintness, dizziness, lightheadedness.
WHAT TO DO:
Overdose unlikely to threaten life. If person uses much larger amount than prescribed or if accidentally swallowed, call doctor or poison control center 1-800-222-1222 for help.

When to take:
Once or twice daily as directed.

If you forget a dose:
Take as soon as you remember. If it is almost time for the next dose, wait for that dose (don't double this dose) and resume regular schedule.

What drug does:
Lowers blood pressure by relaxing the blood vessels to allow improved blood flow in the body.

Time lapse before drug works:
May take several weeks for full effectiveness.

Don't take with:
Any other medicine or any dietary supplement without consulting your doctor or pharmacist.

POSSIBLE ADVERSE REACTIONS OR SIDE EFFECTS

SYMPTOMS	WHAT TO DO
Life-threatening:	
None expected.	
Common:	
Headache.	Continue. Call doctor when convenient.
Infrequent:	
• Dizziness, fever or sore throat (upper respiratory infection).	Continue, but call doctor right away.
• Diarrhea, back pain, cough, fatigue, stuffy nose.	Continue. Call doctor when convenient.
Rare:	
Dry cough, trouble sleeping, muscle cramps, leg pain.	Continue. Call doctor when convenient.

WARNINGS & PRECAUTIONS

Don't take if:
You are allergic to angiotensin II receptor antagonists.

Before you start, consult your doctor if:
- You have any kidney or liver disease.
- You are allergic to any medication, food or other substance.

Over age 60:
No special problems expected.

Pregnancy:
Decide with your doctor if drug benefits justify risks to unborn child. Risk category C for first trimester and category D for second and third trimesters (see page xviii).

Breast-feeding:
One or more of these drugs may pass into milk. Avoid drug or discontinue nursing until you finish medicine. Consult doctor for advice.

Infants & children:
Olmesartan and valsartan approved to treat high blood pressure in ages 6 to 16. For other angiotensin II receptor antagonists, consult doctor.

Prolonged use:
- No special problems expected. Hypertension usually requires life-long treatment.
- Schedule regular doctor visits to determine if drug is continuing to be effective in controlling the hypertension and to check for any kidney problems.

Skin & sunlight:
No special problems expected.

Driving, piloting or hazardous work:
Don't drive or pilot aircraft until you learn how medicine affects you. Don't work around dangerous machinery. Don't climb ladders or work in high places. Danger increases if you drink alcohol or take other medicines affecting alertness and reflexes.

Discontinuing:
Don't discontinue without consulting your doctor, even if you feel well. You can have hypertension without feeling any symptoms. Untreated high blood pressure can cause serious problems.

Others:
- Advise any doctor or dentist whom you consult that you take this medicine. May interfere with the accuracy of some medical tests.
- Follow any special diet your doctor may prescribe. It can help control hypertension.
- Consult doctor if you become ill with vomiting or diarrhea.
- Use caution when exercising or performing activities in hot weather and with excessive sweating. You may experience dizziness, lightheadedness or faintness.

POSSIBLE INTERACTION WITH OTHER DRUGS

GENERIC NAME OR DRUG CLASS	COMBINED EFFECT
Anti-inflammatory drugs, nonsteroidal (NSAIDs)*	Decreased anti-hypertensive effect.
Cyclosporine	Excess potassium levels in the body.
Diuretics*	Increased anti-hypertensive effect.
Diuretics, potassium-sparing*	Excess potassium levels in the body.
Hypotension-causing drugs,* other	Increased anti-hypertensive effect.
Indomethacin	Decreased anti-hypertensive effect.
Potassium-containing medications	Excess potassium levels in the body.
Potassium supplements*	Excess potassium levels in the body.
Sympathomimetics*	Decreased anti-hypertensive effect.

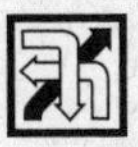

POSSIBLE INTERACTION WITH OTHER SUBSTANCES

INTERACTS WITH	COMBINED EFFECT
Alcohol:	Unknown effect. Consult doctor.
Beverages:	
Low-salt milk.	Possible excess potassium in the body.
Grapefruit juice.	Decreased effect of losartan.
Cocaine:	Unknown effect. Avoid.
Foods:	
Salt substitutes containing potassium.	Excess potassium in the body.
Marijuana:	Increased sedation. Avoid.
Tobacco:	None expected.

***See Glossary**

ANGIOTENSIN-CONVERTING ENZYME (ACE) INHIBITORS

GENERIC AND BRAND NAMES

See full list of generic and brand names in the *Generic and Brand Name Directory*, page 866.

BASIC INFORMATION

Habit forming? No
Prescription needed? Yes
Available as generic? Yes, for some
Drug class: Antihypertensive, angiotensin converting enzyme (ACE) inhibitor

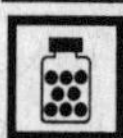

USES

- Treatment for hypertension (high blood pressure) and congestive heart failure.
- Used for kidney disease in diabetic patients.
- Helps prevent complications in patients with stable coronary artery disease.
- Treatment for acute myocardial infarction.

DOSAGE & USAGE INFORMATION

How to take:
Capsule, tablet, long-acting tablet, liquid—Follow directions provided with your prescription.

When to take:
At the same times each day, usually 2-3 times daily. Captopril should be taken on an empty stomach 1 hour before or 2 hours after eating.

If you forget a dose:
Take as soon as you remember. If it is almost time for the next dose, wait for that dose (don't double this dose) and resume regular schedule.

What drug does:
Relaxes artery walls and lowers blood pressure.

Time lapse before drug works:
60 to 90 minutes.

Don't take with:
Any other medicine or any dietary supplement without consulting your doctor or pharmacist.

OVERDOSE

SYMPTOMS:
Low blood pressure, fever, chills, sore throat, fainting, convulsions, coma.
WHAT TO DO:
- **Dial 911 (emergency) for medical help or call poison control center 1-800-222-1222 for instructions.**
- **See emergency information on last 3 pages of this book.**

POSSIBLE ADVERSE REACTIONS OR SIDE EFFECTS

SYMPTOMS	WHAT TO DO
Life-threatening	
Hives, rash, intense itching, faintness, difficulty breathing (anaphylaxis)..	Seek emergency treatment immediately.
Common:	
Rash, loss of taste.	Discontinue. Call doctor right away.
Infrequent:	
• Swelling of mouth, face, hands or feet.	Discontinue. Seek emergency treatment.
• Dizziness, fainting, chest pain, fast or irregular heartbeat, confusion, nervousness, numbness and tingling in hands or feet.	Discontinue. Call doctor right away.
• Diarrhea, headache, tiredness, cough.	Continue. Call doctor when convenient.
Rare:	
• Sore throat, cloudy urine, fever, chills.	Discontinue. Call doctor right away.
• Nausea, vomiting, indigestion, abdominal pain.	Continue. Call doctor when convenient.

WARNINGS & PRECAUTIONS

Don't take if:
- You are allergic to any ACE inhibitor.*
- You are receiving blood from a blood bank.
- You will have surgery within 2 months, including dental surgery, requiring general or spinal anesthesia.

Before you start, consult your doctor if:
- You have had a stroke.
- You have angina or heart or blood vessel disease.
- You have any autoimmune disease, including AIDS or lupus.
- You have high level of potassium in blood.
- You have kidney or liver disease.
- You are on severe salt-restricted diet.
- You have a bone marrow disorder.

Over age 60:
Adverse reactions and side effects may be more frequent and severe than in younger persons.

ANGIOTENSIN-CONVERTING ENZYME (ACE) INHIBITORS

Pregnancy:
Drugs increase risk of birth defects. Risk factors vary for drugs in this group. See category list on page xviii and consult doctor.

Breast-feeding:
Drug passes into milk. Avoid drug or discontinue nursing until you finish medicine. Consult doctor for advice on maintaining milk supply.

Infants & children:
Under close medical supervision only.

Prolonged use:
Request periodic laboratory blood counts and urine tests.

Skin & sunlight:
One or more drugs in this group may cause rash or intensify sunburn in areas exposed to sun or ultraviolet light (photosensitivity reaction). Avoid overexposure. Notify doctor if reaction occurs.

Driving, piloting or hazardous work:
Avoid if you become dizzy or faint. Otherwise, no problems expected.

Discontinuing:
Don't discontinue without consulting doctor. Dose may require gradual reduction if you have taken drug for a long time. Doses of other drugs may also require adjustment.

Others:
- Avoid exercising in hot weather.
- May affect results in some medical tests.
- Advise any doctor or dentist whom you consult that you take this medicine.

POSSIBLE INTERACTION WITH OTHER DRUGS

GENERIC NAME OR DRUG CLASS	COMBINED EFFECT
Amiloride	Possible excessive potassium in blood.
Antihypertensives, other*	Increased anti-hypertensive effect. Dosage of each may require adjustment.
Anti-inflammatory drugs nonsteroidal (NSAIDs), cox-2 inhibitors	May decrease ACE inhibitor effect.
Beta-adrenergic blocking agents*	Increased anti-hypertensive effect. Dosage of each may require adjustment.
Carteolol	Increased anti-hypertensive effects of both drugs. Dosages may require adjustment.
Chloramphenicol	Possible blood disorders.
Diuretics*	Possible severe blood pressure drop with first dose.
Diclofenac	May decrease ACE inhibitor effect.
Guanfacine	Increased effect of both drugs.
Meloxicam	Decreased effect of ACE inhibitor.
Nicardipine	Possible excessive potassium in blood. Dosages may require adjustment.
Nimodipine	Possible excessive potassium in blood. Dangerous blood pressure drop.
Nitrates*	Possible excessive blood pressure drop.
Pentamidine	May increase bone marrow depression or make kidney damage more likely.
Pentoxifylline	Increased anti-hypertensive effect.
Potassium	May raise potassium levels in blood to toxic levels.

Continued on page 899

POSSIBLE INTERACTION WITH OTHER SUBSTANCES

INTERACTS WITH	COMBINED EFFECT
Alcohol:	Possible excessive blood pressure drop.
Beverages: Low-salt milk.	Possible excessive potassium in blood.
Cocaine	Increased risk of heart block and high blood pressure.
Foods: Salt substitutes.	Possible excessive potassium.
Marijuana:	Increased dizziness.
Tobacco:	May decrease ACE inhibitor effect.

***See Glossary**

ANGIOTENSIN-CONVERTING ENZYME (ACE) INHIBITORS & HYDROCHLOROTHIAZIDE

GENERIC AND BRAND NAMES

See full list of generic and brand names in the *Generic and Brand Name Directory*, page 866.

BASIC INFORMATION

Habit forming? No
Prescription needed? Yes
Available as generic? Yes, for some
Drug class: Antihypertensive, diuretic (thiazide), ACE inhibitor

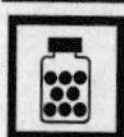

USES

- Treatment for high blood pressure and congestive heart failure.
- Reduces fluid retention.

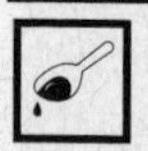

DOSAGE & USAGE INFORMATION

How to take:
Tablet—Swallow with liquid. Instructions to take on empty stomach mean 1 hour before or 2 hours after eating.

When to take:
At the same times each day, usually 2 to 3 times daily. Take first dose at bedtime and lie down immediately.

If you forget a dose:
Take as soon as you remember. If it is almost time for the next dose, wait for the next scheduled dose (don't double this dose).

What drug does:
- Forces sodium and water excretion, thereby reducing body fluid.
- Relaxes muscle cells of small arteries.
- Reduced body fluid and relaxed arteries lower blood pressure.
- Reduces resistance in arteries.
- Strengthens heartbeat.

Continued next column

OVERDOSE

SYMPTOMS:
Cramps, weakness, drowsiness, weak pulse, low blood pressure.
WHAT TO DO:
- **Dial 911 (emergency) for medical help or call poison control center 1-800-222-1222 for instructions.**
- **See emergency information on last 3 pages of this book.**

Don't take with:
Any other medicine or any dietary supplement without consulting your doctor or pharmacist.

POSSIBLE ADVERSE REACTIONS OR SIDE EFFECTS

SYMPTOMS	WHAT TO DO
Life-threatening:	
Irregular heartbeat (fast or uneven); hives, rash, intense itching, faintness soon after a dose (anaphylaxis).	Discontinue. Seek emergency treatment.
Common:	
• Dry mouth, thirst, tiredness, weakness, muscle cramps, vomiting, chest pain, skin rash, coughing, weak pulse.	Discontinue. Call doctor right away.
• Taste loss, dizziness.	Continue. Call doctor when convenient.
Infrequent:	
• Face, mouth, hands swell.	Discontinue. Call doctor right away.
• Nausea, diarrhea.	Continue. Call doctor when convenient.
Rare:	
Jaundice (yellow eyes and skin), bruising, back pain.	Discontinue. Call doctor right away.

WARNINGS & PRECAUTIONS

Don't take if:
- You are allergic to any ACE inhibitor or any thiazide diuretic drug.
- You are receiving blood from a blood bank.
- If you will have surgery within 2 months, including dental surgery, requiring general or spinal anesthesia.

Before you start, consult your doctor if:
- You have had a stroke.
- You have angina, heart or blood vessel disease, a high level of potassium in blood, lupus, gout, liver, pancreas or kidney disorder.
- You have any autoimmune disease, including AIDS or lupus.
- You are on severe salt-restricted diet.
- You are allergic to any sulfa drug.
- You have a bone marrow disorder.

Over age 60:
Adverse reactions and side effects may be more frequent and severe than in younger persons, such as dizziness and excessive potassium loss.

ANGIOTENSIN-CONVERTING ENZYME (ACE) INHIBITORS & HYDROCHLOROTHIAZIDE

Pregnancy:
Drugs increase risk of birth defects. Risk factors vary for drugs in this group. See category list on page xviii and consult doctor.

Breast-feeding:
Drug passes into milk. Avoid drug or discontinue nursing until you finish medicine. Consult doctor for advice on maintaining milk supply.

Infants & children:
Not recommended.

Prolonged use:
Talk to your doctor about the need for follow-up medical examinations or laboratory studies to check blood pressure, ECG,* liver function, kidney function.

Skin & sunlight:
One or more drugs in this group may cause rash or intensify sunburn in areas exposed to sun or ultraviolet light (photosensitivity reaction). Avoid overexposure. Notify doctor if reaction occurs.

Driving, piloting or hazardous work:
Don't drive or pilot aircraft until you learn how medicine affects you. Don't work around dangerous machinery. Don't climb ladders or work in high places. Danger increases if you drink alcohol or take medicine affecting alertness and reflexes, such as antihistamines, tranquilizers, sedatives, pain medicine, narcotics and mind-altering drugs.

Discontinuing:
Don't discontinue without consulting doctor. Dose may require gradual reduction if you have taken drug for a long time. Doses of other drugs may also require adjustment.

Others:
- Hot weather and fever may cause dehydration and drop in blood pressure. Dose may require temporary adjustment. Weigh daily and report any unexpected weight decreases to your doctor.
- May cause rise in uric acid, leading to gout.
- May cause blood-sugar rise in diabetics.

POSSIBLE INTERACTION WITH OTHER DRUGS

GENERIC NAME OR DRUG CLASS	COMBINED EFFECT
Allopurinol	Decreased allopurinol effect.
Amiloride	Possible excessive potassium in blood.
Antidepressants, tricyclic*	Dangerous drop in blood pressure. Avoid combination unless under medical supervision.
Antihypertensives, other*	Increased anti-hypertensive effect. Dosage of each may require adjustment.
Anti-inflammatory drugs nonsteroidal (NSAIDs)*	Decreased captopril effect.
Barbiturates*	Increased hydro-chlorothiazide effect.
Beta-adrenergic blocking agents*	Increased anti-hypertensive effect. Dosage of each may require adjustments.
Carteolol	Increased antihyper-tensive effects of both drugs. Dosages may require adjustment.
Chloramphenicol	Possible blood disorders.
Cholestyramine	Decreased hydro-chlorothiazide effect.
Digitalis preparations*	Excessive potassium loss that causes dan-gerous heart rhythms.

Continued on page 899

POSSIBLE INTERACTION WITH OTHER SUBSTANCES

INTERACTS WITH	COMBINED EFFECT
Alcohol:	Dangerous blood pressure drop. Avoid.
Beverages: Low-salt milk.	Possible excessive potassium in blood.
Cocaine	Increased risk of heart block and high blood pressure.
Foods: Salt substitutes.	Possible excessive potassium.
Marijuana:	Increased dizziness; may increase blood pressure.
Tobacco:	May decrease blood pressure lowering effect.

*See Glossary

ANTACIDS

GENERIC AND BRAND NAMES

See full list of generic and brand names in the *Generic and Brand Name Directory*, page 866.

BASIC INFORMATION

Habit forming? No
Prescription needed? No
Available as generic? Yes, for some
Drug class: Antacid

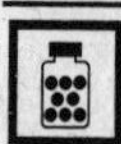

USES

Treatment for hyperacidity in upper gastrointestinal tract, including stomach and esophagus. Symptoms may be heartburn or acid indigestion. Diseases include peptic ulcer, gastritis, esophagitis, hiatal hernia.

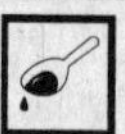

DOSAGE & USAGE INFORMATION

How to take:
Follow package instructions.

When to take:
1 to 3 hours after meals unless directed otherwise by your doctor.

If you forget a dose:
Take as soon as you remember, but not simultaneously with any other medicine.

What drug does:
- Neutralizes some of the hydrochloric acid in the stomach.
- Reduces action of pepsin, a digestive enzyme.

Time lapse before drug works:
15 minutes for antacid effect.

Continued next column

OVERDOSE

SYMPTOMS:
Dry mouth, shallow breathing, diarrhea or constipation, headache, mental confusion, weakness, fatigue, stupor, bone pain.
WHAT TO DO:
- **Overdose unlikely to threaten life. Depending on severity of symptoms and amount taken, dial 911 (emergency) for medical help or call poison control center 1-800-222-1222 for instructions.**
- **See emergency information on last 3 pages of this book.**

Don't take with:
- Any other medicine or any dietary supplement without consulting your doctor or pharmacist.
- Other drugs at the same time. Decreases absorption of that drug. Wait 2 hours.

POSSIBLE ADVERSE REACTIONS OR SIDE EFFECTS

SYMPTOMS	WHAT TO DO
Life-threatening: None expected.	
Common: Chalky taste.	Continue. Tell doctor at next visit.
Infrequent: Mild constipation, increased thirst, laxative effect, unpleasant taste in mouth, stomach cramps, stool color changes (whitish or speckling).	Continue. Call doctor when convenient.
Rare: Bone pain, frequent or urgent urination, muscle weakness or pain, nausea, weight gain, severe constipation, dizziness, headache, appetite loss, mood changes, vomiting, nervousness, swollen feet and ankles, tiredness or weakness.	Discontinue. Call doctor right away.

Note: Side effects are rare unless too much medicine is taken for a long time.

WARNINGS & PRECAUTIONS

Don't take if:
- You are allergic to any antacid.
- You have a high blood-calcium level.

Before you start, consult your doctor if:
You have kidney disease, chronic constipation, colitis, diarrhea, symptoms of appendicitis, stomach or intestinal bleeding, irregular heartbeat.

Over age 60:
Adverse reactions and side effects may be more frequent and severe than in younger persons. Diarrhea or constipation particularly likely.

Pregnancy:
Risk factors vary for drugs in this group. See category list on page xviii and consult doctor.

Breast-feeding:
Drug passes into milk. Consult doctor.

Infants & children:
Use only under medical supervision.

Prolonged use:
- High blood level of calcium (if your antacid contains calcium) which disturbs electrolyte balance.
- Kidney stones, impaired kidney function.
- Talk to your doctor about the need for follow-up medical examinations or laboratory studies to check kidney function, serum calcium, serum potassium.

Skin & sunlight:
No problems expected.

Driving, piloting or hazardous work:
No problems expected.

Discontinuing:
May be unnecessary to finish medicine. Follow doctor's instructions.

Others:
- Don't take longer than 2 weeks unless under medical supervision.
- Advise any doctor or dentist whom you consult that you take this medicine. May affect results in some medical tests.

POSSIBLE INTERACTION WITH OTHER DRUGS

GENERIC NAME OR DRUG CLASS	COMBINED EFFECT
Alendronate	Decreased alendronate effect. Take antacid 30 minutes after alendronate.
Antifungals, azoles	Decreased azole absorption.
Anti-inflammatory drugs nonsteroidal (NSAIDs), COX-2 inhibitors	Decreased pain relief.
Capecitabine	Increased risk of capecitabine toxicity.
Chlorpromazine	Decreased chlorpromazine effect.
Ciprofloxacin	May cause kidney dysfunction.
Dexamethasone	Decreased dexa-methasone effect.
Digitalis preparations*	Decreased digitalis effect.
Iron supplements*	Decreased iron effect.
Isoniazid	Decreased isoniazid effect.
Levodopa	Increased levodopa effect.
Mecamylamine	Increased mecamylamine effect.
Meperidine	Increased meperidine effect.
Methenamine	Reduced methenamine effect.
Nalidixic acid	Decreased nalidixic acid effect.
Nicardipine	Possible decreased nicardipine effect.
Nizatidine	Decreased nizatidine absorption.
Ofloxacin	Decreased ofloxacin effect.
Oxyphenbutazone	Decreased oxyphenbutazone effect.
Para-aminosalicylic acid (PAS)	Decreased PAS effect.
Penicillins*	Decreased penicillin effect.
Prednisone	Decreased prednisone effect.
Pseudoephedrine	Increased pseudo-ephedrine effect.
Salicylates*	Increased salicylate effect.
Tetracyclines	Decreased tetracycline effect.
Ticlopidine	Decreased ticlopidine effect.

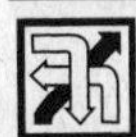

POSSIBLE INTERACTION WITH OTHER SUBSTANCES

INTERACTS WITH	COMBINED EFFECT
Alcohol:	Decreased antacid effect.
Beverages:	No proven problems.
Cocaine:	No proven problems.
Foods:	Decreased antacid effect. Wait 1 hour after eating.
Marijuana:	Decreased antacid effect.
Tobacco:	Decreased antacid effect.

*See Glossary

ANTHELMINTICS

GENERIC AND BRAND NAMES

ALBENDAZOLE
Albenza
IVERMECTIN
Stromectol
PYRANTEL
Antiminth
Aut
Cobantril
Helmex
Lombriareu
Reese's Pinworm Medicine
Trilombrin
PYRVINIUM
Vanquin
Viprynium
THIABENDAZOLE
Foldan
Mintezol
Mintezol Topical
Minzolum
Triasox

BASIC INFORMATION

Habit forming? No
Prescription needed? Yes
Available as generic? Yes
Drug class: Anthelmintics, antiparasitic

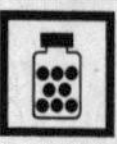

USES

- Treatment of roundworms, pinworms, whipworms, hookworms and other intestinal parasites.
- Treatment of hydatid disease, neurocysticercosis, strongyloidiasis and onchocerciasis.

DOSAGE & USAGE INFORMATION

How to take or apply:
- Tablet—Swallow with liquid or food to lessen stomach irritation.
- Topical suspension—Apply to end of each tunnel or burrow made by worm.
- Chewable tablet—Chew thoroughly before swallowing.
- Oral suspension—Follow package instructions.

Continued next column

When to take:
Morning and evening with food to increase uptake.

If you forget a dose:
Skip dose and begin treatment again. Often only one or two doses are needed to complete treatment.

What drug does:
Kills or paralyzes the parasites. They then pass out of the body in the feces. Usually the type of worm parasite must be identified so the appropriate drug can be prescribed.

Time lapse before drug works:
Some take only hours; others, 1 to 3 days.

Don't take with:
Any other medicine or any dietary supplement without consulting your doctor or pharmacist.

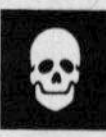

OVERDOSE

SYMPTOMS:
Increased severity of adverse reactions and side effects.
WHAT TO DO:
Overdose unlikely to threaten life. If person uses much larger amount than prescribed or if accidentally swallowed, call doctor or poison control center 1-800-222-1222 for help.

POSSIBLE ADVERSE REACTIONS OR SIDE EFFECTS

SYMPTOMS	WHAT TO DO
Life-threatening: None expected.	
Common: None expected.	
Infrequent:	
• Abdominal pain, diarrhea, dizziness, fever, nausea, rectal itching.	Continue. Call doctor when convenient.
• Red stools, asparagus-like urine smell, bad taste in mouth.	No action necessary.
Rare:	
Skin rash, itching, sore throat and fever, weakness (severe), hair loss, headache, blurred vision, seizures.	Discontinue. Call doctor right away.

WARNINGS & PRECAUTIONS

Don't take if:
You are allergic to any anthelmintic.

Before you start, consult your doctor if:
- You have liver disease.
- You have Crohn's disease.
- You have ulcerative colitis.

Over age 60:
Adverse reactions and side effects may be more frequent and severe than in younger persons. You may need smaller doses for shorter periods of time.

Pregnancy:
Risk factors vary for drugs in this group. See category list on page xviii and consult doctor.

Breast-feeding:
Unknown effect. Consult your doctor.

Infants & children:
No problems expected. Don't give to a child under age 2 without doctor's approval.

Prolonged use:
- Not intended for long-term use.
- Talk to your doctor about the need for follow-up medical examinations or laboratory studies to check stools, cellophane tape swabs pressed against rectal area to check for parasite eggs, complete blood counts (white blood cell count, platelet count, red blood cell count, hemoglobin, hematocrit).

Skin & sunlight:
Thiabendazole may cause rash or intensify sunburn in areas exposed to sun or ultraviolet light (photosensitivity reaction). Avoid overexposure. Notify doctor if reaction occurs.

Driving, piloting or hazardous work:
Use caution if the medicine causes you to feel dizzy or weak. Otherwise, no problems expected.

Discontinuing:
No problems expected.

Others:
- Take full course of treatment. Repeat course may be necessary if follow-up examinations reveal persistent infection.
- Advise any doctor or dentist whom you consult that you take this medicine.
- Wash all bedding after treatment to prevent re-infection.

POSSIBLE INTERACTION WITH OTHER DRUGS

GENERIC NAME OR DRUG CLASS	COMBINED EFFECT
Cimetidine	Increased effect of albendazole.
Corticosteroids*	Increased effect of albendazole.
Praziquantel	Increased effect of albendazole.
Xanthines*	Dosage of xanthine drug may need adjusting.

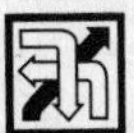

POSSIBLE INTERACTION WITH OTHER SUBSTANCES

INTERACTS WITH	COMBINED EFFECT
Alcohol:	None expected.
Beverages: Grapefruit juice.	May increase effect of anthelmintic.
Cocaine:	None expected.
Foods:	None expected.
Marijuana:	None expected.
Tobacco:	None expected.

*See Glossary

ANTHRALIN (Topical)

BRAND NAMES

Anthra-Derm
Anthraforte
Anthranol
Anthrascalp
Dithranol
Drithocreme
Drithocreme HP
Dritho-Scalp
Lasan
Lasan HP
Lasan Pomade
Lasan Unguent
Micanol

BASIC INFORMATION

Habit forming? No
Prescription needed? Yes
Available as generic? No
Drug class: Antipsoriatic, hair growth stimulant

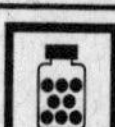

USES

- Treats quiescent or chronic psoriasis.
- Stimulates hair growth in some people (not an approved use by the FDA).

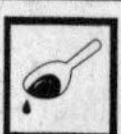

DOSAGE & USAGE INFORMATION

How to use:

- Wear plastic gloves for all applications.
- If directed, apply at night.
- Cream, lotion, ointment—Bathe and dry area before use. Apply small amount and rub gently.
- If for short contact, same as above for cream.
- Leave on 20 to 30 minutes. Then remove medicine by bathing or shampooing.
- If for scalp overnight—Shampoo before use to remove scales or medicine. Dry hair. Part hair several times and apply to scalp. Wear plastic cap on head. Clean off next morning with petroleum jelly, then shampoo.

When to use:
As directed.

If you forget a dose:
Use as soon as you remember.

Continued next column

OVERDOSE

SYMPTOMS:
None expected.
WHAT TO DO:
Not for internal use. If child accidentally swallows, call doctor or poison control center 1-800-222-1222 for help.

What drug does:
Reduces growth activity within abnormal cells by inhibiting enzymes.

Time lapse before drug works:
May require several weeks or more.

Don't use with:
Any other medicine or any dietary supplement without consulting your doctor or pharmacist.

POSSIBLE ADVERSE REACTIONS OR SIDE EFFECTS

SYMPTOMS	WHAT TO DO
Life-threatening: None expected.	
Common: None expected.	
Infrequent: Redness or irritation of skin not present before application, rash.	Discontinue. Call doctor when convenient.
Rare: None expected.	

WARNINGS & PRECAUTIONS

Don't use if:
- You are allergic to anthralin.
- You have infected skin.

Before you start, consult your doctor if:
- You have chronic kidney disease.
- You are allergic to anything.

Over age 60:
No problems expected, but check with doctor.

Pregnancy:
Studies in animals and humans have not been done. Consult doctor. Risk category C (see page xviii).

Breast-feeding:
No problems expected, but check with doctor.

Infants & children:
No problems expected, but check with doctor.

Prolonged use:
No problems expected, but check with doctor.

Skin & sunlight:
May cause rash or intensify sunburn in areas exposed to sun or ultraviolet light (photosensitivity reaction). Avoid overexposure. Notify doctor if reaction occurs.

Driving, piloting or hazardous work:
No problems expected.

Discontinuing:
No problems expected.

Others:
- Keep cool, but don't freeze.
- Apply petroleum jelly to normal skin or scalp to protect areas not being treated.
- Will stain hair, clothing, shower, bathtub or sheets. Wash as soon as possible.
- Advise any doctor or dentist whom you consult that you take this medicine.
- Heat and moisture in bathroom medicine cabinet can cause breakdown of medicine. Store someplace else.

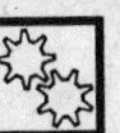

POSSIBLE INTERACTION WITH OTHER DRUGS

GENERIC NAME OR DRUG CLASS	COMBINED EFFECT
Antidiabetic agents*	Increased sensitivity to sun exposure.
Coal tar preparations*	Increased sensitivity to sun exposure.
Diuretics, thiazide*	Increased sensitivity to sun exposure.
Griseofulvin	Increased sensitivity to sun exposure.
Methoxsalen	Increased sensitivity to sun exposure.
Nalidixic acid	Increased sensitivity to sun exposure.
Phenothiazines*	Increased sensitivity to sun exposure.
Sulfa drugs*	Increased sensitivity to sun exposure.
Tetracyclines*	Increased sensitivity to sun exposure.
Trioxsalen	Increased sensitivity to sun exposure.

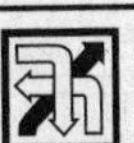

POSSIBLE INTERACTION WITH OTHER SUBSTANCES

INTERACTS WITH	COMBINED EFFECT
Alcohol:	None expected.
Beverages:	None expected.
Cocaine:	None expected.
Foods:	None expected.
Marijuana:	None expected.
Tobacco:	None expected.

*See Glossary

ANTIACNE, CLEANSING (Topical)

GENERIC AND BRAND NAMES

ALCOHOL & ACETONE
Seba-Nil
ALCOHOL & SULFUR
Liquimat
Postacne
SULFURATED LIME
Vlemasque
Vleminckx Solution

BASIC INFORMATION

Habit forming? No
Prescription needed? No
Available as generic? Yes
Drug class: Antiacne agent, Cleansing agent

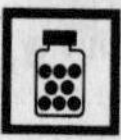

USES

Treats acne or oily skin.

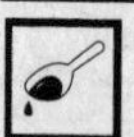

DOSAGE & USAGE INFORMATION

How to use:

- Lotion, gel or pledget—Start with small amount and wipe over face to remove dirt and surface oil. Don't apply to wounds or burns. Don't rinse with water and avoid contact with eyes. Skin may be more sensitive in dry or cold climates.
- Plaster—Follow package instructions.

When to use:
As directed. May increase frequency up to 3 or more times daily as tolerated. Warm, humid weather may allow more frequent use.

If you forget a dose:
Use as soon as you remember and then go back to regular schedule.

Continued next column

OVERDOSE

SYMPTOMS:
None expected.
WHAT TO DO:

- **Not for internal use. If child accidentally swallows, call numbers below.**
- **Dial 911 (emergency) for medical help or call poison control center 1-800-222-1222 for instructions.**
- **See emergency information on last 3 pages of this book.**

What drug does:
Helps remove oil from skin's surface.

Time lapse before drug works:
Works immediately.

Don't use with:
Other topical acne treatments unless directed by doctor.

POSSIBLE ADVERSE REACTIONS OR SIDE EFFECTS

SYMPTOMS	WHAT TO DO
Life-threatening:	
None expected.	
Common:	
None expected.	
Infrequent:	
• Skin infection, pustules or rash; unusual pain, swelling or redness of treated skin.	Discontinue. Call doctor right away.
• Burning, dryness, stinging, peeling of skin.	Continue. Call doctor when convenient.
Rare:	
None expected.	

WARNINGS & PRECAUTIONS

Don't use if:
You have to apply over a wounded or burned area.

Before you start, consult your doctor if:
You use benzoyl peroxide, resorcinol, salicylic acid, sulfur or tretinoin (vitamin A acid).

Over age 60:
No problems expected.

Pregnancy:
Risk category not assigned to this drug group. Consult doctor about use.

Breast-feeding:
No problems expected, but check with doctor.

Infants & children:
No problems expected, but check with doctor. Use only under close medical supervision.

Prolonged use:
Excessive drying of skin.

Skin & sunlight:
No special problems expected.

Driving, piloting or hazardous work:
No problems expected, but check with doctor.

Discontinuing:
No problems expected, but check with doctor.

Others:
Some antiacne agents are flammable. Don't use near fire or while smoking.

POSSIBLE INTERACTION WITH OTHER DRUGS

GENERIC NAME OR DRUG CLASS	COMBINED EFFECT
Abrasive or medicated soaps	Irritation or too much drying.
After-shave lotions	Irritation or too much drying.
Antiacne topical preparations (other)	Irritation or too much drying.
"Cover-up" cosmetics	Irritation or too much drying.
Drying cosmetic soaps	Irritation or too much drying.
Isotretinoin	Irritation or too much drying.
Mercury compounds	May stain skin black and smell bad.
Perfumed toilet water	Irritation or too much drying.
Preparations containing skin-peeling agents such as benzoyl peroxide, resorcinol, salicylic acid, sulfur, tretinoin	Irritation or too much drying.

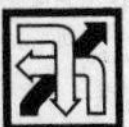

POSSIBLE INTERACTION WITH OTHER SUBSTANCES

INTERACTS WITH	COMBINED EFFECT
Alcohol:	None expected.
Beverages:	None expected.
Cocaine:	None expected.
Foods:	None expected.
Marijuana:	None expected.
Tobacco:	None expected.

*See Glossary

ANTIALLERGIC AGENTS (Ophthalmic)

GENERIC AND BRAND NAMES

ALCAFTADINE
Lastacaft
AZELASTINE (ophthalmic)
Optivar
BEPOTASTINE
Bepreve
EMEDASTINE
Emadine
EPINASTINE
Elestat
KETOTIFEN
Alaway
Claritin Eye
Refresh Eye Itch Relief
Zaditor
Zyrtec Eye Drops
LEVOCABASTINE
Livostin
LODOXAMIDE
Alomide
NEDOCROMIL
Alocril
OLOPATADINE
Pataday
Patanol
PEMIROLAST
Alamast

BASIC INFORMATION

Habit forming? No
Prescription needed? Yes, for some
Available as generic? Yes, for some
Drug class: Ophthalmic antiallergic agents, antihistaminic

USES

Prevention and treatment of seasonal allergic (hay fever) eye disorders. May be referred to as seasonal conjunctivitis, vernal conjunctivitis, vernal keratitis or vernal keratoconjunctivitis.

DOSAGE & USAGE INFORMATION

How to use:
Eye solution
- Wash hands.
- Apply pressure to inside corner of eye with middle finger.
- Continue pressure for 1 minute after placing medicine in eye.

Continued next column

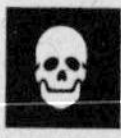

OVERDOSE

SYMPTOMS:
None expected.
WHAT TO DO:
Not intended for internal use. If child accidentally swallows, call doctor or poison control center 1-800-222-1222 for help.

- Tilt head backward. Pull lower lid away from eye with index finger of the same hand.
- Drop eye drops into pouch and close eye. Don't blink.
- Keep eyes closed for 1 to 2 minutes.

When to use:
1 to 2 drops 4 times a day or as directed by doctor or instructions on product.

If you forget a dose:
Use as soon as you remember, then return to regular schedule.

What drug does:
Prevents a hypersensitivity reaction to certain allergens such as pollen.

Time lapse before drug works:
Relief of symptoms may begin immediately, but full benefit might take a few days.

Don't use with:
Any other eye medications without consulting your doctor or pharmacist.

POSSIBLE ADVERSE REACTIONS OR SIDE EFFECTS

SYMPTOMS	WHAT TO DO
Life-threatening: None expected.	
Common: Brief and mild burning or stinging when drops are administered.	No action necessary.
Infrequent: Blurred vision, feeling that something is in the the eye, redness of eye, eye irritation not present before, eye tearing or discharge.	Discontinue. Call doctor right away.
Rare:	
• Aching in eye, crusting in corner of eye or eyelid, dryness of eyes or nose, drowsiness or sleepiness, feeling of heat in eye or body, nausea, stomach discomfort, sneezing, sticky or tired feeling of eye.	Continue. Call doctor when convenient.
• Redness or irritation of eyelid, swelling of eye, pain in eye, sensitivity to light, headache, dizziness, skin rash.	Discontinue. Call doctor right away.

WARNINGS & PRECAUTIONS

Don't use if:
You are allergic to any of the antiallergic ophthalmic drugs.

Before you start, consult your doctor if:
- You wear soft contact lenses.
- You are allergic to any other medications, foods or other substances.

Over age 60:
No special problems expected.

Pregnancy:
Risk category B for azelastine, emedastine, levocabastine, lodoxamide, nedocromil and pemirolast. Risk category C for epinastine, olopatadine and ketotifen. See page xviii for category information. Consult doctor about use.

Breast-feeding:
It is unknown if these drugs placed in the eyes then pass into milk. Consult your doctor.

Infants & children:
No information available on safety or effectiveness for children under age 2 for lodoxamide and under age 12 for levocabastine. Consult doctor. Azelastine approved for children 3 years and older.

Prolonged use:
No special problems expected.

Skin & sunlight:
No special problems expected.

Driving, piloting or hazardous work:
Avoid if you feel dizzy or side effects cause vision problems.

Discontinuing:
No special problems expected.

Others:
- Don't use leftover medicine for other eye problems without your doctor's approval.
- If symptoms don't improve after a few days of use, call your doctor.

POSSIBLE INTERACTION WITH OTHER DRUGS

GENERIC NAME OR DRUG CLASS	COMBINED EFFECT
None significant.	

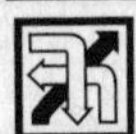

POSSIBLE INTERACTION WITH OTHER SUBSTANCES

INTERACTS WITH	COMBINED EFFECT
Alcohol:	None expected.
Beverages:	None expected.
Cocaine	None expected.
Foods:	None expected.
Marijuana:	None expected.
Tobacco:	None expected.

*See Glossary

ANTIANDROGENS, NONSTEROIDAL

GENERIC AND BRAND NAMES

BICALUTAMIDE
Casodex
FLUTAMIDE
Euflex
Eulexin
NILUTAMIDE
Amandron
Nilandron

BASIC INFORMATION

Habit forming? No
Prescription needed? Yes
Available as generic? No
Drug class: Antineoplastic

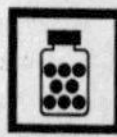

USES

Treatment for prostate cancer. Used in combination with a testosterone lowering measure such as surgery (removal of the testicles) or use of a special monthly injection of luteinizing hormone-releasing hormone (LHRH).

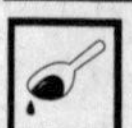

DOSAGE & USAGE INFORMATION

How to take:
Tablet or capsule—Swallow with liquid. May be taken with or without food.

When to take:
According to doctor's instructions. Normally at the same times each day.

If you forget a dose:
Take as soon as you remember. If it is almost time for your next dose, skip the missed dose and return to your regular dosing schedule (don't double this dose).

What drug does:
Interferes with utilization of androgen (male hormone) testosterone by body cells. Prostate cancer cells require testosterone in order to grow and reproduce.

Continued next column

OVERDOSE

SYMPTOMS:
Diarrhea, nausea, vomiting, tiredness, headache, dizziness, breast tenderness.
WHAT TO DO:
Overdose unlikely to threaten life. If person uses much larger amount than prescribed or if accidentally swallowed, call doctor or poison control center 1-800-222-1222 for help.

Time lapse before drug works:
Starts working within two hours, but may take several weeks to be effective.

Don't take with:
Any other medicine or any dietary supplement without consulting your doctor or pharmacist.

POSSIBLE ADVERSE REACTIONS OR SIDE EFFECTS

SYMPTOMS	WHAT TO DO
Life-threatening: None expected.	
Common:	
• Decreased sex drive, diarrhea, appetite loss, nausea, vomiting, cough or hoarseness, fever, runny nose, sneezing, sore throat, tightness in chest or wheezing, constipation, insomnia.	Continue. Call doctor when convenient.
• Hot flashes with mild sweating.	No action necessary.
Infrequent:	
• Hands and feet tingling or numb, painful or swollen breasts, swollen feet and legs, chest pain, shortness of breath.	Continue. Call doctor right away.
• Bloody or black tarry stools, itching, back or side pain, depression, muscle weakness, unusual tiredness, skin rash, bloated feeling, confusion, dry mouth, nervousness, color vision changes (with nilutamide).	Continue. Call doctor when convenient.
Rare:	
• Jaundice (yellow eyes and skin), pain or tenderness in the stomach.	Continue. Call doctor right away.
• Bluish colored lips, skin or nails; dark urine; dizziness or fainting; unusual bleeding or bruising.	Continue. Call doctor when convenient.

Note: Adverse effects that occur may also be due to use of LHRH or symptoms of prostate cancer.

ANTIANDROGENS, NONSTEROIDAL

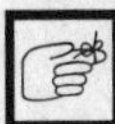

WARNINGS & PRECAUTIONS

Don't take if:
- You are allergic to any of the antiandrogens.
- You are female.

Before you start, consult your doctor if:
- You have liver disease.
- You use tobacco.
- You have lung disease or other breathing problems.
- You have glucose-6-phosphate dehydrogenase (G6PD) deficiency or hemoglobin M disease.
- You are planning on starting a family. May decrease sperm count.

Over age 60:
Adverse reactions and side effects may be more frequent and severe than in younger persons. You may need smaller doses for shorter periods of time.

Pregnancy:
These drugs are not intended for use in women. Risk categories vary for each drug. Bicalutamide is risk category X, flutamide is risk category D and nilutamide is risk category C (see page xviii).

Breast-feeding:
Not intended for use in women.

Infants & children:
Not intended for use in infants and children.

Prolonged use:
Talk to your doctor about the need for follow-up medical examinations or laboratory studies to check liver and pulmonary functions, PSA levels, chest x-rays, and other tests as recommended.

Skin & sunlight:
May cause rash or intensify sunburn in areas exposed to sun or ultraviolet light (photosensitivity reaction). Avoid overexposure. Notify doctor if reaction occurs.

Driving, piloting or hazardous work:
You may experience vision problems when going from a dark area to a lighted area and vice versa (such as driving in and out of tunnels). Use caution.

Discontinuing:
No special problems expected. Don't discontinue drug without doctor's approval.

Others:
- Advise any doctor or dentist whom you consult that you take this medicine.
- May affect results in some medical tests.
- May decrease sperm count.

POSSIBLE INTERACTION WITH OTHER DRUGS

GENERIC NAME OR DRUG CLASS	COMBINED EFFECT
Anticoagulants*	Increased effect of anticoagulant.
Phenytoin	Increased effect of phenytoin with nilutamide.
Theophylline	Increased effect of theophylline.

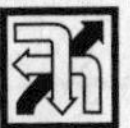

POSSIBLE INTERACTION WITH OTHER SUBSTANCES

INTERACTS WITH	COMBINED EFFECT
Alcohol:	Nilutamide may cause alcohol intolerance reaction. Avoid alcohol while on this drug.
Beverages:	None expected.
Cocaine:	None expected. Best to avoid.
Foods:	None expected.
Marijuana:	None expected. Best to avoid.
Tobacco:	Increased risk of toxicity. Avoid.

*See Glossary

ANTIARRHYTHMICS, BENZOFURAN-TYPE

GENERIC AND BRAND NAMES

AMIODARONE	DRONEDARONE
Cordarone	Multaq

BASIC INFORMATION

Habit forming? No
Prescription needed? Yes
Available as generic? Yes, for amiodarone
Drug class: Antiarrhythmic

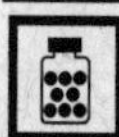

USES

Prevents and treats certain types of life-threatening irregular heart rhythms.

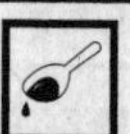

DOSAGE & USAGE INFORMATION

How to take:
Tablet—Swallow whole with liquid or food to lessen stomach irritation. If you can't swallow tablet whole, ask doctor or pharmacist for advice.

When to take:
Amiodarone is usually taken once a day. Dronedarone is usually taken twice daily (with morning and evening meals).

If you forget a dose:
Take as soon as you remember. If it is almost time for the next dose, skip the missed dose and wait for your next scheduled dose (don't double this dose).

What drug does:
Antiarrhythmic drugs slow the electrical impulses in the heart to help restore, maintain or control normal heart rhythm.

Time lapse before drug works:
May take up to 2 weeks for therapeutic effect.

Don't take with:
Any other medicine or any dietary supplement without consulting your doctor or pharmacist.

OVERDOSE

SYMPTOMS:
Weakness, slow heart rate, lightheadedness, or fainting.
WHAT TO DO:
- **Dial 911 (emergency) for medical help or call poison control center 1-800-222-1222 for instructions.**
- **See emergency information on last 3 pages of this book.**

POSSIBLE ADVERSE REACTIONS OR SIDE EFFECTS

SYMPTOMS	WHAT TO DO
Life-threatening:	
Rare allergic reaction (hives, itching, rash, trouble breathing, tightness in chest, swelling of lips or tongue or face).	Seek emergency treatment immediately.
Common:	
• Painful breathing, cough, shortness of breath, coughing up blood.	Continue, but call doctor right away or seek emergency. treatment.
• Dizziness, fainting, lightheadedness, low fever, tingling or numbness in fingers or toes, hands tremble or shake, trouble walking, uncontrolled body movements.	Continue, but call doctor right away.
• Diarrhea, weakness, nausea or vomiting, tiredness, stomach pain, headache, loss of appetite, constipation.	Continue. Call doctor when convenient.
Infrequent:	
• Skin color change to blue-gray, unusual tiredness, difficulty breathing (can occur when lying down or sleeping), eye symptoms (blurred vision or less clarity, dry eyes, sensitive to light, seeing halos, other vision changes), scrotum swelling or pain, swollen feet or ankles or hands, fast or slow or irregular heartbeat, chest pain, weight gain or loss, sweating, sensitive to heat, feeling hot or cold.	Continue, but call doctor right away.
• Odd taste or smell, decreased libido, insomnia, flushed face, nervousness.	Continue. Call doctor when convenient.
Rare:	
• Yellow skin or eyes, severe stomach pain.	Continue, but call doctor right away.
• Skin symptoms (rash, itchy, red or puffy), heartburn, other new symptoms.	Continue. Call doctor when convenient.

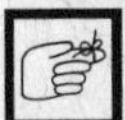

WARNINGS & PRECAUTIONS

Don't take if:
You are allergic to amiodarone or dronedarone.

Before you start, consult your doctor if:
- You have diabetes; liver, kidney, thyroid, lung, or electrolyte (e.g., low potassium) disorder.
- You are pregnant or plan to become pregnant.
- You take herbal or vitamin supplements.
- You have any heart problem or heart disorder (e.g., slow heartbeat, congestive heart failure, high blood pressure, or stroke).

Over age 60:
No problems expected.

Pregnancy:
Drug use may cause fetal harm. Amiodarone is risk category D and dronedarone is risk category X (see page xviii). Consult doctor.

Breast-feeding:
Drug may pass into milk. Avoid drug or discontinue nursing until you finish medicine. Consult doctor for advice on maintaining milk supply.

Infants & children:
Safety and efficacy not established.

Prolonged use:
- Blue-gray discoloration of skin may occur with. amiodarone.
- Talk to your doctor about the need for follow-up medical exams or lab tests.

Skin & sunlight:
May cause rash or intensify sunburn in areas exposed to sun or ultraviolet light (called photosensitivity reaction). Avoid overexposure. Notify doctor if reaction occurs.

Driving, piloting or hazardous work:
Don't drive or pilot aircraft until you learn how medicine affects you. Don't work around dangerous machinery. Don't climb ladders or work in high places. Danger increases if you drink alcohol or take other medicines affecting alertness and reflexes.

Discontinuing:
- Don't discontinue without doctor's advice. Dose may require gradual reduction if you have taken drug for a long time. Doses of other drugs may also require adjustment.
- Notify doctor if cough, fever, breathing difficulty or other symptoms occur after discontinuing the drug.

Others:
- Call doctor right away if you have symptoms of lung toxicity (e.g., cough or painful breathing) or liver toxicity (e.g., yellow skin or eyes, swelling of feet and ankles).
- Advise any doctor or dentist whom you consult that you take this medicine.
- Dronedarone has been linked to increased risk of death, stroke, and heart failure in some patients. Ask your doctor about your risks.
- May interfere with the accuracy of some medical tests.
- It is important that you have regular eye exams before and during treatment.
- Carry or wear medical identification stating that you are taking this drug.

POSSIBLE INTERACTION WITH OTHER DRUGS

GENERIC NAME OR DRUG CLASS	COMBINED EFFECT
Antiarrhythmics, other*	Increased risk of irregular heartbeat.
Anticoagulants*	May increase anticoagulant effect.
Beta-adrenergic blocking agents*	Increased risk of slow heartbeat.
Calcium channel blockers*	Increased risk of slow heartbeat.
Cholestyramine	May decrease amiodarone effect.
Clopidogrel	May decrease effect of clopidogrel.
Cholestyramine	May decrease effect of amiodarone.

Continued on page 899

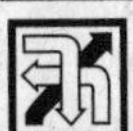

POSSIBLE INTERACTION WITH OTHER SUBSTANCES

INTERACTS WITH	COMBINED EFFECT
Alcohol:	None expected.
Beverages: Grapefruit juice.	Increased risk of benzofuran-type antiarrhythmic toxicity. Avoid.
Cocaine:	Unknown effect Avoid.
Foods: Grapefruit.	Increased risk of benzofuran-type antiarrhythmic toxicity. Avoid.
Marijuana:	Unknown effect. Avoid.
Tobacco:	None expected.

***See Glossary**

ANTIBACTERIALS, ANTIFUNGALS (Topical)

GENERIC AND BRAND NAMES

CLIOQUINOL & HYDROCORTISONE
- Vioform Hydrocortisone Cream
- Vioform Hydrocortisone Lotion
- Vioform Hydrocortisone Mild Cream
- Vioform Hydrocortisone Mild Ointment
- Vioform Hydrocortisone Ointment

SULFADIAZINE
- Flamazine
- Flint SSD
- Sildamac
- Silvadene
- SSD
- SSD AF
- Thermazene

BASIC INFORMATION

Habit forming? No
Prescription needed? Yes
Available as generic? Yes, some are
Drug class: Antibacterial (topical), antifungal (topical)

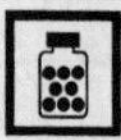

USES

Treats eczema, other inflammatory skin conditions, athlete's foot, skin infections.

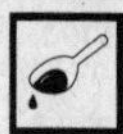

DOSAGE & USAGE INFORMATION

How to use:
- Cream, lotion, ointment—Bathe and dry area before use. Apply small amount and rub gently.
- Keep away from eyes.

When to use:
2 to 4 times a day.

If you forget a dose:
Use as soon as you remember.

Continued next column

OVERDOSE

SYMPTOMS:
Severe nausea, vomiting, diarrhea.
WHAT TO DO:
- **Not for internal use. If child accidentally swallows, call numbers below.**
- **Dial 911 (emergency) for medical help or call poison control center 1-800-222-1222 for instructions.**
- **See emergency information on last 3 pages of this book.**

What drug does:
Kills some types of fungus and bacteria on contact.

Time lapse before drug works:
2 to 4 weeks, sometimes longer.

Don't use with:
Other skin ointments, creams or lotions without consulting your doctor or pharmacist.

POSSIBLE ADVERSE REACTIONS OR SIDE EFFECTS

SYMPTOMS	WHAT TO DO
Life-threatening:	
None expected.	
Common:	
May stain skin around nails.	Continue. Tell doctor at next visit.
Infrequent:	
Stomach cramps; hives; itching, burning, peeling, red, stinging, swelling skin.	Discontinue. Call doctor right away.
Rare:	
None expected.	

WARNINGS & PRECAUTIONS

Don't use if:
You are allergic to clioquinol, iodine or any iodine-containing preparation.

Before you start, consult your doctor if:
You are allergic to anything that touches your skin.

Over age 60:
No problems expected.

Pregnancy:
Risk factors vary for drugs in this group. See category list on page xviii and consult doctor.

Breast-feeding:
No problems expected, but check with doctor.

Infants & children:
No problems expected, but check with doctor.

Prolonged use:
No problems expected, but check with doctor.

Skin & sunlight:
No special problems expected.

Driving, piloting or hazardous work:
No problems expected, but check with doctor.

Discontinuing:
No problems expected, but check with doctor.

Others:
- If not improved in 2 weeks, check with doctor.
- May stain clothing or bed linens.
- May stain hair, skin and nails yellow.
- If accidentally gets into eyes, flush with clear water immediately.
- Tests of thyroid function may yield inaccurate results if you use clioquinol within 1 month before testing.

POSSIBLE INTERACTION WITH OTHER DRUGS

GENERIC NAME OR DRUG CLASS	COMBINED EFFECT
None expected.	

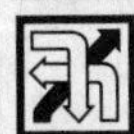

POSSIBLE INTERACTION WITH OTHER SUBSTANCES

INTERACTS WITH	COMBINED EFFECT
Alcohol:	None expected.
Beverages:	None expected.
Cocaine:	None expected.
Foods:	None expected.
Marijuana:	None expected.
Tobacco:	None expected.

ANTIBACTERIALS FOR ACNE (Topical)

GENERIC AND BRAND NAMES

CHLORTETRACYCLINE (topical)
Aureomycin

CLINDAMYCIN (topical)
Acanya
Benzaclin
Cleocin T Gel
Cleocin T Lotion
Cleocin T Topical Solution
Clinda-Derm
ClindaReach
Dalacin T Topical Solution
DUAC Topical Gel
Evoclin Foam
Veltin Gel
Ziana Gel

DOXYCYCLINE (topical)
Adoxa
Adoxa Pak

ERYTHROMYCIN (topical)
Akne-Mycin
A/T/S
Benzamycin
Erycette
EryDerm
EryGel
EryMax
EurySol
Erythro-statin
ETS
Sans-Acne
Staticin
Theramycin Z
T-Stat

MECLOCYCLINE (topical)
Meclan

TETRACYCLINE (topical)
Achromycin
Topicycline

BASIC INFORMATION

Habit forming? No
Prescription needed? Yes
Available as generic? Yes
Drug class: Antibacterial (topical)

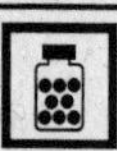

USES

Treats acne by killing skin bacteria that may be part of the cause of acne.

OVERDOSE

SYMPTOMS:
None expected.
WHAT TO DO:
Not for internal use. If child accidentally swallows, call doctor or poison control center 1-800-222-1222 for help.

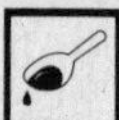

DOSAGE & USAGE INFORMATION

How to use:

- Pledgets and solutions are flammable. Use away from flame or heat.
- Apply drug to entire area, not just to pimples.
- If you use other acne medicines on skin, wait an hour after using erythromycin before applying other medicine.
- Cream, lotion, ointment—Wash and dry area Then apply small amount and rub gently.

When to use:
2 times a day, morning and evening, or as directed by your doctor.

If you forget a dose:
Use as soon as you remember.

What drug does:
Kills bacteria on skin, skin glands or in hair follicles.

Time lapse before drug works:
3 to 4 weeks to begin improvement.

Don't use with:
Other skin medicine without consulting your doctor or pharmacist.

POSSIBLE ADVERSE REACTIONS OR SIDE EFFECTS

SYMPTOMS	WHAT TO DO
Life-threatening: None expected.	
Common: Stinging or burning of skin for a few minutes after application; faint yellow skin color, especially around hair roots (with chlortetracycline, meclocycline or tetracycline).	Continue. Tell doctor at next visit.
Infrequent: Red, peeling, itching, irritated or dry skin.	Continue. Call doctor when convenient.
Rare (extremely): Symptoms of excess medicine absorbed by body—Abdominal pain, diarrhea, fever, nausea, vomiting, bloating, thirst, weakness, weight loss.	Discontinue. Call doctor right away.

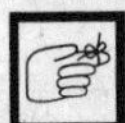

WARNINGS & PRECAUTIONS

Don't use if:
You are allergic to erythromycins, clindamycins or tetracyclines.

Before you start, consult your doctor if:
- You are allergic to any substance that touches your skin.
- You use benzoyl peroxide, resorcinol, salicylic acid, sulfur or tretinoin (vitamin A acid).

Over age 60:
No problems expected.

Pregnancy:
Risk factors vary for drugs in this group. See category list on page xviii and consult doctor.

Breast-feeding:
No problems expected, but check with doctor.

Infants & children:
No problems expected, but check with doctor.

Prolonged use:
Excess irritation to skin.

Skin & sunlight:
No special problems expected.

Driving, piloting or hazardous work:
No problems expected, but check with doctor.

Discontinuing:
No problems expected, but check with doctor.

Others:
- Use water-base cosmetics.
- Keep medicine away from mouth or eyes.
- If accidentally gets into eyes, flush immediately with clear water.
- Keep away from heat or flame.
- Keep cool, but don't freeze.

POSSIBLE INTERACTION WITH OTHER DRUGS

GENERIC NAME OR DRUG CLASS	COMBINED EFFECT
Abrasive or medicated soaps	Irritation or too much drying.
After-shave lotions	Irritation or too much drying.
Antiacne topical preparations (other)	Irritation or too much drying.
"Cover-up" cosmetics	Irritation or too much drying.
Drying cosmetic soaps	Irritation or too much drying.
Isotretinoin	Irritation or too much drying.
Mercury compounds	May stain skin black and smell bad.
Perfumed toilet water	Irritation or too much drying.
Preparations containing skin peeling agents such as benzoyl peroxide, resorcinol, salicylic acid, sulfur, tretinoin	Irritation or too much drying.

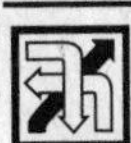

POSSIBLE INTERACTION WITH OTHER SUBSTANCES

INTERACTS WITH	COMBINED EFFECT
Alcohol:	None expected.
Beverages:	None expected.
Cocaine:	None expected.
Foods:	None expected.
Marijuana:	None expected.
Tobacco:	None expected.

ANTIBACTERIALS (Ophthalmic)

GENERIC AND BRAND NAMES

See full list of generic and brand names in the *Generic and Brand Name Directory*, page 867.

BASIC INFORMATION

Habit forming? No
Prescription needed? Yes
Available as generic? Yes, for some
Drug class: Antibacterial (ophthalmic)

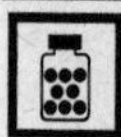

USES

- Helps body overcome eye infections on surface tissues of the eye.
- Treatment for corneal ulcers.

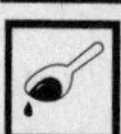

DOSAGE & USAGE INFORMATION

How to use:
Eye drops
- Wash hands.
- Apply pressure to inside corner of eye with middle finger.
- Continue pressure for 1 minute after placing medicine in eye.
- Tilt head backward. Pull lower lid away from eye with index finger of the same hand.
- Drop eye drops into pouch and close eye. Don't blink.
- Keep eyes closed for 1 to 2 minutes.

Eye ointment
- Wash hands.
- Pull lower lid down from eye to form a pouch.
- Squeeze tube to apply thin strip of ointment into pouch.
- Close eye for 1 to 2 minutes.
- Don't touch applicator tip to any surface (including the eye). If you accidentally touch tip, clean with warm soap and water.
- Keep container tightly closed.
- Keep cool, but don't freeze.
- Wash hands immediately after using.

Continued next column

When to use:
As directed. Don't miss doses.

If you forget a dose:
Use as soon as you remember.

What drug does:
Penetrates bacterial cell membrane and prevents cells from multiplying.

Time lapse before drug works:
Begins in 1 hour. May require 7 to 10 days to control infection.

Don't use with:
Any other eye drops or ointment without checking with your doctor or pharmacist.

OVERDOSE

SYMPTOMS:
None expected.
WHAT TO DO:
Not intended for internal use. If child accidentally swallows, call doctor or poison control center 1-800-222-1222 for help.

POSSIBLE ADVERSE REACTIONS OR SIDE EFFECTS

SYMPTOMS	WHAT TO DO
Life-threatening: None expected.	
Common: Ointments cause blurred vision for a few minutes.	Continue. Tell doctor at next visit.
Infrequent:	
• Signs of irritation not present before drug use.	Discontinue. Call doctor right away.
• Burning or stinging of the eye.	Continue. Call doctor when convenient.
Rare (with chloramphenicol): Sore throat, pale skin, fever, unusual bleeding or bruising.	Discontinue. Call doctor right away.

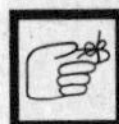

WARNINGS & PRECAUTIONS

Don't use if:
You are allergic to any antibiotic used on skin, ears, vagina or rectum.

Before you start, consult your doctor if:
You have had an allergic reaction to any medicine, food or other substances.

Over age 60:
No problems expected.

Pregnancy:
Risk factors vary for drugs in this group. See category list on page xviii and consult doctor.

Breast-feeding:
No problems expected, but check with doctor.

Infants & children:
No problems expected. Use only under medical supervision.

Prolonged use:
Sensitivity reaction may develop.

Skin & sunlight:
No problems expected.

Driving, piloting or hazardous work:
No problems expected.

Discontinuing:
Possible rare adverse reaction of bone marrow depression that leads to aplastic anemia may occur after discontinuing chloramphenicol.

Others:
- Notify doctor if symptoms fail to improve in 2 to 4 days.
- Keep medicine cool, but don't freeze.

POSSIBLE INTERACTION WITH OTHER DRUGS

GENERIC NAME OR DRUG CLASS	COMBINED EFFECT

Clinically significant interactions with oral or injected medicines unlikely.

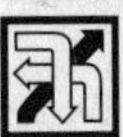

POSSIBLE INTERACTION WITH OTHER SUBSTANCES

INTERACTS WITH	COMBINED EFFECT
Alcohol:	None expected.
Beverages:	None expected.
Cocaine:	None expected.
Foods:	None expected.
Marijuana:	None expected.
Tobacco:	None expected.

*See Glossary

ANTIBACTERIALS (Otic)

GENERIC AND BRAND NAMES

ACETIC ACID
VoSol
ACETIC ACID & ALUMINUM ACETATE
Domeboro
ACETIC ACID & HYDROCORTISONE
Acetasol HC
VoSol HC
CIPROFLOXACIN (otic)
Cetraxal
CIPROFLOXACIN & DEXAMETHASONE
Ciprodex
CIPROFLOXACIN & HYDROCORTISONE
Cipro HC
NEOMYCIN, COLISTIN & HYDRO-CORTISONE
Coly-Mycin S
NEOMYCIN, POLYMIXIN B & HYDROCORTI-SONE (otic)
Antibiotic Ear
Cortatrigen
Cort-Biotic
Drotic
Ear-Eze
LazerSporin
Masporin Otic
Octigen
Oticair
Otimar
Otocidin
Otocort
Pediotic
OFLOXACIN (otic)
Floxin Otic

BASIC INFORMATION

Habit forming? No
Prescription needed? Yes
Available as generic? Yes, for some
Drug class: Antibacterial (otic)

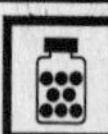

USES

- Treatment for outer ear infection (called swimmer's ear or otitis externa).
- Treats certain acute or chronic middle ear infections (e.g., otitis media).
- Most of these drugs contain an antibacterial to fight the infection and an anti-inflammatory to help provide relief from redness, irritation and discomfort.

OVERDOSE

SYMPTOMS:
None expected.
WHAT TO DO:
Not intended for internal use. If child accidentally swallows, call doctor or poison control center 1-800-222-1222 for help.

DOSAGE & USAGE INFORMATION

How to use:
As directed by your doctor or pharmacist. The following are general instructions.

How to use ear drops:
- Wash and dry hands.
- Warm drops by holding container in your hand for a few minutes.
- Lie down with affected ear up.
- Adults—Pull ear lobe back and up.
- Children—Pull ear lobe down and back.
- Put the correct number of drops into the ear. Do not allow dropper to touch the ear.
- Wipe away any spilled drops.
- Stay lying down for 2 to 5 minutes.

When to use:
As directed on label. The number of daily doses will vary depending on the specific drug.

If you forget a dose:
Use as soon as you remember. If it is almost time for the next dose, wait for next scheduled dose (don't double this dose).

What drug does:
Antibacterials destroy the bacteria causing the infection. Anti-inflammatories reduce symptoms of inflammation.

Time lapse before drug works:
Symptoms should improve within a few days. Complete healing of the infection will take longer.

Don't use with:
Other ear medications unless directed by your doctor or pharmacist.

POSSIBLE ADVERSE REACTIONS OR SIDE EFFECTS

SYMPTOMS	WHAT TO DO
Life-threatening: None expected.	
Common: None expected.	
Infrequent:	
Burning or stinging of the ear.	Continue. Call doctor if symptoms persist.
Rare:	
• Itching, redness, hives, swelling (allergic reaction), hearing changes, bleeding from ear.	Discontinue. Call doctor right away.
• Headache, fever, sore throat, runny or stuffy nose, taste changes, ear ringing.	Continue. Call doctor when convenient.

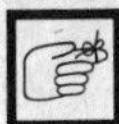

WARNINGS & PRECAUTIONS

Don't use if:
You are allergic to any of the drugs listed or other antibiotics, fluoroquinolones or steroid medications.

Before you start, consult your doctor if:
- Your eardrum is punctured.
- You have tendonitis (if ofloxacin prescribed).
- You have a viral infection such as chickenpox (varicella) or herpes simplex.

Over age 60:
No problems expected.

Pregnancy:
Decide with your doctor if drug benefits justify risk to unborn child. Risk category C for most of these drugs (see page xviii).

Breast-feeding:
Drugs may be absorbed into the body and into milk. Avoid drugs or discontinue nursing until you finish medicine. Consult doctor for advice on maintaining milk supply.

Infants & children:
Follow instructions provided by your doctor. Use the correct dosage for your infant or child's age and weight.

Prolonged use:
- Not intended for prolonged use. Don't use longer than prescribed by your doctor.
- Overuse or unnecessary use of the drug can lead to its decreased effectiveness in fighting infections.

Skin & sunlight:
No problems expected.

Driving, piloting or hazardous work:
Avoid if you experience dizziness or balance problems caused by the ear infection.

Discontinuing:
Don't discontinue without doctor's advice until you complete prescribed dosage.

Others:
- Follow your doctor's instructions for additional ear care at home.
- Call your doctor if ear symptoms worsen or don't improve after a few days of treatment.
- There is a slight risk of a secondary infection (one that occurs during or after treatment of another infection). Consult doctor if new, unexpected symptoms develop.
- Rarely, some of these drugs may increase the risk of hearing or balance problems. Discuss the drug's benefits and risks with your doctor.
- Advise any doctor or dentist whom you consult that you are using this drug.

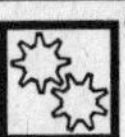

POSSIBLE INTERACTION WITH OTHER DRUGS

GENERIC NAME OR DRUG CLASS	COMBINED EFFECT
None expected.	

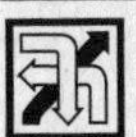

POSSIBLE INTERACTION WITH OTHER SUBSTANCES

INTERACTS WITH	COMBINED EFFECT
Alcohol:	None expected.
Beverages:	None expected.
Cocaine:	None expected.
Foods:	None expected.
Marijuana:	None expected.
Tobacco:	None expected.

ANTIBACTERIALS (Topical)

GENERIC AND BRAND NAMES

CHLORAMPHENICOL (topical)
- Chloromycetin

GENTAMICIN
- Garamycin
- Gentamar
- G-Myticin Antibiotic

MUPIROCIN
- Bactroban
- Bactroban Nasal

NEOMYCIN & POLYMIXIN B
- Neosporin Cream

NEOMYCIN, POLYMIXIN B & BACITRACIN
- Bactine First Aid
- Foille
- Mycitracin
- Neo-Polycin
- Neosporin Ointment
- Topisporin
- Triple Antibiotic

RETAPAMULIN
- Altabax

BASIC INFORMATION

Habit forming? No
Prescription needed? Yes, for some
Available as generic? Yes, for some
Drug class: Antibacterial (topical)

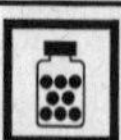

USES

Treats skin infections that may accompany burns, superficial boils, insect bites or stings, skin ulcers, impetigo, minor surgical wounds.

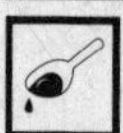

DOSAGE & USAGE INFORMATION

How to use:
- Cream, lotion, ointment—Bathe and dry area before use. Apply small amount and rub gently. May cover with gauze or bandage if desired.
- Nasal ointment—Follow instructions provided with prescription.

Continued next column

When to use:
3 or 4 times daily, or as directed by doctor.

If you forget a dose:
Use as soon as you remember.

What drug does:
Kills susceptible bacteria by interfering with bacterial DNA and RNA.

Time lapse before drug works:
Begins first day. May require treatment for a week or longer to cure infection.

Don't use with:
Any other topical medicine without consulting your doctor or pharmacist.

OVERDOSE

SYMPTOMS:
None expected.
WHAT TO DO:
Not for internal use. If child accidentally swallows, call numbers below.
- **Dial 911 (emergency) for medical help or call poison control center 1-800-222-1222 for instructions.**
- **See emergency information on last 3 pages of this book.**

POSSIBLE ADVERSE REACTIONS OR SIDE EFFECTS

SYMPTOMS	WHAT TO DO
Life-threatening: None expected.	
Common: None expected.	
Infrequent: Itching, swollen or red skin; rash.	Discontinue. Call doctor right away.
Rare: Any sort of hearing loss (with neomycin products); pale skin, sore throat, fever, unusual bleeding or bruising, unusual tiredness or weakness (with chloramphenicol).	Discontinue. Call doctor right away.

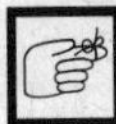

WARNINGS & PRECAUTIONS

Don't use if:
You are allergic to chloramphenicol, gentamicin or related antibiotics (name usually ends with "mycin" or "micin"), mupirocin, neomycin, polymyxins.

Before you start, consult your doctor if:
Any of the lesions on the skin are open sores.

Over age 60:
No problems expected.

Pregnancy:
Risk factors vary for drugs in this group. See category list on page xviii and consult doctor.

Breast-feeding:
No problems expected, but check with doctor.

Infants & children:
No problems expected, but check with doctor.

Prolonged use:
No problems expected, but check with doctor.

Skin & sunlight:
No special problems expected.

Driving, piloting or hazardous work:
No problems expected, but check with doctor.

Discontinuing:
No problems expected, but check with doctor.

Others:
- Heat and moisture in bathroom medicine cabinet can cause breakdown of medicine. Store someplace else.
- Keep cool, but don't freeze.

POSSIBLE INTERACTION WITH OTHER DRUGS

GENERIC NAME OR DRUG CLASS	COMBINED EFFECT
Any other topical medication	Hypersensitivity* reactions more likely to occur.

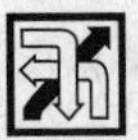

POSSIBLE INTERACTION WITH OTHER SUBSTANCES

INTERACTS WITH	COMBINED EFFECT
Alcohol:	None expected.
Beverages:	None expected.
Cocaine:	None expected.
Foods:	None expected.
Marijuana:	None expected.
Tobacco:	None expected.

*See Glossary

ANTICHOLINERGICS

GENERIC AND BRAND NAMES

See full list of generic and brand names in the *Generic and Brand Name Directory*, page 868.

BASIC INFORMATION

Habit forming? No
Prescription needed?
Low strength: No
High strength: Yes
Available as generic? Yes
Drug class: Antispasmodic, anticholinergic

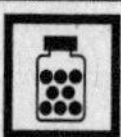

USES

- Reduces spasms of digestive system, bladder and urethra.
- Treatment of bronchial spasms.
- Used as a component in some cough and cold preparations.
- Treatment of peptic ulcers.

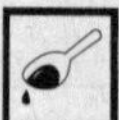

DOSAGE & USAGE INFORMATION

How to take:
- Tablet—Swallow with liquid or food to lessen stomach irritation.
- Aerosol—Dilute in saline and inhale as nebulizer.

When to take:
30 minutes before meals (unless directed otherwise by doctor).

If you forget a dose:
Take as soon as you remember. If it is almost time for the next dose, wait for the next scheduled dose (don't double this dose).

What drug does:
Blocks nerve impulses at parasympathetic nerve endings, preventing muscle contractions and gland secretions of organs involved.

Continued next column

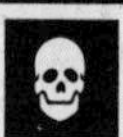

OVERDOSE

SYMPTOMS:
Dilated pupils, rapid pulse and breathing, dizziness, fever, hallucinations, confusion, slurred speech, agitation, flushed face, convulsions, coma.
WHAT TO DO:
- **Dial 911 (emergency) for medical help or call poison control center 1-800-222-1222 for instructions.**
- **See emergency information on last 3 pages of this book.**

Time lapse before drug works:
15 to 30 minutes.

Don't take with:
- Antacids* or antidiarrheals.*
- Any other medicine or any dietary supplement without consulting your doctor or pharmacist.

POSSIBLE ADVERSE REACTIONS OR SIDE EFFECTS

SYMPTOMS	WHAT TO DO
Life-threatening:	
In case of overdose, see previous column.	
Common:	
• Confusion, delirium, rapid heartbeat.	Discontinue. Call doctor right away.
• Nausea, vomiting, decreased sweating.	Continue. Call doctor when convenient.
• Constipation.	Continue. Tell doctor at next visit.
• Dryness in ears, nose, throat, mouth.	No action necessary.
Infrequent:	
• Lightheadedness.	Discontinue. Call doctor right away.
• Headache, difficult or painful urination, nasal congestion, altered taste, increased sensitivity to light.	Continue. Call doctor when convenient.
Rare:	
Rash or hives, eye pain, blurred vision, fever.	Discontinue. Call doctor right away.

WARNINGS & PRECAUTIONS

Don't take if:
- You are allergic to any anticholinergic.
- You have trouble with stomach bloating.
- You have difficulty emptying your bladder completely.
- You have narrow-angle glaucoma.
- You have severe ulcerative colitis.

Before you start, consult your doctor if:
- You have open-angle glaucoma.
- You have angina or any heart disease or heart rhythm problem.
- You have chronic bronchitis or asthma.
- You have liver, kidney or thyroid disease.
- You have hiatal hernia or esophagitis.
- You have enlarged prostate or urinary retention.
- You have myasthenia gravis.
- You have peptic ulcer.
- You will have surgery within 2 months, including dental surgery, requiring general or spinal anesthesia.

Over age 60:
Adverse reactions and side effects may be more frequent and severe than in younger persons.

Pregnancy:
Risk factors vary for drugs in this group. See category list on page xviii and consult doctor.

Breast-feeding:
Drug may pass into milk and could affect milk flow. Avoid drug or discontinue nursing until you finish medicine. Consult doctor for advice on maintaining milk supply.

Infants & children:
Use only under medical supervision.

Prolonged use:
Chronic constipation, possible fecal impaction. Consult doctor immediately.

Skin & sunlight:
No special problems expected.

Driving, piloting or hazardous work:
Use disqualifies you for piloting aircraft. Otherwise, no problems expected.

Discontinuing:
May be unnecessary to finish medicine. Follow doctor's instructions.

Others:
Advise any doctor or dentist whom you consult that you take this medicine.

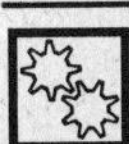

POSSIBLE INTERACTION WITH OTHER DRUGS

GENERIC NAME OR DRUG CLASS	COMBINED EFFECT
Adrenocorticoids, systemic	Possible glaucoma.
Amantadine	Increased anticholinergic effect.
Antacids*	Space doses of the drugs 2 to 3 hours apart.
Anticholinergics, other*	Increased anticholinergic effect.
Antidepressants, tricyclic*	Increased anticholinergic effect. Increased sedation.
Antifungals, azoles	Decreased azole absorption.
Antihistamines*	Increased anticholinergic effect.
Attapulgite	Decreased anticholinergic effect.
Haloperidol	Increased internal eye pressure.
Methylphenidate	Increased anticholinergic effect.
Molindone	Increased anticholinergic effect.
Monoamine oxidase (MAO) inhibitors*	Increased anticholinergic effect.
Narcotics*	Increased risk of severe constipation.
Orphenadrine	Increased anticholinergic effect.
Phenothiazines*	Increased anticholinergic effect.
Potassium supplements*	Possible intestinal ulcers with oral potassium tablets.
Quinidine	Increased anticholinergic effect.

POSSIBLE INTERACTION WITH OTHER SUBSTANCES

INTERACTS WITH	COMBINED EFFECT
Alcohol:	None expected.
Beverages:	None expected.
Cocaine:	Excessively rapid heartbeat. Avoid.
Foods:	None expected.
Marijuana:	Drowsiness and dry mouth.
Tobacco:	None expected.

*See Glossary

ANTICOAGULANTS (Oral)

GENERIC AND BRAND NAMES

WARFARIN
Coumadin
Jantoven

BASIC INFORMATION

Habit forming? No
Prescription needed? Yes
Available as generic? Yes
Drug class: Anticoagulant

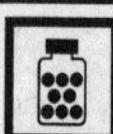

USES

It is used to help prevent harmful blood clots from forming (or growing larger) in the blood vessels or heart. Preventing clots helps reduce the risk of stroke, heart attack or pulmonary embolism.

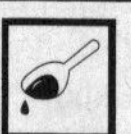

DOSAGE & USAGE INFORMATION

How to take:
Tablet—Swallow with liquid. It may be taken with or without food. If you can't swallow whole, crumble tablet and take with liquid or food.

When to take:
Once a day at the same time each day.

If you forget a dose:
Take as soon as you remember. If it is almost time for the next dose, wait for the next scheduled dose (don't double this dose).

What drug does:
It is in a class of drugs called anticoagulants (blood thinners). It works by decreasing the clotting ability of the blood.

Time lapse before drug works:
It will begin to work within 24 hours, but the full effect may take 3 to 5 days.

Don't take with:
Any other medicine or any dietary supplement without consulting your doctor or pharmacist. Many interactions are possible with warfarin.

OVERDOSE

SYMPTOMS:
Bloody vomit, coughing blood, bloody or black stools, red urine.
WHAT TO DO:

- **Dial 911 (emergency) for medical help or call poison control center 1-800-222-1222 for instructions.**
- **See emergency information on last 3 pages of this book.**

POSSIBLE ADVERSE REACTIONS OR SIDE EFFECTS

SYMPTOMS	WHAT TO DO
Life-threatening:	
Rare allergic reaction (hives, itching, rash, trouble breathing, tightness in chest, swelling of lips or tongue or face).	Seek emergency treatment immediately.
Common:	
None expected.	
Infrequent:	
• Black or red or tarry stools, nosebleeds, bleeding gums, red or brown urine, coughing up blood, vomiting blood or coffee-ground material, easy bruising, heavy menstrual flow, vaginal or rectal bleeding, cuts that won't stop bleeding, purple or red spots under the skin, discomfort or pain or swelling in any part of the body, headaches, dizziness, weakness.	Continue, but call doctor right away.
• Diarrhea, cramps, nausea or vomiting, bloating, rash, itch.	Continue. Call doctor when convenient.
Rare:	
• Purple or dark color of toes or foot; skin tissue death (pain, change in color or temperature in any body area), any bleeding that will not stop.	Seek emergency treatment.
• Yellow skin or eyes.	Continue, but call doctor right away.
• Changes in taste, tiredness, pale skin, loss of hair, feeling cold or having chills, fever, low blood pressure, any unusual symptoms that cause concern.	Continue. Call doctor when convenient.

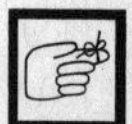

WARNINGS & PRECAUTIONS

Don't take if:
You are allergic to any oral anticoagulant.

ANTICOAGULANTS (Oral)

Before you start, consult your doctor if:

- You have a bleeding disorder.
- You have an active ulcer.
- You have high blood pressure (hypertension).
- You have a stomach or intestinal infection.
- You have congestive heart failure.
- You have had deep venous thrombosis (DVT) or a stroke.
- You drink alcohol or have problems with alcohol abuse.
- You have diabetes.
- You fall often.
- You are a female of reproductive age.
- You have a bladder catheter.
- You have protein C or protein S deficiency.
- You have liver or kidney disease.
- You have memory problems and may not be able to take drug as prescribed.
- You will have surgery in the near future (including eye or dental surgery).

Over age 60:
May have increased risk of bleeding side effects.

Pregnancy:
Use of this drug can cause pregnancy loss, birth defects or fetal death. Risk category X (risk category D for women with mechanical heart valves). See page xviii and consult doctor.

Breast-feeding:
Drug may or may not pass into breast milk. Consult your doctor for advice.

Infants & children:
Use only under doctor's supervision.

Prolonged use:
Your doctor will schedule regular blood tests to monitor drug levels.

Skin & sunlight:
No problems expected.

Driving, piloting or hazardous work:
Avoid hazardous activities that could cause injury. Don't drive if you experience dizziness.

Discontinuing:
Don't discontinue drug without doctor's approval. Stopping the drug can increase the risk of blood clots and their complications.

Others:

- Advise any doctor, dentist or pharmacist whom you consult that you take this drug.
- Get regular blood tests to check your response to the drug.
- Your doctor or dentist may tell you to stop taking warfarin or change the dosage before surgery or a medical procedure.
- Carry or wear medical ID to state that you take this drug.
- Your genetic makeup may affect your response to warfarin. Ask your doctor about genetic testing.
- Use of this drug may cause severe bleeding (can be life-threatening or even cause death).

POSSIBLE INTERACTION WITH OTHER DRUGS

GENERIC NAME OR DRUG CLASS	COMBINED EFFECT
Acetaminophen	Increased risk of bleeding.
Antibiotics*	Increased risk of bleeding.
Anticoagulants,* other	Increased risk of bleeding.
Antifungals*	Increased risk of bleeding.
Anti-inflammatory drugs, nonsteroidal (NSAIDs)*	Increased risk of bleeding.
Antiplatelet drugs*	Increased risk of bleeding.
Aspirin	Increased risk of bleeding.
Cholestyramine	Decreased effect of warfarin.
Dietary supplements or herbal products	Increased risk of bleeding or decrease in warfarin effect.
Enzyme inducers*	Decreased effect of warfarin.
Enzyme inhibitors*	Increased effect of warfarin.
Selective serotonin reuptake inhibitors	Increased risk of bleeding.
Tamoxifen	Increased risk of bleeding.

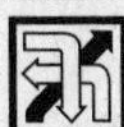

POSSIBLE INTERACTION WITH OTHER SUBSTANCES

INTERACTS WITH	COMBINED EFFECT
Alcohol:	Increase or decrease warfarin effect. Avoid.
Beverages:	None expected.
Cocaine:	May increase risk of bleeding. Avoid.
Foods: High in vitamin K—green, leafy vegetables (e.g., spinach, kale), Brussels sprouts, others.	Decreased anti-coagulant effect.
Marijuana:	May increase risk of bleeding. Avoid.
Tobacco:	Unclear effect.

***See Glossary**

ANTICONVULSANTS, HYDANTOIN

GENERIC AND BRAND NAMES

ETHOTOIN
Peganone

PHENYTOIN
Dilantin
Dilantin 30
Dilantin 125
Dilantin Infatabs
Dilantin Kapseals
Diphenylan

BASIC INFORMATION

Habit forming? No
Prescription needed? Yes
Available as generic? Yes
Drug class: Anticonvulsant (hydantoin)

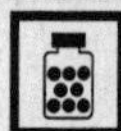

USES

- Prevents some forms of epileptic seizures.
- Stabilizes irregular heartbeat.

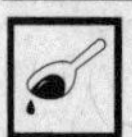

DOSAGE & USAGE INFORMATION

How to take:
- Tablet—Swallow with liquid.
- Chewable tablet—Chew well before swallowing.
- Suspension—Shake solution well before taking with liquid.

When to take:
At the same time each day.

If you forget a dose:
- If drug taken 1 time per day—Take as soon as you remember. If it is almost time for the next dose, wait for the next scheduled dose (don't double this dose).
- If taken several times per day—Take as soon as possible, then return to regular schedule.

Continued next column

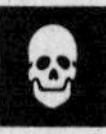

OVERDOSE

SYMPTOMS:
Jerky eye movements; stagger; slurred speech; imbalance; drowsiness; blood pressure drop; slow, shallow breathing; coma.

WHAT TO DO:
- **Dial 911 (emergency) for medical help or call poison control center 1-800-222-1222 for instructions.**
- **See emergency information on last 3 pages of this book.**

What drug does:
Promotes sodium loss from nerve fibers. This lessens excitability and inhibits spread of nerve impulses.

Time lapse before drug works:
7 to 10 days continual use.

Don't take with:
Any other medicine or any dietary supplement without consulting your doctor or pharmacist.

POSSIBLE ADVERSE REACTIONS OR SIDE EFFECTS

SYMPTOMS	WHAT TO DO
Life-threatening:	
Severe allergic reaction (rash, fever, swollen glands, kidney failure).	Seek emergency help.
Common:	
• Bleeding, swollen or tender gums.	Continue, but call doctor right away.
• Mild dizziness or drowsiness, constipation.	Continue. Call doctor when convenient.
Infrequent:	
• Hallucinations, confusion, stagger, fever, uncontrolled eye movements, increase in seizures, rash, change in vision, agitation, sore throat, diarrhea, slurred speech, muscle twitching.	Continue, but call doctor right away.
• Increased body and facial hair, breast swelling, insomnia, enlargement of facial features.	Continue. Call doctor when convenient.
Rare:	
Nausea; vomiting; unusual bleeding or bruising; swollen lymph nodes; stomach pain; yellow skin or eyes; joint pain; light gray stools; loss of appetite; weight loss; trouble breathing; uncontrolled movements of arms, legs, hands, lips, tongue or cheeks; slowed growth; learning problems.	Continue, but call doctor right away.

WARNINGS & PRECAUTIONS

Don't take if:
You are allergic to any hydantoin anticonvulsant.

Before you start, consult your doctor if:
- You have had impaired liver function or disease.
- You will have surgery within 2 months, including dental surgery, requiring general or spinal anesthesia.
- You have diabetes.
- You have a blood disorder.

Over age 60:
Adverse reactions and side effects may be more frequent and severe than in younger persons.

Pregnancy:
Decide with your doctor if drug benefits justify risk to unborn child. Risk category C (see page xviii).

Breast-feeding:
Drug passes into milk. Avoid drug or discontinue nursing until you finish medicine. Consult doctor for advice on maintaining milk supply.

Infants & children:
Use only under medical supervision.

Prolonged use:
- Weakened bones.
- Lymph gland enlargement.
- Possible liver damage.
- Numbness and tingling of hands and feet.
- Continual back-and-forth eye movements.
- Talk to your doctor about the need for follow-up medical examinations or laboratory studies to check complete blood counts (white blood cell count, platelet count, red blood cell count, hemoglobin, hematocrit), liver function, EEG.*

Skin & sunlight:
One or more drugs in this group may cause rash or intensify sunburn in areas exposed to sun or ultraviolet light (photosensitivity reaction). Avoid overexposure. Notify doctor if reaction occurs.

Driving, piloting or hazardous work:
Don't drive or pilot aircraft until you learn how medicine affects you. Don't work around dangerous machinery. Don't climb ladders or work in high places. Danger increases if you drink alcohol or take medicine affecting alertness and reflexes.

Discontinuing:
Don't discontinue without consulting doctor. Dose may require gradual reduction if you have taken drug for a long time. Doses of other drugs may also require adjustment.

Others:
- May cause learning disability.
- Good dental care is important while using this medicine.
- Advise any doctor or dentist whom you consult about the use of this drug.
- Rarely, antiepileptic drugs may lead to suicidal thoughts and behaviors. Call doctor right away if suicidal symptoms or unusual behaviors occur.

POSSIBLE INTERACTION WITH OTHER DRUGS

GENERIC NAME OR DRUG CLASS	COMBINED EFFECT
Adrenocorticoids, systemic	Decreased adreno-corticoid effect.
Amiodarone	Increased anticonvulsant effect.
Antacids*	Decreased anticonvulsant effect.
Antiandrogens, nonsteroidal	Increased effect of phenytoin.
Anticoagulants*	Increased effect of both drugs.
Antidepressants, tricyclic*	May need to adjust anticonvulsant dose.
Antifungals, azoles	Increased anticoagulant effect.
Antivirals, HIV/AIDS*	Increased risk of peripheral neuropathy with phenytoin.
Barbiturates*	Changed seizure pattern.
Calcium	Decreased effects of both drugs.
Carbamazepine	Possible increased anticonvulsant metabolism.
Carbonic anhydrase inhibitors*	Increased chance of bone disease.

Continued on page 900

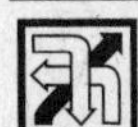

POSSIBLE INTERACTION WITH OTHER SUBSTANCES

INTERACTS WITH	COMBINED EFFECT
Alcohol:	Possible decreased anticonvulsant effect. Use with caution.
Beverages:	None expected.
Cocaine:	Possible seizures.
Foods:	None expected.
Marijuana:	Drowsiness, unsteadiness, decreased anticonvulsant effect.
Tobacco:	None expected.

*See Glossary

ANTICONVULSANTS, SUCCINIMIDE

GENERIC AND BRAND NAMES

ETHOSUXIMIDE	METHSUXIMIDE
Zarontin	Celontin

BASIC INFORMATION

Habit forming? No
Prescription needed? Yes
Available as generic? Yes, for some
Drug class: Anticonvulsant (succinimide)

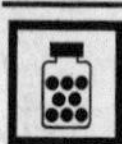

USES

Controls seizures in treatment of some forms of epilepsy.

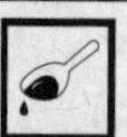

DOSAGE & USAGE INFORMATION

How to take:
Capsule or syrup—Swallow with liquid or food to lessen stomach irritation.

When to take:
Every day in regularly spaced doses, according to prescription.

If you forget a dose:
Take as soon as you remember. If it is almost time for the next dose, wait for the next scheduled dose (don't double this dose).

What drug does:
Depresses nerve transmissions in part of brain that controls muscles.

Time lapse before drug works:
3 hours.

Don't take with:
Any other medicine or any dietary supplement without consulting your doctor or pharmacist.

OVERDOSE

SYMPTOMS:
Severe drowsiness, slow or irregular breathing, coma.
WHAT TO DO:
- **Dial 911 (emergency) for medical help or call poison control center 1-800-222-1222 for instructions.**
- **If person is unconscious, check breathing and pulse. If not breathing, begin mouth-to-mouth rescue breathing. If heart is not beating, begin chest compressions.**
- **See emergency information on last 3 pages of this book.**

POSSIBLE ADVERSE REACTIONS OR SIDE EFFECTS

SYMPTOMS	WHAT TO DO
Life-threatening:	
In case of overdose, see previous column.	
Common:	
• Muscle pain, skin rash or itching, swollen glands, sore throat, fever.	Continue, but call doctor right away.
• Nausea, vomiting, appetite loss, dizziness, drowsiness, hiccups, stomach pain, headache, loss of appetite.	Continue. Call doctor when convenient.
• Change in urine color (pink, red, red-brown).	No action necessary.
Infrequent:	
Nightmares, irritability, mood changes, tiredness, difficulty concentrating.	Continue, but call doctor right away.
Rare:	
Unusual bleeding or bruising, depression, swollen glands, chills, increased seizures, shortness of breath, wheezing, chest pain, sores in mouth or on lips.	Continue, but call doctor right away.

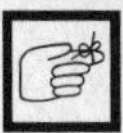

WARNINGS & PRECAUTIONS

Don't take if:
You are allergic to any succinimide anticonvulsant.

Before you start, consult your doctor if:
- You plan to become pregnant within medication period.
- You take other anticonvulsants.
- You have blood disease.
- You have kidney or liver disease.

Over age 60:
Adverse reactions and side effects may be more frequent and severe than in younger persons.

Pregnancy:
Risk factors vary for drugs in this group. See category list on page xviii and consult doctor.

Breast-feeding:
Drug passes into milk. Avoid drug or discontinue nursing. Consult your doctor about maintaining milk supply.

Infants & children:
Use only under medical supervision.

Prolonged use:
Talk to your doctor about the need for follow-up medical examinations or laboratory studies to check complete blood counts (white blood cell count, platelet count, red blood cell count, hemoglobin, hematocrit), liver function, kidney function, urine.

Skin & sunlight:
No problems expected.

Driving, piloting or hazardous work:
Don't drive or pilot aircraft until you learn how medicine affects you. Don't work around dangerous machinery. Don't climb ladders or work in high places. Danger increases if you drink alcohol or take medicine affecting alertness and reflexes, such as antihistamines, tranquilizers, sedatives, pain medicine, narcotics and mind-altering drugs.

Discontinuing:
Don't discontinue without doctor's advice until you complete prescribed dose, even though symptoms diminish or disappear.

Others:
- Your response to medicine should be checked regularly by your doctor. Dose and schedule may have to be altered frequently to fit individual needs.
- Periodic blood cell counts, kidney and liver function studies recommended.
- May discolor urine pink to red-brown. No action necessary.
- Advise any doctor or dentist whom you consult that you use this medicine.
- Rarely, antiepileptic drugs may lead to suicidal thoughts and behaviors. Call doctor right away if suicidal symptoms or unusual behaviors occur.

POSSIBLE INTERACTION WITH OTHER DRUGS

GENERIC NAME OR DRUG CLASS	COMBINED EFFECT
Anticonvulsants, other*	Increased effect of both drugs.
Antidepressants, tricyclic*	May provoke seizures.
Antipsychotics*	May provoke seizures.
Central nervous system (CNS) depressants*	Decreased anticonvulsant effect.
Haloperidol	Decreased haloperidol effect; changed seizure pattern.
Phenytoin	Increased phenytoin effect.

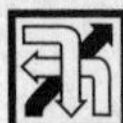

POSSIBLE INTERACTION WITH OTHER SUBSTANCES

INTERACTS WITH	COMBINED EFFECT
Alcohol:	May provoke seizures.
Beverages:	None expected.
Cocaine:	May provoke seizures.
Foods:	None expected.
Marijuana:	May provoke seizures.
Tobacco:	None expected.

*See Glossary

ANTIDEPRESSANTS, TRICYCLIC

GENERIC AND BRAND NAMES

See full list of generic and brand names in the *Generic and Brand Name Directory*, page 868.

BASIC INFORMATION

Habit forming? No
Prescription needed? Yes
Available as generic? Yes
Drug class: Antidepressant (tricyclic)

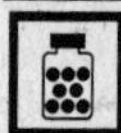

USES

- Gradually relieves symptoms of depression.
- Used to decrease bedwetting in children.
- Pain relief (sometimes).
- Clomipramine is used to treat obsessive-compulsive disorder.
- Treatment for narcolepsy, bulimia, panic attacks, cocaine withdrawal, attention-deficit disorder. Brand name Silenor treats insomnia.
- May be useful for restless leg syndrome.

DOSAGE & USAGE INFORMATION

How to take:
Tablet, capsule or syrup—Swallow with liquid.

When to take:
At the same time each day, usually at bedtime.

If you forget a dose:
Bedtime dose—If you forget your once-a-day bedtime dose, don't take it more than 3 hours late. If more than 3 hours, wait for next scheduled dose. Don't double this dose.

What drug does:
Probably affects part of brain that controls messages between nerve cells.

Continued next column

OVERDOSE

SYMPTOMS:
Hallucinations, drowsiness, enlarged pupils, respiratory failure, fever, cardiac arrhythmias, convulsions, coma.
WHAT TO DO:

- **Dial 911 (emergency) for medical help or call poison control center 1-800-222-1222 for instructions.**
- **If person is unconscious, check breathing and pulse. If not breathing, begin mouth-to-mouth rescue breathing. If heart is not beating, begin chest compressions.**
- **See emergency information on last 3 pages of this book.**

Time lapse before drug works:
2 to 4 weeks. May require 4 to 6 weeks for maximum benefit.

Don't take with:
Any other medicine or any dietary supplement without consulting your doctor or pharmacist.

POSSIBLE ADVERSE REACTIONS OR SIDE EFFECTS

SYMPTOMS	WHAT TO DO
Life-threatening: In case of overdose, see previous column.	
Common:	
• Tremor.	Discontinue. Call doctor right away.
• Headache, dry mouth or unpleasant taste, constipation or diarrhea, nausea, indigestion, fatigue, weakness, drowsiness, nervousness, anxiety, excessive sweating.	Continue. Call doctor when convenient.
• Insomnia, "sweet tooth."	Continue. Tell doctor at next visit.
Infrequent:	
• Convulsions.	Discontinue. Seek emergency treatment.
• Hallucinations, shakiness, dizziness, fainting, blurred vision, eye pain, vomiting, irregular heartbeat or slow pulse, inflamed tongue, abdominal pain, jaundice, hair loss, rash, fever, chills, joint pain, palpitations, hiccups, visual changes.	Discontinue. Call doctor right away.
• Difficult or frequent urination; decreased sex drive; muscle aches; abnormal dreams; nasal congestion; weakness and faintness when arising from bed or chair; back pain.	Continue. Call doctor when convenient.
Rare:	
Itchy skin; sore throat; involuntary movements of jaw, lips and tongue; nightmares; confusion; swollen breasts; swollen testicles.	Discontinue. Call doctor right away.

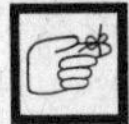

WARNINGS & PRECAUTIONS

Don't take if:
- You are allergic to any tricyclic antidepressant.
- You drink alcohol in excess.
- You have had a heart attack in past 6 weeks.
- You have taken MAO inhibitors* within 2 weeks.
- Patient is younger than age 12.

Before you start, consult your doctor if:
- You will have surgery within 2 months, including dental surgery, requiring anesthesia.
- You have an enlarged prostate or glaucoma.
- You have high blood pressure, heart disease or stomach or intestinal problems.
- You have an overactive thyroid.
- You have asthma or liver disease.

Over age 60:
More likely to develop urination difficulty and serious side effects such as seizures, hallucinations, shaking, dizziness, fainting, headache, insomnia.

Pregnancy:
Risk factors vary for drugs in this group. See category list on page xviii and consult doctor.

Breast-feeding:
Drug may pass into milk. Avoid drug or discontinue nursing until you finish medicine. Consult doctor about maintaining milk supply.

Infants & children:
- Not recommended for ages 12 and under.
- Carefully read information provided with prescription. Contact doctor right away if depression symptoms get worse or there is any talk of suicide or suicide behaviors. Also, read information under Others.

Prolonged use:
Talk to your doctor about the need for follow-up medical examinations or laboratory studies to check complete blood counts (white blood cell count, platelet count, red blood cell count, hemoglobin, hematocrit), blood pressure, eyes, teeth.

Skin & sunlight:
One or more drugs in this group may cause rash or intensify sunburn in areas exposed to sun or ultraviolet light (photosensitivity reaction). Avoid overexposure and use sunscreen. Notify doctor if reaction occurs.

Driving, piloting or hazardous work:
Don't drive or pilot aircraft until you learn how medicine affects you. Don't work around dangerous machinery. Don't climb ladders or work in high places. Danger increases if you drink alcohol or take medicine affecting alertness and reflexes.

Discontinuing:
- Don't discontinue without consulting doctor. Dose may require gradual reduction if you have taken drug for a long time. Doses of other drugs may also require adjustment.
- Physical or emotional withdrawal symptoms may occur once you stop drug. Contact your doctor if any symptoms cause concern.

Others:
- Adults and children taking antidepressants may experience a worsening of the depression symptoms and may have increased suicidal thoughts or behaviors. Call doctor right away if these symptoms or behaviors occur.
- Advise any doctor or dentist whom you consult that you take this medicine.

POSSIBLE INTERACTION WITH OTHER DRUGS

GENERIC NAME OR DRUG CLASS	COMBINED EFFECT
Adrenocorticoids, systemic	Increased risk of mental side effects.
Anticoagulants,* oral	Possible increased anticoagulant effect.
Anticholinergics*	Increased anticholinergic effect.
Antifungals, azoles	Increased effect of antidepressant.
Antiglaucoma agents*	Decreased ocular hypertensive effect.
Antihistamines*	Increased antihistamine effect.
Barbiturates*	Decreased anti-depressant effect. Increased sedation.

Continued on page 901

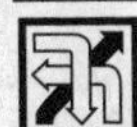

POSSIBLE INTERACTION WITH OTHER SUBSTANCES

Alcohol:	Sedation. Avoid.
Beverages:	Grapefruit juice may increase effect of clomipramine.
Cocaine:	Increased risk of heartbeat irregularity.
Foods:	None expected.
Marijuana:	Drowsiness. Risk of side effects. Avoid.
Tobacco:	Decreased anti-depressant effect.

***See Glossary**

ANTIDYSKINETICS

GENERIC AND BRAND NAMES

See full list of generic and brand names in the *Generic and Brand Name Directory*, page 869.

BASIC INFORMATION

Habit forming? No
Prescription needed? Yes
Available as generic? Yes
Drug class: Antidyskinetic, antiparkinsonism, dopamine agonists

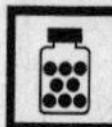

USES

- Treatment of Parkinson's disease.
- Treatment of adverse effects of certain central nervous system drugs.
- Treatment of moderate to severe restless leg syndrome.
- Treatment for Tourette syndrome.

DOSAGE & USAGE INFORMATION

How to take:

- Tablet—Swallow with liquid. If you can't swallow whole, ask doctor or pharmacist for advice.
- Extended-release capsule or tablet—Swallow whole with liquid.
- Elixir—Follow directions on prescription label.
- All forms—Take with, or right after, a meal to lessen stomach irritation (unless otherwise directed by doctor).

When to take:
At the same time(s) each day.

If you forget a dose:
Take as soon as you remember. If it is almost time for the next dose, wait for the next scheduled dose (don't double this dose).

Continued next column

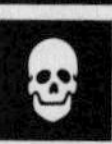

OVERDOSE

SYMPTOMS:
Agitation, dilated pupils, hallucinations, dry mouth, rapid heartbeat, sleepiness.
WHAT TO DO:

- **Dial 911 (emergency) for medical help or call poison control center 1-800-222-1222 for instructions.**
- **If person is unconscious, check breathing and pulse. If not breathing, begin mouth-to-mouth rescue breathing. If heart is not beating, begin chest compressions.**
- **See emergency information on last 3 pages of this book.**

What drug does:

- Balances chemical reactions necessary to send nerve impulses within base of brain.
- Improves muscle control and reduces stiffness.

Time lapse before drug works:
1 to 2 hours. Full effect may take 2 to 3 days.

Don't take with:
Any other medicine or any dietary supplement without consulting your doctor or pharmacist.

POSSIBLE ADVERSE REACTIONS OR SIDE EFFECTS

SYMPTOMS	WHAT TO DO
Life-threatening:	
In case of overdose, see previous column.	
Common:	
• Blurred vision, light sensitivity, unusual body movements, painful or difficult or frequent urination, vomiting, hallucinations.	Continue, but call doctor right away.
• Dry mouth, tiredness, weakness, insomnia or drowsiness, constipation, nausea, lightheadedness.	Continue. Call doctor when convenient.
Infrequent:	
Headache, memory loss, abdominal pain, weakness and faintness when rising from bed or chair, nervousness, impotence, sore throat, cough or wheezing, viral infection, appetite loss, restlessness.	Continue. Call doctor when convenient.
Rare:	
• Rash, hives, eye pain, delusions, amnesia, paranoia, fever, swollen neck glands, vision changes, chest pain, swallowing or breathing difficulty, numbness or tingling or swelling in hands or feet, urine bloody or cloudy, ear buzzing, irregular heartbeat.	Continue, but call doctor right away.
• Confusion, dizziness, sore mouth or tongue, muscle cramps or weakness, depression.	Continue. Call doctor when convenient.

Note: Many symptoms caused by side effects either disappear or decrease when dose is reduced. Consult doctor.

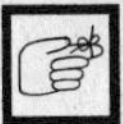

WARNINGS & PRECAUTIONS

Don't take if:
You are allergic to any antidyskinetic.

Before you start, consult your doctor if:
- You have glaucoma or retinal problems.
- You have had high blood pressure, heart disease, impaired liver function.
- You have hypotension or orthostatic hypotension.*
- You have had tardive dyskinesia.*
- You have had kidney disease, urination difficulty, prostatic hypertrophy or intestinal obstruction.
- You have myasthenia gravis.

Over age 60:
More sensitive to drug. Aggravates symptoms of enlarged prostate. Causes impaired thinking, hallucinations, nightmares. Consult doctor about any of these.

Pregnancy:
Decide with your doctor whether drug benefits justify risk to unborn child. Risk category C (see page xviii).

Breast-feeding:
Effects unknown. May inhibit lactation. Consult doctor.

Infants & children:
Use only under doctor's supervision.

Prolonged use:
- Possible glaucoma.
- Talk to your doctor about the need for follow-up medical examinations to assess drug's effectiveness and examination to check eye pressure.

Skin & sunlight:
No special problems expected.

Driving, piloting or hazardous work:
Don't drive or pilot aircraft until you learn how medicine affects you. Don't work around dangerous machinery. Don't climb ladders or work in high places. Danger increases if you drink alcohol or take medicine affecting alertness and reflexes, such as antihistamines, tranquilizers, sedatives, pain medicine, narcotics and mind-altering drugs.

Discontinuing:
- Don't discontinue without consulting doctor. Dose may require gradual reduction if you have taken drug for a long time. Doses of other drugs may also require adjustment.
- After discontinuing, if you experience extrapyramidal reaction* recurrence or worsening, orthostatic hypotension, fast heartbeat, or trouble in sleeping, consult doctor.

Others:
- Internal eye pressure should be measured regularly.
- Avoid becoming overheated.
- Use caution when arising from a sitting or lying position.
- Advise any doctor or dentist whom you consult that you take this medicine.

POSSIBLE INTERACTION WITH OTHER DRUGS

GENERIC NAME OR DRUG CLASS	COMBINED EFFECT
Antacids*	Possible decreased absorption.
Anticholinergics, others*	Increased anti-cholinergic effect.
Antidepressants, tricyclic*	Increased anti-dyskinetic effect.
Antihistamines*	Increased antidyskinetic effect.
Carbidopa	Increased effect of carbidopa.
Central nervous system (CNS) depressants*	May add to any sedative effect.
Chlorpromazine	Decreased effect of chlorpromazine.
Ciprofloxacin	Increased effect of ropinirole.
Dopamine antagonists*	Decreased effect of pramipexole and ropinirole.
Estrogens	Increased effect of ropinirole.

Continued on page 902

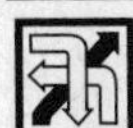

POSSIBLE INTERACTION WITH OTHER SUBSTANCES

INTERACTS WITH	COMBINED EFFECT
Alcohol:	Oversedation. Avoid.
Beverages:	None expected.
Cocaine:	Decreased anti-dyskinetic effect. Avoid.
Foods:	None expected.
Marijuana:	None expected.
Tobacco:	Decreased effect of ropinirole.

***See Glossary**

ANTIFIBRINOLYTIC AGENTS

GENERIC AND BRAND NAMES

AMINOCAPROIC ACID	TRANEXAMIC ACID
Amicar	Cyklokapron
	Lysteda

BASIC INFORMATION

Habit forming? No
Prescription needed? Yes
Available as generic? Yes, for some
Drug class: Antifibrinolytic, antihemorrhagic

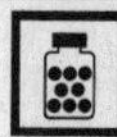

USES

- Treats serious bleeding, especially that occurring after surgery, dental or otherwise.
- Treatment of women with menorrhagia (heavy menstrual bleeding).
- May be used before surgery to help prevent risk of excessive bleeding in patients with disorders that increase the chance of serious bleeding.

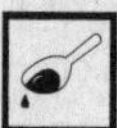

DOSAGE & USAGE INFORMATION

How to take:
- Tablet—Swallow with liquid or food to lessen stomach irritation. If you can't swallow whole, crumble tablet and take with liquid or food.
- Syrup—Take as directed on label.

When to take:
As directed by your doctor.

If you forget a dose:
Take as soon as you remember. Don't double this dose.

What drug does:
Inhibits activation of plasminogen to cause blood clots to disintegrate.

Time lapse before drug works:
Within 2 hours.

Don't take with:
- Thrombolytic chemicals such as streptokinase or urokinase.
- Any other medicine or any dietary supplement without consulting your doctor or pharmacist.

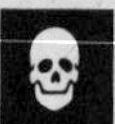

OVERDOSE

SYMPTOMS:
None expected for oral forms. Injectable forms may cause drop in blood pressure or slow heartbeat.
WHAT TO DO:
Follow doctor's instructions.

POSSIBLE ADVERSE REACTIONS OR SIDE EFFECTS

SYMPTOMS	WHAT TO DO
Life-threatening: Shortness of breath, slurred speech, leg or arm numbness.	Seek emergency treatment.
Common: Diarrhea, nausea, vomiting, severe menstrual cramps.	Continue. Call doctor when convenient.
Infrequent: Dizziness; headache; muscular pain and weakness; red eyes; ringing in ears; skin rash; abdominal pain; stuffy nose; decreased urine; swelling of feet, face, legs; rapid weight gain.	Continue. Call doctor when convenient.
Rare: • Signs of thrombosis (sudden, severe headache; pains in chest, groin or legs; loss of coordination; shortness of breath; slurred speech; vision changes; weakness or numbness in arms or leg).	Seek emergency treatment.
• Unusual tiredness, blurred vision, clotting of menstrual flow.	Continue. Call doctor when convenient.

WARNINGS & PRECAUTIONS

Don't take if:
- You are allergic to aminocaproic acid or tranexamic acid.
- You have a diagnosis of disseminated intravascular coagulation (DIC).

Before you start, consult your doctor if:
- You have heart disease.
- You have bleeding from the kidney.
- You have had impaired liver function.
- You have had kidney disease or urination difficulty.
- You have blood clots in parts of the body.

Over age 60:
No changes from other age groups expected.

Pregnancy:
Risk factors vary for drugs in this group. See category list on page xviii and consult doctor.

Breast-feeding:
No problems documented. Consult doctor.

Infants & children:
Use for children only under doctor's supervision.

Prolonged use:
Talk to your doctor about the need for follow-up medical examinations or laboratory studies to check eyes.

Skin & sunlight:
No problems expected.

Driving, piloting or hazardous work:
Don't drive or pilot aircraft until you learn how medicine affects you. Don't work around dangerous machinery. Don't climb ladders or work in high places. Danger increases if you drink alcohol or take medicine affecting alertness and reflexes, such as antihistamines, tranquilizers, sedatives, pain medicine, narcotics and mind-altering drugs.

Discontinuing:
Don't discontinue without consulting doctor. Dose may require gradual reduction if you have taken drug for a long time. Doses of other drugs may also require adjustment.

Others:
- Should not be used in patients with disseminated intravascular coagulation.
- Advise any doctor or dentist whom you consult that you take this medicine.
- Have eyes checked frequently.

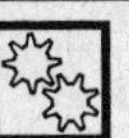

POSSIBLE INTERACTION WITH OTHER DRUGS

GENERIC NAME OR DRUG CLASS	COMBINED EFFECT
Contraceptives, oral*	Increased possibility of blood clotting.
Estrogens*	Increased possibility of blood clotting.
Thrombolytic agents* (alteplase, streptokinase, urokinase)	Decreased effects of both drugs.

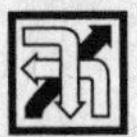

POSSIBLE INTERACTION WITH OTHER SUBSTANCES

INTERACTS WITH	COMBINED EFFECT
Alcohol:	Decreases effectiveness. Avoid.
Beverages:	No problems expected.
Cocaine:	Combined effect unknown. Avoid.
Foods:	No problems expected.
Marijuana:	Combined effect unknown. Avoid.
Tobacco:	Combined effect unknown. Avoid.

***See Glossary**

ANTIFUNGALS, AZOLES

GENERIC AND BRAND NAMES

FLUCONAZOLE
Diflucan
ITRACONAZOLE
Sporanox
KETOCONAZOLE
Nizoral
POSACONAZOLE
Noxafil
VORICONAZOLE
Vfend

BASIC INFORMATION

Habit forming? No
Prescription needed? Yes, for some
Available as generic? Yes, for some
Drug class: Antifungal

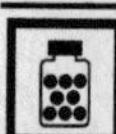

USES

- Treatment for fungal infections.
- Treatment for meningitis.
- Treatment for prostate cancer.

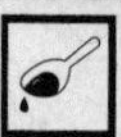

DOSAGE & USAGE INFORMATION

How to take:
- Capsule or tablet—Swallow with liquid. If you can't swallow whole, crumble tablet or open capsule and take with liquid or food.
- Oral suspension—Shake well before using; follow instructions supplied with medication.
- Shampoo or cream—Follow instructions supplied with medication.

When to take:
At the same time each day.

If you forget a dose:
Take as soon as you remember. If it is almost time for the next dose, wait for the next scheduled dose (don't double this dose).

What drug does:
Prevents fungi from growing and reproducing. In treating prostate cancer, ketoconazole decreases male hormone (testosterone) levels.

Continued next column

OVERDOSE

SYMPTOMS:
None expected.
WHAT TO DO:
If person is unconscious, check breathing and pulse. If not breathing, begin mouth-to-mouth rescue breathing. If heart is not beating, begin chest compressions.

Time lapse before drug works:
Several weeks or months for full benefit.

Don't take with:
Any other medicine or any dietary supplement without consulting your doctor or pharmacist.

POSSIBLE ADVERSE REACTIONS OR SIDE EFFECTS

SYMPTOMS	WHAT TO DO
Life-threatening: None expected.	
Common: None expected.	
Infrequent:	
• Skin rash.	Discontinue. Call doctor right away.
• Diarrhea, nausea, vomiting, appetite loss, constipation, headache, abdominal pain.	Continue. Call doctor when convenient.
Rare:	
• Pale stools, yellow skin or eyes, dark or amber urine, unusual tiredness or weakness.	Discontinue. Call doctor right away.
• Diminished sex drive in males, swollen breasts in males, increased sensitivity to light, drowsiness, dizziness, insomnia.	Continue. Call doctor when convenient.

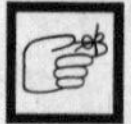

WARNINGS & PRECAUTIONS

Don't take if:
You have had an allergic reaction to any of the azoles.

Before you start, consult your doctor if:
- You have impaired kidney or liver function.
- You have been diagnosed with reduced stomach acidity.

Over age 60:
Adverse reactions and side effects may be more frequent and severe than in younger persons. Dosage may need adjustment if there is age-related kidney impairment.

Pregnancy:
Risk category varies for drugs in this group. See category list on page xviii and consult doctor.

Breast-feeding:
Drug passes into milk. Avoid drug or discontinue nursing until you finish medicine. Consult doctor for advice on maintaining milk supply.

Infants & children:
Use only under close medical supervision.

Prolonged use:
Request periodic liver function studies.

Skin & sunlight:
No problems expected.

Driving, piloting or hazardous work:
Don't drive or pilot aircraft until you learn how medicine affects you. Don't work around dangerous machinery. Don't climb ladders or work in high places. Danger increases if you drink alcohol or take medicine affecting alertness and reflexes, such as antihistamines, tranquilizers, sedatives, pain medicine, narcotics and mind-altering drugs.

Discontinuing:
Don't discontinue without consulting doctor. Dose may require gradual reduction if you have taken drug for a long time. Doses of other drugs may also require adjustment.

Others:
- Advise any doctor or dentist whom you consult that you take this medicine.
- May affect the results of some medical tests.

POSSIBLE INTERACTION WITH OTHER DRUGS

GENERIC NAME OR DRUG CLASS	COMBINED EFFECT
Adrenocorticoids, systemic	Decreased azole effect.
Antacids*	Decreased azole effect.
Anticholinergics*	Decreased azole effect.
Anticoagulants, oral*	Increased effect of anticoagulant.
Antidepressants, tricyclic*	Increased effect of antidepressant.
Antidiabetics, oral*	Increased risk of hypoglycemia.
Antivirals, HIV/AIDS*	Reduced effect of both drugs. Risk of pancreatitis.
Atropine	Decreased azole effect.
Belladonna	Decreased azole effect.
Carbamazepine	Decreased azole effect.
Cimetidine	Decreased azole effect.
Clidinium	Decreased azole absorption.
Contraceptives, oral*	Decreased effect of contraceptive.
Cyclosporine	Increased risk of toxicity to kidney.
Digoxin	Possible toxic levels of digoxin.
Ergot preparations*	Can cause serious or life-threatening problems with blood circulation. Avoid.
Eszopiclone	Decreased effect of ketoconazole.
Famotidine	Reduced antifungal effect. Take 2 hours apart.
Glycopyrrolate	Decreased azole effect.
Hepatotoxic medications*	Increased risk of toxicity to kidney.
Histamine H_2 receptor antagonists	Decreased azole absorption.
HMG-CoA reductase inhibitors	Risk of muscle toxicity.
Hyoscyamine	Decreased azole effect.
Hypoglycemics, oral	Increased effect of oral hypoglycemics.
Isoniazid	Decreased azole effect.

Continued on page 902

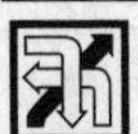

POSSIBLE INTERACTION WITH OTHER SUBSTANCES

INTERACTS WITH	COMBINED EFFECT
Alcohol:	Liver damage risk or disulfiram reaction.*
Beverages: Grapefruit juice.	Decreased effect of drug. Avoid.
Cocaine:	Decreased azole effect. Avoid.
Foods:	None expected.
Marijuana:	Decreased azole effect. Avoid.
Tobacco:	Decreased azole effect. Avoid.

*See Glossary

ANTIFUNGALS (Topical)

GENERIC AND BRAND NAMES

See full list of generic and brand names in the *Generic and Brand Name Directory*, page 869.

BASIC INFORMATION

Habit forming? No
Prescription needed? Yes, for some
Available as generic? Yes, for some
Drug class: Antifungal (topical)

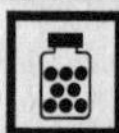

USES

- Treats skin fungus infections such as ringworm of the scalp, athlete's foot, jock itch, "sun fungus," nail fungus and others.
- Treatment of fungus (yeast) infection of the mouth and throat (also called oral thrush).
- Treatment of seborrheic dermatitis (dandruff, cradle cap).

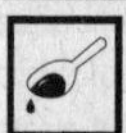

DOSAGE & USAGE INFORMATION

How to use:

- Solution—Apply to affected area once daily for one week.
- Cream, lotion, ointment, gel—Bathe and dry area before use. Apply small amount and rub gently.
- Powder—Apply lightly to skin.
- Shampoo—Follow package instructions.
- Buccal tablet—Follow package instructions.
- Don't bandage or cover treated areas with plastic wrap.
- Follow other instructions from manufacturer listed on label.

When to use:
Follow instructions provided with the product or use as directed by your doctor.

Continued next column

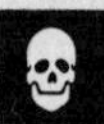

OVERDOSE

SYMPTOMS:
None expected.
WHAT TO DO:

- **Not for internal use. If child accidentally swallows, call poison control center.**
- **Dial 911 (emergency) for medical help or call poison control center 1-800-222-1222 for instructions.**
- **See emergency information on last 3 pages of this book.**

If you forget a dose:
Use as soon as you remember.

What drug does:
Kills fungi by damaging the fungal cell wall.

Time lapse before drug works:
May require 6 to 8 weeks or longer for cure.

Don't use with:
Other skin medicines without consulting your doctor or pharmacist.

POSSIBLE ADVERSE REACTIONS OR SIDE EFFECTS

SYMPTOMS	WHAT TO DO
Life-threatening:	
Rare allergic reaction (hives, itching, rash, wheezing, tightness in chest, swelling of lips or tongue or throat).	Seek emergency treatment immediately.
Common:	
None expected.	
Infrequent:	
Itching, redness, swelling of treated skin not present before treatment.	Discontinue. Call doctor right away.
Rare:	
With buccal form—diarrhea, headache, taste changes, nausea or vomiting, stomach pain.	Discontinue. Call doctor right away.

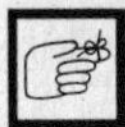

WARNINGS & PRECAUTIONS

Don't use if:
You are allergic to any topical antifungal medicine listed.

Before you start, consult your doctor if:
- You are allergic to anything that touches your skin.
- You are using buccal tablet form of drug and have liver disease or milk protein allergy.

Over age 60:
No problems expected.

Pregnancy:
Risk category varies for drugs in this group. See category list on page xviii and consult doctor.

Breast-feeding:
No problems expected, but check with doctor.

Infants & children:
No problems expected, but read instructions or check with doctor. Some drugs in this group have not been studied in children under age 16.

Prolonged use:
No problems expected, but check with doctor.

Skin & sunlight:
No special problems expected.

Driving, piloting or hazardous work:
No problems expected, but check with doctor.

Discontinuing:
No problems expected, but check with doctor.

Others:
- Avoid contact with eyes.
- Heat and moisture in bathroom medicine cabinet can cause breakdown of medicine. Store someplace else.
- Keep medicine cool, but don't freeze.
- Store away from heat or sunlight.
- Don't use on other members of the family without consulting your doctor.
- If using for jock itch, avoid wearing tight underwear.
- If using for athlete's foot, dry feet carefully after bathing, wear clean cotton socks with sandals or well-ventilated shoes.

POSSIBLE INTERACTION WITH OTHER DRUGS

GENERIC NAME OR DRUG CLASS	COMBINED EFFECT
Other drugs	Consult doctor about interactions if using buccal tablet form.

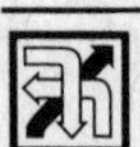

POSSIBLE INTERACTION WITH OTHER SUBSTANCES

INTERACTS WITH	COMBINED EFFECT
Alcohol:	None expected.
Beverages:	None expected.
Cocaine:	None expected.
Foods:	None expected.
Marijuana:	None expected.
Tobacco:	None expected.

*See Glossary

ANTIFUNGALS (Vaginal)

GENERIC AND BRAND NAMES

See full list of generic and brand names in the *Generic and Brand Name Directory*, page 869.

BASIC INFORMATION

Habit forming? No
Prescription needed? Yes, for some
Available as generic? Yes, for some
Drug class: Antifungal (vaginal)

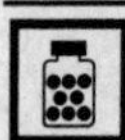

USES

Treats fungus infections of the vagina.

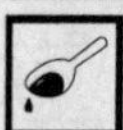

DOSAGE & USAGE INFORMATION

How to use:

- Vaginal cream—Insert into vagina with applicator as illustrated in patient instructions that come with prescription.
- Vaginal tablet—Insert with applicator as illustrated in instructions.
- Vaginal suppository—Insert as illustrated in instructions.

When to use:
According to instructions. Usually once or twice daily.

If you forget a dose:
Use as soon as you remember.

What drug does:
Destroys fungus cell membrane causing loss of essential elements to sustain fungus cell life.

Time lapse before drug works:
Begins immediately. May require 2 weeks of treatment to cure vaginal fungus infections. Recurrence common.

Don't use with:
Other vaginal preparations or douches unless otherwise instructed by your doctor.

OVERDOSE

SYMPTOMS:
None expected.
WHAT TO DO:
Not for internal use. If child accidentally swallows, call doctor or poison control center 1-800-222-1222 for help.

POSSIBLE ADVERSE REACTIONS OR SIDE EFFECTS

SYMPTOMS	WHAT TO DO
Life-threatening: None expected.	
Common: None expected.	
Infrequent: Vaginal burning, itching, irritation, swelling of labia, redness, increased discharge (not present before starting medicine).	Discontinue. Call doctor right away.
Rare: Skin rash, hives, irritation of sex partner's penis.	Discontinue. Call doctor right away.

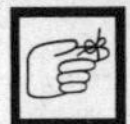

WARNINGS & PRECAUTIONS

Don't use if:
- You are allergic to any of the products listed.
- You have pre-existing liver disease.

Before you start, consult your doctor if:
You are pregnant.

Over age 60:
No problems expected.

Pregnancy:
Risk factors vary for drugs in this group. See category list on page xviii and consult doctor.

Breast-feeding:
No problems expected. Consult doctor.

Infants & children:
Use only under close medical supervision.

Prolonged use:
No problems expected.

Skin & sunlight:
No problems expected.

Driving, piloting or hazardous work:
No problems expected.

Discontinuing:
Recurrence likely if you stop before time suggested.

Others:
- Gentian Violet and some of the other products can stain clothing. Sanitary napkins may protect against staining.
- Keep the genital area clean. Use plain unscented soap.
- Take showers rather than tub baths.
- Wear cotton underpants or pantyhose with a cotton crotch. Avoid underpants made from non-ventilating materials. Wear freshly laundered underpants.
- Don't sit around in wet clothing—especially a wet bathing suit.
- After urination or bowel movements, cleanse by wiping or washing from front to back (vagina to anus).
- Don't douche unless your doctor recommends it.
- If urinating causes burning, urinate through a tubular device, such as a toilet-paper roll or plastic cup with the end cut out.

POSSIBLE INTERACTION WITH OTHER DRUGS

GENERIC NAME OR DRUG CLASS	COMBINED EFFECT
Warfarin	May cause bleeding with miconazole vaginal cream.

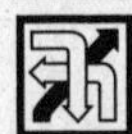

POSSIBLE INTERACTION WITH OTHER SUBSTANCES

INTERACTS WITH	COMBINED EFFECT
Alcohol:	None expected.
Beverages:	None expected.
Cocaine:	None expected.
Foods:	None expected.
Marijuana:	None expected.
Tobacco:	None expected.

*See Glossary

ANTIGLAUCOMA, ADRENERGIC AGONISTS

GENERIC AND BRAND NAMES

APRACLONIDINE
Iopidine
BRIMONIDINE
Alphagan
Alphagan P
Combigan
DIPIVEFRIN
AKPro
DPE
Ophtho-Dipivefrin
Propine
Propine C Cap
EPINEPHRINE
Epifren
Epinal
Eppy/N
Glaucon

BASIC INFORMATION

Habit forming? No
Prescription needed? Yes
Available as generic? Yes, for some
Drug class: Antiglaucoma

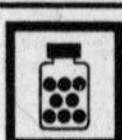

USES

Treats open-angle glaucoma, secondary glaucoma and ocular hypertension. May be used with eye surgery.

DOSAGE & USAGE INFORMATION

How to use:
Eye drops

- Wash hands.
- Apply pressure to inside corner of eye with middle finger.
- Continue pressure for 1 minute after placing medicine in eye.
- Tilt head backward. Pull lower lid away from eye with index finger of the same hand.
- Drop eye drops into pouch and close eye. Don't blink.
- Keep eyes closed for 1 to 2 minutes.
- If using more than one eye solution, wait at least 10 minutes between instillations to avoid a "wash-out" effect.

Continued next column

When to use:
As directed on label.

If you forget a dose:
Apply as soon as you remember. If almost time for next dose, wait and apply at regular time (don't double this dose).

What drug does:
Inactivates enzyme and facilitates movement of fluid (aqueous humor) into and out of the eye.

Time lapse before drug works:
30 minutes to 4 hours.

Don't use with:
Any other eye medicine without consulting your doctor or pharmacist.

OVERDOSE

SYMPTOMS:
Effects unknown.
WHAT TO DO:
Overdose unlikely to threaten life. If person uses much larger amount than prescribed or if accidentally swallowed, call doctor or poison control center 1-800-222-1222 for help.

POSSIBLE ADVERSE REACTIONS OR SIDE EFFECTS

SYMPTOMS	WHAT TO DO
Life-threatening: None expected.	
Common:	
• Allergic reaction (itching, redness, tearing of eye).	Discontinue. Call doctor right away.
• Headache, eye discomfort, dry mouth.	Continue. Call doctor when convenient.
Infrequent:	
Eye symptoms: pain, changes in vision, blurred vision, discharge or swelling, color change in white of eye, feeling of something in the eye, stinging, burning, watering, light sensitivity, crusting on eyelid, paleness of eye or inner eyelid.	Continue. Call doctor right away.
Rare:	
• Symptoms of too much drug absorbed in body: faintness, skin paleness, chest pain, increased or fast or irregular heartbeat, swelling (face, hands, or feet), dizziness, numbness or tingling in fingers or toes, wheezing, troubled breathing.	Discontinue. Call doctor right away.
• Other symptoms of drug absorbed in body: sore throat, muscle aches, nausea, smell or taste changes, anxiety, nervousness, depression, constipation, insomnia or drowsiness.	Continue. Call doctor when convenient.

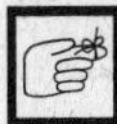

WARNINGS & PRECAUTIONS

Don't use if:
You are allergic to any of the adrenergic agonist antiglaucoma drugs.

Before you start, consult your doctor if:
- You suffer from depression.
- You have any eye disease.
- You have heart problems, high or low blood pressure or thromboangiitis obliterans.
- You have Raynaud's disease.
- You have a history of vasovagal attacks* (if using apraclonidine).
- You have liver or kidney problems.

Over age 60:
No problems expected.

Pregnancy:
Risk factors vary for drugs in this group. See category list on page xviii and consult doctor.

Breast-feeding:
It is not known if drugs pass into milk. Avoid drugs or discontinue nursing until you finish medicine. Consult doctor for advice on maintaining milk supply.

Infants & children:
Use only under close medical supervision.

Prolonged use:
May be necessary.

Skin & sunlight:
No problems expected.

Driving, piloting or hazardous work:
Your vision may be blurred or there may be a change in your near or far vision or night vision for a short time after drug use. Don't drive or pilot aircraft until you learn how medicine affects you. Don't work around dangerous machinery. Don't climb ladders or work in high places.

Discontinuing:
Don't discontinue without consulting your doctor. Dose may require gradual reduction if you have used drug for a long time. Doses of other drugs may also require adjustment.

Others:
- Advise any doctor or dentist whom you consult that you use this medicine.
- Drugs may cause your eyes to become more sensitive to light. Wear sunglasses and avoid too much exposure to bright light.
- Brimonidine contains a preservative that could be absorbed by soft contact lenses. Wait at least 15 minutes after putting eye drops in before you put in your soft contact lenses.
- If you have any eye infection, injury or wound, consult doctor before using this medicine.
- Keep appointments for regular eye examinations to measure pressure in the eye.

POSSIBLE INTERACTION WITH OTHER DRUGS

GENERIC NAME OR DRUG CLASS	COMBINED EFFECT
Antidepressants, tricyclic	May decrease ocular hypertensive effect. Dipivefrin may cause heart rhythm problem, high blood pressure.
Antiglaucoma, beta blockers	May help decrease eye pressure.
Antihypertensives*	May decrease blood pressure.
Central nervous system (CNS) depressants*	May increase CNS depressant effect.
Digitalis preparations*	Increased risk of heart problems.
Maprotiline	Heart rhythm problems, high blood pressure.
Monoamine oxidase (MAO) inhibitors*	Separate use by at least 14 days.

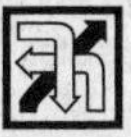

POSSIBLE INTERACTION WITH OTHER SUBSTANCES

INTERACTS WITH	COMBINED EFFECT
Alcohol:	None expected.
Beverages:	None expected.
Cocaine:	None expected. Best to avoid.
Foods:	None expected.
Marijuana:	Unknown effect. Consult doctor.
Tobacco:	None expected.

*See Glossary

ANTIGLAUCOMA, ANTICHOLINESTERASES

GENERIC AND BRAND NAMES

DEMECARIUM
Humorsol

ECHOTHIOPHATE
Phospholine Iodide

BASIC INFORMATION

Habit forming? No
Prescription needed? Yes
Available as generic? No
Drug class: Antiglaucoma

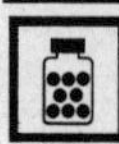

USES

- Treatment for certain types of glaucoma.
- Used for diagnosis and treatment for other eye conditions.

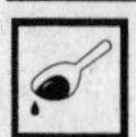

DOSAGE & USAGE INFORMATION

How to use:
Eye drops

- Wash hands. Tilt head back.
- Press finger gently on the skin right under the lower eyelid; pull the eyelid away from the eye to make a space or small pocket.
- Drop the medicine into this pocket, then let go of the skin and gently close the eyes; don't blink.
- Keep the eyes closed and apply pressure to the inner corner of the eye with your finger for 1 to 2 minutes.
- Wash hands again after using the drops.
- To keep the solution germ-free, do not allow the applicator tip to touch the skin or eye.
- If using more than one eye solution, wait at least 10 minutes between instillations to avoid a "wash-out" effect.

Continued next column

When to use:
As directed on label.

If you forget a dose:
Apply as soon as you remember. If almost time for next dose, wait and apply at regular time (don't double this dose).

What drug does:
Inactivates an enzyme to reduce pressure inside the eye.

Time lapse before drug works:
5 to 60 minutes.

Don't use with:
Any other eye medicine without consulting your doctor or pharmacist.

OVERDOSE

SYMPTOMS:
Fast heartbeat, diarrhea, heavy sweating, breathing difficulty, unable to control bladder, shock.

WHAT TO DO:

- **For overdose in the eye, flush with warm tap water and call doctor immediately.**
- **For accidentally ingested overdose or signs of system toxicity, dial 911 (emergency) for medical help or call poison control center 1-800-222-1222 for instructions.**
- **See emergency information on last 3 pages of this book.**

POSSIBLE ADVERSE REACTIONS OR SIDE EFFECTS

SYMPTOMS	WHAT TO DO
Life-threatening: None expected.	
Common: Stinging, burning watery eyes.	Continue. Call doctor when convenient.
Infrequent: Blurred vision, change in vision, change in night vision, eyelids twitch, headache, ache in brow area.	Continue. Call doctor when convenient.
Rare: Decreased vision with veil or curtain appearing in part of vision, eye redness, symptoms of too much of drug absorbed in body (loss of bladder control, slow heartbeat, increased sweating, weakness, difficult breathing, vomiting, nausea, diarrhea, stomach pain or cramping).	Discontinue. Call doctor right away.

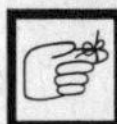

WARNINGS & PRECAUTIONS

Don't use if:
You are allergic to demecarium or echothiophate.

Before you start, consult your doctor if:
- You have eye infection or other eye disease.
- You have ulcers in stomach or duodenum or other stomach disorder.
- You have myasthenia gravis, overactive thyroid or urinary tract blockage.
- You have asthma, epilepsy, Down syndrome, heart disease, high or low blood pressure, Parkinson's disease.

Over age 60:
Adverse reactions and side effects may be more frequent and severe than in younger persons.

Pregnancy:
Risk factors vary for drugs in this group. See category list on page xviii and consult doctor.

Breast-feeding:
It is not known if drug passes into milk. Avoid drugs or discontinue nursing until you finish medicine. Consult doctor for advice on maintaining milk supply.

Infants & children:
Use under medical supervision only. Children are more susceptible to adverse effects.

Prolonged use:
Cataracts or other eye problems may occur. Be sure to see your doctor for regular eye examinations.

Skin & sunlight:
No problems expected.

Driving, piloting or hazardous work:
Your vision may be blurred or there may be a change in your near or far vision or night vision for a short time after drug use. Don't drive or pilot aircraft until you learn how medicine affects you. Don't work around dangerous machinery. Don't climb ladders or work in high places.

Discontinuing:
Don't discontinue without consulting your doctor. Dose may require gradual reduction if you have used drug for a long time. Doses of other drugs may also require adjustment.

Others:
- Advise any doctor or dentist whom you consult that you use this medicine.
- Keep appointments for regular eye examinations to measure pressure in the eye.
- If you have any eye infection, injury or wound, consult doctor before using this medicine.

POSSIBLE INTERACTION WITH OTHER DRUGS

GENERIC NAME OR DRUG CLASS	COMBINED EFFECT
Anticholinergics*	Increased risk of toxicity.
Antimyasthenics*	Increased risk of side effects.
Cholinesterase inhibitors*	Increased risk of toxicity.
Insecticides or pesticides with organic phosphates	Increased toxic absorption of pesticides.
Topical anesthetics	Increased risk of toxic effects of antiglaucoma eye medicines.

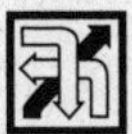

POSSIBLE INTERACTION WITH OTHER SUBSTANCES

INTERACTS WITH	COMBINED EFFECT
Alcohol:	None expected.
Beverages:	None expected.
Cocaine:	None expected. Best to avoid.
Foods:	None expected.
Marijuana:	Unknown effect. Consult doctor.
Tobacco:	None expected.

*See Glossary

ANTIGLAUCOMA, BETA BLOCKERS

GENERIC AND BRAND NAMES

BETAXOLOL (ophthalmic)
- Betoptic
- Betoptic S

CARTEOLOL (ophthalmic)
- Ocupress

LEVOBUNOLOL (ophthalmic)
- AKBeta
- Betagen C Cap B.I.D.
- Betagen C Cap Q.D.
- Betagen Standard Cap

METIPRANOLOL (ophthalmic)
- OptiPranolol

TIMOLOL (ophthalmic)
- Apo-Timop
- Beta-Tim
- Betimol
- Combigan
- Cosopt
- Cosopt PF
- Gen-Timolo
- Istalol
- Med Timolol
- Novo-Timolol
- Nu-Timolol
- Timodal
- Timoptic
- Timoptic in Ocudose
- Timoptic-XE
- Xalcom

BASIC INFORMATION

Habit forming? No
Prescription needed? Yes
Available as generic? Yes, for some
Drug class: Antiglaucoma

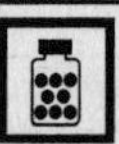

USES

Treatment for glaucoma and ocular hypertension. May be used in eye surgery.

DOSAGE & USAGE INFORMATION

How to take:
Eye drops—Follow directions on prescription.

Continued next column

OVERDOSE

SYMPTOMS:
Slow heartbeat, low blood pressure, bronchospasm, heart failure (these symptoms are what might be expected if similar drugs were taken orally).

WHAT TO DO:
- **For overdose in the eye, flush with warm tap water and call doctor immediately.**
- **For accidentally ingested overdose or signs of system toxicity, dial 911 (emergency) for medical help or call poison control center 1-800-222-1222 for instructions.**
- **See emergency information on last 3 pages of this book.**

When to take:
At the same time each day, usually in the morning. Follow your doctor's instructions.

If you forget a dose:
- Once-a-day dose—Apply as soon as you remember. If almost time for next dose, wait and apply at regular time (don't double this dose).
- More than once-a-day dose—Apply as soon as you remember. If close to time for next dose, wait and apply at regular time (don't double this dose).

What drug does:
Appears to reduce production of aqueous humor (fluid inside eye), thereby reducing pressure inside eye.

Time lapse before drug works:
30 minutes to 1 hour.

Don't take with:
Any other eye medicine without consulting your doctor or pharmacist.

POSSIBLE ADVERSE REACTIONS OR SIDE EFFECTS

SYMPTOMS	WHAT TO DO
Life-threatening:	
In case of overdose, see previous column.	
Common:	
• Redness of eyes or inside of eyelids.	Continue. Call doctor right away.
• Temporary blurred vision, night vision decreased, eye irritation or discomfort when drug is used.	Continue. Call doctor when convenient.
Infrequent:	
Ongoing blurred vision, other vision changes, different size pupils, eyeball discolored, droopy eyelid, eye pain, or swelling or irritation.	Continue. Call doctor when convenient.
Rare:	
• Increased sensitivity to light; sensation of foreign body in eye; dryness, discharge or pain in eye; crusty eyelids; inflammation.	Continue. Call doctor when convenient.
• Symptoms of body absorbing too much of drug include problems with heart, stomach, lungs (breathing difficulties), skin, nervous system, hair loss, and others.	Discontinue. Call doctor right away.

WARNINGS & PRECAUTIONS

Don't take if:
You are allergic to any beta-adrenergic blocking agent taken orally or used in the eye.

Before you start, consult your doctor if:
- You have asthma, a bronchial disorder or pulmonary disease.
- You have any heart disease or heart problem.
- You suffer from depression.
- You have diabetes or low blood sugar, overactive thyroid or myasthenia gravis.

Over age 60:
Adverse reactions and side effects may be more frequent and severe than in younger persons.

Pregnancy:
Decide with your doctor whether drug benefits justify risk to unborn child. Risk category C (see page xviii).

Breast-feeding:
Some of these drugs pass into milk; others are unknown. Avoid drugs or discontinue nursing until you finish medicine. Consult doctor for advice on maintaining milk supply.

Infants & children:
Give only under close medical supervision. Children may be more sensitive to drug and side effects.

Prolonged use:
Talk to your doctor about the need for follow-up medical examinations to check pressure inside eye.

Skin & sunlight:
No special problems expected.

Driving, piloting or hazardous work:
Your vision may be blurred or there may be a change in your near or far vision or night vision for a short time after drug use. Don't drive or pilot aircraft until you learn how medicine affects you. Don't work around dangerous machinery. Don't climb ladders or work in high places.

Discontinuing:
- Don't discontinue without doctor's approval.
- May need to discontinue drug temporarily before major surgery. Your doctor will provide instructions.

Others:
- Advise any doctor or dentist whom you consult that you take this medicine.
- These drugs may affect blood sugar levels in diabetic patients.
- Keep appointments for regular eye examinations to measure pressure in the eye.
- If you have any eye infection, injury or wound, consult doctor before using this medicine.

POSSIBLE INTERACTION WITH OTHER DRUGS

GENERIC NAME OR DRUG CLASS	COMBINED EFFECT

Drug interactions are unlikely unless a significant amount of the eye medication is absorbed into the system. Potential interactions that may occur are similar to those listed in Possible Interactions With Other Drugs under Beta-Adrenergic Blocking Agents.

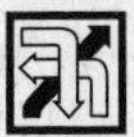

POSSIBLE INTERACTION WITH OTHER SUBSTANCES

INTERACTS WITH	COMBINED EFFECT
Alcohol:	None expected.
Beverages:	None expected.
Cocaine:	Decreased anti-glaucoma effect; heart problems. Avoid.
Foods:	None expected.
Marijuana:	Unknown effect. Consult doctor.
Tobacco:	None expected.

*See Glossary

ANTIGLAUCOMA, CARBONIC ANHYDRASE INHIBITORS

GENERIC AND BRAND NAMES

BRINZOLAMIDE
Azopt

DORZOLAMIDE
Cosopt
Cosopt PF
Trusopt

BASIC INFORMATION

Habit forming? No
Prescription needed? Yes
Available as generic? Yes, for some
Drug class: Antiglaucoma

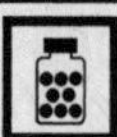

USES

- Treatment for open-angle glaucoma (increased pressure in the eye).
- Treatment for ocular hypertension.

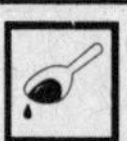

DOSAGE & USAGE INFORMATION

How to use:
Eye drops
- Wash hands. Tilt head back.
- Press finger gently on the skin right under the lower eyelid; pull the eyelid away from the eye to make a space or small pocket.
- Drop the medicine into this pocket, then let go of the skin and gently close the eyes; don't blink.
- Keep the eyes closed and apply pressure to the inner corner of the eye with your finger for 1 to 2 minutes.
- Wash hands again after using the drops.
- To keep the solution germ-free, do not allow the applicator tip to touch the skin or eye.
- If using more than one eye solution, wait at least 10 minutes between instillations to avoid a "wash-out" effect.

When to use:
Normally used 3 times a day (about 8 hours apart). Always use as directed by your doctor.

Continued next column

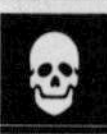

OVERDOSE

SYMPTOMS:
Unknown effect.
WHAT TO DO:
Overdose unlikely to threaten life. If person uses much larger amount than prescribed or if accidentally swallowed, call doctor or poison control center 1-800-222-1222 for help.

If you forget a dose:
Use as soon as you remember. If it is almost time for the next dose, wait for next dose (don't double this dose).

What drug does:
This medicine is a topically applied carbonic anhydrase inhibitor that helps decrease production of aqueous humor (the fluid in the eye) and lowers the pressure inside the eye.

Time lapse before drug works:
30 to 60 minutes.

Don't take with:
Any other eye medicine without consulting your doctor or pharmacist.

POSSIBLE ADVERSE REACTIONS OR SIDE EFFECTS

SYMPTOMS	WHAT TO DO
Life-threatening: None expected.	
Common:	
• Allergic reaction (redness, itching or swelling of eye or eyelid); feeling of something in the eye; continued or severe sensitivity to light.	Discontinue. Call doctor right away.
• Bitter taste; burning, stinging or discomfort when medicine is used; mild sensitivity to light.	Continue. Call doctor when convenient.
Infrequent:	
Blurred vision, dryness or mild tearing of eyes, tiredness or weakness, headache, hair loss.	Continue. Call doctor when convenient.
Rare:	
Blood in urine; continued nausea or vomiting; hives; pain in chest, back, side or abdomen; eye pain; severe or continued tearing; seeing double; skin rash; shortness of breath.	Discontinue. Call doctor right away.

ANTIGLAUCOMA, CARBONIC ANHYDRASE INHIBITORS

WARNINGS & PRECAUTIONS

Don't use if:
You are allergic to ophthalmic carbonic anhydrase inhibitors or any sulfonamide* medications.

Before you start, consult your doctor if:
- You have kidney or liver disease.
- You are allergic to any medication, food, preservatives or other substances.

Over age 60:
No special problems expected.

Pregnancy:
Decide with your doctor whether drug benefits justify risk to unborn child. Risk category C (see page xviii).

Breast-feeding:
It is not known if drug passes into milk. Avoid drugs or discontinue nursing until you finish medicine. Consult doctor for advice on maintaining milk supply.

Infants & children:
- Dorzolamide is used to treat pediatric patients.
- Safety and dosage of other drugs in this group has not been established. Use only under medical supervision.

Prolonged use:
Schedule regular appointments with your eye doctor for eye examinations to be sure the medication is controlling the glaucoma.

Skin & sunlight:
No special problems expected.

Driving, piloting or hazardous work:
Your vision may be blurred or there may be a change in your near or far vision or night vision for a short time after drug use. Don't drive or pilot aircraft until you learn how medicine affects you. Don't work around dangerous machinery. Don't climb ladders or work in high places.

Discontinuing:
Don't discontinue without consulting your doctor.

Others:
- If you have any eye infection, injury or wound, consult doctor before using this medicine.
- Advise any doctor or dentist whom you consult that you use this medicine.
- Keep appointments for regular eye examinations to measure pressure in the eye.
- Wear sunglasses when outside in sunlight.

POSSIBLE INTERACTION WITH OTHER DRUGS

GENERIC NAME OR DRUG CLASS	COMBINED EFFECT
Amphetamines	Increased risk of side effects.
Carbonic anhydrase inhibitors (oral)	Increased effect of both drugs. Avoid.
Mecamylamine	Increased risk of side effects.
Quinidine	Increased risk of side effects.
Salicylates (High doses)	Increased risk of adverse effects.

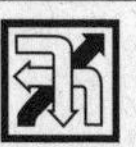

POSSIBLE INTERACTION WITH OTHER SUBSTANCES

INTERACTS WITH	COMBINED EFFECT
Alcohol:	None expected.
Beverages:	None expected.
Cocaine:	None expected. Best to avoid.
Foods:	None expected.
Marijuana:	Unknown effect. Consult doctor.
Tobacco:	None expected.

*See Glossary

ANTIGLAUCOMA, CHOLINERGIC AGONISTS

GENERIC AND BRAND NAMES

CARBACHOL
Carbastat
Carboptic
Miostat

PILOCARPINE
Adsorbocarpine
Akarpine
Almocarpine
Carpine
Isopto Carpine
Minims
Miocarpine
Ocu-Carpine
Ocusert Pilo
Pilocarpine Pilocar
Pilopine HS
Piloptic
Pilostat
P.V. Carpine Liquifilm

BASIC INFORMATION

Habit forming? No
Prescription needed? Yes
Available as generic? Yes, for some
Drug class: Antiglaucoma

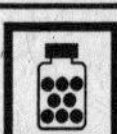

USES

Treatment for glaucoma and other eye conditions. May be used in eye surgery.

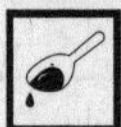

DOSAGE & USAGE INFORMATION

How to take:

- Drops—Apply to eyes. Close eyes for 1 or 2 minutes to absorb medicine.
- Eye insert system—Follow label directions.
- Gel—Follow label directions.

When to use:
As directed on label.

Continued next column

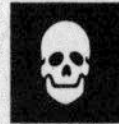

OVERDOSE

SYMPTOMS:
If accidental overdose in eye, flush with water. If swallowed—nausea, vomiting, diarrhea, sweating.
WHAT TO DO:
Overdose unlikely to threaten life. If person uses much larger amount than prescribed or if accidentally swallowed, call doctor or poison control center 1-800-222-1222 for help.

If you forget a dose:

- For eye drops or gel, use as soon as possible. If it is almost time for your next dose, skip the missed dose and return to regular schedule (don't double this dose).
- For eye insert, replace it as soon as possible. Then return to your regular schedule.

What drug does:
Reduces internal eye pressure.

Time lapse before drug works:
75 minutes to 4 hours.

Don't take with:
Any other eye medicine without consulting your doctor or pharmacist.

POSSIBLE ADVERSE REACTIONS OR SIDE EFFECTS

SYMPTOMS	WHAT TO DO
Life-threatening: None expected.	
Common: Blurred or altered vision (near or distant vision), eye stinging or burning.	Continue. Call doctor when convenient.
Infrequent: Headache, eye irritation, redness, of eye, eyelid twitching.	Continue. Call doctor when convenient.
Rare: Eye pain, a veil or curtain appears across part of vision, symptoms of too much of drug absorbed in the body (increased sweating, muscle trembling, nausea, vomiting, diarrhea, troubled breathing or wheezing, mouth watering, stomach cramps, fainting, flushing or redness of face, urge to urinate).	Discontinue. Call doctor right away.

ANTIGLAUCOMA, CHOLINERGIC AGONISTS

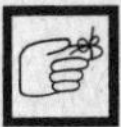

WARNINGS & PRECAUTIONS

Don't take if:
You are allergic to carbachol or pilocarpine.

Before you start, consult your doctor if:
- You have other eye problems.
- You have heart disease, overactive thyroid, Parkinson's disease, ulcers, or urinary blockage problems.
- You have asthma.

Over age 60:
No special problems expected.

Pregnancy:
Decide with your doctor if drug benefits justify risk to unborn child. Risk category C (see page xviii).

Breast-feeding:
It is not known if drugs pass into milk. Avoid drugs or discontinue nursing until you finish medicine. Consult doctor for advice on maintaining milk supply.

Infants & children:
Not recommended.

Prolonged use:
- You may develop tolerance* for drug, making it ineffective. Your doctor may switch antiglaucoma drugs for a period of time to return effectiveness.
- Talk to your doctor about the need for follow-up medical examinations to check eye pressure.

Skin & sunlight:
No problems expected.

Driving, piloting or hazardous work:
Your vision may be blurred or there may be a change in your near or far vision or night vision for a short time after drug use. Don't drive or pilot aircraft until you learn how medicine affects you. Don't work around dangerous machinery. Don't climb ladders or work in high places.

Discontinuing:
Don't discontinue without consulting your doctor.

Others:
- Advise any doctor or dentist whom you consult that you use this medicine.
- Keep appointments for regular eye examinations to measure pressure in the eye.
- If you have any eye infection, injury or wound, consult doctor before using this medicine.

POSSIBLE INTERACTION WITH OTHER DRUGS

GENERIC NAME OR DRUG CLASS	COMBINED EFFECT
Belladonna (ophthalmic)	Decreased antiglaucoma effect.
Cyclopentolate	Decreased antiglaucoma effect.
Flurbiprofen (ophthalmic)	Decreased antiglaucoma effect.

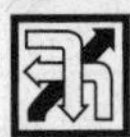

POSSIBLE INTERACTION WITH OTHER SUBSTANCES

INTERACTS WITH	COMBINED EFFECT
Alcohol:	None expected.
Beverages:	None expected.
Cocaine:	None expected. Best to avoid.
Foods:	None expected.
Marijuana:	Unknown effect. Consult doctor.
Tobacco:	None expected.

*See Glossary

ANTIGLAUCOMA, PROSTAGLANDINS

GENERIC AND BRAND NAMES

BIMATOPROST
Latisse
Lumigan
Xalcom
ISOPROPYL UNOPROSTONE
Rescula
LATANOPROST
Xalatan
TAFLUPROST
Zioptan
TRAVOPROST
Travatan
Travatan Z

BASIC INFORMATION

Habit forming? No
Prescription needed? Yes
Available as generic? Yes, for some
Drug class: Antiglaucoma

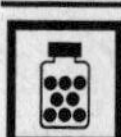

USES

- Treats diseases of the eye like glaucoma and hypertension of the eye.
- Treats hypotrichosis (reduced amount of hair) of the eyelashes.

DOSAGE & USAGE INFORMATION

How to use:
Eye drops
- Wash hands.
- Apply pressure on the skin just beneath the lower eyelid. Pull the lower eyelid away from the eye to make a space.
- Drop the medicine into this space.
- Release eyelid and gently close eyes.
- Don't blink.
- Keep eyes closed for 1 to 2 minutes.
- Remove excess solution from around the eye with a clean tissue, being careful not to touch the eye.
- Don't touch applicator tip to any surface (including the eye). If you accidentally touch tip, clean with warm water and soap.
- Keep container tightly closed.
- Wash hands immediately after using.

When to use:
As directed on label.

Continued next column

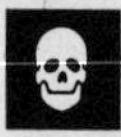

OVERDOSE

SYMPTOMS:
Unknown effect.
WHAT TO DO:
Overdose unlikely to threaten life. If person uses much larger amount than prescribed or if accidentally swallowed, call doctor or poison control center 1-800-222-1222 for help.

If you forget a dose:
Use as soon as you remember. If it is almost time for the next dose, wait for next dose (don't double this dose).

What drug does:
Inactivates enzyme and facilitates movement of fluid (aqueous humor) into and out of the eye.

Time lapse before drug works:
10-30 minutes.

Don't use with:
Any other eye medicine without consulting your doctor or pharmacist.

POSSIBLE ADVERSE REACTIONS OR SIDE EFFECTS

SYMPTOMS	WHAT TO DO
Life-threatening:	
None expected.	
Common:	
Eye symptoms: itching, discomfort, mild pain, redness, feeling of something in eye, vision decreased.	Continue. Call doctor when convenient.
Infrequent:	
Eye tearing or dry, crusting on eyelid, eyes more sensitive to light, eye discharge, color vision or other vision changes, hair growth increased.	Continue. Call doctor when convenient.
Rare:	
• Faintness, increased sweating, irregular or fast heartbeat, chest pain or tightness, shortness of breath, wheezing, unusual tiredness, paleness, heartburn, indigestion, coughing up mucus, fainting, chills or fever, dizziness, pain and stiffness in muscles or joints, headache, urination problems, cold symptoms, back pain, mental and mood changes.	Discontinue. Call doctor right away.

• May cause changes in the treated eye only (color of the iris and eyelid). It may change eyelashes (thicker, longer, color). Changes may take months or years and may be permanent.	Continue. Call doctor when convenient.

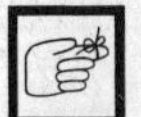

WARNINGS & PRECAUTIONS

Don't take if:
You are allergic to any prostaglandin eye medicine.

Before you start, consult your doctor if:
- You plan to have eye or dental surgery.
- You have any eye disease.
- You have heart problems or high blood pressure.
- You have liver or kidney problems.

Over age 60:
Adverse reactions and side effects may be more frequent and severe than in younger persons. Ask doctor about smaller doses.

Pregnancy:
Risk factors vary for drugs in this group. See category list on page xviii and consult doctor.

Breast-feeding:
It is not known if drugs pass into milk. Avoid drugs or discontinue nursing until you finish medicine. Consult doctor for advice on maintaining milk supply.

Infants & children:
Safety and efficacy not established in this age group.

Prolonged use:
May be necessary.

Skin & sunlight:
No problems expected.

Driving, piloting or hazardous work:
Your vision may be blurred or there may be a change in your near or far vision or night vision for a short time after drug use. Don't drive or pilot aircraft until you learn how medicine affects you. Don't work around dangerous machinery. Don't climb ladders or work in high places.

Discontinuing:
Don't discontinue without consulting your doctor. Dose may require gradual reduction if you have used drug for a long time. Doses of other drugs may also require adjustment.

Others:
- If you have any eye infection, injury or wound, consult doctor before using this medicine.
- Advise any doctor or dentist whom you consult that you use this medicine.
- Keep appointments for regular eye examinations to measure pressure in the eye.

POSSIBLE INTERACTION WITH OTHER DRUGS

GENERIC NAME OR DRUG CLASS	COMBINED EFFECT
None specific	Other drugs may increase or decrease antiglaucoma effect. Consult doctor.

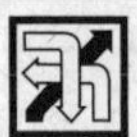

POSSIBLE INTERACTION WITH OTHER SUBSTANCES

INTERACTS WITH	COMBINED EFFECT
Alcohol:	None expected.
Beverages:	None expected.
Cocaine:	None expected. Best to avoid.
Foods:	None expected.
Marijuana:	Unknown effect. Consult doctor.
Tobacco:	None expected.

ANTIGOUT DRUGS

GENERIC AND BRAND NAMES

ALLOPURINOL
- Alloprin
- Apo-Allopurinol
- Lopurin
- Novopural
- Purinol
- Zyloprim

FEBUXOSTAT
- Uloric

BASIC INFORMATION

Habit forming? No
Prescription needed? Yes
Available as generic? Yes, for some
Drug class: Antigout

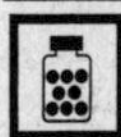

USES

- Treats symptoms of chronic gout.
- Treatment for increased levels of uric acid (hyperuricemia) in the body.
- Prevention of kidney stones caused by uric acid.

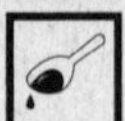

DOSAGE & USAGE INFORMATION

How to take:
Tablet—Swallow with liquid or food to lessen stomach irritation. Drink extra fluids each day.

When to take:
At the same time(s) each day.

If you forget a dose:
Take as soon as you remember. If it is almost time for the next dose, skip the missed dose and wait for your next scheduled dose (don't double this dose).

What drug does:
Slows formation of uric acid by inhibiting enzyme (xanthine oxidase) activity.

Time lapse before drug works:
Reduces blood uric acid in 1 to 3 weeks. May require 6 months to prevent acute gout attacks.

Don't take with:
Any other medicine or any dietary supplement without consulting your doctor or pharmacist.

OVERDOSE

SYMPTOMS:
May have nausea, vomiting and diarrhea.
WHAT TO DO:
Overdose unlikely to threaten life. If person uses much larger amount than prescribed or if accidentally swallowed, call doctor or poison control center 1-800-222-1222 for help.

POSSIBLE ADVERSE REACTIONS OR SIDE EFFECTS

SYMPTOMS	WHAT TO DO
Life-threatening:	
Rare allergic reaction (rash, painful urination, blood in the urine, eye irritation, swelling of mouth or lips).	Discontinue. Seek emergency help.
Common:	
Rash, hives, itch.	Discontinue. Call doctor right away.
Infrequent:	
Drowsiness, diarrhea, stomach ache or pain, nausea or vomiting without other symptoms, headache.	Continue. Call doctor when convenient.
Rare:	
• Sore throat, fever, unusual bleeding or bruising, black or tarry stools, mouth or lips sores, blood in urine or stools, skin problems (redness, peeling, burning, tenderness, scaly, thickened), red or itchy eyes, wheezing or shortness of breath or trouble breathing or swelling (hands, feet, lower legs, fingers), fast weight gain, unusual tiredness or weakness, yellow skin or eyes, abnormal heartbeat, chest pain, dizziness, vision problems, hearing loss, slurred speech, numbness or tingling in face or arm or legs.	Discontinue. Call doctor right away.
• Loose fingernails, pain in lower back or side, unexpected nosebleeds, hair loss.	Continue. Call doctor when convenient.

WARNINGS & PRECAUTIONS

Don't take if:
You are allergic to allopurinol or febuxostat.

Before you start, consult your doctor if:
- You have liver or kidney problems.
- You have history of heart disease or stroke.
- You have diabetes.
- You have hypertension (high blood pressure).
- You are having an acute gout attack.

Over age 60:
No problems expected.

Pregnancy:
Decide with your doctor whether drug benefits justify risk to unborn child. Risk category C (see page xviii).

Breast-feeding:
Allopurinol passes into milk. It is unknown if febuxostat passes into milk. Avoid drug or discontinue nursing. Consult doctor for advice on maintaining milk supply.

Infants & children:
Usually not recommended for ages under 18. Allopurinol may be used to treat certain rare conditions in children.

Prolonged use:
Talk to your doctor about the need for follow-up medical examinations or laboratory studies to check liver function, kidney function and serum uric-acid levels.

Skin & sunlight:
No problems expected.

Driving, piloting or hazardous work:
Avoid if you feel drowsy. Use of this drug may disqualify you for piloting aircraft.

Discontinuing:
Don't discontinue without doctor's advice, even though symptoms diminish or disappear. These drugs are usually prescribed for long-term use to prevent gout attacks.

Others:
- Acute gout attacks may increase during first weeks of use. If so, consult doctor about your symptoms.
- Consult your doctor before taking vitamin C supplement as it can increase the risk for kidney stones.
- Febuxostat may rarely increase the risk for heart attack or stroke.
- Advise any doctor or dentist whom you consult that you use this medicine.

POSSIBLE INTERACTION WITH OTHER DRUGS

GENERIC NAME OR DRUG CLASS	COMBINED EFFECT
Amoxicillin	Risk of skin rash (with allopurinol).
Ampicillin	Risk of skin rash (with allopurinol).
Anticoagulants, oral*	May increase anticoagulant effect (with allopurinol).
Antineoplastics*	Usage needs to be carefully monitored (with allopurinol).
Azathioprine	Increased effect of azathioprine. Don't use with febuxostat.
Chlorpropamide	Increased effect of chlorpropamide (with allopurinol).
Chlorthalidone	Decreased allopurinol effect.
Cyclosporine	Increased cyclosporine effect (with allopurinol).
Diuretics, thiazide*	Risk of adverse effects (with allopurinol).
Mercaptopurine	Increased mercaptopurine effect. Don't use with febuxostat.
Probenecid	Increased allopurinol effect.
Theophylline	Increased effect of theophylline. Don't use with febuxostat.

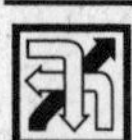

POSSIBLE INTERACTION WITH OTHER SUBSTANCES

INTERACTS WITH	COMBINED EFFECT
Alcohol:	May increase uric acid. Avoid.
Beverages:	None expected.
Cocaine:	Unknown. Avoid.
Foods:	None expected.
Marijuana:	Unknown. Avoid.
Tobacco:	None expected.

***See Glossary**

ANTIHISTAMINES

GENERIC AND BRAND NAMES

See full list of generic and brand names in the *Generic and Brand Name Directory*, page 870.

BASIC INFORMATION

Habit forming? No
Prescription needed?
High strength: Yes
Low strength: No
Available as generic? Yes
Drug class: Antihistamine

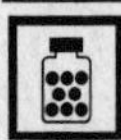

USES

- Reduces allergic symptoms such as hay fever, hives, rash or itching.
- Prevents motion sickness, nausea, vomiting.
- Relieves symptoms associated with the common cold.
- Induces sleep.
- Reduces stiffness and tremors of Parkinson's disease.

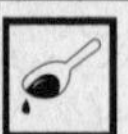

DOSAGE & USAGE INFORMATION

How to take:
Follow label directions.

When to take:
Varies with form. Follow label directions.

If you forget a dose:
Take as soon as you remember. If it is almost time for the next dose, wait for the next scheduled dose (don't double this dose).

What drug does:
- Blocks action of histamine after an allergic response triggers histamine release in sensitive cells. Histamines cause itching, sneezing, runny nose and eyes and other symptoms.
- Appears to work in the vomiting center of the brain to control nausea and vomiting and help prevent motion sickness.

Continued next column

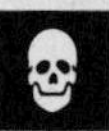

OVERDOSE

SYMPTOMS:
Convulsions, red face, hallucinations, coma.
WHAT TO DO:
- **Dial 911 (emergency) for medical help or call poison control center 1-800-222-1222 for instructions.**
- **See emergency information on last 3 pages of this book.**

Time lapse before drug works:
15 minutes to 1 hour.

Don't take with:
Any other medicine or any dietary supplement without consulting your doctor or pharmacist.

POSSIBLE ADVERSE REACTIONS OR SIDE EFFECTS

SYMPTOMS	WHAT TO DO
Life-threatening: In case of overdose, see previous column.	
Common: Drowsiness; dizziness; dryness of mouth, nose or throat.	Continue. Tell doctor at next visit.
Infrequent:	
• Change in vision, clumsiness, rash.	Discontinue. Call doctor right away.
• Less tolerance for contact lenses, painful or difficult urination.	Continue. Call doctor when convenient.
• Appetite loss.	Continue. Tell doctor at next visit.
Rare: Nightmares, agitation, irritability, sore throat, fever, rapid heartbeat, unusual bleeding or bruising, fatigue, weakness, confusion, fainting, seizures.	Discontinue. Call doctor right away.

WARNINGS & PRECAUTIONS

Don't take if:
You are allergic to any antihistamine.

Before you start, consult your doctor if:
- You have glaucoma.
- You have enlarged prostate.
- You have asthma.
- You have kidney disease.
- You have peptic ulcer.
- You will have surgery within 2 months, including dental surgery, requiring general or spinal anesthesia.

Over age 60:
Don't exceed recommended dose. Adverse reactions and side effects may be more frequent and severe than in younger persons, especially urination difficulty, diminished alertness and other brain and nervous-system symptoms.

Pregnancy:
Risk factors vary for drugs in this group. See category list on page xviii and consult doctor.

Breast-feeding:
Drug passes into milk. Avoid drug or discontinue nursing until you finish medicine. Consult doctor for advice on maintaining milk supply.

Infants & children:
- Read the label on the product to see if it is approved for your child's age. Always follow the directions on product's label about how to use. If unsure, ask your doctor or pharmacist.
- Do not use antihistamines for the purpose of making a child sleepy.

Prolonged use:
Consult your doctor.

Skin & sunlight:
May cause rash or intensify sunburn in areas exposed to sun or sunlamp.

Driving, piloting or hazardous work:
Don't drive or pilot aircraft until you learn how medicine affects you. Don't work around dangerous machinery. Don't climb ladders or work in high places. Danger increases if you drink alcohol or take medicine affecting alertness and reflexes, such as other antihistamines, tranquilizers, sedatives, pain medicine, narcotics and mind-altering drugs.

Discontinuing:
No problems expected.

Others:
- May mask symptoms of hearing damage from aspirin, other salicylates, cisplatin, paromomycin, vancomycin or anticonvulsants. Consult doctor if you use these.
- Advise any doctor or dentist whom you consult that you take this medicine.

POSSIBLE INTERACTION WITH OTHER DRUGS

GENERIC NAME OR DRUG CLASS	COMBINED EFFECT
Anticholinergics*	Increased anti-cholinergic effect.
Anticoagulants, oral*	Decreased anti-histamine effect.
Antidepressants*	Excess sedation. Avoid.
Antihistamines, other*	Excess sedation. Avoid.
Carteolol	Decreased anti-histamine effect.
Central nervous system (CNS) depressants*	May increase sedation.
Clozapine	Toxic effect on the central nervous system.
Dronabinol	Increased effects of both drugs. Avoid.
Hypnotics*	Excess sedation. Avoid.
Mind-altering drugs*	Excess sedation. Avoid.
Molindone	Increased sedative and antihistamine effect.
Monoamine oxidase (MAO) inhibitors*	Increased antihistamine effect.
Nabilone	Greater depression of central nervous system.
Narcotics*	Excess sedation. Avoid.
Procarbazine	May increase sedation.
Sedatives*	Excess sedation. Avoid.
Sertraline	Increased depressive effects of both drugs.
Sleep inducers*	Excess sedation. Avoid.
Sotalol	Increased antihistamine effect.
Tranquilizers*	Excess sedation. Avoid.

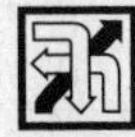

POSSIBLE INTERACTION WITH OTHER SUBSTANCES

INTERACTS WITH	COMBINED EFFECT
Alcohol:	Excess sedation. Avoid.
Beverages: Caffeine drinks.	Less antihistamine sedation.
Cocaine:	Decreased antihistamine effect. Avoid.
Foods:	None expected.
Marijuana:	Excess sedation. Avoid.
Tobacco:	None expected.

***See Glossary**

ANTIHISTAMINES (Nasal)

GENERIC AND BRAND NAMES

AZELASTINE
- Astelin
- Astepro
- Dymista

OLOPATADINE
- Patanase

BASIC INFORMATION

Habit forming? No
Prescription needed? Yes
Available as generic? No
Drug class: Antihistamine

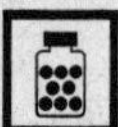

USES

- Reduces allergic symptoms caused by hay fever (seasonal allergic rhinitis), such as sneezing, itching, runny nose and other nasal symptoms of allergies.
- Azelastine is used to treat vasomotor rhinitis (also called nonallergic rhinitis) which is not caused by allergic reactions, but has similar symptoms.

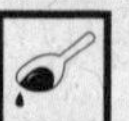

DOSAGE & USAGE INFORMATION

How to use:
Nasal spray—Gently blow nose before using. Prime the pump per package instructions. Use 2 sprays per nostril. Use 1 spray of azelastine in children ages 5 through 11. Avoid eyes.

When to take:
Usually twice a day or according to doctor's instructions. Effects of spray last for 12 hours.

If you forget a dose:
Use as soon as you remember. If it is almost time for next dose, wait for next scheduled dose (don't double this dose).

Continued next column

What drug does:
- Blocks action of histamines which are released in the body during an allergic reaction (such as to seasonal pollens). Histamines cause itching, swollen tissues, sneezing, runny nose and eyes and other symptoms.
- Azelastine also blocks the action of other inflammatory chemicals that cause stuffy and runny nose.

Time lapse before drug works:
Thirty minutes to 1 to 3 hours.

Don't take with:
Any other medicine or any dietary supplement without consulting your doctor or pharmacist.

OVERDOSE

SYMPTOMS:
May include extreme drowsiness, and feeling restless or agitated, but an overdose with this dosage form is unlikely to occur.
WHAT TO DO:
If person uses much larger amount than prescribed, call doctor or poison control center 1-800-222-1222 for help.

POSSIBLE ADVERSE REACTIONS OR SIDE EFFECTS

SYMPTOMS	WHAT TO DO
Life-threatening:	
Rare allergic reaction (hives, itching, rash, trouble breathing, tightness in chest, swelling of lips or tongue or face).	Seek emergency treatment immediately.
Common:	
• Mild drowsiness, bitter taste.	Usually no action needed. If symptoms continue, call doctor.
• Mild nosebleeds, irritation/soreness in the nose, runny nose, headache.	Discontinue. Call doctor when convenient.
Infrequent:	
Dry mouth, sore or painful throat, cough, nausea.	Discontinue. Call doctor when convenient.
Rare:	
• Extreme drowsiness, severe or frequent nosebleeds, rapid or forceful heartbeat, nasal perforation (pain and swelling).	Discontinue. Call doctor right away.
• Fatigue, flu or cold-like symptoms, post nasal drip, sinus infection, dizziness, weight gain, burning or pain when urinating, changes in urination, other unexplained symptoms.	Discontinue. Call doctor when convenient.

ANTIHISTAMINES (Nasal)

WARNINGS & PRECAUTIONS

Don't take if:
You are allergic to azelastine or olopatadine.

Before you start, consult your doctor if:
- You have kidney problems.
- You have any disorder or injury involving the nose (such as a deviated septum).
- You are allergic to any medication, food or other substance.

Over age 60:
No problems expected.

Pregnancy:
Decide with your doctor if drug benefits justify risks to unborn child. Risk category C (see page xviii).

Breast-feeding:
It is not known if drugs pass into milk. Avoid drug or discontinue nursing until you finish medicine. Consult doctor for advice on maintaining milk supply.

Infants & children:
- Azelastine is approved in children 12 years and older for vasomotor rhinitis and in children 5 years and older for allergic rhinitis.
- Olopatadine is approved in children 12 years and older for allergic rhinitis.

Prolonged use:
- Antihistamines are normally used during the hay fever season. They are not intended for long-term uninterrupted use.
- Consult your doctor about long-term use of azelastine for vasomotor rhinitis symptoms.

Skin & sunlight:
No problems expected.

Driving, piloting or hazardous work:
Don't drive or pilot aircraft until you learn how medicine affects you. Don't work around dangerous machinery. Don't climb ladders or work in high places. Danger increases if you drink alcohol or take other medicines affecting alertness and reflexes such as antihistamines, tranquilizers, sedatives, pain medicine, narcotics and mind-altering drugs.

Discontinuing:
No problems expected. Consult your doctor if you have been using the spray for a long time.

Others:
- Don't exceed recommended dose. It could increase the risk of adverse reactions.
- Advise any doctor or dentist whom you consult that you take this medicine.
- Consult doctor if new nasal problems occur.
- Avoid getting the spray in your eyes. Rinse eyes with water if this occurs.

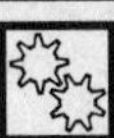

POSSIBLE INTERACTION WITH OTHER DRUGS

GENERIC NAME OR DRUG CLASS	COMBINED EFFECT
Central nervous system (CNS) depressants*	May add to any sedative effect.
Cimetidine	Increased azelastine effect. May result in increased sedation.

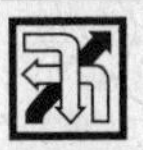

POSSIBLE INTERACTION WITH OTHER SUBSTANCES

INTERACTS WITH	COMBINED EFFECT
Alcohol:	May cause excessive sedation. Avoid.
Beverages:	None expected.
Cocaine:	Decreased antihistamine effect. Avoid.
Foods:	None expected.
Marijuana:	May cause sedation. Avoid.
Tobacco:	None expected.

***See Glossary**

ANTIHISTAMINES, NONSEDATING

GENERIC AND BRAND NAMES

See full list of generic and brand names in the *Generic and Brand Name Directory*, page 872.

BASIC INFORMATION

Habit forming? No
Prescription needed? Yes, for some
Available as generic? Yes, for some
Drug class: Antihistamine

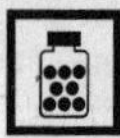

USES

- Reduces allergic symptoms caused by hay fever (seasonal allergic rhinitis) and perennial rhinitis, such as sneezing, runny nose, itchy nose or throat, itchy and watery eyes.
- Treatment for urticaria (hives).
- Used to help relieve some asthma symptoms.
- Other uses as recommended by your doctor.

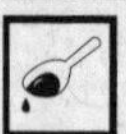

DOSAGE & USAGE INFORMATION

How to take:
- Capsule, tablet, suspension, syrup—Swallow with liquid. Most may be taken with food or milk to lessen stomach irritation.
- Chewable tablet—Chew the tablets well before swallowing.
- Oral disintegrating tablet—Let tablet dissolve in mouth. Don't chew. No need to drink fluid.

When to take:
Varies with form and brand. Follow label directions.

If you forget a dose:
Take as soon as you remember. If it is almost time for the next dose, wait for the next scheduled dose (don't double this dose).

Continued next column

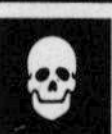

OVERDOSE

SYMPTOMS:
Serious irregular heartbeat, convulsions, being clumsy or unsteady, drowsiness, nausea, severe headache, hallucinations.
WHAT TO DO:
- **Dial 911 (emergency) for medical help or call poison control center 1-800-222-1222 for instructions.**
- **See emergency information on last 3 pages of this book.**

What drug does:
Blocks action of histamine after an allergic response triggers histamine release in sensitive cells. Histamines cause itching, sneezing, runny nose and eyes and other symptoms.

Time lapse before drug works:
1 to 2 hours.

Don't take with:
Any other medicine or any dietary supplement without consulting your doctor or pharmacist.

POSSIBLE ADVERSE REACTIONS OR SIDE EFFECTS

SYMPTOMS	WHAT TO DO
Life-threatening:	
Rare allergic reaction (hives, itching, rash, wheezing, tightness in chest, swelling of lips or tongue or throat).	Seek emergency treatment immediately.
Common:	
Dryness of mouth, nose or throat.	Continue. Tell doctor at next visit.
Infrequent:	
Increased appetite, weight gain, mild stomach or intestinal problems, cold or flu-like symptoms.	Continue. Call doctor when convenient.
Rare:	
• Heart rhythm disturbances, fainting.	Discontinue. Call doctor right away or get emergency care.
• Allergic reaction such as mild skin rash, headache, nausea, dizziness, nervousness, fatigue, muscle aches. Drowsiness may occur even though these drugs are nonsedating.	Discontinue. Call doctor when convenient.

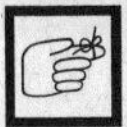

WARNINGS & PRECAUTIONS

Don't take if:
You are allergic to any antihistamine.

Before you start, consult your doctor if:
- You have any type of heart disorder.
- You have glaucoma.
- You have enlarged prostate or urinary retention problems.
- You have asthma or a respiratory disease.
- You have liver or kidney disease.
- You have peptic ulcer.
- You have electrolyte abnormality, such as low potassium (hypokalemia).

Over age 60:
Adverse reactions and side effects may be more frequent and severe than in younger persons.

Pregnancy:
Risk factors vary for drugs in this group. See category list on page xviii and consult doctor.

Breast-feeding:
Drug may pass into milk. Avoid drug or discontinue nursing until you finish medicine. Consult doctor for advice on maintaining milk supply.

Infants & children:
Read the label on the product to see if it is approved for your child's age. Always follow the directions on product's label about how to use. If unsure, ask your doctor or pharmacist.

Prolonged use:
Antihistamines are normally taken during the hay fever season. Longer use may be recommended by your doctor depending on the disorder being treated.

Skin & sunlight:
Rarely, may cause rash or intensify sunburn in areas exposed to sun or ultraviolet light (photosensitivity reaction). Avoid overexposure. Notify doctor if reaction occurs.

Driving, piloting or hazardous work:
No problems expected.

Discontinuing:
No problems expected.

Others:
- Don't exceed recommended dose. This can increase the risk of adverse reactions.
- Advise any doctor or dentist whom you consult that you take this medicine.

POSSIBLE INTERACTION WITH OTHER DRUGS

GENERIC NAME OR DRUG CLASS	COMBINED EFFECT
Anticholinergics	Increased anti-cholinergic effect.
Central nervous system (CNS) depressants*	May add to any sedative effect.
Erythromycins*	Heart rhythm problems. Avoid.
Fluvoxamine	Increased antihistamine effect.
Leukotriene modifiers	Effects unknown. Consult doctor.
Macrolide antibiotics	Increased risk of adverse reactions.
Monoamine oxidase (MAO) inhibitors	Increased sedation. Avoid.

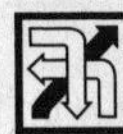

POSSIBLE INTERACTION WITH OTHER SUBSTANCES

INTERACTS WITH	COMBINED EFFECT
Alcohol:	May cause sedation. Avoid.
Beverages:	Grapefruit juice may increase the effect of fexofenadine.
Cocaine:	Decreased antihistamine effect. Avoid.
Foods:	None expected.
Marijuana:	May cause sedation. Avoid.
Tobacco:	None expected.

***See Glossary**

ANTIHISTAMINES, PHENOTHIAZINE-DERIVATIVE

GENERIC AND BRAND NAMES

See full list of generic and brand names in the *Generic and Brand Name Directory*, page 872.

BASIC INFORMATION

Habit forming? No
Prescription needed? Yes
Available as generic? Yes, for most
Drug class: Tranquilizer (phenothiazine), antihistamine

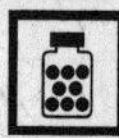

USES

- Relieves itching of hives, skin allergies, chickenpox.
- Treatment for hay fever, motion sickness, vertigo.
- Treatment for nausea and vomiting.

DOSAGE & USAGE INFORMATION

How to take:
- Tablet or syrup—Swallow with liquid or food to lessen stomach irritation.
- Extended-release capsule—Swallow each dose whole. If you take regular tablets, you may chew or crush them.

When to take:
At the same times each day.

If you forget a dose:
Take as soon as you remember. If it is almost time for the next dose, wait for the next scheduled dose (don't double this dose).

Continued next column

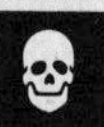

OVERDOSE

SYMPTOMS:
Fast heartbeat, flushed face, shortness of breath, clumsiness, drowsiness, muscle spasms, jerking movements of head and face.
WHAT TO DO:
- **Dial 911 (emergency) for medical help or call poison control center 1-800-222-1222 for instructions.**
- **See emergency information on last 3 pages of this book.**

What drug does:
- Blocks action of histamine after an allergic response triggers histamine release in sensitive cells. Histamines cause itching, sneezing, runny nose and eyes and other symptoms.
- Appears to work in the vomiting center of the brain to control nausea and vomiting and help prevent motion sickness.

Time lapse before drug works:
15 minutes to 1 hour.

Don't take with:
- Antacid or medicine for diarrhea.
- Nonprescription drug for cough, cold or allergy.
- Any other medicine or any dietary supplement without consulting your doctor or pharmacist.

POSSIBLE ADVERSE REACTIONS OR SIDE EFFECTS

SYMPTOMS	WHAT TO DO
Life-threatening:	
In case of overdose, see previous column.	
Common:	
Drowsiness; dryness of mouth, nose or throat; nasal congestion.	Continue. Call doctor when convenient.
Infrequent:	
• Difficult urination; blurred or changed vision; dizziness; ringing in ears; skin rash; uncontrolled, jerky movements (with high doses); slow, snakelike movement of arms; spasm of neck muscles; stiffening of tongue; eyes rolling upward.	Discontinue. Call doctor right away.
• Nightmares, unusual excitement, nervousness, irritability, loss of appetite, sweating.	Continue. Call doctor when convenient.
Rare:	
Sore throat, fever, confusion, yellow skin or eyes, fast heartbeat, feeling faint, unusual tiredness or weakness, unusual bleeding or bruising.	Discontinue. Call doctor right away.

ANTIHISTAMINES, PHENOTHIAZINE-DERIVATIVE

WARNINGS & PRECAUTIONS

Don't take if:
- You are allergic to any phenothiazine.
- You have a blood or bone marrow disease.

Before you start, consult your doctor if:
- You will have surgery within 2 months, including dental surgery, requiring anesthesia.
- You have asthma, emphysema or other lung disorder.
- You take nonprescription ulcer medicine, asthma medicine or amphetamines.

Over age 60:
Adverse reactions and side effects may be more frequent and severe than in younger persons. More likely to develop tardive dyskinesia (involuntary movement of jaws, lips, tongue, chewing). Call doctor right away. Early treatment can help.

Pregnancy:
Decide with your doctor if drug benefits justify risk to unborn child. Risk category C (see page xviii).

Breast-feeding:
Drug passes into milk. Avoid drug or discontinue nursing until you finish medicine. Consult doctor for advice on maintaining milk supply.

Infants & children:
Read the label on the product to see if it is approved for your child's age. Always follow the directions on product's label about how to use. If unsure, ask your doctor or pharmacist.

Prolonged use:
- May lead to tardive dyskinesia (involuntary movement of jaws, lips, tongue, chewing).
- Talk to your doctor about the need for follow-up medical examinations or laboratory studies to check complete blood counts, liver function, and eyes.

Skin & sunlight:
One or more drugs in this group may cause rash or intensify sunburn in areas exposed to sun or ultraviolet light (photosensitivity reaction). Avoid overexposure. Notify doctor if reaction occurs.

Driving, piloting or hazardous work:
Don't drive or pilot aircraft until you learn how medicine affects you. Don't work around dangerous machinery. Don't climb ladders or work in high places. Danger increases if you drink alcohol or take medicine affecting alertness and reflexes.

Discontinuing:
May be unnecessary to finish medicine. Follow doctor's instructions.

Others:
- Advise any doctor or dentist whom you consult that you take this medicine.
- May affect results in some medical tests.

POSSIBLE INTERACTION WITH OTHER DRUGS

GENERIC NAME OR DRUG CLASS	COMBINED EFFECT
Antacids*	Decreased antihistamine effect.
Anticholinergics*	Increased anticholinergic effect.
Anticonvulsants, hydantoin*	Increased anticonvulsant effect.
Antidepressants, tricyclic*	Increased antihistamine effect.
Antihistamines,* other	Increased antihistamine effect.
Antithyroid drugs*	Increased risk of bone marrow depression.
Appetite suppressants*	Decreased appetite suppressant effect.
Barbiturates*	Oversedation.
Carteolol	Decreased antihistamine effect.
Central nervous system (CNS) depressants*	Dangerous degree of sedation.
Cisapride	Decreased antihistamine effect.

Continued on page 903

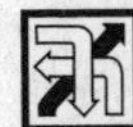

POSSIBLE INTERACTION WITH OTHER SUBSTANCES

INTERACTS WITH	COMBINED EFFECT
Alcohol:	Dangerous oversedation.
Beverages:	None expected.
Cocaine:	Decreased trimeprazine effect. Avoid.
Foods:	None expected.
Marijuana:	Drowsiness.
Tobacco:	None expected.

ANTIHISTAMINES, PIPERAZINE (Antinausea)

GENERIC AND BRAND NAMES

CYCLIZINE	MECLIZINE
Marezine	Antivert
	Antivert/25
	Antivert/50
	Bonamine
	Bonine
	Dramamine II
	D-Vert 15
	D-Vert 30
	Meclicot
	Medivert
	Zentrip

BASIC INFORMATION

Habit forming? No
Prescription needed? Yes, for some
Available as generic? Yes
Drug class: Antihistamine, antiemetic, anti-motion sickness

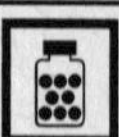

USES

- Prevention and treatment of motion sickness.
- Treats nausea and vomiting after operations or radiation treatment.
- Treatment for vertigo.

DOSAGE & USAGE INFORMATION

How to take:

- Tablet or capsule—Swallow with liquid or food to lessen stomach irritation. If you can't swallow whole, crumble tablet or open capsule and take with liquid or food.
- Chewable tablet—May be chewed, swallowed whole or mixed with food.
- Quick-dissolving strips—Let strip dissolve on the tongue. Water or fluid is not needed.

Continued next column

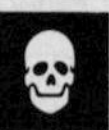

OVERDOSE

SYMPTOMS:
Drowsiness, confusion, incoordination, stupor, coma, weak pulse, blurred vision, shallow breathing, hallucinations, seizures.
WHAT TO DO:

- **Dial 911 (emergency) for medical help or call poison control center 1-800-222-1222 for instructions.**
- **See emergency information on last 3 pages of this book.**

When to take:
30 minutes to 1 hour before traveling, or as directed by doctor, or follow label instructions.

If you forget a dose:
Take as soon as you remember. If it is almost time for the next dose, wait for the next scheduled dose (don't double this dose).

What drug does:
It is not known just how drug works. Appears to reduce sensitivity of nerve endings in inner ear, blocking messages to brain's vomiting center.

Time lapse before drug works:
30 to 60 minutes.

Don't take with:
Any other medicine or any dietary supplement without consulting your doctor or pharmacist.

POSSIBLE ADVERSE REACTIONS OR SIDE EFFECTS

SYMPTOMS	WHAT TO DO
Life-threatening:	
In case of overdose, see previous column.	
Common:	
Drowsiness.	Continue. Tell doctor at next visit.
Infrequent:	
• Headache, diarrhea or constipation, upset stomach.	Continue. Call doctor when convenient.
• Dry mouth, nose, throat.	Continue. Tell doctor at next visit.
Rare:	
Restlessness, insomnia, blurred vision, frequent or difficult urination, hallucinations, dizziness, increased heartbeat, loss of appetite.	Discontinue. Call doctor if symptoms continue or are severe.

WARNINGS & PRECAUTIONS

Don't take if:
You are allergic to meclizine or cyclizine.

Before you start, consult your doctor if:
- You have glaucoma.
- You have an intestinal or bladder blockage.
- You have heart problems.
- You have chronic obstructive pulmonary disease (COPD).
- You have prostate enlargement.

Over age 60:
Adverse reactions and side effects may be more frequent and severe than in younger persons, especially impaired urination from enlarged prostate gland.

Pregnancy:
Usually safe, but decide with your doctor if drug benefits justify any possible risk to unborn child. Risk category B (see page xviii).

Breast-feeding:
Meclizine passes into milk; it is unknown if cyclizine does. Consult doctor.

Infants & children:
Follow doctor's instructions or those on the label if used in children. Children may be more sensitive to side effects. Not recommended for children under age 6.

Prolonged use:
No problems expected.

Skin & sunlight:
No problems expected.

Driving, piloting or hazardous work:
Don't drive or pilot aircraft until you learn how medicine affects you. Don't work around dangerous machinery. Don't climb ladders or work in high places. Danger increases if you drink alcohol or take medicine affecting alertness and reflexes.

Discontinuing:
No problems expected.

Others:
- Advise any doctor or dentist whom you consult that you take this medicine (if using on a regular basis).
- May interfere with some skin allergy tests.
- If you have dry mouth from using this drug, try sugarless candy or gum or small pieces of ice. If dry mouth continues longer than 2 weeks, consult doctor.

POSSIBLE INTERACTION WITH OTHER DRUGS

GENERIC NAME OR DRUG CLASS	COMBINED EFFECT
Anticholinergics*	Increased effect of both drugs.
Central nervous system (CNS) depressants*	Increased depressive effects of both drugs.

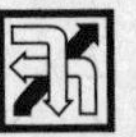

POSSIBLE INTERACTION WITH OTHER SUBSTANCES

INTERACTS WITH	COMBINED EFFECT
Alcohol:	Increased sedation. Avoid.
Beverages:	None expected.
Cocaine:	None expected. Best to avoid.
Foods:	None expected.
Marijuana:	Increased drowsiness, dry mouth.
Tobacco:	None expected.

*See Glossary

ANTI-INFLAMMATORY DRUGS, NONSTEROIDAL (NSAIDs)

GENERIC AND BRAND NAMES

See full list of generic and brand names in the *Generic and Brand Name Directory*, page 873.

BASIC INFORMATION

Habit forming? No
Prescription needed? Yes, for some.
Available as generic? Yes, for some.
Drug class: Anti-inflammatory (nonsteroidal), analgesic, antigout agent, fever-reducer

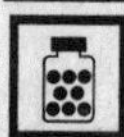

USES

- Treatment for joint pain, stiffness, inflammation and swelling of arthritis, gout, osteoarthritis, juvenile idiopathic arthritis, and others.
- Treatment for pain, fever and inflammation of a variety of disorders, illnesses and injuries.

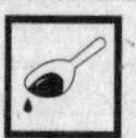

DOSAGE & USAGE INFORMATION

How to take:
- Tablet, capsule, extended-release tablet, delayed-release tablet or extended-release capsule—Swallow with liquid or food to lessen stomach irritation. If you can't swallow whole, crumble tablet and take with liquid or food. Don't crumble delayed- or extended-release tablets.
- Suspension, rectal, oral soluble film, chewable tablet—Take as directed on label.
- Nasal spray—Use one spray into each nostril every 4 to 6 hours.

When to take:
At the same times each day.

If you forget a dose:
Take or use as soon as you remember. If it is almost time for the next dose, wait for next scheduled dose (don't double this dose).

Continued next column

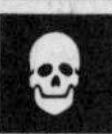

OVERDOSE

SYMPTOMS:
Confusion, agitation, severe headache, incoherence, convulsions, possible hemorrhage from stomach or intestine, coma.
WHAT TO DO:
- **Dial 911 (emergency) for medical help or call poison control center 1-800-222-1222 for instructions.**
- **See emergency information on last 3 pages of this book.**

What drug does:
Reduces tissue concentration of prostaglandins (hormones which produce inflammation and pain).

Time lapse before drug works:
Begins in 4 to 24 hours. May require 3 weeks regular use for maximum benefit.

Don't take with:
Any other medicine or any dietary supplement without consulting your doctor or pharmacist.

POSSIBLE ADVERSE REACTIONS OR SIDE EFFECTS

SYMPTOMS	WHAT TO DO
Life-threatening:	
Hives, rash, intense itching, faintness soon after a dose (anaphylaxis in aspirin-sensitive persons).	Seek emergency treatment immediately.
Common:	
• Diarrhea, skin rash, bleeding from rectum (with suppositories).	Discontinue. Call doctor right away.
• Dizziness, nausea, stomach cramps, headache.	Continue. Call doctor when convenient.
Infrequent:	
• Muscle cramps, numbness or tingling in hands or feet, mouth ulcers, rapid weight gain.	Discontinue. Call doctor right away.
• Depression; drowsiness; ringing in ears; swollen feet, face or legs; constipation; vomiting; gas; dry mouth; tremors; nose pain (spray); insomnia.	Continue. Call doctor when convenient.
Rare:	
• Convulsions; confusion; hives or itching; blurred vision; black, bloody, tarry stool; difficult breathing; tightness in chest; rapid heartbeat; unusual bleeding or bruising; vomiting blood; blood in urine; jaundice; psychosis; frequent, painful urination; fainting; sore throat; fever; chills; diminished hearing; eye pain; nose bleeds; severe or ongoing stomach pain.	Discontinue. Call doctor right away.
• Fatigue, weakness, menstrual irregularities, skin irritation with patch.	Continue. Call doctor if symptoms persist.

ANTI-INFLAMMATORY DRUGS, NONSTEROIDAL (NSAIDs)

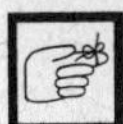

WARNINGS & PRECAUTIONS

Don't take if:
You are allergic to or intolerant of any nonsteroidal, anti-inflammatory drug or aspirin.

Before you start, consult your doctor if:
You have epilepsy, Parkinson's disease, ulcers, gastritis, enteritis, ileitis, ulcerative colitis, heart disease, asthma, high blood pressure, bleeding problems, impaired kidney or liver function, fluid retention, lupus erythematosus, alcohol abuse, hemorrhoids, anemia, mental illness, recent tobacco use, porphyria, temporal arteritis, polymyalgia rheumatica or mouth sores.

Over age 60:
Adverse reactions and side effects may be more frequent and severe than in younger persons.

Pregnancy:
Risk factors vary for drugs in this group. See category list on page xviii and consult doctor.

Breast-feeding:
One or more of these drugs may pass into breast milk. Consult your doctor for advice.

Infants & children:
- Use only as directed by your child's doctor.
- For nonprescription drugs, read labels and use only those approved for your child's age.

Prolonged use:
- Stomach (gastrointestinal) bleeding, ulcers, and may raise risk of heart attack or stroke.
- Talk to your doctor about the need for follow-up medical exams or lab studies.

Skin & sunlight:
One or more drugs in this group may cause rash or intensify sunburn in areas exposed to sun or ultraviolet light (photosensitivity reaction). Avoid overexposure. Notify doctor if reaction occurs.

Driving, piloting or hazardous work:
Don't drive or pilot aircraft until you learn how medicine affects you. Don't work around dangerous machinery. Don't climb ladders or work in high places. Danger increases if you drink alcohol or take medicine affecting alertness and reflexes.

Discontinuing:
No problems expected. If drug has been taken for a long time, consult doctor before stopping.

Others:
- Advise any doctor or dentist whom you consult that you take this medicine. May increase risk of bleeding if any surgery is required.
- May affect the results of some lab tests.
- Consult doctor if symptoms don't improve in 10 days or a fever lasts more than 3 days.

POSSIBLE INTERACTION WITH OTHER DRUGS

GENERIC NAME OR DRUG CLASS	COMBINED EFFECT
Acetaminophen	Risk of renal (kidney) problem (long term use).
Adrenocorticoids, systemic	Risk of stomach problems. Increased adrenocorticoid effect.
Antacids*	Decreased NSAID effect.
Anticoagulants, oral*	Increased risk of bleeding.
Anticonvulsants, hydantoin*	Increased anticonvulsant effect.
Antidiabetics*	Increased risk of low blood sugar.
Antihypertensives*	Decreased effect of antihypertensive.
Anti-inflammatory pain relievers (any combination of)	Increased risk of side effects.
Antiplatelet drugs*	Increased risk of bleeding.
Aspirin	Increased risk of side effects.
Cephalosporins*	Increased risk of bleeding.
Didanosine	Increased risk of pancreatitis (sulindac only).

Continued on page 903

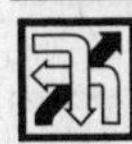

POSSIBLE INTERACTION WITH OTHER SUBSTANCES

INTERACTS WITH	COMBINED EFFECT
Alcohol:	Risk of stomach problems.
Beverages:	None expected.
Cocaine:	Unknown. Avoid.
Foods:	None expected.
Marijuana:	Unknown. Avoid.
Tobacco:	Risk of drug side effects.

*See Glossary

ANTI-INFLAMMATORY DRUGS, NONSTEROIDAL (NSAIDs) COX-2 INHIBITORS

GENERIC AND BRAND NAMES

CELECOXIB
Celebrex

ROFECOXIB

VALDECOXIB

BASIC INFORMATION

Habit forming? No
Prescription needed? Yes
Available as generic? No
Drug class: Anti-inflammatory (nonsteroidal), analgesic, antigout agent, fever-reducer

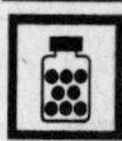

USES

- Treatment for joint pain, stiffness, inflammation and swelling of rheumatoid arthritis, osteoarthritis, ankylosing spondylitis and gout.
- Treatment for pain, fever and inflammation.
- Treatment for dysmenorrhea (painful or difficult menstruation).
- Treatment for colorectal polyps.

Special note: This class of drugs has been linked to an increased risk of heart attack and stroke. Consult doctor before using.

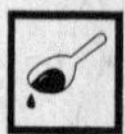

DOSAGE & USAGE INFORMATION

How to take:
- Tablet or capsule—Swallow with liquid. If you can't swallow whole, open capsule or crumble tablet and take with liquid or food.
- Suspension—Shake the bottle well before use. Carefully measure dose with measuring spoon or cup.

When to take:
At the same times each day.

If you forget a dose:
Take as soon as you remember. If it is almost time for the next dose, wait for the next scheduled dose (don't double this dose).

Continued next column

OVERDOSE

SYMPTOMS:
Breathing problems, tightness in chest, decreased urine amount, swelling, thirst, tiredness or weakness, stomach pain, bloody or black stools, dizziness, headache, nausea or vomiting.
WHAT TO DO:
If person takes much larger amount than prescribed, call doctor or poison control center 1-800-222-1222 for help.

What drug does:
Reduces tissue concentration of prostaglandins (hormones which produce inflammation and pain).

Time lapse before drug works:
Begins in 2 to 3 hours. May require 3 weeks of regular use for maximum benefit.

Don't take with:
Any other medicine or any dietary supplement without consulting your doctor or pharmacist.

POSSIBLE ADVERSE REACTIONS OR SIDE EFFECTS

SYMPTOMS	WHAT TO DO
Life-threatening:	
Hives, rash, intense itching, faintness soon after a dose (anaphylaxis in aspirin-sensitive persons).	Seek emergency treatment immediately.
Common:	
• Cough, fever, skin rash, swelling of face, fingers, feet and/or lower legs.	Discontinue. Call doctor right away.
• Back pain, dizziness, gas, headache, nausea, heartburn, burning in throat, sleeplessness, stuffy or runny nose.	Continue. Call doctor when convenient.
Infrequent:	
• Bloody or tarry stools, chills, congestion, diarrhea, fatigue, loss of appetite, muscle pains, blood in urine, pale skin, shortness of breath, severe stomach pain, weight gain, vomiting.	Discontinue. Call doctor right away.
• Anxiety, vision changes, noises in ears, changes in sense of taste, difficulty swallowing, dry mouth, constipation, depression, rapid heartbeat, increased sweating, numbness in fingers or toes, sleepiness.	Continue. Call doctor when convenient.
Rare:	
None expected.	

ANTI-INFLAMMATORY DRUGS, NONSTEROIDAL (NSAIDs) COX-2 INHIBITORS

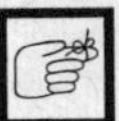

WARNINGS & PRECAUTIONS

Don't take if:
- You are allergic to aspirin or any nonsteroidal, anti-inflammatory drug.
- You are in the third trimester of your pregnancy.
- You have had recent heart surgery.
- You have not read special note under Uses.

Before you start, consult your doctor if:
- You have a history of alcohol abuse.
- You have bleeding problems or ulcers.
- You have used tobacco recently.
- You have impaired kidney or liver function.
- You have anemia, asthma, dehydration or fluid retention.
- You have high blood pressure or heart disease.

Over age 60:
Adverse reactions and side effects may be more frequent and severe than in younger persons.

Pregnancy:
Decide with your doctor whether drug benefits justify risk to unborn child. Risk category C (see page xviii).

Breast-feeding:
Avoid drug or discontinue nursing until you finish medicine. Consult doctor for advice on maintaining milk supply.

Infants & children:
Celecoxib is used to treat juvenile idiopathic arthritis (JIA) in patients age 2 years and older.

Prolonged use:
- Eye damage; reduced hearing.
- Sore throat, fever.
- Weight gain.
- Talk to your doctor about the need for follow-up medical exams or laboratory studies to check complete blood counts, liver function, stools for blood, eyes.

Skin & sunlight:
No problems expected.

Driving, piloting or hazardous work:
Don't drive or pilot aircraft until you learn how medicine affects you. Don't work around dangerous machinery. Don't climb ladders or work in high places. Danger increases if you drink alcohol or take medicine affecting alertness and reflexes, such as antihistamines, tranquilizers, sedatives, pain medicine, narcotics and mind-altering drugs.

Discontinuing:
No problems expected. If drug has been taken for a long time, consult doctor before discontinuing.

Others:
- May affect results in some medical tests.
- Advise any doctor or dentist whom you consult that you take this medicine.

POSSIBLE INTERACTION WITH OTHER DRUGS

GENERIC NAME OR DRUG CLASS	COMBINED EFFECT
Angiotensin-converting enzyme (ACE) inhibitors*	May decrease ACE inhibitor effect.
Antacids*	Decreased pain relief.
Antifungals, azole	Increased risk of side effects.
Anti-inflammatory drugs, nonsteroidal (NSAIDs)* other	Increased risk of side effects.
Aspirin	Increased risk of stomach ulcer.
Dextromethorphan	Increased effect of dextromethorphan.
Diuretics	Decreased diuretic effect.
Lithium	Increased lithium effect.
Methotrexate	Increased methotrexate effect.
Phenytoin	Decreased pain relief.
Rifampin	Decreased rifampin effect.
Warfarin	Increased risk of bleeding problems.

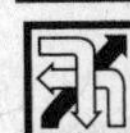

POSSIBLE INTERACTION WITH OTHER SUBSTANCES

INTERACTS WITH	COMBINED EFFECT
Alcohol:	Possible stomach ulcer or bleeding.
Beverages:	None expected.
Cocaine:	None expected.
Foods:	None expected.
Marijuana:	May increase pain relief.
Tobacco:	Possible stomach ulcer or bleeding.

*See Glossary

ANTI-INFLAMMATORY DRUGS, NONSTEROIDAL (NSAIDs) (Ophthalmic)

GENERIC AND BRAND NAMES

BROMFENAC
Xibrom
DICLOFENAC
Voltaren Ophtha
Voltaren Ophthalmic
FLURBIPROFEN
Ocufen
INDOMETHACIN
Indocid
KETOROLAC
Acular
Acular LS
NEPAFENAC
Ilevro
Nevanac
SUPROFEN
Profenal

BASIC INFORMATION

Habit forming? No
Prescription needed? Yes
Available as generic? Yes, for some
Drug class: Ophthalmic anti-inflammatory agents, nonsteroidal

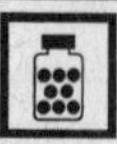

USES

- Used to prevent problems during and following eye surgery, such as cataract removal.
- Treatment for eye itching caused by seasonal allergic conjunctivitis.

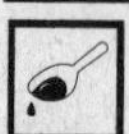

DOSAGE & USAGE INFORMATION

How to use:
Eye solution
- Wash hands.
- Apply pressure to inside corner of eye with middle finger.
- Continue pressure for 1 minute after placing medicine in eye.
- Tilt head backward. Pull lower lid away from eye with index finger of the same hand.
- Drop eye drops into pouch and close eye. Don't blink.
- Keep eyes closed for 1 to 2 minutes.

Continued next column

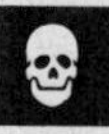

OVERDOSE

SYMPTOMS:
None expected.
WHAT TO DO:
Not intended for internal use. If child accidentally swallows, call doctor or poison control center 1-800-222-1222 for help.

When to use:
As directed by your doctor or on the label. Your doctor or nurse may instill the drug before an eye operation.

If you forget a dose:
Use as soon as you remember.

What drug does:
Blocks prostaglandin production. Prostaglandins cause inflammatory responses and constriction of the pupil.

Time lapse before drug works:
Immediately.

Don't use with:
Any other medicine or any dietary supplement without consulting your doctor or pharmacist.

POSSIBLE ADVERSE REACTIONS OR SIDE EFFECTS

SYMPTOMS	WHAT TO DO
Life-threatening: None expected.	
Common: Brief and mild burning or stinging when drops are administered.	No action necessary.
Infrequent: None expected.	
Rare: Allergic reaction (itching, tearing); redness, swelling or bleeding in eye not present before; eye pain; sensitivity to light.	Discontinue. Call doctor right away.

ANTI-INFLAMMATORY DRUGS, NONSTEROIDAL (NSAIDs) (Ophthalmic)

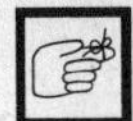

WARNINGS & PRECAUTIONS

Don't use if:
- You are allergic to any eye medication.
- You are allergic to any nonsteroidal anti-inflammatory drugs taken orally, e.g., aspirin.

Before you start, consult your doctor if:
- You have any bleeding disorder such as hemophilia.
- You have or have had herpes simplex keratitis (an inflammation of the cornea).
- You have allergies to any medications, foods or other substances.

Over age 60:
No special problems expected.

Pregnancy:
Risk category C (see page xviii). Decide with your doctor whether drug benefit justifies risk to unborn child.

Breast-feeding:
Unknown if drug passes into breast milk after administration into the eye. Consult doctor.

Infants & children:
No information available on safety or effectiveness. Consult doctor.

Prolonged use:
Not intended for long-term use.

Skin & sunlight:
No special problems expected.

Driving, piloting or hazardous work:
No special problems expected.

Discontinuing:
No special problems expected.

Others:
Don't use leftover medicine for other eye problems without your doctor's approval. Some eye infections could be made worse.

POSSIBLE INTERACTION WITH OTHER DRUGS

GENERIC NAME OR DRUG CLASS	COMBINED EFFECT
Anticoagulants,* oral	May increase bleeding tendency.
Antiglaucoma drugs*	May decrease antiglaucoma effect (with flurbiprofen).
Carbachol	Decreased carbachol effect.

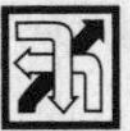

POSSIBLE INTERACTION WITH OTHER SUBSTANCES

INTERACTS WITH	COMBINED EFFECT
Alcohol:	None expected.
Beverages:	None expected.
Cocaine:	None expected.
Foods:	None expected.
Marijuana:	None expected.
Tobacco:	None expected.

*See Glossary

ANTI-INFLAMMATORY DRUGS, STEROIDAL (Ophthalmic)

GENERIC AND BRAND NAMES

See full list of generic and brand names in the *Generic and Brand Name Directory*, page 874.

BASIC INFORMATION

Habit forming? No
Prescription needed? Yes
Available as generic? Yes
Drug class: Adrenocorticoid (ophthalmic); anti-inflammatory, steroidal (ophthalmic)

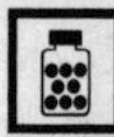

USES

- Relieves redness and irritation due to allergies or other irritants.
- Prevents damage to eye.
- Treatment for anterior uveitis (a type of eye infection).

DOSAGE & USAGE INFORMATION

How to use:
Eye drops
- Wash hands.
- Apply pressure to inside corner of eye with middle finger.
- Continue pressure for 1 minute after placing medicine in eye.
- Tilt head backward. Pull lower lid away from eye with index finger of the same hand.
- Drop eye drops into pouch and close eye. Don't blink.
- Keep eyes closed for 1 to 2 minutes.

Eye ointment
- Wash hands.
- Pull lower lid down from eye to form a pouch.
- Squeeze tube to apply thin strip of ointment into pouch.
- Close eye for 1 to 2 minutes.
- Don't touch applicator tip to any surface (including the eye). If you accidentally touch tip, clean with warm water and soap.
- Keep container tightly closed.

Continued next column

- Keep cool, but don't freeze.
- Wash hands immediately after using.

When to use:
As directed.

If you forget a dose:
Use as soon as you remember.

What drug does:
Affects cell membranes and decreases response to irritating substances.

Time lapse before drug works:
Immediately.

Don't use with:
Medicines for abdominal cramps or glaucoma without first consulting your doctor.

OVERDOSE

SYMPTOMS:
None expected.
WHAT TO DO:
Not intended for internal use. If child accidentally swallows, call doctor or poison control center 1-800-222-1222 for help.

POSSIBLE ADVERSE REACTIONS OR SIDE EFFECTS

SYMPTOMS	WHAT TO DO
Life-threatening: None expected.	
Common: None expected.	
Infrequent:	
Watery, stinging, burning eyes.	Continue. Call doctor when convenient.
Rare:	
• Eye pain, blurred vision, drooping eyelid, halos around lights, enlarged pupils, flashes of light.	Discontinue. Call doctor right away.
• Eye symptoms (discharge, dryness, irritation, tearing, sensation of foreign body); sore throat; runny or stuffy nose.	Continue. Call doctor when convenient.

ANTI-INFLAMMATORY DRUGS, STEROIDAL (Ophthalmic)

WARNINGS & PRECAUTIONS

Don't use if:
You are allergic to any cortisone medicine.

Before you start, consult your doctor if:
- You have or ever have had any eye infection, glaucoma, virus (herpes) or fungus infection of the eye, tuberculosis of the eye.
- You wear contact lenses (may need to discontinue wearing temporarily).

Over age 60:
No problems expected.

Pregnancy:
Risk factors vary for drugs in this group. See category list on page xviii and consult doctor.

Breast-feeding:
Safety not established. Avoid if possible. Consult doctor.

Infants & children:
Use for short periods of time only.

Prolonged use:
- Recheck with eye doctor at regular intervals.
- May develop glaucoma, hypertension of the eye, damage to optic nerve, vision changes, cataracts or infections due to suppressive effects of drug.

Skin & sunlight:
No problems expected.

Driving, piloting or hazardous work:
No problems expected.

Discontinuing:
No problems expected.

Others:
- Cortisone eye medicines should not be used for bacterial, viral, fungal or tubercular infections.
- Keep cool, but don't freeze.
- Notify doctor if condition doesn't improve within 3 days.
- Contact lens wearers have increased risk of infection.

POSSIBLE INTERACTION WITH OTHER DRUGS

GENERIC NAME OR DRUG CLASS	COMBINED EFFECT
Antiglaucoma drugs,* long- and short-acting	Decreased antiglaucoma effect.

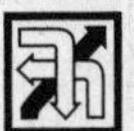

POSSIBLE INTERACTION WITH OTHER SUBSTANCES

INTERACTS WITH	COMBINED EFFECT
Alcohol:	None expected.
Beverages:	None expected.
Cocaine:	None expected.
Foods:	None expected.
Marijuana:	None expected.
Tobacco:	None expected.

***See Glossary**

ANTI-INFLAMMATORY DRUGS, STEROIDAL (Otic)

GENERIC AND BRAND NAMES

BETAMETHASONE (otic)	DEXAMETHASONE (otic)
Betnesol	Decadron

BASIC INFORMATION

Habit forming? No
Prescription needed? Yes
Available as generic? Yes
Drug class: Anti-inflammatory, steroidal (otic); adrenocorticoid (otic)

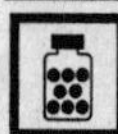

USES

- Treats inflammation symptoms (redness, swelling, itching) of the ear due to allergies or other disorders.
- Treats seborrheic and eczematoid dermatitis involving the ear.

DOSAGE & USAGE INFORMATION

How to use:
As directed by your doctor or pharmacist. The following are general instructions.

How to use ear drops:
- Wash and dry hands.
- Warm drops by holding container in your hand for a few minutes.
- Lie down with affected ear up.
- Adults—Pull ear lobe back and up.
- Children—Pull ear lobe down and back.
- Put the correct number of drops into the ear. Do not allow dropper to touch the ear.
- Wipe away any spilled drops.
- Stay lying down for 2 to 5 minutes.

When to use:
As directed by your doctor.

Continued next column

OVERDOSE

SYMPTOMS:
None expected.
WHAT TO DO:
Not intended for internal use. If child accidentally swallows, call doctor or poison control center 1-800-222-1222 for help.

If you forget a dose:
Use as soon as you remember. If it is almost time for the next dose, wait for next scheduled dose (don't double this dose).

What drug does:
Decreases inflammation.

Time lapse before drug works:
Symptoms should improve within 5 to 7 days. Complete healing may take up to several weeks.

Don't use with:
Other ear medications unless directed by your doctor.

POSSIBLE ADVERSE REACTIONS OR SIDE EFFECTS

SYMPTOMS	WHAT TO DO
Life-threatening:	
None expected.	
Common:	
None expected.	
Infrequent:	
Burning or stinging of the ear.	Continue. Call doctor if symptoms persist.
Rare:	
New or unusual symptoms occur (may be due to drug being absorbed into the body).	Discontinue. Call doctor right away.

ANTI-INFLAMMATORY DRUGS, STEROIDAL (Otic)

WARNINGS & PRECAUTIONS

Don't use if:
You are allergic to any corticosteroid* drugs.

Before you start, consult your doctor if:
- Eardrum is punctured.
- You have diabetes, heart disease, epilepsy, glaucoma, high blood pressure, osteoporosis, or tuberculosis.
- You have a chronic ear infection or other ear problem.
- You have a viral or fungal infection.

Over age 60:
No problems expected.

Pregnancy:
Decide with your doctor if drug benefits justify risk to unborn child. Risk category C (see page xviii).

Breast-feeding:
It is unknown if ear medications are absorbed and then pass into breast milk. Consult doctor.

Infants & children:
Use these drops only if prescribed by your child's doctor.

Prolonged use:
Not intended for prolonged use.

Skin & sunlight:
No problems expected.

Driving, piloting or hazardous work:
No problems expected.

Discontinuing:
No problems expected.

Others:
- Do not increase or decrease dosage without doctor's approval.
- Follow your doctor's instructions for additional ear care at home.
- Call your doctor if ear symptoms worsen or don't improve after a few days of treatment.
- Advise any doctor or dentist whom you consult that you are using this drug.

POSSIBLE INTERACTION WITH OTHER DRUGS

GENERIC NAME OR DRUG CLASS	COMBINED EFFECT
Phenytoin	May decrease effect of anti-inflammatory.

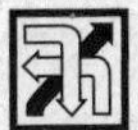

POSSIBLE INTERACTION WITH OTHER SUBSTANCES

INTERACTS WITH	COMBINED EFFECT
Alcohol:	None expected.
Beverages:	None expected.
Cocaine:	None expected.
Foods:	None expected.
Marijuana:	None expected.
Tobacco:	None expected.

*See Glossary

ANTIMALARIAL

GENERIC AND BRAND NAMES

HALOFANTRINE	MEFLOQUINE
Halfan	Lariam

BASIC INFORMATION

Habit forming? No
Prescription needed? Yes
Available as generic? Yes, for some
Drug class: Antiprotozoal, antimalarial, antiparasitic

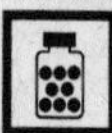

USES

- Treats malaria caused by *plasmodium falciparum* (either chloroquine-sensitive or chloroquine-resistant).
- Treats malaria caused by *plasmodium vivax.*
- Mefloquine helps prevent malaria in people traveling into areas where malaria is prevalent.

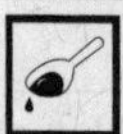

DOSAGE & USAGE INFORMATION

How to take:
- Mefloquine tablet—Swallow with food, milk or water to lessen stomach irritation.
- Halofantrine tablet—Take on an empty stomach.
- Halofantrine suspension—Varies by age and weight; follow physician's directions.

When to take:
- Mefloquine treatment is usually given as 5 tablets in a single dose, while prevention with mefloquine should start a week prior to travel.
- Halofantrine tablets and suspension are taken every 6 hours, 3 times a day for one day on an empty stomach, 1 hour before or 2 hours after a meal.

Continued next column

OVERDOSE

SYMPTOMS:
Seizures, heart rhythm disturbances.
WHAT TO DO:
- **Dial 911 (emergency) for medical help or call poison control center 1-800-222-1222 for instructions.**
- **Induce vomiting and see a doctor immediately because of the potential cardiotoxic effect. Treat vomiting or diarrhea with standard fluid therapy.**
- **See emergency information on last 3 pages of this book.**

If you forget a dose:
Take as soon as you remember, then return to regular dosing schedule.

What drug does:
Exact mechanism unknown. Mefloquine kills parasite in one of its developmental stages, while halofantrine treats malaria in its acute stage.

Time lapse before drug works:
6 to 24 hours.

Don't take with:
- Sulfadoxine and pyrimethamine combination (Fansidar).
- Any other medicines (including over-the-counter drugs such as cough and cold medicines, laxatives, antacids, diet pills, caffeine, nose drops or vitamins) without consulting your doctor or pharmacist.

POSSIBLE ADVERSE REACTIONS OR SIDE EFFECTS

SYMPTOMS	WHAT TO DO
Life-threatening:	
Seizures.	Seek emergency treatment immediately.
Common:	
• Dizziness, headache, lightheadedness, abdominal pain, diarrhea, nausea or vomiting, rash, visual disturbances.	Discontinue. Call doctor right away.
• Insomnia, appetite loss.	Continue. Call doctor when convenient.
Infrequent:	
None expected.	
Rare:	
Change in heart rate, confusion, anxiety, depression, hallucinations, psychosis, black urine or decrease in urine amount, chest or lower back pain, rapid breathing.	Discontinue. Call doctor right away.

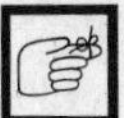

WARNINGS & PRECAUTIONS

Don't take if:
You are allergic to mefloquine, halofantrine, quinine, quinidine or related medications.

Before you start, consult your doctor if:
- You plan to become pregnant within the medication period or 2 months after.
- You have heart trouble, especially heart block.
- You have depression or other emotional problems.
- You are giving this to a child under 40 pounds of body weight.
- You have epilepsy or a seizure disorder.

Over age 60:
Adverse reactions and side effects may be more frequent and severe than in younger persons.

Pregnancy:
Not recommended. If traveling to an area where malaria is endemic, consult your doctor about prophylaxis. Risk category C (see page xviii).

Breast-feeding:
One or more of these drugs may pass into mother's milk. Avoid drug or discontinue nursing.

Infants & children:
- For halofantrine pediatric use, consult your doctor.
- Mefloquine is not recommended for children under 2.

Prolonged use:
Not recommended.

Skin & sunlight:
No problems expected.

Driving, piloting or hazardous work:
Don't drive or pilot aircraft until you learn how medicine affects you. Don't work around dangerous machinery. Don't climb ladders or work in high places. Danger increases if you drink alcohol or take medicine affecting alertness and reflexes.

Discontinuing:
Don't discontinue without doctor's advice until you complete the prescribed dosage.

Others:
- Periodic physical (including eye) examinations and blood studies recommended.
- Resistance to one or more of these drugs by some strains of malaria has been reported, so prevention and treatment of malaria may not be uniformly effective.

POSSIBLE INTERACTION WITH OTHER DRUGS

GENERIC NAME OR DRUG CLASS	COMBINED EFFECT
Anticonvulsants*	Possible lowered seizure control.
Beta-adrenergic blocking agents*	Heartbeat irregularities or cardiac arrest. Avoid.
Calcium channel blockers*	Heartbeat irregularities.
Chloroquine	Increased chance of seizures. Avoid.
Propranolol	Heartbeat irregularities.
Quinidine	Increased chance of seizures and heart rhythm disturbances.
Quinine	Increased chance of seizures and heart rhythm disturbances.
Typhoid vaccine (oral)	Concurrent use may decrease effectiveness of vaccine.

POSSIBLE INTERACTION WITH OTHER SUBSTANCES

INTERACTS WITH	COMBINED EFFECT
Alcohol:	Possible liver toxicity. Avoid.
Beverages: Any alcoholic beverage.	Possible liver toxicity. Avoid.
Cocaine:	No problems expected.
Foods:	No problems expected.
Marijuana:	No problems expected.
Tobacco:	No problems expected.

*See Glossary

ANTIMYASTHENICS

GENERIC AND BRAND NAMES

NEOSTIGMINE	PYRIDOSTIGMINE
Prostigmin	Mestinon
	Mestinon Timespans
	Regonol

BASIC INFORMATION

Habit forming? No
Prescription needed? Yes
Available as generic? Yes, for some
Drug class: Cholinergic, antimyasthenic

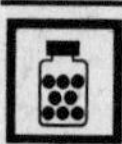

USES

- Diagnosis and treatment of myasthenia gravis.
- Treatment of urinary retention and abdominal distension.
- Antidote to adverse effects of muscle relaxants used in surgery.

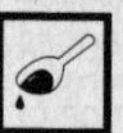

DOSAGE & USAGE INFORMATION

How to take:
- Tablet or syrup—Swallow with liquid or food to lessen stomach irritation.
- Extended-release tablet—Swallow each dose whole. If you take regular tablets, you may chew or crush them.

When to take:
As directed, usually 3 or 4 times a day.

If you forget a dose:
Take as soon as you remember. If it is almost time for the next dose, wait for the next scheduled dose (don't double this dose).

Continued next column

OVERDOSE

SYMPTOMS:
Muscle weakness or paralysis, cramps, twitching or clumsiness; severe diarrhea, nausea, vomiting, stomach cramps or pain; breathing difficulty; confusion, irritability, nervousness, restlessness, fear; unusually slow heartbeat; seizures; blurred vision; extreme fatigue.
WHAT TO DO:
- **Dial 911 (emergency) for medical help or call poison control center 1-800-222-1222 for instructions.**
- **See emergency information on last 3 pages of this book.**

What drug does:
Inhibits the chemical activity of an enzyme (cholinesterase) so nerve impulses can cross the junction of nerves and muscles.

Time lapse before drug works:
Usually takes 10 to 14 days to determine if drug helps relieve symptoms.

Don't take with:
Any other medicine or any dietary supplement without consulting your doctor or pharmacist.

POSSIBLE ADVERSE REACTIONS OR SIDE EFFECTS

SYMPTOMS	WHAT TO DO
Life-threatening:	
In case of overdose, see previous column.	
Common:	
Excess saliva, unusual sweating. mild diarrhea, nausea, vomiting, stomach cramps or pain.	Continue. Call doctor when convenient.
Infrequent:	
Constricted pupils, watery eyes, lung congestion, frequent urge to urinate, confusion, slurred speech.	Continue, but call doctor right away.
Rare:	
Other symptoms.	Continue. Call doctor when convenient.

WARNINGS & PRECAUTIONS

Don't take if:
You are allergic to any cholinergic* or bromide.

Before you start, consult your doctor if:
- You plan to become pregnant within medication period.
- You have bronchial asthma.
- You have heartbeat irregularities.
- You have urinary obstruction or urinary tract infection.

Over age 60:
Adverse reactions and side effects may be more frequent and severe than in younger persons.

Pregnancy:
Decide with your doctor if drug benefits justify risk to unborn child. Risk category C (see page xviii).

Breast-feeding:
Pyridostigmine passes into milk. It is unknown if others pass into milk. Avoid drug or discontinue nursing until you finish medicine. Consult doctor for advice on maintaining milk supply.

Infants & children:
Use only under close medical supervision.

Prolonged use:
Medication may lose effectiveness. Ask your doctor about discontinuing drug for a few days to possibly help restore effect.

Skin & sunlight:
No problems expected.

Driving, piloting or hazardous work:
Don't drive or pilot aircraft until you learn how medicine affects you. Don't work around dangerous machinery. Don't climb ladders or work in high places. Danger increases if you drink alcohol or take medicine affecting alertness and reflexes, such as antihistamines, tranquilizers, sedatives, pain medicine, narcotics and mind-altering drugs.

Discontinuing:
Don't discontinue without doctor's advice until you complete prescribed dose, even though symptoms diminish or disappear.

Others:
- Advise any doctor or dentist whom you consult that you take this medicine.
- Be cautious about participating in hot weather activities since drug may cause excessive sweating.

POSSIBLE INTERACTION WITH OTHER DRUGS

GENERIC NAME OR DRUG CLASS	COMBINED EFFECT
Anesthetics, local or general*	Decreased effect of antimyasthenic.
Antiarrhythmics*	Decreased effect of antimyasthenic.
Anticholinergics*	May mask severe side effects.
Cholinergics,* other	Possible brain and nervous system toxicity.
Guanadrel	Decreased effect of antimyasthenic.
Guanethidine	Decreased effect of antimyasthenic.
Mecamylamine	Decreased effect of antimyasthenic.
Procainamide	Decreased effect of antimyasthenic.
Quinidine	Decreased effect of antimyasthenic.

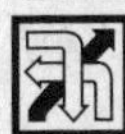

POSSIBLE INTERACTION WITH OTHER SUBSTANCES

INTERACTS WITH	COMBINED EFFECT
Alcohol:	No proven problems with small doses.
Beverages:	None expected.
Cocaine:	Decreased antimyasthenic effect. Avoid.
Foods:	None expected.
Marijuana:	No proven problems.
Tobacco:	No proven problems.

*See Glossary

ANTIPYRINE & BENZOCAINE (Otic)

BRAND NAMES

A/B Otic
Allergen
Analgesic Ear Drops
Antiben
Auralgan
Aurodex
Dolotic
Earache Drops
Earocol
Otiprin
Otocalm

BASIC INFORMATION

Habit forming? No
Prescription needed?
Yes (in US;
No in Canada)
Available as generic? Yes
Drug class: Analgesic (otic); anesthetic

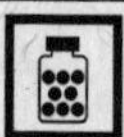

USES

- Relieves symptoms of middle ear infections (otitis media). It does not treat the infection itself.
- Used to soften earwax so it can be removed.

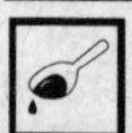

DOSAGE & USAGE INFORMATION

How to use ear drops:

- Wash and dry hands.
- Warm drops by holding container in your hand for a few minutes.
- Lie down with affected ear up.
- Adults—Pull ear lobe back and up.
- Children—Pull ear lobe down and back.
- Put the correct number of drops into the ear. Do not allow dropper to touch the ear.
- Wipe away any spilled drops.
- Stay lying down for 2 to 5 minutes.
- For ear wax removal, follow your doctor's instructions.

When to use:
Every 1 to 2 hours for 4 hours, then 4 times a day when needed for pain.

If you forget a dose:
Use as soon as you remember. If it is almost time for the next dose, wait for next scheduled dose (don't double this dose).

Continued next column

OVERDOSE

SYMPTOMS:
None expected.
WHAT TO DO:
Not intended for internal use. If child accidentally swallows, call doctor or poison control center 1-800-222-1222 for help.

What drug does:
Helps relieve the pain, congestion and swelling of ear infections. It does not cure the infection.

Time lapse before drug works:
10 minutes.

Don't use with:
Any other ear medicine without consulting your doctor or pharmacist.

POSSIBLE ADVERSE REACTIONS OR SIDE EFFECTS

SYMPTOMS	WHAT TO DO
Life-threatening: None expected.	
Common: None expected.	
Infrequent: Itching or burning in ear (probably represents allergic reaction).	Discontinue. Call doctor right away.
Rare: None expected.	

ANTIPYRINE & BENZOCAINE (Otic)

WARNINGS & PRECAUTIONS

Don't use if:
You are allergic to any local anesthetic (name usually ends with "caine").

Before you start, consult your doctor if:
Eardrum is ruptured.

Over age 60:
No problems expected.

Pregnancy:
Decide with your doctor if drug benefits justify risk to unborn child. Risk category C (see page xviii).

Breast-feeding:
No problems expected. Consult doctor.

Infants & children:
No problems expected.

Prolonged use:
Not intended for prolonged use.

Skin & sunlight:
No problems expected.

Driving, piloting or hazardous work:
No problems expected.

Discontinuing:
No problems expected.

Others:
- Keep cool, but don't freeze.
- Don't touch tip of dropper to any other surface.
- Don't rinse the dropper. Wipe with clean cloth and close tightly.

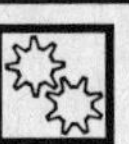

POSSIBLE INTERACTION WITH OTHER DRUGS

GENERIC NAME OR DRUG CLASS	COMBINED EFFECT
None expected.	

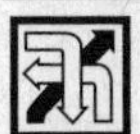

POSSIBLE INTERACTION WITH OTHER SUBSTANCES

INTERACTS WITH	COMBINED EFFECT
Alcohol:	None expected.
Beverages:	None expected.
Cocaine:	None expected.
Foods:	None expected.
Marijuana:	None expected.
Tobacco:	None expected.

ANTISEBORRHEICS (Topical)

GENERIC AND BRAND NAMES

See full list of generic and brand names in the *Generic and Brand Name Directory,* page 874.

BASIC INFORMATION

Habit forming? No
Prescription needed? Yes
Available as generic? Yes
Drug class: Antiseborrheic

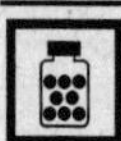

USES

Treats dandruff or seborrheic dermatitis of scalp.

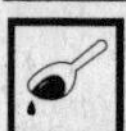

DOSAGE & USAGE INFORMATION

How to use:
- Wet hair and scalp.
- Apply enough medicine to form lather.
- Rub in well. Keep away from eyes.
- Allow to remain on scalp 3 to 5 minutes, then rinse.
- Repeat above steps once.

When to use:
As directed by doctor. Twice a week for shampoo is average.

If you forget a dose:
Use as soon as you remember.

What drug does:
Slows cell growth in scales on scalp.

Time lapse before drug works:
Varies a great deal. If no improvement in 2 weeks, notify doctor.

Don't use with:
Other hair or scalp preparations without consulting your doctor or pharmacist.

OVERDOSE

SYMPTOMS:
None expected.
WHAT TO DO:
- **Not for internal use. If child accidentally swallows, dial 911 (emergency) for medical help or call poison control center 1-800-222-1222 for instructions.**
- **See emergency information on last 3 pages of this book.**

POSSIBLE ADVERSE REACTIONS OR SIDE EFFECTS

SYMPTOMS	WHAT TO DO
Life-threatening: None expected.	
Common: None expected.	
Infrequent:	
• Irritation not present before using, rash.	Discontinue. Call doctor when convenient.
• Dryness or itching scalp.	Continue. Call doctor when convenient.
Rare: None expected.	

WARNINGS & PRECAUTIONS

Don't use if:

- You have had an allergic reaction to chloroxine, clioquinol (iodochlorhydroxyquin), iodoquinol (diiodohydroxyquin) or sodium edate.
- Scalp is blistered or infected with oozing or raw areas.

Before you start, consult your doctor if:
You are allergic to anything.

Over age 60:
No problems expected.

Pregnancy:
Risk factors vary for drugs in this group. See category list on page xviii and consult doctor.

Breast-feeding:
No problems expected, but check with doctor.

Infants & children:
No problems expected, but check with doctor.

Prolonged use:
No problems expected, but check with doctor.

Skin & sunlight:
No special problems expected.

Driving, piloting or hazardous work:
No problems expected, but check with doctor.

Discontinuing:
No problems expected, but check with doctor.

Others:

- If medicine accidentally gets into eyes, flush them immediately with cool water.
- Heat and moisture in bathroom medicine cabinet can cause breakdown of medicine. Store someplace else.
- Keep cool, but don't freeze.

POSSIBLE INTERACTION WITH OTHER DRUGS

GENERIC NAME OR DRUG CLASS	COMBINED EFFECT
Other medicated shampoos	May increase adverse reactions of each medicine.

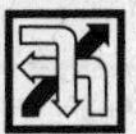

POSSIBLE INTERACTION WITH OTHER SUBSTANCES

INTERACTS WITH	COMBINED EFFECT
Alcohol:	None expected.
Beverages:	None expected.
Cocaine:	None expected.
Foods:	None expected.
Marijuana:	None expected.
Tobacco:	None expected.

ANTITHYROID DRUGS

GENERIC AND BRAND NAMES

METHIMAZOLE	PROPYLTHIOURACIL
Tapazole	Propyl-Thyracil
Thiamazole	

BASIC INFORMATION

Habit forming? No
Prescription needed? Yes
Available as generic? Yes
Drug class: Antihyperthyroid

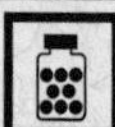

USES

- Treatment of overactive thyroid (hyperthyroidism).
- Treatment of angina in patients who have overactive thyroid.

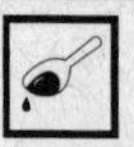

DOSAGE & USAGE INFORMATION

How to take:
Tablet—Swallow with liquid or food to lessen stomach irritation. If you can't swallow whole, crumble tablet and take with liquid or food.

When to take:
At the same times each day.

If you forget a dose:
Take or use as soon as you remember. If it is almost time for the next dose, wait for next scheduled dose (don't double this dose).

What drug does:
Prevents thyroid gland from producing excess thyroid hormone.

Time lapse before drug works:
10 to 20 days.

Don't take with:
Any other medicine or any dietary supplement without consulting your doctor or pharmacist.

OVERDOSE

SYMPTOMS:
Bleeding, spots on skin, jaundice (yellow eyes and skin), loss of consciousness.
WHAT TO DO:
Overdose unlikely to threaten life. If person uses much larger amount than prescribed or if accidentally swallowed, call doctor or poison control center 1-800-222-1222 for help.

POSSIBLE ADVERSE REACTIONS OR SIDE EFFECTS

SYMPTOMS	WHAT TO DO
Life-threatening: None expected.	
Common: Skin symptoms (rash, itching).	Continue, but call doctor right away.
Infrequent:	
• Dizziness, sore, throat. chills, fever, abdominal pain.	Continue, but call doctor right away.
• Taste loss, constipation, diarrhea.	Continue. Call doctor when convenient.
Rare: Headache; enlarged lymph glands; irregular or rapid heartbeat; unusual bruising or bleeding; backache; numbness or tingling in toes, fingers or face; joint pain; muscle aches; menstrual irregularities; jaundice; tiredness or weakness; listless; swollen eyes or feet; black stools; excessive cold feeling; puffy skin; irritability; propylthiouracil may cause severe liver problems (low fever, itching, nausea, stomach pain, loss of appetite, dark urine, clay-colored stools, yellow skin or eyes).	Continue, but call doctor right away.

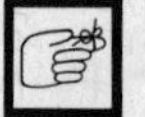

WARNINGS & PRECAUTIONS

Don't take if:
You are allergic to antithyroid medicines.

Before you start, consult your doctor if:
- You have liver disease.
- You have a blood disease.
- You have an infection.
- You take anticoagulants.

Over age 60:
Adverse reactions and side effects may be more frequent and severe than in younger persons.

Pregnancy:
Consult doctor. Risk category D (see page xviii).

Breast-feeding:
Drugs pass into breast milk. Consult doctor.

Infants & children:
Use only under special medical supervision.

Prolonged use:
- Adverse reactions and side effects more common.
- Talk to your doctor about the need for follow-up medical examinations or laboratory studies to check thyroid function, complete blood counts (white blood cell count, platelet count, red blood cell count, hemoglobin, hematocrit).

Skin & sunlight:
No problems expected.

Driving, piloting or hazardous work:
Don't drive or pilot aircraft until you learn how medicine affects you. Don't work around dangerous machinery. Don't climb ladders or work in high places. Danger increases if you drink alcohol or take medicine affecting alertness and reflexes, such as antihistamines, tranquilizers, sedatives, pain medicine, narcotics and mind-altering drugs.

Discontinuing:
Don't discontinue without consulting doctor. Dose may require gradual reduction if you have taken drug for a long time. Doses of other drugs may also require adjustment.

Others:
- Advise any doctor or dentist whom you consult that you take this medicine.
- Ask your doctor about the symptoms of overactive or underactive thyroid and what to do if they occur.

POSSIBLE INTERACTION WITH OTHER DRUGS

GENERIC NAME OR DRUG CLASS	COMBINED EFFECT
Amiodarone	Decreased antithyroid effect.
Anticoagulants*	Increased effect of anticoagulants.
Antineoplastic drugs*	Increased chance to suppress bone marrow.
Chloramphenicol	Increased chance to suppress bone marrow.
Clozapine	Toxic effect on bone marrow.
Digitalis preparations*	Increased digitalis effect.
Iodine	Decreased antithyroid effect.
Levamisole	Increased risk of bone marrow depression.
Lithium	Decreased thyroid activity.
Potassium iodide	Decreased antithyroid effect.
Tiopronin	Increased risk of toxicity to bone marrow.

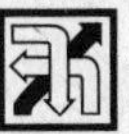

POSSIBLE INTERACTION WITH OTHER SUBSTANCES

INTERACTS WITH	COMBINED EFFECT
Alcohol:	Increased possibility of liver toxicity. Avoid.
Beverages:	No problems expected.
Cocaine:	Increased toxicity potential of medicines. Avoid.
Foods:	No problems expected.
Marijuana:	Increased rapid or irregular heartbeat. Avoid.
Tobacco:	Increased chance of rapid heartbeat. Avoid.

*See Glossary

ANTIVIRALS FOR HERPES VIRUS

GENERIC AND BRAND NAMES

ACYCLOVIR
- Alti-Acyclovir
- Avirax
- Zovirax

FAMCICLOVIR
- Famvir

GANCICLOVIR
- Cytovene

VALACYCLOVIR
- Valtrex

BASIC INFORMATION

Habit forming? No
Prescription needed? Yes
Available as generic? Yes, for some
Drug class: Antiviral

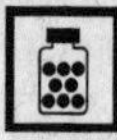

USES

- Treatment for symptoms of herpes virus infections (does not cure the disorders). These infections include herpes simplex, genital herpes and herpes zoster (also known as shingles). Herpes infections may occur on the lips and mouth, genitals, skin and the brain.
- May be used to treat chickenpox and other viral infections as prescribed by your doctor.
- Ganciclovir is used for treatment of cytomegalovirus (CMV) eye infection in persons whose immune system is impaired.

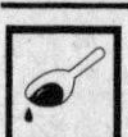

DOSAGE & USAGE INFORMATION

How to take:
Tablet, capsule or oral suspension—Swallow with liquid. If you can't swallow whole, open capsule or crumble tablet and take with liquid or food. Take ganciclovir with food and do not open capsule. Other drugs may be taken with or without food. Measure oral suspension with specially marked measuring device.

Continued next column

When to take:
At the same times each day and night. Drugs work best if started within 48 hours of diagnosis (or when symptoms first appear).

If you forget a dose:
Take as soon as you remember. If it is almost time for the next dose, wait for the next scheduled dose (don't double this dose).

What drug does:
Inhibits the growth and spread of the virus thereby decreasing length of infection and lessening the severity of the symptoms.

Time lapse before drug works:
Begins the first day, but may take several days for symptoms (pain, burning and blisters) to improve.

Don't take with:
Any other medicine or any dietary supplement without consulting your doctor or pharmacist.

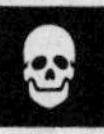

OVERDOSE

SYMPTOMS:
Unknown effects.
WHAT TO DO:
Overdose unlikely to threaten life. If person uses much larger amount than prescribed or if accidentally swallowed, call doctor or poison control center 1-800-222-1222 for help.

POSSIBLE ADVERSE REACTIONS OR SIDE EFFECTS

SYMPTOMS	WHAT TO DO
Life-threatening:	
Hives, rash, intense itching, faintness soon after a dose (anaphylaxis); difficulty breathing.	Seek emergency treatment immediately.
Common:	
General feeling of illness or discomfort.	Continue. Call doctor when convenient.
Infrequent:	
Headache, nausea, diarrhea, vomiting, tiredness, dizziness; with ganciclovir—sore throat and fever, unusual bleeding or bruising, mood changes.	Continue. Call doctor when convenient.
Rare:	
Vision changes, eyes irritated, swelling, agitation, confusion, fever, hallucinations, chills, fever, sore throat or mouth, skin (rash, blister, itch, peel), muscle cramps.	Discontinue. Call doctor right away.

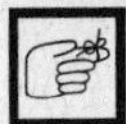

WARNINGS & PRECAUTIONS

Don't take if:
You are allergic to antiviral agents.

Before you start, consult your doctor if:
- You have kidney disease or neurological problems.
- You have any disease of the blood.
- You are allergic to any medication, food or other substance.

Over age 60:
No special problems expected.

Pregnancy:
Risk factors vary for drugs in this group. See category list on page xviii and consult doctor.

Breast-feeding:
Drugs may pass into milk. Avoid nursing until you finish medicine. Consult doctor for advice on maintaining milk supply.

Infants & children:
Use only under medical supervision.

Prolonged use:
See your doctor for regular visits to check effectiveness of the drug and to check for any blood problems.

Skin & sunlight:
No special problems expected.

Driving, piloting or hazardous work:
Avoid if you experience dizziness after taking drug, otherwise no problems expected.

Discontinuing:
Don't discontinue without doctor's advice until you complete prescribed dose, even though symptoms diminish or disappear.

Others:
- Advise any doctor or dentist whom you consult that you take this medicine.
- If symptoms don't improve within a few days, or if they worsen, consult doctor.
- See your eye doctor regularly if you are taking the drug for eye infection.
- If drug is prescribed for genital herpes, be sure you use proper precautions to prevent spreading the disorder to your sexual partner. If unsure, ask your doctor for information.
- Keep affected skin area clean and dry.
- Decrease blister irritation by wearing loose-fitting clothing.

POSSIBLE INTERACTION WITH OTHER DRUGS

GENERIC NAME OR DRUG CLASS	COMBINED EFFECT
Bone marrow depressants*	Increased risk of bone marrow depression with ganciclovir.
Cimetidine	Increased antiviral effect.
Didanosine	Increased didanosine effect with ganciclovir.
Probenecid	Increased effect of antivirals.
Nephrotoxics*	Increased risk of kidney problems.
Nucleotide reverse transcriptase inhibitors	Increased effect of nucleotide reverse transcriptase inhibitor.
Zidovudine	Increased risk of adverse effects.

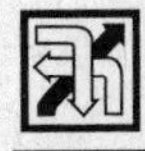

POSSIBLE INTERACTION WITH OTHER SUBSTANCES

INTERACTS WITH	COMBINED EFFECT
Alcohol:	None expected.
Beverages:	None expected.
Cocaine:	None expected. Best to avoid.
Foods:	None expected.
Marijuana:	None expected. Best to avoid.
Tobacco:	None expected.

*See Glossary

ANTIVIRALS FOR INFLUENZA

GENERIC AND BRAND NAMES

AMANTADINE	RIMANTADINE
Symadine	Flumadine
Symmetrel	

BASIC INFORMATION

Habit forming? No
Prescription needed? Yes
Available as generic? Yes
Drug class: Antiviral, antiparkinsonism

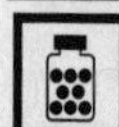

USES

- Prevention and treatment for Type-A flu infections.
- Relief for symptoms of Parkinson's disease (amantadine).

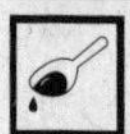

DOSAGE & USAGE INFORMATION

How to take:
- Capsule—Swallow with liquid or food to lessen stomach irritation.
- Syrup—Dilute dose in beverage before swallowing.

When to take:
At the same times each day. For Type-A flu it is especially important to take regular doses as prescribed.

If you forget a dose:
Take as soon as you remember. If it is almost time for the next dose, wait for the next scheduled dose (don't double this dose).

What drug does:
- Type-A flu—May block penetration of tissue cells by infectious material from virus cells.
- Parkinson's disease and drug-induced extrapyramidal* reactions—Improves muscular condition and coordination.

Continued next column

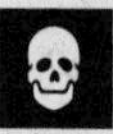

OVERDOSE

SYMPTOMS:
Heart rhythm disturbances, blood pressure drop, convulsions, hallucinations, violent behavior, confusion, slurred speech, rolling eyes.
WHAT TO DO:
- **Dial 911 (emergency) for medical help or call poison control center 1-800-222-1222 for instructions.**
- **See emergency information on last 3 pages of this book.**

Time lapse before drug works:
- Type-A flu—48 hours.
- Parkinson's disease—2 days to 2 weeks.

Don't take with:
- Alcohol.
- Any other medicine or any dietary supplement without consulting your doctor or pharmacist.

POSSIBLE ADVERSE REACTIONS OR SIDE EFFECTS

SYMPTOMS	WHAT TO DO
Life-threatening: In case of overdose, see previous column.	
Common: Headache, difficulty in concentrating, dizziness or lightheadedness, insomnia, irritability, nervousness, nightmares (these side effects infrequent with rimantadine).	Continue. Call doctor when convenient.
Infrequent:	
• With amantadine—Blurred or changed vision, confusion, difficult urination, hallucinations, fainting.	Discontinue. Call doctor right away.
• Constipation; dry mouth, nose or throat; vomiting; appetite loss; nausea.	Continue. Call doctor when convenient.
Rare:	
• With amantadine—Swelling or irritated eyes; depression; swelling of hands, legs or feet; skin rash.	Discontinue. Call doctor right away.
• Seizures (may occur in persons with a history of seizures).	Discontinue. Seek emergency help.

WARNINGS & PRECAUTIONS

Don't take if:
You are allergic to amantadine or rimantadine.

Before you start, consult your doctor if:
- You have had epilepsy or other seizures.
- You have had heart disease or heart failure.
- You have had liver or kidney disease.
- You have had peptic ulcers.
- You have had eczema or skin rashes.
- You have had emotional or mental disorders or taken drugs for them.

Over age 60:
Adverse reactions and side effects may be more frequent and severe than in younger persons.

Pregnancy:
Decide with your doctor whether benefits justify risk to unborn child. Risk category C (see page xviii).

Breast-feeding:
Drug may pass into milk. Avoid drug or discontinue nursing until you finish medicine. Consult doctor for advice on maintaining milk supply.

Infants & children:
Use only under medical supervision.

Prolonged use:
Skin splotches, feet swelling, rapid weight gain, shortness of breath. Consult doctor.

Skin & sunlight:
One or more drugs in this group may cause rash or intensify sunburn in areas exposed to sun or ultraviolet light (photosensitivity reaction). Avoid overexposure. Notify doctor if reaction occurs.

Driving, piloting or hazardous work:
Don't drive or pilot aircraft until you learn how medicine affects you. Don't work around dangerous machinery. Don't climb ladders or work in high places. Danger increases if you drink alcohol or take medicine affecting alertness and reflexes.

Discontinuing:
- Parkinson's disease—Don't discontinue without doctor's advice until you complete prescribed dose, even though symptoms diminish or disappear.
- Type-A flu—Discontinue 48 hours after symptoms disappear.

Others:
- Parkinson's disease—May lose effectiveness in 3 to 6 months. Consult doctor.
- These drugs are not effective for influenza-B virus.
- Drug-resistant strains of the virus may occur within the same household.

POSSIBLE INTERACTION WITH OTHER DRUGS

GENERIC NAME OR DRUG CLASS	COMBINED EFFECT
Acetaminophen	With rimantadine—Decreased antiviral effect.
Anticholinergics*	With amantadine—Increased risk of side effects.
Antidepressants, tricyclic*	With amantadine—Increased risk of side effects.
Antidyskinetics*	With amantadine—Increased risk of side effects.
Antihistamines*	With amantadine—Increased risk of side effects.
Aspirin	With rimantadine—Decreased antiviral effect.
Carbidopa & Levodopa	With amantadine—Increased effect of carbidopa & levodopa.
Central nervous system (CNS) stimulants*	With amantadine—Increased risk of adverse reactions.
Memantine	With amantadine—Adverse effects of either drug.

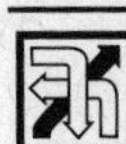

POSSIBLE INTERACTION WITH OTHER SUBSTANCES

INTERACTS WITH	COMBINED EFFECT
Alcohol:	Increased alcohol effect. Possible fainting.
Beverages:	None expected.
Cocaine:	Dangerous overstimulation.
Foods:	None expected.
Marijuana:	None expected.
Tobacco:	None expected.

*See Glossary

ANTIVIRALS FOR INFLUENZA, NEURAMINIDASE INHIBITORS

GENERIC AND BRAND NAMES

OSELTAMIVIR	ZANAMIVIR
Tamiflu	Relenza

BASIC INFORMATION

Habit forming? No
Prescription needed? Yes
Available as generic? No
Drug class: Anti-influenza

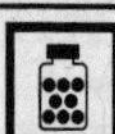

USES

- Shortens the duration of influenza types A and B. It is best to start using this medicine within 2 days of onset of symptoms.
- Used to help prevent influenza types A and B.

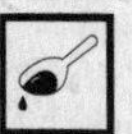

DOSAGE & USAGE INFORMATION

How to take:
- Capsule—Swallow with liquid. If you can't swallow whole, open capsule and take with liquid or food.
- Oral solution—Take as directed on label.
- Powder—This medication is to be used with a device called a Diskhaler. Read and carefully follow the instructions provided with the device. If you are still unsure, consult your pharmacist for detailed instructions.

When to take:
- For oseltamivir, take two doses daily at the same times.
- For zanamivir, take two doses on the first day separated by 2 hours and then two doses daily for 5 days separated by 12 hours.

Continued next column

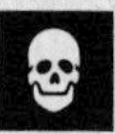

OVERDOSE

SYMPTOMS:
There has been very little experience with overdose; however, relatively large doses have resulted in nausea and vomiting.
WHAT TO DO:
- **Dial 911 (emergency) for medical help or call poison control center 1-800-222-1222 for instructions.**
- **See emergency information on last 3 pages of this book.**

If you forget a dose:
Take as soon as you remember. If it is almost time for the next dose, wait for the next scheduled dose (don't double this dose).

What drug does:
Inhibits the spread of the virus by preventing release of the cells within the respiratory tract.

Time lapse before drug works:
Begins in 2 to 3 days.

Don't take with:
Any other medicine or any dietary supplement without consulting your doctor or pharmacist.

POSSIBLE ADVERSE REACTIONS OR SIDE EFFECTS

SYMPTOMS	WHAT TO DO
Life-threatening:	
Hives, rash, intense itching, faintness soon after a dose (anaphylaxis).	Seek emergency treatment immediately.
Common:	
• Cough, fever, skin rash, swelling (of face, fingers, feet and/or lower legs).	Discontinue. Call doctor right away.
• Back pain, dizziness, gas, headache, nausea, heartburn, burning in throat, sleeplessness, stuffy or runny nose.	Continue. Call doctor when convenient.
Infrequent:	
• Bloody or tarry stools, chills, congestion, diarrhea, fatigue, loss of appetite, muscle pains, shortness of breath, severe stomach pain, weight gain, vomiting.	Discontinue. Call doctor right away.
• Anxiety, vision changes, noises in ears, change in sense of taste, difficulty swallowing, dry mouth, constipation, depression, rapid heartbeat, increased sweating, numbness in fingers or toes, sleepiness.	Continue. Call doctor if symptoms persist.
Rare:	
Abnormal behaviors.	Discontinue. Call doctor right away.

WARNINGS & PRECAUTIONS

Don't take if:
You are allergic to oseltamivir or zanamivir.

Before you start, consult your doctor if:
- You have a history of asthma or chronic obstructive pulmonary disease (zanamivir).
- You have kidney disease (oseltamivir).

Over age 60:
Adverse reactions and side effects may be more frequent and severe than in younger persons.

Pregnancy:
Decide with your doctor whether drug benefits justify risk to unborn child. Risk category B for zanamivir and risk category C for oseltamivir (see page xviii).

Breast-feeding:
It is unknown if oseltamivir or zanamivir pass into milk. Avoid drug or discontinue nursing until you finish medicine. Consult doctor for advice on maintaining milk supply.

Infants & children:
- Oseltamivir is approved for children over age 2 weeks for influenza treatment and over age 1 for influenza prevention.
- Zanamivir is approved for children over age 7 for influenza treatment and over age 5 for influenza prevention.

Prolonged use:
Not intended for long-term use.

Skin & sunlight:
No problems expected.

Driving, piloting or hazardous work:
Don't drive or pilot aircraft until you learn how medicine affects you. Don't work around dangerous machinery. Don't climb ladders or work in high places. Danger increases if you drink alcohol or take medicine affecting alertness and reflexes, such as antihistamines, tranquilizers, sedatives, pain medicine, narcotics and mind-altering drugs.

Discontinuing:
Do not discontinue until you finish all of your medicine; otherwise, symptoms may return.

Others:
- You should continue receiving an annual flu shot according to guidelines on immunization practices or as recommended by your doctor.
- People with the flu (including children and adolescents) may be at increased risk shortly after taking oseltamivir of self-injury, confusion, hallucinations, delirium and abnormal behavior leading to injury which in some cases may have fatal outcomes. Watch patient's behavior closely and call doctor if symptoms develop.
- Use of the drug does not reduce the risk of transmitting influenza to others.
- Advise any doctor or dentist whom you consult that you take this medicine.

POSSIBLE INTERACTION WITH OTHER DRUGS

GENERIC NAME OR DRUG CLASS	COMBINED EFFECT
None expected.	

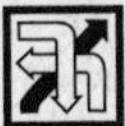

POSSIBLE INTERACTION WITH OTHER SUBSTANCES

INTERACTS WITH	COMBINED EFFECT
Alcohol:	None expected.
Beverages:	None expected.
Cocaine:	None expected.
Foods:	None expected.
Marijuana:	None expected.
Tobacco:	None expected.

ANTIVIRALS (Ophthalmic)

GENERIC AND BRAND NAMES

IDOXURIDINE
Herplex Eye Drops
Stoxil Eye Ointment
GANCICLOVIR (ophthalmic)
Zirgan
TRIFLURIDINE
Trifluorothymidine
Viroptic

BASIC INFORMATION

Habit forming? No
Prescription needed? Yes
Available as generic? No
Drug class: Antiviral (ophthalmic)

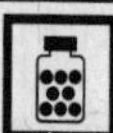

USES

Treats virus infections of the eye (e.g., herpes simplex virus) and acute herpetic keratitis (dendritic ulcers).

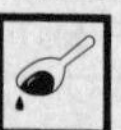

DOSAGE & USAGE INFORMATION

How to use:
Eye drops

- Wash hands.
- Apply pressure to inside corner of eye with middle finger.
- Continue pressure for 1 minute after placing medicine in eye.
- Tilt head backward. Pull lower lid away from eye with index finger of the same hand.
- Drop eye drops into pouch and close eye. Don't blink.
- Keep eyes closed for 1 to 2 minutes.

Eye ointment

- Wash hands.
- Pull lower lid down from eye to form a pouch.
- Squeeze tube to apply thin strip of ointment into pouch.
- Close eye for 1 to 2 minutes.
- Don't touch applicator tip to any surface (including the eye). If you accidentally touch tip, clean with warm water and soap.

Continued next column

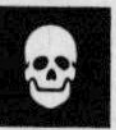

OVERDOSE

SYMPTOMS:
None expected.
WHAT TO DO:
Not intended for internal use. If child accidentally swallows, call doctor or poison control center 1-800-222-1222 for help.

- Keep container tightly closed.
- Keep cool, but don't freeze.
- Wash hands immediately after using.

When to use:
As directed. Usually 1 drop every 2 hours up to maximum of 9 drops daily.

If you forget a dose:
Use as soon as you remember. Then return to regular schedule.

What drug does:
Destroys reproductive capacity of virus.

Time lapse before drug works:
Begins to work immediately. Usual course of treatment is 7 days.

Don't use with:
Other eye drugs or products, boric acid or ointment without consulting doctor or pharmacist.

POSSIBLE ADVERSE REACTIONS OR SIDE EFFECTS

SYMPTOMS	WHAT TO DO
Life-threatening:	
None expected.	
Common:	
Stinging or burning eyes.	Continue. Tell doctor at next visit.
Infrequent:	
Blurred vision for a few minutes (with ointment).	No action necessary.
Rare:	
Itchy, red eyes; swollen eyelid or eye; excess flow of tears; dimming or haziness of vision.	Discontinue. Call doctor right away.

WARNINGS & PRECAUTIONS

Don't use if:
You are allergic to trifluridine, idoxuridine or ganciclovir.

Before you start, consult your doctor if:
- You have had any other eye problems.
- You use eye drops for glaucoma.

Over age 60:
No problems expected.

Pregnancy:
Risk factors vary for drugs in this group. See category list on page xviii and consult doctor.

Breast-feeding:
No problems expected, but safety not established. Consult doctor.

Infants & children:
Use only under close medical supervision.

Prolonged use:
Avoid unless directed by your eye doctor.

Skin & sunlight:
No problems expected.

Driving, piloting or hazardous work:
No problems expected.

Discontinuing:
Don't discontinue without consulting doctor.

Others:
- Don't use more often or longer than prescribed.
- Keep cool, but don't freeze.
- If problem doesn't improve within a week, notify your doctor.

POSSIBLE INTERACTION WITH OTHER DRUGS

GENERIC NAME OR DRUG CLASS	COMBINED EFFECT
Eye products containing boric acid	Increased risk of toxicity to eye.

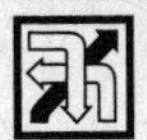

POSSIBLE INTERACTION WITH OTHER SUBSTANCES

INTERACTS WITH	COMBINED EFFECT
Alcohol:	None expected.
Beverages:	None expected.
Cocaine:	None expected.
Foods:	None expected.
Marijuana:	None expected.
Tobacco:	None expected.

ANTIVIRALS (Topical)

GENERIC AND BRAND NAMES

ACYCLOVIR (topical)
Lipsovir
Xerese Cream
Zovirax Ointment

DOCOSANOL (topical)
Abreva

PENCICLOVIR (topical)
Denavir

BASIC INFORMATION

Habit forming? No
Prescription needed? Yes
Available as generic? Yes, for some
Drug class: Antiviral

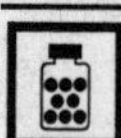

USES

- Treatment of symptoms of herpes infections of the skin, mucous membranes, lips, mouth and genitals.
- May be used for other skin disorders as prescribed by your doctor.

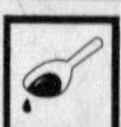

DOSAGE & USAGE INFORMATION

How to take:

- Acyclovir ointment—Apply to skin and mucous membranes every 3 hours (6 times a day) for 7 days. Use rubber glove when applying. Apply 1/2-inch strip to each sore or blister. Wash before using.
- Penciclovir cream—Use only on lips and face. Avoid eye area. Use every 2 hours, while awake, for 4 days.
- Docosanol—Apply directly to the affected area at the first sign of a cold sore. It should be used five times daily until the cold sore or fever blister is completely healed.

When to use:
Use as soon as symptoms begin to appear (burning, pain or blisters).

If you forget a dose:
Apply as soon as you remember, then continue with regular schedule.

Continued next column

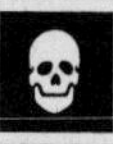

OVERDOSE

SYMPTOMS:
None expected.
WHAT TO DO:
If person accidentally swallows topical form of drug, call doctor or poison control center 1-800-222-1222 for help.

What drug does:

- Inhibits reproduction of virus in cells without killing normal cells.
- Does not cure. Herpes breakout often recurs.

Time lapse before drug works:
2 hours.

Don't take with:
Any other topical medicine without consulting your doctor or pharmacist.

POSSIBLE ADVERSE REACTIONS OR SIDE EFFECTS

SYMPTOMS	WHAT TO DO
Life-threatening: None expected.	
Common: May cause mild pain, burning, itching or stinging.	Continue. Call doctor when convenient.
Infrequent: None expected.	
Rare: Skin rash.	Continue. Call doctor when convenient.

WARNINGS & PRECAUTIONS

Don't take if:
You are allergic to topical acyclovir, docosanol or penciclovir.

Before you start, consult your doctor if:
You are allergic to any medication, food or other substance.

Over age 60:
Adverse reactions and side effects may be more frequent and severe than in younger persons.

Pregnancy:
Decide with your doctor whether drug benefits justify risk to unborn child. Risk category C (see page xviii).

Breast-feeding:
It is unknown if topical antivirals are absorbed and then pass into breast milk. Consult doctor.

Infants & children:
Use only under special medical supervision.

Prolonged use:
Don't use longer than prescribed time.

Skin & sunlight:
No problems expected.

Driving, piloting or hazardous work:
No problems expected.

Discontinuing:
May be unnecessary to finish medicine. Follow doctor's instructions.

Others:

- Women: Get pap smear every 6 months because those with herpes infections are possibly at increased risk to develop cancer of the cervix. Avoid sexual activity until all blisters or sores heal.
- Don't get topical medicine in eyes.
- Check with doctor if no improvement in 1 week.

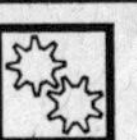

POSSIBLE INTERACTION WITH OTHER DRUGS

GENERIC NAME OR DRUG CLASS	COMBINED EFFECT
None expected.	

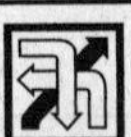

POSSIBLE INTERACTION WITH OTHER SUBSTANCES

INTERACTS WITH	COMBINED EFFECT
Alcohol:	None expected.
Beverages:	None expected.
Cocaine:	None expected.
Foods:	None expected.
Marijuana:	None expected.
Tobacco:	None expected.

APPETITE SUPPRESSANTS

GENERIC AND BRAND NAMES

See full list of generic and brand names in the *Generic and Brand Name Directory*, page 874.

BASIC INFORMATION

Habit forming? Yes
Prescription needed? Yes
Available as generic? Yes, for most
Drug class: Appetite suppressant

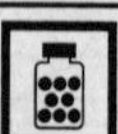

USES

Suppresses appetite. Temporary treatment for overweight and obesity.

DOSAGE & USAGE INFORMATION

How to take:

- Tablet or capsule—Swallow with liquid. You may chew or crush tablet.
- Extended-release tablet or capsule—Swallow each dose whole with liquid; do not chew, crush or open.
- Oral disintegrating tablet—Let dissolve on top of tongue; then swallow with or without water.
- Elixir—Swallow with liquid.

When to take:

- Long-acting forms—10 to 14 hours before bedtime.
- Short-acting forms—1 hour before meals. Last dose no later than 4 to 6 hours before bedtime.

If you forget a dose:
Take as soon as you remember. If it is almost time for the next dose, wait for the next scheduled dose (don't double this dose).

Continued next column

OVERDOSE

SYMPTOMS:
Irritability, overactivity, trembling, insomnia, mood changes, fever, rapid heartbeat, confusion, disorientation, hallucinations, convulsions, coma.
WHAT TO DO:

- **Dial 911 (emergency) for medical help or call poison control center 1-800-222-1222 for instructions.**
- **See emergency information on last 3 pages of this book.**

What drug does:
Apparently stimulates brain's appetite control center.

Time lapse before drug works:
Begins in 1 hour. Short-acting form lasts 4 hours. Long-acting form lasts 14 hours.

Don't take with:
Any other medicine or any dietary supplement without consulting your doctor or pharmacist.

POSSIBLE ADVERSE REACTIONS OR SIDE EFFECTS

SYMPTOMS	WHAT TO DO
Life-threatening: In case of overdose, see previous column.	
Common:	
Irritability, nervousness, insomnia, false sense of well-being.	Continue. Call doctor when convenient.
Infrequent:	
• Irregular or pounding heartbeat, urgent or difficult urination.	Discontinue. Call doctor right away.
• Blurred vision, unpleasant taste or dry mouth, constipation or diarrhea, nausea, vomiting, cramps, changes in sex drive, increased sweating, headache, nightmares, weakness.	Continue. Call doctor when convenient.
Rare:	
• Rash or hives, breathing difficulty.	Discontinue. Call doctor right away.
• Hair loss.	Continue. Call doctor when convenient.

WARNINGS & PRECAUTIONS

Don't take if:

- You are allergic to benzphetamine, diethylpropion, mazindol, phendimetrazine or phentermine.
- You have glaucoma.
- You have taken MAO inhibitors within 2 weeks.
- You plan to become pregnant within medication period.
- You have a history of drug or alcohol abuse.
- You have irregular or rapid heartbeat.

Before you start, consult your doctor if:
- You have high blood pressure or heart disease.
- You have an overactive thyroid, nervous tension or anxiety.
- You have epilepsy.
- You will have surgery within 2 months, including dental surgery, requiring general or spinal anesthesia.
- You take any other nonprescription medicine.

Over age 60:
Adverse reactions and side effects may be more frequent and severe than in younger persons.

Pregnancy:
Risk factors vary for drugs in this group. See category list on page xviii and consult doctor.

Breast-feeding:
Safety not established. Consult doctor.

Infants & children:
Don't give to children younger than 12.

Prolonged use:
- Loses effectiveness. Avoid.
- Talk to your doctor about the need for follow-up medical examinations or laboratory studies.

Skin & sunlight:
No problems expected.

Driving, piloting or hazardous work:
Don't drive or pilot aircraft until you learn how medicine affects you. Don't work around dangerous machinery. Don't climb ladders or work in high places. Danger increases if you drink alcohol or take medicine affecting alertness and reflexes, such as antihistamines, tranquilizers, sedatives, pain medicine, narcotics and mind-altering drugs.

Discontinuing:
- Don't discontinue without consulting doctor. Dose may require gradual reduction if you have taken drug for a long time. Doses of other drugs may also require adjustment.
- Consult doctor if following symptoms occur after stopping the drug—depression, nausea and vomiting, stomach cramps, insomnia, nightmares, extreme tiredness or weakness.

Others:
- Don't increase dose without doctor's approval.
- Advise any doctor or dentist whom you consult that you take this medicine.

POSSIBLE INTERACTION WITH OTHER DRUGS

GENERIC NAME OR DRUG CLASS	COMBINED EFFECT
Antidiabetic agents,* oral or insulin	May require dosage adjustment of anti-diabetic agent.
Antihypertensives*	Decreased anti-hypertensive effect.
Appetite suppressants other*	Dangerous overstimulation.
Caffeine	Increased stimulant effect.
Central nervous system (CNS) depressants*	Increased depressive effects of both drugs.
Central nervous system (CNS) stimulants*	Increased stimulant effects of both drugs.
Guanethidine	Decreased guanethidine effect.
Methyldopa	Decreased methyldopa effect.
Monoamine oxidase (MAO) inhibitors*	Dangerous blood pressure rise.
Phenothiazines*	Decreased appetite suppressant effect.
Rauwolfia alkaloids*	Decreased effect of rauwolfia alkaloids.

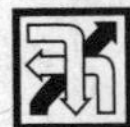

POSSIBLE INTERACTION WITH OTHER SUBSTANCES

INTERACTS WITH	COMBINED EFFECT
Alcohol:	Increased sedation.
Beverages: Caffeine drinks.	Excessive stimulation.
Cocaine:	Convulsions or excessive nervousness.
Foods:	None expected.
Marijuana:	Frequent use—Irregular heartbeat.
Tobacco:	None expected.

*See Glossary

ARIPIPRAZOLE

BRAND NAMES

Abilify
Abilify DiscMelt
Abilify Oral Solution

BASIC INFORMATION

Habit forming? Not expected to be
Prescription needed? Yes
Available as generic? No
Drug class: Antipsychotic

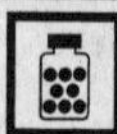

USES

- Treats nervous, mental and emotional conditions. Helps in managing the signs and symptoms of schizophrenia (treats positive symptoms such as hearing voices and negative symptoms such as social withdrawal).
- Treatment for bipolar disorder.
- Treatment for major depressive disorder (MDD).
- Treatment of irritability associated with autistic disorder in children ages 6 to 17 years.
- May be used for treatment of other disorders as determined by your doctor.

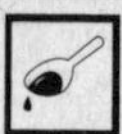

DOSAGE & USAGE INFORMATION

How to take:

- Tablet or capsule—Swallow with liquid. May be taken with or without food.
- Oral disintegrating tablet—Let tablet dissolve in mouth. Do not chew or swallow.
- Oral solution—Use the oral dosing cup provided with the bottle. Store open bottle in a refrigerator; can be used for up to 6 months after opening.
- An injectable form is given by a health care professional.

When to take:
Once a day at the same time each day. Always follow the advice of your doctor.

Continued next column

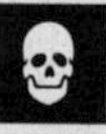

OVERDOSE

SYMPTOMS:
Unknown, possibly drowsiness and vomiting.
WHAT TO DO:
Overdose unlikely to threaten life. If person uses much larger amount than prescribed or if accidentally swallowed, call doctor or poison center control 1-800-222-1222 for help.

If you forget a dose:
Take as soon as you remember. If it is almost time for the next dose, wait for the next scheduled dose (don't double this dose).

What drug does:
The exact mechanism is unknown. It appears to block certain nerve impulses between nerve cells.

Time lapse before drug works:
1-4 weeks. A further increase in the dosage amount may be necessary to relieve symptoms for some patients. Do not increase dosage without your doctor's approval.

Don't take with:
Any other medicine or any dietary supplement without consulting your doctor or pharmacist.

POSSIBLE ADVERSE REACTIONS OR SIDE EFFECTS

SYMPTOMS	WHAT TO DO
Life-threatening:	
High fever, rapid pulse, profuse sweating, muscle rigidity, confusion and irritability, seizures (rare neuroleptic malignant syndrome).	Discontinue. Seek emergency treatment.
Common:	
Anxiety, insomnia, headache, stomach upset, vomiting, constipation, lightheadedness, restlessness (akathisia), weight loss.	Continue. Call doctor when convenient.
Infrequent:	
Runny nose, cough, skin rash, dry mouth, weight gain, drowsiness.	Continue. Call doctor when convenient.
Rare:	
• Tardive dyskinesia (involuntary movements, especially of the face, lips, jaw and tongue; sometimes involves twitching of hands or feet), high blood sugar (thirstiness, frequent urination, increased hunger, weakness).	Discontinue. Call doctor right away.
• Other symptoms causing concern, not listed above.	Continue. Call doctor when convenient.

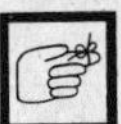

WARNINGS & PRECAUTIONS

Don't take if:
You are allergic to aripiprazole.

Before you start, consult your doctor if:
- You have or have had liver or kidney disease, heart disease or stroke.
- You have irregular heartbeat, problems with blood pressure or a blood disorder.
- You have depression, or a history of alcohol or drug abuse.
- You have a family history of, are at risk for, or have diabetes.
- You have difficulty in swallowing.
- You are allergic to any other medications.
- You have a history of seizures.

Over age 60:
- Adverse reactions and side effects may be more likely than in younger persons.
- Use of antipsychotic drugs in elderly patients with dementia-related psychosis may increase risk of death. Consult doctor.

Pregnancy:
Decide with your doctor if drug benefits justify any possible risk to unborn child. Risk category C (see page xviii).

Breast-feeding:
It is unknown if drug passes into milk. Avoid nursing until you finish medicine.

Infants & children:
- Used in the treatment of schizophrenia in adolescents 13 to 17 years of age.
- Used for treatment of manic and mixed episodes associated with bipolar disorder in ages 10-17.

Prolonged use:
Consult with your doctor on a regular basis while taking this drug to check your progress or to discuss any increase or changes in side effects, blood sugar levels, and the need for continued treatment.

Skin & sunlight:
No problems expected.

Driving, piloting or hazardous work:
Don't drive or pilot aircraft until you learn how medicine affects you. Don't work around dangerous machinery. Don't climb ladders or work in high places. Danger increases if you drink alcohol or take medicine affecting alertness and reflexes.

Discontinuing:
Don't discontinue this drug without consulting doctor even if you feel well. Dosage may require a gradual reduction before stopping.

Others:
- Get up slowly from a sitting or lying position to avoid any dizziness, faintness or lightheadedness.
- The drug may reduce the body's ability to reduce body temperature. Avoid getting overheated or dehydrated.
- Advise any doctor or dentist whom you consult that you take this medicine.
- Take medicine as directed. Do not increase or reduce dosage without doctor's approval.
- Consult doctor if weight loss is a problem.

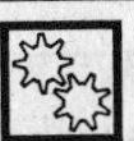

POSSIBLE INTERACTION WITH OTHER DRUGS

GENERIC NAME OR DRUG CLASS	COMBINED EFFECT
Enzyme inducers*	Decreased effect of aripiprazole.
Enzyme inhibitors*	Increased effect of aripiprazole.

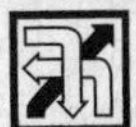

POSSIBLE INTERACTION WITH OTHER SUBSTANCES

INTERACTS WITH	COMBINED EFFECT
Alcohol:	Increased sedative affect. Avoid.
Beverages:	None expected.
Cocaine:	Effect not known. Best to avoid.
Foods:	None expected.
Marijuana:	Effect not known. Best to avoid.
Tobacco:	None expected.

*See Glossary

ASENAPINE

BRAND NAMES

Saphris

BASIC INFORMATION

Habit forming? No
Prescription needed? Yes
Available as generic? No
Drug class: Antipsychotic

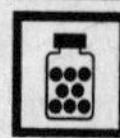

USES

- Treatment for schizophrenia.
- Treatment for acute manic or mixed episodes associated with bipolar disorder (manic-depression).

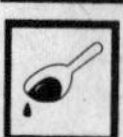

DOSAGE & USAGE INFORMATION

How to take:
Sublingual tablet—Follow prescription instructions to remove tablet from pack. Place tablet under the tongue and allow it to dissolve slowly (takes a few seconds). Don't swallow, crush or chew tablet. Don't eat or drink for 10 minutes after taking drug.

When to take:
Usually twice a day at the same times each day.

If you forget a dose:
Take as soon as you remember. If it is almost time for the next dose, wait for the next scheduled dose (don't double this dose).

What drug does:
The exact way the drug works is unknown. It appears to suppress excess levels of the brain chemicals dopamine and serotonin.

Time lapse before drug works:
Starts working within hours, but can take up to several weeks for full effect.

Don't take with:
Any other medicine or any dietary supplement without consulting your doctor or pharmacist.

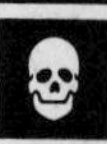

OVERDOSE

SYMPTOMS:
Agitation, confusion, severe dizziness, or uncontrolled muscle movements.
WHAT TO DO:
- **Dial 911 (emergency) for medical help or call poison control center 1-800-222-1222 for instructions.**
- **See emergency information on last 3 pages of this book.**

POSSIBLE ADVERSE REACTIONS OR SIDE EFFECTS

SYMPTOMS	WHAT TO DO
Life-threatening:	
Rare allergic reaction (hives, itching, rash, wheezing, tightness in chest, swelling of lips or tongue or throat).	Seek emergency treatment immediately.
Common:	
Dizziness, headache, drowsiness, unable to sit still, loss of feeling around the mouth, weight gain, restlessness.	Continue. Call doctor when convenient.
Infrequent:	
Dry mouth, tiredness, taste changes, increased appetite, joint aches, toothache, being agitated or anxious, indigestion, trouble sleeping, depression.	Continue. Call doctor when convenient.
Rare:	
• More or less urine output; fainting; loss of consciousness; trouble swallowing; sore throat, fever or chills; muscle pain or weakness or stiffness; fast, slow or irregular heartbeat; mental or mood changes; seizures; uncontrolled body movements (of arms, legs, tongue, jaw or cheeks); tremors; twitching; unusual sweating; high blood sugar symptoms (excess thirst and urination, dry mouth, fatigue); mouth or lip sores; white patches in mouth; sudden and severe headache; problem with speech or vision or balance; sudden numbness or weakness; unusual bleeding or bruising; suicidal thoughts or actions; fainting.	Discontinue. Call doctor right away.
• Other new symptoms that cause concern.	Continue. Call doctor when convenient.

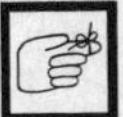

WARNINGS & PRECAUTIONS

Don't take if:
You are allergic to asenapine.

Before you start, consult your doctor if:
- You have or have had liver disease, heart disease, heart rhythm problems, stroke, QT prolongation, heart failure, blood vessel problems, low blood pressure, recent heart attack, breast cancer, Parkinson disease, low blood cell counts, trouble swallowing, hyperprolactinemia or seizures.
- You have or have had suicidal thoughts or attempts or alcohol abuse or dependence.
- Patient has Alzheimer's or dementia.
- You have a family history of, or have diabetes.
- You have tardive dyskinesia.
- You have hypokalemia (low potassium) or hypomagnesemia (low magnesium).
- You have neuroleptic malignant syndrome (serious or fatal problems may occur).

Over age 60:
- Adverse reactions and side effects may be more severe than in younger persons. A lower starting dosage is usually recommended.
- Use of antipsychotic drugs in elderly patients with dementia-related psychosis may increase risk of death. Consult doctor.

Pregnancy:
Decide with your doctor if drug benefits justify any possible risk to unborn child. Risk category C (see page xviii).

Breast-feeding:
It is unknown if drug passes into milk. Consult doctor for advice.

Infants & children:
Safety and efficacy has not been established. Use only under close medical supervision.

Prolonged use:
Consult with your doctor on a regular basis while taking this drug to monitor your progress, check for side effects and for recommended lab tests.

Skin & sunlight:
Drug may affect body's ability to maintain normal temperature. Use caution with strenuous exercising or exposure to extreme heat. Drink plenty of water to avoid dehydration.

Driving, piloting or hazardous work:
Don't drive or pilot aircraft until you learn how medicine affects you. Don't work around dangerous machinery. Don't climb ladders or work in high places. Danger increases if you drink alcohol or take medicine affecting alertness and reflexes.

Discontinuing:
Don't discontinue this drug without consulting doctor. Dosage may require a gradual reduction before stopping.

Others:
- Get up slowly from a sitting or lying position to avoid dizziness, faintness or lightheadedness.
- Advise any doctor or dentist whom you consult that you take this medicine.
- Take medicine only as directed. Do not change the dosage without doctor's approval.

POSSIBLE INTERACTION WITH OTHER DRUGS

GENERIC NAME OR DRUG CLASS	COMBINED EFFECT
Anticholinergics*	Increased risk of side effects of asenapine.
Antihypertensives*	Increased risk of low blood pressure.
Antiparkinsonism drugs*	Decreased effect of antiparkinsonism drug.
Central nervous system (CNS) depressants*	Increased sedative effect.
Enzyme inhibitors*	May increase effect of asenapine and/or enzyme inhibitor.
Metoclopramide	Increased risk of side effects of asenapine.
Fluvoxamine	Increased risk of side effects of asenapine.
QT interval prolongation-causing drugs*	Heart rhythm problems. Avoid.

POSSIBLE INTERACTION WITH OTHER SUBSTANCES

INTERACTS WITH	COMBINED EFFECT
Alcohol:	Increased sedative affect. Avoid.
Beverages: Grapefruit juice.	May increase effect of drug.
Cocaine:	Unknown. Avoid.
Foods: Grapefruit.	May increase effect of drug.
Marijuana:	Sedation. Avoid.
Tobacco:	None expected.

*See Glossary

ASPIRIN

BRAND NAMES

See full list of brand names in the *Generic and Brand Name Directory*, page 875.

BASIC INFORMATION

Habit forming? No
Prescription needed? No
Available as generic? Yes
Drug class: Analgesic, anti-inflammatory (nonsteroidal)

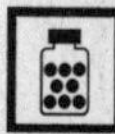

USES

- Reduces pain, fever, inflammation.
- Relieves swelling, stiffness, joint pain of arthritis or rheumatism.
- Antiplatelet effect to reduce chances of heart attack and/or stroke.

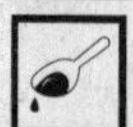

DOSAGE & USAGE INFORMATION

How to take:

- Tablet or capsule—Swallow with liquid or food to lessen stomach irritation.
- Extended-release tablet or capsule—Swallow each dose whole.
- Effervescent tablet—Dissolve in water.
- Chewing gum tablet—Chew completely. Don't swallow whole.
- Dispersible tablet—Dissolve in the mouth before swallowing.
- Chewable tablet—Chew before swallowing or dissolve in liquid before swallowing.

Continued next column

- Crystals—Let them dissolve on tongue.
- Suppository—Remove wrapper and moisten suppository with water. Gently insert into rectum, large end first.

When to take:
Pain, fever, inflammation—As needed, no more often than every 4 hours.

If you forget a dose:
Take as soon as you remember. If it is almost time for the next dose, wait for the next scheduled dose (don't double this dose).

What drug does:

- Affects hypothalamus, the part of the brain which regulates temperature by dilating small blood vessels in skin.
- Prevents clumping of platelets (small blood cells) so blood vessels remain open.
- Decreases prostaglandin effect.
- Suppresses body's pain messages.

Time lapse before drug works:
30 minutes for pain, fever, arthritis.

Don't take with:

- Tetracyclines. Space doses 1 hour apart.
- Any other medicine or any dietary supplement without consulting your doctor or pharmacist.

OVERDOSE

SYMPTOMS:

- **Mild overdose–Confusion, severe diarrhea, stomach pain, increased thirst, vision problems, ringing or buzzing in ears, dizziness, lightheadedness, severe headache.**
- **Severe overdose–Bloody urine; hallucinations; severe nervousness, excitement or confusion; shortness of breath; trouble breathing; convulsions.**
- **In some children–The only symptoms may be behavior changes, severe drowsiness or tiredness, fast or deep breathing.**

WHAT TO DO:

- **Dial 911 (emergency) for medical help or call poison control center 1-800-222-1222 for instructions.**
- **See emergency information on last 3 pages of this book.**

POSSIBLE ADVERSE REACTIONS OR SIDE EFFECTS

SYMPTOMS	WHAT TO DO
Life-threatening:	
Black or bloody vomit; blood in urine; difficulty breathing; hives, rash, intense itching, faintness soon after a dose (anaphylaxis).	Seek emergency treatment immediately.
Common:	
Heartburn, indigestion, mild nausea or vomiting.	Continue. Call doctor when convenient.
Infrequent:	
Trouble sleeping; rectal irritation (with suppository).	Continue. Call doctor when convenient.
Rare:	
Severe headache, convulsions, extreme drowsiness, flushing or other change in skin color, any loss of hearing, severe vomiting, swelling of face, vision problems, bloody or black stools, ringing in ears, severe or ongoing stomach cramps or pain (all symptoms more likely with repeated doses for long periods).	Discontinue. Call doctor right away or seek emergency treatment.

WARNINGS & PRECAUTIONS

Don't take if:

- You are allergic to aspirin or salicylates or nonsteroidal anti-inflammatory drugs.
- Aspirin has a strong vinegar-like odor, which means it has decomposed.

Before you start, consult your doctor if:
You have stomach or duodenal ulcers, gout, asthma, nasal polyps, a bleeding or blood clotting disorder, overactive thyroid, anemia, heart disease, high blood pressure, kidney or liver disease, hemophilia, glucose-6-phosphate dehydrogenase (G6PD) deficiency, hay fever.

Over age 60:

- Adverse reactions and side effects may be more frequent and severe.
- More likely to cause hidden bleeding in stomach or intestines. Watch for dark stools.

Pregnancy:
Risk category C; D in third trimester (see page xviii). Consult doctor.

Breast-feeding:
Drug passes into milk. Avoid drug or discontinue nursing until you finish medicine. Consult doctor for advice on maintaining milk supply.

Infants & children:

- Use only as advised by your child's doctor.
- Do not give to persons under age 18 who have fever and discomfort of viral illness, especially chicken pox and influenza. Aspirin can increase risk of Reye's syndrome.

Prolonged use:

- Talk to your doctor about the need for follow-up medical exams or lab studies.
- Kidney damage may result. Periodic kidney function tests recommended.

Skin & sunlight:
No special problems expected.

Driving, piloting or hazardous work:
No restrictions unless you feel drowsy.

Discontinuing:
For chronic illness, don't discontinue without doctor's advice until you complete prescribed dose, even though symptoms diminish or disappear.

Others:

- Consult doctor before taking aspirin routinely to treat or prevent heart conditions or stroke.
- Advise any doctor or dentist whom you consult about the use of this medicine. This is important if any surgery is planned.
- Consult doctor if you are taking aspirin for pain that lasts longer than 10 days (5 days for children), a fever that lasts more than 3 days, a sore throat lasts for over 2 days, or new or more severe symptoms develop.

*See Glossary

POSSIBLE INTERACTION WITH OTHER DRUGS

GENERIC NAME OR DRUG CLASS	COMBINED EFFECT
Acebutolol	Decreased anti-hypertensive effect of acebutolol.
Acetaminophen	Increased risk of adverse effects of both drugs.
Adrenocorticoids, systemic	Decreased aspirin effect.
Alendronate	Increased risk of stomach irritation.
Allopurinol	Decreased allopurinol effect.
Angiotensin-converting enzyme (ACE) inhibitors*	Decreased ACE inhibitor effect.
Antacids*	Decreased aspirin effect.
Anticoagulants*	Increased anti-coagulant effect. Abnormal bleeding.
Antidiabetic agents, oral*	Low blood sugar.
Anti-inflammatory drugs nonsteroidal (NSAIDs)*	Risk of stomach bleeding and ulcers and adverse effects.
Bumetanide	Possible aspirin toxicity.
Carteolol	Decreased anti-hypertensive effect of carteolol.

Continued on page 904

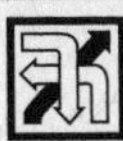

POSSIBLE INTERACTION WITH OTHER SUBSTANCES

INTERACTS WITH	COMBINED EFFECT
Alcohol:	Possible stomach irritation and bleeding. Avoid.
Beverages:	None expected.
Cocaine:	Unknown. Avoid.
Foods:	None expected.
Marijuana:	Unknown. Avoid.
Tobacco:	None expected.

ATOMOXETINE

BRAND NAMES

Strattera

BASIC INFORMATION

Habit forming? Not expected
Prescription needed? Yes
Available as generic? Yes
Drug class: Selective norepinephrine reuptake inhibitor

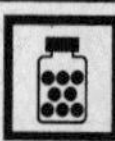

USES

Treatment of symptoms (inattention, hyperactivity and impulsiveness) of attention deficit hyperactivity disorder (ADHD) in children, adolescents and adults. The drug is used as part of a total treatment program for ADHD that may include other therapy measures (psychological, educational and social) for patients.

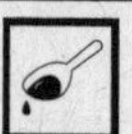

DOSAGE & USAGE INFORMATION

How to take:
Capsule—Swallow whole with liquid. It may be taken with or without food. Do not open capsule.

When to take:
- Once-a-day dose at the same time each day usually in the morning.
- Twice-a-day dose at the same times each day usually in the morning and then late afternoon or early evening.

If you forget a dose:
Take as soon as you remember. If it is almost time for your next dose, skip the missed dose and go back to your regular dosing schedule. Do not double doses.

Continued next column

OVERDOSE

SYMPTOMS:
Sleepiness, agitation, being hyperactive, abnormal behavior, stomach symptoms, blurred vision, fast heartbeat or dry mouth.
WHAT TO DO:
Overdose unlikely to threaten life. If person uses much larger amount than prescribed or if accidentally swallowed, call doctor or poison center control 1-800-222-1222 for help.

What drug does:
The exact mechanism by which the drug works is unknown. It appears to block a chemical (neurotransmitter) in the brain having to do with attention and activity.

Time lapse before drug works:
1 to 2 hours, but full benefits may take up to 4 weeks with possible dosage increases. Don't increase dosage without doctor's approval.

Don't take with:
Any other medicine or any dietary supplement without consulting your doctor or pharmacist.

POSSIBLE ADVERSE REACTIONS OR SIDE EFFECTS

SYMPTOMS	WHAT TO DO
Life-threatening:	
Rare allergic reaction (hives, itching, rash, trouble breathing, tightness in chest, swelling of lips or tongue or face); heart problems (chest pain, trouble breathing, fainting).	Seek emergency treatment immediately.
Common:	
In children—appetite loss, mood swings, nausea, vomiting, upset stomach, dizziness, tiredness, weight loss, runny nose, eyes tearing.	Continue. Call doctor when convenient.
Infrequent:	
In adults—insomnia, dry mouth, stomach pain, constipation, weight loss, loss of libido, impotence, ejaculatory difficulty, problems in urinating, menstrual pain; in adults and children—may feel lightheaded when getting up after sitting or lying down.	Continue. Call doctor when convenient.
Rare:	
Mental problems (hallucinations, manic behavior, becoming suspicious); liver problems (dark urine, itching, yellow skin or eyes, tender abdomen, flu-like symptoms); suicidal thoughts or behaviors.	Discontinue. Call doctor right away.

WARNINGS & PRECAUTIONS

Don't take if:
You are allergic to atomoxetine.

Before you start, consult your doctor if:
- You have liver or kidney disease.
- You have narrow angle glaucoma.
- You take MAO inhibitors* or have taken them in the last 14 days.
- You have heart problems, high or low blood pressure, or blood vessel disorder.
- You have history of mental disorders.
- You have history of alcohol or drug abuse.

Over age 60:
Drug has not been studied in this age group. Consult doctor.

Pregnancy:
Decide with your doctor if drug benefits justify any possible risk to unborn child. Risk category C (see page xviii).

Breast-feeding:
It is unknown if drug passes into breast milk. Avoid drug or discontinue nursing until you finish medicine. Consult doctor for advice on maintaining milk supply.

Infants & children:
- Use only under medical supervision for children 6 or older.
- Regular doctor visits are important to monitor drug's effectiveness and side effects.
- Read the warnings under Others.

Prolonged use:
It is unknown about the long term effects of taking this drug. Talk to your doctor about the need for follow-up medical examinations to check weight and height changes in children and adolescents, and to check the effectiveness of the drug in treating ADHD.

Skin & sunlight:
No problems expected.

Driving, piloting or hazardous work:
Don't drive or pilot aircraft until you learn how medicine affects you. Don't work around dangerous machinery. Don't climb ladders or work in high places. Danger increases if you drink alcohol or take other medicines affecting alertness and reflexes such as antihistamines, tranquilizers, sedatives, pain medicine, narcotics and mind-altering drugs.

Discontinuing:
No problems expected, but talk to your doctor before discontinuing the drug.

Others:
- Consult doctor if your child is not gaining weight or growing at an expected or satisfactory level.
- Will commonly cause a slight increase in blood pressure. Your doctor will monitor your blood pressure on a regular basis.
- In children and teenagers, the drug may increase suicidal thoughts or behaviors. Watch for any new or increased suicidal thoughts, mood or behavioral changes (e.g., becoming irritable or anxious). Call doctor right away if any symptoms occur.
- Rarely, the drug can cause liver damage. Call doctor if you have dark urine, itching, yellowing of skin or eyes, abdominal tenderness or flu-like symptoms.
- Rarely, use of this drug in children, teenagers and adults can lead to serious heart problems, including sudden unexplained death. Adults may have stroke or heart attack. Patients with heart defects or serious heart problems are more at risk. Consult doctor.
- Consult doctor if new mental symptoms occur (e.g., abnormal thoughts or behaviors).
- Follow your doctor's recommendation for any additional measures for treating ADHD.
- Advise any doctor or dentist whom you consult about the use of this medicine.

POSSIBLE INTERACTION WITH OTHER DRUGS

GENERIC NAME OR DRUG CLASS	COMBINED EFFECT
Beta agonists*	Increased risk of heart problems.
Enzyme inhibitors*	May increase effect of atomoxetine.
Monoamine oxidase (MAO) inhibitors*	Serious reactions (potentially fatal). Take at least 2 weeks apart.
Vasoconstrictors* (vasopressors)	May increase heart rate and/or blood pressure.

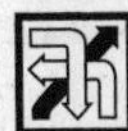

POSSIBLE INTERACTION WITH OTHER SUBSTANCES

INTERACTS WITH	COMBINED EFFECT
Alcohol:	None expected. Best to avoid.
Beverages:	None expected.
Cocaine:	Unknown. Avoid.
Foods:	None expected.
Marijuana:	Unknown. Avoid.
Tobacco:	None expected. Best to avoid.

*See Glossary

ATOVAQUONE

BRAND NAMES

Malarone
Mepron

BASIC INFORMATION

Habit forming? No
Prescription needed? Yes
Available as generic? No
Drug class: Antiprotozoal, antimalarial.

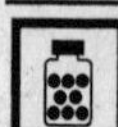

USES

- Treats mild to moderate pneumocystis jiroveci pneumonia.
- May be effective for other parasitic infections such as toxoplasmosis and malaria.

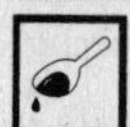

DOSAGE & USAGE INFORMATION

How to take:

- Tablet—Swallow with liquid. Take with a meal. If you cannot swallow whole, crumble tablet and take with liquid or food.
- Suspension—Follow instructions provided with product.

When to take:
At the same times each day. Take with meals that are high in fat (eggs, cheese, butter, milk, meat, pizza, nuts) to increase absorption.

If you forget a dose:
Take as soon as you remember. If it is almost time for the next dose, wait for the next scheduled dose (don't double this dose).

What drug does:
Stops harmful growth of susceptible organisms.

Time lapse before drug works:
3 weeks.

Don't take with:
Any other medicine or any dietary supplement without consulting your doctor or pharmacist.

OVERDOSE

SYMPTOMS:
None expected.
WHAT TO DO:
Overdose unlikely to threaten life. If person uses much larger amount than prescribed or if accidentally swallowed, call doctor or poison control center 1-800-222-1222 for help.

POSSIBLE ADVERSE REACTIONS OR SIDE EFFECTS

SYMPTOMS	WHAT TO DO
Life-threatening: None expected.	
Common:	
• Fever, skin rash.	Discontinue. Call doctor right away.
• Nausea or vomiting, diarrhea, headache, cough, trouble sleeping.	Continue. Call doctor when convenient.
Infrequent: None expected.	
Rare: None expected.	

WARNINGS & PRECAUTIONS

Don't take if:
You are allergic to atovaquone.

Before you start, consult your doctor if:
You have any gastrointestinal disorder.

Over age 60:
No problems expected.

Pregnancy:
Discuss with your doctor whether drug benefits justify risk to unborn child. Risk category C (see page xviii).

Breast-feeding:
Not known if drug passes into breast milk. Avoid drug or discontinue nursing until you finish medicine. Consult doctor for advice on maintaining milk supply.

Infants & children:
Give only under close medical supervision.

Prolonged use:
Not intended for long-term use.

Skin & sunlight:
No problems expected.

Driving, piloting or hazardous work:
No problems expected.

Discontinuing:
No problems expected.

Others:
- Advise any doctor or dentist whom you consult that you take this medicine.
- May affect the results in some medical tests.
- Talk to your doctor about the need for follow-up medical examinations or laboratory studies to check blood counts and liver function.

POSSIBLE INTERACTION WITH OTHER DRUGS

GENERIC NAME OR DRUG CLASS	COMBINED EFFECT
None significant.	

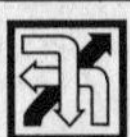

POSSIBLE INTERACTION WITH OTHER SUBSTANCES

INTERACTS WITH	COMBINED EFFECT
Alcohol:	None expected.
Beverages:	None expected.
Cocaine:	None expected.
Foods:	None expected.
Marijuana:	None expected.
Tobacco:	None expected.

ATROPINE, HYOSCYAMINE, METHENAMINE, METHYLENE BLUE, PHENYLSALICYLATE & BENZOIC ACID

BRAND NAMES

Atrosept	Urimed
Dolsed	Urinary Antiseptic No. 2
Hexalol	Urised
Prosed/DS	Uritab
Trac Tabs 2X	Uritab
UAA	Uritin
Uribel	Urogesic-Blue
Uridon Modified	Uro-Ves

BASIC INFORMATION

Habit forming? No
Prescription needed? Yes
Available as generic? No
Drug class: Analgesic (urinary), antispasmodic, anti-infective (urinary)

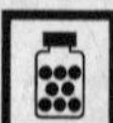

USES

A combination drug to control infection, spasms and pain caused by urinary tract infections.

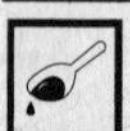

DOSAGE & USAGE INFORMATION

How to take:
Tablet—Swallow with liquid or food to lessen stomach irritation.

When to take:
30 minutes before meals (unless directed otherwise by doctor).

If you forget a dose:
Take as soon as you remember. If it is almost time for the next dose, wait for the next scheduled dose (don't double this dose).

Continued next column

OVERDOSE

SYMPTOMS:
Dilated pupils, rapid pulse and breathing, dizziness, fever, hallucinations, confusion, slurred speech, agitation, flushed face, convulsions, coma.
WHAT TO DO:
- **Dial 911 (emergency) for medical help or call poison control center 1-800-222-1222 for instructions.**
- **See emergency information on last 3 pages of this book.**

What drug does:
Makes urine acid. Blocks nerve impulses at parasympathetic nerve endings, preventing muscle contractions and gland secretions of organs involved. Methenamine destroys some germs.

Time lapse before drug works:
15 to 30 minutes.

Don't take with:
- Antacids* or antidiarrheals* at the same time.
- Any other medicine or any dietary supplement without consulting your doctor or pharmacist.

POSSIBLE ADVERSE REACTIONS OR SIDE EFFECTS

SYMPTOMS	WHAT TO DO
Life-threatening:	
Heartbeat irregularity, shortness of breath or difficulty breathing.	Seek emergency treatment immediately.
Common:	
Dry mouth, throat, ears, nose.	Continue. Call doctor when convenient.
Infrequent:	
• Flushed, red face; drowsiness; difficult urination; nausea and vomiting; abdominal pain; ringing or buzzing in ears; severe drowsiness; back pain; lightheadedness.	Discontinue. Call doctor right away.
• Headache, nasal congestion, altered taste.	Continue. Call doctor when convenient.
Rare:	
Blurred vision; pain in eyes; skin rash, hives.	Discontinue. Seek emergency treatment.

WARNINGS & PRECAUTIONS

Don't take if:
- You are allergic to any of the ingredients or aspirin.
- There is brain damage in a child.
- You have glaucoma.

ATROPINE, HYOSCYAMINE, METHENAMINE, METHYLENE BLUE, PHENYLSALICYLATE & BENZOIC ACID

Before you start, consult your doctor if:
- You are on any special diet such as low-sodium.
- You have had a hiatal hernia, bronchitis, liver disease, asthma, stomach or duodenal ulcers.
- You have asthma, nasal polyps, bleeding disorder, glaucoma or enlarged prostate.
- You will have any surgery within 2 months.
- You have heart disease.

Over age 60:
- Adverse reactions and side effects may be more frequent and severe than in younger persons.
- More likely to cause hidden bleeding in stomach or intestines. Watch for dark stools.

Pregnancy:
Risk factors vary for drugs in this group. See category list on page xviii and consult doctor.

Breast-feeding:
Drug passes into milk. Avoid or discontinue nursing until you finish medicine.

Infants & children:
Side effects more likely. Not recommended in children under 12.

Prolonged use:
May lead to constipation or kidney damage. Request lab studies to monitor effects of prolonged use.

Skin & sunlight:
No problems expected.

Driving, piloting or hazardous work:
May disqualify for piloting aircraft during time you take medicine.

Discontinuing:
May be unnecessary to finish medicine. Follow your symptoms and doctor's advice.

Others:
- Salicylates can complicate surgery, pregnancy, labor and delivery, and illness.
- Urine tests for blood sugar may be inaccurate.
- The generic ingredients in the brand names listed may vary. Read labels.
- Ask doctor about drinking cranberry juice to help make urine more acid.

POSSIBLE INTERACTION WITH OTHER DRUGS

GENERIC NAME OR DRUG CLASS	COMBINED EFFECT
Allopurinol	Decreased allopurinol effect.
Amantadine	Increased atropine and belladonna effect.
Antacids*	Decreased salicylate and methenamine effect.
Anticoagulants*	Increased anti-coagulant effect. Abnormal bleeding.
Anticholinergics, other*	Increased atropine and belladonna effect.
Antidepressants, other*	Increased sedation.
Antidiabetics, oral*	Low blood sugar.
Antifungals, azoles	Reduced azole effect.
Antihistamines*	Increased atropine and hyoscyamine effect.
Anti-inflammatory drugs, nonsteroidal (NSAIDs)*	Risk of stomach bleeding and ulcers.
Aspirin	Likely salicylate toxicity.
Beta-adrenergic blocking agents*	Decreased anti-hypertensive effect.
Carbonic anhydrase inhibitors*	Decreased methenamine effect.

Continued on page 904

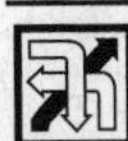

POSSIBLE INTERACTION WITH OTHER SUBSTANCES

INTERACTS WITH	COMBINED EFFECT
Alcohol:	Excessive sedation. Possible stomach irritation and bleeding. Avoid.
Beverages:	None expected.
Cocaine:	Excessively rapid heartbeat. Avoid.
Foods:	None expected.
Marijuana:	Drowsiness and dry mouth. May slow body's recovery.
Tobacco:	Dry mouth.

***See Glossary**

ATTAPULGITE

BRAND NAMES

Diar-Aid
Diasorb
Fowlers Diarrhea Tablets
Kaopectate
Kaopectate Advanced Formula
Kaopectate Maximum Strength
Rheaban
St. Joseph Antidiarrheal

BASIC INFORMATION

Habit forming? No
Prescription needed? No
Available as generic? Yes
Drug class: Antidiarrheal

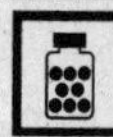

USES

Treats diarrhea. Used in conjunction with fluids, appropriate diet and rest. Treats symptoms only. Does not cure any disorder that causes diarrhea.

DOSAGE & USAGE INFORMATION

How to take:

- Tablet—Swallow with liquid. If you can't swallow whole, crumble tablet and take with liquid or food. Instructions to take on empty stomach mean 1 hour before or 2 hours after eating.
- Chewable tablet—Chew well before swallowing.
- Oral suspension—Follow label instructions.

When to take:
2 hours before or 3 hours after taking any other oral medications. Outside of this restriction, take a dose after each loose bowel movement until diarrhea is controlled.

If you forget a dose:
Take as soon as you remember, then resume regular schedule.

Continued next column

OVERDOSE

SYMPTOMS:
None expected.
WHAT TO DO:
Overdose unlikely to threaten life. If person uses much larger amount than prescribed or if accidentally swallowed, call doctor or poison control center 1-800-222-1222 for help.

What drug does:
Absorbs bacteria and toxins and reduces water loss. Attapulgite does not get absorbed into the body.

Time lapse before drug works:
5 to 8 hours.

Don't take with:
Any other medicine or any dietary supplement without consulting your doctor or pharmacist.

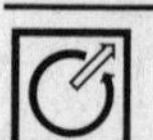

POSSIBLE ADVERSE REACTIONS OR SIDE EFFECTS

SYMPTOMS	WHAT TO DO
Life-threatening: None expected.	
Common: None expected.	
Infrequent: Constipation (usually mild and of short duration).	Continue. Call doctor when convenient.
Rare: None expected.	

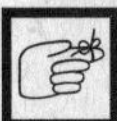

WARNINGS & PRECAUTIONS

Don't take if:
- You are allergic to attapulgite.
- You or your doctor suspects intestinal obstruction.

Before you start, consult your doctor if:
You are dehydrated (signs are a dry mouth, loose skin, sunken eyes and parched lips).

Over age 60:
- Dehydration is more likely in this age group.
- Side effects of constipation are more likely.

Pregnancy:
Risk category not designated. See list on page xviii and consult doctor.

Breast-feeding:
No problems expected, but consult doctor.

Infants & children:
Use only under close medical supervision for children up to 3 years of age. This age group is quite susceptible to fluid and electrolyte loss.

Prolonged use:
Not intended for prolonged use.

Skin & sunlight:
No special problems expected.

Driving, piloting or hazardous work:
No special problems expected.

Discontinuing:
May be unnecessary to finish medicine. Follow doctor's instructions.

Others:
No special problems expected.

POSSIBLE INTERACTION WITH OTHER DRUGS

GENERIC NAME OR DRUG CLASS	COMBINED EFFECT
Digitalis	May decrease effectiveness of digitalis.
Lincomycins*	May decrease effectiveness of lincomycins.
Any other medicine taken by mouth	When taken at the same time, neither drug may be as effective. Take other medicines 2 hours before or 3 hours after attapulgite.

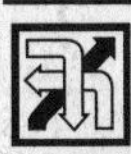

POSSIBLE INTERACTION WITH OTHER SUBSTANCES

INTERACTS WITH	COMBINED EFFECT
Alcohol:	None expected.
Beverages:	None expected.
Cocaine:	None expected.
Foods: Prunes, prune juice and other fruits or foods that may cause diarrhea.	Decreased effect of attapulgite.
Marijuana:	None expected.
Tobacco:	None expected.

*See Glossary

AZATHIOPRINE

BRAND NAMES

Azasan
Imuran

BASIC INFORMATION

Habit forming? No
Prescription needed? Yes
Available as generic? Yes
Drug class: Immunosuppressant, antirheumatic

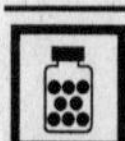

USES

- Protects against rejection of transplanted organs (e.g., kidney, heart).
- Treats severe active rheumatoid arthritis and other immunologic diseases if simpler treatment plans have been ineffective.

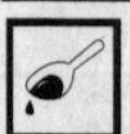

DOSAGE & USAGE INFORMATION

How to take:
Tablet—Swallow with liquid. If you can't swallow whole, crumble tablet and take with liquid or food. Instructions to take on empty stomach mean 1 hour before or 2 hours after eating.

When to take:
Follow your doctor's instructions. Usually once a day.

If you forget a dose:
Take as soon as you remember. If it is almost time for the next dose, wait for the next scheduled dose (don't double this dose).

What drug does:
Unknown; probably inhibits synthesis of DNA and RNA.

Time lapse before drug works:
6 to 8 weeks.

Don't take with:
Any other medicines (including over-the-counter drugs such as cough and cold medicines, laxatives, antacids, diet pills, caffeine, nose drops or vitamins) without consulting your doctor.

OVERDOSE

SYMPTOMS:
None expected.
WHAT TO DO:
Overdose unlikely to threaten life. If person uses much larger amount than prescribed or if accidentally swallowed, call doctor or poison control center 1-800-222-1222 for help.

POSSIBLE ADVERSE REACTIONS OR SIDE EFFECTS

SYMPTOMS	WHAT TO DO
Life-threatening:	
Rapid heart rate, sudden fever, muscle or joint pain, cough, shortness of breath.	Seek emergency treatment immediately.
Common:	
• Infection or low blood count causing fever and chills, back pain, cough, painful urination; anemia (tiredness or weakness); nausea; vomiting.	Discontinue. Call doctor right away.
• Appetite loss.	Continue. Call doctor when convenient.
Infrequent:	
Jaundice (yellow eyes, skin), skin rash.	Discontinue. Call doctor right away.
Rare:	
Low platelet count causing bleeding or bruising, tarry or black stools, bloody urine, red spots under skin; severe abdominal pain; mouth sores.	Discontinue. Call doctor right away.

WARNINGS & PRECAUTIONS

Don't take if:
- You are allergic to azathioprine.
- You have chicken pox.
- You have shingles (herpes zoster).

Before you start, consult your doctor if:
- You have gout.
- You have liver or kidney disease.
- You have an infection.

Over age 60:
Adverse reactions and side effects may be more frequent and severe than in younger persons. You may need smaller doses for shorter periods of time.

Pregnancy:
Risk to unborn child outweighs drug benefits. Don't use. Risk category D (see page xviii).

Breast-feeding:
Drug passes into milk. Avoid drug or discontinue nursing until you finish medicine. Consult doctor for advice on maintaining milk supply.

Infants & children:
No special problems expected.

Prolonged use:
- May increase likelihood of problems upon discontinuing.
- Talk to your doctor about the need for follow-up medical examinations or laboratory studies to check thyroid function, liver function, electrolytes (sodium, potassium, chloride), blood pressure and complete blood counts (white blood count, platelet count, red blood cell count, hemoglobin, hematocrit) every week during first two months, then once a month.

Skin & sunlight:
No special problems expected.

Driving, piloting or hazardous work:
Avoid if you feel confused, drowsy or dizzy.

Discontinuing:
May still experience symptoms of bone marrow depression, such as: blood in stools, fever or chills, blood spots under the skin, back pain, hoarseness, bloody urine. If any of these occur, call your doctor right away.

Others:
- Advise any doctor or dentist whom you consult that you take this medicine.
- May affect results in some medical tests.

POSSIBLE INTERACTION WITH OTHER DRUGS

GENERIC NAME OR DRUG CLASS	COMBINED EFFECT
Allopurinol	Greatly increased azathioprine activity.
Antivirals, HIV/AIDS*	Increased risk of pancreatitis.
Clozapine	Toxic effect on bone marrow.
Immunosuppressants, other*	Higher risk of developing infection or malignancies.
Levamisole	Increased risk of bone marrow depression.
Tiopronin	Increased risk of toxicity to bone marrow.
Vaccines	May decrease effectiveness or cause disease itself.

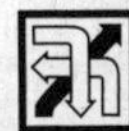

POSSIBLE INTERACTION WITH OTHER SUBSTANCES

INTERACTS WITH	COMBINED EFFECT
Alcohol:	No special problems expected.
Beverages:	No special problems expected.
Cocaine:	Increased likelihood of adverse reactions. Avoid.
Foods:	No special problems expected.
Marijuana:	Increased likelihood of adverse reactions. Avoid.
Tobacco:	No special problems expected.

***See Glossary**

AZELAIC ACID

BRAND NAMES

Azelex
Finacea
Finevin

BASIC INFORMATION

Habit forming? No
Prescription needed? Yes
Available as generic? No
Drug class: Antiacne agent, hypopigmentation agent

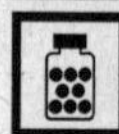

USES

- Topical treatment for mild to moderate acne vulgaris.
- May be used for treatment of melasma (chloasma), a skin condition in which brownish patches of pigmentation appear on the face.

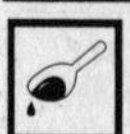

DOSAGE & USAGE INFORMATION

How to use:
Cream—Wash the affected skin area and then apply the prescribed amount of cream and rub it into the skin. Rub it in thoroughly, but gently, to avoid irritation. Wash hands after applying.

When to use:
Usually twice a day (morning and evening).

If you forget a dose:
Use as soon as you remember.

What drug does:
The drug helps prevents the development of new acne lesions (whiteheads), but the exact mechanism is unknown. It appears to have some antibacterial and anti-inflammatory effect, and also helps in skin renewal.

Time lapse before drug works:
Results should be visible in about 4 weeks, but full benefits may take months.

Don't use with:
Other topical medications without consulting your doctor or pharmacist.

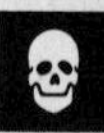

OVERDOSE

SYMPTOMS:
None expected.
WHAT TO DO:
If person accidentally swallows drug, call doctor or poison control center 1-800-222-1222 for help.

POSSIBLE ADVERSE REACTIONS OR SIDE EFFECTS

SYMPTOMS	WHAT TO DO
Life-threatening: None expected.	
Common: Peeling, itching, redness or dryness of skin; tingling, burning or stinging may occur when medicine first used.	Continue. Call doctor when convenient.
Infrequent: None expected.	
Rare: Lightening of skin or white spots in persons with darker complexions.	Discontinue. Call doctor when. convenient.

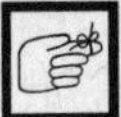

WARNINGS & PRECAUTIONS

Don't use if:
You are sensitive to azelaic acid.

Before you start, consult your doctor if:
- You are allergic to any medicine, food or other substance, or have a family history of allergies.
- You have a dark complexion.

Over age 60:
No special problems expected, however the drug has not been tested extensively in this age group.

Pregnancy:
Consult doctor. Risk category B (see page xviii).

Breast-feeding:
No special problems expected. Consult doctor.

Infants & children:
Normally not used in this age group. Safety and effectiveness in children under age 12 has not been established.

Prolonged use:
No problems expected.

Skin & sunlight:
No problems expected.

Driving, piloting or hazardous work:
No problems expected.

Discontinuing:
No problems expected.

Others:
- Use as directed. Don't increase or decrease dosage without doctor's approval. Using more of the cream or using it more frequently than prescribed won't improve results and may cause excessive skin irritation.
- The side effects involving skin irritation usually go away with continued use. If they continue beyond 4 weeks, or are severe, consult doctor about reducing the dosage to once a day.
- You may use water-based cosmetics while undergoing treatment with this drug.

POSSIBLE INTERACTION WITH OTHER DRUGS

GENERIC NAME OR DRUG CLASS	COMBINED EFFECT
None expected.	

POSSIBLE INTERACTION WITH OTHER SUBSTANCES

INTERACTS WITH	COMBINED EFFECT
Alcohol:	None expected.
Beverages:	None expected.
Cocaine:	None expected.
Foods:	None expected.
Marijuana:	None expected.
Tobacco:	None expected.

BACLOFEN

BRAND NAMES

Kemstro Lioresal

BASIC INFORMATION

Habit forming? No
Prescription needed? Yes
Available as generic? Yes
Drug class: Muscle relaxant

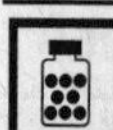

USES

- Relieves spasms, cramps and spasticity of muscles caused by medical problems, including multiple sclerosis and spine injuries.
- Reduces number and severity of trigeminal neuralgia attacks.

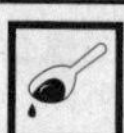

DOSAGE & USAGE INFORMATION

How to take:
- Tablet—Swallow with liquid or food to lessen stomach irritation.
- Oral disintegrating tablet—Dissolves in the mouth.

When to take:
3 or 4 times daily as directed.

If you forget a dose:
Take as soon as you remember. If it is almost time for the next dose, wait for the next scheduled dose (don't double this dose).

What drug does:
Blocks body's pain and reflex messages to brain.

Time lapse before drug works:
Variable. Few hours to weeks.

Don't take with:
Any other medicine or any dietary supplement without consulting your doctor or pharmacist.

OVERDOSE

SYMPTOMS:
Blurred vision, blindness, difficult breathing, vomiting, drowsiness, muscle weakness, convulsive seizures.

WHAT TO DO:
- **Dial 911 (emergency) for medical help or call poison control center 1-800-222-1222 for instructions.**
- **If person is unconscious, check breathing and pulse. If not breathing, begin mouth-to-mouth rescue breathing. If heart is not beating, begin chest compressions.**
- **See emergency information on last 3 pages of this book.**

POSSIBLE ADVERSE REACTIONS OR SIDE EFFECTS

SYMPTOMS	WHAT TO DO
Life-threatening: In case of overdose, see previous column.	
Common: Dizziness, lightheadedness, nausea, drowsiness, confusion.	Continue. Call doctor when convenient.
Infrequent:	
• Rash with itching, numbness or tingling in hands or feet.	Discontinue. Call doctor right away.
• Headache, stomach pain, diarrhea or constipation, loss of appetite, muscle weakness, difficult or painful urination, sexual problems, stuffy nose, clumsiness, slurred speech, insomnia.	Continue. Call doctor when convenient.
Rare:	
• Fainting, weakness, hallucinations, depression, chest or muscle pain, pounding heartbeat.	Discontinue. Call doctor right away.
• Ringing in ears, lowered blood pressure, dry mouth, weight gain, taste change, overexcitement.	Continue. Call doctor when convenient.

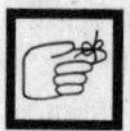

WARNINGS & PRECAUTIONS

Don't take if:
- You are allergic to any muscle relaxant.
- Muscle spasm is due to strain or sprain.

Before you start, consult your doctor if:
- You have Parkinson's disease.
- You have cerebral palsy.
- You have had a recent stroke.
- You have had a recent head injury.
- You have arthritis, diabetes or epilepsy.
- You have psychosis.
- You have kidney disease.
- You will have surgery within 2 months, including dental surgery, requiring general or spinal anesthesia.

Over age 60:
Adverse reactions and side effects may be more frequent and severe than in younger persons.

Pregnancy:
Decide with your doctor if drug benefits justify risk to unborn child. Risk category C (see page xviii).

Breast-feeding:
Avoid nursing or discontinue until you finish medicine. Consult doctor about maintaining milk supply.

Infants & children:
Not recommended.

Prolonged use:
Epileptic patients should be monitored with EEGs. Diabetics should more closely monitor blood sugar levels. Obtain periodic liver function tests.

Skin & sunlight:
No problems expected.

Driving, piloting or hazardous work:
Don't drive or pilot aircraft until you learn how medicine affects you. Don't work around dangerous machinery. Don't climb ladders or work in high places. Danger increases if you drink alcohol or take medicine affecting alertness and reflexes, such as antihistamines, tranquilizers, sedatives, pain medicine, narcotics and mind-altering drugs.

Discontinuing:
Don't discontinue without consulting doctor. Dose may require gradual reduction if you have taken drug for a long time. Doses of other drugs may also require adjustment.

Others:
Advise any doctor or dentist whom you consult that you take this medicine.

POSSIBLE INTERACTION WITH OTHER DRUGS

GENERIC NAME OR DRUG CLASS	COMBINED EFFECT
Anesthetics, general*	Increased sedation. Low blood pressure. Avoid.
Antidiabetic drugs,* insulin or oral	Need to adjust diabetes medicine dosage.
Central nervous system (CNS) depressants*	Increased sedation. Low blood pressure. Avoid.
Clozapine	Toxic effect on the central nervous system.
Ethinamate	Dangerous increased effects of ethinamate. Avoid combining.
Fluoxetine	Increased depressant effects of both drugs.
Guanfacine	May increase depressant effects of either drug.
Leucovorin	High alcohol content of leucovorin may cause adverse effects.
Methyprylon	Increased sedative effect, perhaps to dangerous level. Avoid.
Nabilone	Greater depression of the central nervous system.
Sertraline	Increased depressive effects of both drugs.

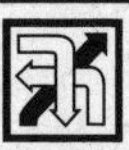

POSSIBLE INTERACTION WITH OTHER SUBSTANCES

INTERACTS WITH	COMBINED EFFECT
Alcohol:	Increased sedation. Low blood pressure. Avoid.
Beverages:	None expected.
Cocaine:	Increased spasticity. Avoid.
Foods:	None expected.
Marijuana:	Increased spasticity. Avoid.
Tobacco:	May interfere with absorption of medicine.

***See Glossary**

BARBITURATES

GENERIC AND BRAND NAMES

See full list of generic and brand names in the *Generic and Brand Name Directory*, page 875.

BASIC INFORMATION

Habit forming? Yes
Prescription needed? Yes
Available as generic? Yes, for some
Drug class: Sedative-hypnotic agent, anticonvulsant

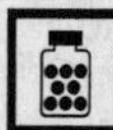

USES

- Reduces likelihood of seizures (tonic-clonic seizure pattern and simple partial) in epilepsy.
- Preventive treatment for febrile seizures.
- Reduces anxiety or nervous tension.
- Used in combination drugs to treat gastro-intestinal disorders, headaches and asthma.
- Aids sleep at night (on a short-term basis).

DOSAGE & USAGE INFORMATION

How to take:

- Capsule—Swallow with liquid. If you can't swallow whole, open capsule and take with liquid or food. Take on empty stomach (1 hour before or 2 hours after eating).
- Elixir—Swallow with liquid.
- Rectal suppository—Remove wrapper and moisten suppository with water. Gently insert into rectum, pointed end first. If suppository is too soft, chill first in refrigerator or cool water.
- Tablet—Swallow with liquid or food to lessen stomach irritation. If you can't swallow whole, crumble tablet and take with liquid or food.

When to take:
At the same times each day.

Continued next column

OVERDOSE

SYMPTOMS:
Deep sleep, trouble breathing, weak pulse, coma.
WHAT TO DO:

- **Dial 911 (emergency) for medical help or call poison control center 1-800-222-1222 for instructions.**
- **If person is unconscious, check breathing and pulse. If not breathing, begin mouth-to-mouth rescue breathing. If heart is not beating, begin chest compressions.**
- **See emergency information on last 3 pages of this book.**

If you forget a dose:
Take as soon as you remember. If it is almost time for the next dose, wait for the next scheduled dose (don't double this dose).

What drug does:
Blocks the transmission of nerve impulses from the brain to other parts of the body.

Time lapse before drug works:
60 minutes, but will take several weeks for maximum antiepilepsy effect.

Don't take with:
Any other medicine or any dietary supplement without consulting your doctor or pharmacist.

POSSIBLE ADVERSE REACTIONS OR SIDE EFFECTS

SYMPTOMS	WHAT TO DO
Life-threatening:	
Rare allergic reaction—may have hives, rash, itching, swelling, trouble breathing, wheezing, chest pain, dizziness, faintness.	Seek emergency treatment immediately.
Common:	
Dizziness, drowsiness, clumsiness, unsteadiness, signs of addiction.*	Continue. Call doctor when convenient.
Infrequent:	
Confusion, headache, irritability, feeling faint, nausea, vomiting, depression, nightmares, trouble sleeping.	Continue, but call doctor right away.
Rare:	
Agitation, slow heartbeat, difficult breathing, bleeding sores on lips, fever, chest pain, unexplained bleeding or bruising, muscle or joint pain, skin rash or hives, thickened or scaly skin, white spots in mouth, tightness in chest, face swelling, sore throat, yellow eyes or skin, hallucinations, unusual tiredness or weakness, sleep-related behaviors.*	Continue, but call doctor right away.

WARNINGS & PRECAUTIONS

Don't take if:

- You are allergic to any barbiturate.
- You have porphyria.

Before you start, consult your doctor if:
- You have epilepsy, kidney or liver problems, asthma, anemia or chronic pain.
- You will have surgery within 2 months, including dental surgery, requiring anesthesia.

Over age 60:
Adverse reactions and side effects may be more frequent and severe than in younger persons. Use small doses.

Pregnancy:
Risk to unborn child outweighs drug benefits. Don't use. Risk category D (see page xviii).

Breast-feeding:
Drug passes into milk. Avoid drug or discontinue nursing until you finish medicine. Consult doctor for advice on maintaining milk supply.

Infants & children:
Use only under doctor's supervision.

Prolonged use:
- May cause addiction, anemia, chronic intoxication. Unlikely to occur with the usual anticonvulsant or sedative dosage levels.
- May lower body temperature, making exposure to cold temperatures hazardous.
- Talk to your doctor about the need for follow-up medical examinations or laboratory studies to check blood sugar, kidney function.

Skin & sunlight:
No problems expected.

Driving, piloting or hazardous work:
Don't drive or pilot aircraft until you learn how medicine affects you. Don't work around dangerous machinery. Don't climb ladders or work in high places. Danger increases if you drink alcohol or take medicine affecting alertness and reflexes.

Discontinuing:
If you become addicted, don't stop taking barbiturates suddenly. Seek medical help for safe withdrawal.

Others:
- May affect results in some medical tests.
- Barbiturate addiction is common. Withdrawal effects may be fatal.
- Advise any doctor or dentist whom you consult that you take this medicine.

POSSIBLE INTERACTION WITH OTHER DRUGS

GENERIC NAME OR DRUG CLASS	COMBINED EFFECT
Adrenocorticoids, systemic	Decreased effect of prednisone.
Anticoagulants, oral*	Decreased effect of anticoagulant.
Anticonvulsants*	Changed seizure patterns.
Antidepressants, tricyclic*	Decreased anti-depressant effect. Possible dangerous oversedation.
Antidiabetic, agents, oral*	Increased effect of barbiturate.
Antihistamines*	Dangerous sedation. Avoid.
Aspirin	Decreased aspirin effect.
Beta-adrenergic blocking agents*	Decreased effect of beta-adrenergic blocker.
Carbamazepine	Decreased carbamazepine effect.
Carteolol	Increased barbiturate effect. Dangerous sedation.
Clozapine	Toxic effect on the central nervous system.
Contraceptives, oral*	Decreased contraceptive effect.
Dextrothyroxine	Decreased barbiturate effect.
Doxycycline	Decreased doxycycline effect.
Griseofulvin	Decreased griseofulvin effect.
Lamotrigine	Decreased lamotrigine effect.
Leukotriene modifiers	Decreased montelukast effect.

Continued on page 905

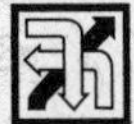

POSSIBLE INTERACTION WITH OTHER SUBSTANCES

INTERACTS WITH	COMBINED EFFECT
Alcohol:	Possible fatal oversedation. Avoid.
Beverages:	None expected.
Cocaine:	Decreased barbiturate effect.
Foods:	None expected.
Marijuana:	Excessive sedation. Avoid.
Tobacco:	None expected.

*See Glossary

BARBITURATES, ASPIRIN & CODEINE (Also contains caffeine)

GENERIC AND BRAND NAMES

See full list of generic and brand names in the *Generic and Brand Name Directory*, page 876.

BASIC INFORMATION

Habit forming? Yes
Prescription needed? Yes
Available as generic? Yes
Drug class: Narcotic, analgesic

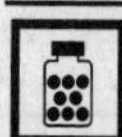

USES

- Reduces anxiety or nervous tension (low dose).
- Reduces pain, fever, inflammation..

DOSAGE & USAGE INFORMATION

How to take:
- Tablet or capsule—Swallow with liquid or food to lessen stomach irritation. If you can't swallow whole, crumble tablet or open capsule and take with liquid or food.
- Extended-release tablet or capsule—Swallow each dose whole. Do not crush, open or chew,

When to take:
When needed. No more often than every 4 hours.

If you forget a dose:
Take as soon as you remember. Wait 4 hours for next dose.

Continued next column

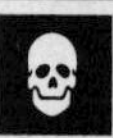

OVERDOSE

SYMPTOMS:
Deep sleep, slow and weak pulse, ringing in ears, nausea, vomiting, dizziness, fever, deep and rapid breathing, hallucinations, convulsions, coma.
WHAT TO DO:
- **Dial 911 (emergency) for medical help or call poison control center 1-800-222-1222 for instructions.**
- **If person is unconscious, check breathing and pulse. If not breathing, begin mouth-to-mouth rescue breathing. If heart is not beating, begin chest compressions.**
- **See emergency information on last 3 pages of this book.**

What drug does:
- May partially block nerve impulses at nerve-cell connections.
- Affects hypothalamus, the part of the brain which regulates temperature by dilating small blood vessels in skin.
- Prevents clumping of platelets (small blood cells) so blood vessels remain open.
- Decreases prostaglandin effect.
- Blocks pain messages to brain and spinal cord.
- Reduces sensitivity of brain's cough-control center.

Time lapse before drug works:
30 minutes.

Don't take with:
Any other medicine or any dietary supplement without consulting your doctor or pharmacist.

POSSIBLE ADVERSE REACTIONS OR SIDE EFFECTS

SYMPTOMS	WHAT TO DO
Life-threatening:	
Rare allergic reaction (hives, itching, rash, wheezing, tightness in chest, swelling of lips or tongue or throat).	Seek emergency treatment immediately.
Common:	
Dizziness, drowsiness, heartburn, flushed face, depression, false sense of well-being, increased urination.	Continue. Call doctor when convenient.
Infrequent:	
Jaundice; vomiting blood; easy bruising; skin rash, hives; confusion; depression; sore throat, fever, mouth sores; difficult urination; hearing loss; slurred speech; blood in urine; decreased vision.	Discontinue. Call doctor right away.
Rare:	
Insomnia, nightmares, constipation, headache, nervousness, flushed face, increased sweating, unusual tiredness, sleep-related behaviors.*	Continue. Call doctor when convenient.

BARBITURATES, ASPIRIN & CODEINE (Also contains caffeine)

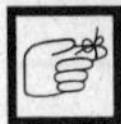

WARNINGS & PRECAUTIONS

Don't take if:
You are allergic to any barbiturate or narcotic or aspirin.

Before you start, consult your doctor if:
- You have had stomach or duodenal ulcers.
- You have asthma, epilepsy, kidney or liver damage, anemia, chronic pain, gout.
- You will have surgery within 2 months, including dental surgery, requiring general or spinal anesthesia.

Over age 60:
- Adverse reactions and side effects may be more frequent and severe than in younger persons.
- More likely to cause hidden bleeding in stomach or intestines. Watch for dark stools.
- More likely to be drowsy, dizzy, unsteady or constipated. Use only if absolutely necessary.

Pregnancy:
Risk factors vary for drugs in this group. See category list on page xviii and consult doctor.

Breast-feeding:
Drug passes into milk. Avoid drug or discontinue nursing until you finish medicine. Consult doctor for advice on maintaining milk supply.

Infants & children:
- Overdose frequent and severe. Keep bottles out of children's reach.
- Use only under doctor's supervision.
- Do not give to persons under age 18 who have fever and discomfort of viral illness, especially chicken pox and influenza. May increase risk of Reye's syndrome.*

Prolonged use:
- Kidney damage. Periodic kidney function test recommended.
- May cause addiction, anemia, chronic intoxication.
- May lower body temperature, making exposure to cold temperatures hazardous.

Skin & sunlight:
One or more drugs in this group may cause rash or intensify sunburn in areas exposed to sun or ultraviolet light (photosensitivity reaction). Avoid overexposure. Notify doctor if reaction occurs.

Driving, piloting or hazardous work:
Don't drive or pilot aircraft until you learn how medicine effects you. Don't work around dangerous machinery. Don't climb ladders or work in high places. Danger increases if you drink alcohol or take medicine affecting alertness and reflexes, such as antihistamines, tranquilizers, sedatives, pain medicine, narcotics and mind-altering drugs.

Discontinuing:
May be unnecessary to finish medicine. Follow doctor's instructions. If you develop withdrawal symptoms of hallucinations, agitation or sleeplessness after discontinuing, call doctor right away.

Others:
- Aspirin can complicate surgery, illness, pregnancy, labor and delivery.
- For arthritis—Don't change dose without consulting doctor.
- Advise any doctor or dentist whom you consult that you take this medicine.
- Urine tests for blood sugar may be inaccurate.
- Great potential for abuse.

POSSIBLE INTERACTION WITH OTHER DRUGS

GENERIC NAME OR DRUG CLASS	COMBINED EFFECT
Adrenocorticoids, systemic	Increased risk of ulcers.
Allopurinol	Decreased allopurinol effect.
Analgesics, other*	Increased analgesic effect.
Antacids*	Decreased aspirin effect.

Continued on page 906

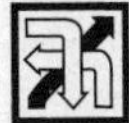

POSSIBLE INTERACTION WITH OTHER SUBSTANCES

INTERACTS WITH	COMBINED EFFECT
Alcohol:	Possible stomach irritation and bleeding, possible fatal oversedation. Avoid.
Beverages:	None expected.
Cocaine:	Increased cocaine toxic effects. Avoid.
Foods:	None expected.
Marijuana:	Possible increased pain relief, but marijuana may slow body's recovery. Impairs physical and mental performance. Avoid.
Tobacco:	None expected.

*See Glossary

BECAPLERMIN

BRAND NAMES

Regranex

BASIC INFORMATION

Habit forming? No
Prescription needed? Yes
Available as generic? No
Drug class: Platelet-derived growth factor

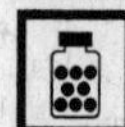

USES

Treatment of skin ulcers in patients with diabetes.

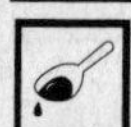

DOSAGE & USAGE INFORMATION

How to use:
Gel—Apply to the affected area. Follow all instructions provided with the prescription. Dosage may change as wound heals.

When to use:
At the same time each day. Change the wound dressing between applications of the medication.

If you forget a dose:
Apply it as soon as possible. If it is almost time for your next dose, skip the missed dose and go back to your regular dosing schedule. Do not double doses.

What drug does:
Stimulates growth of cells involved in wound repair.

Time lapse before drug works:
Up to six months.

Don't use with:
Any other medicine or any dietary supplement without consulting your doctor or pharmacist.

OVERDOSE

SYMPTOMS:
None expected.
WHAT TO DO:
Overdose unlikely to threaten life. If person uses much larger amount than prescribed, call doctor or poison control center 1-800-222-1222 for help.

POSSIBLE ADVERSE REACTIONS OR SIDE EFFECTS

SYMPTOMS	WHAT TO DO
Life-threatening:	
None expected.	
Common:	
None expected.	
Infrequent:	
Rash in area of skin ulcer.	Discontinue. Call doctor right away.
Rare:	
None expected.	

WARNINGS & PRECAUTIONS

Don't take if:
- You are allergic to becaplermin, parabens or metacresol.
- You have any new growths or wounds in the application area.

Before you start, consult your doctor if:
- You have any other medical problem.
- You are allergic to any other substances, such as food preservatives or dyes.
- You have a malignancy or cancer.

Over age 60:
No problems expected.

Pregnancy:
Decide with your doctor if drug benefits justify risk to unborn child. Risk category C (see page xviii).

Breast-feeding:
It is not known if drug passes into milk. Avoid drug or discontinue nursing until you finish medicine. Consult doctor for advice on maintaining milk supply.

Infants & children:
Safety and efficacy in children under age 16 has not been established.

Prolonged use:
No problems expected. Your doctor should periodically evaluate your response to the drug and adjust the dose according to the rate of change in the width and length of the diabetic ulcer.

Skin & sunlight:
No problems expected.

Driving, piloting or hazardous work:
No problems expected.

Discontinuing:
Don't discontinue without consulting doctor.

Others:
- There is an increased risk of cancer death in patients who use 3 or more tubes of this drug. Consult your doctor about your risks.
- Do not place tip of tube onto ulcer or any other object; it may contaminate the medication.
- Be sure you follow application instructions carefully.
- Avoid bearing weight on the affected extremity.
- Wash hands carefully before preparing your dose.
- Keep this medication in refrigerator; do not freeze.
- Advise any doctor or dentist whom you consult that you take this medicine.

POSSIBLE INTERACTION WITH OTHER DRUGS

GENERIC NAME OR DRUG CLASS	COMBINED EFFECT
None expected.	

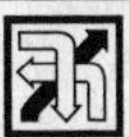

POSSIBLE INTERACTION WITH OTHER SUBSTANCES

INTERACTS WITH	COMBINED EFFECT
Alcohol:	None expected.
Beverages:	None expected.
Cocaine:	Effects unknown. Avoid.
Foods:	None expected.
Marijuana:	Effects unknown. Avoid.
Tobacco:	None expected.

BELLADONNA ALKALOIDS & BARBITURATES

GENERIC AND BRAND NAMES

See full list of generic and brand names in the *Generic and Brand Name Directory*, page 876.

BASIC INFORMATION

Habit forming? Yes
Prescription needed? Yes
Available as generic? Yes, for some
Drug class: Antispasmodic, anticholinergic, sedative

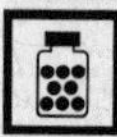

USES

- Reduces spasms of digestive system, bladder and urethra.
- Reduces anxiety or nervous tension.
- Relieves insomnia.

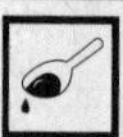

DOSAGE & USAGE INFORMATION

How to take:

- Tablet, liquid or capsule—Swallow with liquid or food to lessen stomach irritation. If you can't swallow whole, crumble tablet or open capsule and take with liquid or food.
- Extended-release tablet or capsule—Swallow each dose whole. Don't crush, open or chew.
- Chewable tablets—Chew well before swallowing.
- Elixir—Take by mouth. Follow directions on the product label. Measure the dose with the special dropper or spoon provided. Take 30 to 60 minutes before meals.
- Drops—Dilute dose in beverage before swallowing.

When to take:
At the same times each day.

Continued next column

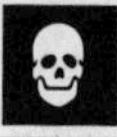

OVERDOSE

SYMPTOMS:
Blurred vision, confusion, convulsions, irregular heartbeat, hallucinations, coma.
WHAT TO DO:

- **Dial 911 (emergency) for medical help or call poison control center 1-800-222-1222 for instructions.**
- **See emergency information on last 3 pages of this book.**

If you forget a dose:
Take as soon as you remember. If it is almost time for the next dose, wait for the next scheduled dose (don't double this dose).

What drug does:

- May partially block nerve impulses at nerve cell connections.
- Blocks nerve impulses at parasympathetic nerve endings, preventing muscle contractions and gland secretions of organs involved.

Time lapse before drug works:
15 to 30 minutes.

Don't take with:

- Antacids* or antidiarrheals* at the same time.
- Any other medicine or any dietary supplement without consulting your doctor or pharmacist.

POSSIBLE ADVERSE REACTIONS OR SIDE EFFECTS

SYMPTOMS	WHAT TO DO
Life-threatening:	
Rare allergic reaction—hives, itching, rash, wheezing, tightness in chest, swelling (lips, tongue or throat).	Seek emergency treatment immediately.
Common:	
• Dry mouth, throat, nose; drowsiness; constipation; dizziness; nausea; vomiting; "hangover" effect; depression; confusion.	Discontinue. Call doctor right away.
• Reduced sweating, slurred speech, agitation, nasal congestion, altered taste.	Continue. Call doctor when convenient.
Infrequent:	
Difficult urination; difficult swallowing; rash or hives; face, lip or eyelid swelling; joint or muscle pain; lightheadedness.	Discontinue. Call doctor right away.
Rare:	
Jaundice; unusual bruising or bleeding; hives, skin rash; pain in eyes; blurred vision; sore throat, fever, mouth sores, sleep-related behaviors.*	Discontinue. Call doctor right away.

WARNINGS & PRECAUTIONS

Don't take if:

- You are allergic to any barbiturate or any anticholinergic.
- You have porphyria, trouble with stomach bloating, difficulty emptying your bladder completely, narrow-angle glaucoma, severe ulcerative colitis.

Before you start, consult your doctor if:

- You have open-angle glaucoma, angina, chronic bronchitis or asthma, hiatal hernia, liver disease, enlarged prostate, myasthenia gravis, peptic ulcer, epilepsy, kidney or liver damage, anemia, chronic pain, thyroid disease.
- You will have surgery within 2 months, including dental surgery, requiring general or spinal anesthesia.

Over age 60:
Adverse reactions and side effects may be more frequent and severe than in younger persons. Ask your doctor about small doses.

Pregnancy:
Risk factors vary for drugs in this group. See category list on page xviii and consult doctor.

Breast-feeding:
Drug passes into milk. Avoid drug or discontinue nursing until you finish medicine.

Infants & children:
Use only under doctor's supervision.

Prolonged use:

- May cause addiction, anemia, chronic intoxication.
- May lower body temperature, making exposure to cold temperatures hazardous.

Skin & sunlight:
One or more drugs in this group may cause rash or intensify sunburn in areas exposed to sun or ultraviolet light (photosensitivity reaction). Avoid overexposure. Notify doctor if reaction occurs.

Driving, piloting or hazardous work:
Don't drive or pilot aircraft until you learn how medicine affects you. Don't work around dangerous machinery. Don't climb ladders or work in high places. Danger increases if you drink alcohol or take medicine affecting alertness and reflexes.

Discontinuing:
May be unnecessary to finish medicine. Follow doctor's instructions. If you develop withdrawal symptoms of hallucinations, agitation or sleeplessness after discontinuing, call doctor right away.

Others:

- Great potential for abuse.
- Advise any doctor or dentist whom you consult that you take this medicine.

POSSIBLE INTERACTION WITH OTHER DRUGS

GENERIC NAME OR DRUG CLASS	COMBINED EFFECT
Acetaminophen	Possible decreased barbiturate effect.
Adrenocorticoids, systemic	Possible glaucoma.
Amantadine	Increased belladonna effect.
Antacids*	Decreased belladonna effect.
Anticholinergics, other*	Increased belladonna effect.
Anticoagulants, oral*	Decreased anticoagulant effect.
Anticonvulsants*	Changed seizure patterns.
Antidepressants, tricyclic*	Possible dangerous oversedation. Avoid.
Antidiabetics, oral*	Increased barbiturate effect.
Antihistamines*	Dangerous sedation. Avoid.
Anti-inflammatory drugs nonsteroidal (NSAIDs)*	Decreased anti-inflammatory effect.
Aspirin	Decreased aspirin effect.

Continued on page 907

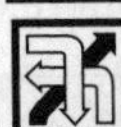

POSSIBLE INTERACTION WITH OTHER SUBSTANCES

INTERACTS WITH	COMBINED EFFECT
Alcohol:	Possible fatal oversedation. Avoid.
Beverages:	None expected.
Cocaine:	Excessively rapid heartbeat. Avoid.
Foods:	None expected.
Marijuana:	Drowsiness and dry mouth. Avoid.
Tobacco:	Decreased effectiveness of acid reduction in stomach.

***See Glossary**

BENZODIAZEPINES

GENERIC AND BRAND NAMES

See full list of generic and brand names in the *Generic and Brand Name Directory*, page 876.

BASIC INFORMATION

Habit forming? Yes
Prescription needed? Yes
Available as generic? Yes, for most
Drug class: Tranquilizer (benzodiazepine), anticonvulsant

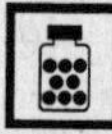

USES

- Treatment for anxiety disorders and panic disorders.
- Treatment for muscle spasm.
- Treatment for seizure disorders.
- Treatment for alcohol withdrawal.
- Treatment for insomnia (short-term).

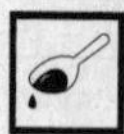

DOSAGE & USAGE INFORMATION

How to take:

- Tablet or capsule—Swallow with liquid. If you can't swallow whole, crumble tablet or open capsule and take with liquid or a bite of food.
- Extended-release capsule—Swallow capsule whole. Do not open or chew.
- Oral suspension—Dilute dose in water, soda or sodalike beverage or small amount of food such as applesauce or pudding.
- Sublingual tablet—Do not chew or swallow. Place under tongue until dissolved.
- Disintegrating tablet—Let dissolve on tongue.
- Rectal gel—Follow instructions provided with prescription or as directed by the doctor.

When to take:
At the same time each day, according to instructions on prescription label.

Continued next column

If you forget a dose:
Take as soon as you remember. If it is almost time for the next dose, wait for that dose (don't double this dose) and resume regular schedule.

What drug does:
Affects limbic system of brain, the part that controls emotions.

Time lapse before drug works:
May take 6 weeks for full benefit; depends on drug when treating anxiety.

Don't take with:
Any other medicine or any dietary supplement without consulting your doctor or pharmacist.

OVERDOSE

SYMPTOMS:
Drowsiness, weakness, tremor, stupor, coma.
WHAT TO DO:

- **Dial 911 (emergency) for medical help or call poison control center 1-800-222-1222 for instructions.**
- **If person is unconscious, check breathing and pulse. If not breathing, begin mouth-to-mouth rescue breathing. If heart is not beating, begin chest compressions.**
- **See emergency information on last 3 pages of this book.**

POSSIBLE ADVERSE REACTIONS OR SIDE EFFECTS

SYMPTOMS	WHAT TO DO
Life-threatening:	
Rare allergic reaction—may have hives, rash, itching, swelling, trouble breathing, wheezing, chest pain, dizziness, faintness.	Seek emergency treatment immediately.
Common:	
Clumsiness, unsteadiness, dizziness, light-headed, drowsiness, slurred speech.	Continue. Call doctor when convenient.
Infrequent:	
• Memory loss, anxiety, depression, fast heartbeat.	Discontinue. Call doctor right away.
• Constipation or diarrhea, nausea, vomiting, urination problems, stomach pain, headache, mouth is dry or watering, muscle spasm, changes in sexual function.	Continue. Call doctor when convenient.
Rare:	
Behavior changes (may be bizarre), delusions, outbursts of anger, loss of reality, infection symptoms (fever, chills), unusual tiredness or weakness, unusual bleeding or bruising, skin rash or itching, sores in mouth, body movements uncontrolled, hallucinations, yellow skin or eyes, sleep-related behaviors.*	Discontinue. Call doctor right away.

WARNINGS & PRECAUTIONS

Don't take if:
You are allergic to any benzodiazepine.

Before you start, consult your doctor if:
- You have myasthenia gravis.
- You have a history of drug or alcohol abuse, or severe depression or mental disorder.
- You have liver, kidney or lung disease.
- You have diabetes, seizure disorder, a swallowing problem (in children), or porphyria.
- You have sleep apnea.
- You have glaucoma.

Over age 60:
Adverse reactions and side effects may be more frequent and severe than in younger persons. May need smaller doses for shorter period.

Pregnancy:
Risk factors vary for drugs in this group. See category list on page xviii and consult doctor.

Breast-feeding:
Drug passes into milk. Avoid drug or discontinue nursing until you finish medicine. Consult doctor for advice on maintaining milk supply.

Infants & children:
Use only under medical supervision.

Prolonged use:
Risk of physical or psychological dependence.

Skin & sunlight:
One or more drugs in this group may cause rash or intensify sunburn in areas exposed to sun or ultraviolet light (photosensitivity reaction). Avoid overexposure and use sunscreen. Notify doctor if reaction occurs.

Driving, piloting or hazardous work:
Don't drive or pilot aircraft until you learn how medicine affects you. Don't work around dangerous machinery. Don't climb ladders or work in high places. Danger increases if you drink alcohol or take medicine affecting alertness and reflexes.

Discontinuing:
- Don't discontinue without consulting doctor. Adverse effects can occur (may be life-threatening) if the drug has been taken for longer periods. Dose may require gradual reduction. Doses of other drugs may also require adjustment.
- If withdrawal symptoms (emotional or physical) occur after stopping the drug, call doctor.

Others:
- Don't use for insomnia more than 4-7 days.
- Hot weather, heavy exercise and sweating may increase risk of heat stroke.
- Advise any doctor or dentist whom you consult that you take this drug.
- Rarely, anticonvulsant (antiepileptic) drugs may lead to suicidal thoughts and behaviors. Call doctor right away if suicidal symptoms or unusual behaviors occur.

POSSIBLE INTERACTION WITH OTHER DRUGS

GENERIC NAME OR DRUG CLASS	COMBINED EFFECT
Antidepressants, tricyclic*	Increased sedative effect of both drugs.
Carbamazepine	Decreased effect of benzodiazepine.
Central nervous system (CNS) depressants*	Increased sedative effect.
Cimetidine	Increased effect of benzodiazepine.
Clozapine	Toxic effect on the central nervous system.
Contraceptives, oral*	Increased effect of benzodiazepine.
Enzyme inhibitors*	Increased effect of benzodiazepine.
Erythromycins*	Increased effect of benzodiazepine.
Fluoxetine	Increased effect of benzodiazepine.
Fluvoxamine	Increased effect of benzodiazepine.
Isoniazid	Increased effect of benzodiazepine.

Continued on page 908

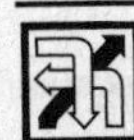

POSSIBLE INTERACTION WITH OTHER SUBSTANCES

INTERACTS WITH	COMBINED EFFECT
Alcohol:	Sedation. Avoid.
Beverages: Grapefruit juice.	Increased effect of benzodiazepine.
Cocaine:	Unknown effect. Avoid.
Foods:	None expected.
Marijuana:	Sedation. Avoid.
Tobacco:	Decreased effect of benzodiazepine.

*See Glossary

BENZOYL PEROXIDE

BRAND NAMES

See full list of brand names in the *Generic and Brand Name Directory*, page 877.

BASIC INFORMATION

Habit forming? No
Prescription needed? No
Available as generic? Yes
Drug class: Antiacne (topical)

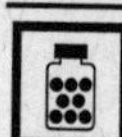

USES

- Treatment for acne.
- Treats pressure sores.

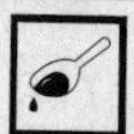

DOSAGE & USAGE INFORMATION

How to use:
Cream, gel, pads, sticks, lotion, cleansing bar, foam or facial mask—Wash affected area with plain soap and water. Dry gently with towel. Apply product as directed into affected areas. Keep away from eyes, nose, mouth. Wash hands after using.

When to use:
Apply as directed on product.

If you forget an application:
Use as soon as you remember.

What drug does:
Slowly releases oxygen from skin, which controls some skin bacteria. Also causes peeling and drying, helping control blackheads and whiteheads.

Time lapse before drug works:
1 to 2 weeks.

Don't use with:
Any other topical medicine without consulting your doctor or pharmacist.

OVERDOSE

SYMPTOMS:
None expected.
WHAT TO DO:
- **If person swallows drug, call doctor or poison control center 1-800-222-1222 for help.**
- **See emergency information on last 3 pages of this book.**

POSSIBLE ADVERSE REACTIONS OR SIDE EFFECTS

SYMPTOMS	WHAT TO DO
Life-threatening: None expected.	
Common: Mild redness and chapping of skin during first few weeks of use.	No action necessary.
Infrequent:	
• Rash, excessive dryness, peeling skin.	Discontinue. Call doctor right away.
• Painful skin irritation.	Continue. Call doctor when convenient.
Rare: None expected.	

WARNINGS & PRECAUTIONS

Don't take if:
You are allergic to benzoyl peroxide.

Before you start, consult your doctor if:
- You plan to become pregnant within medication period.
- You take oral contraceptives.
- You are using any other prescription or nonprescription medicine for acne.
- You are using abrasive skin cleansers or medicated cosmetics.

Over age 60:
No problems expected.

Pregnancy:
Consult doctor. Risk category C (see page xviii).

Breast-feeding:
No proven problems. Consult doctor.

Infants & children:
Not recommended.

Prolonged use:
Permanent rash or scarring.

Skin & sunlight:
May cause rash or intensify sunburn in areas exposed to sun or ultraviolet light (photosensitivity reaction). Avoid overexposure. Notify doctor if reaction occurs.

Driving, piloting or hazardous work:
No problems expected.

Discontinuing:
- May be unnecessary to finish medicine. Discontinue when acne improves.
- If acne doesn't improve in 2 weeks, call doctor.

Others:
- Drug may bleach hair or dyed fabrics, including clothing or carpet.
- Store away from heat in cool, dry place.
- Avoid contact with eyes, lips, nose and sensitive areas of the neck.

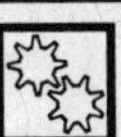

POSSIBLE INTERACTION WITH OTHER DRUGS

GENERIC NAME OR DRUG CLASS	COMBINED EFFECT
Antiacne topical preparations, other	Excessive skin irritation.
Skin-peeling agents (salicylic acid, sulfur, resorcinol, tretinoin)	Excessive skin irritation.

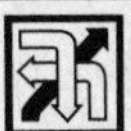

POSSIBLE INTERACTION WITH OTHER SUBSTANCES

INTERACTS WITH	COMBINED EFFECT
Alcohol:	None expected.
Beverages:	None expected.
Cocaine:	None expected.
Foods: Cinnamon, foods with benzoic acid.	Skin rash.
Marijuana:	None expected.
Tobacco:	None expected.

BETA CAROTENE

BRAND NAMES

Solatene
Numerous multiple vitamin and mineral supplements. Check labels.

BASIC INFORMATION

Habit forming? No
Prescription needed? No
Available as generic? Yes
Drug class: Nutritional supplement

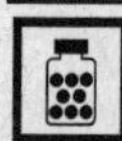

USES

- Used as a nutritional supplement.
- Used as an adjunct to the treatment of steatorrhea, chronic fever, obstructive jaundice, pancreatic insufficiency, protein deficiency, total parenteral nutrition and photosensitivity in photo porphyria.

DOSAGE & USAGE INFORMATION

How to take:
Tablet or capsule—Swallow with liquid. If you can't swallow whole, crumble tablet or open capsule and take with liquid or food.

When to take:
At the same time each day, according to directions on package or prescription label.

If you forget a dose:
Take as soon as you remember (don't double this dose).

What drug does:
Enables the body to manufacture vitamin A, which is essential for the normal functioning of the retina, normal growth and development and normal testicular and ovarian function.

Time lapse before drug works:
Total effect may take several weeks.

Don't take with:
No restrictions unless advised by doctor.

OVERDOSE

SYMPTOMS:
Yellow skin.
WHAT TO DO:
Overdose unlikely to threaten life. If person takes much larger amount than prescribed, call doctor or poison control center 1-800-222-1222 for help.

POSSIBLE ADVERSE REACTIONS OR SIDE EFFECTS

SYMPTOMS	WHAT TO DO
Life-threatening: None expected.	
Common: Yellow palms, hands, soles of feet.	Continue. Call doctor when convenient.
Infrequent: None expected.	
Rare:	
• Joint pain, unusual bleeding or bruising.	Discontinue. Call doctor right away.
• Diarrhea, dizziness.	Continue. Call doctor when convenient.

WARNINGS & PRECAUTIONS

Don't take if:
You are hypersensitive to beta carotene.

Before you start, consult your doctor if:
- You have liver or kidney disease.
- You have hypervitaminosis.*

Over age 60:
No problems expected.

Pregnancy:
Consult doctor. Risk category C (see page xviii).

Breast-feeding:
No problems expected.

Infants & children:
No problems expected.

Prolonged use:
No problems expected.

Skin & sunlight:
No special problems expected.

Driving, piloting or hazardous work:
No special problems expected.

Discontinuing:
No special problems expected.

Others:
- Some researchers claim that beta carotene may reduce the occurrence of some cancers. There is insufficient data to substantiate this claim.
- Advise any doctor or dentist whom you consult that you take this medicine.
- May affect results of some medical tests.

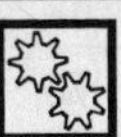

POSSIBLE INTERACTION WITH OTHER DRUGS

GENERIC NAME OR DRUG CLASS	COMBINED EFFECT
Cholestyramine	Decreased absorption of beta carotene.
Colestipol	Decreased absorption of beta carotene.
Mineral oil	Decreased absorption of beta carotene.
Neomycin	Decreased absorption of beta carotene.

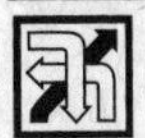

POSSIBLE INTERACTION WITH OTHER SUBSTANCES

INTERACTS WITH	COMBINED EFFECT
Alcohol:	None expected.
Beverages:	None expected.
Cocaine:	None expected.
Foods:	None expected.
Marijuana:	None expected.
Tobacco:	None expected.

***See Glossary**

BETA-ADRENERGIC BLOCKING AGENTS

GENERIC AND BRAND NAMES

See full list of generic and brand names in the *Generic and Brand Name Directory*, page 877.

BASIC INFORMATION

Habit forming? No
Prescription needed? Yes
Available as generic? Yes, for some.
Drug class: Antiadrenergic, antianginal, antiarrhythmic, antihypertensive

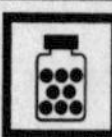

USES

- Treats high blood pressure (hypertension).
- Some beta-blockers are used to relieve angina (chest pain).
- May be used to treat irregular heartbeat.
- May be used to treat anxiety disorders and other conditions as determined by your doctor.
- Treats tremors (some types).
- Reduces frequency of vascular headaches (does not relieve headache pain).

DOSAGE & USAGE INFORMATION

How to take:
Tablet, liquid, capsule, extended-release capsule or extended-release tablet—Swallow with liquid. If you can't swallow whole, crumble tablet or open capsule and take with liquid or food. Don't crush or open extended-release forms.

When to take:
With meals or immediately after.

If you forget a dose:
Take as soon as you remember. Return to regular schedule, but allow 3 hours between doses.

Continued next column

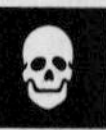

OVERDOSE

SYMPTOMS:
Weakness, slow or weak pulse, blood pressure drop, fainting, difficulty breathing, convulsions, cold and sweaty skin.
WHAT TO DO:
- **Dial 911 (emergency) for medical help or call poison control center 1-800-222-1222 for instructions.**
- **See emergency information on last 3 pages of this book.**

What drug does:
- Blocks certain actions of sympathetic nervous system.
- Lowers heart's oxygen requirements.
- Slows nerve impulses through heart.
- Reduces blood vessel contraction in heart, scalp and other body parts.

Time lapse before drug works:
1 to 4 hours.

Don't take with:
Any other medicine or any dietary supplement without consulting your doctor or pharmacist.

POSSIBLE ADVERSE REACTIONS OR SIDE EFFECTS

SYMPTOMS	WHAT TO DO
Life-threatening:	
Congestive heart failure (severe shortness of breath, rapid heartbeat); severe asthma.	Discontinue. Seek emergency treatment.
Common:	
• Pulse slower than 50 beats per minute.	Discontinue. Call doctor right away.
• Drowsiness, fatigue, numbness or tingling of fingers or toes, dizziness, diarrhea, nausea, weakness.	Continue. Call doctor when convenient.
• Cold hands or feet; dry mouth, eyes and skin.	Continue. Tell doctor at next visit.
Infrequent:	
• Hallucinations, nightmares, insomnia, headache, difficult breathing, joint pain, anxiety, chest pain.	Discontinue. Call doctor right away.
• Confusion, reduced alertness, depression, impotence, abdominal pain.	Continue. Call doctor when convenient.
• Constipation.	Continue. Tell doctor at next visit.
Rare:	
• Rash, sore throat, fever.	Discontinue. Call doctor right away.
• Unusual bleeding and bruising; dry, burning eyes.	Continue. Call doctor when convenient.

BETA-ADRENERGIC BLOCKING AGENTS

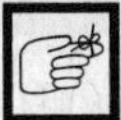

WARNINGS & PRECAUTIONS

Don't take if:

- You are allergic to any beta-adrenergic blocker.
- You have asthma.
- You have hay fever symptoms.
- You have taken a monoamine oxidase (MAO) inhibitor* in the past 2 weeks.

Before you start, consult your doctor if:

- You have heart disease or poor circulation to the extremities.
- You have hay fever, asthma, chronic bronchitis, emphysema.
- You have overactive thyroid function.
- You have impaired liver or kidney function.
- You will have surgery within 2 months, including dental surgery, requiring general or spinal anesthesia.
- You have diabetes or hypoglycemia.

Over age 60:
Adverse reactions and side effects may be more frequent and severe than in younger persons.

Pregnancy:
Risk factors vary for drugs in this group. See category list on page xviii and consult doctor.

Breast-feeding:
Drug passes into milk. Avoid drug or discontinue nursing until you finish medicine. Consult doctor for advice on maintaining milk supply.

Infants & children:
Not recommended.

Prolonged use:
Talk to your doctor about the need for follow-up medical examinations or laboratory studies to check blood pressure, ECG,* kidney function, blood sugar.

Skin & sunlight:
No problems expected.

Driving, piloting or hazardous work:
Don't drive or pilot aircraft until you learn how medicine affects you. Don't work around dangerous machinery. Don't climb ladders or work in high places. Danger increases if you drink alcohol or take medicine affecting alertness and reflexes.

Discontinuing
Don't discontinue without consulting doctor. Dose may require gradual reduction if you have taken drug for a long time. Doses of other drugs may also require adjustment. Angina may result from abrupt discontinuing.

Others:

- May mask diabetic hypoglycemia symptoms.
- May affect results in some medical tests.
- Advise any doctor or dentist whom you consult that you take this medicine.

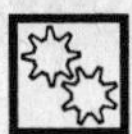

POSSIBLE INTERACTION WITH OTHER DRUGS

GENERIC NAME OR DRUG CLASS	COMBINED EFFECT
Angiotensin-converting (ACE) inhibitors*	Increased anti-hypertensive effects of both drugs. Dosages may require adjustment.
Antidiabetics*	Increased anti-diabetic effect.
Antihistamines*	Decreased antihistamine effect.
Antihypertensives*	Increased anti-hypertensive effect.
Anti-inflammatory drugs, nonsteroidal (NSAIDs)*	Decreased anti-hypertensive effect of beta blocker.
Betaxolol eyedrops	Possible increased beta blocker effect.
Calcium channel blockers*	Additional blood pressure drop.
Clonidine	Additional blood pressure drop. High blood pressure if clonidine stopped abruptly.
Dextrothyroxine	Possible decreased beta blocker effect.

Continued on page 908

POSSIBLE INTERACTION WITH OTHER SUBSTANCES

INTERACTS WITH	COMBINED EFFECT
Alcohol:	Excessive blood pressure drop. Avoid.
Beverages:	None expected.
Cocaine:	Irregular heartbeat; decreased beta-adrenergic effect. Avoid.
Foods:	None expected.
Marijuana:	Daily use—Impaired circulation to hands and feet.
Tobacco:	Possible irregular heartbeat.

***See Glossary**

BETA-ADRENERGIC BLOCKING AGENTS & THIAZIDE DIURETICS

GENERIC AND BRAND NAMES

See full list of generic and brand names in the *Generic and Brand Name Directory*, page 878.

BASIC INFORMATION

Habit forming? No
Prescription needed? Yes
Available as generic? Yes
Drug class: Beta-adrenergic blocker, diuretic (thiazide)

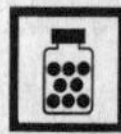

USES

- Controls, but doesn't cure, high blood pressure.
- Reduces fluid retention (edema).
- Reduces angina attacks.
- Stabilizes irregular heartbeat.
- Reduces frequency of migraine headaches. (Does not relieve headache pain.)
- Other uses as determined by your doctor.

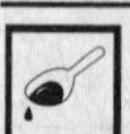

DOSAGE & USAGE INFORMATION

How to take:
- Tablet—Swallow with liquid.
- Extended-release capsule or tablet—Swallow whole with liquid. Do not open, chew or crush.

When to take:
At the same time each day.

If you forget a dose:
Take as soon as you remember. If it is almost time for the next dose, wait for next scheduled dose (don't double this dose).

What drug does:
- Forces sodium and water excretion, reducing body fluid.
- Relaxes muscle cells of small arteries.

Continued next column

- Reduced body fluid and relaxed arteries lower blood pressure.
- Blocks some of the actions of sympathetic nervous system.
- Lowers heart's oxygen requirements.
- Slows nerve impulses through heart.
- Reduces blood vessel contraction in heart, scalp and other body parts.

Time lapse before drug works:
- 1 to 4 hours for beta-blocker effect.
- May require several weeks to lower blood pressure.

Don't take with:
Any other medicines, even over-the-counter drugs such as cough/cold medicines, diet pills, nose drops, or caffeine, without consulting your doctor or pharmacist.

OVERDOSE

SYMPTOMS:
Irregular heartbeat (usually too slow), seizures, confusion, fainting, convulsions, coma.

WHAT TO DO:
- **Dial 911 (emergency) for medical help or call poison control center 1-800-222-1222 for instructions.**
- **See emergency information on last 3 pages of this book.**

POSSIBLE ADVERSE REACTIONS OR SIDE EFFECTS

SYMPTOMS	WHAT TO DO
Life-threatening:	
Wheezing, chest pain, seizures, irregular heartbeat.	Seek emergency treatment immediately.
Common:	
• Dry mouth, weak pulse, vomiting, muscle cramps, increased thirst, mood changes, nausea.	Discontinue. Call doctor right away.
• Weakness, tiredness, dizziness, mental depression, diminished sex drive, constipation, nightmares, insomnia.	Continue. Call doctor when convenient.
Infrequent:	
• Cold feet and hands, chest pain, breathing difficulty, anxiety, nervousness, headache, appetite loss, abdominal pain, numbness and tingling in fingers and toes, slow heartbeat.	Discontinue. Call doctor right away.
• Confusion, diarrhea.	Continue. Call doctor when convenient.
Rare:	
• Hives, skin rash; joint pain; jaundice; fever, sore throat, mouth ulcers.	Discontinue. Call doctor right away.
• Impotence, back pain.	Continue. Call doctor when convenient.

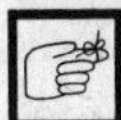

WARNINGS & PRECAUTIONS

Don't take if:
- You are allergic to any beta-adrenergic blocker or any thiazide diuretic drug.
- You have asthma or hay fever symptoms.
- You have taken MAO inhibitors in past two weeks.

Before you start, consult your doctor if:
- You have heart disease or poor circulation to the extremities.
- You have hay fever, asthma, chronic bronchitis, emphysema, overactive thyroid function, impaired liver or kidney function, gout, diabetes, hypoglycemia, pancreas disorder, systemic lupus erythematosus.
- You are allergic to any sulfa drug or tartrazine dye.
- You will have surgery within 2 months, including dental surgery, requiring general or spinal anesthesia.

Over age 60:
Adverse reactions and side effects may be more frequent and severe than in younger persons, especially dizziness and excessive potassium loss.

Pregnancy:
Risk factors vary for drugs in this group. See category list on page xviii and consult doctor.

Breast-feeding:
Drug passes into milk. Avoid drug or discontinue nursing until you finish medicine. Consult doctor for advice on maintaining milk supply.

Infants & children:
Not recommended.

Prolonged use:
- Weakens heart muscle contractions.
- You may need medicine to treat high blood pressure for the rest of your life.
- Talk to your doctor about the need for follow-up medical examinations or laboratory studies.

Skin & sunlight:
One or more drugs in this group may cause rash or intensify sunburn in areas exposed to sun or ultraviolet light (photosensitivity reaction). Avoid overexposure. Notify doctor if reaction occurs.

Driving, piloting or hazardous work:
Don't drive or pilot aircraft until you learn how medicine affects you. Don't work around dangerous machinery. Don't climb ladders or work in high places. Danger increases if you drink alcohol or take medicine affecting alertness and reflexes, such as antihistamines, tranquilizers, sedatives, pain medicine, narcotics and mind-altering drugs.

Discontinuing:
Don't discontinue without consulting doctor. Dose may require gradual reduction if you have taken drug for a long time. Doses of other drugs may also require adjustment.

Others:
- May mask hypoglycemia symptoms.
- Hot weather and fever may cause dehydration and drop in blood pressure. Dose may require temporary adjustment. Weigh daily and report any unexpected weight decreases to your doctor.
- May cause rise in uric acid, leading to gout.
- May cause blood sugar rise in diabetics.

POSSIBLE INTERACTION WITH OTHER DRUGS

GENERIC NAME OR DRUG CLASS	COMBINED EFFECT
Allopurinol	Decreased allopurinol effect.
Aminophylline	Decreased effectiveness of both.
Antidepressants, tricyclic*	Dangerous drop in blood pressure. Avoid combination unless under medical supervision.

Continued on page 909

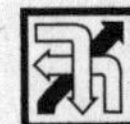

POSSIBLE INTERACTION WITH OTHER SUBSTANCES

INTERACTS WITH	COMBINED EFFECT
Alcohol:	Dangerous blood pressure drop. Avoid.
Beverages:	None expected.
Cocaine:	Irregular heartbeat, decreased beta blocker effect. Avoid.
Foods: Licorice.	Excessive potassium loss that causes dangerous heart rhythms.
Marijuana:	May increase blood pressure.
Tobacco:	May increase blood pressure and make heart work harder. Avoid.

***See Glossary**

BETHANECHOL

BRAND NAMES

Duvoid
Urabeth
Urecholine

BASIC INFORMATION

Habit forming? No
Prescription needed? Yes
Available as generic? Yes
Drug class: Cholinergic

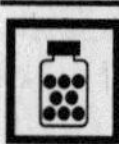

USES

- Helps initiate urination following surgery, or for persons with urinary infections or enlarged prostate.
- Treats reflux esophagitis.

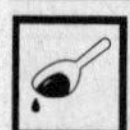

DOSAGE & USAGE INFORMATION

How to take:
Tablet—Swallow with liquid, 1 hour before or 2 hours after eating.

When to take:
At the same times each day.

If you forget a dose:
Take as soon as you remember. If it is almost time for the next dose, wait for the next scheduled dose (don't double this dose).

What drug does:
Affects chemical reactions in the body that strengthen bladder muscles.

Time lapse before drug works:
30 to 90 minutes.

Don't take with:
Any other medicine or any dietary supplement without consulting your doctor or pharmacist.

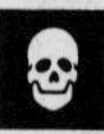

OVERDOSE

SYMPTOMS:
Shortness of breath, wheezing or chest tightness, unconsciousness, coma.
WHAT TO DO:

- **Dial 911 (emergency) for medical help or call poison control center 1-800-222-1222 for instructions.**
- **If person is unconscious, check breathing and pulse. If not breathing, begin mouth-to-mouth rescue breathing. If heart is not beating, begin chest compressions.**
- **See emergency information on last 3 pages of this book.**

POSSIBLE ADVERSE REACTIONS OR SIDE EFFECTS

SYMPTOMS	WHAT TO DO
Life-threatening: In case of overdose, see previous column.	
Common: None expected.	
Infrequent: Dizziness, headache, faintness, blurred or changed vision, diarrhea, nausea, vomiting, stomach discomfort, belching, excessive urge to urinate.	Continue. Call doctor when convenient.
Rare: Shortness of breath, wheezing, tightness in chest.	Discontinue. Call doctor right away.

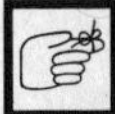

WARNINGS & PRECAUTIONS

Don't take if:
You are allergic to any cholinergic.

Before you start, consult your doctor if:
- You plan to become pregnant within medication period.
- You have asthma.
- You have epilepsy.
- You have heart or blood vessel disease.
- You have high or low blood pressure.
- You have overactive thyroid.
- You have intestinal blockage.
- You have Parkinson's disease.
- You have stomach problems (including ulcer).
- You have had bladder or intestinal surgery within 1 month.

Over age 60:
Adverse reactions and side effects may be more frequent and severe than in younger persons.

Pregnancy:
Decide with your doctor if drug benefits justify risk to unborn child. Risk category C (see page xviii).

Breast-feeding:
Unknown effect. Consult doctor.

Infants & children:
Use only under medical supervision.

Prolonged use:
No problems expected.

Skin & sunlight:
No problems expected.

Driving, piloting or hazardous work:
Don't drive or pilot aircraft until you learn how medicine effects you. Don't work around dangerous machinery. Don't climb ladders or work in high places. Danger increases if you drink alcohol or take medicine affecting alertness and reflexes, such as antihistamines, tranquilizers, sedatives, pain medicine, narcotics and mind-altering drugs.

Discontinuing:
May be unnecessary to finish medicine. Follow doctor's instructions.

Others:
- Be cautious about standing up suddenly.
- Advise any doctor or dentist whom you consult that you take this medicine.
- Interferes with laboratory studies of liver and pancreas function.

POSSIBLE INTERACTION WITH OTHER DRUGS

GENERIC NAME OR DRUG CLASS	COMBINED EFFECT
Cholinergics,* other	Increased effect of both drugs. Possible toxicity.
Ganglionic blockers*	Decreased blood pressure.
Nitrates*	Decreased bethanechol effect.
Procainamide	Decreased bethanechol effect.
Quinidine	Decreased bethanechol effect.

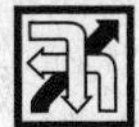

POSSIBLE INTERACTION WITH OTHER SUBSTANCES

INTERACTS WITH	COMBINED EFFECT
Alcohol:	None expected.
Beverages:	None expected.
Cocaine:	None expected.
Foods:	None expected.
Marijuana:	None expected.
Tobacco:	None expected.

*See Glossary

BIOLOGICS FOR PSORIASIS

GENERIC AND BRAND NAMES

USTEKINUMAB
Stelara

BASIC INFORMATION

Habit forming? No
Prescription needed? Yes
Available as generic? No
Drug class: Immunosuppressant; antipsoriatic

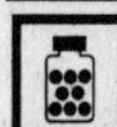

USES

Treatment for adult patients with moderate to severe, chronic, plaque psoriasis. Drug helps treat the cause of psoriasis as well as treating the symptoms.

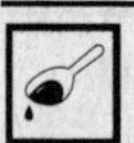

DOSAGE & USAGE INFORMATION

How to take:
Injection—It is injected by a health care provider.

When to take:
Your doctor will determine the schedule.

If you forget a dose:
For an injection given by a health care provider, call the medical office.

What drug does:
The exact mechanism is unknown. The drug blocks certain cells in the body's immune system to help prevent skin inflammation that leads to psoriasis.

Time lapse before drug works:
Improvement may be seen in 4 weeks, but it may take 3 months for maximum benefits.

Don't take with:
Any other medicine or any dietary supplement without consulting your doctor or pharmacist.

OVERDOSE

SYMPTOMS:
Unknown effects.
WHAT TO DO:
If person takes much larger amount than prescribed, call doctor or poison control center 1-800-222-1222 for help.

POSSIBLE ADVERSE REACTIONS OR SIDE EFFECTS

SYMPTOMS	WHAT TO DO
Life-threatening:	
Rare allergic reaction—Breathing difficulty; swelling of hands, feet, face, mouth, neck; skin rash.	Discontinue. Seek emergency treatment.
Common:	
• Chills, fever, cough, urination painful or difficult, lower back or side pain, hoarseness.	Discontinue. Call doctor right away.
• Injection site problems (pain, swelling, rash, bleeding, lumps), tiredness.	Continue. Call doctor when convenient.
Infrequent:	
• Congestion, dry or sore throat, body aches or pain, runny nose, swollen or tender neck glands, signs of infection, swallowing difficulty, voice changes.	Discontinue. Call doctor right away.
• Dizziness, itching skin, painful or swollen joints, muscle aches or stiffness, difficulty in moving, headache.	Continue. Call doctor when convenient.
Rare:	
Chest symptoms (pain, heaviness, tightness, discomfort), arm or jaw pain, fast or irregular heartbeat, shortness of breath, nausea or vomiting, sweating, bloating, dark urine, tiredness or weakness, light color stools, loss of appetite, yellow eyes or skin, flu-like symptoms, neurological disorder (headache, seizures, confusion, vision changes).	Discontinue. Call doctor right away.

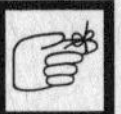

WARNINGS & PRECAUTIONS

Don't take if:
You are allergic to ustekinumab.

Before you start, consult your doctor if:
- You have kidney or liver problems.
- You have heart or blood vessel disorders.
- You have or have had cancer.
- You have any type of infection or have recurrent or chronic infections.
- You have a weak (suppressed) immune system due to illness or drugs.
- You have or have had tuberculosis.
- You have diverticulitis.
- You are getting phototherapy treatment.
- You are allergic to any medication, food or other substance.

Over age 60:
Unknown effect. Adverse reactions and side effects may be more frequent and severe.

Pregnancy:
Decide with your doctor if drug benefits justify risks to unborn child. Risk category B. (see page xviii).

Breast-feeding:
It is unknown if drug passes into milk. Avoid drug or discontinue nursing until you finish medicine. Consult doctor for advice on maintaining milk supply.

Infants & children:
Not recommended for ages under 18.

Prolonged use:
- Long-term use has not been established. Discuss continued use with the doctor.
- Visit the doctor regularly to see if the drug continues to be effective and to monitor your blood and platelet counts. If they get too low, the drug may be stopped on a temporary or permanent basis.

Skin & sunlight:
No special problems expected.

Driving, piloting or hazardous work:
Avoid if you feel dizzy, otherwise no special problems expected.

Discontinuing:
Consult doctor about discontinuing.

Others:
- Advise any doctor or dentist whom you consult about the use of this medicine.
- The drug may increase the risk of developing cancer.
- Because the drug affects the immune system, you are at risk for new infections or reactivation of a chronic infection that has not been active. These include bacterial, viral and fungal infections that can be serious, possibly fatal. Call your doctor right away if symptoms of an infection develop.
- Avoid people with infections and people who have recently had a live virus vaccine.

POSSIBLE INTERACTION WITH OTHER DRUGS

GENERIC NAME OR DRUG CLASS	COMBINED EFFECT
Immunosuppressants,* other	Increased risk of infections or cancer.
Other drugs	Unknown. Consult doctor or pharmacist.
Vaccines, live virus	Unknown. May decrease effect of vaccine or may be harmful.

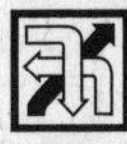

POSSIBLE INTERACTION WITH OTHER SUBSTANCES

INTERACTS WITH	COMBINED EFFECT
Alcohol:	None expected. Best to avoid.
Beverages:	None expected.
Cocaine:	Unknown. Best to avoid.
Foods:	None expected.
Marijuana:	Unknown. Best to avoid.
Tobacco:	None expected.

***See Glossary**

BISMUTH SALTS

GENERIC AND BRAND NAMES

BISKALCITRATE
Pylera

BISMUTH SUBSALICYLATE
Bismatrol
Helidac
Maalox Total Stomach Relief
Pepto-Bismol

BASIC INFORMATION

Habit forming? No
Prescription needed? No
Available as generic? Yes
Drug class: Antidiarrheal; antacid

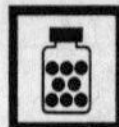

USES

- Treats symptoms of diarrhea, heartburn, nausea, acid indigestion.
- Helps prevent traveler's diarrhea.
- Treats ulcers.
- Used with other medications to treat a stomach infected by the bacteria *H. Pylori*.

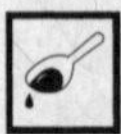

DOSAGE & USAGE INFORMATION

How to take:
- Tablet—Swallow with water.
- Chewable tablet—Chew well before swallowing.
- Liquid—Take as directed on label.

When to take:
As directed on label or by your doctor.

If you forget a dose:
Take as soon as you remember. Don't double this dose.

Continued next column

OVERDOSE

SYMPTOMS:
Hearing loss, ringing or buzzing in the ears, severe drowsiness or tiredness, severe excitement or nervousness, fast or deep breathing, unconsciousness or death.
WHAT TO DO:
- **Dial 911 (emergency) for medical help or call poison control center 1-800-222-1222 for instructions.**
- **See emergency information on last 3 pages of this book.**

What drug does:
- Decreases inflammation and increased motility of the intestinal muscles and lining.
- In combination with other drugs, it works to destroy certain bacterial infections.

Time lapse before drug works:
30 minutes to 1 hour.

Don't take with:
Any other medicine or any dietary supplement without consulting your doctor or pharmacist.

POSSIBLE ADVERSE REACTIONS OR SIDE EFFECTS

SYMPTOMS	WHAT TO DO
Life-threatening: In case of overdose, see previous column.	
Common: Black stools, dark tongue. (These symptoms are normal and medically insignificant).	No action necessary.
Infrequent: None expected.	
Rare: Abdominal pain, increased sweating, muscle weakness, drowsiness, anxiety, trembling, hearing loss, ringing or buzzing in ears, confusion, dizziness, headache, increased thirst, vision problems, severe constipation, continuing diarrhea, trouble breathing (all more likely to occur with high doses or chronic use).	Discontinue. Call doctor right away.

WARNINGS & PRECAUTIONS

Don't take if:
- You are allergic to aspirin, salicylates or other nonsteroidal anti-inflammatory drugs.
- You have stomach ulcers that have ever bled.
- The patient is a child with fever.

Before you start, consult your doctor if:
- You are on a low-sodium, low-sugar or other special diet.
- You have had diarrhea for more than 24 hours. This is especially applicable to infants, children and those over 60.
- You have had kidney disease.

Over age 60:
- Consult doctor before using.
- May cause severe constipation.

Pregnancy:
Decide with your doctor if drug benefits justify risk to unborn child. Risk category C; D in third trimester (see page xviii).

Breast-feeding:
Drug passes into milk. Avoid or discontinue nursing until you finish medicine. Consult doctor about maintaining milk supply.

Infants & children:
Not recommended for children 3 and younger. May cause constipation.

Prolonged use:
May cause constipation.

Skin & sunlight:
No problems expected.

Driving, piloting or hazardous work:
Don't drive or pilot aircraft if you take high or prolonged dose until you learn how medicine affects you. Don't work around dangerous machinery. Don't climb ladders or work in high places. Danger increases if you drink alcohol or take medicine affecting alertness and reflexes, such as antihistamines, tranquilizers, sedatives, pain medicine, narcotics and mind-altering drugs.

Discontinuing:
No problems expected.

Others:
- Pepto-Bismol contains salicylates. When given to children with flu or chicken pox, salicylates may cause a serious illness called Reye's syndrome.* An overdose in children can cause the same problems as aspirin poisoning.
- May cause false urine sugar tests.
- Dehydration can develop if too much body fluid has been lost. Consult doctor if any of the following symptoms occur: decreased urination, dizziness or lightheadedness, dryness of mouth, increased thirst, wrinkled skin.
- Don't store tablet form of drug in bathroom or near kitchen sink. Heat and moisture can cause it to break down.
- Consult doctor if diarrhea doesn't improve within 2 days.
- Read labels of any other drugs being used, such as for pain or inflammation. They may contain salicylates* and can lead to increased risk of side effects and overdose.

POSSIBLE INTERACTION WITH OTHER DRUGS

GENERIC NAME OR DRUG CLASS	COMBINED EFFECT
Anticoagulants*	Increased risk of bleeding.
Insulin or oral antidiabetic drugs*	Increased insulin effect. May require dosage adjustment.
Probenecid	Decreased effect of probenecid.
Salicylates,* other	Increased risk of salicylate toxicity.
Sulfinpyrazone	Decreased effect of sulfinpyrazone.
Tetracyclines*	Decreased absorption of tetracycline.
Thrombolytic agents*	Increased risk of bleeding.

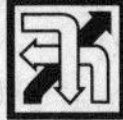

POSSIBLE INTERACTION WITH OTHER SUBSTANCES

INTERACTS WITH	COMBINED EFFECT
Alcohol:	None expected.
Beverages:	None expected.
Cocaine:	Decreased bismuth subsalicylate effect. Avoid.
Foods:	None expected.
Marijuana:	None expected.
Tobacco:	None expected.

BISPHOSPHONATES

GENERIC AND BRAND NAMES

See full list of generic and brand names in the *Generic and Brand Name Directory*, page 878.

BASIC INFORMATION

Habit forming? No
Prescription needed? Yes
Available as generic? Yes, for some
Drug class: Osteoporosis therapy, bisphosphonate; osteopenia therapy

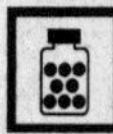

USES

- Prevention and treatment of postmenopausal osteopenia and osteoporosis (thinning of bones). Treatment for osteoporosis in men.
- Treats osteoporosis caused by certain drugs.
- May be used to treat other bone disease or bone cancer as determined by your doctor.
- Treatment for Paget's disease of bone.
- Treatment for hypercalcemia (high calcium).

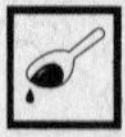

DOSAGE & USAGE INFORMATION

How to take:

- Tablet or extended-release tablet (alendronate or risedronate)—Swallow with a full glass of water (6 to 8 oz.). To help the medicine reach your stomach faster and to prevent throat irritation, stay upright for 30 minutes after you take it. Don't lie down.
- Tablet (etidronate or tiludronate)—Take morning, midday or evening 2 hours before or after any food.
- Tablet (ibandronate)—Take before first meal of the day. Swallow whole with water (6 to 8 oz). Do not lie down for 60 minutes.
- Effervescent tablet (alendronate)—Follow instructions provided with prescription.
- Injection—Etidronate, pamidronate or zoledronic acid are given by a medical person.

Continued next column

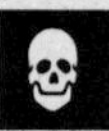

OVERDOSE

SYMPTOMS:
May rarely increase the severity of heartburn, stomach cramps, throat irritation.
WHAT TO DO:
Overdose unlikely to threaten life. If person takes much larger amount than prescribed, call doctor or poison control center 1-800-222-1222 for help.

When to take:

- Daily dose (alendronate or risedronate), take first thing in the morning at least 30 to 60 minutes before eating, drinking or taking any other medications.
- Daily dose (etidronate or tiludronate), take anytime during the day 2 hours before or 2 hours after eating.
- Once-a-week dose, take on the same day each week. Follow instructions as daily dose.
- Once a month dose (ibandronate), take on the same date each month.

If you forget a dose:

- Daily dose taken first thing in morning: skip the missed dose entirely, then resume schedule the next day. Do not double this dose.
- For weekly dose: take the next morning and then return to your regular weekly schedule.
- Daily dose taken anytime: take as soon as you remember. If it is almost time for the next dose, wait for the next scheduled dose (don't double this dose).

What drug does:
Slows down the loss of bone tissue and increases bone mass. Osteoporosis and osteopenia are progressive diseases in which bone breakdown occurs faster than bone formation.

Time lapse before drug works:
Up to 6 months or longer.

Don't take with:

- Any other medicine or any dietary supplement without consulting your doctor or pharmacist.
- Any other medication at the same time as the bisphosphonate. Follow doctor's instructions.

POSSIBLE ADVERSE REACTIONS OR SIDE EFFECTS

SYMPTOMS	WHAT TO DO
Life-threatening:	
None expected.	
Common:	
Stomach pain.	Continue. Call doctor when convenient.
Infrequent:	
Mild bone or muscle pain, nausea, diarrhea, constipation, gas, leg cramps, bloated feeling, anxiety, depression, throat pain or irritation, mild heart-burn, swallowing difficulty, headache, weak muscles.	Continue. Call doctor when convenient.

Rare:

• Chest pain, severe heartburn or throat pain, leg or groin pain, severe muscle pain.	Discontinue. Call doctor right away.
• Skin rash, ankle or leg swelling, eye or dental problems, cold or flu symptoms.	Continue. Call doctor when convenient.

WARNINGS & PRECAUTIONS

Don't take if:
You are allergic to any bisphosphonate.

Before you start, consult your doctor if:
- You currently have a gastrointestinal problem or serious esophageal disease.
- You have low blood levels of calcium (hypocalcemia) or a vitamin D deficiency.
- You have asthma or heart disease.
- You have dental disease or plan dental surgery. Consult your dentist also.
- You have a kidney (renal) disorder.

Over age 60:
No special problems expected.

Pregnancy:
Risk factors vary for drugs in this group. See category list on page xviii and consult doctor.

Breast-feeding:
Unknown if drugs pass into milk. Avoid drug or discontinue nursing until you finish medicine. Consult doctor for advice on maintaining milk supply.

Infants & children:
Not recommended for this age group.

Prolonged use:
Visit your doctor regularly to determine if the drug is continuing to control bone loss.

Skin & sunlight:
No special problems expected.

Driving, piloting or hazardous work:
No special problems expected.

Discontinuing:
No problems expected, but don't discontinue without your doctor's approval. After stopping the drug, it still remains in the body bound to the bone for as long as 10 years in some patients.

Others:
- Bisphosphonates may rarely increase the risk of a femoral (thigh bone) fracture.
- May affect the results of some medical tests.
- To avoid throat (esophagus) problems, carefully follow directions for taking the drug.
- Using zoledronic acid increases risk of kidney failure in certain patients. Consult your doctor.
- Advise any doctor and especially any dentist whom you consult that you take this medicine.
- In addition to the drug, your doctor may recommend exercises, diet changes, and calcium and vitamin D supplements.
- Though rare, bisphosphonates can increase the risk for osteonecrosis (bone destruction), especially of the jaw. Dental disease, oral surgery or tooth removal add to the risk. Talk to your doctor and dentist about your risks.

POSSIBLE INTERACTION WITH OTHER DRUGS

GENERIC NAME OR DRUG CLASS	COMBINED EFFECT
Antacids*	Decreased effect of bisphosphonate. Take 30 minutes after bisphosphonate.
Aspirin-containing products	Increased risk of stomach irritation.
Calcium supplements*	Decreased effect of bisphosphonate. Take 30 minutes after bisphosphonate.
Mineral or vitamin supplements	Decreased effect of bisphosphonate. Take 30 minutes after bisphosphonate

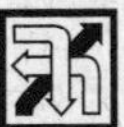

POSSIBLE INTERACTION WITH OTHER SUBSTANCES

INTERACTS WITH	COMBINED EFFECT
Alcohol:	None expected. Alcohol will increase risk for osteoporosis. Try to avoid.
Beverages: Any beverage other than plain water.	Decreased effect of drug. Wait 30 minutes after you take drug.
Cocaine:	No special problems expected.
Foods: Any food.	Decreased effect of drug. Wait 30 minutes to 2 hours after you take drug.
Marijuana:	No special problems expected.
Tobacco:	None expected. Smoking increases risk for osteoporosis. Try to avoid.

*See Glossary

BONE FORMATION AGENTS

GENERIC AND BRAND NAMES

TERIPARATIDE
Forteo

BASIC INFORMATION

Habit forming? No
Prescription needed? Yes
Available as generic? No
Drug class: Osteoporosis therapy

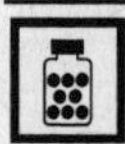

USES

- Treatment of advanced postmenopausal osteoporosis (thinning of bones) in females. Osteoporosis is a cause of bone fractures.
- Treatment of osteoporosis associated with sustained, systemic glucocorticoid therapy in patients at high risk of fracture.
- Treatment for hypogonadal osteoporosis in men at high risk for fracture.

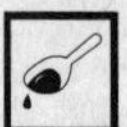

DOSAGE & USAGE INFORMATION

How to take:
Injection—Inject under the skin (subcutaneously) with the pen device provided. Follow your doctor's instructions and the directions provided with the prescription on how, when and where to inject. Do not use the medication unless you are sure about the proper method for injection. Store medication in the refrigerator (do not freeze) until you plan to use it.

When to take:
At the same time each day.

If you forget a dose:
Inject as soon as possible. If it is almost time for your next dose, skip the missed dose and go back to your regular dosing schedule. Do not double doses.

What drug does:
Increases the action of osteoblasts, the body's bone building cells. The bones become more dense and more resistant to fractures.

Continued next column

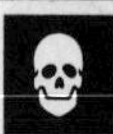

OVERDOSE

SYMPTOMS:
None expected.
WHAT TO DO:
If an overdose is suspected, call doctor or call poison control center 1-800-222-1222 for help.

Time lapse before drug works:
Up to 3 months or longer.

Don't take with:
Any other medicine or any dietary supplement without consulting your doctor or pharmacist.

POSSIBLE ADVERSE REACTIONS OR SIDE EFFECTS

SYMPTOMS	WHAT TO DO
Life-threatening: None expected.	
Common: None expected.	
Infrequent: Injection site discomfort or redness, nausea, headache, stomach cramps, dizziness.	Continue. Call doctor when convenient.
Rare: Leg cramps, lightheadedness when rising after sitting or lying down, syncope (fainting), vertigo.	Continue. Call doctor when convenient.

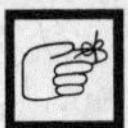

WARNINGS & PRECAUTIONS

Don't take if:
You are allergic to teriparatide or its components.

Before you start, consult your doctor if:
- You have had radiation treatment on the skeleton (bones).
- You have excess calcium in blood (hypercalcemia) or urine (hypercalcuria).
- You have or have had bone cancer/disease.
- You have Paget's disease.
- You have urolithiasis.
- You are allergic to any medication, food or other substance or latex.

Over age 60:
No special problems expected, but caution should be used in the elderly.

Pregnancy:
Normally not used in premenopausal women. Risk category C (see page xviii).

Breast-feeding:
Normally not used in premenopausal women.

Infants & children:
Not recommended for this age group.

Prolonged use:
- Long-term use after 2 years has not been established. Discuss with your doctor.
- Visit your doctor regularly to determine if the drug is continuing to be effective and to monitor your calcium levels.

Skin & sunlight:
No special problems expected.

Driving, piloting or hazardous work:
No special problems expected.

Discontinuing:
No problems expected. Consult doctor.

Others:
- In medical studies on rats injected with teriparatide, a few developed bone cancer (osteosarcoma). Risk in humans is unknown. To date, no women taking the drug have developed the cancer.
- Too much calcium in the blood (hypercalcemia) occurs in some patients using this drug. Consult your doctor about blood tests.
- Other therapies and nondrug routines (e.g., weight-bearing exercise), for treating osteoporosis may be recommended by your doctor. Teriparatide works effectively with certain other drugs for osteoporosis because the drugs work by different mechanisms.
- Advise any doctor or dentist whom you consult that you take this medicine.
- Smoking and alcohol consumption are risk factors for osteoporosis and should be discontinued.

POSSIBLE INTERACTION WITH OTHER DRUGS

GENERIC NAME OR DRUG CLASS	COMBINED EFFECT
Other drugs	Consult doctor or pharmacist.

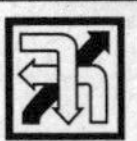

POSSIBLE INTERACTION WITH OTHER SUBSTANCES

INTERACTS WITH	COMBINED EFFECT
Alcohol:	No special problems expected, but alcohol is a risk factor for osteoporosis.
Beverages:	No special problems expected.
Cocaine:	No special problems expected.
Foods:	No special problems expected.
Marijuana:	No special problems expected.
Tobacco:	No special problems expected, but smoking is a risk factor for osteoporosis.

*See Glossary

BOTULINUM TOXIN TYPE A

BRAND NAMES

Botox
Dysport
Myobloc
Xeomin

BASIC INFORMATION

Habit forming? No
Prescription needed? Yes
Available as generic? No
Drug class: Neuromuscular blocking agent

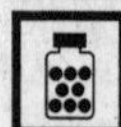

USES

- Provides temporary improvement in appearance in the frown lines between the eyebrows (glabellar lines). May also be used for lines and wrinkles in the forehead, around the eyes, in the lower face area and the neck.
- Treats strabismus (lazy eye) and blepharospasm (uncontrolled eye blinking).
- Treats certain facial nerve disorders and cervical dystonia (neck and shoulder tightness).
- Treatment for migraine, upper limb spasticity, excessive sweating, and urinary incontinence.
- May be used for writer's cramp, tremor, muscle-related disorders, pain, effects of a stroke, and other disorders.

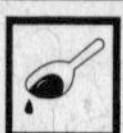

DOSAGE & USAGE INFORMATION

How to take:
Injection—The medicine is administered by your doctor or a health professional. It is injected into the muscle in or around the area being treated.

When to take:
As directed by your doctor.

If you forget a dose:
Injection is done only by scheduled appointment.

What drug does:
It paralyzes, weakens or relaxes the injected muscle by blocking the release of a chemical that normally signals the muscle to contract or tighten. The effect is temporary and most patients will require repeat treatments.

Continued next column

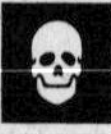

OVERDOSE

SYMPTOMS:
Unknown. May possibly cause body weakness.
WHAT TO DO:
If accidentally injected or swallowed, call doctor or call poison control center 1-800-222-1222 for help.

Time lapse before drug works:
Improvement may be seen in 1-3 days and lasts up to 3-6 months. The degree of improvement will vary from person to person and will depend on the disorder being treated.

Don't take with:
Any other medicine or any dietary supplement without consulting your doctor or pharmacist.

POSSIBLE ADVERSE REACTIONS OR SIDE EFFECTS

SYMPTOMS	WHAT TO DO
Life-threatening:	
Severe problems with swallowing or breathing after treatment (can happen hours to weeks after an injection).	Seek emergency treatment immediately.
Common:	
• With blepharospasm (dry eyes, eyelid does not close completely).	Call doctor right away.
• With blepharospasm or strabismus (eye irritation or watering, eyelid drooping or bruised, light sensitivity).	Call doctor if you are concerned or symptoms continue.
Infrequent:	
• With blepharospasm or strabismus (blinking decreased, cornea irritation, eyelid edge turns in or out, skin rash, eyelid swelling, vision changes, eye pointing up or down).	Call doctor right away.
• With lines/wrinkles (injection site numb, burning or swelling).	Call doctor if you are concerned or symptoms continue.
Rare:	
• Any problems with speech, breathing or swallowing or heart symptoms occur or allergic reaction occurs.	Call doctor right away or seek emergency treatment if symptoms severe.
• With lines/wrinkles (drooping eyelids, redness or bruising at injection site, facial pain, skin rash or itching, headache, nausea, flu or cold symptoms).	Call doctor if you are concerned or symptoms continue.

- Other side effects or adverse reactions may occur depending on the disorder being treated. Drugs injected into muscles can be absorbed by the body and cause symptoms. — Call doctor if you are concerned or symptoms continue or they are severe.

WARNINGS & PRECAUTIONS

Don't take if:
You are allergic to botulinum toxin type A.

Before you start, consult your doctor if:
- You have heart problems.
- You have a nerve or muscle disorder, or a problem with swallowing.
- You have inflammation in the muscle area to be treated.
- You are allergic to any medication, food or other substance.
- You have a history of infection involving botulism poisoning.

Over age 60:
No special problems expected. Currently, for wrinkle treatment, the drug is approved for people between ages 18 and 65.

Pregnancy:
Decide with your doctor if drug benefits justify any possible risk to unborn child. Risk category C (see page xviii). Consult doctor if you become pregnant and have had a botulinum injection.

Breast-feeding:
It is unknown if drug passes into milk. Avoid nursing if you use this medicine. Consult doctor for advice on maintaining milk supply.

Infants & children:
Not approved for children under age 12 for strabismus or blepharospasm treatment, or under age 18 for facial lines or wrinkle treatment.

Prolonged use:
- Long term effects are unknown. Discuss with you doctor about long term use. Benefits and risks will differ depending on the problem being treated.
- Benefits may decrease with continued use.
- For facial lines and wrinkles, the injections should be at least 3 months apart.

Skin & sunlight:
No special problems expected.

Driving, piloting or hazardous work:
Since this medicine may be used for treatment of a variety of disorders (including eye muscle disorders, muscle contraction problems and muscle spasms), always consult your doctor about your individual circumstances.

Discontinuing:
Symptoms and signs of the problem being treated will most likely return.

Others:
- This treatment is given in a medical office and the risks and benefits will be explained to you. The information provided in this topic does not replace the information or special instructions provided by your doctor.
- Patients who have been inactive (sedentary) should resume activities gradually after receiving an injection.
- Very rarely, botulinum toxin may affect areas of the body away from the injection site and cause symptoms of botulism (a serious condition). It can happen hours to weeks after an injection. Symptoms of botulism include: loss of strength and muscle weakness all over the body, double vision, blurred vision and drooping eyelids, hoarseness or change or loss of voice, trouble saying words clearly, loss of bladder control, trouble breathing and swallowing. Call doctor or seek emergency care.
- Advise any doctor or dentist whom you consult (within the few months following the injection) that you have used this medicine.

POSSIBLE INTERACTION WITH OTHER DRUGS

GENERIC NAME OR DRUG CLASS	COMBINED EFFECT
Aminoglycosides*	Increased effect of botulinum toxin type A.

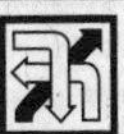

POSSIBLE INTERACTION WITH OTHER SUBSTANCES

INTERACTS WITH	COMBINED EFFECT
Alcohol:	None expected.
Beverages:	None expected.
Cocaine:	None expected. Best to avoid.
Foods:	None expected.
Marijuana:	May contribute to facial lines. Avoid.
Tobacco:	May contribute to facial lines. Avoid.

*See Glossary

BROMOCRIPTINE

BRAND NAMES

Alti-Bromocriptine
Apo-Bromocriptine
Cycloset
Parlodel
Parlodel Snaptabs

BASIC INFORMATION

Habit forming? No
Prescription needed? Yes
Available as generic? Yes
Drug class: Antiparkinsonism; antidiabetic

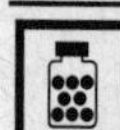

USES

- Controls Parkinson's disease symptoms such as rigidity, tremors and unsteady gait.
- Treats male and female infertility.
- Treats acromegaly (an overproduction of growth hormone).
- Treatment for diabetes type 2 (along with diet and exercise).
- Treats some pituitary tumors.

DOSAGE & USAGE INFORMATION

How to take:
Tablet or capsule—Swallow with liquid or food to lessen stomach irritation. If you can't swallow whole, crumble tablet or open capsule and take with liquid or food.

When to take:
At the same times each day. Take brand name Cycloset with food within 2 hours after waking up in the morning.

Continued next column

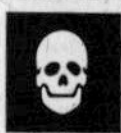

OVERDOSE

SYMPTOMS:

- **Muscle twitch, spastic eyelid closure, nausea, vomiting, diarrhea, irregular and rapid pulse, weakness, fainting, confusion, agitation, hallucination, coma.**
- **Diabetic patients need to be aware of symptoms of low blood sugar.**

WHAT TO DO:

- **Dial 911 (emergency) for medical help or call poison control center 1-800-222-1222 for instructions.**
- **If person is unconscious, check breathing and pulse. If not breathing, begin mouth-to-mouth rescue breathing. If heart is not beating, begin chest compressions.**
- **See emergency information on last 3 pages of this book.**

If you forget a dose:
Take as soon as you remember. If it is almost time for the next dose, wait for the next scheduled dose (don't double this dose).

What drug does:

- Restores chemical balance necessary for normal nerve impulses.
- It is unknown how it works to lower blood sugar in diabetic patients.

Time lapse before drug works:
2 to 3 weeks to improve; several months or longer for maximum benefit.

Don't take with:
Any other medicine or any dietary supplement without consulting your doctor or pharmacist.

POSSIBLE ADVERSE REACTIONS OR SIDE EFFECTS

SYMPTOMS	WHAT TO DO
Life-threatening: In case of overdose, see previous column.	
Common: Dizziness, mild nausea, lightheadedness when getting up, headache.	Continue. Call doctor when convenient.
Infrequent: Constipation, diarrhea, tiredness, drowsiness, dry mouth, depression, tingling and numbness of hands and feet.	Continue. Call doctor when convenient.
Rare:	
• Severe nausea and vomiting (may be bloody), vision changes, nervousness, sudden weakness, unusual headache, excess sweating, seizures, fainting, chest pain, black or tarry stools, uncontrollable body movements.	Discontinue. Call doctor right away.
• Stomach or back pain, runny nose, urinary frequency.	Continue. Call doctor when convenient.

WARNINGS & PRECAUTIONS

Don't take if:
- You are allergic to bromocriptine or ergotamine.
- You have taken a monoamine oxidase (MAO) inhibitor* in the past 2 weeks.
- You have glaucoma (narrow-angle type).

Before you start, consult your doctor if:
- You have diabetes or epilepsy.
- You have had high blood pressure, heart or lung disease.
- You have had liver or kidney disease.
- You have a peptic ulcer.
- You have a history of mental problems.
- You will have surgery within 2 months, requiring general or spinal anesthesia.

Over age 60:
Adverse reactions and side effects may be more frequent and severe than in younger persons.

Pregnancy:
Decide with your doctor if drug benefits justify risk to unborn child. Risk category B (see page xviii).

Breast-feeding:
Drug inhibits milk production. Avoid.

Infants & children:
Not recommended if under 15 years old.

Prolonged use:
- May lead to uncontrolled movements of head, face, mouth, tongue, arms or legs.
- Changes in lung tissue and excess fluid in chest cavity may occur.
- Talk to your doctor about the need for follow-up medical examinations or laboratory studies to check blood pressure, x-rays, growth hormone levels, or blood sugar levels.

Skin & sunlight:
No problems expected.

Driving, piloting or hazardous work:
Don't drive or pilot aircraft until you learn how medicine effects you. Don't work around dangerous machinery. Don't climb ladders or work in high places. Danger increases if you drink alcohol or take medicine affecting alertness and reflexes, such as antihistamines, tranquilizers, sedatives, pain medicine, narcotics and mind-altering drugs.

Discontinuing:
Don't discontinue without doctor's advice until you complete prescribed dose, even though symptoms diminish or disappear.

Others:
- May start treatment with small doses and increase gradually to lessen frequency and severity of adverse reactions.
- For diabetes type 2 patients: you and your family should educate yourselves about diabetes; learn to recognize hypoglycemia and treat it with sugar or glucagon.
- Advise any doctor or dentist whom you consult that you take this medicine.

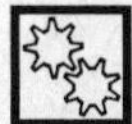

POSSIBLE INTERACTION WITH OTHER DRUGS

GENERIC NAME OR DRUG CLASS	COMBINED EFFECT
Antihypertensives*	May decrease blood pressure.
Antiparkinsonism drugs, other*	Increased bromocriptine effect.
Ergot alkaloids, other	Increased risk of high blood pressure.
Erythromycin	Increased bromocriptine effect.
Haloperidol	Decreased bromocriptine effect.
Levodopa	Decreased antiparkinson effect.
Methyldopa	Decreased bromocriptine effect.
Papaverine	Decreased bromocriptine effect.
Phenothiazines*	Decreased bromocriptine effect.
Risperidone	Increased bromocriptine effect.
Ritonavir	Increased bromocriptine effect.

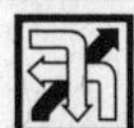

POSSIBLE INTERACTION WITH OTHER SUBSTANCES

INTERACTS WITH	COMBINED EFFECT
Alcohol:	Decreased alcohol tolerance. Avoid.
Beverages:	None expected.
Cocaine:	Decreased bromocriptine effect. Avoid.
Foods:	None expected.
Marijuana:	Increased fatigue, lethargy, fainting. Avoid.
Tobacco:	Interferes with absorption. Avoid.

BRONCHODILATORS, ADRENERGIC

GENERIC AND BRAND NAMES

See full list of generic and brand names in the *Generic and Brand Name Directory*, page 878.

BASIC INFORMATION

Habit forming? No
Prescription needed? Yes, for most
Available as generic? Yes, for some
Drug class: Sympathomimetic

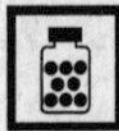

USES

- Relieves bronchial asthma.
- Decreases congestion of breathing passages.
- Suppresses allergic reactions.
- Treats bronchoconstriction in COPD.*
- Relieves exercise-induced bronchospasm.

DOSAGE & USAGE INFORMATION

How to take:
- Tablet or capsule—Swallow with liquid. You may chew or crush tablet.
- Extended-release tablet—Swallow each dose whole.
- Syrup—Take as directed on bottle.
- Drops—Dilute dose in beverage.
- Inhaler—Follow directions in package.

When to take:
As directed by your doctor.

If you forget a dose:
Take as soon as you remember. If it is almost time for the next dose, wait for the next scheduled dose (don't double this dose).

What drug does:
- Prevents cells from releasing allergy-causing chemicals (histamines).
- Relaxes muscles of bronchial tubes.
- Decreases blood-vessel size and blood flow, thus causing decongestion.

Continued next column

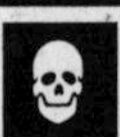

OVERDOSE

SYMPTOMS:
Severe anxiety, confusion, delirium, muscle tremors, rapid and irregular pulse, severe weakness.
WHAT TO DO:
- **Dial 911 (emergency) for medical help or call poison control center 1-800-222-1222 for instructions.**
- **See emergency information on last 3 pages of this book.**

Time lapse before drug works:
30 to 60 minutes.

Don't take with:
- Nonprescription drugs with ephedrine, pseudoephedrine or epinephrine.
- Nonprescription drugs for cough, cold, allergy or asthma without consulting doctor.
- Any other medicine or any dietary supplement without consulting your doctor or pharmacist.

POSSIBLE ADVERSE REACTIONS OR SIDE EFFECTS

SYMPTOMS	WHAT TO DO
Life-threatening: In case of overdose, see previous column.	
Common:	
• Nervousness, restlessness, trembling.	Continue. Call doctor when convenient.
• Dry mouth or throat.	Continue. Tell doctor at next visit.
Infrequent:	
• Fast heartbeat, nausea, vomiting, headache, dizziness, lightheadedness.	Discontinue. Call doctor right away.
• Trouble sleeping, appetite loss, coughing.	Continue. Call doctor when convenient.
Rare:	
• Increased wheezing, difficulty breathing, chest discomfort or pain, irregular heartbeat, painful or difficult urination, allergic reaction (bluish, reddish or flushed skin; rash; itching; hives; swelling of face area; wheezing).	Discontinue. Call doctor right away or seek emergency treatment.
• Smell or taste changes.	No action necessary.

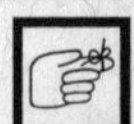

WARNINGS & PRECAUTIONS

Don't take if:
You are allergic to ephedrine, any bronchodilator* drug or sulfites used in some preparations.

Before you start, consult your doctor if:
- You have high blood pressure.
- You have diabetes.
- You have cardiovascular disease.
- You have overactive thyroid gland.
- You have difficulty urinating.
- You have taken any monoamine oxidase (MAO) inhibitor* in past 2 weeks.
- You have taken digitalis preparations* in the last 7 days.

- If you will have surgery within 2 months, including dental surgery, requiring anesthesia.
- If you have pheochromocytoma.

Over age 60:
More likely to develop high blood pressure, heart rhythm disturbances, angina and to feel drug's stimulant effects.

Pregnancy:
Risk factors vary for drugs in this group. See category list on page xviii and consult doctor.

Breast-feeding:
Drug passes into milk. Avoid drug or discontinue nursing until you finish medicine. Consult doctor for advice on maintaining milk supply.

Infants & children:
No problems expected for most. Use only under close medical supervision. Xopenex is not recommended for children under 12.

Prolonged use:
- Excessive doses—Rare toxic psychosis.
- Men with enlarged prostate gland may have more urination difficulty.
- Talk to your doctor about the need for follow-up medical examinations or laboratory studies.

Skin & sunlight:
No problems expected.

Driving, piloting or hazardous work:
Avoid if you feel dizzy. Otherwise, no problems expected.

Discontinuing:
- May be unnecessary to finish medicine. Follow doctor's instructions.
- Don't suddenly discontinue the drug without medical advice.

Others:
- May affect results in some medical tests.
- Advise any doctor or dentist whom you consult that you take this medicine.
- Ask your doctor about specific risks that may involve the drug salmeterol.
- Some of these drugs may increase the chance of severe asthma episodes, and death when those episodes occur. Ask your doctor about your risk for the drug you are using.
- Complications increase if you use more than prescribed. If you need to use the drug more frequently, consult your doctor.

POSSIBLE INTERACTION WITH OTHER DRUGS

GENERIC NAME OR DRUG CLASS	COMBINED EFFECT
Antidepressants, tricyclic*	Increased effect of bronchodilator. Heart and blood pressure problems.
Antihypertensives*	Decreased anti-hypertensive effect.
Beta-adrenergic blocking agents*	Decreased effects of both drugs.
Digitalis preparations*	Serious heart rhythm disturbances.
Epinephrine	Increased bronchodilator effect.
Ergot preparations*	Serious blood pressure rise.
Finasteride	Decreased finasteride effect.
Furazolidone	Increased risk of heart problems.
Maprotiline	Increased risk of heart problems.
Methyldopa	Increased risk of heart problems.
Monoamine oxidase (MAO) inhibitors*	Increased bronchodilator effect. Increased risk of heart problems.
Nicotine	Decreased effect of isoproterenol.
Nitrates*	Decreased effect of both drugs.
Phenothiazines*	Increased risk of heart problems.
Pseudoephedrine	Increased effect of bronchodilator.

Continued on page 910

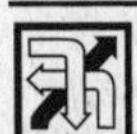

POSSIBLE INTERACTION WITH OTHER SUBSTANCES

INTERACTS WITH	COMBINED EFFECT
Alcohol:	None expected.
Beverages:	
Caffeine drinks.	Nervousness or insomnia.
Grapefruit juice.	Risk of toxicity of theophylline. Avoid.
Cocaine:	Irregular heartbeat and high blood pressure. Avoid.
Foods:	None expected.
Marijuana:	Rapid heartbeat or heart rhythm problem. Avoid.
Tobacco:	None expected.

BRONCHODILATORS, ANTICHOLINERGIC

GENERIC AND BRAND NAMES

ACLIDINIUM	TIOTROPIUM
Tudorza Pressair	Spiriva

BASIC INFORMATION

Habit forming? No
Prescription needed? Yes
Available as generic? No
Drug class: Anticholinergic; bronchodilator

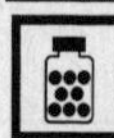

USES

Maintenance treatment for bronchospasms that occur with chronic obstructive pulmonary disease (COPD), including chronic bronchitis and emphysema. These drugs are not used to relieve an acute attack of breathing difficulty.

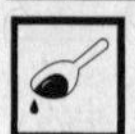

DOSAGE & USAGE INFORMATION

How to take:
Inhalation powder—Carefully follow the instructions provided with each product. Review them often; don't depend on memory. Don't swallow capsule.

When to take:
Once a day for tiotropium or twice a day for aclidinium. Take at the same time(s) each day.

If you forget a dose:
Take as soon as you remember. If it is almost time for your next dose, skip the missed dose and go back to the regular dosing schedule. Do not double doses.

What drug does:
Relaxes the muscles around narrowed airways in the lungs and helps to keep them open and make breathing easier.

Continued next column

OVERDOSE

SYMPTOMS:
Inhaled overdose is unlikely. Dry mouth, conjunctivitis, tremors, stomach pain, confusion may occur. Swallowed capsule is unlikely to cause symptoms as capsule is not well-absorbed by the gastrointestinal tract.
WHAT TO DO:
If person inhales much larger amount than prescribed or someone accidentally swallows a capsule, dial 911 (emergency) for medical help or call poison control center 1-800-222-1222 for instructions.

Time lapse before drug works:
Begins working right away, but will take about 2 to 3 weeks for full maintenance benefits.

Don't take with:
Any other medicine or any dietary supplement without consulting your doctor or pharmacist.

POSSIBLE ADVERSE REACTIONS OR SIDE EFFECTS

SYMPTOMS	WHAT TO DO
Life-threatening:	
Rare allergic reaction (hives, itching, rash, wheezing, tightness in chest, swelling of lips or tongue or throat).	Seek emergency treatment immediately.
Common:	
Dry mouth, cold or sinus infection symptoms (stuffy nose, sneezing, cough, sore throat), headache.	Continue. Call doctor when convenient.
Infrequent:	
• Painful or frequent urination, urinary retention.	Discontinue. Call doctor right away.
• Constipation, upset stomach, diarrhea.	Continue. Call doctor when convenient.
Rare:	
• Increased heart rate, chest pain, bloody nose, breathing problem, induced broncho-spasm (wheezing or cough), eye symptoms (pain, redness, blurred vision, seeing halos or colors around lights).	Discontinue. Call doctor right away.
• Heartburn, rash, vomiting, muscle or bone aches, dizziness.	Continue. Call doctor when convenient.

WARNINGS & PRECAUTIONS

Don't take if:
You are allergic to aclidinium, tiotropium or atropine (or similar drugs).

Before you start, consult your doctor if:
- You have a kidney disorder.
- You have bladder problems, or urinary blockage or trouble urinating.
- You have enlarged prostate gland (prostatic hypertrophy).
- You have eye problems (e.g., glaucoma).
- You are allergic to milk proteins.
- You are allergic to any medications.

Over age 60:
No problems expected.

Pregnancy:
Decide with your doctor whether drug benefits justify risk to unborn child. Risk category C (see page xviii).

Breast-feeding:
It is unknown if drug passes into breast milk. Consult your doctor for advice.

Infants & children:
Not recommended for this age group. COPD does not normally occur in children.

Prolonged use:
See your doctor for regular visits to make sure the drug is working properly and to check for unwanted effects.

Skin & sunlight:
No problems expected.

Driving, piloting or hazardous work:
Don't drive or pilot aircraft until you learn how medicine affects you. Don't work around dangerous machinery. Don't climb ladders or work in high places.

Discontinuing:
No problems expected. Consult your doctor before discontinuing.

Others:
- Advise any doctor, dentist or pharmacist whom you consult that you take this drug.
- Do not increase the dose or use drug more often than prescribed without checking with your doctor.
- The drug should not be used for sudden breathing problems. It is not a rescue inhaler.
- For dry mouth, suck sugarless hard candy or chew sugarless gum. If dry mouth continues, consult your doctor or dentist.

POSSIBLE INTERACTION WITH OTHER DRUGS

GENERIC NAME OR DRUG CLASS	COMBINED EFFECT
Anticholinergics,* other	May increase anticholinergic effect. Consult doctor.

POSSIBLE INTERACTION WITH OTHER SUBSTANCES

INTERACTS WITH	COMBINED EFFECT
Alcohol:	None expected.
Beverages:	None expected.
Cocaine:	Effect unknown. Avoid.
Foods:	None expected.
Marijuana:	Effect unknown. Avoid.
Tobacco:	May decrease effect of drug. People with COPD should not smoke.

*See Glossary

BRONCHODILATORS, XANTHINE

GENERIC AND BRAND NAMES

See full list of generic and brand names in the *Generic and Brand Name Directory*, page 878.

BASIC INFORMATION

Habit forming? No
Prescription needed? Yes
Available as generic? Yes
Drug class: Bronchodilator (xanthine)

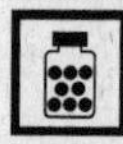

USES

- Treatment for bronchial asthma symptoms.
- Treatment for chronic bronchitis, emphysema and other pulmonary diseases.

DOSAGE & USAGE INFORMATION

How to take:
- Tablet or capsule—Swallow with liquid.
- Extended-release tablet or capsule—Swallow each dose whole. If you take regular tablets, you may chew or crush them.
- Suppository—Remove wrapper and moisten suppository with water. Gently insert larger end into rectum. Push well into rectum with finger.
- Syrup, elixir or oral solution—Take as directed on bottle.
- Enema—Use as directed on label.

When to take:
Most effective taken on empty stomach 1 hour before or 2 hours after eating. However, may take with food to lessen stomach upset.

If you forget a dose:
Take as soon as you remember. If it is almost time for the next dose, wait for the next scheduled dose (don't double this dose).

What drug does:
Relaxes and expands bronchial tubes.

Continued next column

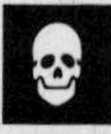

OVERDOSE

SYMPTOMS:
Restlessness, irritability, confusion, black or tarry stool, breathing difficulty, pounding and irregular heartbeat, vomiting blood, delirium, convulsions, rapid pulse, coma.

WHAT TO DO:
- **Dial 911 (emergency) for medical help or call poison control center 1-800-222-1222 for instructions.**
- **See emergency information on last 3 pages of this book.**

Time lapse before drug works:
15 to 30 minutes.

Don't take with:
Any other medicine or any dietary supplement without consulting your doctor or pharmacist.

POSSIBLE ADVERSE REACTIONS OR SIDE EFFECTS

SYMPTOMS	WHAT TO DO
Life-threatening: In case of overdose, see previous column.	
Common: Headache, irritability, nervousness, nausea, restlessness, insomnia, vomiting, stomach pain.	Continue. Call doctor when convenient.
Infrequent: • Rash or hives, flushed face, diarrhea, rapid breathing, irregular heartbeat.	Discontinue. Call doctor right away.
• Dizziness or lightheadedness, appetite loss, trembling, fatigue, weakness.	Continue. Call doctor when convenient.
Rare: Frequent urination.	Continue. Call doctor when convenient.

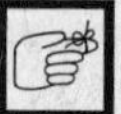

WARNINGS & PRECAUTIONS

Don't take if:
- You are allergic to any bronchodilator.
- You have an active peptic ulcer.

Before you start, consult your doctor if:
- You have had impaired kidney or liver function.
- You have gastritis.
- You have a peptic ulcer.
- You have high blood pressure or heart disease.
- You take medication for gout.

Over age 60:
Adverse reactions and side effects may be more frequent and severe than in younger persons.

Pregnancy:
Decide with your doctor if drug benefits justify risk to unborn child. Risk category C (see page xviii).

Breast-feeding:
Drug passes into milk. Avoid drug or discontinue nursing until you finish medicine. Consult doctor for advice on maintaining milk supply.

Infants & children:
Use only under medical supervision.

Prolonged use:
Stomach irritation may occur.

Skin & sunlight:
No problems expected.

Driving, piloting or hazardous work:
Avoid if lightheaded or dizzy. Otherwise, no problems expected.

Discontinuing:
May be unnecessary to finish medicine. Follow doctor's instructions.

Others:
Advise any doctor or dentist whom you consult that you take this medicine.

POSSIBLE INTERACTION WITH OTHER DRUGS

GENERIC NAME OR DRUG CLASS	COMBINED EFFECT
Allopurinol	Increased theophylline effect.
Aminoglutethimide	Possible decreased bronchodilator effect.
Beta-agonists*	Increased effect of both drugs.
Beta-adrenergic blocking agents*	Decreased bronchodilator effect.
Cimetidine	Increased bronchodilator effect.
Clarithromycin	Increased concentration of theophylline.
Clindamycin	May increase bronchodilator effect.
Corticosteroids*	Possible increased bronchodilator effect.
Erythromycin	Increased bronchodilator effect.
Finasteride	Decreased finasteride effect.
Fluoroquinolones	Increased xanthine bronchodilator in blood. May need dose adjustment.
Fluvoxamine	Increased theophylline effect.
Furosemide	Increased furosemide effect.
Lansoprazole	May require dosage adjustment of theophylline.
Leukotriene modifiers	Unknown effects. Consult doctor.
Lincomycins*	May increase bronchodilator effect.
Lithium	Decreased lithium effect.
Modafinil	Decreased bronchodilator effect.
Moricizine	Decreased bronchodilator effect.
Nicotine	Possible increased bronchodilator effect.
Phenobarbital	Decreased bronchodilator effect.
Phenytoin	Decreased effect of both drugs.
Probenecid	Increased effect of dyphylline.
Ranitidine	Possible increased bronchodilator effect and toxicity.
Rauwolfia alkaloids*	Rapid heartbeat.
Rifampin	Decreased bronchodilator effect.
Sulfinpyrazone	Increased effect of dyphylline.
Sympathomimetics*	Possible increased bronchodilator effect
Tacrine	Increased bronchodilator effect.

Continued on page 910

POSSIBLE INTERACTION WITH OTHER SUBSTANCES

INTERACTS WITH	COMBINED EFFECT
Alcohol:	None expected.
Beverages:	
Caffeine drinks.	Nervousness and insomnia.
Grapefruit juice.	Toxicity risk with theophylline. Avoid.
Cocaine:	Excess stimulation. Avoid.
Foods:	None expected.
Marijuana:	Slightly increased antiasthmatic effect of bronchodilator. Decreased effect with chronic use.
Tobacco:	Decreased bronchodilator effect.

***See Glossary**

BUPRENORPHINE & NALOXONE

BRAND NAMES

Suboxone Film

BASIC INFORMATION

Habit forming? Yes
Prescription needed? Yes
Available as generic? Yes (for tablet)
Drug class: Narcotic

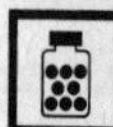

USES

- Treatment for dependence on narcotic (opioid) painkillers including prescription drugs and illicit drugs such as heroin. Should be used in conjunction with an addiction treatment program that involves counseling and/or behavioral therapy. Only certain qualified doctors are able to start in-office treatment and provide prescriptions for ongoing medication.
- A buprenorphine-only tablet may be used in the first few days of treatment.

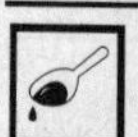

DOSAGE & USAGE INFORMATION

How to take:

- Sublingual film—Follow instructions provided with the prescription.
- Sublingual tablet—Place under your tongue and let tablet dissolve. Do not eat or drink or smoke while it dissolves.

When to take:
Once a day at the same time every day. Do not take more or less than prescribed. Dosage may be adjusted only by your doctor.

If you forget a dose:
Take as soon as you remember. If it is almost time for your next dose, skip the missed dose and go back to your regular dosing schedule. Do not double doses (unless advised by doctor).

Continued next column

OVERDOSE

SYMPTOMS:
Especially if injected—slowed breathing, dizziness, faintness, confusion, pinpoint pupils, low blood pressure (an untreated overdose can lead to death).

WHAT TO DO:

- **Dial 911 (emergency) for medical help or call poison control center 1-800-222-1222 for instructions.**
- **See emergency information on last 3 pages of this book.**

What drug does:

- Reduces withdrawal symptoms and blocks the craving without producing strong narcotic high.
- Naloxone is combined with buprenorphine to guard against the intravenous abuse of buprenorphine. It can produce intense withdrawal symptoms if misused that way. When used as prescribed, naloxone has no effect.

Time lapse before drug works:
Within 30 to 60 minutes of taking the dose. May take 3 to 7 days for the effects of the drug to become stable in the body.

Don't take with:
Any other medicine or any dietary supplement without consulting your doctor or pharmacist.

POSSIBLE ADVERSE REACTIONS OR SIDE EFFECTS

SYMPTOMS	WHAT TO DO
Life-threatening:	
Allergic reaction (hives, facial swelling, sweating, wheezing, loss of blood pressure, and consciousness).	Seek emergency treatment immediately.
Common:	
Constipation, nausea, headache, appetite loss, drowsiness, pain, insomnia, mood swings, cold or flu symptoms, sweating.	Continue. Call doctor when convenient.
Infrequent:	
• Liver problems (yellow skin or eyes, dark urine, stools light in color, stomach pain).	Discontinue. Call doctor right away.
• Withdrawal syndrome (nausea or vomiting, muscle aches, runny nose, teary eyes, enlarged pupils, diarrhea, yawning, fever, insomnia).	Continue, but call doctor right away.
Rare:	
Other unexplained symptoms occur that cause concern.	Continue. Call doctor when convenient.

WARNINGS & PRECAUTIONS

Don't take if:
You are allergic to buprenorphine or naloxone.

Before you start, consult your doctor if:
- You have liver or kidney disease.
- You have gallbladder problems, adrenal gland problems, low thyroid (hypothyroidism) or pancreatitis.
- You have severe mental problems or suffer from hallucinations.
- You are an alcoholic.
- You have respiratory (lung) problems.
- You have problems with urination or constipation, or bowel obstruction.
- You have a head injury or brain problem.
- You have enlarged prostate (males).
- You have scoliosis (causing breathing problems).

Over age 60:
No special problems expected, but caution should be used in the elderly.

Pregnancy:
Decide with your doctor whether drug benefits justify risk to unborn child. Risk category C (see page xviii).

Breast-feeding:
Drug passes into milk. Avoid drug or discontinue nursing until you finish medicine. Consult doctor for advice on maintaining milk supply.

Infants & children:
Not recommended for children under age 16.

Prolonged use:
Talk to your doctor about the need for follow-up medical examinations or laboratory studies to check liver function.

Skin & sunlight:
No problems expected.

Driving, piloting or hazardous work:
Don't drive or pilot aircraft until you learn how medicine affects you. Don't work around dangerous machinery. Don't climb ladders or work in high places. Danger increases if you drink alcohol or take medicine affecting alertness and reflexes.

Discontinuing:
Don't discontinue without consulting doctor. Withdrawal syndrome can occur. Dose may require gradual reduction. Doses of other drugs may also require adjustment.

Others:
- This drug treatment must be given and followed up closely by a specially trained doctor. Be sure to see your doctor as scheduled for office visits. Be compliant with your treatment plan. The information on these pages does not take the place of talking to your doctor.
- Withdrawal syndrome may occur as you are transferred (or switched) from the addicting drug or methadone treatment to this drug. Consult your doctor if symptoms occur.
- Be sure your family members are aware of your drug dependence and that you are taking this drug. They will need to advise medical professionals if an emergency occurs.
- Keep the drug in a safe place, protect from theft and don't let anyone else use it.
- Use only as directed. Deaths have been reported in addicts who have intravenously misused this drug.
- Advise any doctor or dentist whom you consult that you take this medicine.
- Your doctor will discuss the possibility of discontinuing the drug therapy once you are on a maintenance dose or are stabilized.

POSSIBLE INTERACTION WITH OTHER DRUGS

GENERIC NAME OR DRUG CLASS	COMBINED EFFECT
Benzodiazepines	Serious overdose may occur.
CNS depressants,* other	Increased risk of adverse effects.
Enzyme inhibitors*	Increased effect of buprenorphine.
Phenothiazines	Decreased effect of buprenorphine.

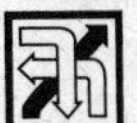

POSSIBLE INTERACTION WITH OTHER SUBSTANCES

INTERACTS WITH	COMBINED EFFECT
Alcohol:	Increased adverse effects including diminished breathing and death. Avoid.
Beverages:	None expected.
Cocaine:	Unpredictable effects. Avoid.
Foods:	None expected.
Marijuana:	Unpredictable effects. Avoid.
Tobacco:	None expected.

*See Glossary

BUPROPION

BRAND NAMES

Aplenzin
Forfivo XL
Wellbutrin
Wellbutrin SR
Wellbutrin XL
Zyban

BASIC INFORMATION

Habit forming? No
Prescription needed? Yes
Available as generic? Yes
Drug class: Antidepressant

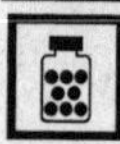

USES

- Relieves severe depression. (Has less effect on sexual functioning than some other antidepressants and may be more acceptable to some patients.)
- May be used in combination with other therapy for smoking cessation.
- Prevention of major depressive episodes in those with seasonal affective disorder (SAD).
- Treatment for other disorders as determined by your doctor.

DOSAGE & USAGE INFORMATION

How to take:
- Tablet—Swallow with liquid. May take with food to lessen stomach irritation. If you can't swallow whole, ask doctor or pharmacist for advice.
- Sustained-release tablet or extended release tablet—Swallow with liquid. Do not crush or crumble tablet.

When to take:
At the same time(s) each day, according to instructions on prescription label.

If you forget a dose:
Take as soon as you remember. If it is almost time for the next dose, wait for the next scheduled dose (don't double this dose).

Continued next column

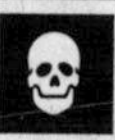

OVERDOSE

SYMPTOMS:
Confusion, agitation, seizures, coma.
WHAT TO DO:
- **Dial 911 (emergency) for medical help or call poison control center 1-800-222-1222 for instructions.**
- **See emergency information on last 3 pages of this book.**

What drug does:
Blocks certain chemicals that are necessary for nerve transmission in the brain. Boosts dopamine and norepinephrine (two brain chemicals) that are also boosted by nicotine.

Time lapse before drug works:
For depression symptoms, about 3 to 4 weeks. For smoking cessation, may take 7-12 weeks.

Don't take with:
Any other medicine or any dietary supplement without consulting your doctor or pharmacist.

POSSIBLE ADVERSE REACTIONS OR SIDE EFFECTS

SYMPTOMS	WHAT TO DO
Life-threatening: In case of overdose, see previous column.	
Common:	
• Agitation, anxiety.	Discontinue. Call doctor right away.
• Dry mouth, dizziness, insomnia, loss of appetite, constipation, stomach or muscle pain, nausea or vomiting, sore throat, unusual weight loss, trembling, increased sweating.	Continue. Call doctor when convenient.
Infrequent:	
• Skin rash or hives or itching, severe headache, hearing noises in ears.	Discontinue. Call doctor right away.
• Drowsiness, change in taste, blurred vision, frequent urination, euphoria.	Continue. Call doctor when convenient.
Rare:	
Fainting, seizures. confusion, delusions, hallucinations, feeling paranoid, unable to concentrate, fast or irregular heartbeat, higher blood pressure, behavior changes, thoughts/talk of suicide.	Discontinue. Call doctor right away.

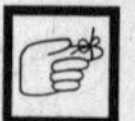

WARNINGS & PRECAUTIONS

Don't take if:
You are allergic to bupropion.

Before you start, consult your doctor if:
- You have or have had any mental illness, a seizure disorder, anorexia nervosa or bulimia.

- You have a history of alcohol or drug abuse.
- You have liver, kidney or heart disease.
- You have had recent head injury.
- You have a brain or spinal cord tumor.

Over age 60:
Adverse reactions and side effects may be more frequent and severe. You may need smaller doses for shorter periods of time.

Pregnancy:
Decide with your doctor whether drug benefits justify risk to unborn child. Risk category B (see page xviii).

Breast-feeding:
Drug passes into milk. May cause adverse reactions. Avoid drug or stop breast-feeding. Consult doctor about maintaining milk supply.

Infants & children:
If prescribed for age under 18, carefully read information provided with prescription. Contact doctor right away if depression symptoms get worse or there is any talk of suicide or suicide behaviors. Also, read information under Others.

Prolonged use:
Talk to your doctor about the need for follow-up medical examinations or laboratory studies to check kidney function, liver function, blood pressure and levels of bupropion in your blood.

Skin & sunlight:
No problems expected.

Driving, piloting or hazardous work:
Don't drive or pilot aircraft until you learn how medicine affects you. Don't work around dangerous machinery. Don't climb ladders or work in high places. Danger increases if you drink alcohol or take drugs affecting alertness and reflexes.

Discontinuing:
Don't discontinue without doctor's advice. Dose may require gradual reduction.

Others:
- If drug is taken to help stop smoking, be sure to follow all medical instructions.
- Use of this drug may lead to serious mental health events. They include worsening or new depression symptoms, changes in behavior (hostility, agitation) and may have increased suicidal thoughts or behaviors. Call doctor right away if these symptoms or behaviors occur.
- Advise any doctor or dentist whom you consult that you take this medicine.

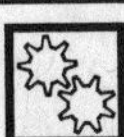

POSSIBLE INTERACTION WITH OTHER DRUGS

GENERIC NAME OR DRUG CLASS	COMBINED EFFECT
Adrenocorticoids (systemic)	Increased risk of seizures.
Antidepressants, tricyclic*	Increased risk of seizures.
Clozapine	Increased risk of seizures.
Enzyme inducers*	Decreased effect of bupropion.
Enzyme inhibitors*	Increased effect of bupropion.
Fluoxetine	Increased risk of seizures.
Haloperidol	Increased risk of seizures.
Levodopa	Increased risk of side effects.
Lithium	Increased risk of seizures.
Loxapine	Increased risk of seizures.
Maprotiline	Increased risk of seizures.
Molindone	Increased risk of seizures.
Monoamine oxidase (MAO) inhibitors*	Increased risk of toxicity. Take at least 14 days apart.
Nicotine	May increase blood pressure.
Phenothiazines*	Increased risk of seizures.
Phenytoin	Increased phenytoin effect and risk of seizures.
Ritonivir	Increased risk of seizures.
Thioxanthenes*	Increased risk of seizures.
Trazodone	Increased risk of seizures.

***See Glossary**

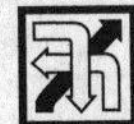

POSSIBLE INTERACTION WITH OTHER SUBSTANCES

INTERACTS WITH	COMBINED EFFECT
Alcohol:	Seizure risk. Avoid.
Beverages: Grapefruit juice.	Toxicity risk. Avoid.
Cocaine:	Unknown. Avoid.
Foods:	None expected.
Marijuana:	Unknown. Avoid.
Tobacco:	None expected.

BUSPIRONE

BRAND NAMES

BuSpar

BASIC INFORMATION

Habit forming? Probably not
Prescription needed? Yes
Available as generic? Yes
Drug class: Antianxiety agent

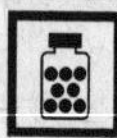

USES

- Treats chronic anxiety disorders with nervousness or tension. Not intended for treatment of ordinary stress of daily living. Causes less sedation than some antianxiety drugs. Not useful for acute anxiety.
- Useful in agitation associated with dementia.
- Reduces aggression and irritability in patients with dementia, brain injury, mental retardation.
- Used for anxiety in alcoholics or substance abusers (buspirone has low abuse potential).
- Reduces frequency of vascular headaches (does not relieve headache pain).
- Not useful in withdrawal from sedatives.

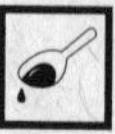

DOSAGE & USAGE INFORMATION

How to take:
Tablet—Swallow with water. Take with or without food, but be consistent and always take it the same way.

When to take:
As directed. Usually 3 times daily. Food increases absorption.

If you forget a dose:
Take as soon as you remember. If it is almost time for your next dose, skip the missed dose and go back to your regular dosing schedule. Do not double doses.

Continued next column

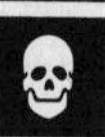

OVERDOSE

SYMPTOMS:
Severe drowsiness or nausea, vomiting, small pupils, unconsciousness.
WHAT TO DO:
- **Dial 911 (emergency) for medical help or call poison control center 1-800-222-1222 for instructions.**
- **See emergency information on last 3 pages of this book.**

What drug does:
Affects certain chemicals in the brain and causes a calming effect.

Time lapse before drug works:
1 to 2 weeks before beneficial effects may be observed.

Don't take with:
- Alcohol, other tranquilizers, antihistamines, muscle relaxants, sedatives or narcotics.
- Any other medicine or any dietary supplement without consulting your doctor or pharmacist.

POSSIBLE ADVERSE REACTIONS OR SIDE EFFECTS

SYMPTOMS	WHAT TO DO
Life-threatening:	
Chest pain; pounding, fast heartbeat (rare).	Discontinue. Seek emergency treatment.
Common:	
Lightheadedness, headache, nausea, restlessness, dizziness.	Continue. Call doctor when convenient.
Infrequent:	
Drowsiness, dry mouth, ringing in ears, nightmares or vivid dreams, unusual fatigue.	Continue. Call doctor when convenient.
Rare:	
Numbness or tingling in feet or hands; sore throat; fever; depression or confusion; uncontrollable movements of tongue, lips, arms and legs; slurred speech; psychosis; blurred vision.	Discontinue. Call doctor right away.

WARNINGS & PRECAUTIONS

Don't take if:
You are allergic to buspirone.

Before you start, consult your doctor if:
- You have ever been addicted to any substance.
- You have chronic kidney or liver disease.
- You are already taking any medicine.

Over age 60:
Adverse reactions and side effects may be more frequent and severe than in younger persons.

Pregnancy:
No problems expected, but better to avoid if possible. Consult doctor. Risk category B (see page xviii).

Breast-feeding:
Unknown if drug passes into milk. Avoid nursing until you finish medicine. Consult doctor for advice on maintaining milk supply.

Infants & children:
Safety and efficacy not established for children under 18 years old.

Prolonged use:
- Not recommended for prolonged use. Adverse side effects more likely.
- Request follow-up studies to check kidney function, blood counts, and platelet counts.

Skin & sunlight:
No problems expected.

Driving, piloting or hazardous work:
Don't drive or pilot aircraft until you learn how medicine affects you. Don't work around dangerous machinery. Don't climb ladders or work in high places. Danger increases if you drink alcohol or take medicine affecting alertness and reflexes, such as antihistamines, tranquilizers, sedatives, pain medicine, narcotics and mind-altering drugs.

Discontinuing:
No problems expected.

Others:
- Before elective surgery requiring local or general anesthesia, tell your dentist, surgeon or anesthesiologist that you take buspirone.
- Advise any doctor or dentist whom you consult that you take this medicine.

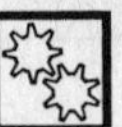

POSSIBLE INTERACTION WITH OTHER DRUGS

GENERIC NAME OR DRUG CLASS	COMBINED EFFECT
Antihistamines*	Increased sedative effect of both drugs.
Barbiturates*	Excessive sedation. Sedative effect of both drugs may be increased.
Benzodiazepines*	Recent use of benzodiazepines may lessen effect of buspirone.
Central nervous system (CNS) depressants*	Increased sedative effect.
Monoamine oxidase MAO inhibitors*	May increase blood pressure.
Narcotics*	Excessive sedation. Sedative effect of both drugs may be increased.

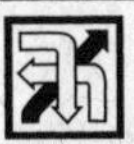

POSSIBLE INTERACTION WITH OTHER SUBSTANCES

INTERACTS WITH	COMBINED EFFECT
Alcohol:	Excess sedation. Use caution.
Beverages:	
Caffeine-containing drinks.	Avoid. Decreased antianxiety effect of buspirone.
Grapefruit juice.	Toxicity risk. Avoid.
Cocaine:	Avoid. Decreased antianxiety effect of buspirone.
Foods:	None expected.
Marijuana:	Avoid. Decreased antianxiety effect of buspirone.
Tobacco:	Avoid. Decreased antianxiety effect of buspirone.

***See Glossary**

BUSULFAN

BRAND NAMES

Myleran

BASIC INFORMATION

Habit forming? No
Prescription needed? Yes
Available as generic? No
Drug class: Antineoplastic, immunosuppressant

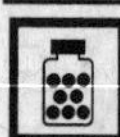

USES

- Treatment for chronic myelogenous leukemia.
- Suppresses immune response after transplant and in immune disorders.

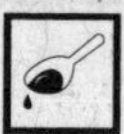

DOSAGE & USAGE INFORMATION

How to take:
Tablet—Swallow with liquid after light meal. Don't drink fluids with meals. Drink extra fluids between meals. Avoid sweet or fatty foods.

When to take:
At the same time each day.

If you forget a dose:
Take as soon as you remember. Never double dose.

What drug does:
Inhibits abnormal cell reproduction. May suppress immune system.

Time lapse before drug works:
Up to 6 weeks for full effect.

Don't take with:
Any other medicine or any dietary supplement without consulting your doctor or pharmacist.

OVERDOSE

SYMPTOMS:
Bleeding, chills, fever, collapse, stupor, seizure.
WHAT TO DO:
- **Dial 911 (emergency) for medical help or call poison control center 1-800-222-1222 for instructions.**
- **If person is unconscious, check breathing and pulse. If not breathing, begin mouth-to-mouth rescue breathing. If heart is not beating, begin chest compressions.**
- **See emergency information on last 3 pages of this book.**

POSSIBLE ADVERSE REACTIONS OR SIDE EFFECTS

SYMPTOMS	WHAT TO DO
Life-threatening: In case of overdose, see previous column.	
Common:	
• Unusual bleeding or bruising, mouth sores with sore throat, chills and fever, black stools, lip sores, menstrual irregularities.	Discontinue. Call doctor right away.
• Hair loss.	Continue. Call doctor when convenient.
• Nausea, vomiting, diarrhea (almost always occurs), tiredness, weakness.	Continue. Tell doctor at next visit.
Infrequent:	
• Mental confusion, shortness of breath.	Continue. Call doctor when convenient.
• Cough, joint pain, dizziness, appetite loss.	Continue. Tell doctor at next visit.
Rare:	
• Jaundice, cataracts, symptoms of myasthenia gravis.*	Discontinue. Call doctor right away.
• Swollen breasts.	Continue. Call doctor when convenient.

WARNINGS & PRECAUTIONS

Don't take if:
- You have had hypersensitivity to alkylating antineoplastic drugs.
- Your physician has not explained the serious nature of your medical problem and risks of taking this medicine.

Before you start, consult your doctor if:
- You have gout.
- You have had kidney stones.
- You have active infection.
- You have impaired kidney or liver function.
- You have taken other antineoplastic drugs or had radiation treatment in last 3 weeks.

Over age 60:
Adverse reactions and side effects may be more frequent and severe than in younger persons.

Pregnancy:
Consult doctor. Risk to child is significant. Risk category D (see page xviii).

Breast-feeding:
Drug passes into milk. Don't nurse.

Infants & children:
Use only under care of medical supervisors who are experienced in anticancer drugs.

Prolonged use:
- Adverse reactions more likely the longer drug is required.
- Talk to your doctor about the need for follow-up medical examinations or laboratory studies to check complete blood counts (white blood cell count, platelet count, red blood cell count, hemoglobin, hematocrit), serum uric acid.

Skin & sunlight:
No problems expected.

Driving, piloting or hazardous work:
No problems expected.

Discontinuing:
Don't discontinue without doctor's advice until you complete prescribed dose, even though symptoms diminish or disappear. Some side effects may follow discontinuing. Report to doctor blurred vision, convulsions, confusion, persistent headache.

Others:
- Advise any doctor or dentist whom you consult that you take this medicine.
- May increase chance of developing lung or blood problems.

POSSIBLE INTERACTION WITH OTHER DRUGS

GENERIC NAME OR DRUG CLASS	COMBINED EFFECT
Antigout drugs*	Decreased antigout effect.
Antineoplastic drugs, other*	Increased effect of all drugs (may be beneficial).
Chloramphenicol	Increased likelihood of toxic effects of both drugs.
Clozapine	Toxic effect on bone marrow.
Lovastatin	Increased heart and kidney damage.
Tiopronin	Increased risk of toxicity to bone marrow.
Vaccines, live or killed	Increased risk of toxicity or reduced effectiveness of vaccine.

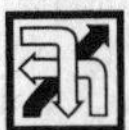

POSSIBLE INTERACTION WITH OTHER SUBSTANCES

INTERACTS WITH	COMBINED EFFECT
Alcohol:	May increase chance of intestinal bleeding.
Beverages:	None expected.
Cocaine:	Increases chance of toxicity.
Foods:	Reduces irritation in stomach.
Marijuana:	None expected.
Tobacco:	Increases lung toxicity.

***See Glossary**

BUTORPHANOL

BRAND NAMES

Butorphanol Tartrate Nasal Spray
Stadol NS

BASIC INFORMATION

Habit forming? Yes
Prescription needed? Yes
Available as generic? No
Drug class: Narcotic analgesic

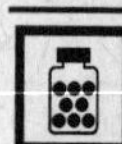

USES

- Treatment for migraine headache pain and postoperative pain.
- Treatment for other types of pain for which a narcotic analgesic is appropriate.

DOSAGE & USAGE INFORMATION

How to take:
Nasal spray—Spray in one nostril using the metered-dose pump.

When to take:
For pain as directed by your doctor. Usual treatment consists of one dose in one nostril followed by a second dose in 60 to 90 minutes if pain persists. Your doctor may direct that the initial 2-dose sequence may be repeated in 3 to 4 hours as needed.

If you forget a dose:
Unlikely to be a problem since the drug is taken for pain and not routinely.

What drug does:
Blocks the pain impulses at specific sites in the brain and spinal cord.

Time lapse before drug works:
Within 15 minutes of the first dose.

Don't take with:
Any other medicine or any dietary supplement without consulting your doctor or pharmacist.

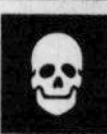

OVERDOSE

SYMPTOMS:
Heartbeat irregularities, breathing difficulty, coma.
WHAT TO DO:
- **Dial 911 (emergency) for medical help or call poison control center 1-800-222-1222 for instructions.**
- **See emergency information on last 3 pages of this book.**

POSSIBLE ADVERSE REACTIONS OR SIDE EFFECTS

SYMPTOMS	WHAT TO DO
Life-threatening:	
In case of overdose, see previous column.	
Common:	
Drowsiness, dizziness, nausea or vomiting, nasal congestion or irritation.	Discontinue. Call doctor when convenient.
Infrequent:	
Constipation (with continued use), faintness, high or low blood pressure.	Discontinue. Call doctor when convenient.
Rare:	
• Taste changes, ear ringing, dry mouth.	No action necessary.
• Difficult breathing, heart palpitations.	Discontinue. Call doctor right away.

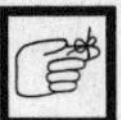

WARNINGS & PRECAUTIONS

Don't take if:
You are allergic to butorphanol or the preservative benzethonium chloride,* which is used in the manufacture of the drug.

Before you start, consult your doctor if:
- You have a respiratory disorder or a central nervous system disease.
- You have had adverse reactions to other narcotics.*
- You have a history of emotional problems.
- You have heart, kidney or liver disease.

Over age 60:
Adverse reactions and side effects (particularly dizziness) may be more frequent and severe than in younger persons.

Pregnancy:
Risk category C (see page xviii). Decide with your doctor if drug benefits justify any possible risk to unborn child.

Breast-feeding:
Drug may pass into milk. Decide with your doctor if you should continue breast-feeding while taking this drug.

Infants & children:
Not recommended for children under age 18. Safety and effectiveness have not been established.

Prolonged use:
Long-term use effects are unknown. Probably habit forming. Consult with your doctor on a regular basis while using this drug.

Skin & sunlight:
No special problems expected.

Driving, piloting or hazardous work:
Don't drive or pilot aircraft until you learn how medicine affects you. Don't work around dangerous machinery. Don't climb ladders or work in high places. Danger increases if you drink alcohol or take medicine affecting alertness and reflexes.

Discontinuing:
Don't discontinue this drug after prolonged use without consulting doctor. Dosage may require a gradual reduction before stopping to avoid any withdrawal symptoms.

Others:
- When first using this drug, get up slowly from a sitting or lying position to avoid any dizziness, faintness or lightheadedness.
- Advise any doctor or dentist whom you consult that you take this medicine.
- Take medicine only as directed. Do not increase or reduce dosage without doctor's approval.

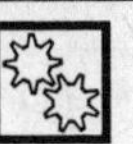

POSSIBLE INTERACTION WITH OTHER DRUGS

GENERIC NAME OR DRUG CLASS	COMBINED EFFECT
Central nervous system (CNS) depressants,* other	Increased sedative effect.
Oxymetazoline	Delays start of butorphanol effect.

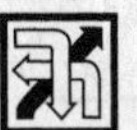

POSSIBLE INTERACTION WITH OTHER SUBSTANCES

INTERACTS WITH	COMBINED EFFECT
Alcohol:	Increased sedative affect. Avoid.
Beverages:	None expected.
Cocaine:	Effect not known. Best to avoid.
Foods:	None expected.
Marijuana:	Effect not known. Best to avoid.
Tobacco:	None expected.

*See Glossary

CAFFEINE

BRAND NAMES

See full list of brand names in the *Generic and Brand Name Directory*, page 879.

BASIC INFORMATION

Habit forming? Yes
Prescription needed? No
Available as generic? Yes
Drug class: Stimulant (xanthine), vasoconstrictor

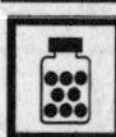

USES

- Treatment for drowsiness and fatigue (occasional use only).
- Treatment for migraine and other vascular headaches in combination with ergot.

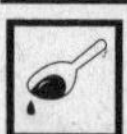

DOSAGE & USAGE INFORMATION

How to take:

- Tablet or liquid—Swallow with liquid or food to lessen stomach irritation. If you can't swallow whole, crumble tablet and take with liquid or food.
- Extended-release capsule—Swallow whole with liquid.
- Powder—Stir powder into water or other liquid. The powder may also be placed on the tongue and then followed by liquid.

When to take:
At the same times each day.

If you forget a dose:
Take as soon as you remember. If it is almost time for the next dose, wait for the next scheduled dose (don't double this dose).

What drug does:

- Constricts blood vessel walls.
- Stimulates central nervous system.

Continued next column

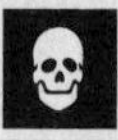

OVERDOSE

SYMPTOMS:
Excitement, insomnia, rapid heartbeat (infants can have slow heartbeat), confusion, fever, hallucinations, convulsions, coma.
WHAT TO DO:

- **Dial 911 (emergency) for medical help or call poison control center 1-800-222-1222 for instructions.**
- **See emergency information on last 3 pages of this book.**

Time lapse before drug works:
30 minutes.

Don't take with:
Any other medicine or any dietary supplement without consulting your doctor or pharmacist.

POSSIBLE ADVERSE REACTIONS OR SIDE EFFECTS

SYMPTOMS	WHAT TO DO
Life-threatening: In case of overdose, see previous column.	
Common:	
• Rapid heartbeat, low blood sugar (hunger, anxiety, cold sweats, rapid pulse) with tremor, irritability (mild).	Discontinue. Call doctor right away.
• Nervousness, insomnia.	Continue. Tell doctor at next visit.
• Increased urination.	No action necessary.
Infrequent:	
• Confusion, irritability (severe).	Discontinue. Call doctor right away.
• Nausea, indigestion, burning feeling in stomach.	Continue. Call doctor when convenient.
Rare: None expected.	

WARNINGS & PRECAUTIONS

Don't take if:
- You are allergic to any stimulant.
- You have heart disease.
- You have active peptic ulcer of stomach or duodenum.

Before you start, consult your doctor if:
- You have irregular heartbeat.
- You have hypoglycemia (low blood sugar).
- You have epilepsy.
- You have a seizure disorder.
- You have high blood pressure.
- You have insomnia.

Over age 60:
Adverse reactions and side effects may be more frequent and severe than in younger persons.

Pregnancy:
Decide with your doctor if drug benefits justify risk to unborn child. Risk category C (see page xviii).

Breast-feeding:
Drug passes into milk. Avoid drug or discontinue nursing until you finish medicine. Consult doctor for advice on maintaining milk supply.

Infants & children:
Not recommended.

Prolonged use:
Can affect people in different ways. Consult your doctor if you are concerned.

Skin & sunlight:
No problems expected.

Driving, piloting or hazardous work:
No problems expected.

Discontinuing:
Will cause withdrawal symptoms of headache, irritability, drowsiness. Discontinue gradually if you use caffeine for a month or more.

Others:
Consult your doctor if drowsiness or fatigue continues, recurs or is not relieved by caffeine.

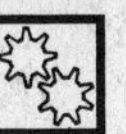

POSSIBLE INTERACTION WITH OTHER DRUGS

GENERIC NAME OR DRUG CLASS	COMBINED EFFECT
Caffeine-containing drugs, other	Increased risk of overstimulation.
Central nervous system (CNS) stimulants*	Increased risk of overstimulation.
Cimetidine	Increased caffeine effect.
Contraceptives, oral*	Increased caffeine effect.
Isoniazid	Increased caffeine effect.
Monoamine oxidase (MAO) inhibitors*	Dangerous blood pressure rise.
Sympathomimetics*	Overstimulation.
Xanthines*	Increased risk of overstimulation.

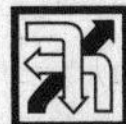

POSSIBLE INTERACTION WITH OTHER SUBSTANCES

INTERACTS WITH	COMBINED EFFECT
Alcohol:	Decreased alcohol effect.
Beverages: Caffeine drinks (coffee, tea or soft drinks).	Increased caffeine effect. Use caution.
Cocaine	Convulsions or excessive nervousness.
Foods:	None expected.
Marijuana:	Increased effect of both drugs. May lead to dangerous, rapid heartbeat. Avoid.
Tobacco:	Increased heartbeat. Avoid. Decreased caffeine effect.

*See Glossary

CALCITONIN

BRAND NAMES

Fortical
Miacalcin

BASIC INFORMATION

Habit forming? No
Prescription needed? Yes
Available as generic? No
Drug class: Osteoporosis therapy

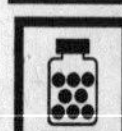

USES

Treatment for postmenopausal osteoporosis (thinning of bones) in females. Osteoporosis is a major cause of bone fractures.

DOSAGE & USAGE INFORMATION

How to take:
Nasal spray—One spray per day in a nostril, alternating nostrils daily. Follow directions on label about activating and using the pump supplied with the medication.

When to take:
At the same time each day.

If you forget a dose:
Take as soon as you remember. If it is almost time for the next dose, wait for the next scheduled dose (don't double this dose).

What drug does:
The exact mechanism is not fully understood. It slows down the loss of bone tissue and increases bone mass in women with osteoporosis.

Time lapse before drug works:
Up to 6 months or longer.

Don't take with:
Any other medicine or any dietary supplement without consulting your doctor or pharmacist.

OVERDOSE

SYMPTOMS:
None reported.
WHAT TO DO:
Overdose unlikely to threaten life. If person uses much larger amount than prescribed or if accidentally swallowed, call doctor or poison control center 1-800-222-1222 for help.

POSSIBLE ADVERSE REACTIONS OR SIDE EFFECTS

SYMPTOMS	WHAT TO DO
Life-threatening:	
Rare allergic reaction—Breathing difficulty; swelling of hands, feet, face, mouth, neck; skin rash.	Discontinue. Seek emergency treatment.
Common:	
Nasal inflammation, dryness, crusting, sores, irritation, itching, redness; swollen, runny, stuffy nose; small amount of nasal bleeding, discomfort, tenderness.	Continue. Call doctor when convenient.
Infrequent:	
Back pain, joint pain, headache, flushing, nausea, sinus infection.	Continue. Call doctor when convenient.
Rare:	
None expected.	

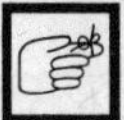

WARNINGS & PRECAUTIONS

Don't take if:
You are allergic to calcitonin.

Before you start, consult your doctor if:
You are allergic to any medication, food or other substance. A skin test may be performed before beginning treatment with calcitonin.

Over age 60:
No special problems expected.

Pregnancy:
Not normally used in premenopausal women. Risk category C (see page xviii).

Breast-feeding:
Not normally used in premenopausal women.

Infants & children:
Not recommended for this age group.

Prolonged use:
- No special problems expected.
- Visit your doctor regularly to determine if the drug is continuing to control bone loss and to have periodic nasal examinations to check for ulceration or irritation.

Skin & sunlight:
No special problems expected.

Driving, piloting or hazardous work:
No special problems expected.

Discontinuing:
Don't discontinue without your doctor's approval.

Others:
- In addition to taking the drug, weight-bearing exercise and adequate dietary intake of calcium and vitamin D are essential in preventing bone loss. Dietary supplements of 1000 mg elemental calcium and 400 I.U. vitamin D daily may be recommended by your doctor.
- Advise any doctor or dentist whom you consult that you take this medicine.
- May affect the results of some medical tests.

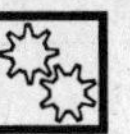

POSSIBLE INTERACTION WITH OTHER DRUGS

GENERIC NAME OR DRUG CLASS	COMBINED EFFECT
None significant.	

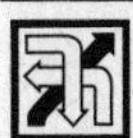

POSSIBLE INTERACTION WITH OTHER SUBSTANCES

INTERACTS WITH	COMBINED EFFECT
Alcohol:	None expected.
Beverages:	None expected.
Cocaine:	None expected.
Foods:	None expected.
Marijuana:	None expected.
Tobacco:	None expected.

CALCIUM CHANNEL BLOCKERS

GENERIC AND BRAND NAMES

See full list of generic and brand names in *Generic and Brand Name Directory*, page 879.

BASIC INFORMATION

Habit forming? No
Prescription needed? Yes
Available as generic? Yes, for most
Drug class: Calcium channel blocker, antiarrhythmic, antianginal

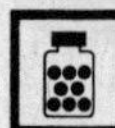

USES

- Used for high blood pressure (hypertension) angina attacks and irregular heartbeat.
- Treats migraines and Raynaud's disease.

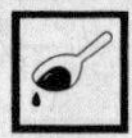

DOSAGE & USAGE INFORMATION

How to take:
- Tablet or capsule—Swallow with liquid. You may chew or crush tablet.
- Extended-release tablet or capsule—Swallow each dose whole with liquid; do not crush tablet or open capsule.

When to take:
At the same times each day. Take verapamil with food.

If you forget a dose:
Take as soon as you remember. If it is almost time for the next dose, wait for the next scheduled dose (don't double this dose).

What drug does:
- Reduces work that heart must perform.
- Reduces normal artery pressure.
- Increases oxygen to heart muscle.

Continued next column

OVERDOSE

SYMPTOMS:
Unusually fast or unusually slow heartbeat, loss of consciousness, cardiac arrest.
WHAT TO DO:
- **Dial 911 (emergency) for medical help or call poison control center 1-800-222-1222 for instructions.**
- **If person is unconscious, check breathing and pulse. If not breathing, begin mouth-to-mouth rescue breathing. If heart is not beating, begin chest compressions.**
- **See emergency information on last 3 pages of this book.**

Time lapse before drug works:
1 to 2 hours.

Don't take with:
Any other medicine or any dietary supplement without consulting your doctor or pharmacist.

POSSIBLE ADVERSE REACTIONS OR SIDE EFFECTS

SYMPTOMS	WHAT TO DO
Life-threatening: In case of overdose, see previous column.	
Common:	
Tiredness.	Continue. Tell doctor at next visit.
Infrequent:	
• Unusually fast or unusually slow heartbeat, wheezing, cough, shortness of breath.	Discontinue. Call doctor right away.
• Dizziness; numbness or tingling in hands and feet; swollen feet, ankles or legs; difficult urination.	Continue. Call doctor when convenient.
• Nausea, constipation.	Continue. Tell doctor at next visit.
Rare:	
• Fainting, depression, psychosis, rash, jaundice.	Discontinue. Call doctor right away.
• Headache, insomnia, vivid dreams, hair loss.	Continue. Tell doctor at next visit.

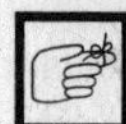

WARNINGS & PRECAUTIONS

Don't take if:
- You are allergic to calcium channel blockers.
- You have very low blood pressure.

Before you start, consult your doctor if:
- You have kidney or liver disease.
- You have high blood pressure.
- You have heart disease other than coronary artery disease.

Over age 60:
Adverse reactions and side effects may be more frequent and severe than in younger persons.

Pregnancy:
Decide with your doctor if drug benefits justify risk to unborn child. Risk category C (see page xviii).

Breast-feeding:
Safety not established. Avoid if possible. Consult doctor.

Infants & children:
Not recommended.

Prolonged use:
Talk to your doctor about the need for follow-up medical examinations or laboratory studies to check blood pressure, liver function, kidney function, ECG.*

Skin & sunlight:
One or more drugs in this group may cause rash or intensify sunburn in areas exposed to sun or ultraviolet light (photosensitivity reaction). Avoid overexposure. Notify doctor if reaction occurs.

Driving, piloting or hazardous work:
Avoid if you feel dizzy. Otherwise, no problems expected.

Discontinuing:
Don't discontinue without doctor's advice until you complete prescribed dose, even though symptoms diminish or disappear.

Others:
- Learn to check your own pulse rate. If it drops to 50 beats per minute or lower, don't take drug until you consult your doctor.
- Advise any doctor or dentist whom you consult that you take this medicine.

POSSIBLE INTERACTION WITH OTHER DRUGS

GENERIC NAME OR DRUG CLASS	COMBINED EFFECT
Angiotensin-converting enzyme (ACE) inhibitors*	Possible excessive potassium in blood. Dosages may require adjustment.
Antiarrhythmics*	Possible increased effect and toxicity of each drug.
Anticoagulants, oral*	Possible increased anticoagulant effect.
Anticonvulsants, hydantoin*	Increased anticonvulsant effect.
Antihypertensives*	Blood pressure drop. Dosages may require adjustment.
Beta-adrenergic blocking agents*	Possible irregular heartbeat and congestive heart failure.
Calcium (large doses)	Possible decreased effect of calcium channel blocker.
Carbamazepine	May increase carbamazepine effect and toxicity.
Cimetidine	Possible increased effect of calcium channel blocker.
Cyclosporine	Increased cyclosporine toxicity.
Digitalis preparations*	Increased digitalis effect. May need to reduce dose.
Disopyramide	May cause dangerously slow, fast or irregular heartbeat.
Diuretics*	Dangerous blood pressure drop. Dosages may require adjustment.
Dofetilide	Increased risk of heart problems.
Encainide	Increased effect of toxicity on heart muscle.
Fluvoxamine	Slow heartbeat (with diltiazem).
HMG-CoA reductase inhibitors	Increased effect of HMG-CoA reductase inhibitor.
Hypokalemia-causing medications*	Increased anti-hypertensive effect.
Leukotriene modifiers	Increased effect of calcium channel blocker.

Continued on page 910

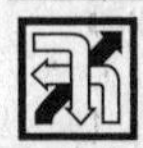

POSSIBLE INTERACTION WITH OTHER SUBSTANCES

INTERACTS WITH	COMBINED EFFECT
Alcohol:	Very low blood pressure. Avoid.
Beverages: Grapefruit juice.	Possible increased drug effect.
Cocaine:	Possible irregular heartbeat. Avoid.
Foods: Grapefruit.	Possible increased drug effect.
Marijuana:	Possible irregular heartbeat. Avoid.
Tobacco:	Possible rapid heartbeat. Avoid.

*See Glossary

CALCIUM SUPPLEMENTS

GENERIC AND BRAND NAMES

See full list of generic and brand names in the *Generic and Brand Name Directory*, page 880.

BASIC INFORMATION

Habit forming? No
Prescription needed? For some
Available as generic? Yes
Drug class: Antihypocalcemic, dietary replacement

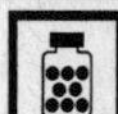

USES

- Treats or prevents osteoporosis (thin, porous, easily fractured bones). Frequently prescribed with estrogen beginning at menopause.
- Helps heart, muscle and nervous system to work properly.
- Dietary supplement when calcium ingestion is insufficient or there is a deficiency such as osteomalacia or rickets.

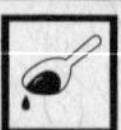

DOSAGE & USAGE INFORMATION

How to take:
- Tablet or capsule—Swallow whole with liquid.
- Chewable tablet—Chew tablet well before swallowing.
- Syrup—Take before meals.
- Powder—Follow directions on label.
- Suspension—Swallow with liquid.

When to take:
Take 1 to 1 1/2 hours after meals (except for syrup) in 3 to 4 daily doses. Try to avoid taking other medicine you take by mouth within 1 to 2 hours of taking calcium.

If you forget a dose:
Use as soon as you remember. Then return to regular schedule.

Continued next column

OVERDOSE

SYMPTOMS:
Confusion, irregular heartbeat, depression, bone pain, coma.
WHAT TO DO:
- **Dial 911 (emergency) for medical help or call poison control center 1-800-222-1222 for instructions.**
- **See emergency information on last 3 pages of this book.**

What drug does:
Calcium helps maintain strong bones and teeth. It also helps heart function, muscle contraction, blood clotting and nerve transmission.

Time lapse before drug works:
Starts within 15 to 30 minutes, but may take months or years to improve certain conditions.

Don't take with:
- Any other oral medicine until 1 to 2 hours have passed since taking calcium.
- Any other medicine or any dietary supplement without consulting your doctor or pharmacist.

POSSIBLE ADVERSE REACTIONS OR SIDE EFFECTS

SYMPTOMS	WHAT TO DO
Life-threatening:	
Irregular or very slow heart rate.	Discontinue. Seek emergency treatment.
Common:	
None expected.	
Infrequent:	
Constipation, diarrhea, drowsiness, headache, appetite loss, dry mouth, weakness.	Discontinue. Call doctor right away.
Rare:	
Frequent, painful or difficult urination; increased thirst; nausea, vomiting; rash; urine frequency increased and volume larger; confusion; high blood pressure; eyes sensitive to light.	Discontinue. Call doctor right away.

WARNINGS & PRECAUTIONS

Don't take if:
- You are allergic to calcium.
- You have a high blood calcium level.

Before you start, consult your doctor if:
You have diarrhea, heart disease, kidney stones, kidney disease, sarcoidosis or malabsorption.

Over age 60:
No problems expected.

Pregnancy:
Consult doctor. Risk category C (see page xviii).

Breast-feeding:
No problems expected. Consult doctor.

Infants & children:
Use correct dose for your child's age and weight.

Prolonged use:
Talk to your doctor about the need for any follow-up laboratory studies to check calcium levels in the body.

Skin & sunlight:
No problems expected.

Driving, piloting or hazardous work:
No problems expected.

Discontinuing:
No problems expected.

Others:
- Exercise, along with vitamin D from sunshine and calcium, helps prevent osteoporosis.
- Advise any doctor or dentist whom you consult that you take this medicine.

POSSIBLE INTERACTION WITH OTHER DRUGS

GENERIC NAME OR DRUG CLASS	COMBINED EFFECT
Alendronate	Decreased alendronate effect. Take calcium 30 minutes after alendronate.
Anticoagulants, oral*	Decreased anticoagulant effect.
Calcitonin	Decreased calcitonin effect.
Calcium-containing medicines, other	Increased calcium effect.
Chlorpromazine	Decreased chlorpromazine effect.
Contraceptives, oral*	May increase absorption of calcium—frequently a desirable combined effect.
Corticosteroids*	Decreased calcium absorption and effect.
Digitalis preparations*	Decreased digitalis effect.
Diuretics, thiazide*	Increased calcium in blood.
Estrogens*	May increase absorption of calcium—frequently a desirable combined effect.
Etidronate	Decreased etidronate absorption. Take drugs 2 hours apart.
Iron supplements*	Decreased iron effect.
Meperidine	Increased meperidine effect.
Mexiletine	May slow elimination of mexiletine and cause need to adjust dosage.
Nalidixic acid	Decreased effect of nalidixic acid.
Nicardipine	Possible decreased nicardipine effect.
Nimodipine	Possible decreased nimodipine effect.
Oxyphenbutazone	Decreased oxyphenbutazone effect.
Para-aminosalicylic acid (PAS)	Decreased PAS effect.
Penicillins*	Decreased penicillin effect.
Pentobarbital	Decreased pentobarbital effect.
Phenylbutazone	Decreased effect of phenylbutazone.
Phenytoin	Decreased phenytoin effect.
Propafenone	Increased effects of both drugs and increased risk of toxicity.
Pseudoephedrine	Increased pseudoephedrine effect.

Continued on page 910

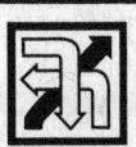

POSSIBLE INTERACTION WITH OTHER SUBSTANCES

INTERACTS WITH	COMBINED EFFECT
Alcohol:	Decreased absorption of calcium.
Beverages:	None expected.
Cocaine:	No proven problems.
Foods:	None expected.
Marijuana:	Decreased absorption of calcium.
Tobacco:	Decreased absorption of calcium.

*See Glossary

CAPECITABINE

BRAND NAMES

Xeloda

BASIC INFORMATION

Habit forming? No
Prescription needed? Yes
Available as generic? No
Drug class: Antineoplastic

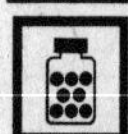

USES

Treatment of cancer of the colon after surgery and colorectal or breast cancer that has spread to other parts of the body (metastatic cancer).

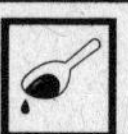

DOSAGE & USAGE INFORMATION

How to take:
Tablet—Swallow with water. If you can't swallow whole, crumble tablet and take with liquid or food.

When to take:
Take in two divided doses every 12 hours after a meal and with water.

If you forget a dose:
Do not take missed dose or double next dose. Continue your regular dosing schedule and consult your doctor.

What drug does:
Capecitabine is converted in the body to the substance 5-fluorouracil. In some patients, this substance kills cancer cells and decreases the size of the tumor.

Time lapse before drug works:
Results may not show for several months.

Don't take with:
Any other medicine or any dietary supplement without consulting your doctor or pharmacist.

OVERDOSE

SYMPTOMS:
Nausea, vomiting, diarrhea, gastrointestinal irritation and bleeding, and bone marrow depression.
WHAT TO DO:
Overdose unlikely to threaten life. If person uses much larger amount than prescribed or if accidentally swallowed, call doctor or poison control center 1-800-222-1222 for help.

POSSIBLE ADVERSE REACTIONS OR SIDE EFFECTS

SYMPTOMS	WHAT TO DO
Life-threatening: None expected.	
Common:	
• Diarrhea (if you have more than 4 bowel movements in a day or any diarrhea at night); vomiting (more than once a day); nausea; loss of appetite; stomatitis (pain, redness or swelling in mouth); hand and foot syndrome (pain, redness or swelling in hands or feet); fever (100.5° or higher).	Discontinue. Call doctor right away.
• Diarrhea, nausea and vomiting, rash, dry or itchy skin, tiredness, weakness, dizziness, headache.	Continue. Call doctor when convenient.
Infrequent:	
Jaundice.	Continue, but call doctor right away.
Rare: None expected.	

WARNINGS & PRECAUTIONS

Don't take if:
You are allergic to capecitabine.

Before you start, consult your doctor if:
- You have an infection or any other medical problem.
- You have heart problems.
- You are taking folic acid.
- You are pregnant or if you plan to become pregnant.
- You have had liver problems.

Over age 60:
Adverse reactions and side effects, especially gastrointestinal, may be more severe and frequent than in younger patients.

Pregnancy:
Animal studies show fetal abnormalities and increased risk of abortion. Discuss with your doctor whether drug benefits justify risk to unborn child. Risk category D (see page xviii).

Breast-feeding:
Not known if drug passes into milk. Avoid drug or discontinue nursing until you finish medicine. Consult doctor for advice on maintaining milk supply.

Infants & children:
Safety and effectiveness of use in children not established.

Prolonged use:
Talk to your doctor about the need for follow-up medical examinations or laboratory studies.

Skin & sunlight:
No problems expected.

Driving, piloting or hazardous work:
Avoid if you feel side effects such as nausea and vomiting.

Discontinuing:
Your doctor will determine the schedule.

Others:
Advise any doctor or dentist whom you consult that you take this medicine.

POSSIBLE INTERACTION WITH OTHER DRUGS

GENERIC NAME OR DRUG CLASS	COMBINED EFFECT
Antacids	Increased risk of capecitabine toxicity.
Leucovorin	Increased risk of capecitabine toxicity.

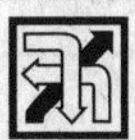

POSSIBLE INTERACTION WITH OTHER SUBSTANCES

INTERACTS WITH	COMBINED EFFECT
Alcohol:	None expected.
Beverages:	None expected.
Cocaine:	Effects unknown. Avoid.
Foods:	None expected.
Marijuana:	Effects unknown. Avoid.
Tobacco:	None expected.

***See Glossary**

CAPSAICIN

BRAND NAMES

ArthriCare
ARTH-RX
Axsain
Capsagel
Dura-Patch
Dura Patch Joint
Methacin
Qutenza
Sinol Nasal Spray
Sinus Buster
WellPatch Capsaicin Pain Patch
Zostrix
Zostrix-HP
Zostrix Neuropathy Cream

BASIC INFORMATION

Habit forming? No
Prescription needed? No
Available as generic? Yes
Drug class: Analgesic (topical)

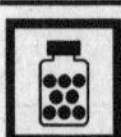

USES

- Treats neuralgias, such as pain that occurs following shingles (herpes zoster) or neuropathy of the feet, ankles and fingers (common in diabetes).
- Nasal spray helps relieves sinus, allergy, and headache symptoms, including migraines.
- Treats discomfort caused by arthritis.

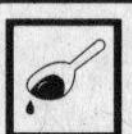

DOSAGE & USAGE INFORMATION

How to use:

- Cream—Apply a small amount and rub carefully on the affected areas. Use every day. Wash hands after applying. Don't apply to irritated skin. Don't bandage over treated areas.
- Nasal spray—Use will depend on condition being treated. Follow package instructions.
- Patch—Follow package instructions for proper application.

When to use:
Apply 3 or 4 times a day.

If you forget a dose:
Use as soon as you remember.

Continued next column

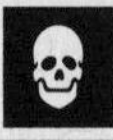

OVERDOSE

SYMPTOMS:
None expected.
WHAT TO DO:
Not intended for internal use. If child accidentally swallows, call doctor or poison control center 1-800-222-1222 for help.

What drug does:
It is made from red chili peppers. When applied to the skin, it appears to decrease a chemical that causes pain. The nasal spray product can help reduce nasal inflammation and desensitize nasal passages to allergens.

Time lapse before drug works:
Begins to work immediately. Frequently takes 2 to 3 weeks for full benefit, but may take up to 6 or 8 weeks.

Don't use with:
No problems expected.

POSSIBLE ADVERSE REACTIONS OR SIDE EFFECTS

SYMPTOMS	WHAT TO DO
Life-threatening:	
None expected.	
Common:	
Stinging or burning sensation at application site.	Nothing. It usually improves in 2 to 3 days or becomes less severe the longer you use the drug.
Infrequent:	
None expected.	
Rare:	
Serious burns or blistering on the skin where product applied.	Discontinue. Call doctor right away.

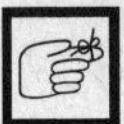

WARNINGS & PRECAUTIONS

Don't use if:
You are allergic to capsaicin or to the fruit of capsaicin plants (for example, hot peppers).

Before you start, consult your doctor if:
You have any allergies.

Over age 60:
No problems expected.

Pregnancy:
Consult doctor. Risk category C (see page xviii).

Breast-feeding:
No problems expected. Consult doctor.

Infants & children:
Not recommended for children under age 2.

Prolonged use:
No problems expected.

Skin & sunlight:
No problems expected.

Driving, piloting or hazardous work:
No problems expected.

Discontinuing:
Discontinue if there are no signs of improvement within a month.

Others:
- Capsaicin is not a local anesthetic.*
- Although capsaicin may help relieve the pain of neuropathy, it does not cure any disorder.
- If you accidentally get some capsaicin in your eye, flush with water.

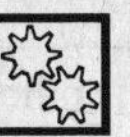

POSSIBLE INTERACTION WITH OTHER DRUGS

GENERIC NAME OR DRUG CLASS	COMBINED EFFECT
None expected.	

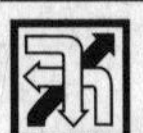

POSSIBLE INTERACTION WITH OTHER SUBSTANCES

INTERACTS WITH	COMBINED EFFECT
Alcohol:	None expected.
Beverages:	None expected.
Cocaine:	None expected.
Foods:	None expected.
Marijuana:	None expected.
Tobacco:	None expected.

***See Glossary**

CARBAMAZEPINE

BRAND NAMES

Apo-Carbamazepine
Carbatrol
Epitol
Equetro
Mazepine
Novocarbamaz
Nu-Carbamazepine
PMS Carbamazepine
Taro-Carbamazepine
Tegretol
Tegretol Chewtabs
Tegretol CR
Tegretol XR

BASIC INFORMATION

Habit forming? No
Prescription needed? Yes
Available as generic? Yes
Drug class: Analgesic, anticonvulsant, antimanic agent

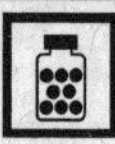

USES

- Treatment for trigeminal neuralgia.
- Treats bipolar (manic-depressive) disorder.
- Used to control certain types of seizures.
- Used for pain relief, restless leg syndrome, alcohol/drug withdrawal and other disorders.

DOSAGE & USAGE INFORMATION

How to take:

- Tablet—Swallow with liquid. Take with food to lessen stomach upset. For chewable tablet, chew well before swallowing.
- Extended-release capsule or tablet or controlled release tablet—Swallow with liquid. May be taken with or without food. Capsule may be opened and sprinkled on food (e.g., teaspoon of applesauce). Do not chew or crush tablet or capsule.
- Oral suspension—Follow label instructions. Do not mix it with other liquid drugs.

Continued next column

OVERDOSE

SYMPTOMS:
Abnormal movements, slurred speech, nausea and vomiting, drowsiness, high or low blood pressure, dilated pupils, flushed skin, irregular heartbeat and breathing, decreased urine, seizures, tremor, fainting, coma.

WHAT TO DO:

- **Dial 911 (emergency) for medical help or call poison control center 1-800-222-1222 for instructions.**
- **See emergency information on last 3 pages of this book.**

When to take:
At the same times each day as directed.

What drug does:
It works by decreasing impulses in nerves that cause seizures and pain.

If you forget a dose:
Take as soon as you remember. If it is almost time for the next dose, wait for that dose (don't double this dose) and resume regular schedule.

Time lapse before drug works:

- Tic douloureux—24 to 72 hours.
- Bipolar disorder—7 to 10 days.
- Seizures—Hours to days in different patients.

Don't take with:
Any other medicine or any dietary supplement without consulting your doctor or pharmacist. May inactivate other medications, such as birth control pills.

POSSIBLE ADVERSE REACTIONS OR SIDE EFFECTS

SYMPTOMS	WHAT TO DO
Life-threatening:	
Rare allergic reaction—Breathing difficulty; closing of the throat; swelling of hands, feet, face, lips or tongue; hives.	Discontinue. Seek emergency treatment.
Common:	
• Back-and-forth eye movements, double or blurred vision.	Discontinue. Call doctor right away.
• Being clumsy or unsteady, mildly dizzy or lightheaded, mild nausea or vomiting.	Continue. Call doctor when convenient.
Infrequent:	
• Behavior changes in a child or in the elderly (e.g., confusion or agitation), ongoing headache, severe diarrhea or nausea or vomiting or drowsiness, increase in seizures, skin rash or hives.	Discontinue. Call doctor right away.
• Mild diarrhea, dry mouth, constipation, impotence, muscle aches, sore tongue or mouth, hair loss, upset stomach, appetite loss, increased sweating.	Continue. Call doctor when convenient.
Rare:	
Breathing difficulty; irregular, pounding or slow heartbeat; chest pain; uncontrollable body	Discontinue. Call doctor right away.

jerks; numbness, weakness or tingling in hands and feet; swollen legs or feet or face; unusual bleeding or bruising, stool changes (black, tarry, bloody, or pale), urine changes (frequent, decreased, bloody, dark or painful), unusual pain, yellow eyes or skin, infection (fever, chills), rapid weight gain, noises in ears, slurred speech, hallucinations, unusual tiredness or weakness.

WARNINGS & PRECAUTIONS

Don't take if:

- You are allergic to carbamazepine or any tricyclic antidepressant.*
- You have taken a monoamine oxidase (MAO) inhibitor* in the past 2 weeks.

Before you start, consult your doctor if:

- You have high blood pressure, heart block, thrombophlebitis or heart disease.
- You have glaucoma.
- You have emotional or mental problems.
- You have diabetes, liver or kidney disease.
- You have a blood disorder (e.g., anemia) or bone marrow depression or disease.
- You have had reactions to other drugs.
- You are of Asian ancestry (a genetic blood test can tell if you are at increased risk of developing a rare, but serious, skin reaction).
- You drink more than 2 alcoholic drinks a day.

Over age 60:
Adverse reactions and side effects may be more frequent and severe than in younger persons.

Pregnancy:
Decide with your doctor whether drug benefits justify risk to unborn child. Risk category C (see page xviii).

Breast-feeding:
Drug passes into milk. Avoid drug or discontinue nursing until you finish medicine. Consult doctor for advice on maintaining milk supply.

Infants & children:
May be used in children. Side effects of behavior changes are more likely in this age group.

Prolonged use:
Talk to your doctor about the need for follow-up medical examinations, blood and urine studies, eye and dental exams, liver and kidney function tests, bone density tests, and others as needed.

Skin & sunlight:
May cause rash or intensify sunburn in areas exposed to sun or ultraviolet light (photosensitivity reaction). Avoid overexposure and use sunscreen. Notify doctor if reaction occurs.

Driving, piloting or hazardous work:
Don't drive or pilot aircraft until you learn how drug effects you. Don't work around dangerous machinery. Don't climb ladders or work in high places. Danger increases if you drink alcohol or take drugs affecting alertness and reflexes.

Discontinuing:
Don't discontinue without doctor's advice until you complete prescribed dose, even though symptoms diminish or disappear.

Others:

- Wear or carry medical identification that states that you take this drug.
- Periodic blood tests are needed.
- Advise any doctor or dentist whom you consult that you take this medicine.
- Rarely, anticonvulsant (antiepileptic) drugs may lead to suicidal thoughts and behaviors. Call doctor right away if suicidal symptoms or unusual behaviors occur.

POSSIBLE INTERACTION WITH OTHER DRUGS

GENERIC NAME OR DRUG CLASS	COMBINED EFFECT
Acetaminophen	Increased risk of liver problems.
Adrenocorticoids, systemic	Decreased adreno-corticoid effect.
Antibiotics, macrolide	Increased effect of carbamazepine.
Anticoagulants, oral*	Decreased anticoagulant effect.
Anticonvulsants, hydantoin* or succinimide*	Decreased effect of both drugs.

Continued on page 910

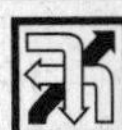

POSSIBLE INTERACTION WITH OTHER SUBSTANCES

INTERACTS WITH	COMBINED EFFECT
Alcohol:	Increased sedative effect. Avoid.
Beverages: Grapefruit juice.	Risk of toxicity. Avoid.
Cocaine:	Increased adverse effects. Avoid.
Foods:	None expected.
Marijuana:	Increased adverse effects. Avoid.
Tobacco:	None expected.

***See Glossary**

CARBIDOPA & LEVODOPA

BRAND NAMES

Parcopa
Sinemet
Sinemet CR
Stalevo

BASIC INFORMATION

Habit forming? No
Prescription needed? Yes
Available as generic? Yes
Drug class: Antiparkinsonism

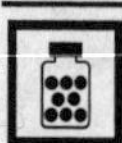

USES

Controls Parkinson's disease symptoms such as rigidity, tremor and unsteady gait.

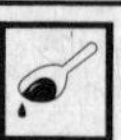

DOSAGE & USAGE INFORMATION

How to take:

- Tablet—Swallow with liquid or food to lessen stomach irritation. If you can't swallow whole, crumble tablet and take with liquid or food. Do not crush, break or chew Stalevo tablet.
- Extended-release tablet—Swallow each dose whole; do not crumble.

When to take:
At the same times each day.

If you forget a dose:
Take as soon as you remember. If it is almost time for the next dose, wait for the next scheduled dose (don't double this dose).

What drug does:
Restores chemical balance necessary for normal nerve impulses.

Continued next column

OVERDOSE

SYMPTOMS:
Muscle twitch, spastic eyelid closure, nausea, vomiting, diarrhea, irregular and rapid pulse, weakness, fainting, confusion, agitation, hallucination, coma.
WHAT TO DO:

- **Dial 911 (emergency) for medical help or call poison control center 1-800-222-1222 for instructions.**
- **If person is unconscious, check breathing and pulse. If not breathing, begin mouth-to-mouth rescue breathing. If heart is not beating, begin chest compressions.**
- **See emergency information on last 3 pages of this book.**

Time lapse before drug works:
2 to 3 weeks to improve; 6 weeks or longer for maximum benefit.

Don't take with:
Any other medicine or any dietary supplement without consulting your doctor or pharmacist.

POSSIBLE ADVERSE REACTIONS OR SIDE EFFECTS

SYMPTOMS	WHAT TO DO
Life-threatening:	
In case of overdose, see previous column.	
Common:	
• Mood changes, uncontrollable body movements, diarrhea.	Continue. Call doctor when convenient.
• Dry mouth, body odor.	No action necessary.
Infrequent:	
• Fainting, severe dizziness, headache, insomnia, nightmares, rash, itch, nausea, vomiting, irregular heartbeat.	Discontinue. Call doctor right away.
• Flushed face, blurred vision, muscle twitching, discolored or dark urine, difficult urination.	Continue. Call doctor when convenient.
• Constipation, tiredness.	Continue. Tell doctor at next visit.
Rare:	
• High blood pressure.	Discontinue. Call doctor right away.
• Upper abdominal pain, anemia.	Continue. Call doctor when convenient.

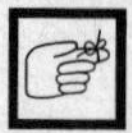

WARNINGS & PRECAUTIONS

Don't take if:

- You are allergic to levodopa or carbidopa.
- You have taken MAO inhibitors in past 2 weeks.
- You have glaucoma (narrow-angle type).

Before you start, consult your doctor if:

- You have diabetes or epilepsy.
- You have had high blood pressure, heart or lung disease.
- You have had liver or kidney disease.
- You have a peptic ulcer.
- You have malignant melanoma.
- You will have surgery within 2 months, including dental surgery, requiring general or spinal anesthesia.

Over age 60:
Adverse reactions and side effects may be more frequent and severe than in younger persons.

Pregnancy:
Decide with your doctor whether drug benefits justify risk to unborn child. Risk category C (see page xviii).

Breast-feeding:
It is unknown if drug passes into milk. Avoid drug or discontinue nursing until you finish medicine. Consult doctor for advice on maintaining milk supply.

Infants & children:
Not recommended.

Prolonged use:
- May lead to uncontrolled movements of head, face, mouth, tongue, arms or legs.
- Talk to your doctor about the need for follow-up medical examinations or laboratory studies.

Skin & sunlight:
No problems expected.

Driving, piloting or hazardous work:
Don't drive or pilot aircraft until you learn how medicine affects you. Don't work around dangerous machinery. Don't climb ladders or work in high places. Danger increases if you drink alcohol or take medicine affecting alertness and reflexes, such as antihistamines, tranquilizers, sedatives, pain medicine, narcotics and mind-altering drugs.

Discontinuing:
Don't discontinue without doctor's advice until you complete prescribed dose, even though symptoms diminish or disappear.

Others:
- Expect to start with small dose and increase gradually to lessen frequency and severity of adverse reactions.
- Advise any doctor or dentist whom you consult that you take this medicine.

POSSIBLE INTERACTION WITH OTHER DRUGS

GENERIC NAME OR DRUG CLASS	COMBINED EFFECT
Anticonvulsants,* hydantoin	Decreased effect of carbidopa and levodopa.
Antidepressants*	Weakness or faintness when arising from bed or chair.
Antihypertensives*	Decreased blood pressure and effect of carbidopa and levodopa.
Antiparkinsonism drugs, other*	Increased effect of carbidopa and levodopa.
Bupropion	Increased levodopa effect.
Haloperidol	Decreased effect of carbidopa and levodopa.
Methyldopa	Decreased effect of carbidopa and levodopa.
Monoamine oxidase (MAO) inhibitors*	Dangerous rise in blood pressure.
Papaverine	Decreased effect of carbidopa and levodopa.
Phenothiazines*	Decreased effect of carbidopa and levodopa.
Phenytoin	Decreased effect of carbidopa and levodopa.
Pyridoxine (Vitamin B-6)	Decreased effect of carbidopa and levodopa.
Rauwolfia alkaloids*	Decreased effect of carbidopa and levodopa.
Selegiline	May require adjustment in dosage of carbidopa and levodopa.

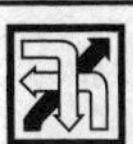

POSSIBLE INTERACTION WITH OTHER SUBSTANCES

INTERACTS WITH	COMBINED EFFECT
Alcohol:	None expected.
Beverages:	None expected.
Cocaine:	Decreased carbidopa and levodopa effect. High rise of heartbeat irregularities. Avoid.
Foods:	None expected.
Marijuana:	Increased fatigue, lethargy, fainting.
Tobacco:	None expected.

CARBONIC ANHYDRASE INHIBITORS

GENERIC AND BRAND NAMES

ACETAZOLAMIDE
Acetazolam
Ak-Zol
Apo Acetazolamide
Dazamide
Diamox
Storzolamide

DICHLORPHENAMIDE
Daranide

METHAZOLAMIDE
MZM
Neptazane

BASIC INFORMATION

Habit forming? No
Prescription needed? Yes
Available as generic? Yes
Drug class: Carbonic anhydrase inhibitor

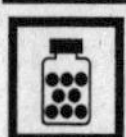

USES

- Treatment of glaucoma.
- Treatment of epileptic seizures.
- Treatment of body fluid retention.
- Treatment for shortness of breath, insomnia and fatigue at high altitudes.
- Treatment for prevention of altitude illness.

DOSAGE & USAGE INFORMATION

How to take:

- Sustained-release tablet—Swallow whole with liquid or food to lessen stomach irritation.
- Extended-release capsule—Swallow whole with liquid.
- Topical—1 drop in the affected eye 3 times a day.

When to take:

- 1 dose per day—At the same time each morning.
- More than 1 dose per day—Take last dose several hours before bedtime.

Continued next column

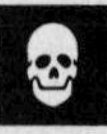

OVERDOSE

SYMPTOMS:
Drowsiness, confusion, excitement, nausea, vomiting, numbness in hands and feet, coma.
WHAT TO DO:

- **Dial 911 (emergency) for medical help or call poison control center 1-800-222-1222 for instructions. Symptoms may not appear until damage has occurred.**
- **See emergency information on last 3 pages of this book.**

If you forget a dose:
Take as soon as you remember. Continue regular schedule.

What drug does:

- Inhibits action of carbonic anhydrase, an enzyme. This lowers the internal eye pressure by decreasing fluid formation in the eye.
- Forces sodium and water excretion, reducing body fluid.

Time lapse before drug works:
2 hours.

Don't take with:
Any other medicine or any dietary supplement without consulting your doctor or pharmacist.

POSSIBLE ADVERSE REACTIONS OR SIDE EFFECTS

SYMPTOMS	WHAT TO DO
Life-threatening:	
Convulsions.	Seek emergency treatment immediately.
Common:	
None expected.	
Infrequent:	
Back pain, sedation, fatigue, weakness, tingling or burning in feet or hands.	Continue. Call doctor when convenient.
Rare:	
• Headache; mood changes; nervousness; clumsiness; trembling; confusion; hives, itch, rash; sores; ringing in ears; hoarseness; dry mouth; thirst; sore throat; fever; appetite change; nausea; vomiting; black, tarry stool; breathing difficulty; irregular or weak heartbeat; easy bleeding or bruising; muscle cramps; painful or frequent urination; blood in urine.	Continue. Call doctor right away.
• Depression, loss of libido.	Continue. Call doctor when convenient.

WARNINGS & PRECAUTIONS

Don't take if:
You are allergic to any carbonic anhydrase inhibitor.

Before you start, consult your doctor if:
- You have gout or lupus.
- You are allergic to any sulfa drug.
- You have liver or kidney disease.
- You have Addison's disease (adrenal gland failure).
- You have diabetes.
- You will have surgery within 2 months, including dental surgery, requiring general or spinal anesthesia.

Over age 60:
- Don't exceed recommended dose.
- If you take a digitalis preparation, eat foods high in potassium content or take a potassium supplement.

Pregnancy:
Avoid if possible, especially first 3 months. Consult doctor. Risk category C (see page xviii).

Breast-feeding:
Avoid drug or don't nurse your infant. Consult doctor about maintaining milk supply.

Infants & children:
Not recommended for children younger than 12.

Prolonged use:
May cause kidney stones, vision change, loss of taste and smell, jaundice or weight loss.

Skin & sunlight:
One or more drugs in this group may cause rash or intensify sunburn in areas exposed to sun or ultraviolet light (photosensitivity reaction). Avoid overexposure. Notify doctor if reaction occurs.

Driving, piloting or hazardous work:
Avoid if you feel drowsy or dizzy. Otherwise, no problems expected.

Discontinuing:
Don't discontinue without medical advice.

Others:
- Medicine may increase sugar levels in blood and urine. Diabetics may need insulin adjustment.
- Advise any doctor or dentist whom you consult that you take this medicine.

POSSIBLE INTERACTION WITH OTHER DRUGS

GENERIC NAME OR DRUG CLASS	COMBINED EFFECT
Adrenocorticoids, systemic	Increased loss of calcium & potassium.
Amphetamines*	Increased amphetamine effect.
Anticonvulsants*	Increased loss of bone minerals.
Antidiabetics, oral*	May need dosage adjustment.
Antiglaucoma, carbonic anhydrase inhibitors	Increased effect of both drugs. Avoid.
Ciprofloxacin	May cause kidney dysfunction.
Digitalis preparations*	Possible digitalis toxicity.
Diuretics*	Increased potassium loss.
Lithium	Decreased lithium effect.
Mecamylamine	Increased mecamylamine effect.
Memantine	Increased effect of memantine.
Methenamine	Decreased methenamine effect.
Mexiletine	May slow elimination of mexiletine and cause need to adjust dosage.
Quinidine	Increased quinidine effect.
Salicylates*	Salicylate toxicity.
Sympathomimetics*	Increased sympathomimetic effect.

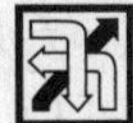

POSSIBLE INTERACTION WITH OTHER SUBSTANCES

INTERACTS WITH	COMBINED EFFECT
Alcohol:	None expected.
Beverages:	None expected.
Cocaine:	Avoid. Decreased carbonic anhydrase inhibitor effect.
Foods: Potassium-rich foods.*	Eat these to decrease potassium loss.
Marijuana:	Avoid. Increased carbonic anhydrase inhibitor effect.
Tobacco:	May decrease effect of carbonic anhydrase inhibitors.

*See Glossary

CENTRAL ALPHA AGONISTS

GENERIC AND BRAND NAMES

CLONIDINE	**METHYLDOPA**
Catapres	Aldoclor
Catapres-TTS	Aldomet
Dixarit	Aldoril
Jenloga	Apo-Methyldopa
Kapvay	Dopamet
Nexiclon XR	Novodoparil
GUANABENZ	Novomedopa
Wytensin	Nu-Medopa
GUANFACINE	PMS Dopazide
Intuniv	Supres
Tenex	

BASIC INFORMATION

Habit forming? No
Prescription needed? Yes
Available as generic? Yes
Drug class: Antihypertensive

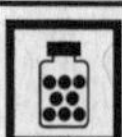

USES

- Control of hypertension (high blood pressure).
- May be used for symptoms of narcotic, alcohol or nicotine withdrawal.
- Prevention of migraine headaches.
- Treatment for menstrual cramps or hot flashes due to menopause.
- Treats attention deficit hyperactivity disorder.

DOSAGE & USAGE INFORMATION

How to take:
- Tablet—Swallow with liquid with or without food.
- Transdermal patch (attaches to skin)—Apply to clean, dry, hairless skin on arm or trunk. Follow all prescription instructions carefully.

Continued next column

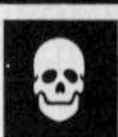

OVERDOSE

SYMPTOMS:
Vomiting, slow heartbeat, weakness, low blood pressure, lightheadedness, cold feeling, extreme tiredness or drowsiness, coma.
WHAT TO DO:
- **Dial 911 (emergency) for medical help or call poison control center 1-800-222-1222 for instructions.**
- **If person is unconscious, check breathing and pulse. If not breathing, begin mouth-to-mouth rescue breathing. If heart is not beating, begin chest compressions.**
- **See emergency information on last 3 pages of this book.**

- Extended-release tablet—Swallow whole with small amount of liquid. Don't crush or chew.
- Solution—Follow label instructions.

When to take:
- Oral form—One to four times a day according to the instructions on your prescription.
- Transdermal patch—Replace as directed, usually once a week.

If you forget a dose:
- Take tablet as soon as you remember. If it is almost time for the next dose, wait for the next scheduled dose (don't double this dose). If you miss 2 doses in a row, call your doctor.
- If the once-a-week patch change is 3 days late, call your doctor for advice.

What drug does:
- Hypertension—Lowers blood pressure by relaxing and dilating (widening) blood vessels. This helps increase flow of blood in the body.
- Withdrawal symptoms—Thought to block nerve impulses in the area of the brain responsible for the symptoms.
- Attention deficit hyperactivity disorder—The way it works is unclear.

Time lapse before drug works:
2 to 3 weeks for full benefit.

Don't take with:
Any other medicine or any dietary supplement without consulting your doctor or pharmacist.

POSSIBLE ADVERSE REACTIONS OR SIDE EFFECTS

SYMPTOMS	WHAT TO DO
Life-threatening:	
Allergic reaction (difficulty breathing, closing of the throat, swelling of the lips or face or tongue, hives).	Seek emergency treatment immediately.
Common:	
Dizziness, constipation, drowsiness, irritated skin (with skin patch), dry mouth, tiredness, headache, insomnia, weakness, low blood pressure.	Continue. Call doctor when convenient.
Infrequent:	
• Darkened skin (with skin patch), light-headedness, dry or burning eyes, anxiety, decreased sex function, nervousness, appetite loss, nausea, vomiting, depression.	Continue. Call doctor when convenient.
• Swollen feet/legs, slow or fast heartbeat, fever.	Continue, but call doctor right away.

Rare:

• Joint pain, pale stools, skin rash or itching, nightmares, confusion.	Continue. Call doctor when convenient.
• Cold fingers and toes, dark urine, chills, breathing difficulty, yellow eyes or skin, stomach pain.	Continue, but call doctor right away.

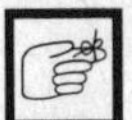

WARNINGS & PRECAUTIONS

Don't take if:
You are allergic to any central alpha agonist.

Before you start, consult your doctor if:
- You will have surgery within 2 months requiring general or spinal anesthesia.
- You have heart, liver or kidney disease.
- You had a recent stroke or heart attack.
- You have a peripheral circulation disorder (intermittent claudication, Raynaud's syndrome, Buerger's disease).
- You have Parkinson's disease.
- You have a history of depression.
- You have a disorder affecting the skin or any skin irritation (with use of transdermal patch).

Over age 60:
Adverse reactions and side effects may be more frequent and severe than in younger persons.

Pregnancy:
Decide with your doctor whether drug benefits justify risk to unborn child. Risk category B for guanfacine and methyldopa; risk category C for clonidine and guanabenz (see page xviii).

Breast-feeding:
Clonidine and methyldopa pass into breast milk. It is unknown if guanabenz or guanfacine pass into breast milk. Consult your doctor.

Infants & children:
One or more of these drugs may be prescribed for attention deficit hyperactivity disorder for ages 6 to 17.

Prolonged use:
Talk to your doctor about the need for follow-up medical or eye exams or laboratory tests.

Skin & sunlight:
None expected.

Driving, piloting or hazardous work:
Don't drive or pilot aircraft until you learn how medicine affects you. Don't work around dangerous machinery. Don't climb ladders or work in high places. Danger increases if you drink alcohol or take medicine affecting alertness and reflexes.

Discontinuing:
- Don't discontinue abruptly. May cause a withdrawal syndrome (anxiety, chest pain, headache, nausea, insomnia, irregular heartbeat, flushed face, sweating). Consult doctor if any symptoms occur after stopping the drug.
- Dose may require gradual reduction if you have taken drug for a long time. Doses of other drugs may also require adjustment.

Others:
- Advise any doctor or dentist whom you consult that you take this medicine.
- For dry mouth, suck sugarless hard candy or chew sugarless gum. If dry mouth continues, consult your dentist.

POSSIBLE INTERACTION WITH OTHER DRUGS

GENERIC NAME OR DRUG CLASS	COMBINED EFFECT
Antidepressants, tricyclic*	Decreased effect of central alpha agonist.
Antihypertensives,* other	Excessive lowering of blood pressure.
Beta-adrenergic blocking agents*	Increased risk of adverse reactions and excessive low blood pressure.

Continued on page 912

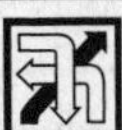

POSSIBLE INTERACTION WITH OTHER SUBSTANCES

INTERACTS WITH	COMBINED EFFECT
Alcohol:	Increased sedative effect of alcohol and very low blood pressure. Avoid.
Beverages:	None expected.
Cocaine:	Increased risk of heart problems and high blood pressure. Avoid.
Foods:	None expected.
Marijuana:	Weakness on standing. Avoid.
Tobacco:	None expected. Persons with high blood pressure should not smoke.

*See Glossary

CEPHALOSPORINS

GENERIC AND BRAND NAMES

CEFACLOR
- Ceclor
- Ceclor CD
- Raniclor

CEFADROXIL
- Duricef
- Ultracef

CEFDINIR
- Omnicef

CEFDITOREN
- Spectracef

CEFIXIME
- Suprax

CEFOTETAN
- Cefotan

CEFPODOXIME
- Vantin

CEFPROZIL
- Cefzil

CEFTIBUTEN
- Cedax

CEFUROXIME
- Ceftin

CEPHALEXIN
- Apo-Cephalex
- Cefanex
- Ceporex
- C-Lexin
- Keflex
- Keftab
- Novolexin
- Nu-Cephalex

CEPHRADINE
- Anspor
- Velosef

BASIC INFORMATION

Habit forming? No
Prescription needed? Yes
Available as generic? Yes
Drug class: Antibacterial

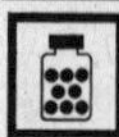

USES

Treatment of bacterial infections. Will not cure viral infections such as cold and flu.

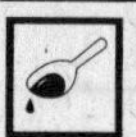

DOSAGE & USAGE INFORMATION

How to take:
- Tablet or capsule—Swallow with liquid. If you can't swallow whole, crumble tablet or open capsule and take with liquid or food.
- Extended-release tablet—Swallow with liquid. Do not crush or chew tablet.

Continued next column

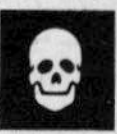

OVERDOSE

SYMPTOMS:
Abdominal cramps, nausea, vomiting, severe diarrhea with mucus or blood in stool, convulsions.
WHAT TO DO:
Overdose unlikely to threaten life. If person uses much larger amount than prescribed or if accidentally swallowed, call doctor or poison control center 1-800-222-1222 for help.

- Chewable tablet—Follow instructions on prescription.
- Liquid and oral suspension—Use measuring spoon. Mix according to package instructions.

When to take:
- At same times each day, 1 hour before or 2 hours after eating.
- Take until gone or as directed.

If you forget a dose:
Take as soon as you remember. If it is almost time for the next dose, wait for the next scheduled dose (don't double this dose).

What drug does:
Kills susceptible bacteria.

Time lapse before drug works:
May require several days to affect infection.

Don't take with:
Any other medicine or any dietary supplement without consulting your doctor or pharmacist.

POSSIBLE ADVERSE REACTIONS OR SIDE EFFECTS

SYMPTOMS	WHAT TO DO
Life-threatening:	
Hives, rash, intense itching, faintness soon after a dose (anaphylaxis); difficulty breathing.	Seek emergency treatment immediately.
Common:	
Mild diarrhea, nausea, vomiting, sore mouth or tongue, mild stomach cramps (all less common with some cephalosporins).	Continue. Call doctor when convenient.
Infrequent:	
None expected.	
Rare:	
• Severe stomach cramps, severe diarrhea with mucus or blood in stool, fever, unusual weakness or tiredness, weight loss, bleeding or bruising, increased thirst, decreased urine, dizziness, joint pain, appetite loss, skin symptoms (rash, itching, redness, swelling), yellow skin or eyes.	Discontinue. Call doctor right away.
• Genital itching or vaginal discharge.	Continue. Call doctor when convenient.

WARNINGS & PRECAUTIONS

Don't take if:
You are allergic to any cephalosporin antibiotic.

Before you start, consult your doctor if:
- You are allergic to any penicillin antibiotic.
- You have a kidney disorder.
- You have colitis or enteritis.

Over age 60:
Adverse reactions and side effects may be more frequent and severe than in younger persons. More likely to itch around rectum and genitals.

Pregnancy:
No proven harm to unborn child. Avoid if possible. Consult doctor. Risk category B (see page xviii).

Breast-feeding:
Drug passes into milk. Avoid drug or discontinue nursing until you finish medicine. Consult doctor for advice on maintaining milk supply.

Infants & children:
No special warnings.

Prolonged use:
- Kills beneficial bacteria that protect body against other germs. Unchecked germs may cause secondary infections.
- Talk to your doctor about the need for follow-up medical examinations or laboratory studies to check prothrombin time.

Skin & sunlight:
No problems expected.

Driving, piloting or hazardous work:
No problems expected.

Discontinuing:
Don't discontinue without doctor's advice until you complete prescribed dose, even though symptoms diminish or disappear.

Others:
- Don't use drug for other medical problems without doctor's approval.
- Advise any doctor or dentist whom you consult that you take this medicine.
- If diarrhea occurs, consult doctor.

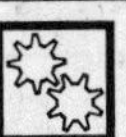

POSSIBLE INTERACTION WITH OTHER DRUGS

GENERIC NAME OR DRUG CLASS	COMBINED EFFECT
Anticoagulants*	Increased anticoagulant effect.
Anti-inflammatory drugs, nonsteroidal (NSAIDs)*	Increased risk of peptic ulcer.
Chloramphenicol	Decreased antibiotic effect of cephalosporin.
Probenecid	Increased cephalosporin effect.
Tetracyclines*	Decreased antibiotic effect of cephalosporin.

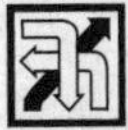

POSSIBLE INTERACTION WITH OTHER SUBSTANCES

INTERACTS WITH	COMBINED EFFECT
Alcohol:	Increased kidney toxicity, likelihood of disulfiram-like* effect.
Beverages:	None expected.
Cocaine:	None expected, but cocaine may slow body's recovery. Avoid.
Foods:	Slow absorption. Take with liquid 1 hour before or 2 hours after eating.
Marijuana:	None expected, but marijuana may slow body's recovery. Avoid.
Tobacco:	None expected.

CHARCOAL, ACTIVATED

BRAND NAMES

Acta-Char
Acta-Char Liquid
Actidose with Sorbitol
Actidose-Aqua
Aqueous Charcodote
Charac-50
Charac-tol 50
Charcoaid
Charcocaps
Charcodote
Charcodote TFS
Insta-Char
Liqui-Char
Pediatric Aqueous Charcodote
Pediatric Charcodote
SuperChar

BASIC INFORMATION

Habit forming? No
Prescription needed? No
Available as generic? Yes
Drug class: Antidote (adsorbent)

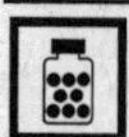

USES

- Treatment of poisonings from medication.
- Treatment (infrequent) for diarrhea or excessive gaseousness.

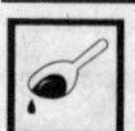

DOSAGE & USAGE INFORMATION

How to take:

- Tablet or capsule—Swallow with liquid. If you can't swallow whole, crumble tablet or open capsule and take with liquid or food.
- Liquid—Take as directed on label. Don't mix with chocolate syrup, ice cream or sherbet.

When to take:

- For poisoning—Take immediately after poisoning. If your doctor or emergency poison control center has also recommended syrup of ipecac, don't take charcoal for 30 minutes or until vomiting from ipecac stops.
- For diarrhea or gas—Take at same times each day.
- Take 2 or more hours after taking other medicines.

Continued next column

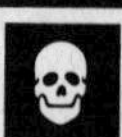

OVERDOSE

SYMPTOMS:
None expected.
WHAT TO DO:
Overdose unlikely to threaten life. If person uses much larger amount than prescribed or if accidentally swallowed, call doctor or poison control center 1-800-222-1222 for help.

If you forget a dose:

- For poisonings—Not applicable.
- For diarrhea or gas—Take as soon as you remember. If it is almost time for the next dose, wait for the next scheduled dose (don't double this dose).

What drug does:

- Helps prevent poison from being absorbed from stomach and intestines.
- Helps absorb gas in intestinal tract.

Time lapse before drug works:
Begins immediately.

Don't take with:
Ice cream or sherbet.

POSSIBLE ADVERSE REACTIONS OR SIDE EFFECTS

SYMPTOMS	WHAT TO DO
Life-threatening: None expected.	
Always: Black bowel movements.	No action necessary.
Infrequent: None expected.	
Rare: Unless taken with cathartic, can cause constipation when taken for overdose of other medicine.	Take a laxative after crisis is over.

WARNINGS & PRECAUTIONS

Don't take if:
The poison was lye or other strong alkali, strong acids (such as sulfuric acid), cyanide, iron, ethyl alcohol or methyl alcohol. Charcoal will not prevent these poisons from causing ill effects.

Before you start, consult your doctor if:
You are taking it as an antidote for poison.

Over age 60:
No problems expected.

Pregnancy:
Consult doctor. Risk category C (see page xviii).

Breast-feeding:
No problems expected. Consult doctor.

Infants & children:
Don't give to children for more than 3 or 4 days for diarrhea. Continuing for longer periods can interfere with normal nutrition.

Prolonged use:
No problems expected.

Skin & sunlight:
No problems expected.

Driving, piloting or hazardous work:
No problems expected.

Discontinuing:
No problems expected.

Others:
No problems expected.

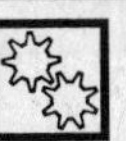

POSSIBLE INTERACTION WITH OTHER DRUGS

GENERIC NAME OR DRUG CLASS	COMBINED EFFECT
Any medicine taken at the same time	May decrease absorption of medicine. Take drugs 2 hours apart.

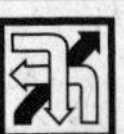

POSSIBLE INTERACTION WITH OTHER SUBSTANCES

INTERACTS WITH	COMBINED EFFECT
Alcohol:	None expected.
Beverages:	None expected.
Cocaine:	None expected.
Foods: Chocolate syrup, ice cream or sherbet.	Decreased charcoal effect.
Marijuana:	None expected.
Tobacco:	None expected.

CHLORAMBUCIL

BRAND NAMES

Leukeran

BASIC INFORMATION

Habit forming? No
Prescription needed? Yes
Available as generic? No
Drug class: Antineoplastic, immunosuppressant

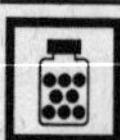

USES

- Treatment for some kinds of cancer.
- Suppresses immune response after transplant and in immune disorders.

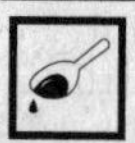

DOSAGE & USAGE INFORMATION

How to take:
Tablet—Swallow with liquid after light meal. Don't drink fluids with meals. Drink extra fluids between meals. Avoid sweet or fatty foods.

When to take:
At the same time each day.

If you forget a dose:
Take as soon as you remember. Never double dose.

What drug does:
Inhibits abnormal cell reproduction. May suppress immune system.

Time lapse before drug works:
Up to 6 weeks for full effect.

Don't take with:
Any other medicine or any dietary supplement without consulting your doctor or pharmacist.

OVERDOSE

SYMPTOMS:
Bleeding, chills, fever, vomiting, abdominal pain, ataxia, collapse, stupor, seizure.
WHAT TO DO:

- **Dial 911 (emergency) for medical help or call poison control center 1-800-222-1222 for instructions.**
- **If person is unconscious, check breathing and pulse. If not breathing, begin mouth-to-mouth rescue breathing. If heart is not beating, begin chest compressions.**
- **See emergency information on last 3 pages of this book.**

POSSIBLE ADVERSE REACTIONS OR SIDE EFFECTS

SYMPTOMS	WHAT TO DO
Life-threatening:	
In case of overdose, see previous column.	
Common:	
• Unusual bleeding or bruising, mouth sores with sore throat, chills and fever, black stools, mouth and lip sores, menstrual irregularities, back pain.	Discontinue. Call doctor right away.
• Hair loss, joint pain.	Continue. Call doctor when convenient.
• Nausea, vomiting, diarrhea, tiredness, weakness.	Continue. Tell doctor at next visit.
Infrequent:	
• Mental confusion, shortness of breath.	Continue. Call doctor when convenient.
• Cough, rash, foot swelling.	Continue. Tell doctor at next visit.
Rare:	
Jaundice, convulsions, hallucinations, muscle twitching.	Discontinue. Call doctor right away.

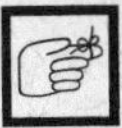

WARNINGS & PRECAUTIONS

Don't take if:
- You have had hypersensitivity to alkylating antineoplastic drugs.
- Your physician has not explained serious nature of your medical problem and risks of taking this medicine.

Before you start, consult your doctor if:
- You have gout.
- You have had kidney stones.
- You have active infection.
- You have impaired kidney or liver function.
- You have taken other antineoplastic drugs or had radiation treatment in last 3 weeks.

Over age 60:
Adverse reactions and side effects may be more frequent and severe than in younger persons.

Pregnancy:
Consult doctor. Risk to unborn child is significant. Risk category D (see page xviii).

Breast-feeding:
Safety not established. Consult doctor.

Infants & children:
Use only under care of doctors who are experienced in anticancer drugs.

Prolonged use:
- Adverse reactions more likely the longer drug is required.
- Talk to your doctor about the need for follow-up medical examinations or laboratory studies to check complete blood counts (white blood cell count, platelet count, red blood cell count, hemoglobin, hematocrit).

Skin & sunlight:
No problems expected.

Driving, piloting or hazardous work:
No problems expected.

Discontinuing:
Don't discontinue without doctor's advice until you complete prescribed dose, even though symptoms diminish or disappear. Some side effects may follow discontinuing. Report to doctor blurred vision, convulsions, confusion, persistent headache.

Others:
- May cause blood problems or cancer.
- Advise any doctor or dentist whom you consult that you take this medicine.
- Consult your doctor before you or a household member gets any immunization.

POSSIBLE INTERACTION WITH OTHER DRUGS

GENERIC NAME OR DRUG CLASS	COMBINED EFFECT
Antigout drugs*	Decreased antigout effect.
Antineoplastic drugs, other*	Increased effect of all drugs (may be beneficial).
Chloramphenicol	Increased likelihood of toxic effects of both drugs.
Clozapine	Toxic effect on bone marrow.
Cyclosporine	May increase risk of infection.
Immuno-suppressants*	Increased chance of infection.
Lovastatin	Increased heart and kidney damage.
Tiopronin	Increased risk of toxicity to bone marrow.

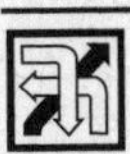

POSSIBLE INTERACTION WITH OTHER SUBSTANCES

INTERACTS WITH	COMBINED EFFECT
Alcohol:	May increase chance of intestinal bleeding.
Beverages:	No problems expected.
Cocaine:	Increases chance of toxicity.
Foods:	Reduces irritation in stomach.
Marijuana:	No problems expected.
Tobacco:	Increases lung toxicity.

***See Glossary**

CHLORAMPHENICOL

BRAND NAMES

Chloromycetin
Novochlorocap

BASIC INFORMATION

Habit forming? No
Prescription needed? Yes
Available as generic? Yes
Drug class: Antibacterial

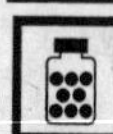

USES

Treatment of infections susceptible to chloramphenicol. Will not treat viral infections such as cold or flu.

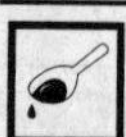

DOSAGE & USAGE INFORMATION

How to take:
Suspension or capsule—Take with a full glass of water.

When to take:
Capsule or suspension—1 hour before or 2 hours after eating.

If you forget a dose:
Take as soon as you remember. If it is almost time for the next dose, wait for the next scheduled dose (don't double this dose).

What drug does:
Prevents bacteria from growing and reproducing. Will not kill viruses.

Time lapse before drug works:
2 to 5 days, depending on type and severity of infection.

Don't take with:
Any other medicine or any dietary supplement without consulting your doctor or pharmacist.

OVERDOSE

SYMPTOMS:
Nausea, vomiting, diarrhea.
WHAT TO DO:
Overdose unlikely to threaten life. If person uses much larger amount than prescribed or if accidentally swallowed, call doctor or poison control center 1-800-222-1222 for help.

POSSIBLE ADVERSE REACTIONS OR SIDE EFFECTS

SYMPTOMS	WHAT TO DO
Life-threatening:	
Hives, rash, intense itching, faintness soon after a dose (anaphylaxis).	Seek emergency treatment immediately.
Common:	
None expected.	
Infrequent:	
• Swollen face or extremities; diarrhea; nausea; vomiting; numbness, tingling, burning pain or weakness in hands and feet; pale skin; unusual bleeding or bruising.	Discontinue. Call doctor right away.
• Headache, confusion.	Continue. Call doctor when convenient.
Rare:	
• Pain, blurred vision, possible vision loss, delirium, rash, sore throat, fever, jaundice, anemia.	Discontinue. Call doctor right away.
• In babies: Bloated stomach, uneven breathing, drowsiness, low temperature, gray skin.	Discontinue. Call doctor right away.

WARNINGS & PRECAUTIONS

Don't take if:
- You are allergic to chloramphenicol.
- It is prescribed for a minor disorder such as flu, cold or mild sore throat.

Before you start, consult your doctor if:
- You have had a blood disorder or bone-marrow disease.
- You have had kidney or liver disease.
- You have diabetes.

Over age 60:
Adverse reactions and side effects may be more frequent and severe than in younger persons, particularly skin irritation around rectum.

Pregnancy:
Decide with your doctor if drug benefits justify risk to unborn child. Risk category C (see page xviii).

Breast-feeding:
Drug passes into milk. Avoid drug or discontinue nursing until you finish medicine. Consult doctor for advice on maintaining milk supply.

Infants & children:
Use only under close medical supervision, especially in infants younger than 2.

Prolonged use:
- You may become more susceptible to infections caused by germs not responsive to chloramphenicol.
- Talk to your doctor about the need for follow-up medical examinations or laboratory studies to check complete blood counts (white blood cell count, platelet count, red blood cell count, hemoglobin, hematocrit), chloramphenicol serum levels.

Skin & sunlight:
No problems expected.

Driving, piloting or hazardous work:
Don't drive or pilot aircraft until you learn how medicine affects you. Don't work around dangerous machinery. Don't climb ladders or work in high places. Danger increases if you drink alcohol or take medicine affecting alertness and reflexes.

Discontinuing:
Don't discontinue without doctor's advice until you complete prescribed dose, even though symptoms diminish or disappear.

Others:
- Chloramphenicol can cause serious anemia. Frequent laboratory blood studies, liver and kidney tests recommended.
- Advise any doctor or dentist whom you consult that you take this medicine.
- Second medical opinion recommended before starting.

POSSIBLE INTERACTION WITH OTHER DRUGS

GENERIC NAME OR DRUG CLASS	COMBINED EFFECT
Anticoagulants*	Increased anticoagulant effect.
Antidiabetics, oral*	Increased antidiabetic effect.
Anticonvulsants*	Increased chance of toxicity to bone marrow.
Antivirals, HIV/AIDS*	Increased risk of peripheral neuropathy.
Cefixime	Decreased antibiotic effect of cefixime.
Cephalosporins*	Decreased chloramphenicol effect.
Clindamycin	Decreased clindamycin effect.
Clozapine	Toxic effect on bone marrow.
Cyclophosphamide	Increased cyclophosphamide effect.
Erythromycins	Decreased erythromycin effect.
Flecainide	Possible decreased blood cell production in bone marrow.
Levamisole	Increased risk of bone marrow depression.
Lincomycin	Decreased lincomycin effect.
Lisinopril	Possible blood disorders.
Penicillins*	Decreased penicillin effect.
Phenobarbital	Increased phenobarbital effect.
Phenytoin	Increased phenytoin effect.
Rifampin	Decreased chloramphenicol effect.
Thioguanine	More likelihood of toxicity of both drugs.
Tiopronin	Increased risk of toxicity to bone marrow.
Tocainide	Possible decreased blood cell production in bone marrow.

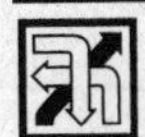

POSSIBLE INTERACTION WITH OTHER SUBSTANCES

INTERACTS WITH	COMBINED EFFECT
Alcohol:	Possible liver problems. Possible disulfiram reaction.*
Beverages:	None expected.
Cocaine:	No proven problems.
Foods:	None expected.
Marijuana:	None expected.
Tobacco:	None expected.

***See Glossary**

CHLORHEXIDINE

BRAND NAMES

Peridex
Periochip
Periogard

BASIC INFORMATION

Habit forming? No
Prescription needed? Yes
Available as generic? Yes
Drug class: Antibacterial (dental)

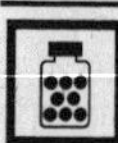

USES

Treatment for gingivitis (inflammation of the gums), periodontal disease and other infections of the mouth.

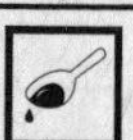

DOSAGE & USAGE INFORMATION

How to use:

- Oral rinse—Swish in mouth for 30 seconds, then spit out. Do not swallow the solution, and do not rinse mouth with water after using. Use product at full strength; do not dilute.
- Implants—Inserted by dentist.

When to use:
Twice a day after brushing and flossing teeth.

If you forget a dose:
Use as soon as you remember, then return to regular schedule.

What drug does:
Kills or prevents growth of susceptible bacteria.

Time lapse before drug works:
Antibacterial action begins within an hour, but full benefit may take several weeks.

Don't use with:
Other mouthwashes without consulting your dentist or pharmacist.

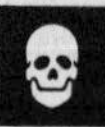

OVERDOSE

SYMPTOMS:
None expected. If a child swallows several ounces of the solution, may have slurred speech, staggering or stumbling walk, sleepiness.
WHAT TO DO:
If symptoms occur, call doctor for instructions. If child weighing under 22 pounds accidentally swallows more than 4 ounces, seek emergency help. Dial 911 (emergency) or poison control center 1-800-222-1222 for help.

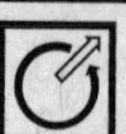

POSSIBLE ADVERSE REACTIONS OR SIDE EFFECTS

SYMPTOMS	WHAT TO DO
Life-threatening: None expected.	
Common: Staining of teeth and other oral surfaces, increased tartar, taste changes, minor mouth irritation.	Continue. Call dentist when convenient.
Infrequent: None expected.	
Rare: Allergic reaction (stuffy nose, shortness of breath, skin rash, hives, itching, face swelling); swollen glands on side of face or neck.	Discontinue. Call doctor right away.

WARNINGS & PRECAUTIONS

Don't take if:
You are allergic to chlorhexidine or skin cleaners that contain chlorhexidine.

Before you start, consult your dentist if:
- You have front tooth fillings (may become discolored).
- You have periodontitis.

Over age 60:
No special problems expected.

Pregnancy:
Consult doctor. Risk category B (see page xviii).

Breast-feeding:
It is unknown if drug passes into milk. Consult doctor.

Infants & children:
Safety in children under age 18 has not been established.

Prolonged use:
See your dentist every 6 months.

Skin & sunlight:
No special problems expected.

Driving, piloting or hazardous work:
No special problems expected.

Discontinuing:
No special problems expected.

Others:
Brush teeth with a tartar-control toothpaste, and floss daily to help reduce tartar buildup.

POSSIBLE INTERACTION WITH OTHER DRUGS

GENERIC NAME OR DRUG CLASS	COMBINED EFFECT
None expected.	

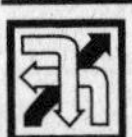

POSSIBLE INTERACTION WITH OTHER SUBSTANCES

INTERACTS WITH	COMBINED EFFECT
Alcohol:	None expected.
Beverages:	Avoid drinking any fluids for several hours after using mouthwash.
Cocaine:	None expected.
Foods:	Avoid eating any foods for several hours after using mouthwash.
Marijuana:	None expected.
Tobacco:	None expected.

CHLOROQUINE

BRAND NAMES

Aralen

BASIC INFORMATION

Habit forming? No
Prescription needed? Yes
Available as generic? Yes
Drug class: Antiprotozoal, antirheumatic

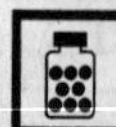

USES

- Treatment for protozoal infections, such as malaria and amebiasis.
- Treatment for some forms of arthritis and lupus.

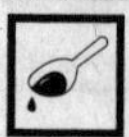

DOSAGE & USAGE INFORMATION

How to take:
Tablet—Swallow with food or milk to lessen stomach irritation.

When to take:
- Depends on condition. Is adjusted during treatment.
- Malaria prevention—Begin taking medicine 2 weeks before traveling to areas where malaria is present and until 8 weeks after return.

If you forget a dose:
- 1 or more doses a day—Take as soon as you remember. If it is almost time for the next dose, wait for the next scheduled dose (don't double this dose).
- 1 dose weekly—Take as soon as possible, then return to regular dosing schedule.

What drug does:
- Inhibits parasite multiplication.
- Decreases inflammatory response in diseased joint.

Continued next column

OVERDOSE

SYMPTOMS:
Severe breathing difficulty, drowsiness, faintness, headache, seizures.
WHAT TO DO:
- **Dial 911 (emergency) for medical help or call poison control center 1-800-222-1222 for instructions.**
- **See emergency information on last 3 pages of this book.**

Time lapse before drug works:
1 to 2 hours. For treatment of arthritis symptoms, may take up to 6 months for maximum effectiveness.

Don't take with:
Any other medicine or any dietary supplement without consulting your doctor or pharmacist.

POSSIBLE ADVERSE REACTIONS OR SIDE EFFECTS

SYMPTOMS	WHAT TO DO
Life-threatening: In case of overdose, see previous column.	
Common:	
Headache, appetite loss, abdominal pain.	Continue. Tell doctor at next visit.
Infrequent:	
• Blurred or changed vision.	Discontinue. Call doctor right away.
• Rash or itch, diarrhea, nausea, vomiting, decreased blood pressure, hair loss, blue-black skin or mouth, dizziness, nervousness.	Continue. Call doctor when convenient.
Rare:	
• Mood or mental changes, seizures, sore throat, fever, unusual bleeding or bruising, muscle weakness, convulsions.	Discontinue. Call doctor right away.
• Ringing or buzzing in ears, hearing loss.	Continue. Call doctor when convenient.

WARNINGS & PRECAUTIONS

Don't take if:
You are allergic to chloroquine or hydroxychloroquine.

Before you start, consult your doctor if:
- You plan to become pregnant within the medication period.
- You have blood disease.
- You have eye or vision problems.
- You have a G6PD deficiency.
- You have liver disease.
- You have nerve or brain disease (including seizure disorders).
- You have porphyria.
- You have psoriasis.
- You have stomach or intestinal disease.
- You drink more than 3 oz. of alcohol daily.

Over age 60:
Adverse reactions and side effects may be more frequent and severe than in younger persons.

Pregnancy:
Decide with your doctor if drug benefits justify risk to unborn child. Risk category C (see page xviii).

Breast-feeding:
Drug passes into milk. Avoid drug or discontinue nursing. Consult doctor about maintaining milk supply.

Infants & children:
Not recommended.

Prolonged use:
- Permanent damage to the retina (back part of the eye) or nerve deafness.
- Talk to your doctor about the need for follow-up medical examinations or laboratory studies to check complete blood counts (white blood cell count, platelet count, red blood cell count, hemoglobin, hematocrit), eyes.

Skin & sunlight:
May cause rash or intensify sunburn in areas exposed to sun or ultraviolet light (photosensitivity reaction). Avoid overexposure. Notify doctor if reaction occurs.

Driving, piloting or hazardous work:
Don't drive or pilot aircraft until you learn how medicine affects you. Don't work around dangerous machinery. Don't climb ladders or work in high places. Danger increases if you drink alcohol or take medicine affecting alertness and reflexes.

Discontinuing:
Don't discontinue without doctor's advice until you complete prescribed dose, even though symptoms diminish or disappear.

Others:
- Periodic physical and blood examinations recommended.
- Advise any doctor or dentist whom you consult that you take this medicine.
- If you are in a malaria area for a long time, you may need to change to another preventive drug every 2 years.

POSSIBLE INTERACTION WITH OTHER DRUGS

GENERIC NAME OR DRUG CLASS	COMBINED EFFECT
Penicillamine	Possible blood or kidney toxicity.

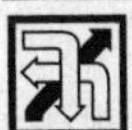

POSSIBLE INTERACTION WITH OTHER SUBSTANCES

INTERACTS WITH	COMBINED EFFECT
Alcohol:	Possible liver toxicity. Avoid.
Beverages:	None expected.
Cocaine:	None expected.
Foods:	None expected.
Marijuana:	None expected.
Tobacco:	None expected.

CHOLESTYRAMINE

BRAND NAMES

Cholybar
Questran
Questran Light

BASIC INFORMATION

Habit forming? No
Prescription needed? Yes
Available as generic? Yes
Drug class: Antihyperlipidemic, antipruritic

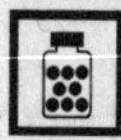

USES

- Removes excess bile acids that occur with some liver problems. Reduces persistent itch caused by bile acids.
- Lowers cholesterol level.
- Treatment for one form of colitis (rare).

DOSAGE & USAGE INFORMATION

How to take:
Powder, granules—Sprinkle into 8 oz. liquid. Let stand for 2 minutes, then mix with liquid before swallowing. Or mix with cereal, soup or pulpy fruit. Don't swallow dry.

When to take:
- 3 or 4 times a day on an empty stomach, 1 hour before or 2 hours after eating.
- If taking other medicines, take 1 hour before or 4 to 6 hours after taking cholestyramine.

If you forget a dose:
Take as soon as you remember. If it is almost time for the next dose, skip the missed dose and wait for your next scheduled dose (don't double this dose).

What drug does:
Binds with bile acids to prevent their absorption.

Time lapse before drug works:
- Cholesterol reduction—1 day.
- Bile-acid reduction—3 to 4 weeks.

Continued next column

OVERDOSE

SYMPTOMS:
Increased side effects and adverse reactions.
WHAT TO DO:
Overdose unlikely to threaten life. If person uses much larger amount than prescribed or if accidentally swallowed, call doctor or poison control center 1-800-222-1222 for help.

Don't take with:
- Another medicine at the same time. Space doses 2 hours apart.
- Any other medicine or any dietary supplement without consulting your doctor or pharmacist.

POSSIBLE ADVERSE REACTIONS OR SIDE EFFECTS

SYMPTOMS	WHAT TO DO
Life-threatening:	
In case of overdose, see previous column.	
Common:	
Constipation.	Continue. Call doctor when convenient.
Infrequent:	
• Belching, bloating, diarrhea, mild nausea, vomiting, stomach pain, rapid weight gain.	Discontinue. Call doctor when convenient.
• Heartburn (mild).	Continue. Call doctor when convenient.
Rare:	
• Severe stomach pain; black, tarry stool.	Discontinue. Seek emergency treatment.
• Rash, hives, hiccups.	Discontinue. Call doctor right away.
• Sore tongue.	Continue. Call doctor when convenient.

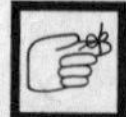

WARNINGS & PRECAUTIONS

Don't take if:
You are allergic to cholestyramine.

Before you start, consult your doctor if:
- You plan to become pregnant within medication period.
- You have angina, heart or blood-vessel disease.
- You have stomach problems (including ulcer).
- You have tartrazine sensitivity.
- You have constipation or hemorrhoids.
- You have kidney disease.

Over age 60:
Adverse reactions and side effects may be more frequent and severe than in younger persons.

Pregnancy:
Decide with your doctor whether drug benefits justify risk to unborn child. Risk category C (see page xviii).

Breast-feeding:
No problems expected, but consult doctor.

Infants & children:
Not recommended.

Prolonged use:
- May decrease absorption of folic acid.
- Talk to your doctor about the need for follow-up medical examinations or laboratory studies to check serum cholesterol and triglycerides.

Skin & sunlight:
No problems expected.

Driving, piloting or hazardous work:
No problems expected.

Discontinuing:
Don't discontinue without doctor's advice until you complete prescribed dose, even though symptoms diminish or disappear.

Others:
Advise any doctor or dentist whom you consult that you take this medicine.

POSSIBLE INTERACTION WITH OTHER DRUGS

GENERIC NAME OR DRUG CLASS	COMBINED EFFECT
Adrenocorticoids, systemic	Decreased adrenocorticoid effect.
Anticoagulants, oral*	Increased anticoagulant effect.
Beta carotene	Decreased absorption of beta carotene.
Dexfenfluramine	May require dosage change as weight loss occurs.
Dextrothyroxine	Decreased dextrothyroxine effect.
Digitalis preparations*	Decreased digitalis effect.
Indapamide	Decreased indapamide effect.
Penicillins*	May decrease penicillin effect.
Raloxifene	Decreased effect of raloxifene.
Thiazides*	Decreased absorption of cholestyramine.
Thyroid hormones*	Decreased thyroid effect.
Trimethoprim	Decreased absorption of cholestyramine.
Ursodiol	Decreased absorption of ursodiol.
Vancomycin	Increased chance of hearing loss or kidney damage. Decreased therapeutic effect of vancomycin.
Vitamins	Decreased absorption of fat-soluble vitamins (A,D,E,K).
All other medicines	Decreased absorption, so dosages or dosage intervals may require adjustment.

POSSIBLE INTERACTION WITH OTHER SUBSTANCES

INTERACTS WITH	COMBINED EFFECT
Alcohol:	None expected.
Beverages:	None expected.
Cocaine:	None expected.
Foods:	Absorption of vitamins in foods decreased. Take vitamin supplements, particularly A, D, E & K.
Marijuana:	None expected.
Tobacco:	None expected.

*See Glossary

CHOLINESTERASE INHIBITORS

GENERIC AND BRAND NAMES

DONEPEZIL
Aricept
Aricept ODT
GALANTAMINE
Razadyne
Razadyne ER
RIVASTIGMINE
Exelon
Exelon Patch

BASIC INFORMATION

Habit forming? No
Prescription needed? Yes
Available as generic? Yes, for some
Drug class: Cholinesterase inhibitor

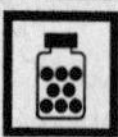

USES

Treats symptoms of mild to moderate dementia (such as problems with memory, judgment, reasoning and other cognitive functions) in patients with Alzheimer's disease or Parkinson's disease.

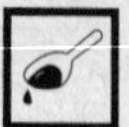

DOSAGE & USAGE INFORMATION

How to take:

- Capsule or tablet—Swallow with liquid. If unable to swallow whole, open capsule or crumble tablet and take with liquid or food.
- Disintegrating tablet—Let dissolve on tongue.
- Patch—Always follow label instructions.
- Oral solution—Take as directed on label.

When to take:

- Donepezil—Once a day at bedtime.
- Rivastigmine or galantamine—At the same times each day.

Continued next column

OVERDOSE

SYMPTOMS:
Severe nausea and vomiting, excessive saliva, sweating, blood pressure decrease, slow heartbeat, collapse, convulsions, muscle weakness (including respiratory muscles, which could lead to death).
WHAT TO DO:

- **Dial 911 (emergency) for medical help or call poison control center 1-800-222-1222 for instructions.**
- **If person is unconscious, check breathing and pulse. If not breathing, begin mouth-to-mouth rescue breathing. If heart is not beating, begin chest compressions.**
- **See emergency information on last 3 pages of this book.**

What drug does:
Slows breakdown of a brain chemical (acetylcholine) that gradually disappears from the brains of people with Alzheimer's disease.

If you forget a dose:
Take as soon as you remember. If it is almost time for the next dose, wait for the next scheduled dose (don't double this dose).

Time lapse before drug works:
May take several weeks or months before beneficial results are observed. Dosage is normally increased over a period of time to help prevent adverse reactions.

Don't take with:
Any other medicine or any dietary supplement without consulting your doctor or pharmacist.

POSSIBLE ADVERSE REACTIONS OR SIDE EFFECTS

SYMPTOMS	WHAT TO DO
Life-threatening: In case of overdose, see previous column.	
Common: Nausea, vomiting, diarrhea, lack of coordination.	Continue. Call doctor when convenient.
Infrequent: Rash, indigestion, headache, muscle aches, loss of appetite, stomach pain, nervousness, chills, dizziness, drowsiness, dry or itching eyes, increased sweating, joint pain, runny nose, sore throat, swelling of feet or legs, insomnia, weight loss, unusual tiredness or weakness, flushing of face.	Continue. Call doctor when convenient.
Rare: Changes in liver function (yellow skin or eyes; black, very dark or light stool color); lack of coordination, convulsions, speech problems, irregular heartbeat, vision changes, increased libido, changes in blood pressure, hot flashes, breathing difficulty.	Continue. Call doctor right away.

WARNINGS & PRECAUTIONS

Don't take if:
You are allergic to cholinesterase inhibitors.

Before you start, consult your doctor if:
- You have heart rhythm problems.
- You have a history of ulcer disease or are at risk of developing ulcers.
- You have a history of liver disease.
- You have a history of urinary tract problems.
- You have epilepsy or seizure disorder.
- You have a history of asthma.
- You have had a head injury with loss of consciousness.
- You have had previous treatment with any cholinesterase inhibitor that caused jaundice (yellow skin and eyes) or elevated bilirubin.

Over age 60:
No problems expected.

Pregnancy:
Unknown effect. Drug is usually not prescribed for women of childbearing age. Risk category C (see page xviii).

Breast-feeding:
Unknown effect. Not recommended for women of childbearing age.

Infants & children:
Not used in this age group.

Prolonged use:
- Drug may lose its effectiveness.
- Talk to your doctor about the need for follow-up medical examinations or laboratory studies to check blood chemistries and liver function.

Skin & sunlight:
No problems expected.

Driving, piloting or hazardous work:
Don't drive or pilot aircraft until you learn how medicine affects you. Don't work around dangerous machinery. Don't climb ladders or work in high places. Danger increases if you drink alcohol or take other medicines affecting alertness and reflexes such as antihistamines, tranquilizers, sedatives, pain medicine, narcotics and mind-altering drugs.

Discontinuing:
Do not discontinue drug unless advised by doctor. Abrupt decreases in dosage may cause a cognitive decline.

Others:
- Advise any doctor or dentist whom you consult that you take this medicine.
- May affect the results in some medical tests.
- Do not increase dosage without doctor's approval.
- Treatment may need to be discontinued or the dosage lowered if weekly blood tests indicate a sensitivity to the drug or liver toxicity develops.

POSSIBLE INTERACTION WITH OTHER DRUGS

GENERIC NAME OR DRUG CLASS	COMBINED EFFECT
Anticholinergics*	Decreased anticholinergic effect.
Anti-inflammatories, nonsteroidal (NSAIDs)	May increase gastric acid secretions.
Enzyme inducers*	May decrease effect of cholinesterase inhibitor.
Ketoconazole	May interact, but effect unknown.
Quinidine	May interact, but effect unknown.
Theophylline	Increased theophylline effect or toxicity.

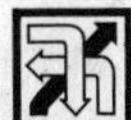

POSSIBLE INTERACTION WITH OTHER SUBSTANCES

INTERACTS WITH	COMBINED EFFECT
Alcohol:	None expected.
Beverages:	None expected.
Cocaine:	None expected.
Foods:	None expected.
Marijuana:	None expected.
Tobacco:	None expected.

*See Glossary

CINOXACIN

BRAND NAMES

Cinobac

BASIC INFORMATION

Habit forming? No
Prescription needed? Yes
Available as generic? Yes
Drug class: Anti-infective (urinary)

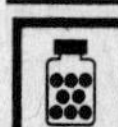

USES

Treatment for urinary tract infections.

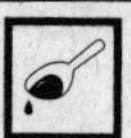

DOSAGE & USAGE INFORMATION

How to take:
Capsule—Swallow with liquid. May be taken with or without food, but be consistent and take it the same way each day.

When to take:
At the same times each day.

If you forget a dose:
Take as soon as you remember. If it is almost time for the next dose, wait for the next scheduled dose (don't double this dose).

What drug does:
Destroys bacteria susceptible to cinoxacin.

Time lapse before drug works:
1 to 2 weeks.

Don't take with:
Any other medicine or any dietary supplement without consulting your doctor or pharmacist.

OVERDOSE

SYMPTOMS:
Lethargy, stomach upset, behavioral changes, convulsions and stupor.
WHAT TO DO:

- **Dial 911 (emergency) for medical help or call poison control center 1-800-222-1222 for instructions.**
- **If person is unconscious, check breathing and pulse. If not breathing, begin mouth-to-mouth rescue breathing. If heart is not beating, begin chest compressions.**
- **See emergency information on last 3 pages of this book.**

POSSIBLE ADVERSE REACTIONS OR SIDE EFFECTS

SYMPTOMS	WHAT TO DO
Life-threatening:	
Hives, rash, intense itching, faintness soon after a dose (anaphylaxis).	Seek emergency treatment immediately.
Common:	
Rash; itch; decreased, blurred or double vision; halos around lights or excess brightness; changes in color vision; nausea; vomiting; diarrhea.	Discontinue. Call doctor right away.
Infrequent:	
Dizziness, drowsiness, headache, ringing in ears, insomnia, appetite loss.	Continue. Call doctor when convenient.
Rare:	
Severe stomach pain, seizures, psychosis, joint pain, numbness or tingling in hands or feet (infants and children).	Discontinue. Call doctor right away.

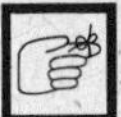

WARNINGS & PRECAUTIONS

Don't take if:
- You are allergic to cinoxacin or nalidixic acid.
- You have a seizure disorder (epilepsy, convulsions).

Before you start, consult your doctor if:
- You plan to become pregnant during medication period.
- You have or have had kidney or liver disease.
- You have impaired circulation to the brain (hardened arteries).

Over age 60:
Adverse reactions and side effects may be more frequent and severe than in younger persons.

Pregnancy:
Decide with your doctor if drug benefits justify risk to unborn child. Risk category C (see page xviii).

Breast-feeding:
Unknown effect. Avoid drug or discontinue nursing until you finish medicine. Consult doctor for advice on maintaining milk supply.

Infants & children:
Give only under close medical supervision.

Prolonged use:
Talk to your doctor about the need for follow-up medical examinations or laboratory studies to check kidney function, liver function.

Skin & sunlight:
No special problems expected.

Driving, piloting or hazardous work:
Avoid if you feel drowsy, dizzy or have vision problems. Otherwise, no problems expected.

Discontinuing:
Don't discontinue without consulting doctor. Dose may require gradual reduction if you have taken drug for a long time. Doses of other drugs may also require adjustment.

Others:
- May interfere with the accuracy of some medical tests.
- Advise any doctor or dentist whom you consult that you take this medicine.

POSSIBLE INTERACTION WITH OTHER DRUGS

GENERIC NAME OR DRUG CLASS	COMBINED EFFECT
Probenecid	Decreased cinoxacin effect.

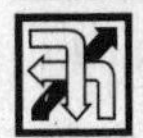

POSSIBLE INTERACTION WITH OTHER SUBSTANCES

INTERACTS WITH	COMBINED EFFECT
Alcohol:	Impaired alertness, judgment and coordination.
Beverages:	None expected.
Cocaine:	Impaired judgment and coordination.
Foods:	None expected.
Marijuana:	Impaired alertness, judgment and coordination.
Tobacco:	None expected.

*See Glossary

CITRATES

GENERIC AND BRAND NAMES

POTASSIUM CITRATE
Citra Forte
Urocit-K
POTASSIUM CITRATE & CITRIC ACID
Polycitra-K
POTASSIUM CITRATE & SODIUM CITRATE
Citrolith
SODIUM CITRATE & CITRIC ACID
Albright's Solution
Bicitra
Modified Shohl's Solution
Oracit
Tussirex with Codeine Liquid
TRICITRATES
Polycitra
Polycitra LC

BASIC INFORMATION

Habit forming? No
Prescription needed? Yes
Available as generic? No
Drug class: Urinary alkalizer, antiurolithic

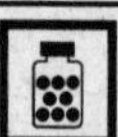

USES

- To make urine more alkaline (less acid).
- To treat or prevent recurrence of some types of kidney stones.

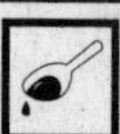

DOSAGE & USAGE INFORMATION

How to take:
- Tablet—Take right after a meal or with a bedtime snack. Swallow tablet whole (do not crush or chew). Take with a full glass of water.
- Solution—Dilute with 6 ounces of water or juice and drink all of the mixture.
- Crystals—Stir into 6 ounces of water or juice and drink all of the mixture.

When to take:
On full stomach, usually after meals or with food.

Continued next column

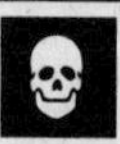

OVERDOSE

SYMPTOMS:
Listlessness, weakness, confusion, tingling in arms or legs, irregular heartbeat, chest pain.
WHAT TO DO:
- **Dial 911 (emergency) for medical help or call poison control center 1-800-222-1222 for instructions.**
- **See emergency information on last 3 pages of this book.**

If you forget a dose:
Take as soon as you remember. If it is almost time for the next dose, skip the missed dose and wait for your next scheduled dose (don't double this dose).

What drug does:
Increases urinary alkalinity by excretion of bicarbonate ions.

Time lapse before drug works:
1 hour.

Don't take with:
Any other medicine or any dietary supplement without consulting your doctor or pharmacist.

POSSIBLE ADVERSE REACTIONS OR SIDE EFFECTS

SYMPTOMS	WHAT TO DO
Life-threatening:	
None expected.	
Common:	
Nausea or mild vomiting, diarrhea, mild stomach cramps.	Continue. Call doctor when convenient.
Infrequent:	
None expected.	
Rare:	
• Black or tarry stools, vomiting (may be bloody), severe stomach cramps.	Discontinue. Seek emergency. treatment.
• Confusion, dizziness, swollen feet and ankles, irritability, depression, muscle pain, nervousness, numbness or tingling in hands or feet, unpleasant taste, unusual weakness or tiredness.	Discontinue. Call doctor right away.

WARNINGS & PRECAUTIONS

Don't take if:
You are allergic to any citrate.

Before you start, consult your doctor if:
You have any disease involving the adrenal glands, diabetes, chronic diarrhea, heart problems, hypertension, kidney disease, stomach ulcer or gastritis, urinary tract infection, intestinal or esophageal blockage or toxemia of pregnancy.

Over age 60:
Adverse reactions and side effects may be more frequent and severe than in younger persons. Ask doctor about smaller doses.

Pregnancy:
Avoid if possible. Consult doctor. Risk category C (see page xviii).

Breast-feeding:
Drug passes into milk. Avoid drug or discontinue nursing until you finish medicine. Consult doctor for advice on maintaining milk supply.

Infants & children:
Use only under close medical supervision.

Prolonged use:
- Adverse reactions more likely.
- Talk to your doctor about the need for follow-up medical examinations or laboratory studies.

Skin & sunlight:
No problems expected.

Driving, piloting or hazardous work:
Don't drive or pilot aircraft until you learn how medicine affects you. Don't work around dangerous machinery. Don't climb ladders or work in high places. Danger increases if you drink alcohol or take medicine affecting alertness and reflexes, such as antihistamines, tranquilizers, sedatives, pain medicine, narcotics and mind-altering drugs.

Discontinuing:
Don't discontinue without consulting doctor. Dose may require gradual reduction if you have taken drug for a long time. Doses of other drugs may also require adjustment.

Others:
- Liquid may be chilled (don't freeze) to improve taste.
- Advise any doctor or dentist whom you consult that you take this medicine.
- Monitor potassium in blood with frequent laboratory studies.

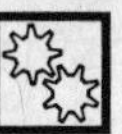

POSSIBLE INTERACTION WITH OTHER DRUGS

GENERIC NAME OR DRUG CLASS	COMBINED EFFECT
Antacids*	Increased risk of side effects.
Angiotensin-converting enzyme (ACE) inhibitors*	Increased risk of side effects.
Anti-inflammatories, nonsteroidal (NSAIDs)	Increased risk of side effects.
Digitalis preparations*	Increased risk of too much potassium in blood.
Diuretics, potassium sparing*	Increased risk of too much potassium in blood.
Methenamine	Decreased effects of methenamine.
Potassium supplements	Increased risk of too much potassium in blood.
Pseudoephedrine	Urinary retention. Increased effect of pseudoephedrine.
Quinidine	Prolonged quinidine effect.

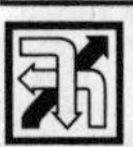

POSSIBLE INTERACTION WITH OTHER SUBSTANCES

INTERACTS WITH	COMBINED EFFECT
Alcohol:	Decreased alertness.
Beverages: Salt-free milk.	Increased risk of side effects.
Cocaine:	None expected.
Foods: Salt substitutes, low salt foods.	Increased risk of side effects.
Marijuana:	None expected.
Tobacco:	Increased risk of stomach irritation.

CLIDINIUM

BRAND NAMES

Apo-Chlorax
Clindex
Clinoxide
Corium
Librax
Lidox
Lodoxide
Quarzan
Zebrax

BASIC INFORMATION

Habit forming? No
Prescription needed?
Low strength: No
High strength: Yes
Available as generic? No
Drug class: Antispasmodic, anticholinergic

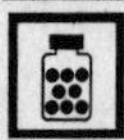

USES

Reduces spasms of digestive system, bladder and urethra.

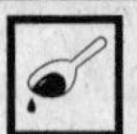

DOSAGE & USAGE INFORMATION

How to take:
Capsule—Swallow with liquid or food to lessen stomach irritation.

When to take:
30 minutes before meals (unless directed otherwise by doctor).

If you forget a dose:
Take as soon as you remember. If it is almost time for the next dose, wait for the next scheduled dose (don't double this dose).

What drug does:
Blocks nerve impulses at parasympathetic nerve endings, preventing muscle contractions and gland secretions of organs involved.

Time lapse before drug works:
15 to 30 minutes.

Continued next column

OVERDOSE

SYMPTOMS:
Dilated pupils, rapid pulse and breathing, dizziness, fever, hallucinations, confusion, slurred speech, agitation, flushed face, convulsions, coma.
WHAT TO DO:
- **Dial 911 (emergency) for medical help or call poison control center 1-800-222-1222 for instructions.**
- **See emergency information on last 3 pages of this book.**

Don't take with:
Any other medicine or any dietary supplement without consulting your doctor or pharmacist.

POSSIBLE ADVERSE REACTIONS OR SIDE EFFECTS

SYMPTOMS	WHAT TO DO
Life-threatening:	
In case of overdose, see previous column.	
Common:	
• Confusion, delirium, rapid heartbeat.	Discontinue. Call doctor right away.
• Nausea, vomiting, decreased sweating.	Continue. Call doctor when convenient.
• Constipation.	Continue. Tell doctor at next visit.
• Dryness in ears, nose, throat, mouth.	No action necessary.
Infrequent:	
• Lightheadedness.	Discontinue. Call doctor right away.
• Nasal congestion, altered taste, difficult urination, headache, impotence.	Continue. Call doctor when convenient.
Rare:	
Rash or hives, eye pain, blurred vision.	Discontinue. Call doctor right away.

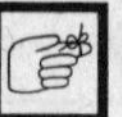

WARNINGS & PRECAUTIONS

Don't take if:
- You are allergic to any anticholinergic.
- You have trouble with stomach bloating.
- You have difficulty emptying your bladder completely (enlarged prostate).
- You have narrow-angle glaucoma.
- You have severe ulcerative colitis.

Before you start, consult your doctor if:
- You have open-angle glaucoma.
- You have angina, chronic bronchitis or asthma, kidney or thyroid disease, hiatal hernia, liver disease, enlarged prostate, myasthenia gravis, peptic ulcer.
- You will have surgery within 2 months, including dental surgery, requiring general or spinal anesthesia.

Over age 60:
Adverse reactions and side effects may be more frequent and severe than in younger persons.

Pregnancy:
Decide with your doctor whether drug benefits justify risk to unborn child. Risk category C (see page xviii).

Breast-feeding:
Drug passes into milk and decreases milk flow. Avoid drug or discontinue nursing until you finish medicine. Consult doctor for advice on maintaining milk supply.

Infants & children:
Use only under medical supervision.

Prolonged use:
Chronic constipation, possible fecal impaction. Consult doctor immediately.

Skin & sunlight:
No problems expected.

Driving, piloting or hazardous work:
Don't drive or pilot aircraft until you learn how medicine affects you. Don't work around dangerous machinery. Don't climb ladders or work in high places. Danger increases if you drink alcohol or take medicine affecting alertness and reflexes, such as antihistamines, tranquilizers, sedatives, pain medicine, narcotics, or mind-altering drugs.

Discontinuing:
May be unnecessary to finish medicine. Follow doctor's instructions.

Others:
Advise any doctor or dentist whom you consult that you take this medicine.

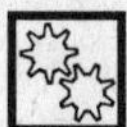

POSSIBLE INTERACTION WITH OTHER DRUGS

GENERIC NAME OR DRUG CLASS	COMBINED EFFECT
Amantadine	Increased clidinium effect.
Antacids*	Decreased clidinium effect.
Anticholinergics, other*	Increased clidinium effect.
Antidepressants, tricyclic*	Increased clidinium effect. Increased sedation.
Antidiarrheals*	Increased clidinium effect.
Antihistamines*	Increased clidinium effect.
Attapulgite	Decreased clidinium effect.
Haloperidol	Increased internal eye pressure.
Ketoconazole	Decreased ketoconazole effect.
Meperidine	Increased clidinium effect.
Methylphenidate	Increased clidinium effect.
Molindone	Increased anticholinergic effect.
Monoamine oxidase (MAO) inhibitors*	Increased clidinium effect.
Nitrates*	Increased internal eye pressure.
Nizatidine	Increased nizatidine effect.
Orphenadrine	Increased clidinium effect.
Pilocarpine	Loss of pilocarpine effect in glaucoma treatment.
Potassium supplements*	Possible intestinal ulcers with oral potassium tablets.
Tranquilizers*	Increased clidinium effect.
Vitamin C	Decreased clidinium effect. Avoid large doses of vitamin C.

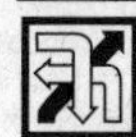

POSSIBLE INTERACTION WITH OTHER SUBSTANCES

INTERACTS WITH	COMBINED EFFECT
Alcohol:	None expected.
Beverages:	None expected.
Cocaine:	Excessively rapid heartbeat. Avoid.
Foods:	None expected.
Marijuana:	Drowsiness and dry mouth.
Tobacco:	None expected.

*See Glossary

CLINDAMYCIN

BRAND NAMES

Cleocin
Cleocin Pediatric
Cleocin (Vaginal)
Clindesse Vaginal Cream
Dalacin C
Dalacin C Palmitate
Dalacin C Phosphate

BASIC INFORMATION

Habit forming? No
Prescription needed? Yes
Available as generic? Yes
Drug class: Antibacterial

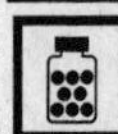

USES

Treatment of bacterial infections that are susceptible to clindamycin.

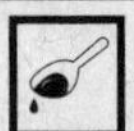

DOSAGE & USAGE INFORMATION

How to take:

- Capsule or liquid—Swallow with liquid. Take with a full glass of water or a meal to avoid gastric irritation.
- Vaginal cream—Use applicator supplied with product to insert cream into vagina. Wash hands immediately after using.

When to take:

- Oral—At the same times each day.
- Vaginal cream—Apply at bedtime unless directed differently by your doctor.

If you forget a dose:
Take as soon as you remember. If it is almost time for the next dose, wait for the next scheduled dose (don't double this dose).

What drug does:
Destroys susceptible bacteria. Does not kill viruses.

Time lapse before drug works:
3 to 5 days.

Continued next column

OVERDOSE

SYMPTOMS:
Severe nausea, vomiting, diarrhea.
WHAT TO DO:
Overdose unlikely to threaten life. If person uses much larger amount than prescribed or if accidentally swallowed, call doctor or poison control center 1-800-222-1222 for help.

Don't take with:
Any other medicine or any dietary supplement without consulting your doctor or pharmacist.

POSSIBLE ADVERSE REACTIONS OR SIDE EFFECTS

SYMPTOMS	WHAT TO DO
Life-threatening:	
Hives, wheezing, faintness, itching, coma.	Seek emergency treatment immediately.
Common:	
Bloating.	Discontinue. Call doctor right away.
Infrequent:	
• Unusual thirst; vomiting; stomach cramps; severe and watery diarrhea with blood or mucus; painful, swollen joints; fever; jaundice; tiredness; weakness.	Discontinue. Call doctor right away.
• White patches in mouth; rash, itch around groin, rectum or armpits; vaginal discharge; dizziness; nausea; mild diarrhea; pain during intercourse.	Continue. Call doctor when convenient.
Rare:	
None expected.	

WARNINGS & PRECAUTIONS

Don't take if:
- You are allergic to lincomycins, clindamycin or doxorubicin.
- You have had ulcerative colitis.

Before you start, consult your doctor if:
- You have had yeast infections of mouth, skin or vagina.
- You will have surgery within 2 months, including dental surgery, requiring general or spinal anesthesia.
- You have kidney or liver disease.
- You have allergies of any kind.
- You have a history of gastrointestinal disorders.

Over age 60:
Adverse reactions and side effects may be more frequent and severe than in younger persons.

Pregnancy:
Decide with your doctor if drug benefits justify risk to unborn child. Risk category B (see page xviii).

Breast-feeding:
Drug passes into milk. Avoid drug or discontinue nursing until you finish medicine. Consult doctor for advice on maintaining milk supply.

Infants & children:
Don't give to infants younger than 1 month. Use for children only under medical supervision.

Prolonged use:
- Severe colitis with diarrhea and bleeding.
- You may become more susceptible to infections caused by germs not responsive to clindamycin.
- Talk to your doctor about the need for follow-up medical examinations or laboratory studies to check stools and perform proctosigmoidoscopy.

Skin & sunlight:
No problems expected.

Driving, piloting or hazardous work:
No problems expected.

Discontinuing:
- Don't discontinue without doctor's advice until you complete prescribed dose, even though symptoms diminish or disappear.
- If vaginal discharge, itching or pain occurs after discontinuing medicine, consult doctor.

Others:
- May interfere with the accuracy of some medical tests. Advise any doctor or dentist whom you consult that you take this medicine.
- Vaginal cream product may decrease the effectiveness of condoms, cervical caps or diaphragms. Wait 72 hours after treatment to use any of these devices.

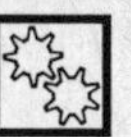

POSSIBLE INTERACTION WITH OTHER DRUGS

GENERIC NAME OR DRUG CLASS	COMBINED EFFECT
Antidiarrheal preparations*	Decreased clindamycin effect.
Antimyasthenics*	Decreased antimyasthenic effect.
Chloramphenicol	Decreased clindamycin effect.
Erythromycins*	Decreased clindamycin effect.
Muscle relaxants*	Increased actions of muscle blockers to unsafe degree. Avoid.
Narcotics*	Increased risk of respiratory problems.

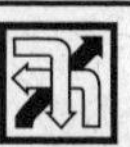

POSSIBLE INTERACTION WITH OTHER SUBSTANCES

INTERACTS WITH	COMBINED EFFECT
Alcohol:	None expected.
Beverages:	None expected.
Cocaine:	None expected.
Foods:	None expected.
Marijuana:	None expected.
Tobacco:	None expected.

*See Glossary

CLOMIPHENE

BRAND NAMES

Clomid
Milophene
Serophene

BASIC INFORMATION

Habit forming? No
Prescription needed? Yes
Available as generic? Yes
Drug class: Gonad stimulant

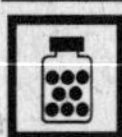

USES

- Treatment for men with low sperm counts.
- Treatment for ovulatory failure in women who wish to become pregnant.

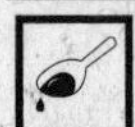

DOSAGE & USAGE INFORMATION

How to take:
Tablet—Swallow with liquid.

When to take:
- Men—Take at the same time each day.
- Women—Follow your doctor's instructions.

If you forget a dose:
Take as soon as you remember. If you forget a day, double next dose. If you miss 2 or more doses, consult doctor.

What drug does:
Antiestrogen effect stimulates ovulation and sperm production.

Time lapse before drug works:
Usually 3 to 6 months. Ovulation may occur 6 to 10 days after last day of treatment in any cycle.

Don't take with:
Any other medicine or any dietary supplement without consulting your doctor or pharmacist.

OVERDOSE

SYMPTOMS:
Increased severity of adverse reactions and side effects.
WHAT TO DO:
Overdose unlikely to threaten life. If person uses much larger amount than prescribed or if accidentally swallowed, call doctor or poison control center 1-800-222-1222 for help.

POSSIBLE ADVERSE REACTIONS OR SIDE EFFECTS

SYMPTOMS	WHAT TO DO
Life-threatening:	
Sudden shortness of breath.	Seek emergency treatment.
Common:	
• Bloating, abdominal pain, pelvic pain.	Discontinue. Call doctor right away.
• Hot flashes.	Continue. Tell doctor at next visit.
Infrequent:	
• Rash, itch, vomiting, jaundice.	Discontinue. Call doctor right away.
• Constipation, diarrhea, increased appetite, heavy menstrual flow, frequent urination, breast discomfort, weight change, hair loss, nausea, eyes sensitive to light.	Continue. Call doctor when convenient.
Rare:	
• Vision changes.	Discontinue. Call doctor right away.
• Dizziness, headache, tiredness, depression, nervousness.	Continue. Call doctor when convenient.

WARNINGS & PRECAUTIONS

Don't take if:
You are allergic to clomiphene.

Before you start, consult your doctor if:
- You have an ovarian cyst, fibroid uterine tumors or unusual vaginal bleeding.
- You have inflamed veins caused by blood clots.
- You have liver disease.
- You are depressed.

Over age 60:
Not recommended.

Pregnancy:
Stop taking at first sign of pregnancy. Consult doctor. Risk category C (see page xviii).

Breast-feeding:
Not used.

Infants & children:
Not used.

Prolonged use:
- Not recommended.
- Talk to your doctor about the need for follow-up medical examinations or laboratory studies to check basal body temperature, endometrial biopsy, kidney function, eyes.

Skin & sunlight:
No special problems expected.

Driving, piloting or hazardous work:
- Avoid if you feel dizzy.
- May cause blurred vision.

Discontinuing:
May be unnecessary to finish medicine. Follow doctor's instructions.

Others:
- Have a complete pelvic examination before treatment.
- Advise any doctor or dentist whom you consult that you take this medicine.
- If you become pregnant, twins or triplets are possible.

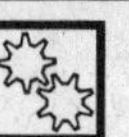

POSSIBLE INTERACTION WITH OTHER DRUGS

GENERIC NAME OR DRUG CLASS	COMBINED EFFECT
Thyroglobulin	May increase serum thyroglobulin.
Thyroxine (T-4)	May increase serum thyroxine.

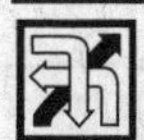

POSSIBLE INTERACTION WITH OTHER SUBSTANCES

INTERACTS WITH	COMBINED EFFECT
Alcohol:	None expected.
Beverages:	None expected.
Cocaine:	None expected.
Foods:	None expected.
Marijuana:	None expected.
Tobacco:	None expected.

CLOTRIMAZOLE (Oral-Local)

BRAND NAMES

Mycelex Troches

BASIC INFORMATION

Habit forming? No
Prescription needed? Yes
Available as generic? Yes
Drug class: Antifungal

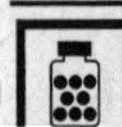

USES

- Treats thrush, white mouth (candidiasis).
- Used primarily in immunosuppressed patients to treat and prevent mouth infection.

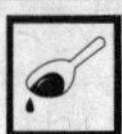

DOSAGE & USAGE INFORMATION

How to take:
Lozenge—Dissolve slowly and completely in the mouth, 5 times a day (usually for 14 days or longer). Swallow saliva during this time. Don't swallow lozenge whole and don't chew.

When to take:
At the same times each day.

If you forget a dose:
Take as soon as you remember. If it is almost time for the next dose, wait for the next scheduled dose (don't double this dose).

What drug does:
Kills fungus by interfering with cell wall membrane and its permeability.

Time lapse before drug works:
1 to 3 hours.

Don't take with:
Any other medicine for your mouth without consulting your doctor or pharmacist.

OVERDOSE

SYMPTOMS:
None expected, but if large dose has been taken, follow instructions below.
WHAT TO DO:

- **Dial 911 (emergency) for medical help or call poison control center 1-800-222-1222 for instructions.**
- **See emergency information on last 3 pages of this book.**

POSSIBLE ADVERSE REACTIONS OR SIDE EFFECTS

SYMPTOMS	WHAT TO DO
Life-threatening: None expected.	
Common: None expected.	
Infrequent: Abdominal pain, diarrhea, nausea, vomiting.	Discontinue. Call doctor right away.
Rare: None expected.	

WARNINGS & PRECAUTIONS

Don't take if:
You have severe liver disease.

Before you start, consult your doctor if:
You have had a recent organ transplant.

Over age 60:
Adverse reactions and side effects may be more frequent and severe than in younger persons. You may need smaller doses for shorter periods of time.

Pregnancy:
Decide with your doctor if drug benefits justify risk to unborn child. Risk category C (see page xviii).

Breast-feeding:
Unknown effect. Consult doctor.

Infants & children:
Use only under medical supervision for children younger than 4 or 5 years.

Prolonged use:
No problems expected.

Skin & sunlight:
No problems expected.

Driving, piloting or hazardous work:
No problems expected.

Discontinuing:
Don't discontinue without consulting doctor. Dose may require gradual reduction if you have taken drug for a long time. Doses of other drugs may also require adjustment.

Others:
- Continue for full term of treatment. May require several months.
- Check with physician if not improved in 1 week.

POSSIBLE INTERACTION WITH OTHER DRUGS

GENERIC NAME OR DRUG CLASS	COMBINED EFFECT
None expected.	

POSSIBLE INTERACTION WITH OTHER SUBSTANCES

INTERACTS WITH	COMBINED EFFECT
Alcohol:	Decreased effects of clotrimazole.
Beverages:	None expected.
Cocaine:	Decreased effects of clotrimazole.
Foods:	None expected.
Marijuana:	Decreased effects of clotrimazole.
Tobacco:	Decreased effects of clotrimazole.

CLOZAPINE

BRAND NAMES

Clozaril
FazaClo
Leponex
Versacloz

BASIC INFORMATION

Habit forming? No
Prescription needed? Yes, prescribed only through a special program.
Available as generic? Yes
Drug class: Antipsychotic

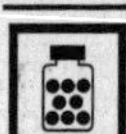

USES

- Treats severe schizophrenia in patients not helped by other medicines.
- Reduces the risk of recurrent suicide behavior in patients with schizophrenia or schizoaffective disorder.

DOSAGE & USAGE INFORMATION

How to take:
- Tablet—Swallow with liquid. If you can't swallow whole, crumble tablet and take with liquid or food.
- Orally disintegrating tablet—Let tablet dissolve in your mouth. Don't chew or swallow it whole.
- Oral suspension—Carefully follow the instructions provided with the prescription.

When to take:
Once or twice daily as directed.

If you forget a dose:
Take as soon as you remember. If it is almost time for the next dose, wait for the next scheduled dose (don't double this dose).

What drug does:
Interferes with binding of dopamine. May produce significant improvement, but may at times also make schizophrenia worse.

Continued next column

OVERDOSE

SYMPTOMS:
Heartbeat fast, slow, irregular; hallucinations; restlessness; excitement; drowsiness; breathing difficulty.
WHAT TO DO:
- **Dial 911 (emergency) for medical help or call poison control center 1-800-222-1222 for instructions.**
- **See emergency information on last 3 pages of this book.**

Time lapse before drug works:
Weeks to months before improvement is evident. Your doctor may increase the dosage to obtain optimal effectiveness.

Don't take with:
Any other medicine or any dietary supplement without consulting your doctor or pharmacist.

POSSIBLE ADVERSE REACTIONS OR SIDE EFFECTS

SYMPTOMS	WHAT TO DO
Life-threatening:	
High fever, rapid pulse, profuse sweating, muscle rigidity, confusion and irritability, seizures, fever, chills, mouth sores.	Discontinue. Seek emergency treatment.
Common:	
Dry mouth, blurred vision, constipation, difficulty urinating, sedation, low blood pressure, dizziness.	Continue. Call doctor when convenient.
Infrequent:	
None expected.	
Rare:	
• Jerky or involuntary movements (especially of the face, lips, jaw, tongue); slow-frequency tremor of head or limbs, (especially while moving); muscle rigidity, lack of facial expression and slow inflexible movements; seizures; high blood sugar (thirstiness, frequent urination, increased hunger, weakness).	Discontinue. Call doctor right away.
• Pacing or restlessness (akathisia), intermittent spasms (of muscles of face, eyes, tongue, jaw, neck, body or limbs).	Continue. Call doctor when convenient.

WARNINGS & PRECAUTIONS

Don't take if:
You are allergic to clozapine.

Before you start, consult your doctor if:
- You are significantly mentally depressed.
- You have bone marrow depression.
- You have a family history of, or have diabetes.
- You have glaucoma or an enlarged prostate.
- You have ever had seizures from any cause.
- You have liver, heart or gastrointestinal disease or any type of blood disorder.

Over age 60:
- May be more at risk of weakness or dizziness upon standing after sitting or lying down and of excitement, confusion or urination difficulty.
- Use of antipsychotic drugs in elderly patients with dementia-related psychosis may increase risk of death. Consult doctor.

Pregnancy:
Risk category B (see page xviii).

Breast-feeding:
May cause sedation, restlessness or irritability in the nursing infant. Avoid.

Infants & children:
Safety not established. Consult doctor.

Prolonged use:
Effects unknown.

Skin & sunlight:
No problems expected.

Driving, piloting or hazardous work:
Don't drive or pilot aircraft until you learn how medicine affects you. Don't work around dangerous machinery. Don't climb ladders or work in high places. Danger increases if you drink alcohol or take medicine affecting alertness and reflexes.

Discontinuing:
Don't discontinue without consulting doctor. Dose may require gradual reduction if you have taken drug for a long time. Doses of other drugs may also require adjustment.

Others:
- This medicine is available only through a special management program for monitoring and distributing this drug.
- You will need laboratory studies each week for white blood cell and differential counts.

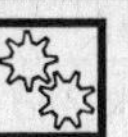

POSSIBLE INTERACTION WITH OTHER DRUGS

GENERIC NAME OR DRUG CLASS	COMBINED EFFECT
Antihypertensives*	Risk of low blood pressure.
Bone marrow depressants*	Toxic bone marrow depression.
Bupropion	Increased risk of seizures.
Carbamazepine	Decreased clozapine effect.
Central nervous system (CNS) depressants*	Toxic effects on the central nervous system.
Fluoxetine	Increased risk of adverse reactions.
Fluvoxamine	Increased risk of adverse reactions.
Haloperidol	Increased risk of seizures.
Lithium	Increased risk of seizures.
Phenytoin	Decreased clozapine effect.
Risperidone	Increased risperidone effect.

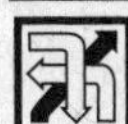

POSSIBLE INTERACTION WITH OTHER SUBSTANCES

INTERACTS WITH	COMBINED EFFECT
Alcohol:	Avoid. Increases toxic effect on the central nervous system.
Beverages: Caffeine drinks.	Excess (more than 3 cups of coffee or equivalent) increases risk of heartbeat irregularities.
Cocaine:	Heartbeat irregularities. Avoid.
Foods:	None expected.
Marijuana:	Heartbeat irregularities. Avoid.
Tobacco:	Decreased effect of clozapine. Avoid.

*See Glossary

COAL TAR (Topical)

BRAND NAMES

See full list of brand names in the *Generic and Brand Name Directory*, page 880.

BASIC INFORMATION

Habit forming? No
Prescription needed? No (for most)
Available as generic? Yes
Drug class: Antiseborrheic, antipsoriatic, keratolytic

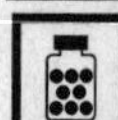

USES

Applied to the skin to treat dandruff, seborrhea, dermatitis, eczema and other skin diseases.

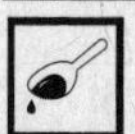

DOSAGE & USAGE INFORMATION

How to use:

- Follow package instructions.
- Don't apply to blistered, oozing, infected or raw skin.
- Keep away from eyes.
- Protect treated area from sunshine for 72 hours.

When to use:
According to package instructions.

If you forget a dose:
Use as soon as you remember.

What drug does:

- Kills bacteria and fungus organisms on contact.
- Suppresses overproduction of skin cells.

Time lapse before drug works:
None. Works immediately. May take several days before maximum effect.

Don't use with:
Any other topical medicine without consulting your doctor or pharmacist.

OVERDOSE

SYMPTOMS:
None expected.
WHAT TO DO:
Overdose unlikely to threaten life. If person uses much larger amount than prescribed or if accidentally swallowed, call doctor or poison control center 1-800-222-1222 for help.

POSSIBLE ADVERSE REACTIONS OR SIDE EFFECTS

SYMPTOMS	WHAT TO DO
Life-threatening:	
None expected.	
Common:	
Skin stinging.	Continue. Call doctor when convenient.
Infrequent:	
Skin more irritated.	Continue. Call doctor when convenient.
Rare:	
Pus forms in lesions on skin.	Continue. Call doctor when convenient.

WARNINGS & PRECAUTIONS

Don't use if:
You have intolerance to coal tar.

Before you start, consult your doctor if:
You have infected skin or open wounds.

Over age 60:
No special problems expected.

Pregnancy:
Consult doctor. Risk category C (see page xviii).

Breast-feeding:
No special problems expected. Consult doctor.

Infants & children:
Don't use on infants.

Prolonged use:
No special problems expected.

Skin & sunlight:
One or more drugs in this group may cause rash or intensify sunburn in areas exposed to sun or ultraviolet light (photosensitivity reaction). Avoid overexposure. Notify doctor if reaction occurs.

Driving, piloting or hazardous work:
No problems expected.

Discontinuing:
No special problems expected.

Others:
- May affect results in some medical tests.
- Protect treated area from direct sunlight for 72 hours.

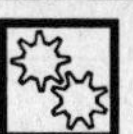

POSSIBLE INTERACTION WITH OTHER DRUGS

GENERIC NAME OR DRUG CLASS	COMBINED EFFECT
Psoralens (methoxsalen, trioxsalen)	Excess sensitivity to sun.

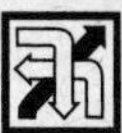

POSSIBLE INTERACTION WITH OTHER SUBSTANCES

INTERACTS WITH	COMBINED EFFECT
Alcohol:	None expected.
Beverages:	None expected.
Cocaine:	None expected.
Foods:	None expected.
Marijuana:	None expected.
Tobacco:	None expected.

COLCHICINE

BRAND NAMES

Colcrys
Col-Probenecid

BASIC INFORMATION

Habit forming? No
Prescription needed? Yes
Available as generic? No
Drug class: Antigout

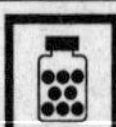

USES

- Used to prevent or treat gout flares.
- Treats familial Mediterranean fever (FMF).
- May be used for dermatitis herpetiformis, calcium pyrophosphate deposition disease, amyloidosis, Paget's disease of bone, recurrent pericarditis, Behcet's syndrome, others.

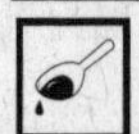

DOSAGE & USAGE INFORMATION

How to take:
Tablet—Swallow with liquid or food to lessen stomach irritation.

When to take:
- For gout prevention, it is usually taken once or twice a day. For gout flares, it is usually taken at first sign of flare and then one hour later. Follow your doctor's advice.
- For other disorders, follow instructions on your prescription label.

If you forget a dose:
If taken daily, take as soon as you remember. If it is almost time for the next dose, wait for the next scheduled dose (don't double this dose).

Continued next column

OVERDOSE

SYMPTOMS:
Bloody urine; severe or bloody diarrhea; burning feeling in the throat, skin or stomach; severe nausea or vomiting; muscle weakness; fever; shortness of breath; stupor; convulsions; coma.

WHAT TO DO:
- **Dial 911 (emergency) for medical help or call poison control center 1-800-222-1222 for instructions.**
- **See emergency information on last 3 pages of this book.**

What drug does:
The exact way it works is unknown. It reduces the inflammatory response and relieves pain caused by gout or familial Mediterranean fever.

Time lapse before drug works:
12 to 24 hours.

Don't take with:
Any other medicine or any dietary supplement without consulting your doctor or pharmacist.

POSSIBLE ADVERSE REACTIONS OR SIDE EFFECTS

SYMPTOMS	WHAT TO DO
Life-threatening:	
Rare allergic reaction (hives, itching, rash, wheezing, tightness in chest, swelling of lips or tongue or throat).	Seek emergency treatment immediately.
Common:	
Diarrhea, nausea, vomiting, abdominal pain.	Discontinue. Call doctor right away.
Infrequent:	
Hair loss with long-term use, appetite loss.	Continue. Call doctor when convenient.
Rare:	
Black or tarry stool, blood in urine, fever, chills, skin symptoms (hives, rash, burning, tingling, peeling, pinpoint red spots, redness), sore throat, muscle weakness or pain, mouth sores, unusual bruising or bleeding, unusual tiredness or weakness, numbness or tingly feeling in fingers or toes, increased infections, pale or gray color of lips or tongue or skin, yellow eyes or skin.	Discontinue. Call doctor right away.

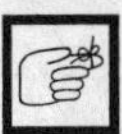

WARNINGS & PRECAUTIONS

Don't take if:
You are allergic to colchicine.

Before you start, consult your doctor if:
- You have stomach problems (e.g., ulcers) or bowel problems (e.g., ulcerative colitis).
- You have heart, liver or kidney disorder.
- You have any blood disorder.
- You have muscle or nerve problems.
- You take herbal or vitamin supplements.
- You drink large amounts of alcohol.

Over age 60:
Increased risk for muscle disorders.

Pregnancy:
Decide with your doctor if drug benefits justify risk to unborn child. Risk category C. (see page xviii).

Breast-feeding:
Drug passes into breast milk. Consult doctor for advice about breast-feeding.

Infants & children:
Used to treat familial Mediterranean fever in children. Follow doctor's instructions.

Prolonged use:
- May increase risk of side effects.
- Talk to your doctor about the need for follow-up medical exams or lab studies.

Skin & sunlight:
No problems expected.

Driving, piloting or hazardous work:
No problems expected.

Discontinuing:
- Follow doctor's instructions.
- Stop taking drug and consult doctor if severe abdominal pain, diarrhea or vomiting occurs.

Others:
- Don't increase dose without medical advice.
- May affect sperm production in males. Consult doctor.
- Advise any doctor or dentist whom you consult that you take this medicine.
- May interfere with the accuracy of some medical tests.

POSSIBLE INTERACTION WITH OTHER DRUGS

GENERIC NAME OR DRUG CLASS	COMBINED EFFECT
Digoxin	Risk of serious muscle disorders—rhabdomyolysis (which can be fatal) or myopathy.
Enzyme inhibitors*	Some enzyme inhibitors increase risk of toxic effect of colchicine (can be fatal). Risk continues 14 days after enzyme inhibitor stopped. Consult doctor or pharmacist.
Fibrates	Risk of serious muscle disorders—rhabdomyolysis (which can be fatal) or myopathy.
Gemfibrozil	Risk of serious muscle disorders—rhabdomyolysis (which can be fatal) or myopathy.
HMG-CoA reductase inhibitors	Risk of serious muscle disorders—rhabdomyolysis (which can be fatal) or myopathy.
P-glycoprotein inhibitors*	Risk of toxic effect of colchicine (can be fatal). Risk continues 14 days after stopping p-glycoprotein inhibitor.
Vitamin B-12	Decreased absorption of vitamin B-12.

POSSIBLE INTERACTION WITH OTHER SUBSTANCES

INTERACTS WITH	COMBINED EFFECT
Alcohol:	Increased risk of gastrointestinal problems. Avoid
Beverages: Grapefruit juice.	Increased colchicine effect. Avoid.
Cocaine:	Unknown effect. Avoid.
Foods: Grapefruit.	Increased colchicine effect. Avoid.
Marijuana:	Unknown effect. Avoid.
Tobacco:	None expected.

*See Glossary

COLESEVELAM

BRAND NAMES

Welchol
Welchol Oral Suspension

BASIC INFORMATION

Habit forming? No
Prescription needed? Yes
Available as generic? No
Drug class: Antihyperlipidemic

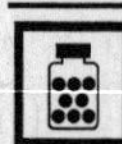

USES

- Reduces low density lipoprotein (LDL) cholesterol. Should be used in addition to diet and exercise.
- Helps lower blood sugar levels in adults with type 2 diabetes.

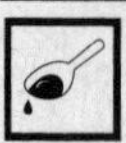

DOSAGE & USAGE INFORMATION

How to take:
- Tablet—Take with food and a full glass of water. If you can't swallow whole, crumble tablet and take with liquid and food.
- Oral suspension—Mix well with 4 to 8 ounces of water. Don't take it in the dry form.

When to take:
As directed by your doctor. Usually once or twice daily with meals.

If you forget a dose:
Take as soon as you remember. If it is almost time for the next dose, wait for the next scheduled dose (don't double this dose).

What drug does:
Attaches to cholesterol and bile fluid in the intestine and passes out of the body without being absorbed.

Time lapse before drug works:
2 to 4 weeks.

Don't take with:
Any other medicine or any dietary supplement without consulting your doctor or pharmacist.

OVERDOSE

SYMPTOMS:
None expected.
WHAT TO DO:
Overdose unlikely to threaten life. If person uses much larger amount than prescribed or if accidentally swallowed, call doctor or poison control center 1-800-222-1222 for help.

POSSIBLE ADVERSE REACTIONS OR SIDE EFFECTS

SYMPTOMS	WHAT TO DO
Life-threatening: None expected.	
Common: Acid or sour stomach, belching, constipation, indigestion, stomach upset or pain.	Continue. Call doctor if condition persists.
Infrequent: Congestion, cough, dry or sore throat, hoarseness, muscle aches or pain, trouble swallowing.	Continue. Call doctor when convenient.
Rare: None expected.	

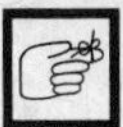

WARNINGS & PRECAUTIONS

Don't take if:
You are allergic to colesevelam.

Before you start, consult your doctor if:
- You have been diagnosed with a bowel obstruction.
- You have had recent gastrointestinal surgery.
- You have had gastrointestinal motility disorders.
- You have a vitamin deficiency.
- You have difficulty swallowing.

Over age 60:
Colesevelam has not been shown to cause different side effects in older adults.

Pregnancy:
Decide with your doctor if drug benefits justify risk to unborn child. Risk category B. (see page xviii).

Breast-feeding:
Drug may pass into milk. Avoid drug or discontinue nursing until you finish medicine. Consult doctor for advice on maintaining milk supply.

Infants & children:
Approved for boys and girls (who have had a menstrual period) ages 10 to 17 years to treat inherited high cholesterol.

Prolonged use:
Talk to your doctor about the need for follow-up medical examinations to determine the effect of colesevelam on your body.

Skin & sunlight:
No problems expected.

Driving, piloting or hazardous work:
No problems expected.

Discontinuing:
Don't discontinue without consulting your doctor.

Others:
- Advise any doctor or dentist whom you consult that you take this medicine.
- May affect the results in some medical tests.

POSSIBLE INTERACTION WITH OTHER DRUGS

GENERIC NAME OR DRUG CLASS	COMBINED EFFECT
Cyclosporine	May affect cyclosporine level. Take 4 hours before colesevelam or as directed.
Glyburide	May affect glyburide level. Take 4 hours before colesevelam or as directed.
Oral contraceptives*	May affect oral contraceptive level. Take 4 hours before colesevelam or as directed.
Phenytoin	May affect phenytoin level. Take 4 hours before colesevelam or as directed.
Thyroid hormones*	May affect thyroid hormone level. Take 4 hours before colesevelam or as directed.
Warfarin	May affect warfarin level. Take 4 hours before colesevelam or as directed.

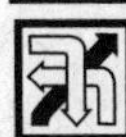

POSSIBLE INTERACTION WITH OTHER SUBSTANCES

INTERACTS WITH	COMBINED EFFECT
Alcohol:	Unknown effect Avoid.
Beverages:	None expected.
Cocaine:	Unknown effect. Avoid.
Foods:	None expected.
Marijuana:	Unknown effect. Avoid.
Tobacco:	None expected.

***See Glossary**

COLESTIPOL

BRAND NAMES

Colestid

BASIC INFORMATION

Habit forming? No
Prescription needed? Yes
Available as generic? Yes
Drug class: Antihyperlipidemic

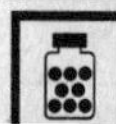

USES

- Reduces cholesterol level in blood in patients with type IIa hyperlipidemia.
- Treats overdose of digitalis.
- Reduces skin itching associated with some forms of liver disease.
- Treats diarrhea after some surgical operations.
- Treatment of one form of colitis (rare).

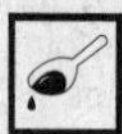

DOSAGE & USAGE INFORMATION

How to take:
Oral suspension—Mix well with 6 ounces or more or water or liquid, or in soups, pulpy fruits, with milk or in cereals. Will not dissolve.

When to take:
- Before meals.
- If taking other medicine, take it 1 hour before or 4 to 6 hours after taking colestipol.

If you forget a dose:
Take as soon as you remember. If it is almost time for the next dose, wait for the next scheduled dose (don't double this dose).

What drug does:
Binds with bile acids in intestines, preventing reabsorption.

Time lapse before drug works:
3 to 12 months.

Don't take with:
Any other medicine or any dietary supplement without consulting your doctor or pharmacist.

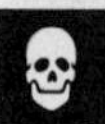

OVERDOSE

SYMPTOMS:
Fecal impaction.
WHAT TO DO:
Overdose unlikely to threaten life. If person uses much larger amount than prescribed or if accidentally swallowed, call doctor or poison control center 1-800-222-1222 for help.

POSSIBLE ADVERSE REACTIONS OR SIDE EFFECTS

SYMPTOMS	WHAT TO DO
Life-threatening: None expected.	
Common: None expected.	
Infrequent:	
• Black, tarry stools from gastrointestinal bleeding.	Discontinue. Seek emergency treatment.
• Severe abdominal pain.	Discontinue. Call doctor right away.
• Constipation, belching, diarrhea, nausea, unexpected weight loss.	Continue. Call doctor when convenient.
Rare: Hives, skin rash, hiccups.	Discontinue. Call doctor right away.

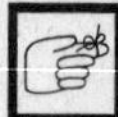

WARNINGS & PRECAUTIONS

Don't take if:
You are allergic to colestipol.

Before you start, consult your doctor if:
- You have liver disease such as cirrhosis.
- You are jaundiced.
- You will have surgery within 2 months, including dental surgery, requiring general or spinal anesthesia.
- You are constipated.
- You have peptic ulcer.
- You have coronary artery disease.

Over age 60:
Constipation more likely. Other adverse effects more likely.

Pregnancy:
Safety not established. Consult doctor. Risk category C (see page xviii).

Breast-feeding:
Unknown if drug passes into milk. Avoid nursing until you finish medicine. Consult doctor for advice on maintaining milk supply.

Infants & children:
Only under expert medical supervision.

Prolonged use:
- Request lab studies to determine serum cholesterol and serum triglycerides.
- May decrease absorption of folic acid.

Skin & sunlight:
No problems expected.

Driving, piloting or hazardous work:
No problems expected.

Discontinuing:
Don't discontinue without consulting doctor. Dose may require gradual reduction if you have taken drug for a long time. Doses of other drugs may also require adjustment, particularly digitalis.

Others:
- This medicine does not cure disorders, but helps to control them.
- May interfere with the accuracy of some medical tests.
- Advise any doctor or dentist whom you consult that you take this drug.

POSSIBLE INTERACTION WITH OTHER DRUGS

GENERIC NAME OR DRUG CLASS	COMBINED EFFECT
Anticoagulants, oral*	Decreased anticoagulant effect.
Beta carotene	Decreased absorption of beta carotene.
Dexfenfluramine	May require dosage change as weight loss occurs.
Dextrothyroxine	Decreased dextrothyroxine effect.
Digitalis preparations*	Decreased absorption of digitalis preparations.
Diuretics, thiazide*	Decreased absorption of thiazide diuretics.
Penicillins*	Decreased absorption of penicillins.
Tetracyclines*	Decreased absorption of tetracyclines.
Thiazides*	Decreased absorption of colestipol.
Thyroid hormones*	Decreased thyroid effect.
Trimethoprim	Decreased absorption of colestipol.
Ursodiol	Decreased absorption of ursodiol.
Vancomycin	Increased chance of hearing loss or kidney damage. Decreased therapeutic effect of vancomycin.
Vitamins	Decreased absorption of fat-soluble vitamins (A,D,E,K).
Other medicines	May delay or reduce absorption.

POSSIBLE INTERACTION WITH OTHER SUBSTANCES

INTERACTS WITH	COMBINED EFFECT
Alcohol:	None expected.
Beverages:	None expected.
Cocaine:	None expected.
Foods:	Interferes with absorption of vitamins. Take supplements.
Marijuana:	None expected.
Tobacco:	None expected.

***See Glossary**

COMT INHIBITORS

GENERIC AND BRAND NAMES

ENTACAPONE
Comtan
Stalevo

TOLCAPONE
Tasmar

BASIC INFORMATION

Habit forming? No
Prescription needed? Yes
Available as generic? Yes (entacapone)
Drug class: Antiparkinsonism

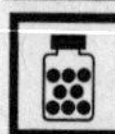

USES

Used in combination with levodopa and carbidopa for the treatment of the symptoms of Parkinson's disease.

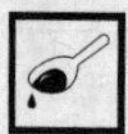

DOSAGE & USAGE INFORMATION

How to take:
Tablet—Swallow whole with water. Do not crush or chew tablet before swallowing. May be taken with or without food.

When to take:
At the same times each day as directed by your doctor.

If you forget a dose:
Take as soon as you remember. If it is almost time for the next dose, wait for the next scheduled dose (don't double this dose).

What drug does:
It inhibits the action of an enzyme called catechol O-methyltransferase (COMT). This action helps prolong the effect of levodopa thereby increasing its effectiveness. The drug has no effect on Parkinson's without taking levodopa.

Time lapse before drug works:
Up to two hours. May take several weeks to get desired effect

Don't take with:
Any other medicine or any dietary supplement without consulting your doctor or pharmacist.

OVERDOSE

SYMPTOMS:
Nausea, vomiting, loose stools and dizziness.
WHAT TO DO:
Overdose unlikely to threaten life. If person takes much larger amount than prescribed or if accidentally swallowed, call doctor or poison control center 1-800-222-1222 for help.

POSSIBLE ADVERSE REACTIONS OR SIDE EFFECTS

SYMPTOMS	WHAT TO DO
Life-threatening:	
Rare allergic reaction (hives, itching, rash, wheezing, tightness in chest, swelling of lips or tongue or throat).	Seek emergency treatment immediately.
Common:	
• Stomach pain, body movements that can't be controlled (new or worsening), nausea or vomiting, twitching, fainting, hyperactivity, headache, diarrhea, hallucinations, sleep problems, feeling dizzy or lightheaded (e.g., when rising after sitting or lying down), drowsiness, infection (cough, fever, runny nose, congestion, sore throat, sneezing).	Continue, but call doctor right away.
• Constipation, fatigue, vivid dreams, excess sweating, dry mouth, muscle cramps.	Continue. Call doctor when convenient.
• Change in urine color to bright yellow or brownish-orange.	No action necessary.
Infrequent:	
• Chest pain, falling, loss of balance control, difficulty breathing, blood in urine, confusion, high fever, lower back or side pain painful or difficult urination, unusual weakness.	Continue, but call doctor right away.
• Heartburn, gas, emotional changes.	Continue. Call doctor when convenient.
Rare:	
• Liver problem (may have yellow skin or eyes, fatigue, light-color stools, appetite loss, dark urine, right-side stomach pain).	Discontinue. Call doctor right away.
• Low blood pressure, muscle stiffness or pain, skin changes, unusual urges (e.g., sexual or gambling), other new symptoms.	Continue, but call doctor right away.

WARNINGS & PRECAUTIONS

Don't take if:
You are allergic to entacapone or tolcapone.

Before you start, consult your doctor if:
- You have any liver problem, alcoholism or have a history of abnormal liver function tests.
- You have kidney problems.
- You have low blood pressure or orthostatic hypotension (lightheadedness or dizziness when rising quickly after sitting or lying down).
- You have uncontrolled muscle movements.
- You suffer from hallucinations.

Over age 60:
May be more at risk for certain side effects such as hallucinations, confusion or drowsiness.

Pregnancy:
Decide with your doctor whether drug benefits justify risk to unborn child. Risk category C (see page xviii).

Breast-feeding:
Drug may pass into breast milk. Consult your doctor for advice.

Infants & children:
Drug is not used in this age group.

Prolonged use:
See your doctor on a regular basis while you take this drug. You may need frequent liver-function blood tests and skin exams.

Skin & sunlight:
No problems expected.

Driving, piloting or hazardous work:
Don't drive or pilot aircraft until you learn how medicine affects you. Don't work around dangerous machinery. Don't climb ladders or work in high places. Danger increases if you drink alcohol or take medicine affecting alertness and reflexes.

Discontinuing:
Don't stop taking drug suddenly. Your doctor may reduce (taper) the dose gradually to avoid withdrawal reaction (e.g., worsening of Parkinson's or fever and confusion). Other drugs you take may require a dosage change.

Others:
- Tolcapone is usually withdrawn if it shows no benefits after 3 weeks of use. Use of this drug may cause severe and fatal liver problems. Ask your doctor about your risks. While taking this drug, consult your doctor if you develop symptoms of liver problems listed under Possible Adverse Reactions or Side Effects.
- Advise any doctor, dentist or pharmacist whom you consult that you take this drug.

POSSIBLE INTERACTION WITH OTHER DRUGS

GENERIC NAME OR DRUG CLASS	COMBINED EFFECT
Apomorphine	Increased risk of side effects.
CNS depressants*	Increased risk of side effects.
Methyldopa	Increased risk of side effects.
Monoamine oxidase (MAO) inhibitors*	Serious adverse effects with some MAO inhibitors. Consult doctor.

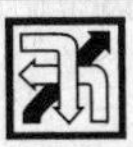

POSSIBLE INTERACTION WITH OTHER SUBSTANCES

INTERACTS WITH	COMBINED EFFECT
Alcohol:	Increased risk of side effects. Avoid.
Beverages:	None expected.
Cocaine:	Increased risk of hallucinations. Avoid.
Foods:	None expected.
Marijuana:	Increased risk of hallucinations. Avoid.
Tobacco:	None expected.

***See Glossary**

CONDYLOMA ACUMINATUM AGENTS

GENERIC AND BRAND NAMES

IMIQUIMOD	PODOFILOX
Aldara	Condylox
Zyclara	PODOPHYLLUM
	Podofin

BASIC INFORMATION

Habit forming? No
Prescription needed? Yes
Available as generic? Yes, for some
Drug class: Cytotoxic (topical)

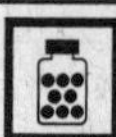

USES

- Treatment for *condylomata acuminata*—external genital and perianal warts.
- Treatment of superficial basal cell carcinoma.
- Treatment for actinic keratoses.
- May be used for other skin disorders as prescribed by your doctor.

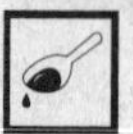

DOSAGE & USAGE INFORMATION

How to use:
For all treatments—Always follow instructions provided with prescription. Wash hands before and after applying medicine. Let the solution dry before allowing other skin surfaces to touch the treated area.

- Imiquimod—Apply a thin film of cream to the wart and rub in well. Leave cream on the treated skin 6 to 10 hours, then wash with soap and water.

Continued next column

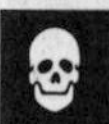

OVERDOSE

SYMPTOMS:
- **Imiquimod: Overdose unlikely. It may increase adverse skin reactions.**
- **Podofilox or podophyllum: The following symptoms may occur when the body absorbs too much—painful urination, breathing difficulty, dizziness, severe nausea or vomiting, fever, heartbeat irregularity, numbness and tingling of hands and feet, abdominal pain, excitement, irritability, seizures, coma.**

WHAT TO DO:
- **Dial 911 (emergency) for medical help or call poison control center 1-800-222-1222 for instructions.**
- **See emergency information on last 3 pages of this book.**

- Podofilox—Apply drug to warts with cotton applicator (supplied with drug). Allow drug to remain on warts for 1 to 6 hours, then remove with soap and water.
- Podophyllum—Apply petroleum jelly on normal skin surrounding warts. With a glass applicator or cotton swab, carefully apply podophyllum to the warts. Allow drug to remain on warts for 1 to 6 hours after application, then remove with soap and water.

When to use:
- Imiquimod cream—Once every other day 3 times a week. Apply at bedtime for up to 16 weeks.
- Podofilox topical solution—Apply twice a day (12 hours apart) for 3 consecutive days, then discontinue use for 4 consecutive days. May repeat this cycle of treatment 4 times (4 weeks).
- Podophyllum topical solution—Once at 1 week intervals for up to 6 weeks.

If you forget a dose:
Apply it as soon as you remember, then return to regular schedule.

What drug does:
Kills cells and erodes tissue.

Time lapse before drug works:
Several weeks.

Don't use with:
Any other topical medicine without consulting your doctor or pharmacist.

POSSIBLE ADVERSE REACTIONS OR SIDE EFFECTS

SYMPTOMS	WHAT TO DO
Life-threatening:	
In case of overdose, see previous column.	
Common:	
Mild skin reactions (slight stinging, mild redness, tenderness or slight swelling in treated area).	No action necessary. If they continue, call doctor.
Infrequent:	
Skin rash, burning, red skin, severe skin reaction. If too much of drug absorbed into body: hallucinations, diarrhea, nausea and vomiting, unusual bleeding, fever, muscle pain, flu-like symptoms.	Discontinue. Call doctor right away.
Rare:	
Lightening of normal skin at application site.	Continue. Call doctor when convenient.

WARNINGS & PRECAUTIONS

Don't use if:
- Warts are crumbled and bleeding.
- If warts have just been biopsied or had other surgery performed on them.
- If you are allergic to condyloma acuminatum agents.

Before you start, consult your doctor if:
You have used one of these drugs previously and have a new outbreak of warts.

Over age 60:
No special problems expected.

Pregnancy:
Consult doctor. Pregnancy risk factor not designated for podophyllum. Imiquimod is risk category B and podofilox is risk category C. See category list on page xviii.

Breast-feeding:
It is not known if drugs pass into milk. Avoid drugs or discontinue nursing until you finish medicine. Consult doctor for advice on maintaining milk supply.

Infants & children:
Efficacy and safety have not been established for all these drugs. Imiquimod is approved for patients 12 and over.

Prolonged use:
Increased risk of adverse reactions.

Skin & sunlight:
No problems expected.

Driving, piloting or hazardous work:
No problems expected.

Discontinuing:
No problems expected. Discontinue medicine once warts are healed.

Others:
- Advise any doctor whom you consult that you are using this medicine.
- Keep medicine away from unaffected skin, eyes, nose and mouth. Wash hands before and after using.
- Don't bandage or cover the treated warts with material that is occlusive. If covering is needed, use cotton gauze or cotton underwear.
- Don't use medicine on moles or birthmarks.
- Don't use near heat or open flame.
- Do not apply more of the medicine than prescribed. It will increase risk of side effects.
- Avoid sexual contact while medicine is on the warts.
- Imiquimod may weaken contraceptive devices such as cervical caps, condoms and diaphragms and reduce their contraceptive effect.
- Recurrence of genital warts is common after treatment.

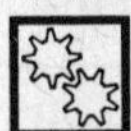

POSSIBLE INTERACTION WITH OTHER DRUGS

GENERIC NAME OR DRUG CLASS	COMBINED EFFECT
Other topical medicines used in same skin area.	Increases risk of side effects. Avoid.

POSSIBLE INTERACTION WITH OTHER SUBSTANCES

INTERACTS WITH	COMBINED EFFECT
Alcohol:	None expected.
Beverages:	None expected.
Cocaine:	None expected.
Foods:	None expected.
Marijuana:	None expected.
Tobacco:	None expected.

CONTRACEPTIVES, ORAL & SKIN

GENERIC AND BRAND NAMES

See full list of generic and brand names in the *Generic and Brand Name Directory*, page 880

BASIC INFORMATION

Habit forming? No
Prescription needed? Yes
Available as generic? Yes, for some
Drug class: Female sex hormone, contraceptive (oral & skin)

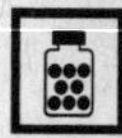

USES

- Prevents pregnancy.
- Helps regulate menstrual periods.
- Treats premenstrual dysphoric disorder.
- May be used to treat acne vulgaris in females.

DOSAGE & USAGE INFORMATION

How to take:
- Tablet—Swallow with liquid or food.
- Chewable tablet—May be swallowed whole or chewed and swallowed. If pill is chewed, drink a full glass of liquid right afterwards.
- Extended-cycle tablet—Take as directed.
- Skin patch—Follow instructions on package.

When to take:
- Tablet—At same time each day, usually for 21 days of 28-day cycle.
- Other forms—Take or use as directed.

If you forget a dose:
Follow instructions provided with your product. May want to call doctor for advice about other protection against pregnancy.

What drug does:
Blocks release of eggs from the ovaries. Alters cervix mucus to resist sperm entry. Alters uterus lining to resist implantation of fertilized egg.

Time lapse before drug works:
10 days or more to provide contraception.

Don't take with:
Any other medicine or any dietary supplement without consulting your doctor or pharmacist.

OVERDOSE

SYMPTOMS:
Drowsiness, nausea, vomiting, bleeding.
WHAT TO DO:
Overdose unlikely to threaten life. If person uses much larger amount than prescribed or if accidentally swallowed, call doctor or poison control center 1-800-222-1222 for help.

POSSIBLE ADVERSE REACTIONS OR SIDE EFFECTS

SYMPTOMS	WHAT TO DO
Life-threatening:	
Blood clot (sudden and severe pain in leg, chest stomach or groin; severe headache; shortness of breath; coughing blood; sudden weakness or numbness or vision changes or slurring speech).	Seek emergency treatment immediately.
Common:	
• Menstrual bleeding changes (during first 3 months of drug use).	Continue, but call doctor right away.
• Cramping or bloating, breast tenderness or swelling, dizziness, fluid retention, acne, nausea or vomiting, feeling tired or weak.	Continue. Call doctor when convenient.
Infrequent:	
• Headache or migraine(increase in number), vaginal discharge or itching or irritation, high blood pressure, higher blood sugar (nausea, sweating, pale skin, faintness).	Continue, but call doctor right away.
• Brown blotches on skin, gain or loss of body hair, weight gain or loss, increase or decrease in sexual desire, skin sensitive to sun, dizziness.	Continue. Call doctor when convenient.
Rare:	
• Breast lumps, pain in stomach or side, yellow eyes or skin, pain or swelling in upper abdomen, depression.	Continue, but call doctor right away.
• Irritated skin from patch, swelling or bleeding gums, increased or decreased appetite, problem wearing contact lenses, other unexplained symptoms.	Continue. Call doctor when convenient.

WARNINGS & PRECAUTIONS

Don't take if:

- You are allergic to any female hormone.
- You have cancer of breast, uterus or ovaries.
- You have or have had a stroke, a history of (or risk of) blood clots, sickle-cell disease, heart attack or heart disease, blood circulation problems, jaundice, liver disease, adrenal problems (Yasmin brand), or unexplained vaginal bleeding.

Before you start, consult your doctor if:

- You have or have had benign breast problems or family history of breast cancer, medical problems in pregnancy, epilepsy, asthma, migraines or other headaches, kidney or gall-bladder disease, high cholesterol, high blood pressure, diabetes or other medical disorders.
- You will have surgery in the near future.
- You are over age 35 or smoke cigarettes.

Over age 60:
Not used in this age group.

Pregnancy:
Stop drug at first sign of pregnancy. See doctor right away. Risk category X (see page xviii).

Breast-feeding:
Drug passes into milk. Avoid drug or discontinue nursing. Consult your doctor.

Infants & children:
Not recommended.

Prolonged use:

- Possibly cause gallstones or gradual blood pressure rise and possible difficulty becoming pregnant after discontinuing.
- Talk to your doctor about the need for follow-up medical examinations or laboratory studies to check blood pressure, liver function, pap smear.

Skin & sunlight:
One or more drugs in this group may cause rash or intensify sunburn in areas exposed to sun or ultraviolet light (photosensitivity reaction). Avoid overexposure. Notify doctor if reaction occurs.

Driving, piloting or hazardous work:
No problems expected.

Discontinuing:

- Use another form of birth control if you want to avoid unintended pregnancy.
- Fertility returns rapidly after discontinuing, but there may be a delay in getting pregnant.

Others:

- Failure to take drug for 1 day may reduce birth control effect. Use backup type of birth control.
- Advise any doctor you consult that you take this drug. Drug use may interfere with the accuracy of some medical tests.
- Risk of severe adverse effects is higher in smokers and in women using the skin patch.
- Drospirenone (a progestin)-containing pills have higher blood clot risk than other pills with progestins. Consult doctor.
- Use of the skin patch exposes you to about 60% more estrogen than typical birth control pills and puts you at higher risk of blood clots and other serious side effects. Consult doctor.

POSSIBLE INTERACTION WITH OTHER DRUGS

GENERIC NAME OR DRUG CLASS	COMBINED EFFECT
Ampicillin	Decreased contraceptive effect.
Antibacterials*	Decreased contraceptive effect.
Anticoagulants*	Decreased anticoagulant effect.
Anticonvulsants, hydantoin*	Decreased contraceptive effect.
Antidepressants, tricyclic*	Increased toxicity of antidepressants.
Antidiabetics* oral	Decreased antidiabetic effect.
Antifibrinolytic agents*	Increased possibility of blood clotting.
Anti-inflammatory drugs nonsteroidal (NSAIDs)*	Decreased contraceptive effect.
Antihistamines*	Decreased contraceptive effect.
Barbiturates*	Decreased contraceptive effect.
Chloramphenicol	Decreased contraceptive effect.

Continued on page 912

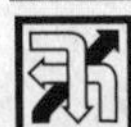

POSSIBLE INTERACTION WITH OTHER SUBSTANCES

INTERACTS WITH	COMBINED EFFECT
Alcohol:	None expected.
Beverages:	None expected.
Cocaine:	None expected.
Foods:	None expected.
Marijuana:	Unknown. Avoid.
Tobacco:	Possible heart attack, blood clots and stroke. *Don't smoke.*

CONTRACEPTIVES, VAGINAL

GENERIC AND BRAND NAMES

See full list of generic and brand names in the *Generic and Brand Name Directory,* page 881.

BASIC INFORMATION

Habit forming? No
Prescription needed? Not for most
Available as generic? Many are available
Drug class: Contraceptive (vaginal)

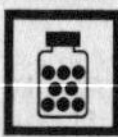

USES

- Provides a degree of protection against pregnancy.
- Spermicides used alone are not recommended for prevention of sexually transmitted diseases including human immunodeficiency virus (HIV).

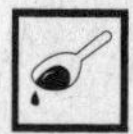

DOSAGE & USAGE INFORMATION

How to take:
Read package insert carefully. Some cautions to remember:
- Do not douche for 6 to 8 hours after intercourse.
- Do not remove sponge, cervical cap or diaphragm for 6 to 8 hours after intercourse.
- Follow product label instructions for storage.
- Plastic ring device—Follow special patient brochure instructions.

When to take:
For barrier forms, use consistently with every sexual exposure. The plastic ring device is replaced every month.

If you forget to use:
Contact your doctor to consider using another form of pregnancy protection, such as the "morning-after" pill.

Continued next column

OVERDOSE

SYMPTOMS:
None expected.
WHAT TO DO:
Not intended for internal use. If child accidentally swallows, call doctor or poison control center 1-800-222-1222 for help.

What drug does:
- Spermicides form a chemical barrier between sperm in semen and the mucous membranes in the vagina. The chemical acts to inactivate viable sperm and also kills some bacteria, viruses, yeast and fungus.
- The plastic ring device releases hormones that go into the bloodstream and provide the same protection as birth control pills.

Time lapse before vaginal contraceptive works:
- Immediate for foam, gels, jellies and sponges.
- 5 to 15 minutes for film and suppositories.
- Plastic ring device takes 7 days to be effective. Use another form of birth control during that time.

Don't use with:
Other vaginal products without consulting your doctor or pharmacist.

POSSIBLE ADVERSE REACTIONS OR SIDE EFFECTS

SYMPTOMS	WHAT TO DO
Life-threatening:	
Toxic shock syndrome—chills, fever, skin rash, muscle aches, extreme weakness, confusion, redness (of vagina, inside of mouth, nose, throat or eyes). (Very rare.)	Seek emergency treatment immediately.
Common:	
None expected.	
Infrequent:	
None expected.	
Rare:	
Vaginal discharge, irritation or rash; painful urination; cloudy or bloody urine.	Discontinue. Call doctor right away.

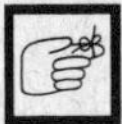

WARNINGS & PRECAUTIONS

Don't take if:
You are allergic to any form of octoxynol, nonoxynol or benzalkonium chloride or female hormones.

Before you start, consult your doctor if:
You desire complete protection against pregnancy. A combination of methods gives better protection than vaginal contraceptives alone.

Over age 60:
Not used in this age group.

Pregnancy:
Risk factor not designated. See categories on page xviii and consult doctor.

Breast-feeding:
Safety not established. Consult doctor.

Infants & children:
Not recommended.

Prolonged use:
Allergic reactions and irritation more likely.

Skin & sunlight:
No problems expected.

Driving, piloting or hazardous work:
No special problems expected.

Discontinuing:
No special problems expected.

Others:

- Failure rate when used alone is relatively high. Therefore a vaginal cream, sponge, suppository, foam, gel, jelly or other product should be used with a mechanical barrier, such as a condom, cervical cap, vaginal diaphragm or other form of pregnancy protection.
- Spermicidal products containing the chemical ingredient nonoxynol 9 (N9) do not provide protection against infection from HIV or other sexually transmitted diseases.
- Nonoxynol 9 (N9) in stand-alone vaginal contraceptives and spermicides can irritate the vagina and rectum, which may increase the risk of contracting HIV/AIDS from an infected partner.
- Don't use a cervical cap, sponge or diaphragm during menstruation. Consider using a condom instead if additional protection is desired.

POSSIBLE INTERACTION WITH OTHER DRUGS

GENERIC NAME OR DRUG CLASS	COMBINED EFFECT
Topical vaginal medications that include any of the following: sulfa drugs, soaps or disinfectants, nitrates,* permanganates, lanolin, hydrogen peroxide, iodides, cotton dressings, aluminum citrates, salicylates*	Spermicidal activity may be reduced or negated. Avoid combinations.
Vaginal douche products	May prevent spermicidal effect. Avoid until 8 hours following intercourse.

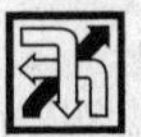

POSSIBLE INTERACTION WITH OTHER SUBSTANCES

INTERACTS WITH	COMBINED EFFECT
Alcohol:	None expected.
Beverages:	None expected.
Cocaine:	None expected.
Foods:	None expected.
Marijuana:	None expected.
Tobacco:	None expected.

***See Glossary**

CROMOLYN

BRAND NAMES

Crolom
Fivent
Gastrocrom
Nalcrom
Nasalcrom
Novo-Cromolyn
Opticrom
PMS-Sodium Cromoglycate
Rynacrom
Sodium Cromoglycate
Vistacrom

BASIC INFORMATION

Habit forming? No
Prescription needed? Yes, for some
Available as generic? Yes, for some
Drug class: Nasal decongestant, anti-inflammatory (nonsteroidal)

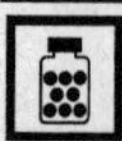

USES

- Powdered form and nebulizer solution prevent asthma attacks. Will not stop an active asthma attack.
- Eye drops treat inflammation of covering to eye and cornea.
- Nasal spray reduces nasal allergic symptoms.
- Capsules may help prevent allergic symptoms.

DOSAGE & USAGE INFORMATION

How to take:

Inhaler

Follow instructions enclosed with inhaler. Don't swallow cartridges for inhaler. Gargle and rinse mouth after inhalations.

Eye drops

- Wash hands.
- Apply pressure to inside corner of eye with middle finger.
- Continue pressure for 1 minute after placing medicine in eye.
- Tilt head backward. Pull lower lid away from eye with index finger of the same hand.
- Drop eye drops into pouch and close eye. Don't blink.

Continued next column

- Keep eyes closed for 1 to 2 minutes.
- Don't touch applicator tip to any surface (including the eye). If you accidentally touch tip, clean with warm water and soap.
- Keep container tightly closed.
- Keep cool, but don't freeze.
- Wash hands immediately after using.

Nasal solution

Follow prescription instructions.

Capsules

Open capsule and dissolve contents in 4 ounces of hot water, then add equal amount of cold water. Drink all the liquid.

When to take:

At the same times each day. If you also use a bronchodilator inhaler, use the bronchodilator before the cromolyn.

If you forget a dose:

Take as soon as you remember. If it is almost time for the next dose, wait for the next scheduled dose (don't double this dose).

What drug does:

Blocks histamine release from mast cells.

Time lapse before drug works:

- For inhaler forms: 4 weeks for prevention of asthma attacks. However, if taken 10-15 minutes before exercise or exposure to known allergens, may prevent wheezing.
- 1 to 2 weeks for nasal symptoms; only a few days for eye symptoms.

Don't take with:

Any other medicine or any dietary supplement without consulting your doctor or pharmacist.

OVERDOSE

SYMPTOMS:
Increased side effects and adverse reactions listed.
WHAT TO DO:
Overdose unlikely to threaten life. If person uses much larger amount than prescribed or if accidentally swallowed, call doctor or poison control center 1-800-222-1222 for help.

POSSIBLE ADVERSE REACTIONS OR SIDE EFFECTS

SYMPTOMS	WHAT TO DO
Life-threatening:	
Hives, rash, intense itching, faintness soon after a dose (anaphylaxis).	Seek emergency treatment immediately.
Common:	
Inhaler—cough, stuffy nose, dry mouth or throat; nasal—burning or stinging inside nose, increased sneezing; oral—diarrhea, headache.	Continue. Call doctor when convenient.
Infrequent:	
Inhaler—hoarseness, watery eyes; nasal—headache, bad taste, postnasal drip; oral—stomach pain, nausea, insomnia, rash.	Continue. Call doctor when convenient.

Rare:

Inhaler—rash, hives, swallowing difficulty, increased wheezing, joint pain or swelling, weakness, muscle pain, difficult or painful urination, difficulty breathing; nasal—difficulty swallowing, hives, itching, skin rash, facial swelling, wheezing, nosebleed; oral—cough, difficulty swallowing, facial swelling, wheezing, breathing difficulty.	Discontinue. Call doctor right away.

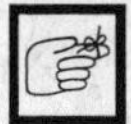

WARNINGS & PRECAUTIONS

Don't take if:
You use the dry powder form of cromolyn and if you are allergic to cromolyn, lactose, milk or milk products.

Before you start, consult your doctor if:
- You plan to become pregnant within medication period.
- You have kidney or liver disease.

Over age 60:
Adverse reactions and side effects may be more frequent and severe than in younger persons.

Pregnancy:
No proven harm to unborn child, but avoid if possible. Consult doctor. Risk category B (see page xviii).

Breast-feeding:
Effects unknown. Confer with your doctor.

Infants & children:
Do not use for children under age two.

Prolonged use:
Consult doctor on a regular basis while using this drug.

Skin & sunlight:
No problems expected.

Driving, piloting or hazardous work:
No problems expected.

Discontinuing:
Don't discontinue without doctor's approval if drug is used to prevent asthma symptoms. Dosages of other drugs may need to be adjusted.

Others:
- Inhaler must be cleaned and work well for drug to be effective.
- Treatment with inhalation cromolyn does not stop an acute asthma attack and may aggravate it.
- Advise any doctor or dentist whom you consult about the use of this medicine.
- Be sure you and the doctor discuss benefits and risks of this drug before starting.
- Call doctor if symptoms worsen or new symptoms develop with use of this medicine.
- Wear a medical identification that indicates the use of this medicine.
- Use medicine only as directed. Don't increase or decrease dosage without doctor's approval.

POSSIBLE INTERACTION WITH OTHER DRUGS

GENERIC NAME OR DRUG CLASS	COMBINED EFFECT
None significant.	

POSSIBLE INTERACTION WITH OTHER SUBSTANCES

INTERACTS WITH	COMBINED EFFECT
Alcohol:	None expected.
Beverages:	None expected.
Cocaine:	None expected.
Foods:	None expected.
Marijuana:	None expected.
Tobacco:	None expected, but tobacco smoke aggravates asthma and eye irritation. Avoid.

CYCLANDELATE

BRAND NAMES

Cyclospasmol   Cyraso-400

BASIC INFORMATION

Habit forming? No
Prescription needed?
U.S.: Yes
Canada: No
Available as generic? Yes
Drug class: Vasodilator

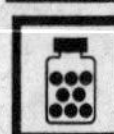

USES

May improve poor blood flow to extremities.

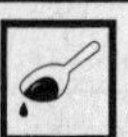

DOSAGE & USAGE INFORMATION

How to take:
Tablet or capsule—Swallow with liquid. If you can't swallow whole, crumble tablet or open capsule and take with liquid or food.

When to take:
At the same time each day.

If you forget a dose:
Take as soon as you remember. If it is almost time for the next dose, wait for the next scheduled dose (don't double this dose).

What drug does:
Increases blood flow by relaxing and expanding blood-vessel walls.

Time lapse before drug works:
3 weeks.

Don't take with:
Any other medicine or any dietary supplement without consulting your doctor or pharmacist.

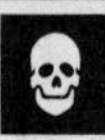

OVERDOSE

SYMPTOMS:
Severe headache, dizziness, nausea, vomiting, face is flushed and hot.
WHAT TO DO:
Overdose unlikely to threaten life. If person uses much larger amount than prescribed or if accidentally swallowed, call doctor or poison control center 1-800-222-1222 for help.

POSSIBLE ADVERSE REACTIONS OR SIDE EFFECTS

SYMPTOMS	WHAT TO DO
Life-threatening: None expected.	
Common: None expected.	
Infrequent:	
• Rapid heartbeat.	Discontinue. Call doctor right away.
• Dizziness; headache; weakness; flushed face; tingling in face, fingers or toes; unusual sweating.	Continue. Call doctor when convenient.
• Belching, heartburn, nausea or stomach pain.	Continue. Tell doctor at next visit.
Rare: None expected.	

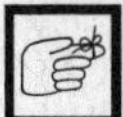

WARNINGS & PRECAUTIONS

Don't take if:
You have had an allergic reaction to cyclandelate.

Before you start, consult your doctor if:
- You have glaucoma.
- You have had a heart attack or stroke.

Over age 60:
Adverse reactions and side effects may be more frequent and severe than in younger persons.

Pregnancy:
Consult doctor. Risk category C (see page xviii).

Breast-feeding:
No proven problems. Consult doctor.

Infants & children:
Not recommended.

Prolonged use:
No problems expected.

Skin & sunlight:
No problems expected.

Driving, piloting or hazardous work:
Avoid if you feel dizzy or weak. Otherwise, no problems expected.

Discontinuing:
Don't discontinue without doctor's advice until you complete prescribed dose, even though symptoms diminish or disappear.

Others:
Response to drug varies. If your symptoms don't improve after 3 weeks of use, consult doctor.

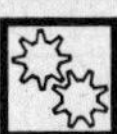

POSSIBLE INTERACTION WITH OTHER DRUGS

GENERIC NAME OR DRUG CLASS	COMBINED EFFECT
None expected.	

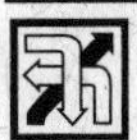

POSSIBLE INTERACTION WITH OTHER SUBSTANCES

INTERACTS WITH	COMBINED EFFECT
Alcohol:	None expected.
Beverages:	None expected.
Cocaine:	Decreased cyclandelate effect. Avoid.
Foods:	None expected.
Marijuana:	None expected.
Tobacco:	May decrease cyclandelate effect.

CYCLOBENZAPRINE

BRAND NAMES

Amrix
Cycoflex
Flexeril

BASIC INFORMATION

Habit forming? No
Prescription needed? Yes
Available as generic? Yes
Drug class: Muscle relaxant

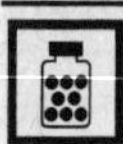

USES

Treatment for pain and limited motion caused by spasms in voluntary muscles.

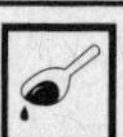

DOSAGE & USAGE INFORMATION

How to take:

- Tablet—Swallow with liquid. Take with food if stomach upset occurs.
- Extended-release tablet—Swallow whole with liquid.

When to take:
Take as directed on label.

If you forget a dose:
Take as soon as you remember. If it is almost time for the next dose, wait for that dose (don't double this dose) and resume regular schedule.

What drug does:
Blocks body's pain messages to brain.

Time lapse before drug works:
30 to 60 minutes.

Don't take with:
Any other medicine or any dietary supplement without consulting your doctor or pharmacist.

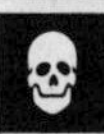

OVERDOSE

SYMPTOMS:
Drowsiness, confusion, difficulty concentrating, visual problems, vomiting, blood pressure drop, low body temperature, weak and rapid pulse, convulsions, coma.
WHAT TO DO:

- **Dial 911 (emergency) for medical help or call poison control center 1-800-222-1222 for instructions.**
- **If person is unconscious, check breathing and pulse. If not breathing, begin mouth-to-mouth rescue breathing. If heart is not beating, begin chest compressions.**
- **See emergency information on last 3 pages of this book.**

POSSIBLE ADVERSE REACTIONS OR SIDE EFFECTS

SYMPTOMS	WHAT TO DO
Life-threatening: In case of overdose, see previous column.	
Common: Drowsiness, dizziness, dry mouth.	Continue. Call doctor when convenient.
Infrequent:	
• Blurred vision, fast heartbeat.	Discontinue. Call doctor right away.
• Insomnia, numbness in extremities, bad taste in mouth, fatigue, nausea, sweating.	Continue. Call doctor when convenient.
Rare:	
• Unsteadiness, confusion, depression, hallucinations, rash, itch, swelling, breathing difficulty.	Discontinue. Call doctor right away.
• Difficult urination.	Continue. Call doctor when convenient.

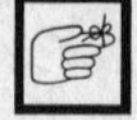

WARNINGS & PRECAUTIONS

Don't take if:

- You are allergic to any skeletal muscle relaxant.*
- You have taken a monoamine oxidase (MAO) inhibitor* in last 2 weeks.
- You have had a heart attack within 6 weeks, or suffer from congestive heart failure.
- You have an overactive thyroid.

Before you start, consult your doctor if:

- You have a heart problem.
- You have reacted to tricyclic antidepressants.
- You have glaucoma.
- You have a prostate condition and urination difficulty.
- You intend to pilot aircraft.

Over age 60:
Adverse reactions and side effects may be more frequent and severe than in younger persons. Avoid extremes of heat and cold.

Pregnancy:
No problems expected. Consult doctor. Risk category B (see page xviii).

Breast-feeding:
Drug may pass into milk. Avoid drug or discontinue nursing until you finish medicine. Consult doctor for advice on maintaining milk supply.

Infants & children:
Don't use for children younger than 15.

Prolonged use:
Do not take for longer than 2 to 3 weeks.

Skin & sunlight:
No special problems expected.

Driving, piloting or hazardous work:
Don't drive or pilot aircraft until you learn how medicine affects you. Don't work around dangerous machinery. Don't climb ladders or work in high places. Danger increases if you drink alcohol or take medicine affecting alertness and reflexes.

Discontinuing:
May be unnecessary to finish medicine. Follow doctor's instructions.

Others:
No problems expected.

POSSIBLE INTERACTION WITH OTHER DRUGS

GENERIC NAME OR DRUG CLASS	COMBINED EFFECT
Anticholinergics*	Increased anticholinergic effect.
Antidepressants*	Increased sedation.
Antihistamines*	Increased antihistamine effect.
Barbiturates*	Increased sedation.
Central nervous system (CNS) depressants*	Increased sedation.
Cimetidine	Possible increased cyclobenzaprine effect.
Cisapride	Decreased cyclobenzaprine effect.
Clonidine	Decreased clonidine effect.
Dronabinol	Increased effect of dronabinol on central nervous system. Avoid combination.
Guanethidine	Decreased guanethidine effect.
Methyldopa	Decreased methyldopa effect.
Mind-altering drugs*	Increased mind-altering effect.
Monoamine oxidase (MAO) inhibitors*	High fever, convulsions, possible death.
Narcotics*	Increased sedation.
Pain relievers*	Increased pain reliever effect.
Procainamide	Possible increased conduction disturbance.
Quinidine	Possible increased conduction disturbance.
Rauwolfia alkaloids*	Decreased effect of rauwolfia alkaloids.
Sedatives*	Increased sedative effect.
Sleep inducers*	Increased sedation.
Tranquilizers*	Increased tranquilizer effect.

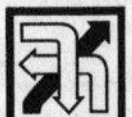

POSSIBLE INTERACTION WITH OTHER SUBSTANCES

INTERACTS WITH	COMBINED EFFECT
Alcohol:	Depressed brain function. Avoid.
Beverages:	None expected.
Cocaine:	Decreased cyclobenzaprine effect.
Foods:	None expected.
Marijuana:	Occasional use—Drowsiness. Frequent use—Severe mental and physical impairment.
Tobacco:	None expected.

*See Glossary

CYCLOPENTOLATE (Ophthalmic)

BRAND NAMES

Ak-Pentolate
Cyclogyl
I-Pentolate
Minims Cyclopentolate
Ocu-Pentolate
Pentolair
Spectro-Pentolate

BASIC INFORMATION

Habit forming? No
Prescription needed? Yes
Available as generic? Yes
Drug class: Cycloplegic, mydriatic

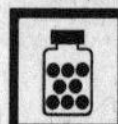

USES

- Enlarges (dilates) pupil.
- Temporarily paralyzes the normal pupil accommodation to light before eye examinations and to treat some eye conditions.

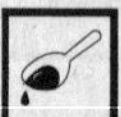

DOSAGE & USAGE INFORMATION

How to use:

Eye drops

- Wash hands.
- Apply pressure to inside corner of eye with middle finger.
- Continue pressure for 1 minute after placing medicine in eye.
- Tilt head backward. Pull lower lid away from eye with index finger of the same hand.
- Drop eye drops into pouch and close eye. Don't blink.
- Keep eyes closed for 1 to 2 minutes.
- Don't touch applicator tip to any surface (including the eye). If you accidentally touch tip, clean with warm water and soap.
- Keep container tightly closed.
- Keep cool, but don't freeze.
- Wash hands immediately after using.

When to use:
As directed on bottle.

Continued next column

If you forget a dose:
Use as soon as you remember.

What drug does:
Blocks sphincter muscle of the iris and ciliary body.

Time lapse before drug works:
Within 30 to 60 minutes. Effects usually disappear in 24 hours.

Don't use with:
Other eye medicines such as carbachol, demecarium, echothiophate, isoflurophate, physostigmine, pilocarpine without doctor's approval.

OVERDOSE

SYMPTOMS:
None expected.
WHAT TO DO:
Not intended for internal use. If child accidentally swallows, call doctor or poison control center 1-800-222-1222 for help.

POSSIBLE ADVERSE REACTIONS OR SIDE EFFECTS

SYMPTOMS	WHAT TO DO
Life-threatening: None expected.	
Common:	
• Increased sensitivity to light.	Continue. Call doctor when convenient.
• Burning eyes.	Continue. Tell doctor at next visit.
Infrequent: None expected.	
Rare (extremely):	
Symptoms of excess medicine absorbed by the body—Clumsiness, confusion, fever, flushed face, hallucinations, rash, slurred speech, swollen stomach (children), drowsiness, fast heartbeat.	Discontinue. Call doctor right away.

WARNINGS & PRECAUTIONS

Don't use if:
You are allergic to cyclopentolate.

Before you start, consult your doctor if:
- Medicine is for a brain-damaged child or child with Down syndrome.
- Prescribed for a child with spastic paralysis.

Over age 60:
No problems expected.

Pregnancy:
Avoid if possible. Consult doctor. Risk category C (see page xviii).

Breast-feeding:
Safety not established. Avoid if possible. Consult doctor.

Infants & children:
Use only under close medical supervision.

Prolonged use:
Avoid. May increase absorption into body.

Skin & sunlight:
No special problems expected.

Driving, piloting or hazardous work:
Don't drive or pilot aircraft until you learn how medicine affects you. Don't work around dangerous machinery. Don't climb ladders or work in high places. Danger increases if you drink alcohol or take medicine affecting alertness and reflexes, such as antihistamines, tranquilizers, sedatives, pain medicine, narcotics and mind-altering drugs.

Discontinuing:
If effects last longer than 36 hours after last drops, consult doctor.

Others:
Wear sunglasses to protect eyes from sunlight and bright light.

POSSIBLE INTERACTION WITH OTHER DRUGS

GENERIC NAME OR DRUG CLASS	COMBINED EFFECT
Antiglaucoma agents*	Decreased antiglaucoma effect.

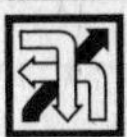

POSSIBLE INTERACTION WITH OTHER SUBSTANCES

INTERACTS WITH	COMBINED EFFECT
Alcohol:	None expected.
Beverages:	None expected.
Cocaine:	None expected.
Foods:	None expected.
Marijuana:	None expected.
Tobacco:	None expected.

*See Glossary

CYCLOPHOSPHAMIDE

BRAND NAMES

Neosar

Procytox

BASIC INFORMATION

Habit forming? No
Prescription needed? Yes
Available as generic? Yes
Drug class: Immunosuppressant, antineoplastic

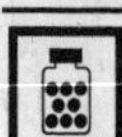

USES

- Treatment for cancer.
- Treatment for severe rheumatoid arthritis, blood-vessel disease and for skin disease.

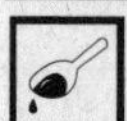

DOSAGE & USAGE INFORMATION

How to take:
Tablet—Swallow with liquid. If you can't swallow tablet whole, crumble tablet and take with liquid or food.

When to take:
Works best if taken first thing in morning. Should be taken on an empty stomach. However, may take with food to lessen stomach irritation. Don't take at bedtime.

If you forget a dose:
Take as soon as you remember up to 12 hours late. If more than 12 hours, wait for next scheduled dose (don't double this dose).

What drug does:
- Kills cancer cells.
- Suppresses spread of cancer cells.
- Suppresses immune system.

Time lapse before drug works:
7 to 10 days continual use.

Don't take with:
Any other medicine or any dietary supplement without consulting your doctor or pharmacist.

OVERDOSE

SYMPTOMS:
Bloody urine, water retention, weight gain, severe infection.
WHAT TO DO:
Overdose unlikely to threaten life. If person uses much larger amount than prescribed or if accidentally swallowed, call doctor or poison control center 1-800-222-1222 for help.

POSSIBLE ADVERSE REACTIONS OR SIDE EFFECTS

SYMPTOMS	WHAT TO DO
Life-threatening:	
Hives, rash, intense itching, faintness soon after a dose (anaphylaxis).	Seek emergency treatment immediately.
Common:	
• Sore throat, fever.	Continue, but call doctor right away.
• Dark skin, nails; nausea; appetite loss; vomiting; missed menstrual period.	Continue. Call doctor when convenient.
Infrequent:	
• Rash, hives, itch; shortness of breath; rapid heartbeat; cough; blood in urine; painful urination; pain in side; bleeding, bruising; increased sweating; hoarseness; foot or ankle swelling.	Continue, but call doctor right away.
• Confusion, agitation, headache, dizziness, flushed face, stomach pain, joint pain, fatigue, weakness, diarrhea.	Continue. Call doctor when convenient.
Rare:	
• Mouth, lip sores; black stool; unusual thirst; jaundice.	Continue, but call doctor right away.
• Blurred vision, increased urination, hair loss.	Continue. Call doctor when convenient.

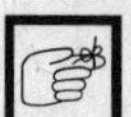

WARNINGS & PRECAUTIONS

Don't take if:
- You are allergic to any alkylating agent.
- You have an infection.
- You have bloody urine.
- You will have surgery within 2 months, including dental surgery, requiring general or spinal anesthesia.

Before you start, consult your doctor if:
- You have impaired liver or kidney function.
- You have impaired bone marrow or blood cell production.
- You have had chemotherapy or x-ray therapy.
- You have taken cortisone drugs in the past year.
- You plan to become pregnant.

Over age 60:
Adverse reactions and side effects may be more frequent and severe than in younger persons. To reduce risk of chemical bladder inflammation, drink 8 to 10 glasses of water daily.

Pregnancy:
Risk to unborn child outweighs drug benefits. Don't use. Risk category D (see page xviii).

Breast-feeding:
Drug passes into milk. Avoid drug or discontinue nursing until you finish medicine. Consult doctor for advice on maintaining milk supply.

Infants & children:
Use only under medical supervision.

Prolonged use:
- Development of fibrous lung tissue.
- Possible jaundice.
- Swelling of feet, lower legs.
- Cancer.
- Infertility in men.
- Talk to your doctor about the need for follow-up medical examinations or laboratory studies to check complete blood counts (white blood cell count, platelet count, red blood cell count, hemoglobin, hematocrit), urine, liver function.

Skin & sunlight:
No problems expected.

Driving, piloting or hazardous work:
Avoid if you feel dizzy or have blurred vision. Otherwise, no problems expected.

Discontinuing:
Don't discontinue without consulting doctor. Dose may require gradual reduction if you have taken drug for a long time. Doses of other drugs may also require adjustment.

Others:
- Frequently causes hair loss. After treatment ends, hair should grow back.
- Avoid vaccinations.
- You will need to drink extra fluids so you will pass more urine. Follow doctor's instructions.

POSSIBLE INTERACTION WITH OTHER DRUGS

GENERIC NAME OR DRUG CLASS	COMBINED EFFECT
Allopurinol or other medicines to treat gout	Possible anemia; decreased antigout effect.
Antidiabetics, oral*	Increased antidiabetic effect.
Bone marrow depressants,* other	Increased bone marrow depressant effect.
Clozapine	Toxic effect on bone marrow.
Cyclosporine	May increase risk of infection.
Digoxin	Possible decreased digoxin absorption.
Immuno-suppressants,* other	Increased risk of infection.
Insulin	Increased insulin effect.
Levamisole	Increased risk of bone marrow depression.
Lovastatin	Increased heart and kidney damage.
Phenobarbital	Increased cyclophosphamide effect.
Probenecid	Increased blood uric acid.
Sulfinpyrazone	Increased blood uric acid.
Tiopronin	Increased risk of toxicity to bone marrow.

POSSIBLE INTERACTION WITH OTHER SUBSTANCES

INTERACTS WITH	COMBINED EFFECT
Alcohol:	None expected.
Beverages:	None expected. Drink plenty of fluids every day.
Cocaine:	Increased danger of brain damage.
Foods:	None expected.
Marijuana:	Increased impairment of immunity.
Tobacco:	None expected.

***See Glossary**

CYCLOPLEGIC, MYDRIATIC (Ophthalmic)

GENERIC AND BRAND NAMES

ATROPINE (ophthalmic)
Atropair
Atropine Care Eye Drops & Ointment
Atropine Sulfate S.O.P.
Atropisol
Atrosulf
Isopto Atropine
I-Tropine
Minims Atropine
Ocu-Tropine

HOMATROPINE (ophthalmic)
AK Homatropine
I-Homatrine
I-Homatropine
Minims Homatropine
Spectro Homatropine

BASIC INFORMATION

Habit forming? No
Prescription needed? Yes
Available as generic? Yes, for some
Drug class: Cycloplegic, mydriatic

USES

- Dilates pupil of the eye.
- Used before some eye examinations, before and after some eye surgical procedures and, rarely, to treat some eye problems such as glaucoma.

DOSAGE & USAGE INFORMATION

How to use:
Eye drops
- Wash hands.
- Apply pressure to inside corner of eye with middle finger.
- Continue pressure for 1 minute after placing medicine in eye.
- Tilt head backward. Pull lower lid away from eye with index finger of the same hand.
- Drop eye drops into pouch and close eye. Don't blink.
- Keep eyes closed for 1 to 2 minutes.

Continued next column

OVERDOSE

SYMPTOMS:
None expected.
WHAT TO DO:
Not intended for internal use. If child accidentally swallows, call doctor or poison control center 1-800-222-1222 for help.

Eye ointment
- Wash hands.
- Pull lower lid down from eye to form a pouch.
- Squeeze tube to apply thin strip of ointment into pouch.
- Close eye for 1 to 2 minutes.
- Don't touch applicator tip to any surface (including the eye). If you accidentally touch tip, clean with warm water and soap.
- Keep container tightly closed.
- Keep cool, but don't freeze.
- Wash hands immediately after using.

When to use:
As directed on label.

If you forget a dose:
Use as soon as you remember.

What drug does:
Blocks normal response to sphincter muscle of the iris of the eye and the accommodative muscle of the ciliary body.

Time lapse before drug works:
Begins within 1 minute. Residual effects may last up to 14 days.

Don't use with:
Other eye medicines such as carbachol, demecarium, echothiophate, isoflurophate, physostigmine, pilocarpine.

POSSIBLE ADVERSE REACTIONS OR SIDE EFFECTS

SYMPTOMS	WHAT TO DO
Life-threatening: None expected.	
Common:	
• Increased sensitivity to light.	Continue. Call doctor when convenient.
• Burning eyes.	Continue. Tell doctor at next visit.
Infrequent: None expected.	
Rare (extremely):	
Symptoms of excess medicine absorbed by the body—Clumsiness, confusion, fever, flushed face, hallucinations, rash, slurred speech, swollen stomach (children), unusual drowsiness, fast heartbeat.	Discontinue. Call doctor right away.

CYCLOPLEGIC, MYDRIATIC (Ophthalmic)

WARNINGS & PRECAUTIONS

Don't use if:
You are allergic to any mydriatic cycloplegic drug.

Before you start, consult your doctor if:
- Medicine is for a brain-damaged child or child with Down syndrome.
- Prescribed for a child with spastic paralysis.

Over age 60:
No problems expected.

Pregnancy:
Decide with your doctor if drug benefits justify risk to unborn child. Risk category C (see page xviii).

Breast-feeding:
Safety not established. Avoid if possible.

Infants & children:
Use only under close medical supervision.

Prolonged use:
Avoid. May increase absorption into body.

Skin & sunlight:
No special problems expected.

Driving, piloting or hazardous work:
Don't drive or pilot aircraft until you learn how medicine affects you. Don't work around dangerous machinery. Don't climb ladders or work in high places. Danger increases if you drink alcohol or take medicine affecting alertness and reflexes, such as antihistamines, tranquilizers, sedatives, pain medicine, narcotics and mind-altering drugs.

Discontinuing:
Effects may last up to 14 days later.

Others:
Wear sunglasses to protect eyes from sunlight and bright light.

POSSIBLE INTERACTION WITH OTHER DRUGS

GENERIC NAME OR DRUG CLASS	COMBINED EFFECT

Clinically significant interactions with oral or injected medicines unlikely.

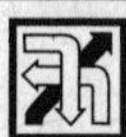

POSSIBLE INTERACTION WITH OTHER SUBSTANCES

INTERACTS WITH	COMBINED EFFECT
Alcohol:	None expected.
Beverages:	None expected.
Cocaine:	None expected.
Foods:	None expected.
Marijuana:	None expected.
Tobacco:	None expected.

CYCLOSERINE

BRAND NAMES

Seromycin

BASIC INFORMATION

Habit forming? No
Prescription needed? Yes
Available as generic? No
Drug class: Antibacterial

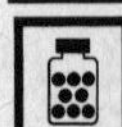

USES

- Treats urinary tract infections.
- Treats tuberculosis.

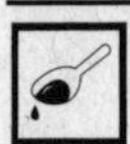

DOSAGE & USAGE INFORMATION

How to take:
Capsule—Swallow with liquid or food to lessen stomach irritation. If you can't swallow whole, open capsule and take with liquid or food.

When to take:
- Once or twice daily as prescribed.
- At the same times each day after meals to prevent stomach irritation.

If you forget a dose:
Take as soon as you remember. If it is almost time for the next dose, wait for the next scheduled dose (don't double this dose).

What drug does:
Interferes with bacterial wall synthesis and keeps germs from multiplying.

Time lapse before drug works:
3 to 4 hours.

Don't take with:
Any other medicine or any dietary supplement without consulting your doctor or pharmacist.

OVERDOSE

SYMPTOMS:
Seizures.
WHAT TO DO:
- **Dial 911 (emergency) for medical help or call poison control center 1-800-222-1222 for instructions.**
- **See emergency information on last 3 pages of this book.**

POSSIBLE ADVERSE REACTIONS OR SIDE EFFECTS

SYMPTOMS	WHAT TO DO
Life-threatening:	
Seizures, muscle twitching or trembling.	Seek emergency treatment immediately.
Common:	
Gum inflammation, pale skin, depression, confusion, dizziness, restlessness, anxiety, nightmares, severe headache, drowsiness.	Continue, but call doctor right away.
Infrequent:	
Visual changes; skin rash; numbness, tingling or burning in hands and feet; jaundice; eye pain.	Continue. Call doctor when convenient.
Rare:	
Seizures, thoughts of suicide.	Discontinue. Seek emergency treatment.

WARNINGS & PRECAUTIONS

Don't take if:
- You are a frequent user of alcohol.
- You have a convulsive disorder.

Before you start, consult your doctor if:
- You are depressed.
- You have kidney disease.
- You have severe anxiety.

Over age 60:
Adverse reactions and side effects may be more frequent and severe than in younger persons. You may need smaller doses for shorter periods of time.

Pregnancy:
Decide with your doctor if drug benefits justify risk to unborn child. Risk category C (see page xviii).

Breast-feeding:
Drug passes into milk. Avoid drug or discontinue nursing until you finish medicine. Consult doctor for advice on maintaining milk supply.

Infants & children:
Use only under close medical supervision.

Prolonged use:
- May cause liver or kidney damage.
- May cause anemia.

Skin & sunlight:
No special problems expected.

Driving, piloting or hazardous work:
Don't drive or pilot aircraft until you learn how medicine affects you. Don't work around dangerous machinery. Don't climb ladders or work in high places. Danger increases if you drink alcohol or take medicine affecting alertness and reflexes.

Discontinuing:
Don't discontinue without consulting doctor. Dose may require gradual reduction if you have taken drug for a long time. Doses of other drugs may also require adjustment.

Others:
- May have to take anticonvulsants, sedatives and/or pyridoxine to prevent or minimize toxic effects on the brain.
- If you must take more than 500 mg per day, toxicity is much more likely to occur.
- Talk to your doctor about taking pyridoxine as a supplement.

POSSIBLE INTERACTION WITH OTHER DRUGS

GENERIC NAME OR DRUG CLASS	COMBINED EFFECT
Ethionamide	Increased risk of seizures.
Isoniazid	Increased risk of central nervous system effects.
Pyridoxine	Reduces effects of pyridoxine. Since pyridoxine is a vital vitamin, patients on cycloserine require pyridoxine supplements to prevent anemia or peripheral neuritis.

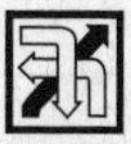

POSSIBLE INTERACTION WITH OTHER SUBSTANCES

INTERACTS WITH	COMBINED EFFECT
Alcohol:	Toxic. May increase risk of seizures. Avoid.
Beverages:	None expected.
Cocaine:	Toxic. Avoid.
Foods:	None expected.
Marijuana:	May increase risk of seizures.
Tobacco:	May decrease effect of cycloserine.

CYCLOSPORINE

BRAND NAMES

Gengraf
Neoral
Sandimmune

BASIC INFORMATION

Habit forming? No
Prescription needed? Yes
Available as generic? Yes
Drug class: Immunosuppressant

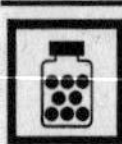

USES

- Suppresses the immune response in patients who have transplants of the heart, lung, kidney, liver, pancreas. Cyclosporine treats rejection as well as helps prevent it.
- Treatment for severe psoriasis when regular treatment is ineffective or not appropriate.

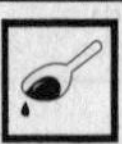

DOSAGE & USAGE INFORMATION

How to take:
- Oral solution—Take after meals with liquid to decrease stomach irritation. May mix with milk, chocolate milk or orange juice. Don't mix in Styrofoam cups. Use special dropper for exact dosage.
- Capsule—Take with water or other fluid. Don't break capsule open.

When to take:
At the same time each day, according to instructions on prescription label.

If you forget a dose:
Take as soon as you remember. If it is almost time for the next dose, wait for the next scheduled dose (don't double this dose).

What drug does:
Exact mechanism is unknown, but believed to inhibit interleuken II to affect T-lymphocytes.

Time lapse before drug works:
3 to 3-1/2 hours.

Continued next column

OVERDOSE

SYMPTOMS:
Irregular heartbeat, seizures, coma.
WHAT TO DO:
- **Dial 911 (emergency) for medical help or call poison control center 1-800-222-1222 for instructions.**
- **See emergency information on last 3 pages of this book.**

Don't take with:
Any other medicine or any dietary supplement without consulting your doctor or pharmacist.

POSSIBLE ADVERSE REACTIONS OR SIDE EFFECTS

SYMPTOMS	WHAT TO DO
Life-threatening:	
Seizures, wheezing with shortness of breath, convulsions.	Discontinue. Seek emergency treatment.
Common:	
• Gum inflammation, blood in urine, jaundice, tremors.	Continue. Call doctor when convenient.
• Increased hair growth.	Continue. Tell doctor at next visit.
Infrequent:	
• Fever, chills, sore throat, shortness of breath.	Continue, but call doctor right away.
• Frequent urination, headache, leg cramps.	Continue. Call doctor when convenient.
Rare:	
• Confusion, irregular heartbeat, numbness of hands and feet, nervousness, face flushing, severe abdominal pain, weakness.	Continue, but call doctor right away.
• Acne, headache.	Continue. Call doctor when convenient.

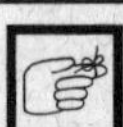

WARNINGS & PRECAUTIONS

Don't take if:
- You have chicken pox.
- You have shingles (herpes zoster).

Before you start, consult your doctor if:
- You have liver problems.
- You have an infection.
- You have kidney disease.

Over age 60:
No special problems expected.

Pregnancy:
Decide with your doctor if drug benefits justify risk to unborn child. Risk category C (see page xviii).

Breast-feeding:
Drug passes into milk. Avoid drug or discontinue nursing until you finish medicine. Consult doctor for advice on maintaining milk supply.

Infants & children:
No problems expected.

Prolonged use:
- Can cause reduced function of kidney.
- Talk to your doctor about the need for follow-up medical examinations or laboratory studies to check blood pressure, kidney function, liver function.

Skin & sunlight:
No problems expected.

Driving, piloting or hazardous work:
Don't drive or pilot aircraft until you learn how medicine affects you. Don't work around dangerous machinery. Don't climb ladders or work in high places. Danger increases if you drink alcohol or take medicine affecting alertness and reflexes.

Discontinuing:
Don't discontinue without consulting doctor. You probably will require this medicine for the remainder of your life.

Others:
- Request regular laboratory studies to measure levels of potassium and cyclosporine in blood and to evaluate liver and kidney function.
- Use of the drug may increase the risk of developing an infection or cancer (e.g., lymphoma or skin cancer). Call doctor right away if new symptoms occur.
- Check blood pressure regularly. Cyclosporine sometimes causes hypertension.
- Don't store solution in the refrigerator.
- Avoid any immunizations except those specifically recommended by your doctor.
- Maintain good dental hygiene. Cyclosporine can cause gum problems.
- Kidney toxicity occurs commonly after 12 months of taking cyclosporine.
- Immunosuppressed patients are at increased risk for opportunistic infections, such as activation of latent viral infections, including BK virus-associated nephropathy.
- Don't mix drug in Styrofoam cups.

POSSIBLE INTERACTION WITH OTHER DRUGS

GENERIC NAME OR DRUG CLASS	COMBINED EFFECT
Androgens	Increased effect of cyclosporine.
Anticonvulsants*	Decreased effect of cyclosporine.
Cimetidine	Increased effect of cyclosporine.
Danazol	Increased effect of cyclosporine.
Diltiazem	Increased effect of cyclosporine.
Diuretics, potassium-sparing	Increased effect of cyclosporine.
Erythromycin	Increased effect of cyclosporine.
Estrogens	Increased effect of cyclosporine.
Fluconazole	Increased effect of cyclosporine. Cyclosporine dosage must be adjusted.
HMG-CoA reductase inhibitors	Increased risk of muscle and kidney problems.
Imatinib	Increased effect of cyclosporine.
Immunosuppressants,* other	Increased risk of adverse effects.
Itraconazole	Increased cyclosporine toxicity.
Ketoconazole	Increased risk of toxicity to kidney.
Leukotriene modifiers	Increased effect of cyclosporine.
Losartan	Increased potassium levels.
Lovastatin	Increased heart and kidney damage.
Nephrotoxic drugs*	Increased risk of toxicity to kidneys.

Continued on page 913

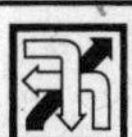

POSSIBLE INTERACTION WITH OTHER SUBSTANCES

INTERACTS WITH	COMBINED EFFECT
Alcohol:	May increase possibility of toxic effects. Avoid.
Beverages: Grapefruit juice.	Increased cyclosporine effect.
Cocaine:	May increase possibility of toxic effects. Avoid.
Foods:	None expected.
Marijuana:	May increase possibility of toxic effects. Avoid.
Tobacco:	May increase possibility of toxic effects. Avoid.

***See Glossary**

DABIGATRAN

BRAND NAMES

Pradaxa

BASIC INFORMATION

Habit forming? No
Prescription needed? Yes
Available as generic? No
Drug class: Anticoagulant

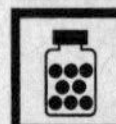

USES

- Used for the prevention of blood clots and stroke in patients with abnormal heart rhythm (atrial fibrillation).
- Other uses as recommended by your doctor.

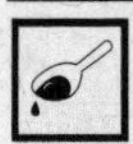

DOSAGE & USAGE INFORMATION

How to take:
Capsule—Swallow whole with liquid. May be taken with or without food. Do not crush, chew, break open or empty the pellets from the capsule.

When to take:
Twice a day at the same times each day or as directed by your doctor.

If you forget a dose:
Take as soon as you remember. If the next dose is less than 6 hours away, skip the missed dose and return to regular schedule (don't double this dose).

What drug does:
It blocks thrombin (a substance in the blood) that is involved in the process of blood clotting thereby reducing the risk of blood clots.

Time lapse before drug works:
One to two hours.

Don't take with:
Any other medicine or any dietary supplement without consulting your doctor or pharmacist.

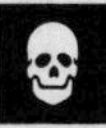

OVERDOSE

SYMPTOMS:
Bleeding problems that may be severe (e.g., vomiting blood, nosebleed, bright-red blood in stool).
WHAT TO DO:
Dial 911 (emergency) for medical help or call poison control center 1-800-222-1222 for instructions.

POSSIBLE ADVERSE REACTIONS OR SIDE EFFECTS

SYMPTOMS	WHAT TO DO
Life-threatening:	
Rare allergic reaction (hives, itching, rash, trouble breathing, tightness in chest, swelling of lips or tongue or face).	Seek emergency treatment immediately.
Common:	
• Bleeding from gums, frequent nosebleeds, vaginal bleeding, heavy menstrual period, pink or brown urine, red or black or tarry stools, coughing up blood, vomiting blood or coffee ground-like material, unusual pain or swelling, joint pain, unexpected bruising, headaches, feeling dizzy or weak.	Continue, but call doctor right away.
• Nausea, upset stomach, diarrhea, indigestion, stomach pain or burning, cuts or scrapes that take a long time to stop bleeding.	Continue. Call doctor when convenient.
Infrequent:	
None expected.	
Rare:	
Other unexpected symptoms.	Continue. Call doctor when convenient.

WARNINGS & PRECAUTIONS

Don't take if:
- You are allergic to dabigatran.
- You have mechanical heart valves.

Before you start, consult your doctor if:
- You have any kidney (renal) problems.
- You have or have had stomach ulcers.
- You have or have had any bleeding problems.
- You have plans for surgery or any invasive procedure in the next few months.
- You are allergic to any food, medicine or other substance.

Over age 60:
Risk of stroke and bleeding increases with age. Consult doctor about your risks.

Pregnancy:
Decide with your doctor whether drug benefits justify risk to unborn child. Risk category C (see page xviii).

Breast-feeding:
It is unknown if drug passes into breast milk. Consult doctor for advice.

Infants & children:
Safety and effectiveness in children under age 18 has not been established.

Prolonged use:
Consult with your doctor on a regular basis while taking this drug to monitor your progress, check for side effects, check your renal (kidney) function, and for recommended lab tests.

Skin & sunlight:
No problems expected.

Driving, piloting or hazardous work:
No problems expected.

Discontinuing:
Do not stop taking drug without first talking with your doctor. Stopping drug may increase risk of stroke.

Others:
- Store capsules in original container and keep it tightly closed. Do not put capsules in a pill box or pill organizer.
- Safely throw away any unused capsules after 4 months (or as directed by doctor) and start using a new container.
- Advise any doctor or dentist whom you consult that you take this drug.
- Your doctor may have you stop taking drug for a short time if you plan to have surgery or a medical or a dental procedure. You will be advised when to stop and when to resume taking the drug.
- Drug lessens the ability of your blood to clot. You may bruise more easily and it may take longer for any bleeding to stop.

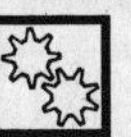

POSSIBLE INTERACTION WITH OTHER DRUGS

GENERIC NAME OR DRUG CLASS	COMBINED EFFECT
Anticoagulants,* other	Increased anti-coagulant effect (bleeding or bruising).
Anti-inflammatory drugs, nonsteroidal (NSAIDs)*	Increased risk of bleeding.
Mifepristone	Increased risk of vaginal bleeding.
P-glycoprotein inducers*	May decrease dabigatran effect.
P-glycoprotein inhibitors*	May increase dabigatran effect.
Platelet inhibitors	Increased risk of bleeding.

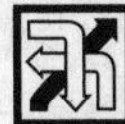

POSSIBLE INTERACTION WITH OTHER SUBSTANCES

INTERACTS WITH	COMBINED EFFECT
Alcohol:	None expected.
Beverages:	None expected.
Cocaine:	Unknown. Avoid.
Foods:	None expected.
Marijuana:	Unknown. Avoid.
Tobacco:	No interaction, but smoking is a risk factor for blood clots. Avoid.

*See Glossary

DANAZOL

BRAND NAMES

Cyclomen
Danocrine

BASIC INFORMATION

Habit forming? No
Prescription needed? Yes
Available as generic? Yes
Drug class: Gonadotropin inhibitor

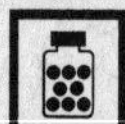

USES

Treatment of endometriosis, fibrocystic breast disease, angioneurotic edema except in pregnant women, gynecomastia, infertility, excessive menstruation, precocious puberty.

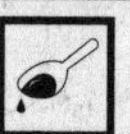

DOSAGE & USAGE INFORMATION

How to take:
Capsule—Swallow with liquid or food to lessen stomach irritation. If you can't swallow whole, open capsule and take with liquid or food.

When to take:
At the same times each day.

If you forget a dose:
Take as soon as you remember (don't double dose).

What drug does:
Partially prevents output of pituitary follicle-stimulating hormone and leuteinizing hormone reducing estrogen production.

Time lapse before drug works:
- 2 to 3 months to treat endometriosis.
- 1 to 2 months to treat other disorders.

Don't take with:
- Birth control pills.
- Any other medicine or any dietary supplement without consulting your doctor or pharmacist.

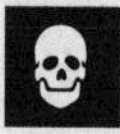

OVERDOSE

SYMPTOMS:
None expected.
WHAT TO DO:
Overdose unlikely to threaten life. If person uses much larger amount than prescribed or if accidentally swallowed, call doctor or poison control center 1-800-222-1222 for help.

POSSIBLE ADVERSE REACTIONS OR SIDE EFFECTS

SYMPTOMS	WHAT TO DO
Life-threatening: None expected.	
Common: Menstrual irregularities.	Continue. Call doctor when convenient.
Infrequent:	
• Unnatural hair growth in women, nosebleeds, bleeding gums, sore throat and chills.	Discontinue. Call doctor right away.
• Dizziness; deepened voice; hoarseness; flushed or red skin; muscle cramps; enlarged clitoris; decreased testicle size; vaginal burning, itching; swollen feet; decreased breast size; increased or decreased sex drive.	Continue. Call doctor when convenient.
• Headache, acne, weight gain, vision changes.	Continue. Tell doctor at next visit.
Rare: Jaundice, flushing, sweating, vaginitis, rash, nausea, vomiting, constipation, abdominal pain.	Discontinue. Call doctor right away.

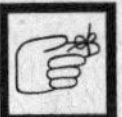

WARNINGS & PRECAUTIONS

Don't take if:
- You become pregnant.
- You have breast cancer.

Before you start, consult your doctor if:
- You take birth control pills.
- You have diabetes.
- You have heart disease.
- You have epilepsy.
- You have kidney disease.
- You have liver disease.
- You have migraine headaches.

Over age 60:
Adverse reactions and side effects may be more frequent and severe than in younger persons.

Pregnancy:
Risk to unborn child outweighs drug benefits. Don't use. Stop if you get pregnant. Risk category X (see page xviii).

Breast-feeding:
Unknown whether medicine filters into milk. Consult doctor.

Infants & children:
Not recommended.

Prolonged use:
- Required for full effect. Don't discontinue without consulting doctor.
- Talk to your doctor about the need for follow-up medical examinations or laboratory studies to check liver function; mammogram.

Skin & sunlight:
No problems expected.

Driving, piloting or hazardous work:
No problems expected.

Discontinuing:
Don't discontinue without consulting doctor. Menstrual periods may be absent for 2 to 3 months after discontinuation.

Others:
- May alter blood sugar levels in persons with diabetes.
- Advise any doctor or dentist whom you consult that you take this medicine.
- May interfere with the accuracy of some medical tests.

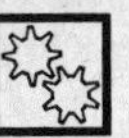

POSSIBLE INTERACTION WITH OTHER DRUGS

GENERIC NAME OR DRUG CLASS	COMBINED EFFECT
Anticoagulants, oral*	Increased anti-coagulant effect.
Antidiabetic agents, oral*	Decreased anti-diabetic effect.
Cyclosporine	Increased risk of kidney damage.
Insulin	Decreased insulin effect.

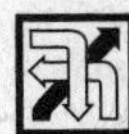

POSSIBLE INTERACTION WITH OTHER SUBSTANCES

INTERACTS WITH	COMBINED EFFECT
Alcohol:	Excessive nervous system depression. Avoid.
Beverages: Caffeine.	Rapid, irregular heartbeat. Avoid.
Cocaine:	May interfere with expected action of danazol. Avoid.
Foods:	None expected.
Marijuana:	May interfere with expected action of danazol. Avoid.
Tobacco:	Rapid, irregular heartbeat. Increased leg cramps. Avoid.

*See Glossary

DANTROLENE

BRAND NAMES

Dantrium

BASIC INFORMATION

Habit forming? No
Prescription needed? Yes
Available as generic? Yes
Drug class: Muscle relaxant, antispastic

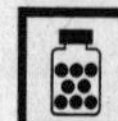

USES

- Relieves muscle spasticity caused by diseases such as multiple sclerosis, cerebral palsy, stroke.
- Relieves muscle spasticity caused by injury to spinal cord.
- Relieves or prevents excess body temperature brought on by some surgical procedures.

DOSAGE & USAGE INFORMATION

How to take:
Capsule—Swallow with liquid.

When to take:
One to 4 times a day as prescribed for muscle spasticity. For excess body temperature, follow label instructions.

If you forget a dose:
Take as soon as you remember. If it is almost time for the next dose, wait for the next scheduled dose (don't double this dose).

What drug does:
Acts directly on muscles to prevent excess contractions.

Time lapse before drug works:
1 or more weeks.

Continued next column

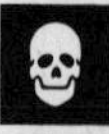

OVERDOSE

SYMPTOMS:
Shortness of breath, bloody urine, chest pain, convulsions.
WHAT TO DO:

- **Dial 911 (emergency) for medical help or call poison control center 1-800-222-1222 for instructions.**
- **If person is unconscious, check breathing and pulse. If not breathing, begin mouth-to-mouth rescue breathing. If heart is not beating, begin chest compressions.**
- **See emergency information on last 3 pages of this book.**

Don't take with:
Any other medicine or any dietary supplement without consulting your doctor or pharmacist.

POSSIBLE ADVERSE REACTIONS OR SIDE EFFECTS

SYMPTOMS	WHAT TO DO
Life-threatening:	
Seizure.	Seek emergency treatment immediately.
Common:	
Drowsiness, dizziness, weakness.	Discontinue. Call doctor right away.
Infrequent:	
• Rash, hives; black or bloody stools; chest pain; fast heartbeat; backache; blood in urine; painful, swollen feet; chills; fever; shortness of breath.	Discontinue. Call doctor right away.
• Depression, confusion, headache, slurred speech, insomnia, nervousness, diarrhea, blurred vision, difficult swallowing, appetite loss, difficult urination, decreased sexual function in males.	Continue. Call doctor when convenient.
Rare:	
• Jaundice, abdominal cramps, double vision.	Discontinue. Call doctor right away.
• Constipation.	Continue. Call doctor when convenient.

WARNINGS & PRECAUTIONS

Don't take if:
You are allergic to dantrolene or any muscle relaxant or antispastic medication.

Before you start, consult your doctor if:
- You have liver disease.
- You have heart disease.
- You have lung disease (especially emphysema).
- You are over age 35.
- You will have surgery within 2 months, including dental surgery, requiring general or spinal anesthesia.

Over age 60:
Adverse reactions and side effects may be more frequent and severe than in younger persons.

Pregnancy:
Decide with your doctor if drug benefits justify risk to unborn child. Risk category C (see page xviii).

Breast-feeding:
Avoid nursing or discontinue until you finish drug. Consult doctor.

Infants & children:
Use only under close medical supervision.

Prolonged use:
Recommended periodically during prolonged use—Blood counts, G6PD* tests, liver function studies.

Skin & sunlight:
No special problems expected.

Driving, piloting or hazardous work:
Don't drive or pilot aircraft until you learn how medicine affects you. Don't work around dangerous machinery. Don't climb ladders or work in high places. Danger increases if you drink alcohol or take medicine affecting alertness and reflexes, such as antihistamines, tranquilizers, sedatives, pain medicine, narcotics and mind-altering drugs.

Discontinuing:
Don't discontinue without consulting doctor. Dose may require gradual reduction if you have taken drug for a long time. Doses of other drugs may also require adjustment.

Others:
- No problems expected.
- Advise any doctor or dentist whom you consult that you take this medicine.

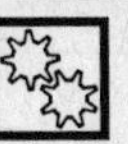

POSSIBLE INTERACTION WITH OTHER DRUGS

GENERIC NAME OR DRUG CLASS	COMBINED EFFECT
Central nervous system (CNS) depressants *	Increased risk of side effects.
Estrogens	Increased dantrolene effect.

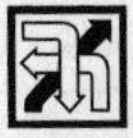

POSSIBLE INTERACTION WITH OTHER SUBSTANCES

INTERACTS WITH	COMBINED EFFECT
Alcohol:	Increased sedation, low blood pressure. Avoid.
Beverages:	None expected.
Cocaine:	Increased spasticity. Avoid.
Foods:	None expected.
Marijuana:	Increased spasticity. Avoid.
Tobacco:	May interfere with absorption of medicine.

*See Glossary

DAPSONE

BRAND NAMES

Aczone
Avlosulfon
DDS

BASIC INFORMATION

Habit forming? No
Prescription needed? Yes
Available as generic? Yes
Drug class: Antibacterial (antileprosy), sulfone

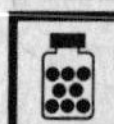

USES

- Treatment of dermatitis herpetiformis.
- Treatment of leprosy.
- Prevention and treatment of *Pneumocystis carinii* pneumonia.
- Gel form of the drug treats acne vulgaris.
- Other uses include granuloma annulare, pemphigoid, pyoderma gangrenosum, polychondritis, eye ulcerations, systemic lupus erythematosus.

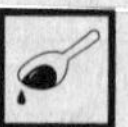

DOSAGE & USAGE INFORMATION

How to take:

- Tablet—Swallow with liquid or food to lessen stomach irritation.
- Topical gel—Follow directions provided with prescription.

When to take:
Once a day at same time.

If you forget a dose:
Take as soon as you remember. If it is almost time for the next dose, wait for the next scheduled dose (don't double this dose).

Continued next column

OVERDOSE

SYMPTOMS:
Bleeding, vomiting, seizures, cyanosis, coma.
WHAT TO DO:

- **Dial 911 (emergency) for medical help or call poison control center 1-800-222-1222 for instructions.**
- **If person is unconscious, check breathing and pulse. If not breathing, begin mouth-to-mouth rescue breathing. If heart is not beating, begin chest compressions.**
- **See emergency information on last 3 pages of this book.**

What drug does:
It helps destroy or inhibit the growth of bacteria that causes leprosy. It is unknown how it works to help dermatitis herpetiformis.

Time lapse before drug works:

- 3 years for leprosy.
- 1 to 2 weeks for dermatitis herpetiformis.

Don't take with:
Any other medicine or any dietary supplement without consulting your doctor or pharmacist.

POSSIBLE ADVERSE REACTIONS OR SIDE EFFECTS

SYMPTOMS	WHAT TO DO
Life-threatening: In case of overdose, see previous column.	
Common:	
• Rash, abdominal pain.	Discontinue. Call doctor right away.
• Appetite loss.	Continue. Call doctor when convenient.
Infrequent:	
Pale skin.	Discontinue. Call doctor right away.
Rare:	
• Dizziness; mental changes; sore throat; fever; difficult breathing; bleeding; jaundice; numbness, tingling, pain or burning in hands or feet; swelling of feet, hands, eyelids; blurred vision; anemia; peeling skin.	Discontinue. Call doctor right away.
• Headache, itching, nausea, vomiting, blue fingernails or lips. Gel form of the drug may cause skin symptoms (oily, peeling dryness, redness).	Continue. Call doctor when convenient.

WARNINGS & PRECAUTIONS

Don't take if:
- You have G6PD* deficiency.
- You are allergic to dapsone, furosemide, thiazide diuretics, sulfonylureas, carbonic anhydrase inhibitors, sulfonamides.

Before you start, consult your doctor if:
- You take any other medicine.
- You are anemic.
- You have liver or kidney disease.
- You are of Mediterranean heritage.
- You will have surgery within 2 months, including dental surgery, requiring general or spinal anesthesia.

Over age 60:
Adverse reactions and side effects may be more frequent and severe than in younger persons.

Pregnancy:
Decide with your doctor if drug benefits justify risk to unborn child. Risk category C (see page xviii).

Breast-feeding:
Drug passes into breast milk. Avoid drug or discontinue nursing until you finish medicine. Consult doctor for advice.

Infants & children:
Use under close medical supervision only.

Prolonged use:
- Request liver function studies.
- Talk to your doctor about the need for follow-up medical examinations or laboratory studies to check complete blood counts (white blood cell count, platelet count, red blood cell count, hemoglobin, hematocrit).

Skin & sunlight:
May cause rash or intensify sunburn in areas exposed to sun or ultraviolet light (photosensitivity reaction). Avoid overexposure. Notify doctor if reaction occurs.

Driving, piloting or hazardous work:
Don't drive or pilot aircraft until you learn how medicine affects you. Don't work around dangerous machinery. Don't climb ladders or work in high places. Danger increases if you drink alcohol or take medicine affecting alertness and reflexes, such as antihistamines, tranquilizers, sedatives, pain medicine, narcotics and mind-altering drugs.

Discontinuing:
Don't discontinue without consulting doctor. Dose may require gradual reduction if you have taken drug for a long time. Doses of other drugs may also require adjustment.

Others:
- This drug has been associated with serious, and sometimes fatal blood or liver problems.
- Contact your doctor right away if you develop a rash while using the gel. In rare cases it has been associated with serious, and sometimes fatal, skin reactions.
- For full effect you may need to take dapsone for many months or years.

POSSIBLE INTERACTION WITH OTHER DRUGS

GENERIC NAME OR DRUG CLASS	COMBINED EFFECT
Aminobenzoic acid (PABA)	Decreased dapsone effect. Avoid.
Antivirals, HIV/AIDS*	Increased risk of peripheral neuropathy. Reduced absorption of both drugs.
Dideoxyinosine (ddI)	Decreased dapsone effect.
Hemolytics*	May increase adverse effects on blood cells.
Methotrexate	May increase blood toxicity.
Probenecid	Increased toxicity of dapsone.
Pyrimethamine	May increase blood toxicity.
Rifampin	Decreased effect of dapsone.
Trimethoprim	May increase blood toxicity.

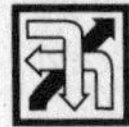

POSSIBLE INTERACTION WITH OTHER SUBSTANCES

INTERACTS WITH	COMBINED EFFECT
Alcohol:	Increased chance of toxicity to liver.
Beverages:	None expected.
Cocaine:	Increased chance of toxicity. Avoid.
Foods:	None expected.
Marijuana:	Increased chance of toxicity. Avoid.
Tobacco:	May interfere with absorption of medicine.

***See Glossary**

DECONGESTANTS (Ophthalmic)

GENERIC AND BRAND NAMES

ANTAZOLINE
Vasocon-A
NAPHAZOLINE
Ak-Con
Albalon
Albalon Liquifilm
Allerest
Clear Eyes
Comfort Eye Drops
Degest 2
Estivin II
I-Naphline
Murine Plus
Muro's Opcon
Nafazair
Naphcon
Naphcon A
Naphcon Forte
Ocu-Zoline
Vasoclear
Vasoclear A
Vasocon
Vasocon Regular
OXYMETAZOLINE
OcuClear
Visine L.R.
TETRAHYDROZOLINE
Visine

BASIC INFORMATION

Habit forming? No
Prescription needed? Yes, for some
Available as generic? Yes
Drug class: Decongestant (ophthalmic)

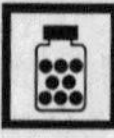

USES

Treats eye redness, itching, burning or other irritation due to dust, colds, allergies, rubbing eyes, wearing contact lenses, swimming or eye strain from close work, watching TV, reading.

OVERDOSE

SYMPTOMS:
None expected.
WHAT TO DO:
Not intended for internal use. If child accidentally swallows, call poison control center 1-800-222-1222 for help.

DOSAGE & USAGE INFORMATION

How to use:
Eye drops

- Wash hands.
- Apply pressure to inside corner of eye with middle finger.
- Tilt head backward. Pull lower lid away from eye with index finger of the same hand.
- Drop eye drops into pouch and close eye. Don't blink.
- Keep eyes closed for 1 to 2 minutes.
- Continue pressure for 1 minute after placing medicine in eye.
- Don't touch applicator tip to any surface (including the eye). If you accidentally touch tip, clean with warm water and soap.
- Keep container tightly closed.
- Keep cool, but don't freeze.
- Wash hands immediately after using.

When to use:
As directed. Usually every 3 or 4 hours.

If you forget a dose:
Use as soon as you remember.

What drug does:
Acts on small blood vessels to make them constrict or become smaller.

Time lapse before drug works:
2 to 10 minutes.

Don't use with:
Other eye drops without consulting your doctor.

POSSIBLE ADVERSE REACTIONS OR SIDE EFFECTS

SYMPTOMS	WHAT TO DO
Life-threatening:	
None expected.	
Common:	
Increased eye irritation.	Discontinue. Call doctor right away.
Infrequent:	
None expected.	
Rare:	
Blurred vision, large pupils, weakness, drowsiness, decreased body temperature, slow heartbeat, dizziness, headache, nervousness, nausea.	Discontinue. Call doctor right away.

WARNINGS & PRECAUTIONS

Don't use if:
You are allergic to any decongestant eye drops.

Before you start, consult your doctor if:
- You take antidepressants or maprotiline.
- You have glaucoma, eye disease, infection or injury.
- You have heart disease, high blood pressure, thyroid disease.

Over age 60:
No problems expected.

Pregnancy:
Decide with your doctor if drug benefits justify risk to unborn child. Risk category C (see page xviii).

Breast-feeding:
No problems expected, but check with doctor.

Infants & children:
Don't use.

Prolonged use:
Don't use for more than 3 or 4 days.

Skin & sunlight:
No problems expected.

Driving, piloting or hazardous work:
No problems expected.

Discontinuing:
May not need all the medicine in container. If symptoms disappear, stop using.

Others:
- Check with your doctor if eye irritation continues or becomes worse.
- Store product out of the reach of children.

POSSIBLE INTERACTION WITH OTHER DRUGS

GENERIC NAME OR DRUG CLASS	COMBINED EFFECT

Clinically significant interactions with oral or injected medicines unlikely.

POSSIBLE INTERACTION WITH OTHER SUBSTANCES

INTERACTS WITH	COMBINED EFFECT
Alcohol:	None expected.
Beverages:	None expected.
Cocaine:	None expected.
Foods:	None expected.
Marijuana:	None expected.
Tobacco:	Smoke may increase eye irritation. Avoid.

DEHYDROEPIANDROSTERONE (DHEA)

BRAND NAMES

Numerous brand names are available

BASIC INFORMATION

Habit forming? No
Prescription needed? No
Available as generic? Yes
Drug class: Adrenal steroid

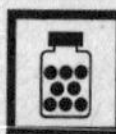

USES

DHEA is a steroid produced in the human body by the adrenal glands (which sit on top of each kidney). DHEA concentration peaks at about age 20 and then decreases progressively with age. Supplements are sold as an antiaging remedy claimed by some to improve energy, strength, and immunity. DHEA is also said to increase muscle and decrease fat. Studies to date do not provide a clear picture of the risks and benefits of DHEA.

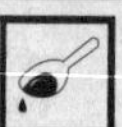

DOSAGE & USAGE INFORMATION

How to take:
For tablet or capsule—Follow instructions on the label or consult your doctor or pharmacist. Different brands supply different doses. DHEA, as a product, is marketed as a dietary supplement and is not reviewed by the U.S. Food & Drug Administration (FDA) for effectiveness and safety. The best dosage amounts are unknown. Use with caution.

When to take:
At the same times each day according to label directions.

If you forget a dose:
Follow label instructions for your particular brand of DHEA. Usually, take it as soon as you remember. If it is almost time for the next dose, wait for the next scheduled dose (don't double this dose).

Continued next column

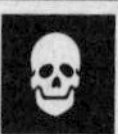

OVERDOSE

SYMPTOMS:
It is unknown what symptoms may occur.
WHAT TO DO:
If person takes much larger amount than prescribed, call doctor or poison control center 1-800-222-1222 for help.

What drug does:

- Although it is not known whether DHEA itself causes hormonal effects, the body breaks DHEA down into two hormones—estrogen and testosterone. Some people's bodies make large amounts of estrogen and testosterone from DHEA, while others make smaller amounts.
- Hormone supplements may not have the same effects on the body as naturally produced hormones have, because the body processes them differently. Higher doses of supplements may result in higher amounts of hormones in the blood than are healthy.

Time lapse before drug works:
Effectiveness will vary from person to person and will also depend on the reason for taking DHEA, such as for a chronic health problem.

Don't take with:
Any other medicine or any dietary supplement without consulting your doctor or pharmacist.

POSSIBLE ADVERSE REACTIONS OR SIDE EFFECTS

SYMPTOMS	WHAT TO DO
Life-threatening: None expected.	
Common: Unknown.	
Infrequent: In women: acne, hair loss, facial hair growth (hirsutism), deepening of voice (the last two may be irreversible).	Discontinue. Call doctor when convenient.
Rare: Unknown. If symptoms occur that you are concerned about, talk to your doctor or pharmacist. Further research may uncover other side effects.	

WARNINGS & PRECAUTIONS

Don't use if:
You are allergic to DHEA.

Before you start, consult your doctor if:
- You have any chronic health problem.
- You have a family history of cancer.
- You are allergic to any medication, food or other substance.
- You have or have had prostate, ovarian, breast, cervical or uterine cancer.

Over age 60:
A lower starting dosage may be recommended until a response is determined.

Pregnancy:
Decide with your doctor if any possible benefits of DHEA justify risk to unborn child. Risk category is unknown since DHEA is not regulated by the FDA (see page xviii).

Breast-feeding:
It is unknown if DHEA passes into milk. Avoid it or discontinue nursing until you finish medicine. Consult doctor for advice on maintaining milk supply.

Infants & children:
Not recommended for children.

Prolonged use:
Effects are unknown. More research is needed to determine long-term effects of DHEA use.

Skin & sunlight:
No problems expected.

Driving, piloting or hazardous work:
No problems expected.

Discontinuing:
No problems expected, but effects after long-term use are unknown.

Others:
- Advise any doctor or dentist whom you consult that you take DHEA.
- DHEA is not researched carefully as yet for use in humans. Most research has been performed on animals. Studies are ongoing to find more definite answers about its effect on aging, muscles, and the immune system. Studies in men and women have shown an improvement in the feeling of well being. Studies in AIDS patients and those with multiple sclerosis also have shown improvement in well being, but without an outcome change.
- Researchers are concerned that DHEA supplements may cause high levels of estrogen or testosterone in some people. The body's own testosterone plays a role in prostate cancer and high levels of naturally produced estrogen are suspected of increasing breast cancer risk. The effect of DHEA is unknown.

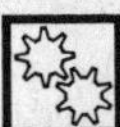

POSSIBLE INTERACTION WITH OTHER DRUGS

GENERIC NAME OR DRUG CLASS	COMBINED EFFECT
All medications	Effects are unknown. Talk to your doctor or pharmacist.

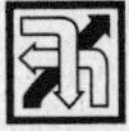

POSSIBLE INTERACTION WITH OTHER SUBSTANCES

INTERACTS WITH	COMBINED EFFECT
Alcohol:	Unknown.
Beverages:	None expected.
Cocaine:	Problems not known. Best to avoid.
Foods:	None expected.
Marijuana:	Problems not known. Best to avoid.
Tobacco:	Unknown.

*See Glossary

DESMOPRESSIN

BRAND NAMES

DDAVP
Stimate

BASIC INFORMATION

Habit forming? No
Prescription needed? Yes
Available as generic? Yes
Drug class: Antidiuretic, antihemorrhagic

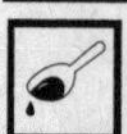

USES

- Prevents and controls symptoms associated with central diabetes insipidus.
- The tablet form (not the nasal spray) of the drug is used to treat primary nocturnal enuresis (bedwetting during sleep).

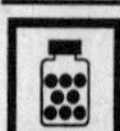

DOSAGE & USAGE INFORMATION

How to take:

- Tablet—Swallow with liquid.
- Nasal spray—Fill the rhinyle (a flexible, calibrated catheter) with a measured dose of the nasal spray. Blow on the other end of the catheter to deposit the solution deep in the nasal cavity.

When to take:
At the same time each day, according to instructions on prescription label. Be sure to restrict fluid intake from 1 hour before to 8 hours after taking drug.

If you forget a dose:
Take as soon as you remember. If it is almost time for the next dose, wait for the next scheduled dose (don't double this dose).

What drug does:
Increases water reabsorption in the kidney and decreases urine output.

Time lapse before drug works:
Within 1 hour. Effect may last from 6 to 24 hours.

Don't take with:
Any other medicine or any dietary supplement without consulting your doctor or pharmacist.

OVERDOSE

SYMPTOMS:
Confusion, coma, seizures.
WHAT TO DO:
Overdose unlikely to threaten life. If person uses much larger amount than prescribed or if accidentally swallowed, call doctor or poison control center 1-800-222-1222 for help.

POSSIBLE ADVERSE REACTIONS OR SIDE EFFECTS

SYMPTOMS	WHAT TO DO
Life-threatening:	
Rare allergic reaction (hives, itching, rash, trouble breathing, tightness in chest, swelling of lips or tongue or face).	Seek emergency treatment immediately.
Common:	
None expected.	
Infrequent:	
Flushing or redness of skin, headache, nausea, nasal congestion.	Continue. Call doctor when convenient.
Rare:	
Water intoxication—confusion, drowsiness, headache, seizures, rapid weight gain, decreased urination (very rare); low sodium level in the body (symptoms include nausea, vomiting, muscle cramps, fatigue, weakness).	Discontinue. Seek emergency treatment.

WARNINGS & PRECAUTIONS

Don't take if:
You or your child is allergic to desmopressin.

Before you start, consult your doctor if:
- You have allergic rhinitis.
- You have nasal congestion.
- You have a cold or other upper respiratory infection or are dehydrated.
- You have heart disease or high blood pressure.
- You have a history of hyponatremia, which is low sodium (salt) levels in the body.
- You have polydipsia (excessive or abnormal thirstiness).
- You have cystic fibrosis.

Over age 60:
Increased risk of water intoxication.

Pregnancy:
No proven harm to unborn child, but avoid if possible. Consult doctor. Risk category B (see page xviii).

Breast-feeding:
Drug passes into milk. Avoid drug or discontinue nursing until you finish medicine. Consult doctor for advice on maintaining milk supply.

Infants & children:
More sensitive to effect. Use only under close medical supervision.

Prolonged use:
May require increasing dosage for same effect.

Skin & sunlight:
No special problems expected.

Driving, piloting or hazardous work:
Don't drive or pilot aircraft until you learn how medicine affects you. Don't work around dangerous machinery. Don't climb ladders or work in high places. Danger increases if you drink alcohol or take medicine affecting alertness and reflexes.

Discontinuing:
No special problems expected.

Others:
- Advise any doctor or dentist whom you consult that you take this medicine.
- Be sure to carefully follow all instructions for use of intranasal desmopressin.
- Consult doctor if the amount of water the patient is drinking changes.
- Treatment with desmopressin tablets for primary nocturnal enuresis should be stopped during illnesses with symptoms of fever, recurrent vomiting, or diarrhea that may lead to fluid and/or electrolyte imbalance.
- If sodium levels fall too much causing hyponatremia, the patient could have seizures and in extreme cases, may die.
- The drug should be used cautiously in patients who may be drinking a lot of fluids (such as during hot weather or when doing vigorous exercising) due to a higher risk of hyponatremia.

POSSIBLE INTERACTION WITH OTHER DRUGS

GENERIC NAME OR DRUG CLASS	COMBINED EFFECT
Antidepressants, tricyclic (TCA)*	Increased risk of thirstiness which may lead to drinking excess fluids.
Carbamazepine	May increase desmopressin effect.
Chlorpropamide	May increase desmopressin effect.
Clofibrate	May increase desmopressin effect.
Demeclocycline	May decrease desmopressin effect.
Lithium	May decrease desmopressin effect.
Norepinephrine	May decrease desmopressin effect.
Selective serotonin reuptake inhibitors (SSRIs)	Increased risk of thirstiness which may lead to drinking excess fluids.

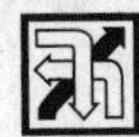

POSSIBLE INTERACTION WITH OTHER SUBSTANCES

INTERACTS WITH	COMBINED EFFECT
Alcohol:	May decrease desmopressin effect.
Beverages: Caffeine drinks.	May decrease desmopressin effect.
Cocaine:	May decrease desmopressin effect.
Foods:	None expected.
Marijuana:	May decrease desmopressin effect.
Tobacco:	May decrease desmopressin effect.

*See Glossary

DEXTROMETHORPHAN

BRAND NAMES

See full list of brand names in the *Generic and Brand Name Directory*, page 881.

BASIC INFORMATION

Habit forming? No
Prescription needed? No
Available as generic? Yes
Drug class: Cough suppressant, antitussive

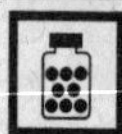

USES

Suppresses cough associated with allergies or infections such as colds, bronchitis, flu and lung disorders. Used in many cough, cold and allergy combination medicines.

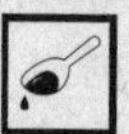

DOSAGE & USAGE INFORMATION

How to take:

- Chewable tablet—Chew well, then swallow.
- Oral suspension, lozenge or syrup—Take as directed on label.
- Thin strip—Allow strips to dissolve on the tongue. Water or other fluid is not needed.
- Capsule—Swallow with liquid.

When to take:
As needed, no more often than every 4 hours or as directed on label.

If you forget a dose:
Take as soon as you remember. If it is almost time for the next dose, wait for the next scheduled dose (don't double this dose).

What drug does:
Reduces sensitivity of brain's cough control center, suppressing urge to cough.

Continued next column

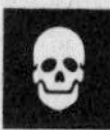

OVERDOSE

SYMPTOMS:
Euphoria, overactivity, sense of intoxication, hallucinations, lack of coordination, stagger, stupor, shallow breathing.
WHAT TO DO:

- **Dial 911 (emergency) for medical help or call poison control center 1-800-222-1222 for instructions.**
- **See emergency information on last 3 pages of this book.**

Time lapse before drug works:
15 to 30 minutes.

Don't take with:
Any other medicine or any dietary supplement without consulting your doctor or pharmacist.

POSSIBLE ADVERSE REACTIONS OR SIDE EFFECTS

SYMPTOMS	WHAT TO DO
Life-threatening: None expected.	
Common: None expected.	
Infrequent: Mild dizziness or drowsiness, nausea or vomiting, stomach cramps, constipation, headache.	Discontinue. Call doctor if symptoms persist.
Rare: None expected.	

WARNINGS & PRECAUTIONS

Don't take if:
You are allergic to dextromethorphan.

Before you start, consult your doctor if:
- You have asthma attacks.
- You have impaired liver function.

Over age 60:
Adverse reactions and side effects may be more frequent and severe than in younger persons. You may require smaller doses for shorter periods of time.

Pregnancy:
Decide with your doctor if drug benefits justify risk to unborn child. Risk category C (see page xviii).

Breast-feeding:
No proven problems. Consult doctor.

Infants & children:
Read the label on the product to see if it is approved for your child's age. Always follow the directions on product's label about how to use. If unsure, ask your doctor or pharmacist.

Prolonged use:
No problems expected.

Skin & sunlight:
No problems expected.

Driving, piloting or hazardous work:
Don't drive or pilot aircraft until you learn how medicine affects you. Don't work around dangerous machinery. Don't climb ladders or work in high places. Danger increases if you drink alcohol or take medicine affecting alertness and reflexes, such as antihistamines, tranquilizers, sedatives, pain medicine, narcotics and mind-altering drugs.

Discontinuing:
May be unnecessary to finish medicine. Follow doctor's instructions.

Others:
- If cough persists or if you cough blood or brown-yellow, thick mucus, call your doctor.
- Excessive use may lead to functional dependence.*

POSSIBLE INTERACTION WITH OTHER DRUGS

GENERIC NAME OR DRUG CLASS	COMBINED EFFECT
Doxepin (topical)	Increased risk of toxicity of both drugs.
Memantine	May lead to adverse effects of either drug.
Monoamine oxidase (MAO) inhibitors*	Disorientation, high fever, drop in blood pressure and loss of consciousness.
Sedatives* and other central nervous system (CNS) depressants*	Increased sedative effect of both drugs.

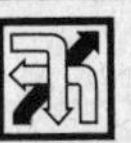

POSSIBLE INTERACTION WITH OTHER SUBSTANCES

INTERACTS WITH	COMBINED EFFECT
Alcohol:	None expected.
Beverages: Grapefruit juice.	Risk of toxicity. Avoid.
Cocaine:	Decreased dextromethorphan effect. Avoid.
Foods:	None expected.
Marijuana:	None expected.
Tobacco:	Smoking increases mucus in lungs. Avoid.

*See Glossary

DICLOFENAC (Topical)

BRAND NAMES

Flector Patch
Pennsaid
Voltaren Gel

BASIC INFORMATION

Habit forming? No
Prescription needed? Yes
Available as generic? No
Drug class: Nonsteroidal anti-inflammatory drug (NSAID), topical

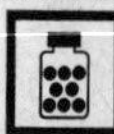

USES

- Used for joint pain in the hands, wrists, elbows, knees, ankles or feet caused by osteoarthritis.
- Patch is used to treat pain due to minor strains, sprains and bruises.
- May be used for treatment of other disorders as determined by your doctor.
- A brand named Solaraze is used to treat actinic keratosis. It is not covered in this topic.

DOSAGE & USAGE INFORMATION

How to use:

- Gel—Follow instructions provided with the prescription. The gel comes with dosing cards that show you how much to use for a 2-gram- or a 4-gram dose. Do not use more than 4 times a day on a single joint. Do not wear gloves for at least 10 minutes after applying gel to the hands. Wait at least 10 minutes before dressing. Do not bathe or shower for at least 1 hour after application. Don't use drug on wounded or sore skin. Don't cover treated area with bandage.
- Patch—Apply to most painful area twice daily. Wash hands after applying patch. Do not wear patch in bath or shower.
- Solution—Apply as directed on label.

When to take:
Follow your doctor's or label's instructions.

Continued next column

OVERDOSE

SYMPTOMS:
May have lethargy, drowsiness, nausea, vomiting, stomach pain.
WHAT TO DO:
If person uses much larger amount than prescribed or if accidentally swallowed, call doctor or poison control center 1-800-222-1222 for help.

If you forget a dose:
Apply as soon as you remember. If it is almost time for next treatment, wait and apply at regular time (don't double this dose).

What drug does:
It is applied to and absorbed by the affected joint. It works by reducing certain hormones that cause inflammation and pain in the body.

Time lapse before drug works:
It may take several weeks or more of treatment to determine full benefit of the drug.

Don't take with:

- Any other medicine or diet supplement without consulting your doctor or pharmacist.
- Other skin products (cosmetics, sunscreen, lotions, insect repellant or other topical drugs) not prescribed by your doctor.

POSSIBLE ADVERSE REACTIONS OR SIDE EFFECTS

SYMPTOMS	WHAT TO DO
Life-threatening:	
Rare allergic reaction if too much absorbed by body (hives; difficulty breathing; swelling of face, lips, tongue, throat).	Seek emergency treatment immediately.
Common:	
Skin reaction where product is applied.	Continue. Call doctor when convenient.
Infrequent:	
None expected.	
Rare:	
These side effects may occur if drug is absorbed into blood-stream: chest pain, shortness of breath, weakness, slurred speech, vision changes loss of balance, stool changes (black, bloody, tarry or clay-color), vomiting blood or what looks like coffee grounds, swelling, rapid weight gain, change in urination, dark urine, nausea, stomach pain, appetite loss, yellow skin or eyes, sore throat and headache, severe skin rash (blistering, red, peeling), bruising, severe tingling, numbness, fever, muscle weakness, any skin rash.	Discontinue. Call doctor right away.

WARNINGS & PRECAUTIONS

Don't take if:
You are allergic to diclofenac or have had an allergic reaction after taking aspirin or any non-steroidal anti-inflammatory drug (NSAID).

Before you start, consult your doctor if:
- You have had or will have heart bypass surgery.
- You have a history of asthma.
- You have a history of stomach ulcer or gastrointestinal bleeding.
- You have kidney or liver disease.
- You have high blood pressure, congestive heart failure or other heart or blood vessel disorder.

Over age 60:
Adverse reactions and side effects may be more frequent and severe than in younger persons.

Pregnancy:
Decide with your doctor if drug benefits justify risk to unborn child. Risk category C (see page xviii).

Breast-feeding:
Drug may be absorbed into body and pass into breast milk. Consult doctor.

Infants & children:
Not approved for children under age 18.

Prolonged use:
- Talk to your doctor about the need for follow-up medical exams and/or blood tests and liver and kidney function studies.
- Long-term continuous use may increase the risk of heart attack or stroke. Consult doctor.

Skin & sunlight:
Avoid exposure of treated skin areas to sunlight or artificial UV rays (sunlamps or tanning beds).

Driving, piloting or hazardous work:
No special problems expected.

Discontinuing:
No special problems expected.

Others:
- Though rare, the drug may be absorbed into your bloodstream and increase the risk of life-threatening heart or circulation problems, including heart attack or stroke. There is also increased risk of serious gastrointestinal problems (e.g., bleeding, ulcers and perforation of the stomach or intestines) which may be fatal.
- Rarely, serious liver problems (necrosis, jaundice, hepatitis, failure) may occur with use of this drug. May lead to need for liver transplant or even death. Consult doctor about the risks.
- Advise any doctor or dentist whom you consult that you use this medicine.
- Avoid getting the drug in your mouth or eyes. If it does get into these areas, rinse with water. Do not apply to wounded or broken skin. Follow product instructions for proper disposal of gel dose cards and patches.
- Do not expose treated areas to heat from a hot tub, heating pad, sauna, or heated water bed. Heat can increase the amount of drug absorbed through the skin and may cause adverse effects.

POSSIBLE INTERACTION WITH OTHER DRUGS

GENERIC NAME OR DRUG CLASS	COMBINED EFFECT
Angiotensin-converting enzyme (ACE) inhibitors*	May decrease ACE inhibitor effect.
Anticoagulants*	May increase risk of internal bleeding.
Anti-inflammatory drugs, nonsteroidal (NSAIDs)* oral	May increase risk of side effects.
Aspirin	May increase risk of side effects.
Cyclosporine	May increase effect of cyclosporine.
Diuretics*	May decrease effect of diuretic.
Hepatotoxics*	Increased risk of liver problems.
Lithium	May increase effect of lithium.
Methotrexate	May increase effect of methotrexate.
Topical skin products	Unknown effect. Consult doctor

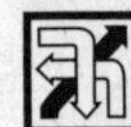

POSSIBLE INTERACTION WITH OTHER SUBSTANCES

INTERACTS WITH	COMBINED EFFECT
Alcohol:	May increase risk of side effects.
Beverages:	None expected.
Cocaine:	Unknown. Avoid.
Foods:	None expected.
Marijuana:	Unknown. Avoid.
Tobacco:	May increase risk of side effects.

***See Glossary**

DICYCLOMINE

BRAND NAMES

See full list of brand names in the *Generic and Brand Name Directory*, page 883.

BASIC INFORMATION

Habit forming? No
Prescription needed? Yes
Available as generic? Yes
Drug class: Antispasmodic, anticholinergic

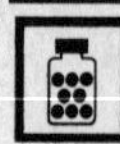

USES

- Reduces spasms of digestive system, bladder and urethra.
- Treats irritable bowel syndrome.

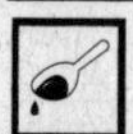

DOSAGE & USAGE INFORMATION

How to take:
Tablet, syrup or capsule—Swallow with liquid or food to lessen stomach irritation.

When to take:
30 minutes before meals (unless directed otherwise by doctor).

If you forget a dose:
Take as soon as you remember. If it is almost time for the next dose, wait for the next scheduled dose (don't double this dose).

What drug does:
Blocks nerve impulses at parasympathetic nerve endings, preventing muscle contractions and gland secretions of organs involved.

Time lapse before drug works:
15 to 30 minutes.

Don't take with:
Any other medicine or any dietary supplement without consulting your doctor or pharmacist.

OVERDOSE

SYMPTOMS:
Dilated pupils, blurred vision, rapid pulse and breathing, dizziness, fever, hallucinations, confusion, slurred speech, agitation, flushed face, convulsions, coma.
WHAT TO DO:
- **Dial 911 (emergency) for medical help or call poison control center 1-800-222-1222 for instructions.**
- **See emergency information on last 3 pages of this book.**

POSSIBLE ADVERSE REACTIONS OR SIDE EFFECTS

SYMPTOMS	WHAT TO DO
Life-threatening:	
Hives, rash, intense itching, faintness soon after a dose (anaphylaxis).	Seek emergency treatment immediately.
Common:	
• Confusion, delirium, rapid heartbeat.	Discontinue. Call doctor right away.
• Nausea, vomiting.	Discontinue. Call doctor when convenient.
• Constipation, loss of taste, decreased sweating.	Continue. Tell doctor at next visit.
• Dry ears, nose, throat, mouth.	No action necessary.
Infrequent:	
• Lightheadedness.	Discontinue. Call doctor right away.
• Headache, difficult urination, nasal congestion, altered taste.	Continue. Call doctor when convenient.
Rare:	
Rash or hives, eye pain, blurred vision.	Discontinue. Call doctor right away.

WARNINGS & PRECAUTIONS

Don't take if:
- You are allergic to any anticholinergic.
- You have trouble with stomach bloating.
- You have difficulty emptying your bladder completely.
- You have narrow-angle glaucoma.
- You have severe ulcerative colitis.

Before you start, consult your doctor if:
- You have open-angle glaucoma.
- You have angina, chronic bronchitis or asthma.
- You have hiatal hernia, liver disease, kidney or thyroid disease, enlarged prostate, myasthenia gravis, peptic ulcer.
- You will have surgery within 2 months, including dental surgery, requiring general or spinal anesthesia.

Over age 60:
Adverse reactions and side effects may be more frequent and severe than in younger persons.

Pregnancy:
Decide with your doctor whether drug benefits justify risk to unborn child. Risk category C (see page xviii).

Breast-feeding:
Drug passes into milk and decreases milk flow. Avoid drug or discontinue nursing until you finish medicine. Consult doctor for advice on maintaining milk supply.

Infants & children:
Use only under medical supervision.

Prolonged use:
Chronic constipation, possible fecal impaction. Consult doctor immediately.

Skin & sunlight:
No problems expected.

Driving, piloting or hazardous work:
Use disqualifies you for piloting aircraft. Otherwise, no problems expected.

Discontinuing:
May be unnecessary to finish medicine. Follow doctor's instructions.

Others:
Advise any doctor or dentist whom you consult that you take this medicine.

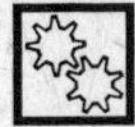

POSSIBLE INTERACTION WITH OTHER DRUGS

GENERIC NAME OR DRUG CLASS	COMBINED EFFECT
Adrenocorticoids, systemic	Possible glaucoma.
Amantadine	Increased dicyclomine effect.
Antacids*	Decreased dicyclomine effect.
Anticholinergics, other*	Increased dicyclomine effect.
Antidepressants, tricyclic*	Increased dicyclomine effect. Increased sedation.
Antidiarrheals*	Decreased dicyclomine effect.
Antihistamines*	Increased dicyclomine effect.
Attapulgite	Decreased dicyclomine effect.
Buclizine	Increased dicyclomine effect.
Digitalis	Possible decreased absorption of digitalis.
Haloperidol	Increased internal eye pressure.
Ketoconazole	Decreased ketoconazole effect.
Meperidine	Increased dicyclomine effect.
Methylphenidate	Increased dicyclomine effect.
Monoamine oxidase (MAO) inhibitors*	Increased dicyclomine effect.
Nitrates*	Increased internal eye pressure.
Nizatidine	Increased nizatidine effect.
Orphenadrine	Increased dicyclomine effect.
Phenothiazines*	Increased dicyclomine effect.
Pilocarpine	Loss of pilocarpine effect in glaucoma treatment.
Potassium supplements*	Possible intestinal ulcers with oral potassium tablets.
Quinidine	Increased dicyclomine effect.
Sedatives* or central nervous system (CNS) depressants*	Increased sedative effect of both drugs.
Vitamin C	Decreased dicyclomine effect. Avoid large doses of vitamin C.

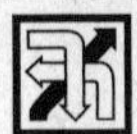

POSSIBLE INTERACTION WITH OTHER SUBSTANCES

INTERACTS WITH	COMBINED EFFECT
Alcohol:	None expected.
Beverages:	None expected.
Cocaine:	Excessively rapid heartbeat. Avoid.
Foods:	None expected.
Marijuana:	Drowsiness and dry mouth.
Tobacco:	None expected.

DIFENOXIN & ATROPINE

BRAND NAMES

Motofen

BASIC INFORMATION

Habit forming? Yes
Prescription needed? Yes
Available as generic? No
Drug class: Antidiarrheal

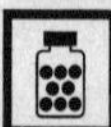

USES

- Reduces spasms of digestive system.
- Treats severe diarrhea.

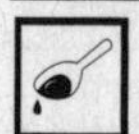

DOSAGE & USAGE INFORMATION

How to take:
Tablet—Swallow with liquid or food to lessen stomach irritation.

When to take:
After each loose stool or every 3 to 4 hours. No more than 5 tablets in 12 hours.

If you forget a dose:
Take as soon as you remember. Don't double this dose.

What drug does:
- Blocks nerve impulses at parasympathetic nerve endings, preventing muscle contractions and gland secretions of organs involved.
- Acts on brain to decrease spasm of smooth muscle.

Time lapse before drug works:
40 to 60 minutes.

Continued next column

OVERDOSE

SYMPTOMS:
Dilated pupils, rapid pulse and breathing, dizziness, fever, hallucinations, confusion, slurred speech, agitation, flushed face, convulsions, coma.
WHAT TO DO:
- **Dial 911 (emergency) for medical help or call poison control center 1-800-222-1222 for instructions.**
- **See emergency information on last 3 pages of this book.**

Don't take with:
Any medicine that will decrease mental alertness or reflexes, such as alcohol, other mind-altering drugs, cough/cold medicines, antihistamines, allergy medicine, sedatives, tranquilizers (sleeping pills or "downers") barbiturates, seizure medicine, narcotics, other prescription medicines for pain, muscle relaxants, anesthetics.

POSSIBLE ADVERSE REACTIONS OR SIDE EFFECTS

SYMPTOMS	WHAT TO DO
Life-threatening:	
Shortness of breath, agitation, nervousness.	Discontinue. Seek emergency treatment.
Common:	
Dizziness, drowsiness.	Continue. Call doctor when convenient.
Infrequent:	
• Bloating; constipation; appetite loss; abdominal pain; blurred vision; warm, flushed skin; fast heartbeat; dry mouth.	Discontinue. Call doctor right away.
• Frequent urination, lightheadedness, dry skin, headache, insomnia.	Continue. Call doctor when convenient.
Rare:	
Weakness, confusion, fever.	Continue. Call doctor when convenient.

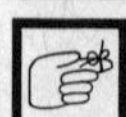

WARNINGS & PRECAUTIONS

Don't take if:
- You are allergic to any anticholinergic.
- You have trouble with stomach bloating, difficulty emptying your bladder completely, narrow-angle glaucoma, severe ulcerative colitis.
- You are dehydrated.

Before you start, consult your doctor if:
- You have open-angle glaucoma, angina, chronic bronchitis, asthma, liver disease, hiatal hernia, enlarged prostate, myasthenia gravis, peptic ulcer.
- You will have surgery within 2 months, including dental surgery, requiring general or spinal anesthesia.

Over age 60:
Adverse reactions and side effects may be more frequent and severe than in younger persons.

Pregnancy:
Decide with your doctor whether drug benefits justify risk to unborn child. Risk category C (see page xviii).

Breast-feeding:
Drug passes into milk. Avoid drug or discontinue nursing until you finish medicine. Consult doctor for advice on maintaining milk supply.

Infants & children:
Use only under medical supervision.

Prolonged use:
- Chronic constipation, possible fecal impaction. Consult doctor immediately.
- Talk to your doctor about the need for follow-up medical examinations or laboratory studies to check liver function.

Skin & sunlight:
No problems expected.

Driving, piloting or hazardous work:
Use disqualifies you for piloting aircraft. Don't drive until you learn how medicine affects you. Don't work around dangerous machinery. Don't climb ladders or work in high places. Danger increases if you drink alcohol or take medicine affecting alertness and reflexes, such as antihistamines, tranquilizers, sedatives, pain medicine, narcotics and mind-altering drugs.

Discontinuing:
May be unnecessary to finish medicine. Follow doctor's instructions.

Others:
Atropine included at doses below therapeutic level to prevent abuse.

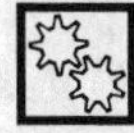

POSSIBLE INTERACTION WITH OTHER DRUGS

GENERIC NAME OR DRUG CLASS	COMBINED EFFECT
Addictive substances (narcotics,* others)	Increased chance of abuse.
Amantadine	Increased atropine effect.
Anticholinergics, other*	Increased atropine effect.
Antidepressants, tricyclic (TCA)*	Increased atropine effect. Increased sedation.
Antihistamines*	Increased atropine effect.
Antihypertensives*	Increased sedation.
Clozapine	Toxic effect on the central nervous system.
Cortisone drugs*	Increased internal eye pressure.
Ethinamate	Dangerous increased effects of ethinamate. Avoid combining.
Fluoxetine	Increased depressant effects of both drugs.
Guanfacine	May increase depressant effects of either drug.
Haloperidol	Increased internal eye pressure.
Leucovorin	High alcohol content of leucovorin may cause adverse effects.
Meperidine	Increased atropine effect.
Methylphenidate	Increased atropine effect.
Methyprylon	Increased sedative effect, perhaps to dangerous level. Avoid.
Monoamine oxidase (MAO) inhibitors*	Increased atropine effect.
Nabilone	Greater depression of central nervous system.
Naltrexone	Triggers withdrawal symptoms.
Narcotics*	Increased sedation. Avoid.

Continued on page 913

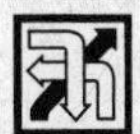

POSSIBLE INTERACTION WITH OTHER SUBSTANCES

INTERACTS WITH	COMBINED EFFECT
Alcohol:	Increased sedation. Avoid.
Beverages:	None expected.
Cocaine:	Excessively rapid heartbeat. Avoid.
Foods:	None expected.
Marijuana:	Drowsiness and dry mouth.
Tobacco:	May increase diarrhea. Avoid.

*See Glossary

DIGITALIS PREPARATIONS (Digitalis Glycosides)

GENERIC AND BRAND NAMES

DIGITOXIN
Crystodigin

DIGOXIN
Lanoxicaps
Lanoxin
Novodigoxin

BASIC INFORMATION

Habit forming? No
Prescription needed? Yes
Available as generic? Yes
Drug class: Digitalis preparation

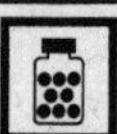

USES

- Strengthens weak heart muscle contractions to prevent congestive heart failure.
- Corrects irregular heartbeat.

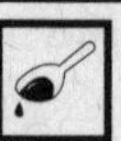

DOSAGE & USAGE INFORMATION

How to take:
- Tablet or capsule—Swallow with liquid. If you can't swallow whole, crumble tablet or open capsule and take with liquid or food.
- Liquid—Dilute dose in beverage before swallowing.

When to take:
At the same time each day.

If you forget a dose:
Take as soon as you remember. If it is almost time for the next dose, wait for the next scheduled dose (don't double this dose).

What drug does:
- Strengthens heart muscle contraction.
- Delays nerve impulses to heart.

Time lapse before drug works:
May require regular use for a week or more.

Continued next column

OVERDOSE

SYMPTOMS:
Nausea, vomiting, diarrhea, vision disturbances, halos around lights, fatigue, irregular heartbeat, confusion, hallucinations, convulsions.
WHAT TO DO:
- **Dial 911 (emergency) for medical help or call poison control center 1-800-222-1222 for instructions.**
- **See emergency information on last 3 pages of this book.**

Don't take with:
Any other medicine or any dietary supplement without consulting your doctor or pharmacist.

POSSIBLE ADVERSE REACTIONS OR SIDE EFFECTS

SYMPTOMS	WHAT TO DO
Life-threatening: In case of overdose, see previous column.	
Common:	
Appetite loss, diarrhea.	Continue. Call doctor when convenient.
Infrequent:	
Extreme drowsiness, lethargy, disorientation, headache, fainting.	Discontinue. Call doctor right away.
Rare:	
• Rash, hives, cardiac arrhythmias, hallucinations, psychosis.	Discontinue. Call doctor right away.
• Double or yellow-green vision; enlarged, sensitive male breasts; tiredness; weakness; depression; decreased sex drive.	Continue. Call doctor when convenient.

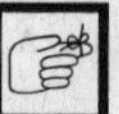

WARNINGS & PRECAUTIONS

Don't take if:
- You are allergic to any digitalis preparation.
- Your heartbeat is slower than 50 beats per minute.

Before you start, consult your doctor if:
- You have taken another digitalis preparation in past 2 weeks.
- You have taken a diuretic within 2 weeks.
- You have liver or kidney disease.
- You have a thyroid disorder.
- You will have surgery within 2 months, including dental surgery, requiring general or spinal anesthesia.

Over age 60:
Adverse reactions and side effects may be more frequent and severe than in younger persons.

Pregnancy:
Decide with your doctor if drug benefits justify risk to unborn child. Risk category C (see page xviii).

Breast-feeding:
Drug filters into milk. May harm child. Avoid.

Infants & children:
Use only under medical supervision.

DIGITALIS PREPARATIONS (Digitalis Glycosides)

Prolonged use:
Talk to your doctor about the need for follow-up medical examinations or laboratory studies to check ECG,* liver function, kidney function, serum electrolytes.

Skin & sunlight:
No problems expected.

Driving, piloting or hazardous work:
Possible vision disturbances. Otherwise, no problems expected.

Discontinuing:
Don't stop without doctor's advice.

Others:
Some digitalis products contain tartrazine dye. Avoid, especially if you are allergic to aspirin.

POSSIBLE INTERACTION WITH OTHER DRUGS

GENERIC NAME OR DRUG CLASS	COMBINED EFFECT
Adrenocorticoids, systemic	Dangerous potassium depletion. Possible digitalis toxicity.
Amiodarone	Increased digitalis effect.
Amphotericin B	Decreased potassium. Increased toxicity of amphotericin B.
Antacids*	Decreased digitalis effect.
Anticonvulsants, hydantoin*	Increased digitalis effect at first, then decreased.
Anticholinergics*	Possible increased digitalis effect.
Attapulgite	May decrease effectiveness of digitalis.
Beta-adrenergic blocking agents*	Increased digitalis effect.
Beta-agonists*	Increased risk of heartbeat irregularity.
Calcium supplements*	Decreased digitalis effects.
Carteolol	Can either increase or decrease heart rate. Improves irregular heartbeat.
Cholestyramine	Decreased digitalis effect.
Colestipol	Decreased digitalis effect.
Dextrothyroxine	Decreased digitalis effect.
Disopyramide	Possible decreased digitalis effect.
Diuretics*	Excessive potassium loss that may cause irregular heartbeat.
DPP-4 inhibitors	Digoxin dosage may need to be adjusted.
Ephedrine	Disturbed heart rhythm. Avoid.
Epinephrine	Disturbed heart rhythm. Avoid.
Erythromycins*	May increase digitalis absorption.
Flecainide	May increase digitalis blood level.
Fluoxetine	Confusion, agitation, convulsions and high blood pressure. Avoid combining.
Hydroxychloroquine	Possible increased digitalis toxicity.
Itraconazole	Possible toxic levels of digitalis.
Laxatives*	Decreased digitalis effect.
Metformin	Increased metformin effect.

Continued on page 913

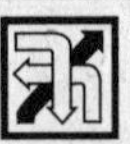

POSSIBLE INTERACTION WITH OTHER SUBSTANCES

INTERACTS WITH	COMBINED EFFECT
Alcohol:	None expected.
Beverages: Caffeine drinks.	Irregular heartbeat. Avoid.
Cocaine:	Irregular heartbeat. Avoid.
Foods: Prune juice, bran cereals, foods high in fiber.	Decreased digitalis effect.
Marijuana:	Decreased digitalis effect.
Tobacco:	Irregular heartbeat. Avoid.

***See Glossary**

DIPHENIDOL

BRAND NAMES

Vontrol

BASIC INFORMATION

Habit forming? No
Prescription needed? Yes
Available as generic? No
Drug class: Antiemetic, antivertigo

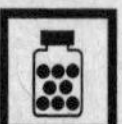

USES

- Prevents motion sickness.
- Controls nausea and vomiting (do not use during pregnancy).

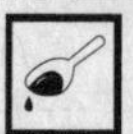

DOSAGE & USAGE INFORMATION

How to take:
Tablet—Swallow with liquid or food to lessen stomach irritation. If you can't swallow whole, crumble tablet and chew or take with liquid or food.

When to take:
30 to 60 minutes before traveling.

If you forget a dose:
Take as soon as you remember. If it is almost time for the next dose, wait for the next scheduled dose (don't double this dose).

What drug does:
Reduces sensitivity of nerve endings in inner ear, blocking messages to brain's vomiting center.

Time lapse before drug works:
30 to 60 minutes.

Don't take with:
Any other medicine or any dietary supplement without consulting your doctor or pharmacist.

OVERDOSE

SYMPTOMS:
Drowsiness, confusion, incoordination, weak pulse, shallow breathing, stupor, coma.
WHAT TO DO:

- **Dial 911 (emergency) for medical help or call poison control center 1-800-222-1222 for instructions.**
- **See emergency information on last 3 pages of this book.**

POSSIBLE ADVERSE REACTIONS OR SIDE EFFECTS

SYMPTOMS	WHAT TO DO
Life-threatening: In case of overdose, see previous column.	
Common:	
Drowsiness.	Continue. Tell doctor at next visit.
Infrequent:	
• Headache, diarrhea or constipation, heartburn.	Continue. Call doctor when convenient.
• Dry mouth, nose or throat; dizziness.	Continue. Tell doctor at next visit.
Rare:	
• Hallucinations, confusion.	Discontinue. Seek emergency treatment.
• Rash or hives, depression, jaundice.	Discontinue. Call doctor right away.
• Restlessness; excitement; insomnia; blurred vision; urgent, painful or difficult urination.	Continue. Call doctor when convenient.
• Appetite loss, nausea, weakness.	Continue. Tell doctor at next visit.

WARNINGS & PRECAUTIONS

Don't take if:
- You have severe kidney disease.
- You are allergic to diphenidol or meclizine.

Before you start, consult your doctor if:
- You have prostate enlargement.
- You have glaucoma.
- You have heart disease.
- You have intestinal obstruction or ulcers in the gastrointestinal tract.
- You have kidney disease.
- You have low blood pressure.
- You will have surgery within 2 months, including dental surgery, requiring general or spinal anesthesia.

Over age 60:
Adverse reactions and side effects may be more frequent and severe than in younger persons.

Pregnancy:
Decide with your doctor whether drug benefits justify risk to unborn child. Risk category C (see page xviii).

Breast-feeding:
Drug passes into milk. Avoid drug or discontinue nursing until you finish medicine. Consult doctor for advice on maintaining milk supply.

Infants & children:
No problems expected.

Prolonged use:
No problems expected.

Skin & sunlight:
No problems expected.

Driving, piloting or hazardous work:
Don't fly aircraft. Don't drive until you learn how medicine affects you. Don't work around dangerous machinery. Don't climb ladders or work in high places. Danger increases if you drink alcohol or take medicine affecting alertness and reflexes, such as antihistamines, tranquilizers, sedatives, pain medicine, narcotics and mind-altering drugs.

Discontinuing:
No problems expected.

Others:
Advise any doctor or dentist whom you consult that you use this medicine.

POSSIBLE INTERACTION WITH OTHER DRUGS

GENERIC NAME OR DRUG CLASS	COMBINED EFFECT
Anticonvulsants*	Increased effect of both drugs.
Antidepressants, tricyclic*	Increased sedative effect of both drugs.
Antihistamines*	Increased sedative effect of both drugs.
Atropine	Increased chance of toxic effect of atropine and atropine-like medicines.
Narcotics*	Increased sedative effect of both drugs.
Sedatives*	Increased sedative effect of both drugs.
Tranquilizers*	Increased sedative effect of both drugs.

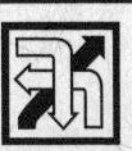

POSSIBLE INTERACTION WITH OTHER SUBSTANCES

INTERACTS WITH	COMBINED EFFECT
Alcohol:	Increased sedation. Avoid.
Beverages: Caffeine.	May decrease drowsiness.
Cocaine:	Increased chance of toxic effects of cocaine. Avoid.
Foods:	None expected.
Marijuana:	Increased drowsiness, dry mouth.
Tobacco:	None expected.

*See Glossary

DIPHENOXYLATE & ATROPINE

BRAND NAMES

Diphenatol	Lomotil
Lofene	Lonox
Logen	Lo-Trol
Lomanate	Nor-Mil

BASIC INFORMATION

Habit forming? Yes
Prescription needed? Yes
Available as generic? Yes
Drug class: Antidiarrheal

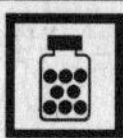

USES

Relieves diarrhea and intestinal cramps.

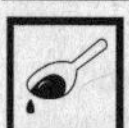

DOSAGE & USAGE INFORMATION

How to take:

- Tablet—Swallow with liquid or food to lessen stomach irritation.
- Drops or liquid—Follow label instructions and use marked dropper.

When to take:
No more often than directed on label.

If you forget a dose:
Take as soon as you remember. If it is almost time for the next dose, wait for the next scheduled dose (don't double this dose).

What drug does:
Blocks digestive tract's nerve supply, which reduces propelling movements.

Time lapse before drug works:
May require 12 to 24 hours of regular doses to control diarrhea.

Continued next column

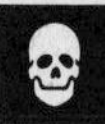

OVERDOSE

SYMPTOMS:
Excitement, constricted pupils, shallow breathing, coma.
WHAT TO DO:

- **Dial 911 (emergency) for medical help or call poison control center 1-800-222-1222 for instructions.**
- **If person is unconscious, check breathing and pulse. If not breathing, begin mouth-to-mouth rescue breathing. If heart is not beating, begin chest compressions.**
- **See emergency information on last 3 pages of this book.**

Don't take with:
Any other medicine or any dietary supplement without consulting your doctor or pharmacist.

POSSIBLE ADVERSE REACTIONS OR SIDE EFFECTS

SYMPTOMS	WHAT TO DO
Life-threatening:	
Hives, rash, intense itching, faintness soon after a dose (anaphylaxis).	Seek emergency treatment immediately.
Common:	
None expected.	
Infrequent:	
Dry mouth or skin, numbness of hands or feet, dizziness, depression, rash or itch, blurred vision, decreased urination, drowsiness, headache, swollen gums (these symptoms usually mean too much of the drug has been taken).	Discontinue. Call doctor right away.
Rare:	
Severe stomach pain, nausea, vomiting, constipation, bloating, loss of appetite.	Discontinue. Call doctor right away.

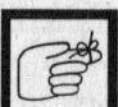

WARNINGS & PRECAUTIONS

Don't take if:

- You are allergic to diphenoxylate and atropine or any narcotic or anticholinergic.
- You have jaundice.
- You have infectious diarrhea or antibiotic-associated diarrhea.
- Patient is younger than 2.

Before you start, consult your doctor if:

- You have had liver problems.
- You have ulcerative colitis.
- You plan to become pregnant within medication period.
- You have any medical disorder.
- You take any medication, including nonprescription drugs.

Over age 60:
Adverse reactions and side effects may be more frequent and severe than in younger persons.

Pregnancy:
Decide with your doctor if drug benefits justify risk to unborn child. Risk category C (see page xviii).

Breast-feeding:
Drug passes into milk. Avoid drug or discontinue nursing until you finish medicine. Consult doctor for advice on maintaining milk supply.

Infants & children:
Don't give to children under 2 years of age. Use only under doctor's supervision for children older than 2.

Prolonged use:
- May be habit forming if larger doses than recommended are taken for a long period of time.
- Talk to your doctor about the need for follow-up medical examinations or laboratory studies to check liver function.

Skin & sunlight:
No problems expected.

Driving, piloting or hazardous work:
Don't drive or pilot aircraft until you learn how medicine affects you. Don't work around dangerous machinery. Don't climb ladders or work in high places. Danger increases if you drink alcohol or take medicine affecting alertness and reflexes.

Discontinuing:
- May be unnecessary to finish medicine. Follow doctor's instructions.
- After discontinuing, consult doctor if you experience muscle cramps, nausea, vomiting, trembling, stomach cramps or unusual sweating.

Others:
If diarrhea lasts longer than 2 days, discontinue and call doctor.

POSSIBLE INTERACTION WITH OTHER DRUGS

GENERIC NAME OR DRUG CLASS	COMBINED EFFECT
Barbiturates*	Increased effect of both drugs.
Clozapine	Toxic effect on the central nervous system.
Ethinamate	Dangerous increased effects of ethinamate. Avoid combining.
Fluoxetine	Increased depressant effects of both drugs.
Guanfacine	May increase depressant effects of either drug.
Leucovorin	High alcohol content of leucovorin may cause adverse effects.
Methyprylon	Increased sedative effect, perhaps to dangerous level. Avoid.
Monoamine oxidase (MAO) inhibitors*	May increase blood pressure excessively.
Naltrexone	Triggers withdrawal symptoms.
Narcotics*	Increased sedation. Avoid.
Sedatives*	Increased effect of both drugs.
Sertraline	Increased depressive effects of both drugs.
Tranquilizers*	Increased effect of both drugs.

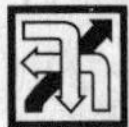

POSSIBLE INTERACTION WITH OTHER SUBSTANCES

INTERACTS WITH	COMBINED EFFECT
Alcohol:	Depressed brain function. Avoid.
Beverages:	None expected.
Cocaine:	Decreased effect of diphenoxylate and atropine.
Foods:	None expected.
Marijuana:	None expected.
Tobacco:	None expected.

DIPYRIDAMOLE

BRAND NAMES

Aggrenox
Apo-Dipyridamole
Dipimol
Dipridacot
Novodipiradol
Persantine
Pyridamole

BASIC INFORMATION

Habit forming? No
Prescription needed?
U.S.: Yes
Canada: No
Available as generic? Yes
Drug class: Platelet aggregation inhibitor

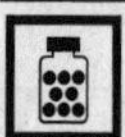

USES

- May reduce frequency and intensity of angina attacks.
- May reduce the risk of blood clots after heart surgery.

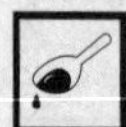

DOSAGE & USAGE INFORMATION

How to take:
Tablet—Swallow with a full glass of water. If you can't swallow whole, crumble tablet and take with liquid.

When to take:
1 hour before or 2 hours after meals.

If you forget a dose:
Take as soon as you remember. If it is almost time for the next dose, wait for the next scheduled dose (don't double this dose).

Continued next column

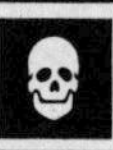

OVERDOSE

SYMPTOMS:
Decreased blood pressure; weak, rapid pulse; cold, clammy skin; collapse.
WHAT TO DO:
- **Dial 911 (emergency) for medical help or call poison control center 1-800-222-1222 for instructions.**
- **If person is unconscious, check breathing and pulse. If not breathing, begin mouth-to-mouth rescue breathing. If heart is not beating, begin chest compressions.**
- **See emergency information on last 3 pages of this book.**

What drug does:
- Probably dilates blood vessels to increase oxygen to heart.
- May reduce platelet clumping, which causes blood clots.

Time lapse before drug works:
3 months of continual use.

Don't take with:
Any other medicine or any dietary supplement without consulting your doctor or pharmacist.

POSSIBLE ADVERSE REACTIONS OR SIDE EFFECTS

SYMPTOMS	WHAT TO DO
Life-threatening:	
In case of overdose, see previous column.	
Common:	
Dizziness.	Continue. Call doctor when convenient.
Infrequent:	
• Fainting, headache.	Discontinue. Call doctor right away.
• Red flush, rash, nausea, vomiting, cramps, weakness.	Continue. Call doctor when convenient.
Rare:	
Chest pain.	Discontinue. Call doctor right away.

WARNINGS & PRECAUTIONS

Don't take if:
- You are allergic to dipyridamole.
- You are recovering from a heart attack.

Before you start, consult your doctor if:
- You have low blood pressure.
- You have liver disease.

Over age 60:
Begin treatment with small doses.

Pregnancy:
No proven harm to unborn child. Avoid if possible. Consult doctor. Risk category B (see page xviii).

Breast-feeding:
No proven problems. Consult doctor.

Infants & children:
Not recommended.

Prolonged use:
Talk to your doctor about the need for follow-up medical examinations or laboratory studies.

Skin & sunlight:
No problems expected.

Driving, piloting or hazardous work:
Avoid if you feel dizzy. Otherwise, no problems expected.

Discontinuing:
Don't discontinue without doctor's advice until you complete prescribed dose, even though symptoms diminish or disappear.

Others:
- Drug increases your ability to be active without angina pain. Avoid excessive physical exertion that might injure heart.
- Advise any doctor or dentist whom you consult that you take this medicine.

POSSIBLE INTERACTION WITH OTHER DRUGS

GENERIC NAME OR DRUG CLASS	COMBINED EFFECT
Anticoagulants, oral*	Increased anticoagulant effect. Bleeding tendency.
Aspirin and combination drugs containing aspirin	Increased dipyridamole effect. Dose may need adjustment.

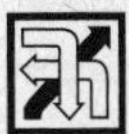

POSSIBLE INTERACTION WITH OTHER SUBSTANCES

INTERACTS WITH	COMBINED EFFECT
Alcohol:	May lower blood pressure excessively.
Beverages:	None expected.
Cocaine:	No proven problems.
Foods:	Decreased dipyridamole absorption unless taken 1 hour before eating.
Marijuana:	Daily use—Decreased dipyridamole effect.
Tobacco: Nicotine.	May decrease dipyridamole effect.

*See Glossary

DISOPYRAMIDE

BRAND NAMES

Norpace
Norpace CR
Rythmodan
Rythmodan-LA

BASIC INFORMATION

Habit forming? No
Prescription needed? Yes
Available as generic? Yes
Drug class: Antiarrhythmic

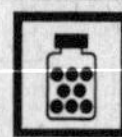

USES

Corrects heart rhythm disorders.

DOSAGE & USAGE INFORMATION

How to take:

- Extended-release tablet or capsule—Swallow with liquid. Do not crush tablet or open capsule.
- Capsule—Swallow with liquid. If you can't swallow whole, ask your pharmacist to prepare a liquid suspension for your use.

When to take:
At the same times each day.

If you forget a dose:
Take as soon as you remember. If it is almost time for the next dose, wait for the next scheduled dose (don't double this dose).

What drug does:
Delays nerve impulses to heart to regulate heartbeat.

Time lapse before drug works:
Begins in 30 to 60 minutes. Must use for 5 to 7 days to determine effectiveness.

Continued next column

OVERDOSE

SYMPTOMS:
Blood-pressure drop, irregular heartbeat, apnea, loss of consciousness.
WHAT TO DO:

- **Dial 911 (emergency) for medical help or call poison control center 1-800-222-1222 for instructions.**
- **If person is unconscious, check breathing and pulse. If not breathing, begin mouth-to-mouth rescue breathing. If heart is not beating, begin chest compressions.**
- **See emergency information on last 3 pages of this book.**

Don't take with:
Any other medicine or any dietary supplement without consulting your doctor or pharmacist.

POSSIBLE ADVERSE REACTIONS OR SIDE EFFECTS

SYMPTOMS	WHAT TO DO
Life-threatening:	
Hives, rash, intense itching, faintness soon after a dose (anaphylaxis).	Seek emergency treatment immediately.
Common:	
• Hypoglycemia (cold sweats, fast heartbeat, extreme hunger, shakiness and nervousness, anxiety, cool and pale skin, drowsiness, headache).	Discontinue. Call doctor right away.
• Dry mouth, constipation, painful or difficult urination, rapid weight gain, blurred vision.	Continue. Call doctor when convenient.
Infrequent:	
• Dizziness, fainting, confusion, chest pain, nervousness, depression, slow or fast heartbeat.	Discontinue. Call doctor right away.
• Swollen feet.	Continue. Call doctor when convenient.
Rare:	
• Shortness of breath, psychosis.	Discontinue. Seek emergency treatment.
• Rash, sore throat, fever, headache, jaundice, muscle weakness.	Discontinue. Call doctor right away.
• Eye pain, diminished sex drive, numbness or tingling of hands and feet, bleeding tendency.	Continue. Call doctor when convenient.

WARNINGS & PRECAUTIONS

Don't take if:

- You are allergic to disopyramide or any antiarrhythmic.
- You have second- or third-degree heart block.
- You have heart failure.

Before you start, consult your doctor if:

- You react unfavorably to other antiarrhythmic drugs.
- You have had heart disease.
- You have low blood pressure.
- You have liver disease.
- You have glaucoma.
- You have enlarged prostate.
- You have myasthenia gravis.
- You take digitalis preparations or diuretics.

Over age 60:

- May require reduced dose.
- More likely to have difficulty urinating or be constipated.
- More likely to have blood pressure drop.

Pregnancy:
Decide with your doctor if drug benefits justify risk to unborn child. Risk category C (see page xviii).

Breast-feeding:
Drug passes into milk. Avoid drug or discontinue nursing until you finish medicine. Consult doctor for advice on maintaining milk supply.

Infants & children:
Safety not established. Don't use.

Prolonged use:
Talk to your doctor about the need for follow-up medical examinations or laboratory studies to check liver function, kidney function, ECG,* blood pressure, serum potassium.

Skin & sunlight:
May cause rash or intensify sunburn in areas exposed to sun or ultraviolet light (photosensitivity reaction). Avoid overexposure. Notify doctor if reaction occurs.

Driving, piloting or hazardous work:
Don't drive or pilot aircraft until you learn how medicine affects you. Don't work around dangerous machinery. Don't climb ladders or work in high places. Danger increases if you drink alcohol or take medicine affecting alertness and reflexes, such as antihistamines, tranquilizers, sedatives, pain medicine, narcotics, or mind-altering drugs.

Discontinuing:
Don't discontinue without doctor's advice until you complete prescribed dose, even though symptoms diminish or disappear.

Others:
If new illness, injury or surgery occurs, tell doctors of disopyramide use.

POSSIBLE INTERACTION WITH OTHER DRUGS

GENERIC NAME OR DRUG CLASS	COMBINED EFFECT
Antiarrhythmics*	May increase effect and toxicity of each drug.
Anticholinergics*	Increased anticholinergic effect.
Anticoagulants, oral*	Possible increased anticoagulant effect.
Antihypertensives*	Increased anti-hypertensive effect.
Cisapride	Decreased disopyramide effect.
Encainide	Increased effect of toxicity on the heart muscle.
Flecainide	Possible irregular heartbeat.
Nicardipine	May cause dangerously slow, fast or irregular heartbeat.
Nimodipine	May cause dangerous irregular, slow or fast heartbeat.
Phenobarbital	Increased metabolism, decreased disopyramide effect.
Phenytoin	Increased metabolism, decreased disopyramide effect.
Propafenone	Increased effect of both drugs and increased risk of toxicity.
Rifampin	Increased metabolism, decreased disopyramide effect.
Tocainide	Increased likelihood of adverse reactions with either drug.

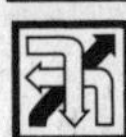

POSSIBLE INTERACTION WITH OTHER SUBSTANCES

INTERACTS WITH	COMBINED EFFECT
Alcohol:	Decreased blood pressure and blood sugar. Use caution.
Beverages:	None expected.
Cocaine:	Irregular heartbeat.
Foods:	None expected.
Marijuana:	Unpredictable. May decrease disopyramide effect.
Tobacco:	May decrease disopyramide effect.

DISULFIRAM

BRAND NAMES

Antabuse

BASIC INFORMATION

Habit forming? No
Prescription needed? Yes
Available as generic? Yes
Drug class: Antialcoholic agent

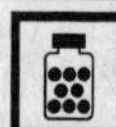

USES

Treatment for alcoholism. Will not cure alcoholism, but is a powerful deterrent to drinking.

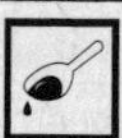

DOSAGE & USAGE INFORMATION

How to take:
Tablet—Swallow with liquid.

When to take:
Morning or bedtime. Avoid if you have used *any* alcohol, tonics, cough syrups, fermented vinegar, after-shave lotion or backrub solutions within 12 hours.

If you forget a dose:
Take as soon as you remember up to 12 hours late. If more than 12 hours, wait for next scheduled dose (don't double this dose).

What drug does:
In combination with alcohol, produces a metabolic change that causes severe, temporary toxicity.

Time lapse before drug works:
3 to 12 hours.

Continued next column

OVERDOSE

SYMPTOMS:
Memory loss, behavior disturbances, lethargy, confusion and headaches; nausea, vomiting, stomach pain and diarrhea; weakness and unsteady walk; temporary paralysis.
WHAT TO DO:
- **Dial 911 (emergency) for medical help or call poison control center 1-800-222-1222 for instructions.**
- **See emergency information on last 3 pages of this book.**

Don't take with:
- Nonprescription drugs that contain *any* alcohol.
- Any other medicine or any dietary supplement without consulting your doctor or pharmacist.
- Any other central nervous system (CNS) depressant drugs.*

POSSIBLE ADVERSE REACTIONS OR SIDE EFFECTS

SYMPTOMS	WHAT TO DO
Life-threatening: In case of overdose, see previous column.	
Common: Drowsiness.	Continue. Tell doctor at next visit.
Infrequent:	
• Eye pain, vision changes, abdominal discomfort, throbbing headache, numbness in hands and feet.	Continue. Call doctor when convenient.
• Mood change, decreased sexual ability in men, tiredness.	Continue. Tell doctor at next visit.
• Bad taste in mouth (metal or garlic).	No action necessary.
Rare: Rash, jaundice.	Discontinue. Call doctor right away.

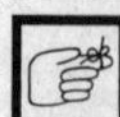

WARNINGS & PRECAUTIONS

Don't take if:
- You are allergic to disulfiram (alcohol-disulfiram combination is not an allergic reaction).
- You have used alcohol in any form or amount within 12 hours.
- You have taken paraldehyde within 1 week.
- You have heart disease.

Before you start, consult your doctor if:
- You have allergies.
- You plan to become pregnant within medication period.
- No one has explained to you how disulfiram reacts with alcohol.
- You think you cannot avoid drinking.
- You have diabetes, epilepsy, liver or kidney disease.
- You take other drugs.

Over age 60:
Adverse reactions and side effects may be more frequent and severe than in younger persons.

Pregnancy:
Decide with your doctor if drug benefits justify risk to unborn child. Risk category C (see page xviii).

Breast-feeding:
Studies inconclusive. Consult your doctor.

Infants & children:
Not recommended.

Prolonged use:
Periodic blood cell counts and liver function tests recommended if you take this drug a long time.

Skin & sunlight:
No problems expected.

Driving, piloting or hazardous work:
Avoid if you feel drowsy or have vision side effects. Otherwise, no restrictions.

Discontinuing:
Don't discontinue without consulting doctor. Dose may require gradual reduction if you have taken drug for a long time. Doses of other drugs may also require adjustment. Avoid alcohol at least 14 days following last dose.

Others:
- Check all liquids that you take or rub on for presence of alcohol.
- Advise any doctor or dentist whom you consult that you take this medicine.

POSSIBLE INTERACTION WITH OTHER DRUGS

GENERIC NAME OR DRUG CLASS	COMBINED EFFECT
Anticoagulants*	Possible unexplained bleeding.
Anticonvulsants*	Excessive sedation.
Barbiturates*	Excessive sedation.
Central nervous system (CNS) depressants*	Increased depressive effect.
Clozapine	Toxic effect on the central nervous system.
Guanfacine	May increase depressant effects of either drug.
Isoniazid	Unsteady walk and disturbed behavior.
Leucovorin	High alcohol content of leucovorin may cause disulfiram reaction.*
Methyprylon	Increased sedative effect, perhaps to dangerous level. Avoid.
Metronidazole	Disulfiram reaction.*
Nabilone	Greater depression of central nervous system.
Sedatives*	Excessive sedation.
Theophylline	Increased theophylline effect; possibly toxic levels.

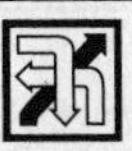

POSSIBLE INTERACTION WITH OTHER SUBSTANCES

INTERACTS WITH	COMBINED EFFECT
Alcohol: *Any* form or amount.	Possible life-threatening toxicity. See disulfiram reaction.*
Beverages: Punch or fruit drink that may contain alcohol.	Disulfiram reaction.*
Cocaine:	Increased disulfiram effect.
Foods: Sauces, fermented vinegar, marinades, desserts or other foods prepared with *any* alcohol.	Disulfiram reaction.*
Marijuana:	None expected.
Tobacco:	None expected.

*See Glossary

DIURETICS, LOOP

GENERIC AND BRAND NAMES

BUMETANIDE
Bumex
ETHACRYNIC ACID
Edecrin
FUROSEMIDE
Apo-Furosemide
Furoside
Lasix
Lasix Special
Myrosemide
Novosemide
Uritol
TORSEMIDE
Demadex

BASIC INFORMATION

Habit forming? No
Prescription needed? Yes
Available as generic? Yes
Drug class: Diuretic (loop), antihypertensive

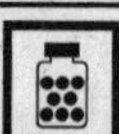

USES

- Lowers high blood pressure.
- Decreases fluid retention.

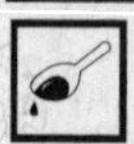

DOSAGE & USAGE INFORMATION

How to take:
Tablet or liquid—Swallow with liquid. If you can't swallow tablet whole, crumble tablet and take with liquid or food.

When to take:
- 1 dose a day—Take after breakfast.
- More than 1 dose a day—Take last dose no later than 6 p.m. unless otherwise directed.

If you forget a dose:
- 1 dose a day—Take as soon as you remember up to 12 hours late. If more than 12 hours, wait for next scheduled dose (don't double this dose).

Continued next column

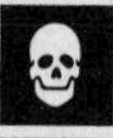

OVERDOSE

SYMPTOMS:
Weakness, lethargy, dizziness, confusion, nausea, vomiting, leg muscle cramps, thirst, stupor, deep sleep, weak and rapid pulse, cardiac arrest.
WHAT TO DO:
- **Dial 911 (emergency) for medical help or call poison control center 1-800-222-1222 for instructions.**
- **See emergency information on last 3 pages of this book.**

- More than 1 dose a day—Take as soon as you remember. If it is almost time for the next dose, wait for the next scheduled dose (don't double this dose).

What drug does:
Increases elimination of sodium, potassium and water from body. Decreased body fluid reduces blood pressure.

Time lapse before drug works:
1 hour to increase water loss. Requires 2 to 3 weeks to lower blood pressure.

Don't take with:
- Nonprescription drugs with aspirin.
- Any other medicine or any dietary supplement without consulting your doctor or pharmacist.

POSSIBLE ADVERSE REACTIONS OR SIDE EFFECTS

SYMPTOMS	WHAT TO DO
Life-threatening: In case of overdose, see previous column.	
Common: Dizziness.	Continue. Call doctor when convenient.
Infrequent: Mood change, fatigue, appetite loss, diarrhea, irregular heartbeat, muscle cramps, low blood pressure, pain in abdomen, weakness.	Discontinue. Call doctor right away.
Rare: Rash or hives, yellow vision, ringing in ears, hearing loss, sore throat, fever, dry mouth, thirst, side or stomach pain, nausea, vomiting, unusual bleeding or bruising, joint pain, jaundice, numbness or tingling in hands or feet.	Discontinue. Call doctor right away.

WARNINGS & PRECAUTIONS

Don't take if:
You are allergic to loop diuretics.

Before you start, consult your doctor if:
- You are taking any other prescription or nonprescription medicine.
- You are allergic to any sulfa drug.
- You have liver or kidney disease.
- You have gout, diabetes or impaired hearing.
- You will have surgery within 2 months, including dental surgery, requiring general or spinal anesthesia.

Over age 60:
Adverse reactions and side effects may be more frequent and severe than in younger persons.

Pregnancy:
Risk factors vary for drugs in this group. See category list on page xviii and consult doctor.

Breast-feeding:
Drug filters into milk. May harm child. Avoid.

Infants & children:
Use only under medical supervision.

Prolonged use:
- Impaired balance of water and salt, with low potassium level in blood and body tissues.
- Possible diabetes.

Skin & sunlight:
One or more drugs in this group may cause rash or intensify sunburn in areas exposed to sun or ultraviolet light (photosensitivity reaction). Avoid overexposure. Notify doctor if reaction occurs.

Driving, piloting or hazardous work:
Avoid if you feel dizzy; otherwise no problems expected.

Discontinuing:
Don't discontinue without doctor's advice until you complete prescribed dose, even though symptoms diminish or disappear.

Others:
Frequent laboratory studies to monitor potassium level in blood recommended. Eat foods rich in potassium or take potassium supplements. Consult doctor.

POSSIBLE INTERACTION WITH OTHER DRUGS

GENERIC NAME OR DRUG CLASS	COMBINED EFFECT
Adrenocorticoids, systemic	Potassium depletion.
Allopurinol	Decreased allopurinol effect.
Amiodarone	Increased risk of heartbeat irregularity due to low potassium.
Angiotensin-converting enzyme (ACE) inhibitors*	Possible excessive potassium in blood.
Anticoagulants*	Abnormal clotting.
Antidepressants, tricyclic*	Excessive blood pressure drop.
Antidiabetics, oral*	Decreased antidiabetic effect.
Antihypertensives*	Increased anti-hypertensive effect. Dosages may require adjustment.
Anti-inflammatory drugs, nonsteroidal (NSAIDs)*	Decreased diuretic effect.
Antivirals, HIV/AIDS*	Increased risk of pancreatitis with furosemide.
Barbiturates*	Low blood pressure.
Beta-adrenergic blocking agents*	Increased anti-hypertensive effect. Dosages may require adjustment.
Corticosteroids*	Decreased potassium.
Digitalis preparations*	Excessive potassium loss could lead to serious heart rhythm disorders.
Diuretics, other*	Increased diuretic effect.
Hypokalemia-causing medicines*	Increased risk of excessive potassium loss.
Insulin	Decreased insulin effect.
Lithium	Increased lithium toxicity.
Meloxicam	Decreased effect of diuretic.
Metformin	Increased metformin effect with furosemide.

Continued on page 914

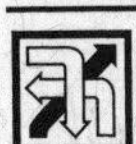

POSSIBLE INTERACTION WITH OTHER SUBSTANCES

INTERACTS WITH	COMBINED EFFECT
Alcohol:	Blood pressure drop. Avoid.
Beverages:	None expected.
Cocaine:	Dangerous blood pressure drop. Avoid.
Foods:	None expected.
Marijuana:	Increased thirst and urinary frequency, fainting.
Tobacco:	Decreased furosemide effect.

*See Glossary

DIURETICS, POTASSIUM-SPARING

GENERIC AND BRAND NAMES

AMILORIDE
Midamor
SPIRONOLACTONE
Aldactone
Novospiroton
TRIAMTERENE
Dyrenium

BASIC INFORMATION

Habit forming? No
Prescription needed? Yes
Available as generic? Yes
Drug class: Diuretic, antihypertensive, antihypokalemic

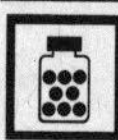

USES

- Treatment for high blood pressure (hypertension) and congestive heart failure. Decreases fluid retention and prevents potassium loss.
- Treatment for hypokalemia (low potassium), polycystic ovary syndrome and hirsutism in women.

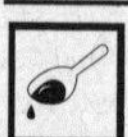

DOSAGE & USAGE INFORMATION

How to take:
Capsule or tablet—Swallow with liquid. If you can't swallow whole, open capsule or crush tablet and take with liquid or food. May take with meal to lessen stomach irritation.

When to take:
At the same times each day. May interfere with sleep if taken after 6 p.m.

Continued next column

OVERDOSE

SYMPTOMS:
Rapid, irregular heartbeat; confusion; shortness of breath; nervousness; extreme weakness; stupor; coma.
WHAT TO DO:
- **Dial 911 (emergency) for medical help or call poison control center 1-800-222-1222 for instructions.**
- **If person is unconscious, check breathing and pulse. If not breathing, begin mouth-to-mouth rescue breathing. If heart is not beating, begin chest compressions.**
- **See emergency information on last 3 pages of this book.**

If you forget a dose:
Take as soon as you remember. If it is almost time for the next dose, wait for next scheduled dose (don't double this dose).

What drug does:
- Blocks exchange of certain chemicals in the kidneys so sodium and water are excreted. Conserves potassium.
- In polycystic ovary syndrome and hirsutism, blocks androgen hormones.

Time lapse before drug works:
2 to 4 hours.

Don't take with:
Any other medicine or any dietary supplement without consulting your doctor or pharmacist.

POSSIBLE ADVERSE REACTIONS OR SIDE EFFECTS

SYMPTOMS	WHAT TO DO
Life-threatening:	
In case of overdose, see previous column.	
Common:	
Headache, nausea, appetite loss, vomiting, mild diarrhea.	Continue. Call doctor when convenient.
Infrequent:	
Dizziness, muscle cramps, dry mouth, decreased sexual drive, constipation.	Continue. Call doctor when convenient.
Rare:	
Shortness of breath, skin rash or itch (with amiloride); cough or hoarseness, painful urination, back or side pain (with triamterene and spironolactone); potassium changes (confusion, dry mouth, breathing difficulty, irregular heartbeat, unusual tiredness or weakness, mood or mental changes, muscle cramps, tingling in body); red, burning, inflamed feeling of tongue (with triamterene).	Discontinue. Call doctor right away.

WARNINGS & PRECAUTIONS

Don't take if:
- You are allergic to potassium-sparing diuretics.
- Your serum potassium level is high.

Before you start, consult your doctor if:

- You have diabetes.
- You have heart disease, kidney or liver disease or gout.

Over age 60:
Adverse reactions and side effects may be more frequent and severe than in younger persons. More likely to exceed safe potassium blood levels.

Pregnancy:
Avoid if possible. Consult doctor. Risk category B (see page xviii).

Breast-feeding:
Drug may pass into milk. Avoid drug or discontinue nursing until you finish medicine. Consult doctor for advice on maintaining milk supply.

Infants & children:
No special problems expected.

Prolonged use:
Talk to your doctor about the need for follow-up medical examinations or laboratory studies to check blood pressure, kidney function, ECG* and serum electrolytes.

Skin & sunlight:
One or more of these drugs may cause increased sensitivity to sunlight (photosensitivity reaction). Avoid overexposure. If reaction occurs, notify doctor.

Driving, piloting or hazardous work:
Don't drive or pilot aircraft until you learn how medicine affects you. Don't work around dangerous machinery. Don't climb ladders or work in high places. Danger increases if you drink alcohol or take medicine affecting alertness and reflexes.

Discontinuing:
Don't discontinue without doctor's advice until you complete prescribed dose, even though symptoms diminish or disappear.

Others:

- Periodic physical checkups and potassium-level tests recommended.
- Advise any doctor or dentist whom you consult that you take this medicine.
- If you experience an illness with severe vomiting and diarrhea, consult doctor.
- A special diet may be recommended in addition to this medicine. Follow doctor's advice.

POSSIBLE INTERACTION WITH OTHER DRUGS

GENERIC NAME OR DRUG CLASS	COMBINED EFFECT
Amantadine	Increased effect of amantadine (with triamterene).
Angiotensin-converting enzyme (ACE) inhibitors*	Possible excessive potassium in blood.
Anticoagulants,* oral	Decreased anticoagulant effect.
Antigout drugs*	Decreased antigout effect.
Antihypertensives*	Increased effect of both drugs.
Anti-inflammatory drugs, nonsteroidal (NSAIDs)*	Increased potassium levels.
Cyclosporine	Increased potassium levels.
Digoxin	Increased digoxin effect (with spironolactone).
Diuretics,* other	Increased effect of both drugs.
Dofetilide	Increased risk of heart problems.
Folic acid	Decreased effect of folic acid.
Lithium	Possible lithium toxicity.
Memantine	Increased effect of memantine or triamterene.
Metformin	Increased metformin effect.
Potassium supplements*	Increased potassium levels.

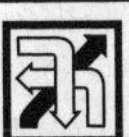

POSSIBLE INTERACTION WITH OTHER SUBSTANCES

INTERACTS WITH	COMBINED EFFECT
Alcohol:	Increased blood pressure drop. Avoid.
Beverages: Low-salt milk.	Possible excess potassium levels. Low-salt milk has extra potassium.
Cocaine:	Blood pressure rise. Avoid.
Foods: Salt substitutes.	Possible excess potassium levels.
Marijuana:	None expected.
Tobacco:	None expected.

*See Glossary

DIURETICS, POTASSIUM-SPARING & HYDROCHLOROTHIAZIDE

GENERIC AND BRAND NAMES

AMILORIDE & HYDROCHLOROTHIAZIDE
- Moduret
- Moduretic

SPIRONOLACTONE & HYDROCHLOROTHIAZIDE
- Aldactazide
- Spirozide

TRIAMTERENE & HYDROCHLOROTHIAZIDE
- Apo-Triazide
- Diazide
- Maxzide
- Novo-Triamzide

BASIC INFORMATION

Habit forming? No
Prescription needed? Yes
Available as generic? Yes
Drug class: Diuretic, antihypertensive, antihypokalemic

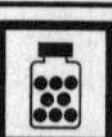

USES

- Treats, but does not cure, high blood pressure (hypertension) and congestive heart failure. Decreases fluid retention and prevents potassium loss.
- Treatment for hypokalemia (low potassium).

DOSAGE & USAGE INFORMATION

How to take:
Capsule or tablet—Swallow with liquid. Take with meals or milk if stomach irritation occurs.

When to take:
At the same time or times each day. May interfere with sleep if taken after 6 p.m.

Continued next column

OVERDOSE

SYMPTOMS: Rapid, irregular heartbeat; confusion; shortness of breath; nervousness; extreme weakness.

WHAT TO DO:
- **Dial 911 (emergency) for medical help or call poison control center 1-800-222-1222 for instructions.**
- **If person is unconscious, check breathing and pulse. If not breathing, begin mouth-to-mouth rescue breathing. If heart is not beating, begin chest compressions.**
- **See emergency information on last 3 pages of this book.**

If you forget a dose:
Take as soon as you remember. If it is almost time for the next dose, wait for next scheduled dose (don't double this dose).

What drug does:
This is a combination of 2 diuretics that blocks exchange of certain chemicals in the kidneys so sodium and water are excreted. Conserves potassium.

Time lapse before drug works:
Starts in 2 to 4 hours; several days for full effect.

Don't take with:
Any other medicine or any dietary supplement without consulting your doctor or pharmacist. This includes any nonprescription medicines for colds, coughs, hay fever, sinus problems, appetite control or asthma.

POSSIBLE ADVERSE REACTIONS OR SIDE EFFECTS

SYMPTOMS	WHAT TO DO
Life-threatening: In case of overdose, see previous column.	
Common:	
Nausea or mild vomiting, appetite loss, stomach cramps, mild diarrhea, constipation (with amiloride).	Continue. Call doctor when convenient.
Infrequent:	
Dizziness, muscle cramps, headache, skin sensitive to sun, dry mouth, decreased interest in sex. With spironolactone—tender breasts, deepening of voice, menstrual changes, and increased hair growth in females; breast enlargement in males; increased sweating in both sexes.	Continue. Call doctor when convenient.
Rare:	
Black, tarry or bloody stools; blood in urine; pain or difficulty in urinating; fever or chills; pain in back, side or joints; spots, rash or hives on skin; severe stomach pain; unusual bleeding or bruising; yellow skin or eyes; potassium changes (confusion, dry mouth, breathing difficulty,	Discontinue. Call doctor right away.

irregular heartbeat, unusual tiredness or weakness, mood or mental changes, muscle cramps, tingling in body); red, burning, inflamed feeling of tongue (with triamterene).

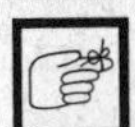

WARNINGS & PRECAUTIONS

Don't take if:
- You are allergic to potassium-sparing or thiazide diuretics* or sulfa drugs.*
- Your serum potassium level is high.

Before you start, consult your doctor if:
- You have diabetes or lupus erythematosus.
- You have menstrual problems (in females) or enlarged breast (in males).
- You have heart or blood vessel disease, kidney or liver disease, pancreatitis or gout.

Over age 60:
Adverse reactions and side effects may be more frequent and severe than in younger persons. More likely to exceed safe potassium blood levels.

Pregnancy:
Does not control pregnancy symptoms of swollen hands and feet. Avoid if possible.
Consult doctor. Risk category B (see page xviii).

Breast-feeding:
Drug passes into milk. Avoid drug or discontinue nursing until you finish medicine. Consult doctor for advice on maintaining milk supply.

Infants & children:
Unknown effect. Use only with doctor's approval.

Prolonged use:
Talk to your doctor about the need for follow-up medical examinations or laboratory studies to check blood pressure, kidney function, ECG* and serum electrolytes.

Skin & sunlight:
One or more of these drugs may cause increased sensitivity to sunlight (photosensitivity reaction). Avoid overexposure. If reaction occurs, notify doctor.

Driving, piloting or hazardous work:
Don't drive or pilot aircraft until you learn how medicine affects you. Don't work around dangerous machinery. Don't climb ladders or work in high places. Danger increases if you drink alcohol or take medicine affecting alertness and reflexes, such as antihistamines, tranquilizers, sedatives, pain medicine, narcotics and mind-altering drugs.

Discontinuing:
Don't discontinue without doctor's approval, even though symptoms diminish or disappear.

Others:
- Your doctor may prescribe a special diet.
- Advise any doctor or dentist whom you consult that you take this medicine.
- If you experience an illness with severe vomiting or diarrhea, consult doctor.

POSSIBLE INTERACTION WITH OTHER DRUGS

GENERIC NAME OR DRUG CLASS	COMBINED EFFECT
Amantadine	Increased effect of amantadine (with triamterene).
Angiotensin-converting enzyme (ACE) inhibitors*	Possible excessive potassium in blood.
Anticoagulants,* oral	Decreased anticoagulant effect.
Antigout drugs*	Decreased antigout effect.
Antihypertensives*	Increased effect of both drugs.
Anti-inflammatory drugs, nonsteroidal (NSAIDs)*	Increased potassium levels.

Continued on page 914

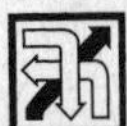

POSSIBLE INTERACTION WITH OTHER SUBSTANCES

INTERACTS WITH	COMBINED EFFECT
Alcohol:	Increased blood pressure drop. Avoid.
Beverages: Low-salt milk.	Possible excess potassium levels. Low-salt milk has extra potassium.
Cocaine:	Blood pressure rise. Avoid.
Foods: Salt substitutes.	Possible excess potassium levels.
Marijuana:	None expected.
Tobacco:	None expected.

DIURETICS, THIAZIDE

GENERIC AND BRAND NAMES

See full list of generic and brand names in the *Generic and Brand Name Directory*, page 883.

BASIC INFORMATION

Habit forming? No
Prescription needed? Yes
Available as generic? Yes, for some.
Drug class: Antihypertensive, diuretic (thiazide)

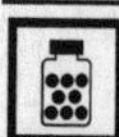

USES

- Controls, but doesn't cure, high blood pressure.
- Reduces fluid retention (edema) caused by conditions such as heart disorders and liver disease.

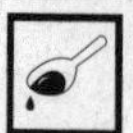

DOSAGE & USAGE INFORMATION

How to take:
Tablet, capsule or liquid—Swallow with liquid. If you can't swallow whole, crumble tablet or open capsule and take with liquid or food. Don't exceed dose.

When to take:
At the same time each day.

If you forget a dose:
Take as soon as you remember. If it is almost time for the next dose, wait for the next scheduled dose (don't double this dose).

What drug does:
- Forces sodium and water excretion, reducing body fluid.
- Relaxes muscle cells of small arteries.
- Reduced body fluid and relaxed arteries lower blood pressure.

Continued next column

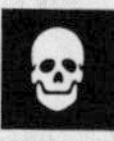

OVERDOSE

SYMPTOMS:
Cramps, weakness, drowsiness, weak pulse, coma.
WHAT TO DO:
- **Dial 911 (emergency) for medical help or call poison control center 1-800-222-1222 for instructions.**
- **See emergency information on last 3 pages of this book.**

Time lapse before drug works:
4 to 6 hours. May require several weeks to lower blood pressure.

Don't take with:
Any other medicine or any dietary supplement without consulting your doctor or pharmacist.

POSSIBLE ADVERSE REACTIONS OR SIDE EFFECTS

SYMPTOMS	WHAT TO DO
Life-threatening: In case of overdose, see previous column.	
Common:	
Muscle cramps.	Discontinue. Call doctor right away.
Infrequent:	
• Blurred vision, severe abdominal pain, nausea, vomiting, irregular heartbeat, weak pulse.	Discontinue. Call doctor right away.
• Dizziness, mood changes, headaches, weakness, tiredness, weight changes, decreased sex drive, diarrhea.	Continue. Call doctor when convenient.
• Dry mouth, thirst.	Continue. Tell doctor at next visit.
Rare:	
• Rash or hives.	Discontinue. Seek emergency treatment.
• Jaundice, joint pain, black stools.	Discontinue. Call doctor right away.
• Sore throat, fever.	Continue. Tell doctor at next visit.

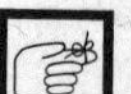

WARNINGS & PRECAUTIONS

Don't take if:
You are allergic to any thiazide diuretic drug.

Before you start, consult your doctor if:
- You are allergic to any sulfa drug or tartrazine dye.
- You have systemic lupus erythematosus.
- You have gout, diabetes or a liver, pancreas or kidney disorder.

Over age 60:
Adverse reactions and side effects may be more frequent and severe than in younger persons, especially dizziness and excessive potassium loss.

Pregnancy:
Risk factors vary for drugs in this group. See category list on page xviii and consult doctor.

Breast-feeding:
Drug passes into milk. Avoid drug or discontinue nursing.

Infants & children:
No problems expected.

Prolonged use:
- You may need medicine to treat high blood pressure for the rest of your life.
- Talk to your doctor about the need for follow-up medical examinations or laboratory studies to check blood sugar, kidney function, blood pressure, serum electrolytes.

Skin & sunlight:
One or more drugs in this group may cause rash or intensify sunburn in areas exposed to sun or ultraviolet light (photosensitivity reaction). Avoid overexposure. Notify doctor if reaction occurs.

Driving, piloting or hazardous work:
Don't drive or pilot aircraft until you learn how medicine affects you. Don't work around dangerous machinery. Don't climb ladders or work in high places. Danger increases if you drink alcohol or take medicine affecting alertness and reflexes, such as antihistamines, tranquilizers, sedatives, pain medicine, narcotics and mind-altering drugs.

Discontinuing:
Don't discontinue without medical advice.

Others:
- Hot weather and fever may cause dehydration and drop in blood pressure. Dose may require temporary adjustment. Weigh daily and report any unexpected weight decreases to your doctor.
- May cause rise in uric acid, leading to gout.
- May cause blood-sugar rise in diabetics.
- May affect results in some medical tests.
- Advise any doctor or dentist whom you consult that you take this medicine.

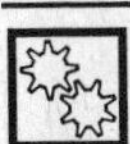

POSSIBLE INTERACTION WITH OTHER DRUGS

GENERIC NAME OR DRUG CLASS	COMBINED EFFECT
Adrenocorticoids, systemic	Potassium depletion.
Allopurinol	Decreased allopurinol effect.
Amiodarone	Increased risk of heartbeat irregularity due to low potassium.
Amphotericin B	Increased potassium.
Angiotensin-converting enzyme (ACE) inhibitors*	Decreased blood pressure.
Antidepressants, tricyclic*	Dangerous drop in blood pressure. Avoid combination unless under medical supervision.
Antidiabetic agents, oral*	Increased blood sugar.
Antihypertensives*	Increased hypertensive effect.
Antivirals, HIV/AIDS*	Increased risk of pancreatitis.
Barbiturates*	Increased anti-hypertensive effect.
Beta-adrenergic blocking agents*	Increased anti-hypertensive effect. Dosages of both drugs may require adjustments.
Calcium supplements*	Increased calcium in blood.
Carteolol	Increased anti-hypertensive effect.
Cholestyramine	Decreased anti-hypertensive effect.
Colestipol	Decreased anti-hypertensive effect.
Digitalis preparations*	Excessive potassium loss that causes dangerous heart rhythms.
Diuretics, thiazide,* other	Increased effect of other thiazide diuretics.

Continued on page 915

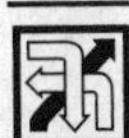

POSSIBLE INTERACTION WITH OTHER SUBSTANCES

INTERACTS WITH	COMBINED EFFECT
Alcohol:	Dangerous blood pressure drop.
Beverages:	None expected.
Cocaine	Increased risk of heart block and high blood pressure.
Foods: Licorice.	Excessive potassium loss that causes dangerous heart rhythms.
Marijuana:	May increase blood pressure.
Tobacco:	None expected.

***See Glossary**

DIVALPROEX

BRAND NAMES

Depakote
Depakote ER
Depakote Sprinkle
Epival

BASIC INFORMATION

Habit forming? No
Prescription needed? Yes
Available as generic? Yes
Drug class: Anticonvulsant

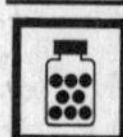

USES

- Treatment of epilepsy.
- Treatment of bipolar disorder.
- Treats migraine headaches.

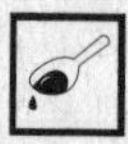

DOSAGE & USAGE INFORMATION

How to take:
Delayed-release tablet/capsule or extended-release tablet—Swallow whole with liquid or food to lessen stomach irritation. Do not crush or chew capsule or tablets. You may open capsule and sprinkle contents on food (such as a teaspoon of applesauce), then swallow right away.

When to take:
Delayed form 2-3 times each day; extended form one time a day. The two different forms (delayed or extended) have different actions in the body.

If you forget a dose:
Take as soon as you remember. If it is almost time for the next dose, wait for the next scheduled dose (don't double this dose).

What drug does:
It helps stabilize electrical activity in the brain.

Time lapse before drug works:
1 to 4 hours, but full effect may take weeks.

Don't take with:
Any other medicine or any dietary supplement without consulting your doctor or pharmacist.

OVERDOSE

SYMPTOMS:
Extreme drowsiness, heart problems, loss of consciousness.
WHAT TO DO:

- **Dial 911 (emergency) for medical help or call poison control center 1-800-222-1222 for instructions.**
- **See emergency information on last 3 pages of this book.**

POSSIBLE ADVERSE REACTIONS OR SIDE EFFECTS

SYMPTOMS	WHAT TO DO
Life-threatening:	
Rare allergic reaction (hives, itching, rash, wheezing, tightness in chest, swelling of lips or tongue or throat).	Seek emergency treatment immediately.
Common:	
Loss of appetite, indigestion, nausea, vomiting, stomach cramps, diarrhea, tremor, headache, weight gain or loss, menstrual changes.	Continue. Call doctor when convenient.
Infrequent:	
Clumsiness or unsteadiness, constipation, mild skin rash, dizziness, drowsiness, irritable or excited, hair loss.	Continue. Call doctor when convenient.
Rare:	
Mood or behavior changes; continued nausea, vomiting and appetite loss; increase in number of seizures; swelling of face, feet or legs; yellow skin or eyes; tiredness or weakness; back-and-forth eye movements (nystagmus); seeing spots/seeing double; unusual bleeding or bruising; dark urine; clay-colored stools; low grade fever; severe stomach cramps; confusion.	Continue, but call doctor right away.

WARNINGS & PRECAUTIONS

Don't take if:
You are allergic to divalproex or valproic acid.

Before you start, consult your doctor if:

- You have liver, kidney, blood or brain disorder, pancreatitis or urea cycle disorder.
- Drug is to be used for a young child.
- You have a history of depression or suicide thoughts or suicidal behavior.
- You are a woman of childbearing age.

Over age 60:
Adverse reactions and side effects may be more frequent and severe than in younger persons.

Pregnancy:
Risk of birth defects to unborn child exists. Use only if benefits of drug greatly exceed fetal risk. Risk category D (see page xviii).

Breast-feeding:
Unknown effect. Consult doctor.

Infants & children:
Increased risk for side effects and adverse reactions. Use under close medical supervision only.

Prolonged use:
Request periodic blood tests, liver and kidney function tests. These tests are necessary for safe and effective use.

Skin & sunlight:
No problems expected.

Driving, piloting or hazardous work:
Don't drive or pilot aircraft until you learn how medicine affects you. Don't work around dangerous machinery. Don't climb ladders or work in high places. Danger increases if you drink alcohol or take medicine affecting alertness and reflexes.

Discontinuing:
Don't discontinue without consulting doctor. Dose may require gradual reduction if you have taken drug for a long time. Doses of other drugs may also require adjustment.

Others:
- Advise any doctor or dentist whom you consult that you take this medicine.
- Be sure you and your doctor discuss benefits and risks of this drug before starting.
- Wear a medical identification that indicates your disorder and the use of this medicine.
- Read and carefully follow the prescription instructions. Use as directed. Don't increase or decrease dosage without doctor's approval.
- In rare cases, the drug can cause life-threatening liver failure (especially in children under age 2) or life-threatening pancreatitis (inflammation of the pancreas).
- Rarely, antiepileptic (anticonvulsant) drugs may lead to suicidal thoughts and behaviors. Call doctor right away if suicidal symptoms or unusual behaviors occur.

POSSIBLE INTERACTION WITH OTHER DRUGS

GENERIC NAME OR DRUG CLASS	COMBINED EFFECT
Anticoagulants,* oral	Increased risk of bleeding problems.
Anticonvulsants,* other	Each drug may need dosage adjusted.
Anti-inflammatory drugs, nonsteroidal* (NSAIDs)	Increased risk of bleeding problems.
Aspirin	Increased effect of divalproex.
Carbamazepine	Decreased effect of divalproex.
Central nervous system (CNS) depressants*	Increased sedative effect.
Clonazepam	May prolong seizure.
Diazepam	Increased effect of diazepam.
Enzyme inducers*	May Increase effect of some enzyme inducers and decrease effect of divalproex.
Felbamate	Increased effect of divalproex.
Hepatotoxics*	Increased risk of liver problems.
Lamotrigine	Increased effect of lamotrigine and risk of life-threatening rash.
Phenobarbital	Increased effect of phenobarbital and decreased effect of divalproex.
Phenytoin	Increased phenytoin effect; decreased divalproex effect.
Primidone	Increased effect of primidone.
Rifampin	Decreased effect of divalproex.
Salicylates*	Increased effect of divalproex.
Zidovudine	Increased effect of zidovudine.

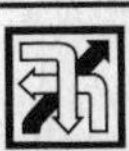

POSSIBLE INTERACTION WITH OTHER SUBSTANCES

INTERACTS WITH	COMBINED EFFECT
Alcohol:	Deep sedation. Avoid.
Beverages:	None expected.
Cocaine:	Unknown. Avoid.
Foods:	None expected.
Marijuana:	Unknown. Avoid.
Tobacco:	None expected.

***See Glossary**

DOFETILIDE

BRAND NAMES

Tikosyn

BASIC INFORMATION

Habit forming? No
Prescription needed? Yes
Available as generic? No
Drug class: Antiarrhythmic

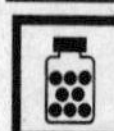

USES

Corrects irregular heartbeats to a normal rhythm.

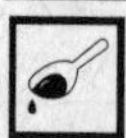

DOSAGE & USAGE INFORMATION

How to take:
Capsule—This drug is first used in a hospital or other setting where the patient can be monitored for any heart problems. Read the information provided with the prescription.

When to take:
At the same times each day.

If you forget a dose:
Skip the missed dose and go back to your regular dosing schedule (don't double this dose).

What drug does:
Slows the nerve impulses in the heart.

Time lapse before drug works:
2 to 3 hours.

Don't take with:
Any other medicine or any dietary supplement without consulting your doctor or pharmacist.

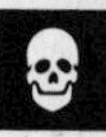

OVERDOSE

SYMPTOMS:
Cardiac arrest, irregular heartbeat, fainting, shortness of breath, unusual tiredness or weakness.
WHAT TO DO:
Dial 911 (emergency) for medical help or call poison control center 1-800-222-1222 for instructions.

POSSIBLE ADVERSE REACTIONS OR SIDE EFFECTS

SYMPTOMS	WHAT TO DO
Life-threatening: In case of overdose, see previous column.	
Common:	
Dizziness, fainting, fast or irregular heartbeat.	Discontinue. Seek emergency evaluation right away.
Infrequent:	
• Unusual swelling of the extremities, chest pain, slow heartbeat, sudden numbness or tingling (hands, feet or face), paralysis, confusion, weakness, slurred speech, shortness of breath, yellow eyes or skin.	Discontinue. Call doctor right away.
• Abdominal pain, back pain, diarrhea, chills, cough, fever, general feeling of illness, joint pain, headache, nausea, runny nose, sore throat, vomiting, sleeplessness, rash.	Continue. Call doctor if symptoms persist.
Rare: None expected.	

WARNINGS & PRECAUTIONS

Don't take if:
You are allergic to dofetilide.

Before you start, consult your doctor if:
- You are using any other medication.
- You have electrolyte disorders, such as low potassium or magnesium levels.
- You have been diagnosed with kidney or liver disease.

Over age 60:
Side effects or problems experienced with this medication appear to be the same in older people as in younger adults; however, older patients are more likely to have kidney problems and should be monitored regularly for possible dosage adjustment.

Pregnancy:
Decide with your doctor if drug benefits justify risk to unborn child. Risk category C (see page xviii).

Breast-feeding:
Drug may pass into milk. Avoid drug or discontinue nursing until you finish medicine. Consult doctor for advice on maintaining milk supply.

Infants & children:
Studies on this medicine have been done only in adult patients. Consult doctor before giving this medicine to persons under age 18.

Prolonged use:
Talk to your doctor about the need for follow up laboratory studies to determine the effect of the medicine on your body.

Skin & sunlight:
None expected.

Driving, piloting or hazardous work:
Don't drive or pilot aircraft until you learn how medicine affects you. Don't work around dangerous machinery. Don't climb ladders or work in high places. Danger increases if you drink alcohol or take medicine affecting alertness and reflexes.

Discontinuing:
Don't discontinue without consulting doctor.

Others:
Advise any doctor or dentist whom you consult that you take this medicine.

POSSIBLE INTERACTION WITH OTHER DRUGS

GENERIC NAME OR DRUG CLASS	COMBINED EFFECT
Antiarrhythmics, other*	Increased dofetilide effect.
Antidepressants, tricyclic*	Increased risk of heart problems.
Calcium channel blockers*	Increased risk of heart problems.
Cimetidine	Increased risk of heart problems.
Diuretics*	Increased risk of heart problems.
Enzyme inhibitors*	Increased dofetilide effect.
Ketoconazole	Increased risk of heart problems.
Macrolides, oral*	Increased risk of heart problems.
Megestrol	Increased dofetilide effect.
Metformin	Increased dofetilide effect.
Norfloxacin	Increased dofetilide effect.
Phenothiazines*	Increased risk of heart problems.
Progestins*	Increased risk of heart problems.
Selective serotonin reuptake inhibitors*	Increased dofetilide effect.
Trimethoprim	Increased dofetilide effect.
Zafirlukast	Increased dofetilide effect.

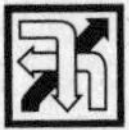

POSSIBLE INTERACTION WITH OTHER SUBSTANCES

INTERACTS WITH	COMBINED EFFECT
Alcohol:	Increases the chance of liver problems.
Beverages: Grapefruit juice.	May increase effect of dofetilide.
Cocaine:	Effect unknown. Avoid.
Foods: Grapefruit.	May increase effect of dofetilide.
Marijuana:	Effect unknown. Avoid.
Tobacco:	None expected.

*See Glossary

DOPAMINE AGONISTS, NONERGOT

GENERIC AND BRAND NAMES

PRAMIPEXOLE
- Mirapex
- Mirapex ER

ROPINIROLE
- Repreve
- Requip
- Requip XL

ROTIGOTINE
- Neupro

BASIC INFORMATION

Habit forming? No
Prescription needed? Yes
Available as generic? Yes, for some
Drug class: Dopamine agonist

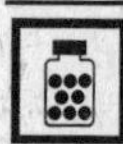

USES

- Treats symptoms of Parkinson's disease.
- Treats restless legs syndrome (RLS); also known as Willis-Ekbom disease.

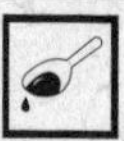

DOSAGE & USAGE INFORMATION

How to take:
- Tablet—Swallow with liquid. May take with or without food (food may lessen stomach upset).
- Extended-release tablet—Swallow whole with liquid. Do not break, crush or chew tablet. Take with or without food (food stops upset stomach).
- Skin (transdermal) patch—Carefully follow instructions provided with the product.

When to take:
- Parkinson's—tablet is taken 3 times a day at same times each day; extended-release tablet is taken once daily at same time each day; skin patch is changed every 24 hours.
- RLS—take a tablet1 to 3 hours before bedtime.
- Skin patch is changed every 24 hours.

If you forget a dose:
Take or use as soon as you remember. If it is almost time for the next dose, wait for the next scheduled dose (don't double this dose).

Continued next column

OVERDOSE

SYMPTOMS:
Agitation, weakness, confusion, cough, chest pain, increased body movements, sweating, hallucinations, low blood pressure.
WHAT TO DO:
Overdose unlikely to threaten life. If person takes much larger amount than prescribed or if accidentally swallowed, call doctor or poison control center 1-800-222-1222 for help.

What drug does:
The drug mimics the action of dopamine in the brain to help improve the symptoms of Parkinson's and RLS. Dopamine is a brain chemical that helps control body movements.

Time lapse before drug works:
May take several weeks for full benefit. Drug dosage starts low and is gradually increased.

Don't take with:
Any other medicine or any dietary supplement without consulting your doctor or pharmacist.

POSSIBLE ADVERSE REACTIONS OR SIDE EFFECTS

SYMPTOMS	WHAT TO DO
Life-threatening:	
Rare allergic reaction (hives, itching, rash, wheezing, tightness in chest, swelling of lips or tongue or throat).	Seek emergency treatment immediately.
Common:	
• Confusion, dizziness or lightheadedness, faintness, falling, hallucinations, skin reaction from patch, drowsiness, swelling (ankles, feet, legs, hands), unusual body movements, twitching, nausea, unusual tiredness or weakness, loss of appetite, vomiting, trouble sleeping.	Continue, but call doctor right away.
• Constipation, dry mouth, indigestion.	Continue. Call doctor when convenient.
Infrequent:	
• Abdominal pain or bloating, blurred or changed vision, cold or flu symptoms, falling asleep without warning, urination is painful or difficult or frequent, blood in urine, muscle or joint pain, muscle weakness, mental changes, difficulty swallowing, headache, high or low blood pressure, slow or fast heartbeat, chest pain, nervousness, memory problems, depression, noises in the ears, rapid weight gain, restlessness, shortness of breath.	Continue, but call doctor right away.

• Decreased libido, increased sweating, abnormal dreams, skin rash or itching, weight loss.	Continue. Call doctor when convenient.
Rare:	
Abnormal thinking, anxiety, unusual urges (e.g., sexual or gambling).	Continue, but call doctor right away.

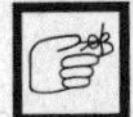

WARNINGS & PRECAUTIONS

Don't take if:
You are allergic to pramipexole, ropinirole or rotigotine.

Before you start, consult your doctor if:
- You have a sleep disorder other than restless legs syndrome (e.g., sleep apnea, insomnia or narcolepsy).
- You have a kidney or liver disorder.
- You have heart problem, high or low blood pressure or orthostatic hypotension (feeling lightheaded or dizzy when rising quickly after sitting or lying down).
- You have uncontrolled muscle movements.
- You have lung disorder such as asthma.
- You have sulfite sensitivity (for drug patch).
- You have a mental or mood disorder.
- You have a problem with alcohol abuse.
- You suffer from hallucinations.

Over age 60:
May be more at risk for certain side effects such as hallucinations.

Pregnancy:
Decide with your doctor whether drug benefits justify risk to unborn child. Risk category C (see page xviii).

Breast-feeding:
It is unknown if drug passes into breast milk. Consult your doctor for advice.

Infants & children:
Drug is not approved for ages under 18.

Prolonged use:
See your doctor on a regular basis while you take this drug to monitor effectiveness, dosage, any unwanted effects, and for skin check.

Skin & sunlight:
For skin patch, avoid exposing patch to sunlight.

Driving, piloting or hazardous work:
Don't drive or pilot aircraft until you learn how medicine affects you. Don't work around dangerous machinery. Don't climb ladders or work in high places. Danger increases if you drink alcohol or take medicine affecting alertness and reflexes.

Discontinuing:
Don't stop taking or using drug suddenly. Your doctor may reduce (taper) the dose gradually to avoid withdrawal symptoms. Other drugs you take may require a dosage change.

Others:
- Advise any doctor, dentist or pharmacist whom you consult that you take/use this drug.
- Use of this drug may cause a person to fall asleep without warning during activities of daily living (e.g., working, talking, eating or driving [which has resulted in accidents]). Use caution where needed.
- Get up slowly from a lying or sitting position to avoid dizziness, lightheadedness or fainting.

POSSIBLE INTERACTION WITH OTHER DRUGS

GENERIC NAME OR DRUG CLASS	COMBINED EFFECT
Antipsychotic drugs*	May decrease effect of both drugs.
Central nervous system (CNS) depressants*	Increased risk of side effects of both drugs.
Dopamine antagonists*	May decrease effect of nonergot dopamine agonist.
Enzyme inhibitors*	May increase effect of ropinirole.
Estrogens*	May increase effect of ropinirole.
Levodopa	Increased risk of side effects of levodopa.

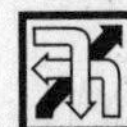

POSSIBLE INTERACTION WITH OTHER SUBSTANCES

INTERACTS WITH	COMBINED EFFECT
Alcohol:	Increased risk of side effects. Avoid.
Beverages:	None expected.
Cocaine:	Increased risk of hallucinations. Avoid.
Foods:	None expected.
Marijuana:	Increased risk of hallucinations. Avoid.
Tobacco:	May affect drug dosage of ropinirole. Consult doctor.

*See Glossary

DOXEPIN (Topical)

BRAND NAMES

Prudoxin   Zonalon

BASIC INFORMATION

Habit forming? No
Prescription needed? Yes
Available as generic? No
Drug class: Antipruritic (topical)

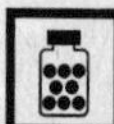

USES

- Treats itching of the skin caused by certain types of eczema (an inflammation of the skin).
- Treatment of moderate itching of atopic dermatitis and lichen simplex chronicus in adult patients.

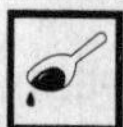

DOSAGE & USAGE INFORMATION

How to use:
Cream—Apply a thin layer to the affected area of skin and gently rub it in. Do not cover the treated area with a bandage or other dressing.

When to use:
Up to 4 times a day. Allow 3 to 4 hours between applications. Not to be used longer than 8 days.

If you forget a dose:
Use as soon as you remember. If it is almost time for the next dose, wait for the next scheduled dose (don't double this dose).

Continued next column

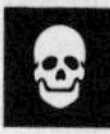

OVERDOSE

SYMPTOMS:
An overdose of topical medicine is unlikely to occur, but if too much is applied, it can be absorbed into the system.

- **Mild effects include blurred vision, drowsiness, very dry mouth, decreased awareness or responsiveness.**
- **More severe effects include irregular or fast heartbeat, enlarged pupils, jerking movements, dizziness, fainting, abdominal pain or swelling, weak or feeble pulse, high fever or low temperature, vomiting, incurable constipation, seizures, breathing difficulty, unconsciousness.**

WHAT TO DO:

- **Dial 911 (emergency) for medical help or call poison control center 1-800-222-1222 for instructions.**
- **See emergency information on last 3 pages of this book.**

What drug does:
The exact mechanism is unknown. It appears to block histamine* reactions, which can cause the itching. The drug also has a sedating effect on some people, which can help to relieve the itching symptoms. Variable and sometimes significant amounts of the drug are absorbed through the skin.

Time lapse before drug works:
May take up to 8 days for maximum benefit.

Don't take with:
Any other oral or topical medication without consulting your doctor or pharmacist. This includes nonprescription drugs such as cold or allergy remedies that may contain alcohol or antihistamines. They increase the risk of drowsiness.

POSSIBLE ADVERSE REACTIONS OR SIDE EFFECTS

SYMPTOMS	WHAT TO DO
Life-threatening:	
In case of overdose, see previous column.	
Common:	
• Swelling of the skin where drug is applied; worsening of the itching; burning, tingling or crawling feeling in the skin.	Discontinue. Call doctor right away.
• Stinging of skin where drug is applied, dryness or tightness of skin, taste changes, dizziness, drowsiness, dry mouth or lips, thirst, emotional changes, fatigue, headache.	Continue. Call doctor when convenient.
Infrequent:	
Scaling or cracking of the skin, nausea, anxiety, irritation.	Continue. Call doctor when convenient.
Rare:	
Fever.	Discontinue. Call doctor right away.

Note: **Though the drug is applied topically, it is absorbed into the bloodstream and can cause systemic reactions. Adverse reactions are more likely in patients who use the drug on more than 10% of their body surface.**

WARNINGS & PRECAUTIONS

Don't use if:
You are allergic to doxepin.

Before you start, consult your doctor if:
- You have narrow-angle glaucoma.
- You are allergic to any other medications.
- You have a problem with urinary retention.

Over age 60:
No special problems expected.

Pregnancy:
Consult doctor. Risk category B (page xviii).

Breast-feeding:
Drug passes into milk. Avoid drug or discontinue nursing until you finish medicine. Consult doctor for advice on maintaining milk supply.

Infants & children:
Safety in children has not been established. Use only under close medical supervision.

Prolonged use:
Don't use for more than 8 days unless directed by doctor. Longer use can increase the risk of side effects or adverse reactions.

Skin & sunlight:
No special problems expected.

Driving, piloting or hazardous work:
Don't drive or pilot aircraft until you learn how medicine affects you. Don't work around dangerous machinery. Don't climb ladders or work in high places. Danger increases if you drink alcohol or take medicine affecting alertness and reflexes.

Discontinuing:
To be sure of maximum benefit, don't discontinue this medicine before the treatment has been completed unless advised to do so by your doctor.

Others:
- Use medicine only on affected area. It is not to be used in the mouth, the eyes or the vagina.
- Advise any doctor or dentist whom you consult that you are using this medicine.
- If your skin condition doesn't improve within 8 days, consult doctor.
- Use medicine only as directed. Do not increase or reduce dosage without doctor's approval.

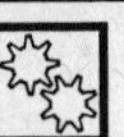

POSSIBLE INTERACTION WITH OTHER DRUGS

GENERIC NAME OR DRUG CLASS	COMBINED EFFECT
Antidepressants*	Increased risk of toxicity of both drugs.
Carbamazepine	Increased risk of toxicity of both drugs.
Central nervous system (CNS) depressants*	Increased sedation. May need dosage adjustment.
Cimetidine	Increased risk of doxepin toxicity.
Dextromethorphan	Increased risk of toxicity of both drugs.
Flecainide	Increased risk of toxicity of both drugs.
Monoamine oxidase (MAO) inhibitors*	Potentially life-threatening. Allow 14 days between use of the 2 drugs.
Phenothiazines*	Increased risk of toxicity of both drugs.
Propafenone	Increased risk of toxicity of both drugs.
Quinidine	Increased risk of toxicity of both drugs.

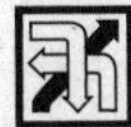

POSSIBLE INTERACTION WITH OTHER SUBSTANCES

INTERACTS WITH	COMBINED EFFECT
Alcohol:	Increased sedative effect. Avoid.
Beverages:	None expected.
Cocaine:	Problems not known. Best to avoid.
Foods:	None expected.
Marijuana:	Problems not known. Best to avoid.
Tobacco:	None expected.

*See Glossary

DPP-4 INHIBITORS

GENERIC AND BRAND NAMES

ALOGLIPTIN
- **Kazano**
- **Nesina**
- **Oseni**

LINAGLIPTIN
- **Jentadueto**
- **Tradjenta**

SAXAGLIPTIN
- **Kombiglyze XR**
- **Onglyza**

SITAGLIPTIN
- **Janumet**
- **Janumet XR**
- **Januvia**
- **Juvisync**

BASIC INFORMATION

Habit forming? No
Prescription needed? Yes
Available as generic? No
Drug class: Antidiabetic; incretin enhancer

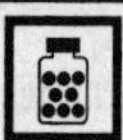

USES

Used in addition to diet and exercise to improve blood sugar levels in patients with type 2 diabetes. It may be prescribed alone or along with other oral diabetes drugs. (Note: The drug is not used for treating type 1 diabetes or diabetic ketoacidosis.)

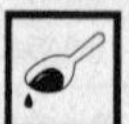

DOSAGE & USAGE INFORMATION

How to take:
- Tablet—Swallow with liquid. May be taken with or without food or as directed by your doctor.
- Extended-release tablet—Swallow whole with liquid. Do not cut, chew or crush tablet.

Continued next column

When to take:
Usually once a day at the same time each day.

If you forget a dose:
Take tablet as soon as you remember. If it is almost time for the next dose, wait for the next scheduled dose (don't double this dose).

What drug does:
It works by increasing incretins. Incretins increase insulin release when blood sugar levels are high, especially after meals. They also decrease the amount of sugar made by the liver.

Time lapse before drug works:
One to four hours.

Don't take with:
Any other medicine or diet supplement without consulting your doctor or pharmacist.

OVERDOSE

SYMPTOMS:
Rarely may cause hypoglycemia (low blood sugar)—See list of symptoms in next column under Rare.
WHAT TO DO:
- **Eat some type of sugar immediately, such as a glucose product, orange juice (add some sugar), nondiet sodas, candy (such as 5 Lifesavers), honey.**
- **If patient loses consciousness, give glucagon if you have it and know how to use it.**
- **Dial 911 (emergency) for medical help or call poison control center 1-800-222-1222 for instructions.**
- **See emergency information on last 3 pages of this book.**

POSSIBLE ADVERSE REACTIONS OR SIDE EFFECTS

SYMPTOMS	WHAT TO DO
Life-threatening:	
Rare allergic reaction (hives, itching, rash, trouble breathing, tightness in chest, swelling of lips or tongue or throat).	Seek emergency treatment immediately.
Common:	
Sore throat, headache, runny or stuffy nose, upper respiratory infection (e.g., cold).	Continue. Call doctor if symptoms persist.
Infrequent:	
Nausea, mild stomach pain, diarrhea, joint pain, urinary tract infection, swelling of hands or feet.	Continue. Call doctor if symptoms persist.
Rare:	
• Symptoms of low blood sugar—nervousness; hunger (excessive); cold sweats, rapid pulse, anxiety, cold skin, chills; confusion, drowsiness, loss of concentration; headache, nausea, weakness, shakiness, vision changes.	Seek treatment (eat some form of quick-acting sugar—glucose tablets, sugar, fruit juice, corn syrup, honey).

• Symptoms of high blood sugar—increased urination; unusual thirst, dry mouth; drowsiness, flushed or dry skin; fruit-like breath odor, appetite loss, stomach pain or vomiting; tiredness, trouble breathing, increased blood sugar level.	Check your blood sugar immediately. Call doctor right away.
• Other symptoms that cause concern.	Continue. Call doctor when convenient.

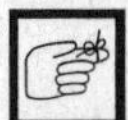

WARNINGS & PRECAUTIONS

Don't take if:
You are allergic to DPP-4 inhibitors.

Before you start, consult your doctor if:
- You have any kidney problems.
- You have HIV or a long-term infection.
- You are pregnant or plan to become pregnant.
- You are an alcoholic.

Over age 60:
A reduced drug dosage may be recommended for patients with decreased kidney function.

Pregnancy:
Decide with your doctor if drug benefits justify risk to unborn child. Risk category B (see page xviii).

Breast-feeding:
Drug may pass into milk. Consult your doctor for advice.

Infants & children:
Safety and effectiveness in children under age 18 has not been established. Consult doctor.

Prolonged use:
Talk to your doctor about the need for follow-up medical examinations and/or laboratory studies to determine continued effectiveness of drug.

Skin & sunlight:
No problems expected.

Driving, piloting or hazardous work:
No problems expected. You do need to be cautious for symptoms of hypoglycemia.

Discontinuing:
Don't discontinue without doctor's advice, even though symptoms diminish or disappear.

Others:
- Along with taking drugs for diabetes, be sure to follow your doctor's instructions for lifestyle changes such as a proper diet, weight control measures and a regular exercise program.
- Notify your doctor if you have a fever, infection, diarrhea, or experience vomiting.
- Advise any doctor or dentist whom you consult that you take this medicine.
- Wear or carry medical identification that indicates you have type 2 diabetes and the drugs you take.
- See your diabetes doctor regularly to review your treatment and check for complications.
- You and your family should educate yourselves about diabetes; learn to recognize the symptoms of hypoglycemia and how to treat it. Hypoglycemia may occur in the treatment of diabetes as a result of skipped meals,
excessive exercise, or alcohol consumption. Carry non-dietetic candy or glucose tablets to treat episodes of low blood sugar.
- Inflammation of the pancreas (acute pancreatitis) may occur with use of sitagliptin. Call doctor right away if symptoms develop (severe abdominal pain, nausea, vomiting).

POSSIBLE INTERACTION WITH OTHER DRUGS

GENERIC NAME OR DRUG CLASS	COMBINED EFFECT
Digoxin	Digoxin dosage may need to be adjusted.
Enzyme inhibitors*	Increased effect of saxagliptin.
Hypoglycemia-causing medications*	May increase risk of low blood sugar or side effects.

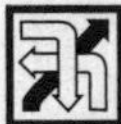

POSSIBLE INTERACTION WITH OTHER SUBSTANCES

INTERACTS WITH	COMBINED EFFECT
Alcohol:	May cause severe low blood sugar. Avoid.
Beverages:	None expected.
Cocaine:	Unknown. Avoid.
Foods:	None expected.
Marijuana:	Unknown. Avoid.
Tobacco:	No drug interaction. Tobacco use does raise risk of diabetes complications. Avoid smoking.

*See Glossary

DRONABINOL (THC, Marijuana)

BRAND NAMES

Marinol

BASIC INFORMATION

Habit forming? Yes
Prescription needed? Yes
Available as generic? Yes
Drug class: Antiemetic

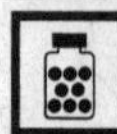

USES

- Prevents nausea and vomiting that may accompany taking anticancer medication (cancer chemotherapy). Should not be used unless other antinausea medicines fail.
- Appetite stimulant. Used to treat appetite loss in AIDS patients.

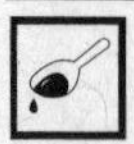

DOSAGE & USAGE INFORMATION

How to take:
Capsule—Swallow with liquid.

When to take:
Under supervision, a total of no more than 4 to 6 doses per day, every 2 to 4 hours after cancer chemotherapy for prescribed number of days.

If you forget a dose:
Take as soon as you remember. If it is almost time for the next dose, wait for the next scheduled dose (don't double this dose).

What drug does:
Affects nausea and vomiting center in brain to make it less irritable following cancer chemotherapy. Exact mechanism is unknown.

Time lapse before drug works:
2 to 4 hours.

Don't take with:
Any other medicine or any dietary supplement without consulting your doctor or pharmacist.

OVERDOSE

SYMPTOMS:
Pounding, rapid heart rate; high or low blood pressure; confusion; hallucinations; drastic mood changes; nervousness or anxiety.
WHAT TO DO:
Overdose unlikely to threaten life. If person uses much larger amount than prescribed or if accidentally swallowed, call doctor or poison control center 1-800-222-1222 for help.

POSSIBLE ADVERSE REACTIONS OR SIDE EFFECTS

SYMPTOMS	WHAT TO DO
Life-threatening: In case of overdose, see previous column.	
Common:	
• Rapid, pounding heartbeat.	Discontinue. Call doctor right away.
• Dizziness, irritability, drowsiness, euphoria, decreased coordination.	Continue. Call doctor when convenient.
• Red eyes, dry mouth.	No action necessary.
Infrequent:	
Depression, anxiety, nervousness, headache, hallucinations, dramatic mood changes, blurred or changed vision.	Discontinue. Call doctor right away.
Rare:	
• Rapid heartbeat, fainting, frequent or difficult urination, convulsions, shortness of breath, paranoia.	Discontinue. Call doctor right away.
• Nausea, loss of appetite, dizziness when standing after sitting or lying down, diarrhea.	Continue. Call doctor when convenient.

WARNINGS & PRECAUTIONS

Don't take if:
- Your nausea and vomiting is caused by anything other than cancer chemotherapy.
- You are sensitive or allergic to any form of marijuana or sesame oil.
- Your cycle of chemotherapy is longer than 7 consecutive days. Harmful side effects may occur.

Before you start, consult your doctor if:
- You have heart disease or high blood pressure.
- You are an alcoholic or drug addict.
- You are pregnant or intend to become pregnant.
- You are nursing an infant.
- You have schizophrenia or a manic-depressive disorder.

Over age 60:
Adverse reactions and side effects may be more frequent and severe than in younger persons.

Pregnancy:
Decide with your doctor if drug benefits justify risk to unborn child. Risk category C (see page xviii).

Breast-feeding:
Drug passes into milk. Avoid drug or discontinue nursing until you finish medicine. Consult doctor about maintaining milk supply.

Infants & children:
Not recommended.

Prolonged use:
- Avoid. Habit forming.
- Talk to your doctor about the need for follow-up medical examinations or laboratory studies to check heart function.

Skin & sunlight:
No problems expected.

Driving, piloting or hazardous work:
Don't drive or pilot aircraft until you learn how medicine affects you. Don't work around dangerous machinery. Don't climb ladders or work in high places. Danger increases if you drink alcohol or take medicine affecting alertness and reflexes, such as antihistamines, tranquilizers, sedatives, pain medicine, narcotics and mind-altering drugs.

Discontinuing:
Withdrawal effects such as irritability, insomnia, restlessness, sweating, diarrhea, hiccups, loss of appetite and hot flashes may follow abrupt withdrawal within 12 hours. Should they occur, these symptoms will probably subside within 96 hours.

Others:
- Store in refrigerator.
- Advise any doctor or dentist whom you consult that you take this medicine.

POSSIBLE INTERACTION WITH OTHER DRUGS

GENERIC NAME OR DRUG CLASS	COMBINED EFFECT
Anesthetics*	Oversedation.
Anticonvulsants*	Oversedation.
Antidepressants, tricyclic*	Oversedation.
Antihistamines*	Oversedation.
Barbiturates*	Oversedation.
Clozapine	Toxic effect on the central nervous system.
Ethinamate	Dangerous increased effects of ethinamate. Avoid combining.
Fluoxetine	Increased depressant effects of both drugs.
Guanfacine	May increase depressant effects of either drug.
Leucovorin	High alcohol content of leucovorin may cause adverse effects.
Methyprylon	Increased sedative effect, perhaps to dangerous level. Avoid.
Molindone	Increased effects of both drugs. Avoid.
Muscle relaxants*	Oversedation.
Nabilone	Greater depression of central nervous system.
Narcotics*	Oversedation.
Sedatives*	Oversedation.
Sertraline	Increased depressive effects of both drugs.
Tranquilizers*	Oversedation.

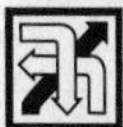

POSSIBLE INTERACTION WITH OTHER SUBSTANCES

INTERACTS WITH	COMBINED EFFECT
Alcohol:	Oversedation.
Beverages:	None expected.
Cocaine:	None expected.
Foods:	None expected.
Marijuana:	Oversedation.
Tobacco:	None expected.

*See Glossary

EFLORNITHINE (Topical)

BRAND NAMES

Vaniqa

BASIC INFORMATION

Habit forming? No
Prescription needed? Yes
Available as generic? No
Drug class: Enzyme inhibitor (topical)

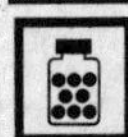

USES

Treatment for unwanted facial hair (hirsutism is the medical term) on women.

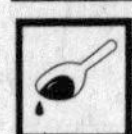

DOSAGE & USAGE INFORMATION

How to take:
Cream—Follow directions on package label. Usually requires twice-daily application. Limit application to facial area and avoid getting medication in eyes, nose or mouth. Apply at least five minutes after hair removal technique (shaving). Do not apply cosmetics until the medication dries. Do not wash face for at least four hours after applying medication.

When to take:
At the same times each day at least 8 hours apart.

If you forget a dose:
Use as soon as possible. Do not use if it is almost time for your next application. Do not double dose.

What drug does:
Inhibits an enzyme that encourages hair growth.

Time lapse before drug works:
4-8 weeks for improvement to be seen.

Don't take with:
Any other medicine or any dietary supplement without consulting your doctor or pharmacist.

OVERDOSE

SYMPTOMS:
None expected.
WHAT TO DO:
Not intended for internal use. If child accidentally swallows, call doctor or poison control center 1-800-222-1222 for help.

POSSIBLE ADVERSE REACTIONS OR SIDE EFFECTS

SYMPTOMS	WHAT TO DO
Life-threatening: None expected.	
Common: Stinging skin, acne breakout.	Continue. Call doctor if condition persists.
Infrequent: Skin symptoms (tingling, redness, chapped, swollen, burning, bleeding, rash, hair bumps, continued acne).	Continue. Call doctor when convenient.
Rare: None expected.	

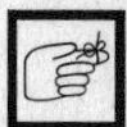

WARNINGS & PRECAUTIONS

Don't take if:
You are allergic to eflornithine.

Before you start, consult your doctor if:
You have facial abrasions, cuts or scrapes.

Over age 60:
No problems expected.

Pregnancy:
Consult doctor. Risk category C (see page xviii).

Breast-feeding:
It is unknown if eflornithine passes into breast milk. Avoid drug or discontinue nursing until you finish medicine. Consult doctor for advice on maintaining milk supply.

Infants & children:
Safety and efficacy has not been established in children under 12 years of age.

Prolonged use:
If no improvement is seen after six months of using this medicine, consult doctor.

Skin & sunlight:
No problems expected. However, if skin irritation occurs after prolonged exposure to sun, consult doctor.

Driving, piloting or hazardous work:
No problems expected.

Discontinuing:
- Consult doctor before discontinuing.
- In about 8 weeks, your hair growth will probably return to the same as it was before you started the medication.

Others:
Advise any doctor or dentist whom you consult that you use this drug.

POSSIBLE INTERACTION WITH OTHER DRUGS

GENERIC NAME OR DRUG CLASS	COMBINED EFFECT
None significant.	

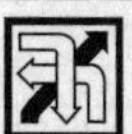

POSSIBLE INTERACTION WITH OTHER SUBSTANCES

INTERACTS WITH	COMBINED EFFECT
Alcohol:	None expected.
Beverages:	None expected.
Cocaine:	None expected.
Foods:	None expected.
Marijuana:	None expected.
Tobacco:	None expected.

ENDOTHELIN RECEPTOR ANTAGONIST

GENERIC AND BRAND NAMES

AMBRISENTAN	BOSENTAN
Letairis	Tracleer

BASIC INFORMATION

Habit forming? No
Prescription needed? Yes
Available as generic? No
Drug class: Antihypertensive (pulmonary)

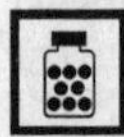

USES

Treats the symptoms of pulmonary arterial hypertension (PAH), which is high blood pressure in the lungs. It improves the breathing and exercise capacity of patients with PAH. The drug does not cure the disorder. These drugs are available only through restricted programs which will be explained by your doctor.

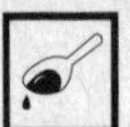

DOSAGE & USAGE INFORMATION

How to take:
Tablet—Swallow with liquid. Take with or without food. Do not break, crush or chew the tablet.

When to take:
Usually once or twice daily at the same times each day. Follow your doctor's instructions.

If you forget a dose:
Take as soon as you remember. If it is almost time for the next dose, wait for next scheduled dose (don't double this dose).

What drug does:
It works by blocking the effect of endothelin (a substance made by the body). In patients with PAH, the blood vessels become narrowed (constricted) due to an excess production of endothelin.

Continued next column

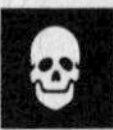

OVERDOSE

SYMPTOMS:
Dizziness or faintness, confusion, blurred vision, sweating, increased heart rate, unusual tiredness or weakness, vomiting.
WHAT TO DO:
Overdose unlikely to threaten life. If person uses much larger amount than prescribed or if accidentally swallowed, call doctor or poison control center 1-800-222-1222 for help.

Time lapse before drug works:
It may take 1 to 2 months or longer to notice effects. The dosage may be increased after 4 weeks if there are no problems in taking the drug.

Don't take with:
Any other medicine or any dietary supplement without consulting your doctor or pharmacist.

POSSIBLE ADVERSE REACTIONS OR SIDE EFFECTS

SYMPTOMS	WHAT TO DO
Life-threatening:	
Rare allergic reaction (hives, itching, rash, trouble breathing, tightness in chest, swelling of lips or tongue or throat).	Seek emergency treatment immediately.
Common:	
Feeling of warmth, flushing, stuffy or sore nose, sore throat, stomach upset, swelling of legs and ankles, mild dizziness.	Continue. Call doctor when convenient.
Infrequent:	
• Difficult breathing, irregular heartbeat, unusual tiredness or weakness, ongoing dizziness or lightheadedness, wheezing or unusual coughing.	Discontinue. Call doctor right away.
• Stomach pain, heartburn, mild heart palpitations, constipation, hoarseness, headache, low blood pressure.	Continue. Call doctor when convenient.
Rare:	
Liver problems (symptoms include loss of appetite, nausea, vomiting, light colored stools, fever, extreme tiredness, right upper stomach pain, yellow skin or eyes, dark urine, itching).	Discontinue. Call doctor right away.

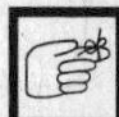

WARNINGS & PRECAUTIONS

Don't take if:

- You are allergic to endothelin receptor antagonists.
- You have moderate or severe liver (hepatic) impairment.
- You are pregnant or plan to become pregnant.
- You are of childbearing age and have not had a negative pregnancy test or you are not willing to use two reliable methods of birth control.

Before you start, consult your doctor if:

- You have mild liver impairment.
- You have not had a liver function test.
- You have anemia or edema (swelling in hands, lower legs or feet).

Over age 60:
Adverse reactions and side effects may be more frequent and severe than in younger persons.

Pregnancy:

- Using this drug while you are pregnant can cause very serious birth defects. Risk category X (see page xviii).
- If this drug is used during pregnancy, or if you become pregnant while taking this drug, you need to talk to your doctor about the potential hazard to the fetus.

Breast-feeding:
It is unknown if drug passes into milk. Avoid drug or discontinue nursing. Consult doctor.

Infants & children:
Not approved for ages under 18.

Prolonged use:

- Your doctor will check your progress at regular visits to make sure this drug is working properly and to check for unwanted effects.
- Your doctor will advise you about any liver function tests needed before you start the drug and while taking the drug.

Skin & sunlight:
No problems expected.

Driving, piloting or hazardous work:
Use caution if you experience dizziness.

Discontinuing:
Consult doctor before discontinuing. The dosage may need to be slowly reduced before stopping.

Others:

- Females of childbearing age will be required to have a pregnancy test every month during treatment. If you miss a menstrual period while using this drug, call your doctor right away. Use two forms of effective birth control to keep from getting pregnant while you are using this drug (even if the drug is temporarily stopped), and for at least one month after you stop taking the drug.
- Use of bosentan may lead to liver problems. Follow your doctor's advice about periodic liver function studies. Call doctor right away if symptoms of liver problems develop (see list in Possible Adverse Reactions or Side Effects).
- These drugs may decrease hemoglobin* and hematocrit.* Follow doctor's advice about routine blood testing.
- Advise any doctor or dentist whom you consult that you take this drug.
- The drug may decrease the amount of sperm men make and affect their ability to have children. Consult doctor.

POSSIBLE INTERACTION WITH OTHER DRUGS

GENERIC NAME OR DRUG CLASS	COMBINED EFFECT
Cyclosporine A	Increased endothelin receptor antagonist effect; decreased cyclosporine effect. Avoid use with bosentan.
Enzyme inducers*	Decreased endothelin receptor antagonist effect.
Enzyme inhibitors*	Increased endothelin receptor antagonist effect.
Glyburide	Decreased effect of both glyburide and endothelin receptor antagonist. May increase risk of liver problems. Avoid with bosentan.
Contraceptives, hormonal*	Decreased birth control effect.

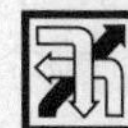

POSSIBLE INTERACTION WITH OTHER SUBSTANCES

INTERACTS WITH	COMBINED EFFECT
Alcohol:	No interaction, but patients should avoid heavy alcohol use.
Beverages:	No proven problems.
Cocaine:	Unknown. Avoid.
Foods:	No proven problems.
Marijuana:	Unknown. Avoid.
Tobacco:	No interaction, but patients with PAH should not smoke.

***See Glossary**

EPHEDRINE

BRAND NAMES

Ami-Rax
Broncholate
Marax
Marax D.F.
Rynatuss
Rynatuss Pediatric

BASIC INFORMATION

Habit forming? No
Prescription needed? Yes
Available as generic? Yes, for some
Drug class: Sympathomimetic

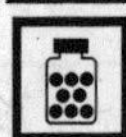

USES

- Relieves bronchial asthma.
- Decreases congestion of breathing passages.
- Suppresses allergic reactions.

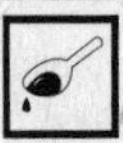

DOSAGE & USAGE INFORMATION

How to take:
- Tablet or capsule—Swallow with liquid. You may chew or crush tablet.
- Extended-release tablet or capsule—Swallow each dose whole.
- Syrup—Take as directed on bottle.
- Drops—Dilute dose in beverage.

When to take:
As needed, no more often than every 4 hours. To prevent insomnia, take last dose at least 2 hours before bedtime.

If you forget a dose:
Take as soon as you remember. If it is almost time for the next dose, wait for the next scheduled dose (don't double this dose).

What drug does:
- Prevents cells from releasing allergy-causing chemicals (histamines).
- Relaxes muscles of bronchial tubes.
- Decreases blood vessel size and blood flow, thus causing decongestion.

Continued next column

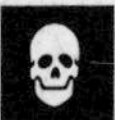

OVERDOSE

SYMPTOMS:
Severe anxiety, confusion, delirium, muscle tremors, rapid and irregular pulse.
WHAT TO DO:
- **Dial 911 (emergency) for medical help or call poison control center 1-800-222-1222 for instructions.**
- **See emergency information on last 3 pages of this book.**

Time lapse before drug works:
30 to 60 minutes.

Don't take with:
- Nonprescription drugs with ephedrine, pseudoephedrine or epinephrine.
- Any other medicine or any dietary supplement without consulting your doctor or pharmacist.

POSSIBLE ADVERSE REACTIONS OR SIDE EFFECTS

SYMPTOMS	WHAT TO DO
Life-threatening: In case of overdose, see previous column.	
Common:	
• Nervousness, headache, paleness, rapid heartbeat.	Continue. Call doctor when convenient.
• Insomnia.	Continue. Tell doctor at next visit.
Infrequent:	
• Irregular heartbeat.	Discontinue. Call doctor right away.
• Dizziness, appetite loss, nausea, vomiting, painful or difficult urination.	Continue. Call doctor when convenient.
Rare: None expected.	

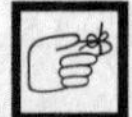

WARNINGS & PRECAUTIONS

Don't take if:
You are allergic to ephedrine or any sympathomimetic* drug.

Before you start, consult your doctor if:
- You have high blood pressure.
- You have diabetes.
- You have overactive thyroid gland.
- You have difficulty urinating.
- You have taken any MAO inhibitor in past 2 weeks.
- You have taken digitalis preparations in the last 7 days.
- You will have surgery within 2 months, including dental surgery, requiring general or spinal anesthesia.

Over age 60:
More likely to develop high blood pressure, heart-rhythm disturbances, angina and to feel drug's stimulant effects.

Pregnancy:
Decide with your doctor if drug benefits justify risk to unborn child. Risk category C (see page xviii).

Breast-feeding:
Drug passes into milk. Avoid drug or discontinue nursing until you finish medicine. Consult doctor for advice on maintaining milk supply.

Infants & children:
Read label on product to determine if it is approved for your child's age.

Prolonged use:
- Excessive doses—Rare toxic psychosis.
- Men with enlarged prostate gland may have more urination difficulty.

Skin & sunlight:
No problems expected.

Driving, piloting or hazardous work:
Avoid if you feel dizzy. Otherwise, no problems expected.

Discontinuing:
May be unnecessary to finish medicine. Follow doctor's instructions.

Others:
No problems expected.

POSSIBLE INTERACTION WITH OTHER DRUGS

GENERIC NAME OR DRUG CLASS	COMBINED EFFECT
Adrenocorticoids, systemic	Decreased adrenocorticoid effect.
Antidepressants, tricyclic*	Increased effect of ephedrine. Excessive stimulation of heart and blood pressure.
Antihypertensives*	Decreased anti-hypertensive effect.
Beta-adrenergic blocking agents*	Decreased effects of both drugs.
Dextrothyroxine	Increased ephedrine effect.
Digitalis preparations*	Serious heart rhythm disturbances.
Epinephrine	Increased epinephrine effect.
Ergot preparations*	Serious blood pressure rise.
Furazolidone	Sudden, severe increase in blood pressure.
Guanadrel	Decreased effect of both drugs.
Guanethidine	Decreased effect of both drugs.
Methyldopa	Possible increased blood pressure.
Monoamine oxidase (MAO) inhibitors*	Increased ephedrine effect. Dangerous blood pressure rise.
Nitrates*	Possible decreased effects of both drugs.
Phenothiazines*	Possible increased ephedrine toxicity. Possible decreased ephedrine effect.
Pseudoephedrine	Increased pseudoephedrine effect.
Rauwolfia	Decreased rauwolfia effect.
Sympathomimetics*	Increased ephedrine effect.
Terazosin	Decreased effectiveness of terazosin.
Theophylline	Increased gastro-intestinal intolerance.

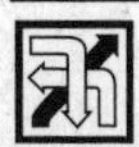

POSSIBLE INTERACTION WITH OTHER SUBSTANCES

INTERACTS WITH	COMBINED EFFECT
Alcohol:	None expected.
Beverages: Caffeine drinks.	Nervousness or insomnia.
Cocaine:	High risk of heartbeat irregularities and high blood pressure.
Foods:	None expected.
Marijuana:	Rapid heartbeat, possible heart rhythm disturbance.
Tobacco:	None expected.

*See Glossary

EPLERENONE

BRAND NAMES

Inspra

BASIC INFORMATION

Habit forming? No
Prescription needed? Yes
Available as generic? Yes
Drug class: Antihypertensive; selective aldosterone blocker

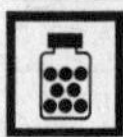

USES

- Treatment for hypertension (high blood pressure). May be used alone or along with other antihypertensive medications.
- Used to treat further complications after a myocardial infarction.
- May be used for treatment of other disorders as determined by your doctor.

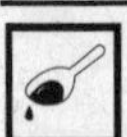

DOSAGE & USAGE INFORMATION

How to take:
Tablet—Swallow with liquid. May be taken with or without food.

When to take:
Once or twice daily as directed by your doctor.

If you forget a dose:
Take as soon as you remember. If it is almost time for the next dose, then skip the missed dose and wait for your next scheduled dose (don't double this dose).

What drug does:
It blocks aldosterone, a hormone in the body that increases blood pressure by causing fluid and salt retention. The drug causes the kidneys to remove the excess water and salt from the body.

Time lapse before drug works:
May take several weeks for full effectiveness.

Don't take with:
Any other medicine or any dietary supplement without consulting your doctor or pharmacist.

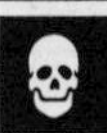

OVERDOSE

SYMPTOMS:
Unknown. Could cause very low blood pressure (hypotension).
WHAT TO DO:
Overdose unlikely to threaten life. If person uses much larger amount than prescribed or if accidentally swallowed, call doctor or poison control center 1-800-222-1222 for help.

POSSIBLE ADVERSE REACTIONS OR SIDE EFFECTS

SYMPTOMS	WHAT TO DO
Life-threatening: None expected.	
Common: Dizziness.	Continue. Call doctor when convenient.
Infrequent: Diarrhea, flu-like, symptoms, cough, fatigue, headache, stomach pain.	Continue. Call doctor when convenient.
Rare:	
• Abnormal vaginal bleeding in women, enlarged breasts or breast pain in men.	Continue. Call doctor when convenient.
• Hyperkalemia (too much potassium in the body; symptoms include confusion, shortness of breath, feeling very weak and tired, numbness and tingling, irregular heartbeat, nervousness, low blood pressure).	Discontinue. Call doctor right away or seek emergency help if symptoms are severe.

WARNINGS & PRECAUTIONS

Don't take if:
You are allergic to eplerenone.

Before you start, consult your doctor if:
- You have any kidney or liver disease.
- You have high blood potassium levels or low blood sodium levels.
- You are on any special diet using low salt or salt substitutes.
- You have diabetes.
- You have high cholesterol or heart disease.
- You are allergic to any medication, food or other substance.

Over age 60:
No special problems expected.

Pregnancy:
Usually safe, but decide with your doctor if drug benefits justify any possible risk to unborn child. Risk category B (see page xviii).

Breast-feeding:
It is unknown if drug passes into milk. Avoid nursing until you finish medicine. Consult doctor for advice on maintaining milk supply.

Infants & children:
Not approved for children under age 18.

Prolonged use:
- No special problems expected. Hypertension usually requires life-long treatment.
- Schedule regular doctor visits to determine if drug is continuing to be effective in controlling the hypertension and to check your potassium levels and kidney function.

Skin & sunlight:
No special problems expected.

Driving, piloting or hazardous work:
Use caution if you feel dizzy or are experiencing other side effects.

Discontinuing:
Don't discontinue without consulting your doctor, even if you feel well. You can have hypertension without feeling any symptoms. Untreated high blood pressure can cause serious problems.

Others:
- Advise any doctor or dentist whom you consult that you take this medicine. May interfere with the accuracy of some medical tests.
- See your doctor regularly, especially when you first start taking this drug.
- Follow any diet or exercise plan your doctor prescribes. It can help control hypertension.
- Get up slowly from a sitting or lying position to avoid any dizziness, faintness or lightheadedness.
- Can elevate triglycerides and cholesterol; these may need to be monitored regularly.
- Consult doctor if you become ill with vomiting or diarrhea.

POSSIBLE INTERACTION WITH OTHER DRUGS

GENERIC NAME OR DRUG CLASS	COMBINED EFFECT
Angiotensin-converting enzyme (ACE) inhibitors*	Decreased anti-hypertensive effect.
Angiotensin II receptor antagonists	Decreased anti-hypertensive effect.
Diuretics, potassium-sparing*	Excess potassium levels in the body.
Enzyme inhibitors*	Increased effect of eplerenone.
Potassium supplements*	Excess potassium levels in the body.
St. Johns Wort	Decreased antihypertensive effect.

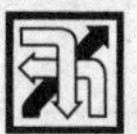

POSSIBLE INTERACTION WITH OTHER SUBSTANCES

INTERACTS WITH	COMBINED EFFECT
Alcohol:	Increased risk of side effects. Avoid.
Beverages: Grapefruit juice.	Increased effect of eplerenone.
Cocaine:	Unknown effect. Avoid.
Foods: Salt substitutes containing potassium or foods high in potassium (e.g., bananas).	Excess potassium in the body. Avoid.
Marijuana:	Unknown effect. Avoid.
Tobacco:	None expected. Best to avoid.

*See Glossary

ERECTILE DYSFUNCTION AGENTS

GENERIC AND BRAND NAMES

AVANAFIL
Stendra
SILDENAFIL
Revatio
Viagra
TADALAFIL
Cialis
VARDENAFIL
Levitra
Staxyn

BASIC INFORMATION

Habit forming? No
Prescription needed? Yes
Available as generic? No
Drug class: Impotence therapy

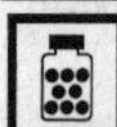

USES

- Treats male sexual function (erection) problems.
- Tadalafil is used for treatment of signs and symptoms of benign prostatic hyperplasia.
- Brand name Revatio treats adult pulmonary arterial hypertension (rare fatal lung disorder).

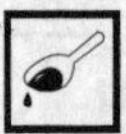

DOSAGE & USAGE INFORMATION

How to take:
- Tablet—Swallow with water. If you can't swallow whole, crumble tablet and take with liquid or food.
- Orally disintegrating tablet—Place on your tongue. It will dissolve rapidly. Do not swallow, crush or split tablet. Do not take it with liquid.

When to take:
- As directed; usually 30 minutes to 1 hour before sexual activity.
- Daily dose tadalafil, take as directed on label.

If you forget a dose:
- Does not apply for the tablet taken before sexual activity.
- For once daily tadalafil, take as soon as you remember. If it is almost time for the next dose, wait for the next scheduled dose (don't double this dose).

Continued next column

What drug does:
- Increases blood flow to the penis that may help men develop and sustain an erection. Sexual stimulation is still needed for these drugs to be effective.
- In pulmonary arterial hypertension, the drug works by dilating (widening) blood vessels, thereby lowering blood pressure in the lungs.

Time lapse before drug works:
- Sildenafil, 30-60 minutes, lasts up to 4 hours.
- Vardenafil, 25-30 minutes, lasts up to 4-5 hours.
- Tadalafil, 16-60 minutes, lasts up to 36 hours.

Don't take with:
Any other medicine or any dietary supplement without consulting your doctor or pharmacist.

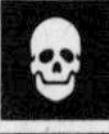

OVERDOSE

SYMPTOMS:
May include nausea, irregular heartbeat, chest pain, faintness, lightheadedness.
WHAT TO DO:
If person takes much larger amount than prescribed, dial 911 (emergency) for medical help or call poison control center 1-800-222-1222 for instructions.

POSSIBLE ADVERSE REACTIONS OR SIDE EFFECTS

SYMPTOMS	WHAT TO DO
Life-threatening: Fatalities have been reported when used with nitrate medications.	
Common:	
Headache, flushing, stomach upset, stuffy or runny nose, back pain, muscle aches.	Continue. Call doctor if symptoms persist.
Infrequent:	
• Urination problems, blurred vision, changes in color perception, light sensitivity, skin rash, dizziness, prolonged erection (lasting more than 4 hours).	Discontinue. Call doctor right away.
• Diarrhea.	Continue. Call doctor if symptoms persist.
Rare:	
• Chest pain, fainting, foot or ankle swelling, allergic reaction, (shortness of breath, skin rash, hives, itching, face swelling), changes in hearing, ringing or buzzing in the ears.	Discontinue. Call doctor right away.
• Unexpected symptoms occur while having sexual intercourse.	Discontinue. Call doctor when convenient.

WARNINGS & PRECAUTIONS

Don't take if:
You are allergic to sildenafil, vardenafil, or tadalafil.

Before you start, consult your doctor if:
- You have any other medical problem.
- You have or have had heart, blood pressure or blood cell problems or have had a stroke.
- You have a stomach ulcer.
- You have vision problems.
- You have retinitis pigmentosa.
- You have a deformed shape of the penis or have had an erection last more than 4 hours.
- You use drugs like amyl nitrate or butyl nitrate recreationally.
- You have liver or kidney disease.

Over age 60:
No problems expected unless person has an increased sensitivity to medications.

Pregnancy:
Not indicated for use in females. Risk category B (see page xviii).

Breast-feeding:
Not indicated for use in females.

Infants & children:
Safety and effectiveness of use in children not established. Not recommended or indicated.

Prolonged use:
Talk to your doctor about the need for follow-up medical examinations or laboratory studies to determine drug's effectiveness.

Skin & sunlight:
No problems expected.

Driving, piloting or hazardous work:
No problems expected.

Discontinuing:
No problems expected.

Others:
- Advise any doctor or dentist whom you consult that you take this medicine.
- Do not increase dose without doctor's approval.
- Consult doctor if there are any significant changes in your vision. A small number of men taking one or more of these drugs have developed NAION (non-arteritic ischemic optic neuropathy) a loss of vision that is frequently irreversible. Ask your doctor about your risks.
- Do not combine the drug with any other impotence therapy unless approved by your doctor.
- These drugs do not protect against sexually transmitted diseases.
- There are many causes of impotence. Your doctor should perform a complete exam before prescribing this medication.
- Call doctor right away in the event of sudden decrease or loss of hearing. You may be also experience tinnitus (ringing/buzzing in the ears) and dizziness.

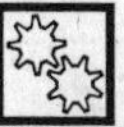

POSSIBLE INTERACTION WITH OTHER DRUGS

GENERIC NAME OR DRUG CLASS	COMBINED EFFECT
Alpha adrenergic receptor blockers	Sudden drop in blood pressure. Do not use together.
Enzyme inhibitors*	Increased effect of erectile dysfunction agent.
Protease inhibitors	Increased effect of erectile dysfunction agent.
Nitrates	Sudden drop in blood pressure. Do not use together.
Rifampin	Decreased effect of erectile dysfunction agent.

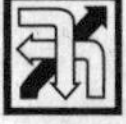

POSSIBLE INTERACTION WITH OTHER SUBSTANCES

INTERACTS WITH	COMBINED EFFECT
Alcohol:	May decrease effect of erectile dysfunction agents.
Beverages:	Grapefruit juice may increase blood levels of erectile dysfunction agents.
Cocaine:	Effects unknown. Avoid.
Foods:	None expected.
Marijuana:	Effects unknown. Avoid.
Tobacco:	None expected.

***See Glossary**

ERGOLOID MESYLATES

BRAND NAMES

Gerimal
Hydergine
Hydergine LC
Niloric

BASIC INFORMATION

Habit forming? No
Prescription needed? Yes
Available as generic? Yes
Drug class: Ergot preparation

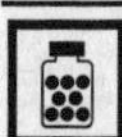

USES

Treatment for reduced alertness, poor memory, confusion, depression or lack of motivation in the elderly.

DOSAGE & USAGE INFORMATION

How to take:
- Tablet or capsule—Swallow with liquid. If you can't swallow whole, crumble tablet or open capsule and take with liquid or food.
- Liquid—Take as directed on label.
- Sublingual tablet—Dissolve tablet under tongue.

When to take:
At the same times each day.

If you forget a dose:
Take as soon as you remember. If it is almost time for the next dose, wait for the next scheduled dose (don't double this dose).

What drug does:
Stimulates brain-cell metabolism to increase use of oxygen and nutrients.

Time lapse before drug works:
Gradual improvements over 3 to 4 months.

Continued next column

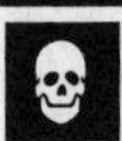

OVERDOSE

SYMPTOMS:
Headache, flushed face, nasal congestion, nausea, vomiting, blood pressure drop, blurred vision, weakness, collapse, coma.
WHAT TO DO:
- **Dial 911 (emergency) for medical help or call poison control center 1-800-222-1222 for instructions.**
- **See emergency information on last 3 pages of this book.**

Don't take with:
- Nonprescription drugs containing alcohol without consulting doctor.
- Any other medicine or any dietary supplement without consulting your doctor or pharmacist.

POSSIBLE ADVERSE REACTIONS OR SIDE EFFECTS

SYMPTOMS	WHAT TO DO
Life-threatening:	
In case of overdose, see previous column.	
Common:	
Runny nose, skin flushing, headache.	Continue. Tell doctor at next visit.
Infrequent:	
Slow heartbeat, tingling fingers, blurred vision.	Discontinue. Call doctor right away.
Rare:	
• Fainting.	Discontinue. Seek emergency treatment.
• Rash, nausea, vomiting, stomach cramps, dizziness when getting up, drowsiness, soreness under tongue, appetite loss.	Continue. Call doctor when convenient.

WARNINGS & PRECAUTIONS

Don't use if:
- If you are allergic to any ergot preparation.
- Your heartbeat is less than 60 beats per minute.
- Your systolic blood pressure is consistently below 100.

Before you start, consult your doctor if:
- You have had low blood pressure.
- You have liver disease.
- You have severe mental illness.

Over age 60:
Primarily used in persons older than 60. Results unpredictable, but many patients show improved brain function.

Pregnancy:
Generally not used in this age group.

Breast-feeding:
Risk to nursing child outweighs drug benefits. Don't use.

Infants & children:
Not recommended.

Prolonged use:
Talk to your doctor about the need for follow-up medical examinations or laboratory studies.

Skin & sunlight:
No problems expected.

Driving, piloting or hazardous work:
Avoid if you feel dizzy, faint or have blurred vision. Otherwise, no problems expected.

Discontinuing:
No problems expected.

Others:
- May lessen your body's ability to adjust to cold temperatures.
- Advise any doctor or dentist whom you consult that you use this medicine.

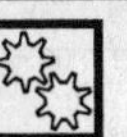

POSSIBLE INTERACTION WITH OTHER DRUGS

GENERIC NAME OR DRUG CLASS	COMBINED EFFECT
Ergot preparations,* other	May cause serious side effects. Avoid.
Sympathomimetics*	May cause decreased circulation to arms, legs, feet and hands. Avoid.

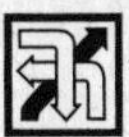

POSSIBLE INTERACTION WITH OTHER SUBSTANCES

INTERACTS WITH	COMBINED EFFECT
Alcohol:	Use caution. May drop blood pressure excessively.
Beverages:	None expected.
Cocaine:	Overstimulation. Avoid.
Foods:	None expected.
Marijuana:	Decreased effect of ergoloid mesylate.
Tobacco:	Decreased ergoloid effect. Don't smoke.

***See Glossary**

ERGOT ALKALOIDS

GENERIC AND BRAND NAMES

ERGONOVINE
- Ergometrine
- Ergotrate
- Ergotrate Maleate

METHYL-ERGONOVINE
- Methylergometrine

BASIC INFORMATION

Habit forming? No
Prescription needed? Yes
Available as generic? Yes
Drug class: Ergot preparation (uterine stimulant)

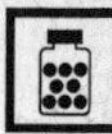

USES

Retards excessive post-delivery bleeding.

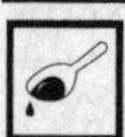

DOSAGE & USAGE INFORMATION

How to take:
Tablet—Swallow with liquid or food to lessen stomach irritation.

When to take:
At the same times each day.

If you forget a dose:
Don't take missed dose and don't double next one. Wait for next scheduled dose.

What drug does:
Causes smooth muscle cells of uterine wall to contract and surround bleeding blood vessels of relaxed uterus.

Time lapse before drug works:
20 to 30 minutes.

Don't take with:
Any other medicine or any dietary supplement without consulting your doctor or pharmacist.

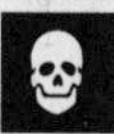

OVERDOSE

SYMPTOMS:
Vomiting, diarrhea, weak pulse, low blood pressure, difficult breathing, angina, convulsions.

WHAT TO DO:
- **Dial 911 (emergency) for medical help or call poison control center 1-800-222-1222 for instructions.**
- **If person is unconscious, check breathing and pulse. If not breathing, begin mouth-to-mouth rescue breathing. If heart is not beating, begin chest compressions.**
- **See emergency information on last 3 pages of this book.**

POSSIBLE ADVERSE REACTIONS OR SIDE EFFECTS

SYMPTOMS	WHAT TO DO
Life-threatening: In case of overdose, see previous column.	
Common:	
Nausea, vomiting, severe lower abdominal menstrual-like cramps.	Discontinue. Call doctor right away.
Infrequent:	
• Confusion, ringing in ears, diarrhea, muscle cramps.	Discontinue. Call doctor right away.
• Unusual sweating.	Continue. Call doctor when convenient.
Rare:	
Sudden, severe headache; shortness of breath; chest pain; numb, cold hands and feet.	Discontinue. Seek emergency treatment.

WARNINGS & PRECAUTIONS

Don't take if:
You are allergic to any ergot alkaloid.

Before you start, consult your doctor if:
- You have coronary artery or blood vessel disease.
- You have liver or kidney disease.
- You have high blood pressure.
- You have postpartum infection.

Over age 60:
Not used in this age group.

Pregnancy:
Consult doctor.

Breast-feeding:
Drug passes into milk. Avoid drug or discontinue nursing until you finish medicine. Consult doctor for advice on maintaining milk supply.

Infants & children:
Not recommended.

Prolonged use:
Talk to your doctor about the need for follow-up medical exams or lab studies.

Skin & sunlight:
No problems expected.

Driving, piloting or hazardous work:
No problems expected.

Discontinuing:
May be unnecessary to finish medicine. Follow doctor's instructions.

Others:
Drug should be used for short time only following childbirth or miscarriage.

POSSIBLE INTERACTION WITH OTHER DRUGS

GENERIC NAME OR DRUG CLASS	COMBINED EFFECT
Antifungals, azoles	Can cause serious or life-threatening problems with blood circulation. Avoid.
Beta-adrenergic blocking agents*	Possible vasospasm (peripheral and cardiac).
Ergot preparations,* other	May cause serious side effects. Avoid.
Macrolide antibiotics	Can cause serious or life-threatening problems with blood circulation. Avoid.
Protease Inhibitors	Can cause serious or life-threatening problems with blood circulation. Avoid.
Sympathomimetics*	May cause decreased circulation to arms, legs, feet and hands. Avoid.
Triptans	May cause serious side effects if taken within 24 hours of ergot alkaloid.

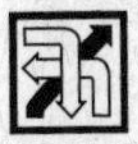

POSSIBLE INTERACTION WITH OTHER SUBSTANCES

INTERACTS WITH	COMBINED EFFECT
Alcohol:	None expected.
Beverages:	None expected.
Cocaine:	None expected.
Foods:	None expected.
Marijuana:	None expected.
Tobacco:	Decreased ergot alkaloid effect. Don't smoke.

*See Glossary

ERGOT DERIVATIVES

GENERIC AND BRAND NAMES

ERGOTAMINE
Cafergot
Ergomar
Migergot
Wigraine

DIHYDRO-ERGOTAMINE
Levadex
Migranal

BASIC INFORMATION

Habit forming? Unlikely
Prescription needed? Yes
Available as generic? Yes, for some
Drug class: Antimigraine

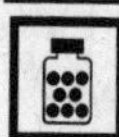

USES

- Treatment for migraine (with or without aura) and cluster headaches.
- Treats other disorders as determined by doctor.

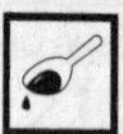

DOSAGE & USAGE INFORMATION

How to take:

- Tablet—Swallow with liquid.
- Sublingual tablet—Don't swallow whole. Let dissolve under tongue. Don't eat or drink while tablet is dissolving.
- Suppository—Remove wrapper and use finger to gently push into rectum.
- Nasal spray or oral inhaler—Use only as directed on prescription label.
- Injection (dihydroergotamine)—Normally given by a healthcare provider.

When to take:
Take or use drug at the first warning sign or symptom of the headache. Lie down in a quiet, dark room. If headache persists, follow your doctor's instructions as to when you should take or use additional dosages.

Continued next column

If you forget a dose:
The drug is taken or used as needed and not on a regular schedule.

What drug does:
It constricts (narrows) blood vessels in the head that have become dilated (widened). This action helps abort (stop) an impending headache or stops a headache in progress.

Time lapse before drug works:
15 to 60 minutes (depends on dosage form).

Don't take with:
Any other medicine or any dietary supplement without consulting your doctor or pharmacist.

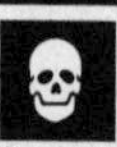

OVERDOSE

SYMPTOMS:
Nausea, vomiting, numbness of fingers and toes, tingling, confusion, drowsiness, headache, shock, convulsions, coma.

WHAT TO DO:

- **Dial 911 (emergency) for medical help or call poison control center 1-800-222-1222 for instructions.**
- **See emergency information on last 3 pages of this book.**

POSSIBLE ADVERSE REACTIONS OR SIDE EFFECTS

SYMPTOMS	WHAT TO DO
Life-threatening:	
Rare allergic reaction (hives, itching, rash, wheezing, tightness in chest, swelling of lips or tongue or throat).	Seek emergency treatment immediately.
Common:	
• Feet and ankle swelling.	Discontinue. Call doctor right away.
• Dizziness, nausea, diarrhea, vomiting, drowsiness, dry mouth.	Continue. Call doctor when convenient.
Infrequent:	
• Itchy or swollen skin; cold, pale hands or fingers or feet; pain or weakness (in arms, legs, back).	Discontinue. Call doctor right away.
• Headaches increase or are more severe, nose irritation or taste changes (with nasal spray), drug aftertaste (with oral inhaler).	Continue. Call doctor when convenient.
Rare:	
Anxiety or confusion; changes in vision; stomach pain; fast or slow heartbeat; chest pain; numbness or tingling in face, fingers, toes; high or low blood pressure; shortness of breath; problems with speech or balance.	Discontinue. Call doctor right away.

Note: Side effects vary depending on dosage form, or possible overuse, of the drug. Some symptoms may result from the headache itself (e.g., nausea).

WARNINGS & PRECAUTIONS

Don't take if:
You are allergic to any ergot derivative.

Before you start, consult your doctor if:
- You have angina, heart problems, high blood pressure, coronary artery disease, peripheral artery disease, blood circulation problem, high cholesterol, or have had a heart attack or stroke.
- You have diabetes, kidney or liver disease.
- You smoke cigarettes.
- You plan to become pregnant.
- You have a serious infection.
- You are allergic to other spray inhalants.

Over age 60:
Adverse reactions and side effects may be more frequent and severe than in younger persons.

Pregnancy:
Risk to unborn child outweighs drug benefits. Don't use. Risk category X (see page xviii).

Breast-feeding:
Drug passes into breast milk and may cause vomiting, diarrhea or other symptoms in nursing infant. Discuss with your doctor about whether to discontinue nursing or discontinue drug.

Infants & children:
Safety and effectiveness not established. Consult your child's doctor.

Prolonged use:
To avoid risk of serious adverse effects, do not exceed prescribed dosage or overuse the drug. It is not intended for chronic daily use. There have been reports of psychological dependence and drug abuse.

Skin & sunlight:
No problems expected.

Driving, piloting or hazardous work:
Don't drive or pilot aircraft until you learn how drug affects you. Don't work around dangerous machinery. Don't climb ladders or work in high places. Danger increases if you drink alcohol or take drugs affecting alertness and reflexes.

Discontinuing:
If drug is used for long period of time or is overused, rebound headaches (also called medication overuse headaches) may occur when drug is stopped. Consult doctor for advice.

Others:
- Advise any doctor, dentist or pharmacist whom you consult that you take this drug.
- Do not exceed the prescribed maximum dose.
- These drugs constrict blood vessels which can lead to serious adverse effects (possibly fatal) due to decrease in blood flow. The drugs can cause fibrosis (scarring) in lungs, heart or kidneys. Consult doctor about your risks.
- It may take several episodes of using the drug to determine full effectiveness.
- The drug product may also contain caffeine. Read the Caffeine Drug Chart for complete information about the drug.

POSSIBLE INTERACTION WITH OTHER DRUGS

GENERIC NAME OR DRUG CLASS	COMBINED EFFECT
Enzyme inhibitors*	Dangerous risk of blood circulation problem. Must avoid.
Ergot preparations,* other	Increased risk of side effects. Take drugs 24 hours apart.
Sympathomimetics*	Risk of dangerous high blood pressure.
Triptans	Increased risk of side effects. Take drugs 24 hours apart.

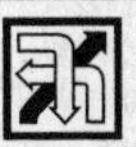

POSSIBLE INTERACTION WITH OTHER SUBSTANCES

INTERACTS WITH	COMBINED EFFECT
Alcohol:	Increased risk of side effects. Avoid.
Beverages: Grapefruit juice.	Increased risk of side effects. Consult doctor.
Cocaine:	Increased risk of side effects. Avoid.
Foods: Grapefruit.	Increased risk of side effects. Consult doctor.
Marijuana:	Increased risk of side effects. Avoid.
Tobacco:	Increased risk of blood circulation problems. Avoid.

*See Glossary

ERYTHROMYCINS

GENERIC AND BRAND NAMES

See full list of generic and brand names in the *Generic and Brand Name Directory*, page 884.

BASIC INFORMATION

Habit forming? No
Prescription needed? Yes
Available as generic? Yes
Drug class: Antibacterial; antiacne agent

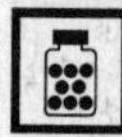

USES

- Treatment of a variety of bacterial infections.
- Treatment for acne.
- May be used to treat other disorders as determined by your doctor.

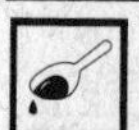

DOSAGE & USAGE INFORMATION

How to take:

- Table, capsule, extended-release tablet or extended-release capsule—Swallow each dose whole with liquid. Do not crush or chew.
- Oral suspension or pediatric drop—Shake well before using. Use dropper supplied with prescription or use a special measuring device to measure dose.
- Chewable tablet—Crush or chew completely and then swallow.

When to take:
At the same times each day, 1 hour before or 2 hours after eating. May be taken with food if stomach upset occurs. Enteric-coated tablets may be taken with or without food.

If you forget a dose:
Take as soon as you remember. If it is almost time for the next dose, wait for that dose (don't double this dose) and resume regular schedule.

Continued next column

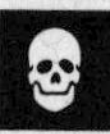

OVERDOSE

SYMPTOMS:
Nausea, vomiting, abdominal discomfort, diarrhea.
WHAT TO DO:
Overdose unlikely to threaten life. If person uses much larger amount than prescribed or if accidentally swallowed, call doctor or poison control center 1-800-222-1222 for help.

What drug does:
Prevents growth and reproduction of susceptible bacteria.

Time lapse before drug works:
Depends on the type of infection or acne symptoms; may take 7 to 21 days or longer.

Don't take with:
Any other medicine or any dietary supplement without consulting your doctor or pharmacist.

POSSIBLE ADVERSE REACTIONS OR SIDE EFFECTS

SYMPTOMS	WHAT TO DO
Life-threatening:	
Rare allergic reaction (hives, itching, rash, wheezing, tightness in chest, swelling of lips or tongue or throat).	Seek emergency treatment immediately.
Common:	
Mild nausea.	Continue. Call doctor when convenient.
Infrequent:	
• Fever with severe nausea and vomiting, severe stomach pain, unusual tiredness or weakness, yellow eyes or skin, pale stools, skin rash (redness and itching).	Discontinue. Call doctor right away.
• Mild diarrhea, stomach cramps or vomiting, sore mouth or tongue or have white patches.	Continue. Call doctor when convenient.
Rare:	
Irregular or slow heartbeat, any hearing loss, fainting.	Discontinue. Call doctor right away.

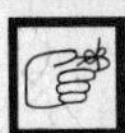

WARNINGS & PRECAUTIONS

Don't take if:
You are allergic to any erythromycin or macrolide antibiotics.

Before you start, consult your doctor if:
- You have had liver disease or impaired liver function or stomach problems.
- You have a hearing loss.
- You have a history of heart rhythm problems, a history of long QT syndrome or myasthenia gravis or an electrolyte imbalance .

Over age 60:
You may have increased risk of hearing loss.

Pregnancy:
Decide with your doctor if drug benefits justify risk to unborn child. Risk category B (see page xviii).

Breast-feeding:
Drug passes into milk. Avoid drug or discontinue nursing until you finish medicine. Consult doctor for advice on maintaining milk supply.

Infants & children:
Use only under close medical supervision.

Prolonged use:
- You may become more susceptible to infections caused by germs not responsive to erythromycin.
- Talk to your doctor about the need for follow-up medical examinations or laboratory studies to check liver function.

Skin & sunlight:
No problems expected.

Driving, piloting or hazardous work:
No problems expected.

Discontinuing:
- Don't discontinue without doctor's advice until you complete prescribed dose, even though symptoms diminish or disappear.
- Diarrhea may occur 2 months or more after you stop using this drug. Consult doctor if it occurs.

Others:
- Advise any doctor or dentist whom you consult that you take this medicine.
- If infection symptoms don't start to improve in a few days or they worsen, call your doctor.

POSSIBLE INTERACTION WITH OTHER DRUGS

GENERIC NAME OR DRUG CLASS	COMBINED EFFECT
Benzodiazepines*	Increased effect of benzodiazepine.
Carbamazepine	Increased effect of carbamazepine.
Chloramphenicol	Decreased effect of chloramphenicol.
Cyclosporine	May increase cyclosporin toxicity.
Digoxins*	Increased effect of digoxin.
Enzyme inhibitors*	Increased effect of erythromycin. Avoid.
Hepatotoxics*	Increased risk of liver problems.
HMG-CoA reductase inhibitors	Increased risk of muscle and kidney problems (with lovastatin).
Leukotriene modifiers	Decreased effect of zafirlukast.
Lincomycins*	Decreased lincomycin effect.
Penicillins*	Decreased penicillin effect.
Sibutramine	Increased effect of sibutramine.
Sildenafil	Increased effect of sildenafil.
Xanthines*	Increased effect of xanthine.
Warfarin	Increased risk of bleeding.

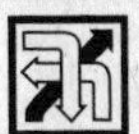

POSSIBLE INTERACTION WITH OTHER SUBSTANCES

INTERACTS WITH	COMBINED EFFECT
Alcohol:	Possible liver damage. Avoid.
Beverages: Grapefruit juice.	May increase effect of erythromycin.
Cocaine:	None expected.
Foods: Grapefruit.	May increase effect of erythromycin.
Marijuana:	None expected.
Tobacco:	None expected.

*See Glossary

ESTRAMUSTINE

BRAND NAMES

Emcyt

BASIC INFORMATION

Habit forming? No
Prescription needed? Yes
Available as generic? No
Drug class: Antineoplastic

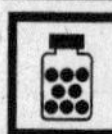

USES

Treats prostate cancer.

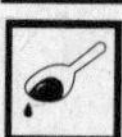

DOSAGE & USAGE INFORMATION

How to take:
Capsule—Swallow with liquid. If you can't swallow whole, open capsule and take with liquid or food. Instructions to take on empty stomach mean 1 hour before or 2 hours after eating.

When to take:
According to doctor's instructions. Try to take 1 hour before or 2 hours after eating or drinking any milk products.

If you forget a dose:
If it is almost time for the next dose, wait for the next scheduled dose (don't double this dose).

What drug does:
Suppresses growth of cancer cells.

Time lapse before drug works:
Within 20 hours.

Don't take with:
Any other medicines (including over-the-counter drugs such as cough and cold medicines, laxatives, antacids, diet pills, caffeine, nose drops or vitamins) without consulting your doctor or pharmacist.

OVERDOSE

SYMPTOMS:
None expected.
WHAT TO DO:
Overdose unlikely to threaten life. If person uses much larger amount than prescribed or if accidentally swallowed, call doctor or poison control center 1-800-222-1222 for help.

POSSIBLE ADVERSE REACTIONS OR SIDE EFFECTS

SYMPTOMS	WHAT TO DO
Life-threatening:	
Sudden headaches, chest pain, shortness of breath, leg pain, vision changes, slurred speech.	Seek emergency treatment immediately.
Common:	
• Skin rash, itching.	Discontinue. Call doctor right away.
• Increased sun sensitivity.	Decrease sun exposure. Call doctor when convenient.
• Diarrhea, dizziness, nausea, vomiting, headache, swelling in hands or feet.	Continue. Call doctor when convenient.
Infrequent:	
• Joint or muscle pain, difficulty swallowing, sore throat and fever, peeling skin, jaundice.	Discontinue. Call doctor right away.
• Mouth or tongue irritation, breast tenderness or enlargement, decreased interest in sex.	Continue. Call doctor when convenient.
Rare:	
Bloody urine, hearing loss, back pain, abdominal pain.	Discontinue. Call doctor right away.

WARNINGS & PRECAUTIONS

Don't take if:
- You are allergic to estramustine, estrogens or mechlorethamine. (Estramustine is a combination of an estrogen and mechlorethamine.)
- You have active thromboembolic disorder.

Before you start, consult your doctor if:
- You have jaundice or hepatitis.
- You have history of thrombophlebitis or blood clots.
- You have an ulcer.
- You have asthma.
- You have epilepsy.
- You have bone disease or depressed bone marrow.
- You have kidney or gallbladder disease.
- You have mental depression.
- You suffer from migraine headaches.
- You have or recently had chicken pox.
- You have shingles (herpes zoster).
- You have had a recent heart attack or stroke or have heart or blood vessel disease.

Over age 60:
Adverse reactions and side effects may be more frequent and severe than in younger persons. You may need smaller doses for shorter periods of time.

Pregnancy:
Used in men only. If a male is taking this drug at the time of conception, there may be a risk of birth defects.

Breast-feeding:
Used in men only.

Infants & children:
Not used in this age group.

Prolonged use:
- Talk to your doctor about the need for follow-up medical examinations or laboratory studies to check complete blood counts (white blood cell count, platelet count, red blood cell count, hemoglobin, hematocrit), blood pressure, liver function, serum acid, serum calcium and alkaline phosphatase.
- The drug may cause permanent sterility after it has been taken for a while. Discuss with your doctor any future plans you have for having children.

Skin & sunlight:
No problems expected.

Driving, piloting or hazardous work:
No problems expected.

Discontinuing:
No problems expected.

Others:
- Advise any doctor or dentist whom you consult that you take this medicine.
- May affect results in some medical tests.
- May decrease sperm count in males.
- Do not get any immunizations (vaccinations) while taking this drug unless approved by your doctor.
- Persons in your household should not take an oral polio vaccine while you are taking this drug. They could pass the polio virus on to you. Avoid any persons who have recently taken oral polio vaccine.

POSSIBLE INTERACTION WITH OTHER DRUGS

GENERIC NAME OR DRUG CLASS	COMBINED EFFECT
Adrenocorticoids, systemic	Increased effect of adrenocorticoid.
Calcium supplements*	Decreased absorption of estramustine.
Hepatotoxic medications*	Increased risk of liver toxicity.
Vaccines (killed virus)	Decreased vaccine effect.

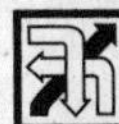

POSSIBLE INTERACTION WITH OTHER SUBSTANCES

INTERACTS WITH	COMBINED EFFECT
Alcohol:	Increased "hangover effect" and other gastrointestinal symptoms.
Beverages: Milk and milk products.	Decreased absorption of estramustine. Take drug 1 hour before or 2 hours after milk product.
Cocaine:	None expected.
Foods: Foods high in calcium.	Decreased absorption of estramustine. Take drug 1 hour before or 2 hours after milk product.
Marijuana:	None expected.
Tobacco:	Increased risk of heart attack and blood clots.

ESTROGENS

GENERIC AND BRAND NAMES

See full list of generic and brand names in *Generic and Brand Name Directory*, page 884.

BASIC INFORMATION

Habit forming? No
Prescription needed? Yes
Available as generic? Yes
Drug class: Female sex hormone (estrogen)

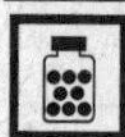

USES

- Treatment for estrogen deficiency.
- Treatment for symptoms of menopause and menstrual cycle irregularity.
- Treatment for estrogen-deficiency osteoporosis (bone softening from calcium loss).
- Treatment for vulvar or vaginal atrophy.
- Treatment for certain breast or prostate cancers.

DOSAGE & USAGE INFORMATION

How to take:

- Tablet or capsule—Take with or after food to reduce nausea. Swallow with liquid. If you can't swallow whole, crumble tablet or open capsule and take with liquid or food.
- Vaginal cream or suppository—Use as directed on label.
- Gel or emulsion—Apply to skin as directed on product's label.
- Injection—Given by medical professional.
- Transdermal patch or transdermal spray—Follow label instructions.
- Vaginal insert—Follow label instructions.

When to take:

- Oral estrogen—Take at the same time each day.
- Other forms—Follow label instructions for correct dosage schedule.

Continued next column

OVERDOSE

SYMPTOMS:
Nausea, vomiting, fluid retention, breast enlargement and discomfort, abnormal vaginal bleeding, headache, drowsiness.
WHAT TO DO:
Overdose unlikely to threaten life. If person uses much larger amount than prescribed or if accidentally swallowed, call doctor or poison control center 1-800-222-1222 for help.

If you forget a dose:
For oral dosage, take as soon as you remember. If it is almost time for the next dose, wait for the next scheduled dose (don't double this dose). For other forms, follow label instructions.

What drug does:

- Increases estrogen levels in the body.
- Combined with progestins for contraception.

Time lapse before drug works:
10 to 20 days.

Don't take with:
Any other medicine or any dietary supplement without consulting your doctor or pharmacist.

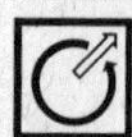

POSSIBLE ADVERSE REACTIONS OR SIDE EFFECTS

SYMPTOMS	WHAT TO DO
Life-threatening:	
Profuse bleeding.	Seek emergency treatment.
Common:	
• Painful or swollen breasts, swollen feet or ankles, rapid weight gain.	Discontinue. Call doctor right away.
• Appetite loss, nausea, stomach, cramps or bloating, skin irritation in patch or spray users.	Continue. Call doctor when convenient.
Infrequent:	
• Breast lumps or discharge, changes in vaginal bleeding (more, less, spotting, prolonged), migraine headache.	Continue, but call doctor right away.
• Dizziness, contact lens intolerance, vomiting, mild diarrhea, headache, increased or decreased sexual desire, slow weight gain, other unusual symptoms.	Continue. Call doctor when convenient.
Rare:	
• Stomach or side pain, joint or muscle pain, jaundice (yellow skin or eyes).	Discontinue. Call doctor right away.
• Blood clots (severe or sudden headache, severe pain in calf or chest or other body parts, shortness of breath, slurred speech, weakness or numbness, sudden vision changes).	Discontinue. Seek emergency help.

WARNINGS & PRECAUTIONS

Don't take if:
You are allergic to any estrogen-containing drugs.

Before you start, consult your doctor if:
- You have or have had cancer of the breast or reproductive organs, fibrocystic breast disease, fibroid tumors of the uterus or endometriosis, unexplained vaginal bleeding.
- You have migraine headaches, epilepsy or porphyria.
- You have had blood clots, stroke, high blood pressure, congestive heart failure or heart attack.
- You have diabetes, asthma, kidney, liver or gallbladder disease.
- You plan to become pregnant within 3 months.

Over age 60:
Controversial. You and your doctor must decide if risks of drug outweigh benefits.

Pregnancy:
Risk to unborn child outweighs benefits of drug. Don't use. Risk category X (see page xviii).

Breast-feeding:
Drug filters into milk. Consult doctor.

Infants & children:
Not recommended.

Prolonged use:
- Increased growth of fibroid tumors of uterus.
- Talk to your doctor about the need for follow-up medical examinations or laboratory studies to check for drug's effectiveness.

Skin & sunlight:
One or more drugs in this group may cause rash or intensify sunburn in areas exposed to sun or ultraviolet light (photosensitivity reaction). Avoid overexposure. Notify doctor if reaction occurs.

Driving, piloting or hazardous work:
No problems expected.

Discontinuing:
Consult your doctor before discontinuing.

Others:
- For postmenopausal women, the use of hormone replacement therapy (HRT) which combines estrogen and progestin increases slightly the risk for breast cancer, heart attacks and stroke. HRT does not prevent heart disease. HRT is effective for menopause symptoms (used short term), and helps protect against osteoporosis and colon cancer. Other treatments are available for osteoporosis. Discuss with your doctor if HRT is the right treatment for you.
- May interfere with the accuracy of some medical tests.
- Carefully read the paper called "Information for the Patient" that was given to you with your first prescription or a refill. If you lose it, ask your pharmacist for a copy.
- Advise any doctor or dentist whom you consult that you take this medicine.

POSSIBLE INTERACTION WITH OTHER DRUGS

GENERIC NAME OR DRUG CLASS	COMBINED EFFECT
Adrenocorticoids	Increased effect of adrenocorticoid.
Anticoagulants, oral*	Decreased anti-coagulant effect.
Anticonvulsants, hydantoin*	Decreased estrogen effect.
Antidepressants, tricyclic*	Increased toxicity of antidepressants.
Antidiabetics, oral*	Unpredictable increase or decrease in blood sugar.
Antivirals, HIV/AIDS*	Increased risk of pancreatitis.
Bromocriptine	May need to adjust bromocriptine dose.
Cyclosporine	Increased effect of cyclosporine.
Hepatotoxics*	Increased risk of liver problems.
Tamoxifen	Decreased effect of tamoxifen.

POSSIBLE INTERACTION WITH OTHER SUBSTANCES

INTERACTS WITH	COMBINED EFFECT
Alcohol:	None expected.
Beverages: Grapefruit juice.	Possible increased estrogen effect.
Cocaine:	None expected.
Foods:	None expected.
Marijuana:	Possible menstrual irregularities and bleeding between periods.
Tobacco:	Increased risk of blood clots leading to stroke or heart attack.

***See Glossary**

ESZOPICLONE

BRAND NAMES

Lunesta

BASIC INFORMATION

Habit forming? Yes
Prescription needed? Yes
Available as generic? No
Drug class: Sedative-hypnotic agent

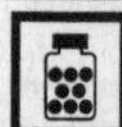

USES

Treatment for insomnia symptoms such as trouble falling asleep, waking up too often during the night and waking up too early in the morning.

DOSAGE & USAGE INFORMATION

How to take:
Tablet—Swallow whole with liquid.

When to take:
Take immediately before bedtime. For best results do not take with or right after a heavy meal.

If you forget a dose:
Take as soon as you remember. Take drug only when you are able to get 7 hours of sleep before your daily activity begins. Do not exceed prescribed dosage.

What drug does:
The exact mechanism is not known. Acts as a central nervous system depressant which helps decrease sleep problems.

Time lapse before drug works:
Usually within 1 hour. The sleep-inducing affect should last for 6 to 8 hours.

Don't take with:
Any other medicine or any dietary supplement without consulting your doctor or pharmacist.

OVERDOSE

SYMPTOMS:
Drowsiness, weakness, stupor (not able to respond), coma.
WHAT TO DO:
- **Dial 911 (emergency) for medical help or call poison control center 1-800-222-1222 for instructions.**
- **See emergency information on last 3 pages of this book.**

POSSIBLE ADVERSE REACTIONS OR SIDE EFFECTS

SYMPTOMS	WHAT TO DO
Life-threatening:	
Rare allergic reaction—may have hives, rash, itching, swelling, trouble breathing, wheezing, chest pain, dizziness, faintness.	Seek emergency treatment immediately.
Common:	
Headache, unpleasant taste, drowsiness in the daytime, dizziness.	Continue. Call doctor when convenient.
Infrequent:	
Indigestion, nausea, nervousness, dry mouth, diarrhea, depression, cold-like symptoms or infection, problems with coordination, lightheadedness, anxiety.	Continue. Call doctor when convenient.
Rare:	
• Behavioral changes, (agitation, confusion, aggressiveness, suicidal thoughts, other bizarre behaviors), hallucinations, chest pain, swelling of arms or legs, enlarged breasts in men, depression worsens, painful menstruation, sleep-related behaviors.*	Discontinue. Call doctor right away.
• Memory problems (may occur if you wake before the effect of drug is gone), any other symptoms occur that cause concern (they may be due to the drug, an underlying disorder or the effects of lack of sleep).	Continue. Call doctor when convenient.

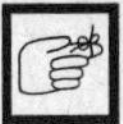

WARNINGS & PRECAUTIONS

Don't take if:
You are allergic to eszopiclone or zopiclone.

Before you start, consult your doctor if:
- You have respiratory problems.
- You have liver disease.
- You suffer from depression or psychiatric disorder.
- You are an active or recovering alcoholic or drug or substance abuser.

Over age 60:
Side effects may be more frequent and severe than in younger persons. You may need smaller doses for shorter periods of time.

Pregnancy:
Decide with your doctor if drug benefits justify any possible risk to unborn child. Risk category C (see page xviii).

Breast-feeding:
It is unknown if drug passes into milk. Avoid drug or discontinue nursing until you finish medicine. Consult doctor for advice on maintaining milk supply.

Infants & children:
Safety and effectiveness for children under age 18 has not been established.

Prolonged use:
You and your doctor will decide if there is a need to take the drug for prolonged period for chronic insomnia (insomnia at least three nights a week for a period of one month or longer).

Skin & sunlight:
No special problems expected.

Driving, piloting or hazardous work:
Don't drive or pilot aircraft until you learn how medicine affects you. Don't work around dangerous machinery. Don't climb ladders or work in high places. Danger increases if you drink alcohol or take other medicines affecting alertness and reflexes.

Discontinuing:
- Don't discontinue without consulting doctor. Dose may require gradual reduction if you have taken drug for a long time.
- You may have sleeping problems for 1 or 2 nights after stopping drug.
- Withdrawal symptoms may occur after you stop the drug. Consult your doctor if any emotional or physical symptoms do occur.

Others:
- Advise any doctor or dentist whom you consult that you take this medicine.
- Don't take drug if you are traveling on an overnight airplane trip of less than 7 or 8 hours. A temporary memory loss may occur (called traveler's amnesia).

POSSIBLE INTERACTION WITH OTHER DRUGS

GENERIC NAME OR DRUG CLASS	COMBINED EFFECT
Central nervous system (CNS) depressants*	Increased sedative effect.
Enzyme inducers*	Decreased effect of eszopiclone.
Enzyme inhibitors*	Increased effect of eszopiclone.
Ketoconazole	Increased effect of eszopiclone.
Olanzapine	Decreased alertness.

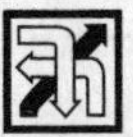

POSSIBLE INTERACTION WITH OTHER SUBSTANCES

INTERACTS WITH	COMBINED EFFECT
Alcohol:	Increased sedation. Avoid.
Beverages:	None expected.
Cocaine:	Unknown. Avoid.
Foods:	Decreased drug effect if taken with a heavy meal.
Marijuana:	Unknown. Avoid.
Tobacco:	None expected.

***See Glossary**

ETHIONAMIDE

BRAND NAMES

Trecator

BASIC INFORMATION

Habit forming? No
Prescription needed? Yes
Available as generic? No
Drug class: Antimycobacterial (antituberculosis)

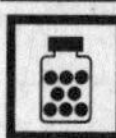

USES

Treats tuberculosis. Used in combination with other antituberculosis drugs such as isoniazid, streptomycin, rifampin, ethambutol.

DOSAGE & USAGE INFORMATION

How to take:
Tablet—Swallow with liquid or food to lessen stomach irritation. If you can't swallow whole, crumble tablet and take with liquid or food.

When to take:
Usually every 8 to 12 hours, with or after meals.

If you forget a dose:
Take as soon as you remember. If it is almost time for the next dose, wait for that dose (don't double this dose) and resume regular schedule.

What drug does:
Kills germs that cause tuberculosis.

Time lapse before drug works:
Within 3 hours.

Don't take with:
Any other medicine or any dietary supplement without consulting your doctor or pharmacist.

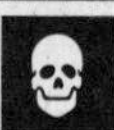

OVERDOSE

SYMPTOMS:
None expected.
WHAT TO DO:
Overdose unlikely to threaten life. If person uses much larger amount than prescribed or if accidentally swallowed, call doctor or poison control center 1-800-222-1222 for help.

POSSIBLE ADVERSE REACTIONS OR SIDE EFFECTS

SYMPTOMS	WHAT TO DO
Life-threatening: None expected.	
Common:	
• Vomiting.	Discontinue. Call doctor right away.
• Dizziness, sore mouth, nausea, metallic taste.	Continue. Call doctor when convenient.
Infrequent:	
Jaundice (yellow eyes and skin); numbness, tingling, pain in hands or feet; depression; confusion.	Discontinue. Call doctor right away.
Rare:	
• Hunger, shakiness, rapid heartbeat, blurred vision or other changes in vision, skin rash.	Discontinue. Call doctor right away.
• Gradual swelling in the neck (thyroid gland).	Continue. Call doctor when convenient.
• Enlargement of breasts (male).	No action necessary.

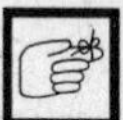

WARNINGS & PRECAUTIONS

Don't take if:
You know you are hypersensitive to ethionamide.

Before you start, consult your doctor if:
- You have diabetes.
- You have liver disease.

Over age 60:
No information available.

Pregnancy:
Decide with your doctor if drug benefits justify risk to unborn child. Risk category C (see page xviii).

Breast-feeding:
Effect not documented. Consult your family doctor or pediatrician.

Infants & children:
Effect not documented. Consult your family doctor or pediatrician.

Prolonged use:
No special problems expected.

Skin & sunlight:
No special problems expected.

Driving, piloting or hazardous work:
Don't drive or pilot aircraft until you learn how medicine affects you. Don't work around dangerous machinery. Don't climb ladders or work in high places. Danger increases if you drink alcohol or take medicine affecting alertness and reflexes.

Discontinuing:
Don't discontinue without consulting doctor.

Others:
- Advise any doctor or dentist whom you consult that you take this medicine.
- Request occasional laboratory studies for liver function.
- Request occasional eye examinations.
- Treatment may take months or years.
- You should take pyridoxine (vitamin B-6) supplements while taking ethionamide.

POSSIBLE INTERACTION WITH OTHER DRUGS

GENERIC NAME OR DRUG CLASS	COMBINED EFFECT
Antivirals, HIV/AIDS*	Increased risk of peripheral neuropathy.
Cycloserine	Increased risk of seizures.
Pyridoxine	Increased excretion by kidney. (Should take pyridoxine supplements while on ethionamide to prevent development of neuritis in feet and hands).

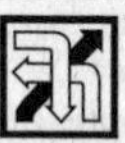

POSSIBLE INTERACTION WITH OTHER SUBSTANCES

INTERACTS WITH	COMBINED EFFECT
Alcohol:	Increased incidence of liver diseases.
Beverages: Any alcoholic beverage.	Increased incidence of liver diseases.
Cocaine:	None expected.
Foods:	None expected.
Marijuana:	No interaction expected, but may slow body's recovery.
Tobacco:	No interaction expected, but may slow body's recovery.

*See Glossary

ETOPOSIDE

BRAND NAMES

VePesid VP-16

BASIC INFORMATION

Habit forming? No
Prescription needed? Yes
Available as generic? No
Drug class: Antineoplastic

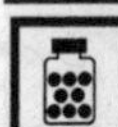

USES

- Treats testicular, lung and bladder cancer.
- Treats Hodgkin's disease and some other forms of cancer.

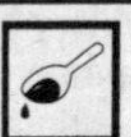

DOSAGE & USAGE INFORMATION

How to take:
- Capsule—Swallow with liquid. If you can't swallow whole, open capsule and take with liquid or food. Instructions to take on empty stomach mean 1 hour before or 2 hours after eating.
- Injection—Given under doctor's supervision.

When to take:
According to your doctor's instructions.

If you forget a dose:
Skip this dose. Never double dose. Resume regular schedule.

What drug does:
Inhibits DNA in cancer cells.

Time lapse before drug works:
Unpredictable.

Don't take with:
Any other medicines (including over-the-counter drugs such as cough and cold medicines, laxatives, antacids, diet pills, caffeine, nose drops or vitamins) without consulting your doctor or pharmacist.

OVERDOSE

SYMPTOMS:
Rapid pulse, shortness of breath, wheezing, fainting, coma.
WHAT TO DO:
- **Dial 911 (emergency) for medical help or call poison control center 1-800-222-1222 for instructions.**
- **See emergency information on last 3 pages of this book.**

POSSIBLE ADVERSE REACTIONS OR SIDE EFFECTS

SYMPTOMS	WHAT TO DO
Life-threatening: In case of overdose, see previous column.	
Common:	
• Appetite loss, nausea, vomiting.	Continue. Call doctor when convenient.
• Loss of hair.	No action necessary.
Infrequent:	
Symptoms of low white blood cell count and low platelet count: black, tarry stools; bloody urine; cough; chills or fever; low back pain; bruising.	Discontinue. Call doctor right away.
Rare:	
Mouth sores.	Continue. Call doctor when convenient.

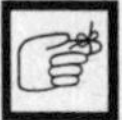

WARNINGS & PRECAUTIONS

Don't take if:
- You have chicken pox.
- You have shingles (herpes zoster).

Before you start, consult your doctor if:
You have liver or kidney disease.

Over age 60:
No special problems expected.

Pregnancy:
Risk to unborn child outweighs drug benefits. Don't use. Risk category D (see page xviii).

Breast-feeding:
Drug passes into milk. Avoid drug or discontinue nursing until you finish medicine. Consult doctor for advice on maintaining milk supply.

Infants & children:
Effect not documented. Consult your doctor.

Prolonged use:
- Talk to your doctor about the need for follow-up medical examinations or laboratory studies to check complete blood counts (white blood cell count, platelet count, red blood cell count, hemoglobin, hematocrit).
- Check mouth frequently for ulcers.

Skin & sunlight:
No problems expected.

Driving, piloting or hazardous work:
Avoid if you feel confused, drowsy or dizzy.

Discontinuing:
May still experience symptoms of bone marrow depression, such as blood in stools, fever or chills, blood spots under the skin, back pain, hoarseness, bloody urine. If any of these occur, call your doctor right away.

Others:
- Advise any doctor or dentist whom you consult that you take this medicine.
- May affect results in some medical tests.
- Etoposide may be used in combinations with other antineoplastic treatment plans. The incidence and severity of side effects may be different when used in combinations such as doxorubicin, procarbazine and etoposide (APE); etoposide, cyclophosphamide, doxorubicin and vincristine (CAVE, ECHO, CAPO, EVAC or VOCA); cyclophosphamide, doxorubicin and etoposide (CAE or ACE); cisplatin, bleomycin, doxorubicin and etoposide; cisplatin, bleomycin and etoposide; cisplatin and etoposide. For further information regarding these combinations, consult your doctor.

POSSIBLE INTERACTION WITH OTHER DRUGS

GENERIC NAME OR DRUG CLASS	COMBINED EFFECT
Angiotensin-converting enzyme (ACE) inhibitors*	May increase bone marrow depression or make kidney damage more likely.
Antineoplastic (cancer-treating) drugs*	May increase bone marrow depression or make kidney damage more likely.
Clozapine	Toxic effect on bone marrow.
Tiopronin	Increased risk of toxicity to bone marrow.
Vaccines, live or killed virus	Increased likelihood of toxicity or reduced effectiveness of vaccine. Wait 3 months to 1 year after etoposide treatment before getting vaccine.

POSSIBLE INTERACTION WITH OTHER SUBSTANCES

INTERACTS WITH	COMBINED EFFECT
Alcohol:	Increased likelihood of adverse reactions. Avoid.
Beverages: Grapefruit juice.	Decreased effect of etoposide. Avoid.
Cocaine:	Increased likelihood of adverse reactions. Avoid.
Foods:	None expected.
Marijuana:	Increased likelihood of adverse reactions. Avoid.
Tobacco:	None expected.

***See Glossary**

EZETIMIBE

BRAND NAMES

Vytorin
Zetia

BASIC INFORMATION

Habit forming? No
Prescription needed? Yes
Available as generic? No
Drug class: Antihyperlipidemic

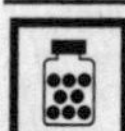

USES

Lowers blood cholesterol levels caused by low-density lipoproteins (LDL) in persons who haven't improved by exercising, dieting or using other measures. May be used alone or with other cholesterol lowering drugs (e.g., HMG-CoA reductase inhibitors).

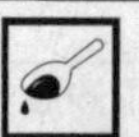

DOSAGE & USAGE INFORMATION

How to take:
Tablet—Swallow with liquid. May be taken on an empty stomach or with food.

When to take:
Once a day at the same time each day.

If you forget a dose:
Take as soon as you remember. If it is almost time for your next dose, skip the missed dose and go back to your regular dosing schedule. Do not double doses.

What drug does:
It lowers the amount of cholesterol your body absorbs from your diet by reducing absorption in the intestines. Other cholesterol lowering drugs alter the production and metabolism of cholesterol in the liver.

Time lapse before drug works:
2 to 4 weeks.

Don't take with:
- A high-fat diet.
- Any other medicine or any dietary supplement without consulting your doctor or pharmacist.

OVERDOSE

SYMPTOMS:
None expected.
WHAT TO DO:
Overdose unlikely to threaten life. If person uses much larger amount than prescribed or if accidentally swallowed, call doctor or poison control center 1-800-222-1222 for help.

POSSIBLE ADVERSE REACTIONS OR SIDE EFFECTS

SYMPTOMS	WHAT TO DO
Life-threatening: None expected.	
Common: None expected.	
Infrequent: Headache, cold or other upper respiratory infection, muscle aches, chest pains, fatigue, dizziness, diarrhea.	Continue. Call doctor when convenient.
Rare: None expected.	

WARNINGS & PRECAUTIONS

Don't take if:
You are allergic to ezetimibe or its components.

Before you start, consult your doctor if:
- You have liver disease.
- You are allergic to any medication, food or other substance.

Over age 60:
No special problems expected.

Pregnancy:
Discuss with your doctor whether drug benefits justify risk to unborn child. Risk category C (see page xviii).

Breast-feeding:
It is unknown if drug passes into breast milk. Avoid drug or discontinue nursing until you finish medicine. Consult doctor for advice on maintaining milk supply.

Infants & children:
Not recommended for children under age 10.

Prolonged use:
Talk to your doctor about the need for follow-up medical examinations or laboratory studies to check liver function and serum cholesterol.

Skin & sunlight:
No problems expected.

Driving, piloting or hazardous work:
No special problems expected.

Discontinuing:
No special problems expected.

Others:
- Advise any doctor or dentist whom you consult that you take this medicine.
- Continue to follow your doctor's instructions about dietary intake, reduced intake of saturated fats, increased fiber intake, weight reduction, and increased physical activity.
- Cholesterol lowering drugs may cause muscle problems or rhabdomyolysis (muscle injury). If you develop persistent muscle aches, pain or weakness or urine turns dark, call the doctor right away.

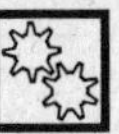

POSSIBLE INTERACTION WITH OTHER DRUGS

GENERIC NAME OR DRUG CLASS	COMBINED EFFECT
Cholestyramine	Take ezetimibe 2 hours before or 4 hours after.
Colestipol	Take ezetimibe 2 hours before or 4 hours after.
Colesevelam	Take ezetimibe 2 hours before or 4 hours after.
Cyclosporine	Increased effect of ezetimibe.
Fibrates	May require dosage adjustment of either drug.
Gemfibrozil	Increased effect of ezetimibe.

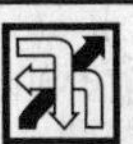

POSSIBLE INTERACTION WITH OTHER SUBSTANCES

INTERACTS WITH	COMBINED EFFECT
Alcohol:	None expected.
Beverages:	None expected.
Cocaine:	None expected.
Foods:	None expected.
Marijuana:	None expected.
Tobacco:	None expected.

FACTOR Xa INHIBITORS

GENERIC AND BRAND NAMES

APIXABAN	RIVAROXABAN
Eliquis	Xarelto

BASIC INFORMATION

Habit forming? No
Prescription needed? Yes
Available as generic? No
Drug class: Anticoagulant

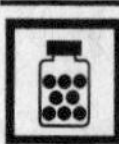

USES

- Used to treat and prevent blood clots (e.g., deep venous thrombosis [DVT]) that can form in blood vessels. Blood clots can travel to the brain and cause a stroke or to the lungs causing pulmonary embolism.
- Used for patients with atrial fibrillation (heart rhythm disorder) to reduce risk of stroke.

DOSAGE & USAGE INFORMATION

How to take:
Tablet—Swallow whole with water. May be taken with or without food. If it is prescribed for atrial fibrillation, take it with your evening meal.

When to take:
Once a day at the same time each day.

If you forget a dose:
Take as soon as you remember as long as it is taken the same day. If you don't remember until the next day, skip the missed dose and wait for the next scheduled dose (don't double this dose).

What drug does:
It works by decreasing the clotting ability of the blood and helps prevent harmful clots from forming in the blood vessels or heart.

Time lapse before drug works:
It starts working within 2 to 4 hours.

Don't take with:
Any other medicine or dietary supplement without consulting your doctor or pharmacist.

OVERDOSE

SYMPTOMS:
Increased risk of dangerous bleeding (may be internal bleeding).
WHAT TO DO:
If person takes much larger amount than prescribed or if accidentally swallowed, call doctor or poison control center 1-800-222-1222 for help.

POSSIBLE ADVERSE REACTIONS OR SIDE EFFECTS

SYMPTOMS	WHAT TO DO
Life-threatening:	
Rare allergic reaction (hives, itching, rash, wheezing, tightness in chest, swelling of lips or tongue or throat).	Seek emergency treatment immediately.
Common:	
Bleeding following surgery, surgical wound oozing or bleeding, anemia (pale skin, shortness of breath, weakness).	Continue, but call doctor right away.
Infrequent:	
• Unusual bleeding from the gums or vagina or rectum or eyes, black or tarry stools, red or brown urine, coughing up blood or coffee-ground material, unusual bruising, purple or red spots under the skin, fast or irregular heartbeat, chest pain.	Continue, but call doctor right away.
• Dizziness, faintness, headache, diarrhea, upset stomach, fever, unusual tiredness or weakness, pain (in back, legs, arms), dry mouth, muscle spasms, swelling in arms or legs, rash or itchy skin, low blood pressure.	Continue. Call doctor when convenient.
Rare:	
• Bleeding in the brain (may have symptoms of sudden numbness or weakness on one side of the body, sudden and severe headache, confusion, balance or vision problems).	Continue, but seek emergency help.
• Liver problem (yellow skin or eyes, nausea, vomiting, weight loss), skin peels or blisters or loosens.	Continue, but call doctor right away.

WARNINGS & PRECAUTIONS

Don't take if:
You are allergic to factor Xa inhibitors.

Before you start, consult your doctor if:
- You have a history of intracranial hemorrhage (bleeding in the brain), spinal deformity or spinal surgery.
- You have a liver or kidney disorder.
- You have or have had conditions that have an increased risk of bleeding (e.g., ulcers, recent surgery, retinopathy or stroke).
- You have rare inherited disorders of lactose or galactose intolerance.
- You have a spinal or epidural catheter.
- You plan on having surgery (including dental surgery) in the near future.

Over age 60:
May have increased risk of side effects.

Pregnancy:
Decide with your doctor whether drug benefits justify risk to unborn child. Risk category C (see page xviii).

Breast-feeding:
It is unknown if drug passes into breast milk. Breast-feeding is not recommended while taking this drug. Consult your doctor for advice.

Infants & children:
Safety and efficacy have not been established for ages under 18.

Prolonged use:
Talk to your doctor about the need for follow-up medical exams or laboratory studies to check the effectiveness of the treatment.

Skin & sunlight:
No problems expected.

Driving, piloting or hazardous work:
Avoid if you experience dizziness or faintness, otherwise no problems expected.

Discontinuing:
Don't discontinue without doctor's approval. Stopping the drug can increase the risk of blood clots and stroke. If drug used for atrial fibrillation, be sure to refill prescription before you run out.

Others:
- Advise any doctor, dentist or pharmacist whom you consult that you take this drug.
- While taking this drug you will likely bruise and bleed more easily than usual or bleed for longer than usual. Avoid rough sports or other situations where you could be bruised, cut or injured. Be extra careful when using sharp objects. Bleeding complications can be serious or fatal. Consult doctor if you have any concerns or questions about side effects.
- Use of this drug in patients who undergo certain spinal procedures (e.g., lumbar puncture or epidural injections for pain) increases risk for hematoma (trapped blood). Consult doctor about your risk and possible complications.
- Drug use may increase risk of serious bleeding during a surgery, other medical procedures or some types of dental work. You may be advised to stop using this drug at least 24 hours before a surgery, medical procedure or dental work.

POSSIBLE INTERACTION WITH OTHER DRUGS

GENERIC NAME OR DRUG CLASS	COMBINED EFFECT
Anticoagulants,* other	Increased risk of bleeding.
Anti-inflammatory drugs, nonsteroidal (NSAIDs)*	Increased risk of bleeding.
Antiplatelet drugs*	Increased risk of bleeding.
Enzyme inducers*	Decreased effect of rivaroxaban.
Enzyme inhibitors*	Increased effect of rivaroxaban.

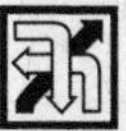

POSSIBLE INTERACTION WITH OTHER SUBSTANCES

INTERACTS WITH	COMBINED EFFECT
Alcohol:	None expected.
Beverages: Grapefruit juice.	May increase effect of rivaroxaban.
Cocaine:	Unknown effect. Avoid.
Foods: Grapefruit.	May increase effect of rivaroxaban.
Marijuana:	Unknown effect. Avoid.
Tobacco:	None expected, but people with heart disorders should not smoke.

*See Glossary

FELBAMATE

BRAND NAMES

FBM
Felbatol

BASIC INFORMATION

Habit forming? No
Prescription needed? Yes
Available as generic? Yes
Drug class: Anticonvulsant

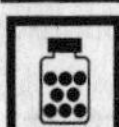

USES

- Treatment for partial epileptic seizures.
- Treatment for Lennox-Gastaut syndrome (a severe form of epilepsy in children).

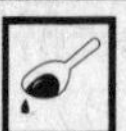

DOSAGE & USAGE INFORMATION

How to take:

- Tablet—Swallow with liquid. May be taken with food to lessen stomach upset unless the doctor has directed taking on an empty stomach.
- Oral suspension—Shake bottle well before measuring. Use specially marked measuring device to measure each dose accurately. Don't measure with a regular household teaspoon.

When to take:
At the same times each day. Your doctor will determine the best schedule. Dosages will gradually be increased over the first 3 weeks.

If you forget a dose:
Take as soon as you remember. If it is almost time for the next dose, wait for that dose (don't double this dose) and resume regular schedule.

What drug does:

- Decreases the frequency of partial seizures that start in a localized part of the brain, including those that progress into more generalized grand mal seizures.
- Decreases seizure activity and improves quality of life in children with Lennox-Gastaut syndrome.

Continued next column

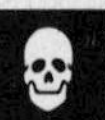

OVERDOSE

SYMPTOMS:
Gastric distress, increased heart rate.
WHAT TO DO:
Overdose unlikely to threaten life. If person uses much larger amount than prescribed or if accidentally swallowed, call doctor or poison control center 1-800-222-1222 for help.

Time lapse before drug works:
May take several weeks for maximum effectiveness.

Don't take with:
Any other medicine or any dietary supplement without consulting your doctor or pharmacist.

POSSIBLE ADVERSE REACTIONS OR SIDE EFFECTS

SYMPTOMS	WHAT TO DO
Life-threatening: None expected.	
Common:	
• Fever, red or purple spots on skin, walking in unusual manner.	Continue, but call doctor right away.
• Abdominal pain, taste changes, constipation, sleeping difficulty, dizziness, headache, nausea or vomiting, indigestion, appetite loss.	Continue. Call doctor when convenient.
Infrequent:	
• Mood or mental changes, clumsiness, skin rash, tremor.	Continue, but call doctor right away.
• Vision changes, diarrhea, drowsiness, coughing or sneezing, ear pain or fullness, runny nose, weight loss.	Continue. Call doctor when convenient.
Rare:	
Black or tarry stools, bloody or dark-colored urine, unusual bruising or bleeding, breathing difficulty, wheezing, pain or tightness in chest, sore throat, mouth or lip sores, swollen face, swollen or painful glands or lymph nodes, yellow skin or eyes, chills, general tired feeling, continuing headache or abdominal pain, hives, itching, muscle cramps, stuffy nose, skin reaction to sunlight.	Continue, but call doctor right away.

WARNINGS & PRECAUTIONS

Don't take if:
You are allergic to felbamate.

Before you start, consult your doctor if:
- You have a sensitivity to other carbamate drugs,* other medications or other substances.
- You have any blood disorder.
- You have a history of bone marrow depression.
- You have or have had any liver disease.

Over age 60:
Adverse reactions and side effects may be more frequent and severe than in younger persons.

Pregnancy:
Decide with your doctor if drug benefits justify risks to unborn child. Risk category B (see page xviii).

Breast-feeding:
Drug passes into milk. Unknown effect. Consult your doctor.

Infants & children:
Give only under close medical supervision.

Prolonged use:
Talk to your doctor about the need for follow-up medical examinations or laboratory studies to check complete blood counts (white blood cell count, platelet count, red blood cell count, hemoglobin, hematocrit), iron concentrations and liver function studies.

Skin & sunlight:
No problems expected.

Driving, piloting or hazardous work:
Don't drive or pilot aircraft until you learn how medicine affects you. Don't work around dangerous machinery. Don't climb ladders or work in high places. Danger increases if you drink alcohol or take other medicines affecting alertness and reflexes such as antihistamines, tranquilizers, sedatives, pain medicine, narcotics and mind-altering drugs.

Discontinuing:
Don't discontinue without doctor's approval due to risk of increased seizure activity.

Others:
- Felbamate may cause serious side effects including blood problems and liver problems (rarely fatal). Decide with your doctor if drug benefits justify risks.
- Advise any doctor or dentist whom you consult that you take this medicine.
- Felbamate may be used alone or combined with other antiepileptic drugs. The dosages of other antiepileptic drugs you currently use will be reduced to minimize side effects and adverse reactions due to interactions.
- Rarely, antiepileptic drugs may lead to suicidal thoughts and behaviors. Call doctor right away if suicidal symptoms or unusual behaviors occur.
- Wear medical identification that indicates the use of this medicine.

POSSIBLE INTERACTION WITH OTHER DRUGS

GENERIC NAME OR DRUG CLASS	COMBINED EFFECT
Carbamazepine	Increased side effects and adverse reactions.
Phenytoin	Increased side effects and adverse reactions.
Valproic acid*	Increased effect of valproic acid.

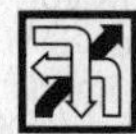

POSSIBLE INTERACTION WITH OTHER SUBSTANCES

INTERACTS WITH	COMBINED EFFECT
Alcohol:	None expected.
Beverages:	None expected.
Cocaine:	None expected.
Foods:	None expected.
Marijuana:	None expected.
Tobacco:	None expected.

*See Glossary

FIBRATES

GENERIC AND BRAND NAMES

CLOFIBRATE	FENOFIBRATE
Abitrate	Antara
Atromid-S	Fenoglide
Claripex	Lipidil
Novofibrate	Lipofen
	Lofibra
	Tricor
	Triglide
	FENOFIBRIC ACID
	Fibricor
	TriLipix

BASIC INFORMATION

Habit forming? No
Prescription needed? Yes
Available as generic? Yes
Drug class: Antihyperlipidemic

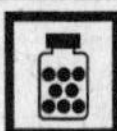

USES

Used in addition to diet changes to help control levels of blood fats (e.g., lipid disorders such as elevated levels of cholesterol and triglycerides).

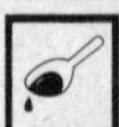

DOSAGE & USAGE INFORMATION

How to take:

- Capsule or tablet—Swallow with liquid. Follow the instructions provided with your prescription about taking the drug with or without food.
- Delayed-release capsule—Swallow with liquid. Do not crush or chew capsule. Take with or without food.

When to take:
At the same time(s) each day. Follow directions on prescription as to when to take each day.

If you forget a dose:
Take as soon as you remember. If it is almost time for the next dose, wait for that dose (don't double this dose) and resume regular schedule.

Continued next column

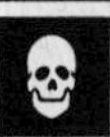

OVERDOSE

SYMPTOMS:
Diarrhea, headache, muscle pain.
WHAT TO DO:
Overdose unlikely to threaten life. If person uses much larger amount than prescribed or if accidentally swallowed, call doctor or poison control center 1-800-222-1222 for help.

What drug does:
Helps break down the fats in the blood.

Time lapse before drug works:
3 months or more as measured by laboratory testing.

Don't take with:
Any other medicine or any dietary supplement without consulting your doctor or pharmacist.

POSSIBLE ADVERSE REACTIONS OR SIDE EFFECTS

SYMPTOMS	WHAT TO DO
Life-threatening: None expected.	
Common: None expected.	
Infrequent:	
• Chest pain, shortness of breath, irregular heartbeat.	Discontinue. Seek emergency treatment.
• Severe symptoms that include nausea, flu-like illness, vomiting.	Discontinue. Call doctor right away.
• Diarrhea, abdominal pain, belching, constipation, muscle aches and pains.	Continue. Call doctor when convenient.
Rare:	
• Cardiac arrhythmias, angina.	Discontinue. Seek emergency treatment.
• Rash, itch; mouth or lip sores; sore throat; swollen feet, legs; blood in urine; painful urination; fever; chills; anemia.	Discontinue. Call doctor right away.
• Dizziness, weakness, drowsiness, muscle cramps, headache, diminished sex drive, hair loss, dry mouth, bloating or stomach pain, chronic indigestion, loss of appetite, unusual bleeding or bruising, unusual tiredness, mild vomiting, yellow eyes or skin.	Continue. Call doctor when convenient.

WARNINGS & PRECAUTIONS

Don't take if:
- You are allergic to any fibrates.
- You have had serious liver disease.

Before you start, consult your doctor if:
- You have had liver or kidney disease.
- You have had peptic ulcer disease.
- You have had gallbladder disease or gallstones.
- You have diabetes.

Over age 60:
Adverse reactions and side effects may be more frequent and severe than in younger persons. May develop flu-like symptoms.

Pregnancy:
Decide with your doctor if drug benefits justify risk to unborn child. Risk category C (see page xviii).

Breast-feeding:
It is unknown if drug passes into milk. Avoid drug or discontinue nursing until you finish medicine. Consult doctor for advice on maintaining milk supply.

Infants & children:
Not recommended.

Prolonged use:
- May cause gallbladder infection.
- Possible cause of stomach cancer.
- Talk to your doctor about the need for follow-up medical examinations or laboratory studies to check cholesterol and triglyceride levels.

Skin & sunlight:
May cause rash or intensify sunburn in areas exposed to sun or ultraviolet light (photosensitivity reaction). Avoid overexposure. Notify doctor if reaction occurs.

Driving, piloting or hazardous work:
Avoid if you feel drowsy or dizzy. Otherwise, no problems expected.

Discontinuing:
Don't discontinue without doctor's advice until you complete prescribed dose, even though symptoms diminish or disappear.

Others:
- Advise any doctor or dentist whom you consult that you take this medicine.
- Periodic blood cell counts and liver-function studies recommended if you take clofibrate for a long time.
- Some medical studies question effectiveness. A number of medical studies warn of toxicity.

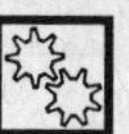

POSSIBLE INTERACTION WITH OTHER DRUGS

GENERIC NAME OR DRUG CLASS	COMBINED EFFECT
Anticoagulants, oral*	Increased anticoagulant effect. Dose reduction of anticoagulant necessary.
Antidiabetics, oral*	Increased antidiabetic effect.
Contraceptives, oral*	Decreased fibrate effect.
Cyclosporine	May cause or worsen kidney problems.
Desmopressin	May decrease desmopressin effect.
Dexfenfluramine	Dose may need to be adjusted.
Estrogens*	Decreased fibrate effect.
Furosemide	Possible toxicity of both drugs.
HMG-CoA reductase inhibitors	May cause muscle or kidney problems or make them worse.
Insulin	Increased insulin effect.
Insulin lispro	May need decreased dosage of insulin.
Probenecid	Increased effect and toxicity of fibrate.
Thyroid hormones*	Increased fibrate effect.
Ursodiol	Decreased effect of ursodiol.

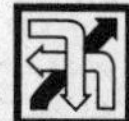

POSSIBLE INTERACTION WITH OTHER SUBSTANCES

INTERACTS WITH	COMBINED EFFECT
Alcohol:	None expected.
Beverages:	None expected.
Cocaine:	None expected.
Foods: Fatty foods.	Decreased fibrate effect.
Marijuana:	None expected.
Tobacco:	None expected.

***See Glossary**

FLAVOXATE

BRAND NAMES

Urispas

BASIC INFORMATION

Habit forming? No
Prescription needed? Yes
Available as generic? Yes
Drug class: Antispasmodic (urinary tract)

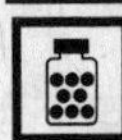

USES

Relieves urinary pain, urgency, nighttime urination, unusual frequency of urination associated with urinary system disorders,

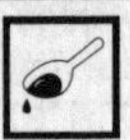

DOSAGE & USAGE INFORMATION

How to take:
Tablet—Swallow with liquid or food to lessen stomach irritation.

When to take:
30 minutes before meals (unless directed otherwise by doctor).

If you forget a dose:
Take as soon as you remember. If it is almost time for the next dose, wait for that dose (don't double this dose) and resume regular schedule.

What drug does:
Blocks nerve impulses at smooth muscle nerve endings, preventing muscle contractions and gland secretions of organs involved.

Time lapse before drug works:
15 to 30 minutes.

Don't take with:
Any other medicine or any dietary supplement without consulting your doctor or pharmacist.

OVERDOSE

SYMPTOMS:
Dilated pupils, rapid pulse and breathing, dizziness, fever, hallucinations, confusion, slurred speech, agitation, flushed face, convulsions, coma.
WHAT TO DO:

- **Dial 911 (emergency) for medical help or call poison control center 1-800-222-1222 for instructions.**
- **See emergency information on last 3 pages of this book.**

POSSIBLE ADVERSE REACTIONS OR SIDE EFFECTS

SYMPTOMS	WHAT TO DO
Life-threatening:	
In case of overdose, see previous column.	
Common:	
• Confusion, delirium, rapid heartbeat.	Discontinue. Call doctor right away.
• Nausea, vomiting, less perspiration, drowsiness.	Continue. Call doctor when convenient.
• Constipation.	Continue. Tell doctor at next visit.
• Dry ears, nose or throat.	No action necessary.
Infrequent:	
• Unusual excitement, irritability, restlessness, clumsiness, hallucinations.	Discontinue. Call doctor right away.
• Headache, increased sensitivity to light, painful or difficult urination.	Continue. Call doctor when convenient.
Rare:	
• Shortness of breath.	Discontinue. Seek emergency treatment.
• Rash or hives, eye pain, blurred vision, sore throat, fever, mouth sores, abdominal pain.	Discontinue. Call doctor right away.
• Dizziness.	Continue. Call doctor when convenient.

WARNINGS & PRECAUTIONS

Don't take if:

- You are allergic to any anticholinergic.
- You have trouble with stomach bloating.
- You have difficulty emptying your bladder completely.
- You have narrow-angle glaucoma.
- You have severe ulcerative colitis.

Before you start, consult your doctor if:

- You have open-angle glaucoma.
- You have angina.
- You have chronic bronchitis or asthma.
- You have liver disease.
- You have hiatal hernia.
- You have enlarged prostate.
- You have myasthenia gravis.
- You have peptic ulcer.
- You will have surgery within 2 months, including dental surgery, requiring general or spinal anesthesia.

Over age 60:
Adverse reactions and side effects, particularly mental confusion, may be more frequent and severe than in younger persons.

Pregnancy:
Consult doctor. Risk category B (see page xviii).

Breast-feeding:
Drug passes into milk. Avoid drug or discontinue nursing until you finish medicine. Consult doctor for advice on maintaining milk supply.

Infants & children:
Use only under medical supervision.

Prolonged use:
Chronic constipation, possible fecal impaction. Consult doctor immediately.

Skin & sunlight:
No problems expected.

Driving, piloting or hazardous work:
Use disqualifies you for piloting aircraft. Don't drive until you learn how medicine affects you. Don't work around dangerous machinery. Don't climb ladders or work in high places. Danger increases if you drink alcohol or take medicine affecting alertness and reflexes, such as antihistamines, tranquilizers, sedatives, pain medicine, narcotics and mind-altering drugs.

Discontinuing:
May be unnecessary to finish medicine. Follow doctor's instructions.

Others:
Advise any doctor or dentist whom you consult that you take this medicine.

POSSIBLE INTERACTION WITH OTHER DRUGS

GENERIC NAME OR DRUG CLASS	COMBINED EFFECT
Antimuscarinics*	Increased effect of flavoxate.
Central nervous system (CNS) depressants, other*	Increased effect of both drugs.
Clozapine	Toxic effect on the central nervous system.
Ethinamate	Dangerous increased effects of ethinamate. Avoid combining.
Fluoxetine	Increased depressant effects of both drugs.
Guanfacine	May increase depressant effects of either drug.
Leucovorin	High alcohol content of leucovorin may cause adverse effects.
Methyprylon	Increased sedative effect, perhaps to dangerous level. Avoid.
Nabilone	Greater depression of central nervous system.
Nizatidine	Increased nizatidine effect.
Sertraline	Increased depressive effects of both drugs.

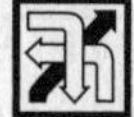

POSSIBLE INTERACTION WITH OTHER SUBSTANCES

INTERACTS WITH	COMBINED EFFECT
Alcohol:	None expected.
Beverages:	None expected.
Cocaine:	Excessively rapid heartbeat. Avoid.
Foods:	None expected.
Marijuana:	Drowsiness, dry mouth.
Tobacco:	None expected.

*See Glossary

FLECAINIDE ACETATE

BRAND NAMES

Tambocor

BASIC INFORMATION

Habit forming? No
Prescription needed? Yes
Available as generic? Yes
Drug class: Antiarrhythmic

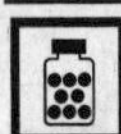

USES

Stabilizes irregular heartbeat.

DOSAGE & USAGE INFORMATION

How to take:
Tablet—Swallow with liquid. If you can't swallow whole, crumble tablet and take with liquid or food.

When to take:
At the same time each day, according to instructions on prescription label. Take tablets approximately 12 hours apart.

If you forget a dose:
Take as soon as you remember. If it is almost time for the next dose, wait for that dose (don't double this dose) and resume regular schedule.

What drug does:
Decreases conduction of abnormal electrical activity in the heart muscle or its regulating systems.

Time lapse before drug works:
1 to 6 hours. May take 3 to 5 days for maximum effect.

Continued next column

OVERDOSE

SYMPTOMS:
Low blood pressure or unconsciousness, irregular or rapid heartbeat, sleepiness, tremor, sweating.
WHAT TO DO:

- **Dial 911 (emergency) for medical help or call poison control center 1-800-222-1222 for instructions.**
- **If person is unconscious, check breathing and pulse. If not breathing, begin mouth-to-mouth rescue breathing. If heart is not beating, begin chest compressions.**
- **See emergency information on last 3 pages of this book.**

Don't take with:
Any other medicine or any dietary supplement without consulting your doctor or pharmacist.

POSSIBLE ADVERSE REACTIONS OR SIDE EFFECTS

SYMPTOMS	WHAT TO DO
Life-threatening:	
In case of overdose, see previous column.	
Common:	
Blurred vision, dizziness.	Continue. Call doctor when convenient.
Infrequent:	
• Chest pain, irregular heartbeat.	Discontinue. Seek emergency treatment.
• Shakiness, rash, nausea, vomiting.	Continue, but call doctor right away.
• Anxiety; depression; weakness; headache; appetite loss; weakness in muscles, bones, joints; swollen feet, ankles or legs; loss of taste; numbness or tingling in hands or feet, abdominal pain.	Continue. Call doctor when convenient.
• Constipation.	Continue. Tell doctor at next visit.
Rare:	
• Shortness of breath.	Discontinue. Seek emergency treatment.
• Sore throat, jaundice, fever.	Continue, but call doctor right away.

WARNINGS & PRECAUTIONS

Don't take if:
You are allergic to flecainide or a local anesthetic such as novocaine, lidocaine or other drug whose generic name ends with "caine."

Before you start, consult your doctor if:

- You have kidney disease.
- You have liver disease.
- You have had a heart attack in past 3 weeks.
- You have a pacemaker.

Over age 60:
Adverse reactions and side effects may be more frequent and severe than in younger persons.

Pregnancy:
Decide with your doctor whether drug benefits justify risk to unborn child. Risk category C (see page xviii).

Breast-feeding:
Drug passes into milk. Avoid drug or discontinue nursing until you finish medicine. Consult doctor for advice on maintaining milk supply.

Infants & children:
Not recommended. Safety and dosage have not been established.

Prolonged use:
Talk to your doctor about the need for follow-up medical examinations or laboratory studies to check complete blood counts (white blood cell count, platelet count, red blood cell count, hemoglobin, hematocrit), ECG.*

Skin & sunlight:
No problems expected.

Driving, piloting or hazardous work:
Don't drive or pilot aircraft until you learn how medicine affects you. Don't work around dangerous machinery. Don't climb ladders or work in high places. Danger increases if you drink alcohol or take medicine affecting alertness and reflexes, such as antihistamines, tranquilizers, sedatives, pain medicine, narcotics and mind-altering drugs.

Discontinuing:
Don't discontinue without consulting doctor. Dose may require gradual reduction if you have taken drug for a long time. Doses of other drugs may also require adjustment.

Others:
- Wear identification bracelet or carry an identification card with inscription of medicine you take.
- Advise any doctor or dentist whom you consult that you take this medicine.

POSSIBLE INTERACTION WITH OTHER DRUGS

GENERIC NAME OR DRUG CLASS	COMBINED EFFECT
Antacids* (high dose)	Possible increased flecainide acetate effect.
Antiarrhythmics, other*	Possible irregular heartbeat.
Beta-adrenergic blocking agents*	Possible decreased efficiency of heart muscle contraction, leading to congestive heart failure.
Bone marrow depressants*	Possible decreased production of blood cells in bone marrow.
Carbonic anhydrase inhibitors*	Possible increased flecainide acetate effect.
Cimetidine	Increased effect of flecainide.
Digitalis preparations*	Possible increased digitalis effect. Possible irregular heartbeat.
Disopyramide	Possible decreased efficiency of heart muscle contraction, leading to congestive heart failure.
Doxepin (topical)	Increased risk of toxicity of both drugs.
Enzyme inhibitors*	Increased effect of flecainide acetate.
Nicardipine	Possible increased effect and toxicity of each drug.
Paroxetine	Increased effect of both drugs.
Propafenone	Increased effect of both drugs and increased risk of toxicity.
Sodium bicarbonate	Possible increased flecainide acetate effect.
Verapamil	Possible decreased efficiency of heart muscle contraction, leading to congestive heart failure.

POSSIBLE INTERACTION WITH OTHER SUBSTANCES

INTERACTS WITH	COMBINED EFFECT
Alcohol:	May further depress normal heart function.
Beverages: Caffeine-containing beverages.	Possible decreased flecainide effect.
Cocaine:	Possible decreased flecainide effect.
Foods:	None expected.
Marijuana:	Possible decreased flecainide effect.
Tobacco:	Possible decreased flecainide effect.

*See Glossary

FLUOROQUINOLONES

GENERIC AND BRAND NAMES

CIPROFLOXACIN	**MOXIFLOXACIN**
Cipro	**Avelox**
Cipro XR	**NORFLOXACIN**
Proquin XR	**Noroxin**
ENOXACIN	**OFLOXACIN**
Penetrex	**Floxin**
GEMIFLOXACIN	**SPARFLOXACIN**
Factive	**Zagam**
LEVOFLOXACIN	**TROVAFLOXACIN**
Levaquin	**Trovan**
LOMEFLOXACIN	
Maxaquin	

BASIC INFORMATION

Habit forming? No
Prescription needed? Yes
Available as generic? Yes, for some
Drug class: Antibacterial

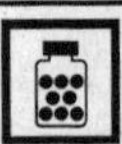

USES

- Treats a wide range of bacteria that may cause diarrhea, pneumonia, skin and soft tissue infections, urinary tract infections, conjunctivitis and bone infections.
- Treatment for specific agents that could be used in biologic warfare.

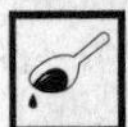

DOSAGE & USAGE INFORMATION

How to take:
- Tablet—Take with full glass of water. Take enoxacin and ofloxacin on an empty stomach. Others may be taken with or without meals.
- Extended release tablet—Swallow whole. Do not crush, break or chew tablet.
- Oral and otic suspension—Take as directed on label.

Continued next column

OVERDOSE

SYMPTOMS:
Confusion and hallucinations, headache, abdominal pain, convulsions.
WHAT TO DO:
- **Dial 911 (emergency) for medical help or call poison control center 1-800-222-1222 for instructions.**
- **See emergency information on last 3 pages of this book.**

When to take:
As directed by your doctor.

If you forget a dose:
Take as soon as you remember. If it is almost time for the next dose, wait for that dose (don't double this dose) and resume regular schedule.

What drug does:
Destroys bacteria that is infecting the body.

Time lapse before drug works:
1 to 2 weeks for most infections, but some infections may take 6 weeks or more for cure.

Don't take with:
Any other medicine or any dietary supplement without consulting your doctor or pharmacist.

POSSIBLE ADVERSE REACTIONS OR SIDE EFFECTS

SYMPTOMS	WHAT TO DO
Life-threatening:	
Hives, rash, intense itching, faintness soon after a dose (anaphylaxis).	Seek emergency treatment immediately.
Common:	
• Sparfloxacin may cause fainting, slow, irregular heart rate.	Discontinue. Call doctor right away.
• Mild stomach discomfort, nausea, dizziness, drowsiness, nervousness, insomnia, headache, vaginal discharge or pain, lightheadedness, mild diarrhea.	Continue. Call doctor when convenient.
Infrequent:	
Skin (itching, red, blisters, burning, rash, swelling, peeling).	Discontinue. Call doctor right away.
Rare:	
• Abdominal pain or cramps or tenderness, agitation, confusion, hallucinations, tremors, shortness of breath, sweating, swelling (neck, face, calves or legs), pale stools, bloody or dark or cloudy urine, joint or calf pain, diarrhea, tired or weak feeling, tendon problems (inflammation, pain, rupture), yellow eyes or skin, seizures, fast or irregular heartbeat, vomiting, fever.	Discontinue. Call doctor right away.

• Appetite loss, dreams abnormal, muscle or back pain, skin sensitive to sun, sore mouth or tongue, vision problems, vaginal infection, taste changes, flushing.	Continue. Call doctor when convenient.

WARNINGS & PRECAUTIONS

Don't take if:
You are allergic to fluoroquinolones or quinolone derivatives.

Before you start, consult your doctor if:
- You have any disorder of the central nervous system such as epilepsy or stroke.
- You have had sun sensitivity or tendinitis.
- You have diabetes or liver, kidney or heart disease.

Over age 60:
Risk of tendinitis or tendon rupture (see Others).

Pregnancy:
Decide with your doctor if drug benefits justify risk to unborn child. Risk category C (see page xviii).

Breast-feeding:
Drug passes into milk. Avoid drug or discontinue nursing until you finish medicine. Consult doctor for advice on maintaining milk supply.

Infants & children:
Normally not recommended for ages under 18.

Prolonged use:
Usually not prescribed for long-term use.

Skin & sunlight:
One or more drugs in this group may cause rash or intensify sunburn in areas exposed to sun or ultraviolet light (photosensitivity reaction). Avoid overexposure. Notify doctor if reaction occurs.

Driving, piloting or hazardous work:
Don't drive or pilot aircraft until you learn how medicine affects you. Don't work around dangerous machinery. Don't climb ladders or work in high places. Risk increases if you drink alcohol or take medicine affecting alertness.

Discontinuing:
Don't discontinue without consulting doctor or completing prescribed dosage. Call doctor if symptoms occur after you stop drug (such as stomach cramps, fever, swelling, calf pain, diarrhea that is watery or bloody).

Others:
- Advise any doctor or dentist whom you consult that you take this medicine.
- These drugs increase the risk of tendinitis or tendon rupture in some patients. If tendon pain or inflammation occurs, stop exercising, discontinue drug and call doctor.
- May affect accuracy of some medical tests.
- Drink plenty of fluids while taking drug.
- Serious liver problems associated with use of trovafloxacin; can lead to liver transplantation and/or death. Consult your doctor about risks.

POSSIBLE INTERACTION WITH OTHER DRUGS

GENERIC NAME OR DRUG CLASS	COMBINED EFFECT
Aminophylline	Increased effect of aminophylline.
Antacids*	Decreased fluoroquinolone effect.
Antidiabetic agents*	Adverse diabetic reactions.
Anti-inflammatory drugs, nonsteroidal (NSAIDs)*	Increased risk of central nervous system problems.
Caffeine	Increased risk of central nervous system problems.
Calcium supplements	Decreased fluoroquinolone effect.
Citrates	Decreased trovafloxacin effect.

Continued on page 915

POSSIBLE INTERACTION WITH OTHER SUBSTANCES

INTERACTS WITH	COMBINED EFFECT
Alcohol:	Increased possibility of central nervous system side effects.
Beverages: Caffeine drinks.	Increased effect of caffeine. Don't use with enoxacin.
Cocaine:	Increased possibility of central nervous system side effects.
Foods: Dairy foods.	Decreased effect of fluoroquinolone. Take 2 hours apart.
Marijuana:	Increased possibility of central nervous system side effects.
Tobacco:	Increased possibility of central nervous system side effects.

FLUOROURACIL (Topical)

BRAND NAMES

5-FU
Efudex
Fluoroplex

BASIC INFORMATION

Habit forming? No
Prescription needed? Yes
Available as generic? No
Drug class: Antineoplastic (topical)

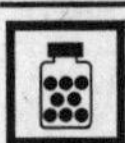

USES

- Treats precancerous actinic keratoses on skin.
- Treats superficial basal cell carcinomas (skin cancers that don't spread to distant organs and, therefore, do not threaten life).

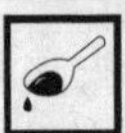

DOSAGE & USAGE INFORMATION

How to use:
- Apply with cotton-tipped applicator.
- Cream, lotion, ointment—Bathe and dry area before use. Apply small amount and rub gently.
- Wash hands (if fingertips are used to apply) after applying medicine to other parts of body.

When to use:
Once or twice a day or as directed by doctor.

If you forget a dose:
Apply as soon as you remember. Resume basic schedule.

What drug does:
Selectively destroys actively proliferating cells.

Time lapse before drug works:
2 to 3 days.

Don't use with:
Other topical medications unless prescribed by your doctor.

OVERDOSE

SYMPTOMS:
None expected.
WHAT TO DO:
Not for internal use. If child accidentally swallows, dial 911 (emergency) for medical help or call poison control center 1-800-222-1222 for instructions.

POSSIBLE ADVERSE REACTIONS OR SIDE EFFECTS

SYMPTOMS	WHAT TO DO
Life-threatening	
None expected.	
Common	
• Skin redness or swelling.	Discontinue. Call doctor right away.
• After 1 or 2 weeks of use—Skin itching or oozing; rash, tenderness, soreness.	Continue. Call doctor when convenient.
Infrequent	
Skin darkening or scaling.	Continue. Call doctor when convenient.
Rare	
Watery eyes.	Discontinue. Call doctor right away.

WARNINGS & PRECAUTIONS

Don't use if:
You are allergic to fluorouracil.

Before you start, consult your doctor if:
- You have chloasma or acne rosacea.
- You have any other skin problems.

Over age 60:
No problems expected.

Pregnancy:
Consult doctor. Risk category X (see page xviii).

Breast-feeding:
Avoid drug or discontinue nursing until you finish medicine. Consult doctor for advice on maintaining milk supply.

Infants & children:
No problems expected, but check with doctor.

Prolonged use:
No problems expected, but check with doctor.

Skin & sunlight:
May cause rash or intensify sunburn in areas exposed to sun or ultraviolet light (photosensitivity reaction). Avoid overexposure. Notify doctor if reaction occurs.

Driving, piloting or hazardous work:
No problems expected, but check with doctor.

Discontinuing:
Pink, smooth area remains after treatment (usually fades in 1 to 2 months).

Others:
- Skin lesions may need biopsy before treatment.
- Keep medicine out of eyes or mouth.
- Heat and moisture in bathroom medicine cabinet can cause breakdown of medicine. Store someplace else.

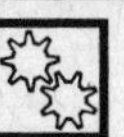

POSSIBLE INTERACTION WITH OTHER DRUGS

GENERIC NAME OR DRUG CLASS	COMBINED EFFECT
None significant.	

POSSIBLE INTERACTION WITH OTHER SUBSTANCES

INTERACTS WITH	COMBINED EFFECT
Alcohol:	None expected.
Beverages:	None expected.
Cocaine:	None expected.
Foods:	None expected.
Marijuana:	None expected.
Tobacco:	None expected.

FOLIC ACID (Vitamin B-9)

BRAND NAMES

Apo-Folic
Beyaz
Folvite
Novo-Folacid
Safyral
Numerous brands of single vitamin and multivitamin combinations may be available.

BASIC INFORMATION

Habit forming? No
Prescription needed?
High strength: Yes
Vitamin mixtures: No
Available as generic? Yes
Drug class: Vitamin supplement

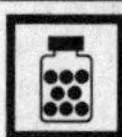

USES

- Dietary supplement to promote normal growth, development and good health.
- Dietary supplement during pregnancy to prevent spinal defects.
- Treatment for anemias due to folic acid deficiency occurring from alcoholism, liver disease, hemolytic anemia, sprue, infants on artificial formula, pregnancy, breast feeding and use of oral contraceptives.
- Some studies have found that folic acid supplementation alone or in combination with other vitamins taken before conception and during early pregnancy may reduce the incidence of neural tube defects in infants.

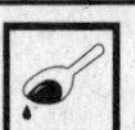

DOSAGE & USAGE INFORMATION

How to take:
Tablet—Swallow with liquid or food to lessen stomach irritation. If you can't swallow whole, crumble tablet and take with liquid or food.

When to take:
At the same time each day.

If you forget a dose:
Take when you remember. Don't double next dose. Resume regular schedule.

Continued next column

OVERDOSE

SYMPTOMS:
None expected.
WHAT TO DO:
Overdose unlikely to threaten life. If child accidentally swallows, dial 911 (emergency) for medical help or call poison control center 1-800-222-1222 for instructions.

What drug does:
Essential to normal red blood cell formation.

Time lapse before drug works:
Not determined.

Don't take with:
Any other medicine or any dietary supplement without consulting your doctor or pharmacist.

POSSIBLE ADVERSE REACTIONS OR SIDE EFFECTS

SYMPTOMS	WHAT TO DO
Life-threatening: None expected.	
Common: Large dose may produce yellow urine.	Continue. Tell doctor at next visit.
Infrequent: None expected.	
Rare: Rash, itching, bronchospasm.	Discontinue. Call doctor right away.

WARNINGS & PRECAUTIONS

Don't take if:
You are allergic to any B vitamin.

Before you start, consult your doctor if:
- You have liver disease.
- You have pernicious anemia. (Folic acid corrects anemia, but nerve damage of pernicious anemia continues.)

Over age 60:
No problems expected.

Pregnancy:
No problems expected. Consult doctor. Risk category A (see page xviii).

Breast-feeding:
No problems expected. Consult doctor.

Infants & children:
No problems expected.

Prolonged use:
No problems expected.

Skin & sunlight:
No problems expected.

Driving, piloting or hazardous work:
No problems expected.

Discontinuing:
Don't discontinue without doctor's advice until you complete prescribed dose, even though symptoms diminish or disappear.

Others:
- Folic acid removed by kidney dialysis. Dialysis patients should increase intake to 300% of RDA or take as directed.
- A balanced diet should provide all the folic acid a healthy person needs and make supplements unnecessary. Best sources are green, leafy vegetables; fruits; liver and kidney.

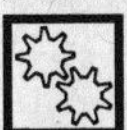

POSSIBLE INTERACTION WITH OTHER DRUGS

GENERIC NAME OR DRUG CLASS	COMBINED EFFECT
Analgesics*	Decreased effect of folic acid.
Anticonvulsants, hydantoin*	Decreased effect of folic acid. Possible increased seizure frequency.
Chloramphenicol	Possible decreased folic acid effect.
Contraceptives, oral*	Decreased effect of folic acid.
Cortisone drugs*	Decreased effect of folic acid.
Methotrexate	Decreased effect of folic acid.
Para-aminosalicylic acid (PAS)	Decreased effect of folic acid.
Pyrimethamine	Decreased effect of folic acid.
Sulfasalazine	Decreased dietary absorption of folic acid.
Triamterene	Decreased effect of folic acid.
Trimethoprim	Decreased effect of folic acid.
Zinc supplements	Increased need for zinc.

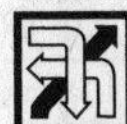

POSSIBLE INTERACTION WITH OTHER SUBSTANCES

INTERACTS WITH	COMBINED EFFECT
Alcohol:	None expected.
Beverages:	None expected.
Cocaine:	None expected.
Foods:	None expected.
Marijuana:	None expected.
Tobacco:	None expected.

FURAZOLIDONE

BRAND NAMES

Furoxone
Furoxone Liquid

BASIC INFORMATION

Habit forming? No
Prescription needed? Yes
Available as generic? No
Drug class: Antiprotozoal, antibacterial (antibiotic)

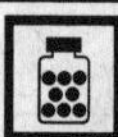

USES

- As an adjunct in treating most germs that infect the gastrointestinal tract such as cholera, salmonellosis, E. coli, proteus infections, and other bacterial causes of diarrhea.
- Treats giardiasis.

DOSAGE & USAGE INFORMATION

How to take:
- Liquid—Use a measuring spoon to ensure correct dose.
- Tablet—Swallow with liquid or food to lessen stomach irritation. If you can't swallow whole, crumble tablet and take with liquid or food.

When to take:
At the same time each day, according to instructions on prescription label.

If you forget a dose:
Take as soon as you remember. If it is almost time for the next dose, wait for that dose (don't double this dose) and resume regular schedule.

What drug does:
Kills microscopic germs.

Time lapse before drug works:
Immediate.

Don't take with:
Any other medicine or any dietary supplement without consulting your doctor or pharmacist.

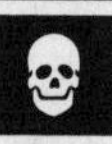

OVERDOSE

SYMPTOMS:
None expected.
WHAT TO DO:
Overdose unlikely to threaten life. If person uses much larger amount than prescribed or if accidentally swallowed, call doctor or poison control center 1-800-222-1222 for help.

POSSIBLE ADVERSE REACTIONS OR SIDE EFFECTS

SYMPTOMS	WHAT TO DO
Life-threatening:	
None expected except when taken with forbidden foods (see Possible Interaction with Other Substances).	
Common:	
• Nausea, vomiting.	Continue. Call doctor when convenient.
• Dark yellow or brown urine.	No action necessary.
Infrequent:	
• Abdominal pain.	Discontinue. Call doctor right away.
• Headache.	Continue. Call doctor when convenient.
Rare:	
Sore throat, fever, skin rash, itching, joint pain.	Discontinue. Call doctor right away.

WARNINGS & PRECAUTIONS

Don't take if:

- You have G6PD* deficiency.
- You have hypersensitivity to furazolidone, nitrofurantoin (Furadantin), or nitrofurazone (Furacin).

Before you start, consult your doctor if:
You are taking any other prescription or nonprescription medicine.

Over age 60:
No special problems expected.

Pregnancy:
Decide with your doctor if drug benefits justify risk to unborn child. Risk category C (see page xviii).

Breast-feeding:
Drug may pass into milk. Avoid drug or discontinue nursing until you finish medicine. Consult doctor for advice on maintaining milk supply.

Infants & children:
Don't use for infants without specific instructions from your doctor.

Prolonged use:
No special problems expected.

Skin & sunlight:
No special problems expected.

Driving, piloting or hazardous work:
No special problems expected.

Discontinuing:
Food restrictions outlined in Possible Interaction with Other Substances must be continued for at least 2 weeks after furazolidone is discontinued.

Others:

- Should not be taken with foods or drinks high in tyramine (see Possible Interaction with Other Substances).
- Advise any doctor or dentist whom you consult that you take this medicine.

POSSIBLE INTERACTION WITH OTHER DRUGS

GENERIC NAME OR DRUG CLASS	COMBINED EFFECT
Antidepressants, tricyclic*	Sudden, severe increase in blood pressure.
Monoamine oxidase (MAO) inhibitors*	Sudden, severe increase in blood pressure.
Sumatriptan	Adverse effects unknown. Avoid.
Sympathomimetics*	Sudden, severe increase in blood pressure.

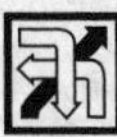

POSSIBLE INTERACTION WITH OTHER SUBSTANCES

INTERACTS WITH	COMBINED EFFECT
Alcohol:	Flushed face, shortness of breath, fever, tightness in chest. Avoid.
Beverages: Any alcoholic beverage.	Flushed face, shortness of breath, fever, tightness in chest. Avoid.
Cocaine:	High blood pressure. Avoid.
Foods: Aged cheese; dark beer; red wine (especially Chianti); sherry; liqueurs; caviar; yeast or protein extracts; fava beans; smoked or pickled meat, poultry, fish; pepperoni, salami, summer sausage; over-ripe fruit.	Sudden, severe high blood pressure that may be life-threatening. Avoid.
Marijuana:	High blood pressure. Avoid.
Tobacco:	No special problems expected.

*See Glossary

FUSION INHIBITOR

GENERIC AND BRAND NAMES

ENFUVIRTIDE
Fuzeon

BASIC INFORMATION

Habit forming? No
Prescription needed? Yes
Available as generic? No
Drug class: Fusion inhibitor

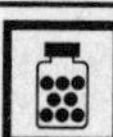

USES

For treatment of HIV and AIDS patients. Used in combination with one or more of the other HIV and AIDS drugs. It is used when other anti-HIV drugs are not effective.

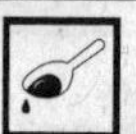

DOSAGE & USAGE INFORMATION

How to take:
Injection—The drug is injected under the skin using small hypodermic needles. Follow all instructions carefully on the prescription label. Dispose of all needles and syringes as instructed by your doctor.

When to take:
Two shots a day; one taken in the morning and the other 12 hours later at night.

If you forget a dose:
Take as soon as you remember. If it is almost time for your next dose, skip the missed dose and go back to the regular dosing schedule. Do not double doses.

What drug does:
It stops HIV from entering healthy cells. It helps slow the progress of HIV disease, but does not cure it.

Time lapse before drug works:
May require several weeks or months before full benefits are apparent.

Continued next column

OVERDOSE

SYMPTOMS:
Unknown effects.
WHAT TO DO:
If person takes much larger amount than prescribed, dial 911 (emergency) for medical help or call poison control center 1-800-222-1222 for instructions.

Don't take with:
Any other medicine or any dietary supplement without consulting your doctor or pharmacist. This is very important with antiviral drugs.

POSSIBLE ADVERSE REACTIONS OR SIDE EFFECTS

SYMPTOMS	WHAT TO DO
Life-threatening:	
Rare allergic reaction—Breathing difficulty; swelling of hands, feet, face, mouth, neck; skin rash.	Discontinue. Seek emergency treatment.
Common:	
• Peripheral neuropathy (burning, tingling, numbness, pain or weakness in arms, hands, feet or legs), pain around cheeks or eyes, fever, chills, runny or stuffy nose, cough, wheezing, tightness in chest.	Continue, but call doctor right away.
• Anxiety, weakness, depression, sores on skin, cold sores, trouble sleeping, weight loss, skin symptoms at site of drug injections, muscle pain, itching.	Continue. Call doctor when convenient.
Infrequent:	
• Eye inflammation (swelling, red and painful), stomach or back pain, dark urine, constipation, appetite loss, nausea or vomiting, indigestion, yellow skin or eyes, skin lump or growth.	Continue, but call doctor right away.
• General ill feeling, diarrhea, headache, joint pain, changes in taste, swollen or painful lymph glands.	Continue. Call doctor when convenient.
Rare:	
Pneumonia symptoms (rapid breathing, shortness of breath, cough with fever). Any other unusual symptoms that occur (may be due to the illness, this drug or other drugs being taken).	Continue, but call doctor right away.

WARNINGS & PRECAUTIONS

Don't take if:
You are allergic to fusion inhibitors.

Before you start, consult your doctor if:
- You have or have had lung disease.
- You have high viral load or low CD4 cell count.
- You use intravenous (IV) drugs.
- You smoke.

Over age 60:
The drug has not been studied in this age group.

Pregnancy:
Decide with your doctor if drug benefits justify risks to unborn child. Risk category B (see page xviii).

Breast-feeding:
It is unknown if drug passes into milk. It is not recommended that HIV-infected mothers breast-feed. Consult your doctor.

Infants & children:
Safety and efficacy have not been established in children under age 6. Use only under close medical supervision for any children.

Prolonged use:
- Long-term effects have not been established.
- Talk to your doctor about frequent blood counts and liver function studies.

Skin & sunlight:
No problems expected.

Driving, piloting or hazardous work:
Don't drive or pilot aircraft until you learn how medicine affects you. Don't work around dangerous machinery. Don't climb ladders or work in high places. Danger increases if you drink alcohol or take medicine affecting alertness and reflexes.

Discontinuing:
Don't discontinue without doctor's advice. Doses of other drugs may require adjustment.

Others:
- Advise any doctor or dentist whom you consult that you take this medicine.
- Avoid sexual intercourse or use condoms to help prevent the transmission of HIV. Don't share needles or equipment for injections with other persons.
- This drug is combined with others for the best treatment. This increases the risk of side effects or adverse reactions.
- May interfere with results of some blood tests.
- Numerous medical studies are ongoing concerning the use of these and other anti-HIV drugs. Full safety and effectiveness are still being determined.

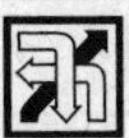

POSSIBLE INTERACTION WITH OTHER DRUGS

GENERIC NAME OR DRUG CLASS	COMBINED EFFECT
None expected.	

POSSIBLE INTERACTION WITH OTHER SUBSTANCES

INTERACTS WITH	COMBINED EFFECT
Alcohol:	None expected.
Beverages:	None expected.
Cocaine:	Unknown effect. Best to avoid.
Foods:	None expected.
Marijuana:	Unknown effect. Best to avoid.
Tobacco:	None expected.

GABAPENTIN

BRAND NAMES

Gralise
Horizant
Neurontin

BASIC INFORMATION

Habit forming? No
Prescription needed? Yes
Available as generic? Yes
Drug class: Anticonvulsant, antiepileptic

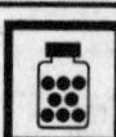

USES

- Treatment for partial (focal) epileptic seizures. Used in combination with other antiepileptic drugs.
- Treats restless legs syndrome (Willis-Ekbom disease).
- Treats postherpetic neuralgia.

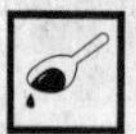

DOSAGE & USAGE INFORMATION

How to take:

- Capsule or tablet—Swallow with liquid. May be taken with or without food.
- Oral solution—Follow directions on your prescription label.
- Extended-release tablet—Swallow whole with liquid. Do not split, chew or crush tablet. Take with food.

When to take:

- For seizure treatment, your doctor will determine the best schedule. Dosages will be increased rapidly over the first 3 days of use. Further increases may be necessary to achieve maximum benefits.
- For restless legs syndrome, take once a day with food at about 5:00 p.m.

If you forget a dose:
Take as soon as you remember. If it is almost time for the next dose, skip the missed dose and wait for your next scheduled dose (don't double this dose).

Continued next column

OVERDOSE

SYMPTOMS:
Double vision, slurred speech, drowsiness, tiredness, diarrhea.
WHAT TO DO:
Overdose unlikely to threaten life. If person uses much larger amount than prescribed or if accidentally swallowed, call doctor or poison control center 1-800-222-1222 for help.

What drug does:

- The exact mechanism in treating seizures is unknown. The anticonvulsant action may result from an altered transport of brain amino acids. Amino acids play an important part in chemical reactions within the cells
- It is unknown just how the drug works to treat restless legs syndrome.

Time lapse before drug works:
May take several weeks for effectiveness.

Don't take with:
Any other medicine or any dietary supplement without consulting your doctor or pharmacist.

POSSIBLE ADVERSE REACTIONS OR SIDE EFFECTS

SYMPTOMS	WHAT TO DO
Life-threatening:	
None expected.	
Common:	
Sleepiness, dizziness, fatigue, clumsiness, lack of coordination.	Continue. Call doctor when convenient.
Infrequent:	
Rapid eye movement (nystagmus), double or blurred vision.	Continue. Call doctor when convenient.
Rare:	
Rash; nervousness; depression; twitching or swelling in hands, feet or legs; runny nose; dry or sore throat; nausea; vomiting; coughing; dry mouth; constipation; impotence; increased appetite; weight gain; muscle or back ache; forgetfulness; indigestion.	Continue. Call doctor when convenient.

WARNINGS & PRECAUTIONS

Don't take if:
You are allergic to gabapentin.

Before you start, consult your doctor if:
You have kidney disease.

Over age 60:
No special problems expected.

Pregnancy:
Decide with your doctor if drug benefits justify risks to unborn child. Risk category C (see page xviii).

Breast-feeding:
It is unknown if drug passes into milk. Consult your doctor.

Infants & children:
Not recommended for children under age 12.

Prolonged use:
No special problems expected. Follow-up laboratory blood studies may be recommended by your doctor.

Skin & sunlight:
No problems expected.

Driving, piloting or hazardous work:
Don't drive or pilot aircraft until you learn how medicine affects you. Don't work around dangerous machinery. Don't climb ladders or work in high places. Danger increases if you drink alcohol or take other medicines affecting alertness and reflexes such as antihistamines, tranquilizers, sedatives, pain medicine, narcotics and mind-altering drugs.

Discontinuing:
Don't discontinue without doctor's approval due to risk of increased seizure activity.

Others:
- Advise any doctor or dentist whom you consult that you take this medicine.
- The brand name Horizant is not interchangeable with other gabapentin brand names. Consult your doctor or pharmacist if you have any concerns.
- Side effects of gabapentin are usually mild to moderate. Because it is normally used with other anticonvulsant drugs, additional side effects may also occur. If they do, discuss them with your doctor.
- Rarely, antiepileptic drugs may lead to suicidal thoughts and behaviors. Call doctor right away if suicidal symptoms or unusual behaviors occur.

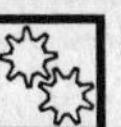

POSSIBLE INTERACTION WITH OTHER DRUGS

GENERIC NAME OR DRUG CLASS	COMBINED EFFECT
Antacids*	Allow at least 2 hours between the 2 drugs.
Central nervous system (CNS) depressants*	Increased sedation.

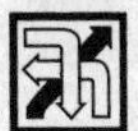

POSSIBLE INTERACTION WITH OTHER SUBSTANCES

INTERACTS WITH	COMBINED EFFECT
Alcohol:	Increased sedation.
Beverages:	None expected.
Cocaine:	None expected.
Foods:	None expected.
Marijuana:	None expected.
Tobacco:	None expected.

GEMFIBROZIL

BRAND NAMES

Lopid

BASIC INFORMATION

Habit forming? No
Prescription needed? Yes
Available as generic? Yes
Drug class: Antihyperlipidemic

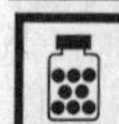

USES

Reduces fatty substances in the blood (triglycerides) and raises high-density lipoprotein (HDL) cholesterol levels.

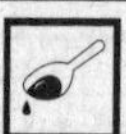

DOSAGE & USAGE INFORMATION

How to take:
Tablet or capsule—Swallow with liquid or food to lessen stomach irritation.

When to take:
Take 30 minutes before morning and evening meals.

If you forget a dose:
Take as soon as you remember. If it is almost time for the next dose, wait for that dose (don't double this dose) and resume regular schedule.

What drug does:
Inhibits formation of fatty substances.

Time lapse before drug works:
3 months or more.

Don't take with:
Any other medicine or any dietary supplement without consulting your doctor or pharmacist.

OVERDOSE

SYMPTOMS:
Diarrhea, headache, muscle pain.
WHAT TO DO:
Overdose unlikely to threaten life. If person uses much larger amount than prescribed or if accidentally swallowed, call doctor or poison control center 1-800-222-1222 for help.

POSSIBLE ADVERSE REACTIONS OR SIDE EFFECTS

SYMPTOMS	WHAT TO DO
Life-threatening: None expected.	
Common: Indigestion.	Continue. Call doctor when convenient.
Infrequent: Chest pain, shortness of breath, irregular heartbeat, nausea, vomiting, diarrhea, stomach pain.	Discontinue. Call doctor right away.
Rare:	
• Rash, itch; sores in mouth, on lips; sore throat; swollen feet, legs; blood in urine; painful urination; fever; chills.	Discontinue. Call doctor right away.
• Dizziness, headache, drowsiness, muscle cramps, dry skin, backache, unusual tiredness, decreased sex drive.	Continue. Call doctor when convenient.

WARNINGS & PRECAUTIONS

Don't take if:
You are allergic to any antihyperlipidemic.

Before you start, consult your doctor if:
- You have had liver or kidney disease.
- You have gallstones or gallbladder disease.
- You have had peptic-ulcer disease.
- You have diabetes.

Over age 60:
Adverse reactions and side effects may be more frequent and severe than in younger persons.

Pregnancy:
Decide with your doctor if drug benefits justify risks to unborn child. Risk category C (see page xviii).

Breast-feeding:
It is not known if drug passes into milk. Avoid drug or discontinue nursing until you finish medicine. Consult doctor for advice on maintaining milk supply.

Infants & children:
Not recommended.

Prolonged use:
Periodic blood cell counts and liver function studies recommended if you take gemfibrozil for a long time.

Skin & sunlight:
No problems expected.

Driving, piloting or hazardous work:
Avoid if you feel drowsy or dizzy. Otherwise, no problems expected.

Discontinuing:
Don't discontinue without doctor's advice until you complete prescribed dose.

Others:
- May affect results in some medical tests.
- Advise any doctor or dentist whom you consult that you take this medicine.

POSSIBLE INTERACTION WITH OTHER DRUGS

GENERIC NAME OR DRUG CLASS	COMBINED EFFECT
Anticoagulants, oral*	Increased anticoagulant effect. Dose reduction of anticoagulant necessary.
Antidiabetics, oral*	Increased antidiabetic effect.
Contraceptives, oral*	Decreased gemfibrozil effect.
Dexfenfluramine	May require dosage change as weight loss occurs.
Estrogens*	Decreased gemfibrozil effect.
Furosemide	Possible toxicity of both drugs.
HMG-CoA reductase inhibitors	Increased risk of muscle inflammation and kidney failure.
Insulin	Increased insulin effect.
Lovastatin	Increased risk of kidney problems.
Thyroid hormones*	Increased gemfibrozil effect.

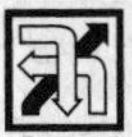

POSSIBLE INTERACTION WITH OTHER SUBSTANCES

INTERACTS WITH	COMBINED EFFECT
Alcohol:	None expected.
Beverages:	None expected.
Cocaine:	Decreased effect of gemfibrozil. Avoid.
Foods: Fatty foods.	Decreased gemfibrozil effect.
Marijuana:	None expected.
Tobacco:	Decreased gemfibrozil absorption. Avoid.

***See Glossary**

GLP-1 RECEPTOR AGONISTS

GENERIC AND BRAND NAMES

EXENATIDE	LIRAGLUTIDE
Bydureon	Victoza
Byetta	

BASIC INFORMATION

Habit forming? No
Prescription needed? Yes
Available as generic? No
Drug class: Antidiabetic; incretin mimetic

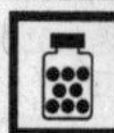

USES

Used alone or in combination with other antidiabetic agents to control blood sugar levels in adults who have type 2 diabetes.

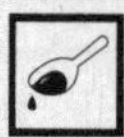

DOSAGE & USAGE INFORMATION

How to take:
Self injection—Injected under the skin (subcutaneous) of the upper leg (thigh), stomach area (abdomen), or upper arm. The drug comes in a prefilled pen that is used with a small needle. Read and follow the instructions provided with the prescription.

When to take:

- Inject Byetta (exenatide) twice a day, at any time within the 60 minutes before morning and evening meals. Do not inject it after eating the meal.
- Inject Bydureon (exenatide) once a week (each 7 days) any time of day with or without food.
- Inject liraglutide once daily at any time of day, independently of meals.

Continued next column

OVERDOSE

SYMPTOMS:
Low blood sugar (hypoglycemia)—See list of symptoms in next column under Infrequent.
WHAT TO DO:

- **Eat some type of sugar immediately, such as glucose product, orange juice (add some sugar), nondiet sodas, candy (such as 5 Lifesavers), honey.**
- **If patient loses consciousness, give glucagon if you have it and know how to use it.**
- **Dial 911 (emergency) for medical help or call poison control center 1-800-222-1222 for instructions.**
- **See emergency information on last 3 pages of this book.**

If you forget a dose:

- If you forget to inject Byetta (exenatide) before a meal, skip that dose and inject next dose as scheduled. Inject Bydureon (exenatide) as soon as you remember. If next dose is due in less than 3 days, skip missed dose and resume schedule. Don't double any doses.
- Inject liraglutide as soon as you remember. If more than 12 hours late, skip the missed dose and resume schedule. Don't double next dose.

What drug does:

- Helps the pancreas produce insulin in response to rising blood sugar levels; inhibits the liver's production of sugar; reduces the rate at which sugar enters the bloodstream by slowing the release of food from the stomach.
- It appears to decrease appetite, which may lead to weight loss.

Time lapse before drug works:
The effects begin right after it is injected.

Don't take with:
Any other medicine or any dietary supplement without consulting your doctor or pharmacist.

POSSIBLE ADVERSE REACTIONS OR SIDE EFFECTS

SYMPTOMS	WHAT TO DO
Life-threatening:	
Rare allergic reaction (hives, itching, rash, trouble breathing, tightness in chest, swelling of lips or tongue or face).	Seek emergency treatment immediately.
Common:	
Nausea, vomiting.	Continue. Call doctor if symptoms persist.
Infrequent:	
• Stomach symptoms (acid, sour, upset, ache, belching), diarrhea, feeling jittery, loss of strength, headache, heartburn, appetite decreased, sweating, dizziness, constipation, injection site soreness, upper respiratory infection.	Continue. Call doctor when convenient.
• Symptoms of low blood sugar–hunger, (excessive), cold sweats and skin, rapid pulse, anxiety, nervousness, chills, confusion, drowsiness, loss of concentration, headache, nausea, weakness, shakiness, vision changes.	Seek treatment (eat some form of quick-acting sugar—glucose tablets, sugar, fruit juice, corn syrup, honey).

• Symptoms of high blood sugar—increased urination, unusual thirst, dry mouth, drowsiness, flushed or dry skin, fruit-like breath odor, appetite loss, stomach pain or vomiting, tiredness, trouble breathing, increased blood sugar level.	Check your blood sugar immediately. Call doctor right away.
Rare:	
• Abdominal pain (persistent, severe, may have vomiting), neck swelling or lump, hoarseness, difficulty breathing or swallowing.	Discontinue. Call doctor right away.
• Other symptoms that cause concern.	Continue. Call doctor when convenient.

WARNINGS & PRECAUTIONS

Don't take if:
You are allergic to exenatide or liraglutide.

Before you start, consult your doctor if:
- You have type 1 diabetes.
- You require insulin for diabetes treatment.
- You have any kidney or liver problems.
- You have a history of pancreatitis.
- You have a personal or family history of multiple endocrine neoplasia syndrome type 2 or medullary thyroid carcinoma (for liraglutide).
- You have severe gastrointestinal disease.

Over age 60:
No special problems expected.

Pregnancy:
Decide with your doctor if drug benefits justify risk to unborn child. Risk category C (see page xviii).

Breast-feeding:
It is unknown if drug passes into milk. Its use is not recommended during breast-feeding. Consult doctor for advice.

Infants & children:
Safety and effectiveness in children has not been established. Consult your child's doctor.

Prolonged use:
Talk to your doctor about the need for follow-up medical examinations and/or laboratory studies to determine continued effectiveness of drug.

Skin & sunlight:
No problems expected.

Driving, piloting or hazardous work:
No problems expected.

Discontinuing:
Don't discontinue without doctor's advice, even though symptoms diminish or disappear.

Others:
- Notify your doctor if you have a fever, infection, diarrhea or experience vomiting.
- Advise any doctor or dentist whom you consult that you take this medicine.
- You and your family should educate yourselves about diabetes; learn to recognize the symptoms of hypoglycemia and how to treat it.
- Wear or carry medical identification that indicates you have type 2 diabetes and the drugs you take.
- Follow your prescribed diet, medication, and exercise routines closely. Changing any of these things can affect blood sugar levels.
- Liraglutide has potential risk for certain thyroid tumors or cancer. Consult doctor about risks.

POSSIBLE INTERACTION WITH OTHER DRUGS

GENERIC NAME OR DRUG CLASS	COMBINED EFFECT
Digoxin	May decrease effect of digoxin.
Drugs taken by mouth that need to pass quickly through the stomach (such as oral contraceptives or antibiotics).	May need to take them 1 hour before injecting GLP-1 receptor agonist. Consult doctor or pharmacist.
Hypoglycemia-causing medications*	Risk of low blood sugar.
Hypoglycemics*	Risk of low blood sugar.

Continued on page 915

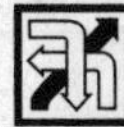

POSSIBLE INTERACTION WITH OTHER SUBSTANCES

INTERACTS WITH	COMBINED EFFECT
Alcohol:	May cause low blood sugar. Avoid.
Beverages:	None expected.
Cocaine:	Unknown effect. Avoid.
Foods:	None expected. Follow your diabetic diet instructions.
Marijuana:	Possible increase in blood sugar. Avoid.
Tobacco:	None expected.

***See Glossary**

GLUCAGON

BRAND NAMES

Glucagon for Injection

BASIC INFORMATION

Habit forming? No
Prescription needed? Yes
Available as generic? Yes
Drug class: Antihypoglycemic, diagnostic aid

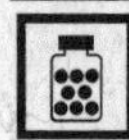

USES

- Treats low blood sugar (hypoglycemia) in diabetics.
- Used as antidote for overdose of beta-adrenergic blockers, quinidine and tricyclic antidepressants.

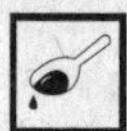

DOSAGE & USAGE INFORMATION

How to take:
Injection—As directed by your doctor.

When to take:
When there are signs of low blood sugar (anxiety; chills; cool, pale skin; hunger; nausea; tremors; sweating; weakness; stomach pain; confusion; drowsiness; fast heartbeat; continuing headache; unsteady walk; unusual tiredness or weakness; vision changes; unconsciousness) in diabetics who don't respond to eating some form of sugar.

If you forget a dose:
Single dose only.

What drug does:
Forces liver to make more sugar and release it into the bloodstream.

Time lapse before drug works:
- For hypoglycemic condition—5 to 20 minutes.
- For muscle relaxant—1 to 10 minutes.

Continued next column

OVERDOSE

SYMPTOMS:
Nausea, vomiting, severe weakness, irregular heartbeat, hoarseness, cramps.
WHAT TO DO:
- **Dial 911 (emergency) for medical help or call poison control center 1-800-222-1222 for instructions.**
- **See emergency information on last 3 pages of this book.**

Don't take with:
Any other medicines (including over-the-counter drugs such as cough and cold medicines, laxatives, antacids, diet pills, caffeine, nose drops or vitamins) without consulting your doctor or pharmacist.

POSSIBLE ADVERSE REACTIONS OR SIDE EFFECTS

SYMPTOMS	WHAT TO DO
Life-threatening:	
Unconsciousness.	Seek emergency treatment immediately.
Common:	
Nausea.	Continue. Call doctor when convenient.
Infrequent:	
Lightheadedness, breathing difficulty, skin rash.	Discontinue. Call doctor right away.
Rare:	
None expected.	

WARNINGS & PRECAUTIONS

Don't take if:
You can't tolerate glucagon.

Before you start, consult your doctor if:
- You are allergic to beef or pork.
- You have pheochromocytoma.*

Over age 60:
No special problems expected.

Pregnancy:
No proven harm to unborn child, but avoid if possible. Consult doctor. Risk category B (see page xviii).

Breast-feeding:
No special problems expected. Consult doctor.

Infants & children:
No special problems expected.

Prolonged use:
To be used intermittently and not for prolonged periods.

Skin & sunlight:
No problems expected.

Driving, piloting or hazardous work:
Don't drive or pilot aircraft until you learn how medicine affects you. Don't work around dangerous machinery. Don't climb ladders or work in high places. Danger increases if you drink alcohol or take medicine affecting alertness and reflexes.

Discontinuing:
No special problems expected.

Others:
- May affect results in some medical tests.
- Explain to other family members how to inject glucagon.
- Before injecting, try to eat some form of sugar, such as glucose tablets, corn syrup, honey, orange juice, hard candy or sugar cubes.
- Store unmixed glucagon at room temperature. Store mixed glucagon in refrigerator, but don't freeze. Mixed solution is only good for 48 hours.
- Check expiration date regularly and replace drug before it expires.

POSSIBLE INTERACTION WITH OTHER DRUGS

GENERIC NAME OR DRUG CLASS	COMBINED EFFECT
Anticoagulants*	Increased anticoagulant effect.

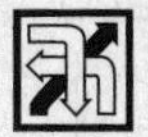

POSSIBLE INTERACTION WITH OTHER SUBSTANCES

INTERACTS WITH	COMBINED EFFECT
Alcohol:	Decreased glucagon effect.
Beverages:	None expected.
Cocaine:	Increased adverse reactions.
Foods: Sugar, fruit juice, candy.	Enhances glucagon effect.
Marijuana:	Increased adverse reactions.
Tobacco:	None expected.

*See Glossary

GLYCOPYRROLATE

BRAND NAMES

Robinul
Robinul Forte

BASIC INFORMATION

Habit forming? No
Prescription needed? Yes
Available as generic? Yes
Drug class: Antispasmodic, anticholinergic

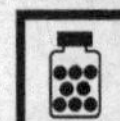

USES

- Reduces spasms of digestive system.
- Reduces production of saliva during dental procedures.
- Treats peptic ulcer by reducing gastric acid secretion.

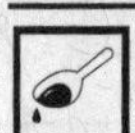

DOSAGE & USAGE INFORMATION

How to take:
Tablet—Swallow with liquid. If you can't swallow whole, crumble tablet and take with small amount of liquid or food.

When to take:
30 minutes before meals (unless directed otherwise by doctor).

If you forget a dose:
Wait for next scheduled dose (don't double this dose).

What drug does:
Blocks nerve impulses at parasympathetic nerve endings, preventing smooth (involuntary) muscle contractions and gland secretions of organs involved.

Time lapse before drug works:
15 to 30 minutes.

Don't take with:
Any other medicine or any dietary supplement without consulting your doctor or pharmacist.

OVERDOSE

SYMPTOMS:
Dry mouth, blurred vision, low blood pressure, decreased breathing rate, rapid heartbeat, flushed skin, drowsiness.
WHAT TO DO:
- **Dial 911 (emergency) for medical help or call poison control center 1-800-222-1222 for instructions.**
- **See emergency information on last 3 pages of this book.**

POSSIBLE ADVERSE REACTIONS OR SIDE EFFECTS

SYMPTOMS	WHAT TO DO
Life-threatening:	
Hives, rash, intense itching, faintness soon after a dose (anaphylaxis).	Seek emergency treatment immediately.
Common:	
Dry mouth, loss of taste, constipation, difficult urination.	Continue. Call doctor when convenient.
Infrequent:	
• Confusion; dizziness; drowsiness; eye pain; headache; rash; sleep disturbance such as nightmares, frequent waking; nausea; vomiting; rapid heartbeat; lightheadedness.	Discontinue. Call doctor right away.
• Insomnia, blurred vision, diminished sex drive, decreased sweating, nasal congestion, altered taste.	Continue. Call doctor when convenient.
Rare:	
Rash, hives.	Discontinue. Call doctor right away.

WARNINGS & PRECAUTIONS

Don't take if:
- You are allergic to any anticholinergic.
- You have trouble with stomach bloating.
- You have difficulty emptying your bladder completely.
- You have narrow-angle glaucoma.
- You have severe ulcerative colitis.

Before you start, consult your doctor if:
- You have open-angle glaucoma.
- You have angina, chronic bronchitis or asthma, liver disease, hiatal hernia, enlarged prostate, myasthenia gravis, peptic ulcer, kidney or thyroid disease.
- You will have surgery within 2 months, including dental surgery, requiring general or spinal anesthesia.

Over age 60:
Adverse reactions and side effects may be more frequent and severe than in younger persons.

Pregnancy:
Consult doctor. Risk category B (see page xviii).

Breast-feeding:
Drug passes into milk and decreases milk flow. Avoid drug or discontinue nursing until you finish medicine. Consult doctor for advice on maintaining milk supply.

Infants & children:
Use only under medical supervision.

Prolonged use:
Chronic constipation, possible fecal impaction. Consult doctor immediately.

Skin & sunlight:
No problems expected.

Driving, piloting or hazardous work:
No problems expected.

Discontinuing:
May be unnecessary to finish medicine. Follow doctor's instructions.

Others:
- Heatstroke more likely if you become overheated during exertion.
- Advise any doctor or dentist whom you consult that you take this medicine.

POSSIBLE INTERACTION WITH OTHER DRUGS

GENERIC NAME OR DRUG CLASS	COMBINED EFFECT
Adrenocorticoids, systemic	Possible glaucoma.
Antacids*	Decreased glycopyrrolate absorption effect.
Amantadine	Increased glycopyrrolate effect.
Anticholinergics, other*	Increased glycopyrrolate effect.
Antidepressants, tricyclic*	Increased glycopyrrolate effect.
Antidiarrheals*	Decreased glycopyrrolate absorption effect.
Attapulgite	Decreased effect of anticholinergic.
Buclizine	Increased glycopyrrolate effect.
Digitalis	Possible decreased absorption of digitalis.
Haloperidol	Increased internal eye pressure.
Ketoconazole	Decreased ketoconazole effect.
Meperidine	Increased glycopyrrolate effect.
Methylphenidate	Increased anticholinergic effect.
Molindone	Increased nizatidine effect.
Monoamine oxidase (MAO) inhibitors*	Increased glycopyrrolate effect.
Orphenadrine	Increased glycopyrrolate effect.
Phenothiazines	Increased glycopyrrolate effect.
Pilocarpine	Increased glycopyrrolate effect. Loss of pilocarpine effect in glaucoma treatment.
Potassium chloride tabs	Increased side effects of potassium tablets.
Quinidine	Increased glycopyrrolate effect.
Sedatives* or central nervous system (CNS) depressants*	Increased sedative effect of both drugs.
Vitamin C	Increased glycopyrrolate effect. Avoid large vitamin C doses.

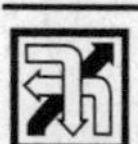

POSSIBLE INTERACTION WITH OTHER SUBSTANCES

INTERACTS WITH	COMBINED EFFECT
Alcohol:	None expected.
Beverages:	None expected.
Cocaine:	Excessively rapid heartbeat.
Foods:	None expected.
Marijuana:	Drowsiness and dry mouth.
Tobacco:	None expected.

*See Glossary

GOLD COMPOUNDS

GENERIC AND BRAND NAMES

AURANOFIN
Ridaura-Oral

GOLD SODIUM THIOMALATE
Myocrisin

BASIC INFORMATION

Habit forming? No
Prescription needed? Yes
Available as generic? No
Drug class: Gold compounds

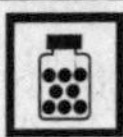

USES

Treatment for rheumatoid arthritis and juvenile idiopathic arthritis.

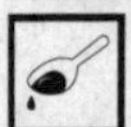

DOSAGE & USAGE INFORMATION

How to take:

- Capsule—Swallow with full glass of fluid. Follow prescription directions. Taking too much can cause serious adverse reactions.
- Injection—Under medical supervision.

When to take:
Once or twice daily, morning and night.

If you forget a dose:
Take as soon as you remember up to 6 hours late, then go back to usual schedule.

What drug does:
Modifies disease activity of rheumatoid arthritis by mechanisms not yet understood.

Time lapse before drug works:
3 to 6 months.

Don't take with:
Any other medicine or any dietary supplement without consulting your doctor or pharmacist.

OVERDOSE

SYMPTOMS:
Confusion, delirium, numbness and tingling in feet and hands.
WHAT TO DO:

- **Dial 911 (emergency) for medical help or call poison control center 1-800-222-1222 for instructions.**
- **See emergency information on last 3 pages of this book.**

POSSIBLE ADVERSE REACTIONS OR SIDE EFFECTS

SYMPTOMS	WHAT TO DO
Life-threatening:	
Hives, rash, intense itching, faintness soon after a dose (anaphylaxis).	Seek emergency treatment immediately.
Common:	
• Itch; hives; sores or white spots in mouth, throat; appetite loss; diarrhea; vomiting; skin rashes; fever.	Discontinue. Call doctor right away.
• Indigestion, constipation.	Continue. Call doctor when convenient.
Infrequent:	
• Excessive fatigue; sore tongue, mouth or gums; metallic or odd taste; unusual bleeding or bruising; blood in urine; vaginal discharge; flushing; fainting; dizziness; sweating after injection.	Discontinue. Call doctor right away.
• Hair loss; pain in muscles, bones and joints (with injections).	Continue. Call doctor when convenient.
Rare:	
• Blood in stool, difficult breathing, coughing, seizures.	Discontinue. Seek emergency treatment.
• Abdominal pain, jaundice, numbness or tingling in hands or feet, muscle weakness.	Discontinue. Call doctor right away.
• "Pink eye."	Continue. Call doctor when convenient.

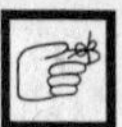

WARNINGS & PRECAUTIONS

Don't take if:
- You have a history of allergy to gold or other metals.
- You have any blood disorder.
- You have kidney disease.

Before you start, consult your doctor if:
- You are pregnant or may become pregnant.
- You have lupus erythematosus.
- You have Sjögren's syndrome.
- You have chronic skin disease.
- You are debilitated.
- You have blood dyscrasias.

Over age 60:
Adverse reactions and side effects may be more frequent and severe than in younger persons.

Pregnancy:
Decide with your doctor if drug benefits justify risks to unborn child. Risk category C (see page xviii).

Breast-feeding:
Drug may filter into milk, causing side effects in infants. Avoid. Consult doctor.

Infants & children:
Not recommended. Safety and dosage have not been established.

Prolonged use:
Request periodic laboratory studies of blood counts, urine and liver function. These should be done before use and at least once a month during treatment.

Skin & sunlight:
- One or more drugs in this group may cause rash or intensify sunburn in areas exposed to sun or ultraviolet light (photosensitivity reaction). Avoid overexposure. Notify doctor if reaction occurs.
- Blue-gray pigmentation in skin exposed to sunlight.

Driving, piloting or hazardous work:
Avoid if you have serious adverse reactions or side effects. Otherwise, no problems expected.

Discontinuing:
Don't discontinue without doctor's advice until you complete prescribed dose.

Others:
- Side effects and adverse reactions may appear during treatment or for many months after discontinuing.
- Gold has been shown to cause kidney tumors and kidney cancer in animals given excessive doses.
- May interfere with the accuracy of some medical tests.

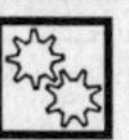

POSSIBLE INTERACTION WITH OTHER DRUGS

GENERIC NAME OR DRUG CLASS	COMBINED EFFECT
Bone marrow depressants*	Increased risk of toxicity of both drugs.
Hepatotoxics*	Increased risk of toxicity of both drugs.
Nephrotoxics*	Increased risk of toxicity of both drugs.
Penicillamine	Increased likelihood of kidney damage.
Phenytoin	Increased phenytoin blood levels. Phenytoin dosage may require adjustment.

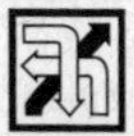

POSSIBLE INTERACTION WITH OTHER SUBSTANCES

INTERACTS WITH	COMBINED EFFECT
Alcohol:	None expected.
Beverages:	None expected.
Cocaine:	None expected.
Foods:	None expected.
Marijuana:	None expected.
Tobacco:	None expected.

***See Glossary**

GRISEOFULVIN

BRAND NAMES

Fulvicin P/G
Fulvicin U/F
Grifulvin V
Grisactin
Grisactin Ultra
Grisovin-FP
Gris-PEG

BASIC INFORMATION

Habit forming? No
Prescription needed? Yes
Available as generic? Yes
Drug class: Antifungal

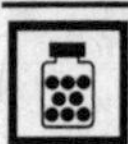

USES

Treatment for fungal infections susceptible to griseofulvin.

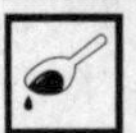

DOSAGE & USAGE INFORMATION

How to take:

- Tablet or capsule—Swallow with liquid or food to lessen stomach irritation. If you can't swallow whole, crumble tablet or open capsule and take with liquid or food.
- Liquid—Follow label instructions.

When to take:
With or immediately after meals.

If you forget a dose:
Take as soon as you remember. If it is almost time for the next dose, wait for that dose (don't double this dose) and resume regular schedule.

What drug does:
Prevents fungi from growing and reproducing.

Time lapse before drug works:
2 to 10 days for skin infections. 2 to 4 weeks for infections of fingernails or toenails. Complete cure of either may require several months.

Don't take with:
Any other medicine or any dietary supplement without consulting your doctor or pharmacist.

OVERDOSE

SYMPTOMS:
Nausea, vomiting, diarrhea. In sensitive individuals, severe diarrhea may occur without overdosing.
WHAT TO DO:
Overdose unlikely to threaten life. If person uses much larger amount than prescribed or if accidentally swallowed, call doctor or poison control center 1-800-222-1222 for help.

POSSIBLE ADVERSE REACTIONS OR SIDE EFFECTS

SYMPTOMS	WHAT TO DO
Life-threatening:	
Allergic reaction (hives, facial swelling, sweating, wheezing, loss of blood pressure, and consciousness).	Seek emergency treatment immediately.
Common:	
Headache.	Continue. Tell doctor at next visit.
Infrequent:	
• Confusion; rash, hives, itch; mouth or tongue irritation; soreness; nausea; vomiting; diarrhea; stomach pain.	Discontinue. Call doctor right away.
• Insomnia, tiredness.	Continue. Call doctor when convenient.
Rare:	
Sore throat, fever, numbness or tingling in hands or feet, cloudy urine, yellow skin or eyes, sensitivity of skin to sunlight (these symptoms are more likely to occur with high doses taken for long periods).	Discontinue. Call doctor right away.

WARNINGS & PRECAUTIONS

Don't take if:
- You are allergic to any antifungal medicine.
- You are allergic to penicillin.
- You have liver disease.
- You have porphyria.
- The infection is minor and will respond to less potent drugs.

Before you start, consult your doctor if:
- You plan to become pregnant within medication period.
- You have lupus.

Over age 60:
Adverse reactions and side effects may be more frequent and severe than in younger persons.

Pregnancy:
Risk to unborn child outweighs drug benefits. Don't use. Risk category X (see page xviii).

Breast-feeding:
No problems expected, but consult your doctor.

Infants & children:
Not recommended for children younger than 2.

Prolonged use:
- You may become susceptible to infections caused by germs not responsive to griseofulvin.
- Talk to your doctor about the need for follow-up medical examinations or laboratory studies to check complete blood counts (white blood cell count, platelet count, red blood cell count, hemoglobin, hematocrit), liver function, kidney function.

Skin & sunlight:
May cause rash or intensify sunburn in areas exposed to sun or ultraviolet light (photosensitivity reaction). Avoid overexposure. Notify doctor if reaction occurs.

Driving, piloting or hazardous work:
Don't drive or pilot aircraft until you learn how medicine affects you. Don't work around dangerous machinery. Don't climb ladders or work in high places. Danger increases if you drink alcohol or take medicine affecting alertness and reflexes.

Discontinuing:
Don't discontinue without doctor's advice until you complete prescribed dose, even though symptoms diminish or disappear.

Others:
- Periodic laboratory blood studies and liver and kidney function tests recommended.
- Advise any doctor or dentist whom you consult that you take this medicine.

POSSIBLE INTERACTION WITH OTHER DRUGS

GENERIC NAME OR DRUG CLASS	COMBINED EFFECT
Anticoagulants, oral*	Decreased anticoagulant effect.
Barbiturates*	Decreased griseofulvin effect.
Contraceptives, oral*	Decreased contraceptive effect.
Photosensitizing medications*	Increased sun hazard.

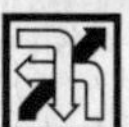

POSSIBLE INTERACTION WITH OTHER SUBSTANCES

INTERACTS WITH	COMBINED EFFECT
Alcohol:	Increased intoxication. Possible disulfiram reaction.*
Beverages:	None expected.
Cocaine:	None expected.
Foods:	None expected, but foods high in fat will improve drug absorption.
Marijuana:	None expected.
Tobacco:	None expected.

GUAIFENESIN

BRAND NAMES

See full list of brand names in the *Generic and Brand Name Directory*, page 884.

BASIC INFORMATION

Habit forming? No
Prescription needed? No
Available as generic? Yes
Drug class: Expectorant

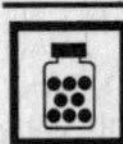

USES

Loosens mucus in respiratory passages from allergies and infections (hay fever, cough or cold). Guaifenesin may be a single ingredient or it can be combined with other drugs, such as in a cough and cold product.

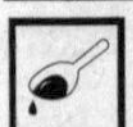

DOSAGE & USAGE INFORMATION

How to take:

- Tablet or capsule—Swallow with liquid. If you can't swallow whole, crumble tablet or open capsule and take with liquid or food.
- Extended-release tablet or extended-release capsule—Swallow whole with liquid.
- Syrup, oral solution or lozenge—Take as directed on label. Follow with 8 oz. water.
- Soft chew—Take as directed on label.

When to take:
As needed, no more often than every 4 hours for regular forms. The extended-release forms are usually taken every 12 hours.

If you forget a dose:
Take as soon as you remember. If it is almost time for the next dose, wait for that dose (don't double this dose) and resume regular schedule.

Continued next column

OVERDOSE

SYMPTOMS:
Drowsiness, mild weakness, nausea, vomiting.
WHAT TO DO:
Overdose unlikely to threaten life. If person uses much larger amount than prescribed or if accidentally swallowed, call doctor or poison control center 1-800-222-1222 for help.

What drug does:
Increases production of watery fluids to thin mucus so it can be coughed out or absorbed.

Time lapse before drug works:
15 to 30 minutes. Regular use for 5 to 7 days may be necessary for maximum benefit.

Don't take with:
Any other medicine or any dietary supplement without consulting your doctor or pharmacist.

POSSIBLE ADVERSE REACTIONS OR SIDE EFFECTS

SYMPTOMS	WHAT TO DO
Life-threatening: None expected.	
Common: None expected.	
Infrequent: Drowsiness, rash, stomach pain, diarrhea, nausea, vomiting, dizziness, headache, hives.	Discontinue. Call doctor if symptoms persist.
Rare: None expected.	

WARNINGS & PRECAUTIONS

Don't take if:
You are allergic to any cough or cold preparation containing guaifenesin.

Before you start, consult your doctor if:
You are allergic to any medicine, food or other substance.

Over age 60:
Adverse reactions and side effects may be more frequent and severe than in younger persons. For drug to work, you should drink 8 to 10 glasses of fluid per day.

Pregnancy:
Decide with your doctor if drug benefits justify risks to unborn child. Risk category C (see page xviii).

Breast-feeding:
No proven problems. Consult your doctor.

Infants & children:
Read the label on the product to see if it is approved for your child's age. Always follow the directions on product's label about how to use. If unsure, ask your doctor or pharmacist.

Prolonged use:
No problems expected.

Skin & sunlight:
No problems expected.

Driving, piloting or hazardous work:
Avoid if you feel drowsy. Otherwise, no problems expected.

Discontinuing:
May be unnecessary to finish medicine. Discontinue when symptoms disappear. If symptoms persist more than 1 week, consult doctor.

Others:
- Some guaifenesin syrup products contain alcohol. Read labels for alcohol content if you want to avoid these products.
- Advise any doctor or dentist whom you consult that you take this medicine.

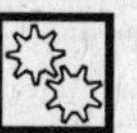

POSSIBLE INTERACTION WITH OTHER DRUGS

GENERIC NAME OR DRUG CLASS	COMBINED EFFECT
Anticoagulants*	Possible risk of bleeding.

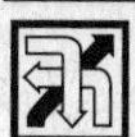

POSSIBLE INTERACTION WITH OTHER SUBSTANCES

INTERACTS WITH	COMBINED EFFECT
Alcohol:	None expected.
Beverages:	You should drink 8 to 10 glasses of fluid per day for drug to work.
Cocaine:	None expected.
Foods:	None expected.
Marijuana:	None expected.
Tobacco:	None expected.

***See Glossary**

GUANADREL

BRAND NAMES

Hylorel

BASIC INFORMATION

Habit forming? No
Prescription needed? Yes
Available as generic? No
Drug class: Antihypertensive

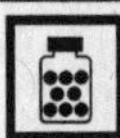

USES

Controls, but doesn't cure, high blood pressure.

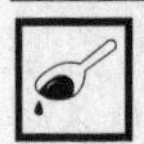

DOSAGE & USAGE INFORMATION

How to take:
Tablet—Swallow with liquid or food to lessen stomach irritation. If you can't swallow whole, crumble tablet and take with liquid or food.

When to take:
At the same time each day.

If you forget a dose:
Take as soon as you remember. If it is almost time for the next dose, wait for that dose (don't double this dose) and resume regular schedule.

What drug does:
Relaxes muscle cells of small arteries.

Time lapse before drug works:
4 to 6 hours. May need to take for lifetime.

Don't take with:
Any other medicine or any dietary supplement without consulting your doctor or pharmacist.

OVERDOSE

SYMPTOMS:
Severe blood pressure drop; fainting; blurred vision; slow, weak pulse; cold, sweaty skin; loss of consciousness.
WHAT TO DO:
- **Dial 911 (emergency) for medical help or call poison control center 1-800-222-1222 for instructions.**
- **See emergency information on last 3 pages of this book.**

POSSIBLE ADVERSE REACTIONS OR SIDE EFFECTS

SYMPTOMS	WHAT TO DO
Life-threatening: In case of overdose, see previous column.	
Common:	
• Diarrhea, more bowel movements, fatigue, weakness.	Continue. Call doctor when convenient.
• Dizziness, lower sex drive, feet and ankle swelling, drowsiness.	Continue. Tell doctor at next visit.
• Stuffy nose, dry mouth.	No action necessary.
Infrequent:	
• Rash, blurred vision, drooping eyelids, chest pain or shortness of breath, muscle pain or tremor.	Discontinue. Call doctor right away.
• Nausea or vomiting, headache.	Continue. Call doctor when convenient.
• Impotence, nighttime urination.	Continue. Tell doctor at next visit.
Rare:	
Decreased white blood cells causing sore throat, fever.	Discontinue. Call doctor right away.

WARNINGS & PRECAUTIONS

Don't take if:
- You are allergic to guanadrel.
- You have taken MAO inhibitors* within 2 weeks.

Before you start, consult your doctor if:
- You have had a stroke or have heart disease.
- You have asthma.
- You have had kidney disease.
- You have peptic ulcer or chronic acid indigestion.
- You will have surgery within 2 months, including dental surgery, requiring general or spinal anesthesia.

Over age 60:
Adverse reactions and side effects may be more frequent and severe than in younger persons. Start with small doses and monitor blood pressure frequently.

Pregnancy:
No proven harm to unborn child. Avoid if possible. Consult doctor. Risk category B (see page xviii).

Breast-feeding:
No proven harm to nursing infant. Avoid if possible. Consult doctor.

Infants & children:
Not recommended.

Prolonged use:
- Due to drug's cumulative effect, dose will require adjustment to prevent wide fluctuations in blood pressure.
- Talk to your doctor about the need for follow-up medical examinations or laboratory studies.

Skin & sunlight:
No problems expected.

Driving, piloting or hazardous work:
Don't drive or pilot aircraft until you learn how medicine affects you. Don't work around dangerous machinery. Don't climb ladders or work in high places. Danger increases if you drink alcohol or take medicine affecting alertness and reflexes, such as antihistamines, tranquilizers, sedatives, pain medicine, narcotics and mind-altering drugs.

Discontinuing:
Don't discontinue without consulting doctor. Dose may require gradual reduction if you have taken drug for a long time. Doses of other drugs may also require adjustment.

Others:
- Hot weather further lowers blood pressure, particularly in patients over 60.
- Advise any doctor or dentist whom you consult that you take this medicine.

POSSIBLE INTERACTION WITH OTHER DRUGS

GENERIC NAME OR DRUG CLASS	COMBINED EFFECT
Angiotensin-converting enzyme (ACE) inhibitors*	Possible excessive potassium in blood.
Antidepressants, tricyclic*	Decreased effect of guanadrel.
Antihypertensives, other*	Increased effect of guanadrel.
Beta-adrenergic blocking agents*	Increased likelihood of dizziness and fainting.
Carteolol	Increased anti-hypertensive effect.
Contraceptives, oral*	Increased side effects of oral contraceptives.
Central nervous system (CNS) depressants* (anticonvulsants,* antihistamines,* muscle relaxants,* narcotics,* sedatives,* tranquilizers*)	Decreased effect of guanadrel.
Diuretics*	Increased likelihood of dizziness and fainting.
Haloperidol	Decreased effect of guanadrel.
Insulin	Increased insulin effect.
Loxapine	Decreased effect of guanadrel.
Monoamine oxidase (MAO) inhibitors*	Severe high blood pressure. Avoid.
Nicardipine	Blood pressure drop. Dosages may require adjustment.
Nimodipine	Dangerous blood pressure drop.
Phenothiazines*	Decreased effect of guanadrel.
Rauwolfia alkaloids*	Increased likelihood of dizziness and fainting.
Sotalol	Increased anti-hypertensive effect.
Sympathomimetics*	Decreased effect of guanadrel.
Terazosin	Decreases effectiveness of terazosin.
Thioxanthenes*	Decreased effect of guanadrel.
Trimeprazine	Decreased effect of guanadrel.

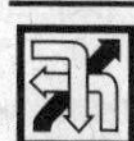

POSSIBLE INTERACTION WITH OTHER SUBSTANCES

INTERACTS WITH	COMBINED EFFECT
Alcohol:	Decreased effect of guanadrel. Avoid.
Beverages: Caffeine.	Decreased effect of guanadrel.
Cocaine:	Increased risk of heart block and high blood pressure.
Foods:	None expected.
Marijuana:	Higher blood pressure. Avoid.
Tobacco:	Higher blood pressure. Avoid.

*See Glossary

HALOPERIDOL

BRAND NAMES

Apo-Haloperidol
Haldol
Haldol Decanoate
Haldol LA
Halperon
Novo-Peridol
Peridol
PMS Haloperidol

BASIC INFORMATION

Habit forming? No
Prescription needed? Yes
Available as generic? Yes
Drug class: Antipsychotic

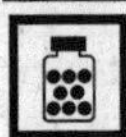

USES

- Reduces severe anxiety, agitation and psychotic behavior.
- Treatment for Tourette's syndrome.
- Treatment for infantile autism.
- Treatment for Huntington's chorea.

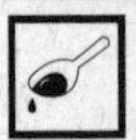

DOSAGE & USAGE INFORMATION

How to take:
- Tablet—Swallow with liquid. If you can't swallow whole, crumble tablet and take with liquid or food.
- Drops—Dilute dose in beverage before swallowing.

When to take:
At the same times each day.

If you forget a dose:
Take as soon as you remember. If it is almost time for the next dose, wait for that dose (don't double this dose) and resume regular schedule.

Continued next column

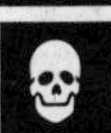

OVERDOSE

SYMPTOMS:
Weak, rapid pulse; shallow, slow breathing; tremor or muscle weakness; very low blood pressure; convulsions; deep sleep ending in coma.

WHAT TO DO:
- **Dial 911 (emergency) for medical help or call poison control center 1-800-222-1222 for instructions.**
- **If person is unconscious, check breathing and pulse. If not breathing, begin mouth-to-mouth rescue breathing. If heart is not beating, begin chest compressions.**
- **See emergency information on last 3 pages of this book.**

What drug does:
Corrects an imbalance in nerve impulses from brain; blocks effect of dopamine.*

Time lapse before drug works:
Up to 4 weeks.

Don't take with:
Any other medicine or any dietary supplement without consulting your doctor or pharmacist.

POSSIBLE ADVERSE REACTIONS OR SIDE EFFECTS

SYMPTOMS	WHAT TO DO
Life-threatening:	
High fever, rapid pulse, profuse sweating, muscle rigidity, confusion and irritability, seizures.	Discontinue. Seek emergency treatment.
Common:	
• Jerky or involuntary movements, especially of the face, lips, jaw, tongue; slow-frequency tremor of head or limbs, especially while moving; lack of facial expression and slow inflexible movements.	Discontinue. Call doctor right away.
• Pacing or restlessness; intermittent spasms of muscles of face, eyes, tongue, jaw, neck, body or limbs.	Continue. Call doctor when convenient.
Infrequent:	
Dry mouth, blurred vision, constipation, difficulty urinating, sedation, low blood pressure, dizziness.	Continue. Call doctor when convenient.
Rare:	
Other symptoms not listed above.	Continue. Call doctor when convenient.

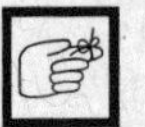

WARNINGS & PRECAUTIONS

Don't take if:
- You have ever been allergic to haloperidol.
- You are depressed.
- You have Parkinson's disease.
- Patient is younger than 3 years old.

Before you start, consult your doctor if:
- You have a history of mental depression.
- You have had kidney or liver problems.
- You have diabetes, epilepsy, glaucoma, prostate trouble or asthma.
- You have high blood pressure, heart disease or cardiac abnormalities.
- You have QT-prolonging conditions, including electrolyte imbalance (particularly hypokalemia and hypomagnesemia) or familial long QT syndrome.
- You have hyper- or hypothyroidism.
- You drink alcoholic beverages frequently.

Over age 60:
- Adverse reactions and side effects may be more frequent and severe than in younger persons.
- Use of antipsychotic drugs in elderly patients with dementia-related psychosis may increase risk of death. Consult doctor.

Pregnancy:
Decide with your doctor if drug benefits justify risk to unborn child. Risk category C (see page xviii).

Breast-feeding:
Drug passes into milk. Avoid drug or discontinue nursing until you finish medicine. Consult doctor about maintaining milk supply.

Infants & children:
Safety and efficacy have not been established.

Prolonged use:
- May develop tardive dyskinesia (involuntary movements of jaws, lips and tongue).
- Talk to your doctor about the need for follow-up medical examinations or laboratory studies to check blood pressure, liver function.

Skin & sunlight:
- May cause rash or intensify sunburn in areas exposed to sun or ultraviolet light (photosensitivity). Avoid overexposure and use sunscreen. Consult doctor if reaction occurs.
- Avoid getting overheated. The drug affects body temperature and sweating.

Driving, piloting or hazardous work:
Don't drive or pilot aircraft until you learn how medicine affects you. Don't work around dangerous machinery. Don't climb ladders or work in high places. Danger increases if you drink alcohol or take medicine affecting alertness and reflexes.

Discontinuing:
Don't discontinue without consulting doctor. Dose may require gradual reduction if you have taken drug for a long time. Doses of other drugs may also require adjustment.

Others:
- For dry mouth, suck on sugarless hard candy or chew sugarless gum. If dry mouth persists, consult your dentist.
- Higher doses of this drug may increase risk of serious heart rhythm problems (including cases of sudden death). Call doctor right away if heart symptoms occur.
- Advise any doctor or dentist whom you consult that you take this medicine.

POSSIBLE INTERACTION WITH OTHER DRUGS

GENERIC NAME OR DRUG CLASS	COMBINED EFFECT
Anticholinergics*	Increased anti-cholinergic effect. May cause elevated pressure within the eye.
Anticonvulsants*	Changed seizure pattern.
Antidepressants*	Excessive sedation.
Antihistamines*	Excessive sedation.
Antihypertensives*	May cause severe blood pressure drop.
Barbiturates*	Excessive sedation.
Bupropion	Increased risk of seizures.
Central nervous system (CNS) depressants*	Increased CNS depression; increased blood pressure drop.
Clozapine	Toxic effect on the nervous system.

Continued on page 915

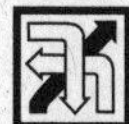

POSSIBLE INTERACTION WITH OTHER SUBSTANCES

INTERACTS WITH	COMBINED EFFECT
Alcohol:	Excessive sedation and depressed brain function. Avoid.
Beverages:	None expected.
Cocaine:	Decreased effect of haloperidol. Avoid.
Foods:	None expected.
Marijuana:	Occasional use—Increased sedation. Frequent use—Possible toxic psychosis.
Tobacco:	None expected.

***See Glossary**

HISTAMINE H_2 RECEPTOR ANTAGONISTS

GENERIC AND BRAND NAMES

CIMETIDINE
Apo-Cimetidine
Liquid Tagamet
Novocimetine
Peptol
Tagamet
Tagamet HB

FAMOTIDINE
Duexis
Fluxid
Mylanta-AR
Pepcid
Pepcid AC
Pepcid Complete
Pepcid RPD
Tums Dual Action
Ulcidine

NIZATIDINE
Axid

RANITIDINE
Apo-Ranitidine
Zantac
Zantac 75
Zantac-C
Zantac Efferdose
Zantac Geldose

BASIC INFORMATION

Habit forming? No
Prescription needed? Yes, for some
Available as generic? Yes, for some
Drug class: Histamine H_2 antagonist

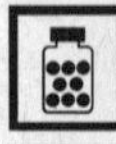

USES

- Treatment for duodenal, gastric and peptic ulcers and other conditions in which stomach produces excess acid.
- Treatment for and prevention of heartburn.
- Maintenance of healing of erosive esophagitis.

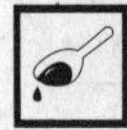

DOSAGE & USAGE INFORMATION

How to take:
- Tablet, capsule or liquid—Swallow with liquid.
- Chewable tablet—Chew thoroughly and swallow with water.
- Disintegrating tablet—Let dissolve on tongue.
- Oral suspension or effervescent tablets for oral solution—Follow instructions on prescription.

Continued next column

When to take:
- 1 dose per day—Take at bedtime.
- 2 or more doses per day—Take at the same times each day.

If you forget a dose:
Take as soon as you remember. If it is almost time for the next dose, wait for that dose (don't double this dose) and resume regular schedule.

What drug does:
Blocks histamine release so stomach secretes less acid.

Time lapse before drug works:
- Begins in 30 minutes. May require several days to relieve pain.
- Lower dosages in nonprescription medicines may take 45 minutes to relieve heartburn.

Don't take with:
Any other medicine or any dietary supplement without consulting your doctor or pharmacist.

OVERDOSE

SYMPTOMS:
Confusion, slurred speech, breathing difficulty, rapid heartbeat, delirium.
WHAT TO DO:
Overdose unlikely to threaten life. If person uses much larger amount than prescribed or if accidentally swallowed, call doctor or poison control center 1-800-222-1222 for help.

POSSIBLE ADVERSE REACTIONS OR SIDE EFFECTS

SYMPTOMS	WHAT TO DO
Life-threatening: None expected.	
Common: None expected.	
Infrequent:	
• Dizziness or headache, diarrhea.	Continue. Call doctor when convenient.
• Diminished sex drive, unusual milk flow in females, hair loss.	Continue. Tell doctor at next visit.
Rare:	
• Confusion; rash, hives; sore throat, fever; slow, fast or irregular heartbeat; unusual bleeding or bruising; muscle cramps or pain; fatigue; weakness.	Discontinue. Call doctor right away.
• Constipation.	Continue. Call doctor when convenient.

WARNINGS & PRECAUTIONS

Don't take if:
You are allergic to any histamine H_2 antagonist.

Before you start, consult your doctor if:
- You plan to become pregnant while on medication.
- You take aspirin. Aspirin may irritate stomach.

Over age 60:
Adverse reactions and side effects may be more frequent and severe than in younger persons.

HISTAMINE H_2 RECEPTOR ANTAGONISTS

Pregnancy:
Risk factors vary for drugs in this group. See category list on page xviii and consult doctor.

Breast-feeding:
Drug passes into milk. Avoid drug or discontinue nursing until you finish medicine. Consult doctor about maintaining milk supply.

Infants & children:
Not recommended.

Prolonged use:
- Possible liver damage.
- Talk to your doctor about the need for follow-up medical examinations or laboratory studies.

Skin & sunlight:
No problems expected.

Driving, piloting or hazardous work:
Don't drive or pilot aircraft until you learn how medicine affects you. Don't work around dangerous machinery. Don't climb ladders or work in high places. Danger increases if you drink alcohol or take medicine affecting alertness and reflexes, such as antihistamines, tranquilizers, sedatives, pain medicine, narcotics and mind-altering drugs.

Discontinuing:
Don't discontinue without consulting a doctor. Dose may require gradual reduction if you have taken drug for a long time. Doses of other drugs may also require adjustment.

Others:
- Patients on kidney dialysis—Take at end of dialysis treatment.
- May interfere with the accuracy of some medical tests.
- Advise any doctor or dentist whom you consult that you take this medicine.

POSSIBLE INTERACTION WITH OTHER DRUGS

GENERIC NAME OR DRUG CLASS	COMBINED EFFECT
Alprazolam	Increased effect and toxicity of alprazolam.
Antacids*	Decreased absorption of histamine H_2 receptor antagonist.
Anticoagulants, oral*	Increased anticoagulant effect.
Anticholinergics*	Increased histamine H_2 receptor antagonist effect.
Antivirals, HIV/AIDS*	Increased antiviral effect with cimetidine.
Azelastine	Increased azelastine effect.
Bupropion	Increased bupropion effect.
Carbamazepine	Increased effect and toxicity of carbamazepine.
Carmustine (BCNU)	Severe impairment of red blood cell production; some interference with white blood cell formation.
Chlordiazepoxide	Increased effect and toxicity of chlordiazepoxide.
Cisapride	Decreased histamine H_2 receptor effect.
Citalopram	Increased effect of citalopram.

Continued on page 916

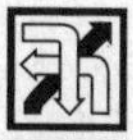

POSSIBLE INTERACTION WITH OTHER SUBSTANCES

INTERACTS WITH	COMBINED EFFECT
Alcohol:	No interactions expected, but alcohol may slow body's recovery. Avoid.
Beverages:	
Milk.	Enhanced effectiveness. Small amounts useful for taking medication.
Caffeine drinks.	May increase acid secretion and delay healing.
Cocaine:	Decreased effect of histamine H_2 receptor antagonist.
Foods:	Enhanced effectiveness. Protein-rich foods should be eaten in moderation to minimize secretion of stomach acid.
Marijuana:	Increased chance of low sperm count. Marijuana may slow body's recovery. Avoid.
Tobacco:	Reversed effect of histamine H_2 receptor antagonist. Tobacco may slow body's recovery. Avoid.

***See Glossary**

HMG-CoA REDUCTASE INHIBITORS

GENERIC AND BRAND NAMES

ATORVASTATIN
- Caduet
- Lipitor

FLUVASTATIN
- Lescol
- Lescol XL

LOVASTATIN
- Advicor
- Altocor
- Mevacor
- Mevinolin

PITAVASTATIN
- Livalo

PRAVASTATIN
- Eptastatin
- Pravachol
- Pravigard PAC

ROSUVASTATIN
- Crestor

SIMVASTATIN
- Epistatin
- Juvisync
- Simcor
- Synvinolin
- Vytorin
- Zocor

BASIC INFORMATION

Habit forming? No
Prescription needed? Yes
Available as generic? Yes, for some
Drug class: Antihyperlipidemic

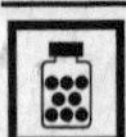

USES

- Lowers blood cholesterol levels caused by low-density lipoproteins (LDL) in persons who haven't improved by exercising, dieting or using other measures. It raises high density lipoproteins (HDL).
- Used along with a low-fat diet to slow the progression of atherosclerosis in patients with coronary heart disease and high cholesterol.
- Reduces risk of heart attacks and strokes in certain patients.
- Lowers triglyceride levels.

DOSAGE & USAGE INFORMATION

How to take:
- Tablet or capsule—Swallow with liquid. If you can't swallow whole, crumble tablet and take with liquid or food.
- Extended release tablet—Swallow with liquid. Do not crumble or chew tablet.

Continued next column

When to take:
According to directions on prescription.

If you forget a dose:
Take as soon as you remember. If it is almost time for the next dose, wait for that dose (don't double this dose) and resume regular schedule.

What drug does:
Inhibits an enzyme in the liver.

Time lapse before drug works:
2 to 4 weeks.

Don't take with:
- A high-fat diet.
- Any other medicine or any dietary supplement without consulting your doctor or pharmacist.

OVERDOSE

SYMPTOMS:
None expected.
WHAT TO DO:
Overdose unlikely to threaten life. If person uses much larger amount than prescribed or if accidentally swallowed, call doctor or poison control center 1-800-222-1222 for help.

POSSIBLE ADVERSE REACTIONS OR SIDE EFFECTS

SYMPTOMS	WHAT TO DO
Life-threatening: None expected.	
Common: None expected.	
Infrequent:	
• Aching muscles, fever, blurred vision.	Discontinue. Call doctor right away.
• Constipation, nausea, dizziness, skin rash, headache, diarrhea, heartburn.	Continue. Call doctor when convenient.
Rare:	
• Muscle or stomach pain, unusual tiredness or weakness.	Discontinue. Call doctor right away.
• Impotence, insomnia, memory loss, forgetfulness, confusion.	Continue. Call doctor when convenient.

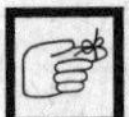

WARNINGS & PRECAUTIONS

Don't take if:
You are allergic to HMG-CoA reductase inhibitor.

Before you start, consult your doctor if:
- You take immunosuppressive drugs, particularly following an organ transplant.
- You have low blood pressure.
- You have hormone abnormalities.
- You have an active infection, active liver disease, or a seizure disorder.
- You have a history of alcohol abuse.
- You have had recent surgery.

Over age 60:
May be more sensitive to drug's side effects.

Pregnancy:
Consult doctor. Risk category X (see page xviii).

Breast-feeding:
Discontinue nursing until you finish medicine. Consult doctor for advice about milk supply.

Infants & children:
Use only as directed by doctor.

Prolonged use:
Talk to your doctor about the need for follow-up medical examinations or laboratory studies.

Skin & sunlight:
No problems expected.

Driving, piloting or hazardous work:
No special problems expected.

Discontinuing:
Don't discontinue without consulting doctor. Dose may require gradual reduction if you have taken drug for a long time. Doses of other drugs may also require adjustment.

Others:
- Advise any doctor or dentist whom you consult that you take this medicine.
- Drugs to lower cholesterol may cause muscle problems or rhabdomyolysis (muscle injury). If you have persistent muscle aches, weakness, pain, or dark urine, call doctor right away.
- Taking these drugs may slightly increase the risk of raised blood sugar and diabetes type 2.
- Use an effective form of birth control while taking this drug. Notify your doctor right away if you do become pregnant.

POSSIBLE INTERACTION WITH OTHER DRUGS

GENERIC NAME OR DRUG CLASS	COMBINED EFFECT
Amiodarone	Risk of muscle injury and kidney failure.
Anticoagulants*	May increase bleeding risk.
Antifungals, azole*	Increased effect of HMG-CoA reductase inhibitor.
Cholestyramine	Decreased HMG-CoA reductase inhibitor effect if taken at same time.
Colestipol	Decreased effect of HMG-CoA reductase inhibitor if taken at same time.
Cyclosporine	Increased risk of muscle and kidney problems.
Digoxin	Increased digoxin effect.
Enzyme inhibitors*	Increased effect of HMG-CoA reductase inhibitor.
Erythromycins*	Risk of muscle injury and kidney failure.
Fibrates	Risk of muscle injury and kidney failure.
Gemfibrozil	Risk of muscle injury and kidney failure.
Macrolides*	Risk of muscle injury and kidney failure.
Immunosuppressants*	Risk of muscle injury and kidney failure.
Niacin	Risk of muscle injury and kidney failure.
Contraceptives, oral*	May increase levels of oral contraceptive with atorvastatin.
Orlistat	Increased effect of HMG-CoA reductase inhibitor.
Protease inhibitors	Risk of muscle injury and kidney failure. Consult doctor.
Ranolazine	Increased effect of simvastatin.
Telithromycin	Increased effect of HMG-CoA reductase inhibitor.

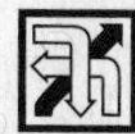

POSSIBLE INTERACTION WITH OTHER SUBSTANCES

INTERACTS WITH	COMBINED EFFECT
Alcohol:	Avoid alcohol while taking this drug.
Beverages: Grapefruit juice.	May increase effect of HMG-CoA reductase inhibitor.
Cocaine:	None expected.
Foods: Grapefruit.	May increase effect of HMG-CoA reductase inhibitor.
Marijuana:	None expected.
Tobacco:	None expected.

*See Glossary

HYDRALAZINE

BRAND NAMES

Apresoline
BiDil
Novo-Hylazin

BASIC INFORMATION

Habit forming? No
Prescription needed? Yes
Available as generic? Yes
Drug class: Antihypertensive

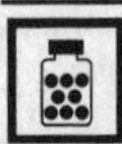

USES

- Treatment for high blood pressure and congestive heart failure.
- The brand name BiDil is approved to treat heart failure specifically in African Americans.

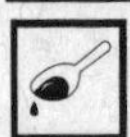

DOSAGE & USAGE INFORMATION

How to take:
Tablet—Swallow with liquid. If you can't swallow whole, crumble tablet and take with liquid or food.

When to take:
At the same time each day. Should be taken with food.

If you forget a dose:
Take as soon as you remember. If it is almost time for the next dose, wait for that dose (don't double this dose) and resume regular schedule.

What drug does:
Relaxes and expands blood vessel walls, lowering blood pressure.

Time lapse before drug works:
Regular use for several weeks may be necessary to determine drug's effectiveness.

Continued next column

OVERDOSE

SYMPTOMS:
Rapid and weak heartbeat, fainting, extreme weakness, cold and sweaty skin, flushing.
WHAT TO DO:
- **Dial 911 (emergency) for medical help or call poison control center 1-800-222-1222 for instructions.**
- **If person is unconscious, check breathing and pulse. If not breathing, begin mouth-to-mouth rescue breathing. If heart is not beating, begin chest compressions.**
- **See emergency information on last 3 pages of this book.**

Don't take with:
- Nonprescription drugs containing alcohol without consulting doctor.
- Any other medicine or any dietary supplement without consulting your doctor or pharmacist.

POSSIBLE ADVERSE REACTIONS OR SIDE EFFECTS

SYMPTOMS	WHAT TO DO
Life-threatening: In case of overdose, see previous column.	
Common:	
• Nausea or vomiting, rapid or irregular heartbeat.	Discontinue. Call doctor right away.
• Headache, diarrhea, appetite loss, painful or difficult urination.	Continue. Tell doctor at next visit.
Infrequent:	
• Hives or rash, flushed face, sore throat, fever, chest pain, swelling of lymph glands, skin blisters, swelling in feet or legs.	Discontinue. Call doctor right away.
• Confusion, dizziness, anxiety, depression, joint pain, general discomfort or weakness, muscle pain.	Continue. Call doctor when convenient.
• Watery and irritated eyes, constipation.	Continue. Tell doctor at next visit.
Rare:	
• Weakness and faintness when arising from bed or chair, jaundice.	Discontinue. Call doctor right away.
• Numbness or tingling in hands or feet, nasal congestion, impotence.	Continue. Call doctor when convenient.

WARNINGS & PRECAUTIONS

Don't take if:
- You are allergic to hydralazine or tartrazine dye.
- You have a history of coronary artery disease or rheumatic heart disease.

Before you start, consult your doctor if:

- You feel pain in chest, neck or arms on physical exertion.
- You have had lupus.
- You have had a stroke.
- You have had kidney disease or impaired kidney function.
- You will have surgery within 2 months, including dental surgery, requiring general or spinal anesthesia.

Over age 60:
Adverse reactions and side effects may be more frequent and severe than in younger persons.

Pregnancy:
Decide with your doctor if drug benefits justify risk to unborn child. Risk category C (see page xviii).

Breast-feeding:
Drug passes into milk. Avoid drug or discontinue nursing until you finish medicine. Consult doctor about maintaining milk supply.

Infants & children:
Not recommended.

Prolonged use:

- May cause lupus (arthritis-like illness).
- Possible psychosis.
- May cause numbness, tingling in hands or feet.
- Talk to your doctor about the need for follow-up medical examinations or laboratory studies to check blood pressure, complete blood counts (white blood cell count, platelet count, red blood cell count, hemoglobin, hematocrit), ANA titers.*

Skin & sunlight:
No problems expected.

Driving, piloting or hazardous work:
Don't drive or pilot aircraft until you learn how medicine affects you. Don't work around dangerous machinery. Don't climb ladders or work in high places. Danger increases if you drink alcohol or take medicine affecting alertness and reflexes, such as antihistamines, tranquilizers, sedatives, pain medicine, narcotics and mind-altering drugs.

Discontinuing:
Don't discontinue without doctor's advice until you complete prescribed dose, even though symptoms diminish or disappear.

Others:

- Vitamin B-6 diet supplement may be advisable. Consult doctor.
- Some products contain tartrazine dye. Avoid, especially if you are allergic to aspirin.
- May interfere with the accuracy of some medical tests.
- Advise any doctor or dentist whom you consult that you take this medicine.

POSSIBLE INTERACTION WITH OTHER DRUGS

GENERIC NAME OR DRUG CLASS	COMBINED EFFECT
Amphetamines*	Decreased hydralazine effect.
Antihypertensives, other*	Increased anti-hypertensive effect.
Anti-inflammatory drugs, nonsteroidal (NSAIDs)*	Decreased effect of hydralazine.
Antivirals, HIV/AIDS*	Increased risk of peripheral neuropathy.
Carteolol	Increased anti-hypertensive effect.
Diazoxide & other anti-hypertensive drugs	Increased anti-hypertensive effect.
Diuretics, oral*	Increased effects of both drugs. When monitored carefully, combination may be beneficial in controlling hypertension.
Guanfacine	Increased effects of both drugs.

Continued on page 917

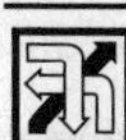

POSSIBLE INTERACTION WITH OTHER SUBSTANCES

INTERACTS WITH	COMBINED EFFECT
Alcohol:	May lower blood pressure excessively. Use extreme caution.
Beverages:	None expected.
Cocaine:	Increased risk of heart block and high blood pressure.
Foods:	Increased hydralazine absorption.
Marijuana:	Weakness on standing.
Tobacco:	Possible angina attacks.

***See Glossary**

HYDRALAZINE & HYDROCHLOROTHIAZIDE

BRAND NAMES

Apresazide
Apresoline-Esidrix
Aprozide
Hydra-Zide

BASIC INFORMATION

Habit forming? No
Prescription needed? Yes
Available as generic? Yes
Drug class: Antihypertensive, diuretic

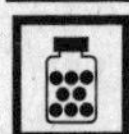

USES

- Controls, but doesn't cure, high blood pressure.
- Reduces fluid retention (edema).

DOSAGE & USAGE INFORMATION

How to take:
Tablet or capsule—Swallow with liquid. If you can't swallow whole, crumble tablet or open capsule and take with liquid or food.

When to take:
At the same time each day.

If you forget a dose:
Take as soon as you remember. If it is almost time for the next dose, wait for that dose (don't double this dose) and resume regular schedule.

What drug does:
- Forces sodium and water excretion, reducing body fluid.
- Relaxes and expands blood vessel walls, lowering blood pressure.
- Reduced body fluid and relaxed arteries lower blood pressure.

Continued next column

OVERDOSE

SYMPTOMS:
Cramps, drowsiness, weak pulse, rapid and weak heartbeat, fainting, extreme weakness, cold and sweaty skin, coma.
WHAT TO DO:
- **Dial 911 (emergency) for medical help or call poison control center 1-800-222-1222 for instructions.**
- **If person is unconscious, check breathing and pulse. If not breathing, begin mouth-to-mouth rescue breathing. If heart is not beating, begin chest compressions.**
- **See emergency information on last 3 pages of this book.**

Time lapse before drug works:
Regular use for several weeks may be necessary to determine drug's effectiveness.

Don't take with:
- Nonprescription drugs containing alcohol without consulting doctor.
- Any other medicine or any dietary supplement without consulting your doctor or pharmacist.

POSSIBLE ADVERSE REACTIONS OR SIDE EFFECTS

SYMPTOMS	WHAT TO DO
Life-threatening:	
Chest pain, irregular and fast heartbeat, weak pulse.	Discontinue. Seek emergency treatment.
Common:	
• Nausea, vomiting.	Discontinue. Call doctor right away.
• Headache, diarrhea, appetite loss, frequent urination, dry mouth, thirst.	Continue. Call doctor when convenient.
Infrequent:	
• Rash; black, bloody or tarry stool; red or flushed face; sore throat, fever, mouth sores; constipation; lymph glands swelling; blurred vision; skin blisters; swelling in feet or legs.	Discontinue. Call doctor right away.
• Dizziness; confusion; watery eyes; weight gain or loss; joint, muscle or chest pain; depression; anxiety; fever.	Continue. Call doctor when convenient.
Rare:	
• Weakness and faintness when arising from bed or chair, jaundice.	Discontinue. Call doctor right away.
• Numbness or tingling in hands or feet, nasal congestion, impotence.	Continue. Call doctor when convenient.

WARNINGS & PRECAUTIONS

Don't take if:
- You are allergic to hydralazine, any thiazide diuretic drug or tartrazine dye.
- You have history of coronary artery disease or rheumatic heart disease.

HYDRALAZINE & HYDROCHLOROTHIAZIDE

Before you start, consult your doctor if:
- You feel pain in chest, neck or arms on physical exertion.
- You are allergic to any sulfa drug.
- You have had lupus or a stroke.
- You have gout, liver, pancreas or kidney disorder.
- You will have surgery within 2 months, including dental surgery, requiring general or spinal anesthesia.

Over age 60:
Adverse reactions and side effects may be more frequent and severe than in younger persons, especially dizziness and excessive potassium loss.

Pregnancy:
Decide with your doctor if drug benefits justify risk to unborn child. Risk category C (see page xviii).

Breast-feeding:
Drug passes into milk. Avoid drug or discontinue nursing until you finish medicine. Consult doctor for advice on maintaining milk supply.

Infants & children:
Not recommended.

Prolonged use:
- May cause lupus (arthritis-like illness).
- Possible psychosis.
- May cause numbness, tingling in hands or feet.
- Talk to your doctor about the need for follow-up medical examinations or laboratory studies to check blood pressure, complete blood counts (white blood cell count, platelet count, red blood cell count, hemoglobin, hematocrit), ANA titers.*

Skin & sunlight:
One or more drugs in this group may cause rash or intensify sunburn in areas exposed to sun or ultraviolet light (photosensitivity reaction). Avoid overexposure. Notify doctor if reaction occurs.

Driving, piloting or hazardous work:
Don't drive or pilot aircraft until you learn how medicine affects you. Don't work around dangerous machinery. Don't climb ladders or work in high places. Danger increases if you drink alcohol or take medicine affecting alertness and reflexes, such as antihistamines, tranquilizers, sedatives, pain medicine, narcotics and mind-altering drugs.

Discontinuing:
Don't discontinue without consulting doctor's advice until you complete prescribed dose, even though symptoms diminish or disappear.

Others:
- Vitamin B-6 diet supplement may be advisable. Consult doctor.
- Hot weather and fever may cause dehydration and drop in blood pressure. Dose may require temporary adjustment. Weigh daily and report any unexpected weight loss to your doctor.
- May cause rise in uric acid, leading to gout.
- May cause blood sugar rise in diabetics.
- Advise any doctor or dentist whom you consult that you take this medicine.

POSSIBLE INTERACTION WITH OTHER DRUGS

GENERIC NAME OR DRUG CLASS	COMBINED EFFECT
Acebutolol	Decreased anti-hypertensive effect of acebutolol.
Allopurinol	Decreased allopurinol effect.
Amphetamines*	Decreased hydralazine effect.
Antidepressants, tricyclic*	Dangerous drop in blood pressure. Avoid combination unless under medical supervision.
Antihypertensives,* other	Increased anti-hypertensive effect.

Continued on page 917

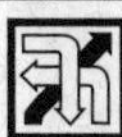

POSSIBLE INTERACTION WITH OTHER SUBSTANCES

INTERACTS WITH	COMBINED EFFECT
Alcohol:	May lower blood pressure excessively. Use extreme caution.
Beverages:	None expected.
Cocaine:	Dangerous blood pressure rise. Avoid.
Foods: Licorice.	Excessive potassium loss that causes dangerous heart rhythms.
Marijuana:	Weakness on standing. May increase blood pressure.
Tobacco:	Possible angina attacks.

*See Glossary

HYDROCORTISONE (Rectal)

BRAND NAMES

Anamantle HC Cream Kit
Anucort
Cort-Dome High Potency
Corticaine
Cortiment-10
Cortiment-40
Dermolate
Hemril-HC
Peranex HC Cream
ProCort
Proctocort
Rectocort
Xyralid RC

BASIC INFORMATION

Habit forming? No
Prescription needed? Yes
Available as generic? Yes, for some
Drug class: Anti-inflammatory, steroidal (rectal); anesthetic (rectal)

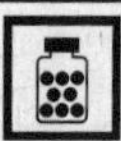

USES

In or around the rectum to relieve swelling, itching and pain from hemorrhoids (piles) and other rectal conditions. Frequently used after hemorrhoid surgery.

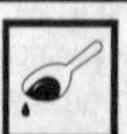

DOSAGE & USAGE INFORMATION

How to use:

- Rectal cream or ointment—Apply to surface of rectum with fingers. Insert applicator into rectum no farther than halfway and apply inside. Wash applicator with warm soapy water or discard. Review instructions if unsure.
- Suppository—Remove wrapper and moisten with water. Lie on side. Push blunt end of suppository into rectum with finger. If suppository is too soft, run cold water over it or put in refrigerator for 15 to 45 minutes before using. Review instructions if unsure.
- Aerosol foam—Read patient instructions. Don't insert into rectum. Use the special applicator and wash carefully after using.

When to use:
Follow instructions in package or when needed.

Continued next column

OVERDOSE

SYMPTOMS:
None expected.
WHAT TO DO:
Not intended for internal use. If child accidentally swallows, dial 911 (emergency) for medical help or call poison control center 1-800-222-1222 for instructions.

If you forget a dose:
Use as soon as you remember.

What drug does:

- Reduces inflammation.
- Relieves pain and itching.

Time lapse before drug works:
5 to 15 minutes.

Don't use with:
Other rectal medicines without consulting your doctor or pharmacist.

POSSIBLE ADVERSE REACTIONS OR SIDE EFFECTS

SYMPTOMS	WHAT TO DO
Life-threatening	
None expected.	
Common	
None expected.	
Infrequent	
• Nervousness, trembling, hives, rash, itch, inflammation or tenderness not present before application, slow heartbeat.	Discontinue. Call doctor right away.
• Dizziness, blurred vision, swollen feet.	Continue. Call doctor when convenient.
Rare	
• Blood in urine.	Discontinue. Call doctor right away.
• Increased or painful urination.	Continue. Call doctor when convenient.

WARNINGS & PRECAUTIONS

Don't use if:
You are allergic to any topical anesthetic.

Before you start, consult your doctor if:
- You have skin infection at site of treatment.
- You have had severe or extensive skin disorders such as eczema or psoriasis.
- You have bleeding hemorrhoids.

Over age 60:
Adverse reactions and side effects may be more frequent and severe than in younger persons.

Pregnancy:
Decide with your doctor if drug benefits justify risk to unborn child. Risk category C (see page xviii).

Breast-feeding:
No problems expected. Consult doctor.

Infants & children:
Don't use without careful medical supervision. Rarely, too much may be absorbed into the blood stream and affect growth.

Prolonged use:
Possible excess absorption. Don't use longer than 3 days for any one problem.

Skin & sunlight:
No problems expected.

Driving, piloting or hazardous work:
No problems expected.

Discontinuing:
May be unnecessary to finish medicine. Follow doctor's instructions.

Others:
- Report any rectal bleeding to your doctor.
- Keep cool, but don't freeze.

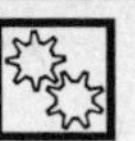

POSSIBLE INTERACTION WITH OTHER DRUGS

GENERIC NAME OR DRUG CLASS	COMBINED EFFECT
Sulfa drugs*	Decreased antiinfective effect of sulfa drugs.

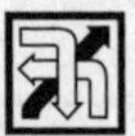

POSSIBLE INTERACTION WITH OTHER SUBSTANCES

INTERACTS WITH	COMBINED EFFECT
Alcohol:	None expected.
Beverages:	None expected.
Cocaine:	Possible nervous system toxicity. Avoid.
Foods:	None expected.
Marijuana:	None expected.
Tobacco:	None expected.

HYDROXYCHLOROQUINE

BRAND NAMES

Plaquenil

BASIC INFORMATION

Habit forming? No
Prescription needed? Yes
Available as generic? No
Drug class: Antiprotozoal, antirheumatic

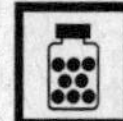

USES

- Treatment for protozoal infections, such as malaria and amebiasis.
- Treatment for some forms of arthritis and lupus.

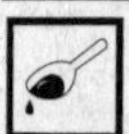

DOSAGE & USAGE INFORMATION

How to take:
Tablet—Swallow with food or milk to lessen stomach irritation.

When to take:
- Depends on condition. Is adjusted during treatment.
- Malaria prevention—Begin taking medicine 2 weeks before entering areas where malaria is present and until 8 weeks after return.

If you forget a dose:
- 1 or more doses a day—Take as soon as you remember. If it is almost time for the next dose, wait for that dose (don't double this dose) and resume regular schedule.
- 1 dose weekly—Take as soon as possible, then return to regular dosing schedule.

What drug does:
- Inhibits parasite multiplication.
- Decreases inflammatory response in diseased joint.

Time lapse before drug works:
1 to 2 hours.

Continued next column

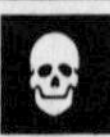

OVERDOSE

SYMPTOMS:
Severe breathing difficulty, drowsiness, faintness, headache, seizures.
WHAT TO DO:
- **Dial 911 (emergency) for medical help or call poison control center 1-800-222-1222 for instructions.**
- **See emergency information on last 3 pages of this book.**

Don't take with:
Any other medicine or any dietary supplement without consulting your doctor or pharmacist.

POSSIBLE ADVERSE REACTIONS OR SIDE EFFECTS

SYMPTOMS	WHAT TO DO
Life-threatening:	
In case of overdose, see previous column.	
Common:	
Headache, appetite loss, abdominal pain.	Continue. Tell doctor at next visit.
Infrequent:	
• Blurred vision, changes in vision.	Discontinue. Call doctor right away.
• Rash or itch, diarrhea, nausea, vomiting, hair loss, blue-black skin or mouth, dizziness, nervousness.	Continue. Call doctor when convenient.
Rare:	
• Mood or mental changes, seizures, sore throat, fever, unusual bleeding or bruising, muscle weakness, convulsions.	Discontinue. Call doctor right away.
• Ringing or buzzing in ears, hearing loss.	Continue. Call doctor when convenient.

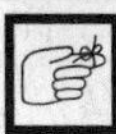

WARNINGS & PRECAUTIONS

Don't take if:
You are allergic to chloroquine or hydroxychloroquine.

Before you start, consult your doctor if:
- You plan to become pregnant within the medication period.
- You have blood disease.
- You have eye or vision problems.
- You have a G6PD* deficiency.
- You have liver disease.
- You have nerve or brain disease (including seizure disorders).
- You have porphyria.
- You have psoriasis.
- You have stomach or intestinal disease.
- You drink more than 3 oz. of alcohol daily.

Over age 60:
Adverse reactions and side effects may be more frequent and severe than in younger persons.

Pregnancy:
Decide with your doctor if drug benefits justify risk to unborn child. Risk category C (see page xviii).

Breast-feeding:
Drug passes into milk. Avoid drug or discontinue nursing. Consult doctor for advice on maintaining milk supply.

Infants & children:
Not recommended. Dangerous.

Prolonged use:
- Permanent damage to the retina (back part of the eye) or nerve deafness.
- Talk to your doctor about the need for follow-up medical examinations or laboratory studies to check complete blood counts (white blood cell count, platelet count, red blood cell count, hemoglobin, hematocrit), eyes.

Skin & sunlight:
No special problems expected.

Driving, piloting or hazardous work:
Don't drive or pilot aircraft until you learn how medicine affects you. Don't work around dangerous machinery. Don't climb ladders or work in high places. Danger increases if you drink alcohol or take medicine affecting alertness and reflexes.

Discontinuing:
Don't discontinue without doctor's advice until you complete prescribed dose, even though symptoms diminish or disappear.

Others:
- Periodic physical and blood examinations recommended.
- If you are in a malaria area for a long time, you may need to change to another preventive drug every 2 years.

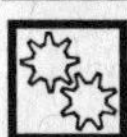

POSSIBLE INTERACTION WITH OTHER DRUGS

GENERIC NAME OR DRUG CLASS	COMBINED EFFECT
Estrogens*	Possible liver toxicity.
Gold compounds*	Risk of severe rash and itch.
Kaolin	Decreased absorption of hydroxychloroquine.
Magnesium trisilicate	Decreased absorption of hydroxychloroquine.
Penicillamine	Possible blood or kidney toxicity.

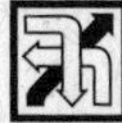

POSSIBLE INTERACTION WITH OTHER SUBSTANCES

INTERACTS WITH	COMBINED EFFECT
Alcohol:	Possible liver toxicity. Avoid.
Beverages:	None expected.
Cocaine:	None expected.
Foods:	None expected.
Marijuana:	None expected.
Tobacco:	None expected.

*See Glossary

HYDROXYUREA

BRAND NAMES

Droxia
Hydrea

BASIC INFORMATION

Habit forming? No
Prescription needed? Yes
Available as generic? Yes
Drug class: Antineoplastic

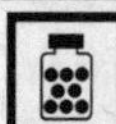

USES

- Treats head, neck, ovarian and cervical cancer.
- Treats leukemia, melanoma and polycythemia vera.
- Treats sickle cell disease.

DOSAGE & USAGE INFORMATION

How to take:
Capsule—Swallow with liquid. If you can't swallow whole, open capsule and take with liquid or food. Instructions to take on empty stomach mean 1 hour before or 2 hours after eating.

When to take:
According to doctor's instructions.

If you forget a dose:
Skip this dose. Never double dose. Resume regular schedule.

What drug does:
Probably interferes with synthesis of DNA.

Time lapse before drug works:
2 hours.

Don't take with:
Any other medicines (including over-the-counter drugs such as cough and cold medicines, laxatives, antacids, diet pills, caffeine, nose drops or vitamins) without consulting your doctor or pharmacist.

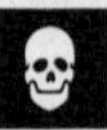

OVERDOSE

SYMPTOMS:
Black, tarry stools; fainting; seizures.
WHAT TO DO:

- **Dial 911 (emergency) for medical help or call poison control center 1-800-222-1222 for instructions.**
- **See emergency information on last 3 pages of this book.**

POSSIBLE ADVERSE REACTIONS OR SIDE EFFECTS

SYMPTOMS	WHAT TO DO
Life-threatening: In case of overdose, see previous column.	
Common:	
• Skin rash, fever, chills, cough, back pain.	Discontinue. Call doctor right away.
• Diarrhea, drowsiness, nausea, vomiting.	Continue. Call doctor when convenient.
Infrequent:	
Mouth sores, bruising, constipation, red skin.	Discontinue. Call doctor right away.
Rare:	
Confusion, hallucinations, headache, swollen feet.	Continue. Call doctor when convenient.

WARNINGS & PRECAUTIONS

Don't take if:
You are allergic to hydroxyurea.

Before you start, consult your doctor if:
- You have chicken pox.
- You have shingles (herpes zoster).
- You have anemia or blood disorder.
- You have gout.
- You have an infection.
- You have kidney disease or kidney stones.
- You have taken interferon in the past.

Over age 60:
Adverse reactions and side effects may be more frequent and severe than in younger persons. You may need smaller doses for shorter periods of time.

Pregnancy:
Decide with your doctor if drug benefits justify risk to unborn child. Risk category C (see page xviii).

Breast-feeding:
Drug passes into milk. Avoid drug or discontinue nursing until you finish medicine. Consult doctor for advice on maintaining milk supply.

Infants & children:
Effect not documented. Consult your pediatrician.

Prolonged use:
Talk to your doctor about the need for follow-up medical examinations or laboratory studies to check kidney function, complete blood counts (white blood cell count, platelet count, red blood cell count, hemoglobin, hematocrit) and serum uric acid.

Skin & sunlight:
No problems expected.

Driving, piloting or hazardous work:
Avoid if you feel confused, drowsy or dizzy.

Discontinuing:
May still experience symptoms of bone marrow depression, such as: blood in stools, fever or chills, blood spots under the skin, back pain, hoarseness, bloody urine. If any of these occur, call your doctor right away.

Others:
- Advise any doctor or dentist whom you consult that you take this medicine.
- May affect results in some medical tests.

POSSIBLE INTERACTION WITH OTHER DRUGS

GENERIC NAME OR DRUG CLASS	COMBINED EFFECT
Bone marrow depressants, other*	Dangerous suppression of bone marrow activity.
Clozapine	Toxic effect on bone marrow.
Levamisole	Increased risk of bone marrow depression.
Probenecid	May require increased dosage to treat gout.
Sulfinpyrazone	May require increased dosage to treat gout.
Tiopronin	Increased risk of toxicity to bone marrow.
Vaccines, live or killed virus	Increased risk of side effects.

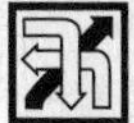

POSSIBLE INTERACTION WITH OTHER SUBSTANCES

INTERACTS WITH	COMBINED EFFECT
Alcohol:	None expected.
Beverages:	None expected.
Cocaine:	None expected.
Foods:	None expected.
Marijuana:	None expected.
Tobacco:	None expected.

***See Glossary**

HYDROXYZINE

BRAND NAMES

Ami Rax
Anxanil
Apo-Hydroxyzine
Atarax
Marax
Marax D.F.
Multipax
Novo-Hydroxyzin
Vistaril

BASIC INFORMATION

Habit forming? No
Prescription needed? Yes
Available as generic? Yes
Drug class: Tranquilizer, antihistamine

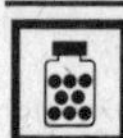

USES

- Treatment for anxiety, tension and agitation.
- Relieves itching from allergic reactions.

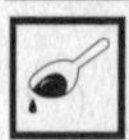

DOSAGE & USAGE INFORMATION

How to take:

- Tablet, syrup or capsule—Swallow with liquid. If you can't swallow whole, crumble tablet or open capsule and take with liquid or food.
- Liquid—If desired, dilute dose in beverage before swallowing.

When to take:
At the same times each day.

If you forget a dose:
Take as soon as you remember. If it is almost time for the next dose, wait for that dose (don't double this dose) and resume regular schedule.

What drug does:
Blocks action of histamine after an allergic response triggers histamine release. Histamines cause itching, sneezing, runny nose and eyes and other symptoms.

Time lapse before drug works:
15 to 30 minutes.

Continued next column

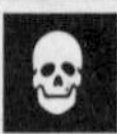

OVERDOSE

SYMPTOMS:
Drowsiness, unsteadiness, agitation, purposeless movements, tremor, convulsions.
WHAT TO DO:

- **Dial 911 (emergency) for medical help or call poison control center 1-800-222-1222 for instructions.**
- **See emergency information on last 3 pages of this book.**

Don't take with:
Any other medicine or any dietary supplement without consulting your doctor or pharmacist.

POSSIBLE ADVERSE REACTIONS OR SIDE EFFECTS

SYMPTOMS	WHAT TO DO
Life-threatening: In case of overdose, see previous column.	
Common: Drowsiness; dizziness; dryness of mouth, nose or throat; nausea.	Continue. Call doctor when convenient.
Infrequent:	
• Change in vision, clumsiness, rash.	Discontinue. Call doctor right away.
• Less tolerance for contact lenses, painful or difficult urination.	Continue. Call doctor when convenient.
• Appetite loss.	Continue. Tell doctor at next visit.
Rare: Nightmares, agitation, irritability, sore throat, fever, rapid heartbeat, unusual bleeding or bruising, fatigue, weakness, confusion, fainting, seizures.	Discontinue. Call doctor right away.

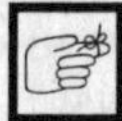

WARNINGS & PRECAUTIONS

Don't take if:
You are allergic to any antihistamine.

Before you start, consult your doctor if:

- You have asthma or kidney disease.
- You will have surgery within 2 months, including dental surgery, requiring general or spinal anesthesia.

Over age 60:

- Adverse reactions and side effects may be more frequent and severe than in younger persons.
- Drug likely to increase urination difficulty caused by enlarged prostate gland.

Pregnancy:
Decide with your doctor if drug benefits justify risk to unborn child. Risk category C (see page xviii).

Breast-feeding:
Drug passes into milk. Avoid drug or discontinue nursing until you finish medicine. Consult doctor for advice on maintaining milk supply.

Infants & children:
Use only under medical supervision.

Prolonged use:
Tolerance* may develop and reduce effectiveness.

Skin & sunlight:
No problems expected.

Driving, piloting or hazardous work:
Don't drive or pilot aircraft until you learn how medicine affects you. Don't work around dangerous machinery. Don't climb ladders or work in high places. Danger increases if you drink alcohol or take medicine affecting alertness and reflexes, such as antihistamines, tranquilizers, sedatives, pain medicine, narcotics and mind-altering drugs.

Discontinuing:
Don't discontinue without consulting doctor. Dose may require gradual reduction if you have taken drug for a long time. Doses of other drugs may also require adjustment.

Others:
Advise any doctor or dentist whom you consult that you take this medicine.

POSSIBLE INTERACTION WITH OTHER DRUGS

GENERIC NAME OR DRUG CLASS	COMBINED EFFECT
Antidepressants, tricyclic*	Increased effects of both drugs.
Antihistamines*	Increased hydroxyzine effect.
Attapulgite	Decreased hydroxyzine effect.
Carteolol	Decreased antihistamine effect.
Central nervous system (CNS) depressants*	Greater depression of central nervous system.
Clozapine	Toxic effect on the central nervous system.
Fluoxetine	Increased depressant effects of both drugs.
Guanfacine	May increase depressant effects of either drug.
Leucovorin	High alcohol content of leucovorin may cause adverse effects.
Narcotics*	Increased effects of both drugs.
Pain relievers*	Increased effects of both drugs.
Sertraline	Increased depressive effects of both drugs.
Sotalol	Increased antihistamine effect.

POSSIBLE INTERACTION WITH OTHER SUBSTANCES

INTERACTS WITH	COMBINED EFFECT
Alcohol:	Increased sedation and intoxication. Use with caution.
Beverages: Caffeine drinks.	Decreased tranquilizer effect of hydroxyzine.
Cocaine:	Decreased hydroxyzine effect. Avoid.
Foods:	None expected.
Marijuana:	None expected.
Tobacco:	None expected.

*See Glossary

HYOSCYAMINE

BRAND NAMES

Anaspaz	Kinesed
Anaspaz PB	Levbid
Barbidonna	Levsin
Barbidonna 2	Levsin S/L
Belladenal	Levsinex
Cystospaz	Levsinex Timecaps
Cystospaz-M	Neoquess
Gastrosed	Nulev

BASIC INFORMATION

Habit forming? No
Prescription needed?
Low strength: No
High strength: Yes
Available as generic? Yes
Drug class: Antispasmodic, anticholinergic

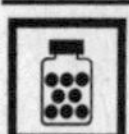

USES

Reduces spasms of digestive system, bladder and urethra.

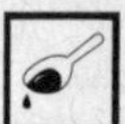

DOSAGE & USAGE INFORMATION

How to take:

- Tablet or liquid—Swallow with liquid or food to lessen stomach irritation. You may chew or crush tablets.
- Extended-release capsule or tablet—Swallow each dose whole.
- Drops—Dilute dose in beverage before swallowing.

When to take:
30 minutes before meals (unless directed otherwise by doctor).

Continued next column

OVERDOSE

SYMPTOMS:
Dilated pupils, rapid pulse and breathing, dizziness, fever, hallucinations, confusion, slurred speech, agitation, flushed face, convulsions, coma.

WHAT TO DO:

- **Dial 911 (emergency) for medical help or call poison control center 1-800-222-1222 for instructions.**
- **See emergency information on last 3 pages of this book.**

If you forget a dose:
Take as soon as you remember. If it is almost time for the next dose, wait for that dose (don't double this dose) and resume regular schedule.

What drug does:
Blocks nerve impulses at parasympathetic nerve endings, preventing muscle contractions and gland secretions of organs involved.

Time lapse before drug works:
15 to 30 minutes.

Don't take with:

- Antacids* or antidiarrheals* at the same time.
- Any other medicine or any dietary supplement without consulting your doctor or pharmacist.

POSSIBLE ADVERSE REACTIONS OR SIDE EFFECTS

SYMPTOMS	WHAT TO DO
Life-threatening: In case of overdose, see previous column.	
Common:	
• Confusion, delirium, rapid heartbeat.	Discontinue. Call doctor right away.
• Nausea, vomiting, decreased sweating.	Continue. Call doctor when convenient.
• Constipation.	Continue. Tell doctor at next visit.
• Dryness in ears, nose, throat, mouth.	No action necessary.
Infrequent:	
• Headache, painful or difficult urination, nasal congestion, altered taste.	Continue. Call doctor when convenient.
• Lightheadedness.	Discontinue. Call doctor right away.
Rare:	
Rash or hives, eye pain, blurred vision.	Discontinue. Call doctor right away.

WARNINGS & PRECAUTIONS

Don't take if:

- You are allergic to any anticholinergic.
- You have trouble with stomach bloating.
- You have difficulty emptying your bladder completely.
- You have narrow-angle glaucoma.
- You have severe ulcerative colitis.

Before you start, consult your doctor if:

- You have open-angle glaucoma.
- You have angina.
- You have chronic bronchitis or asthma.
- You have hiatal hernia.
- You have liver, kidney or thyroid disease.
- You have enlarged prostate.
- You have myasthenia gravis.
- You have peptic ulcer.
- You will have surgery within 2 months, including dental surgery, requiring general or spinal anesthesia.

Over age 60:
Adverse reactions and side effects may be more frequent and severe than in younger persons.

Pregnancy:
Decide with your doctor if drug benefits justify risk to unborn child. Risk category C (see page xviii).

Breast-feeding:
Drug passes into milk and decreases milk flow. Avoid drug or discontinue nursing until you finish medicine. Consult doctor for advice on maintaining milk supply.

Infants & children:
Use only under medical supervision.

Prolonged use:
Chronic constipation, possible fecal impaction. Consult doctor immediately.

Skin & sunlight:
No problems expected.

Driving, piloting or hazardous work:
Use disqualifies you for piloting aircraft. Otherwise, no problems expected.

Discontinuing:
May be unnecessary to finish medicine. Follow doctor's instructions.

Others:
Advise any doctor or dentist whom you consult that you take this medicine.

POSSIBLE INTERACTION WITH OTHER DRUGS

GENERIC NAME OR DRUG CLASS	COMBINED EFFECT
Amantadine	Increased hyoscyamine effect.
Anticholinergics, other*	Increased hyoscyamine effect.
Antidepressants, tricyclic*	Increased hyoscyamine effect.
Antihistamines*	Increased hyoscyamine effect.
Cortisone drugs*	Increased internal eye pressure.
Haloperidol	Increased internal eye pressure.
Ketoconazole	Decreased ketoconazole effect.
Meperidine	Increased hyoscyamine effect.
Methylphenidate	Increased hyoscyamine effect.
Molindone	Increased anticholinergic effect.
Monoamine oxidase (MAO) inhibitors*	Increased hyoscyamine effect.
Nizatidine	Increased nizatidine effect.
Orphenadrine	Increased hyoscyamine effect.
Phenothiazines*	Increased hyoscyamine effect.
Pilocarpine	Loss of pilocarpine effect in glaucoma treatment.
Sedatives* or central nervous system (CNS) depressants*	Increased sedative effect of both drugs.
Vitamin C	Decreased hyoscyamine effect. Avoid large doses of vitamin C.

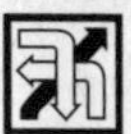

POSSIBLE INTERACTION WITH OTHER SUBSTANCES

INTERACTS WITH	COMBINED EFFECT
Alcohol:	None expected.
Beverages:	None expected.
Cocaine:	Excessively rapid heartbeat. Avoid.
Foods:	None expected.
Marijuana:	Drowsiness and dry mouth.
Tobacco:	None expected.

***See Glossary**

IMATINIB

BRAND NAMES

Gleevec

BASIC INFORMATION

Habit forming? No
Prescription needed? Yes
Available as generic? No
Drug class: Antineoplastic

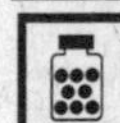

USES

- Treatment for some types of leukemia (cancer of white blood cells).
- Treatment for gastrointestinal stomal tumors.
- Treatment for certain rare cancers and blood diseases.

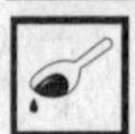

DOSAGE & USAGE INFORMATION

How to take:
Capsule—Swallow with large glass of water to minimize the risk of stomach and gastrointestinal irritation.

When to take:
Usually once a day at mealtime or according to doctor's instructions.

If you forget a dose:
Do not take the missed dose at all. Return to your regular dosing schedule at the prescribed time. Never double a dose to make up for a missed dose. Consult your doctor.

What drug does:
Reduces substantially the level of cancerous cells in the bone marrow and blood of treated patients.

Time lapse before drug works:
Starts working in 2-4 hours, but effectiveness may take 1-3 months.

Don't take with:
Any other medicines (including over-the-counter drugs such as cough and cold medicines, laxatives, antacids, diet pills, caffeine, nose drops or vitamins) without consulting your doctor or pharmacist.

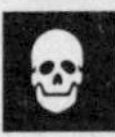

OVERDOSE

SYMPTOMS:
Unknown effect.
WHAT TO DO:
If person takes much larger amount than prescribed, dial 911 (emergency) for medical help or call poison control center 1-800-222-1222 for instructions.

POSSIBLE ADVERSE REACTIONS OR SIDE EFFECTS

SYMPTOMS	WHAT TO DO
Life-threatening:	
Some adverse effects from advanced cancer and/or the medicine can be serious or life threatening.	Seek emergency treatment for any symptoms that appear severe or critical.
Common:	
• Chest pain, shortness of breath, swelling (face, hands, legs. feet), black tarry stools, nausea or vomiting, muscle pain or cramps, blood in urine, decreased or painful urination, fever, chills, pale skin, quick weight gain, stomach cramps, sore throat, sores on body, ulcers or white spots on lips or in mouth, swollen glands, unusual bleeding or tiredness or weakness.	Continue. Call doctor right away.
• Joint or bone pain, diarrhea, skin rash. fatigue.	Continue. Call doctor when convenient.
Infrequent:	
• Convulsions, irregular heartbeat, wheezing, tightness in chest, numbness or tingling (in hands, feet, or lips), pinpoint red spots on skin.	Continue. Call doctor right away.
• Bloody nose, mood changes, slow weight gain, weight loss, sneezing, joint pain, constipation, loss of appetite, headache, increased thirst, dry mouth.	Continue. Call doctor when convenient.
Rare:	
Acid indigestion or upset stomach, stuffy nose, itchy skin.	Continue. Call doctor when convenient.

Note: Side effects are often unavoidable with drugs used to treat cancer. Discuss any concerns or questions or other symptoms with your doctor.

WARNINGS & PRECAUTIONS

Don't take if:
You are allergic to imatinib.

Before you start, consult your doctor if:
- You have any infection.
- You have anemia.
- You have leukopenia, neutropenia or thrombocytopenia.
- You have bone marrow depression.
- You have recent chickenpox or herpes zoster.
- You have liver problems.

Over age 60:
Other than a higher incidence of edema, studies to date have not shown problems that would limit the usefulness of imatinib.

Pregnancy:
Not recommended. Consult doctor. Risk category D (see page xviii).

Breast-feeding:
It is unknown if drug passes into milk. Avoid drug or discontinue nursing until you finish medicine. Consult doctor for advice on maintaining milk supply.

Infants & children:
Safety and efficacy have not been established in children under 18 years of age.

Prolonged use:
- Talk to your doctor about the need for follow-up medical examinations or laboratory studies to check your response to the drug, blood studies, weight gain and liver function.
- The long term effects of the drug are not yet known.

Skin & sunlight:
No problems expected.

Driving, piloting or hazardous work:
No problems expected.

Discontinuing:
No special problems expected. Don't discontinue drug without doctor's approval.

Others:
- Advise any doctor or dentist whom you consult that you take this medicine. Consult doctor before having dental work.
- Do not have any immunizations without your doctor's approval. Imatinib may lower your resistance to the infection that you are getting the immunization for.
- Avoid persons who have recently taken the oral polio virus vaccine; they may pass the virus on to you.
- Avoid people with infections, because you have an increased chance of getting the infection. Advise your doctor of any unusual symptoms, infections or injuries.
- Be careful when brushing or flossing teeth, or using a razor or other sharp object to avoid being injured.
- May affect results in some medical tests.
- Avoid contact sports or activities that could cause, injury, bruising or bleeding.

POSSIBLE INTERACTION WITH OTHER DRUGS

GENERIC NAME OR DRUG CLASS	COMBINED EFFECT
Anticoagulants*	Blood clotting problems.
Blood dyscrasia-causing medications*	Increased risk of adverse effects of imatinib.
Bone marrow depressants, other*	Increased bone marrow suppression.
Cyclosporine	Increased effect of cyclosporine.
Enzyme inducers*	Decreased effect of imatinib.
Enzyme inhibitors*	Increased effect of imatinib.
HMG-CoA reductase inhibitors	Increased effect of HMG-CoA reductase inhibitor.
Pimozide	Increased effect of pimozide.
Vaccines (killed)	Decreased effectiveness of vaccine.
Vaccines (live)	Increased risk of getting the disease the vaccine prevents.

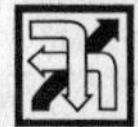

POSSIBLE INTERACTION WITH OTHER SUBSTANCES

INTERACTS WITH	COMBINED EFFECT
Alcohol:	None expected.
Beverages:	None expected.
Cocaine:	None expected. Best to avoid.
Foods:	None expected.
Marijuana:	None expected. Best to avoid.
Tobacco:	None expected.

***See Glossary**

IMMUNOSUPPRESSIVE AGENTS

GENERIC AND BRAND NAMES

MYCOPHENOLATE	TACROLIMUS
Myfortic	Prograf
Myfortic Delayed Release	

BASIC INFORMATION

Habit forming? No
Prescription needed? Yes
Available as generic? Yes
Drug class: Immunosuppressant

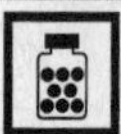

USES

Helps to suppress the immune system and prevent rejection in patients who have undergone organ transplants.

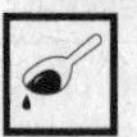

DOSAGE & USAGE INFORMATION

How to take:

- Capsule—Swallow with liquid. Do not open capsule.
- Tablet—Swallow with liquid. Do not crush tablet.
- Delayed-release tablet—Swallow whole with liquid. Do not crush or chew tablet.
- Oral suspension—Take as directed on label.

When to take:
At the same times each day, according to prescription label. Take mycophenolate on an empty stomach (1 hour before or 2 hours after a meal). Tacrolimus may be taken with or without food.

If you forget a dose:
Take as soon as you remember. If it is almost time for the next dose, wait for next scheduled dose (don't double this dose). Consult doctor if you are unsure about dosing schedule.

Continued next column

OVERDOSE

SYMPTOMS:
Increased severity of adverse reactions, coma, delirium.
WHAT TO DO:

- **Dial 911 (emergency) for medical help or call poison control center 1-800-222-1222 for instructions.**
- **See emergency information on last 3 pages of this book.**

What drug does:
Tacrolimus and mycophenolate are 2 different types of immunosuppressive drugs. They suppress immune reactions (to transplanted organs) in certain cells by inhibiting their growth.

Time lapse before drug works:
3 to 3-1/2 hours. May take several weeks to evaluate effectiveness against organ rejection.

Don't take with:
Any other medicine or any dietary supplement without consulting your doctor or pharmacist.

POSSIBLE ADVERSE REACTIONS OR SIDE EFFECTS

SYMPTOMS	WHAT TO DO
Life-threatening: In case of overdose, see previous column.	
Common:	
• Infections (fever, chills, hoarseness, cough, trouble urinating, back or side pain); headache; tingling or numbness of hands or feet; chest pain; blood in urine; trouble sleeping; trembling of hands; shortness of breath.	Continue, but call doctor right away.
• Mild back pain, constipation or diarrhea, stomach pain, heartburn.	Continue. Call doctor when convenient.
Infrequent:	
• Bloody vomit; anxiety; nervousness; white patches on mouth, tongue or throat; weakness; seizures.	Continue, but call doctor right away.
• Hair loss or excess hair growth, nausea, mild vomiting, skin rash or itch, muscle or joint pain, dizziness.	Continue. Call doctor when convenient.
Rare:	
• Bloody, black or tarry stools; small red spots on skin; unusual bleeding or bruising; irregular heartbeat.	Continue, but call doctor right away.
• Mood or mental changes.	Continue. Call doctor when convenient.

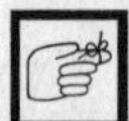

WARNINGS & PRECAUTIONS

Don't take if:
You are allergic to mycophenolate or tacrolimus.

Before you start, consult your doctor if:
- You have liver or kidney disease.
- You have a digestive system disease.
- You have an infection.
- You have chickenpox (or have recently been exposed) or herpes zoster (shingles).
- You are female and planning pregnancy or are able to bear children.

Over age 60:
No special problems expected.

Pregnancy:
- Mycophenolate is pregnancy risk category D. Avoid use. It increases risk of pregnancy loss and congenital malformations. (see page xviii).
- Tacrolimus is pregnancy risk category C. Decide with your doctor if drug benefits justify risk to unborn child (see page xviii).

Breast-feeding:
Tacrolimus passes into milk; mycophenolate may pass into milk. Avoid drugs or discontinue nursing until you finish medicine. Consult doctor for advice on maintaining milk supply.

Infants & children:
Safety and effectiveness of mycophenolate are not established. Tacrolimus has been used in liver transplants in pediatric patients.

Prolonged use:
- Can cause reduced function of kidneys.
- Can increase risk of developing lymphoma (cancer of lymph glands).
- Talk to your doctor about the need for follow-up medical examinations or laboratory studies to check blood concentration of drug, kidney function, liver function, potassium levels, drug's effectiveness and adverse reactions.

Skin & sunlight:
No special problems expected.

Driving, piloting or hazardous work:
Don't drive or pilot aircraft until you learn how medicine affects you. Don't work around dangerous machinery. Don't climb ladders or work in high places. Danger increases if you drink alcohol or take drugs affecting alertness and reflexes.

Discontinuing:
Don't discontinue without consulting doctor. You will usually require this drug for your lifetime.

Others:
- Advise any doctor or dentist whom you consult that you take this drug. May interfere with results of some medical tests.
- Wear medical identification stating that you have had a transplant and take this drug.
- Check blood pressure routinely at home. Drug may sometimes cause hypertension.
- Immunosuppressed patients are at increased risk for opportunistic infections, such as activation of latent viral infections, including BK virus-associated nephropathy.
- Avoid any immunizations except those specifically recommended by your doctor.
- Maintain good dental hygiene. Immunosuppression can cause gum problems.
- Talk to your doctor about forms of birth control before starting treatment with mycophenolate.

POSSIBLE INTERACTION WITH OTHER DRUGS

GENERIC NAME OR DRUG CLASS	COMBINED EFFECT
Acyclovir	Increased effect of mycophenolate.
Antacids*	Decreased effect of mycophenolate.
Cholestyramine	Decreased effect of mycophenolate.
Diuretics, potassium-sparing*	Increased risk of potassium toxicity.
Enzyme inducers*	Decreased effect of tacrolimus.
Enzyme inhibitors*	Increased effect of tacrolimus.
Ganciclovir	Increased effect of mycophenolate.
Immunosuppressants,* other	Increased risk of adverse effects.
Nephrotoxics*	Increased risk of kidney problems.
Nitroimidazoles	Increased tacrolimus effect.
Potassium supplements	Increased risk of potassium toxicity.

Continued on page 918

POSSIBLE INTERACTION WITH OTHER SUBSTANCES

INTERACTS WITH	COMBINED EFFECT
Alcohol:	Increased risk of toxic effects. Avoid.
Beverages: Grapefruit juice.	Increased effect of drug. Avoid.
Cocaine:	Unknown. Avoid.
Foods: Grapefruit.	Increased effect of drug. Avoid.
Marijuana:	Unknown. Avoid.
Tobacco:	None expected.

***See Glossary**

INDAPAMIDE

BRAND NAMES

Lozide
Lozol

BASIC INFORMATION

Habit forming? No
Prescription needed? Yes
Available as generic? Yes
Drug class: Antihypertensive, diuretic

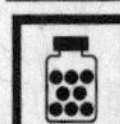

USES

- Controls, but doesn't cure, high blood pressure.
- Reduces fluid retention (edema) caused by conditions such as heart disorders.

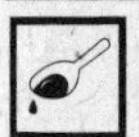

DOSAGE & USAGE INFORMATION

How to take:
Tablet—Swallow with liquid or food to lessen stomach irritation.

When to take:
At the same times each day, usually at bedtime.

If you forget a dose:
Bedtime dose—If you forget your once-a-day bedtime dose, don't take it more than 3 hours late. Never double dose.

What drug does:
Forces kidney to excrete more sodium and causes excess salt and fluid to be excreted.

Time lapse before drug works:
2 hours for effect to begin. May require 1 to 4 weeks for full effects.

Don't take with:
Any other medicine or any dietary supplement without consulting your doctor or pharmacist.

OVERDOSE

SYMPTOMS:
Nausea, vomiting, diarrhea, very dry mouth, thirst, weakness, excessive fatigue, very rapid heart rate, weak pulse.
WHAT TO DO:
- **Dial 911 (emergency) for medical help or call poison control center 1-800-222-1222 for instructions.**
- **If person is unconscious, check breathing and pulse. If not breathing, begin mouth-to-mouth rescue breathing. If heart is not beating, begin chest compressions.**
- **See emergency information on last 3 pages of this book.**

POSSIBLE ADVERSE REACTIONS OR SIDE EFFECTS

SYMPTOMS	WHAT TO DO
Life-threatening: In case of overdose, see previous column.	
Common:	
• Excessive tiredness or weakness, muscle cramps.	Discontinue. Call doctor right away.
• Frequent urination.	Continue. Tell doctor at next visit.
Infrequent:	
Insomnia, mood change, dizziness on changing position, headache, excessive thirst, diarrhea, appetite loss, nausea, dry mouth, decreased sex drive.	Continue. Call doctor when convenient.
Rare:	
• Weak pulse.	Discontinue. Seek emergency treatment.
• Itching, rash, hives, irregular heartbeat.	Discontinue. Call doctor right away.

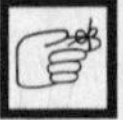

WARNINGS & PRECAUTIONS

Don't take if:
You are allergic to indapamide or to any sulfa drug or thiazide diuretic.*

Before you start, consult your doctor if:
- You have severe kidney disease.
- You have diabetes.
- You have gout.
- You have liver disease.
- You will have surgery within 2 months, including dental surgery, requiring general or spinal anesthesia.
- You have lupus erythematosus.
- You are pregnant or plan to become pregnant.

Over age 60:
Adverse reactions and side effects may be more frequent and severe than in younger persons.

Pregnancy:
Consult doctor. Risk category B (see page xviii).

Breast-feeding:
Unknown effect on child. Consult doctor.

Infants & children:
Use only under close medical supervision.

Prolonged use:
Request laboratory studies for blood sugar, BUN,* uric acid and serum electrolytes (potassium and sodium).

Skin & sunlight:
May cause rash or intensify sunburn in areas exposed to sun or ultraviolet light (photosensitivity reaction). Avoid overexposure. Notify doctor if reaction occurs.

Driving, piloting or hazardous work:
Don't drive or pilot aircraft until you learn how medicine affects you. Don't work around dangerous machinery. Don't climb ladders or work in high places. Danger increases if you drink alcohol or take medicine affecting alertness and reflexes, such as antihistamines, tranquilizers, sedatives, pain medicine, narcotics and mind-altering drugs.

Discontinuing:
Don't discontinue without consulting doctor. Dose may require gradual reduction if you have taken drug for a long time. Doses of other drugs may also require adjustment.

Others:
Advise any doctor or dentist whom you consult that you take this medicine.

POSSIBLE INTERACTION WITH OTHER DRUGS

GENERIC NAME OR DRUG CLASS	COMBINED EFFECT
Adrenocorticoids, systemic	Possible excessive potassium loss.
Allopurinol	Decreased allopurinol effect.
Amiodarone	Increased risk of heartbeat irregularity due to low potassium.
Amphotericin B	Increased potassium.
Angiotensin-converting enzyme (ACE) inhibitors*	Decreased blood pressure. Possible excessive potassium in blood.
Antidepressants, tricyclic*	Dangerous drop in blood pressure.
Antidiabetic agents, oral*	Increased blood sugar.
Antihypertensives, other*	Increased anti-hypertensive effect.
Barbiturates*	Increased indapamide effect.
Beta-adrenergic blocking agents*	Increased effect of indapamide.
Calcium supplements*	Increased calcium in blood.
Carteolol	Increased anti-hypertensive effect.
Cholestyramine	Decreased indapamide effect.
Colestipol	Decreased indapamide effect.
Digitalis preparations*	Excessive potassium loss that may cause dangerous heart rhythms.
Diuretics, thiazide*	Increased effect of thiazide diuretics.
Indomethacin	Decreased indapamide effect.
Lithium	High risk of lithium toxicity.
Monoamine oxidase (MAO) inhibitors*	Increased indapamide effect.
Nicardipine	Dangerous blood pressure drop. Dosages may require adjustment.
Nimodipine	Dangerous blood pressure drop.
Opiates*	Weakness and faintness when arising from bed or chair.

Continued on page 918

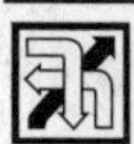

POSSIBLE INTERACTION WITH OTHER SUBSTANCES

INTERACTS WITH	COMBINED EFFECT
Alcohol:	Dangerous blood pressure drop. Avoid.
Beverages:	No problems expected.
Cocaine:	Increased risk of heart block and high blood pressure.
Foods: Licorice.	Excessive potassium loss that may cause dangerous heart rhythms.
Marijuana:	Reduced effectiveness of indapamide. Avoid.
Tobacco:	Reduced effectiveness of indapamide. Avoid.

***See Glossary**

INSULIN

BRAND NAMES

See full list of brand names in the *Generic and Brand Name Directory*, page 886.

BASIC INFORMATION

Habit forming? No
Prescription needed? No
Available as generic? Yes
Drug class: Antidiabetic

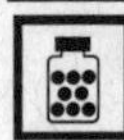

USES

Treats diabetes, a metabolic disorder, in which patients have high levels of sugar in their blood.

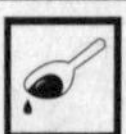

DOSAGE & USAGE INFORMATION

How to take:

- Injection—Injected under the skin. Use disposable, sterile needles. Rotate injection sites.
- Inhaled powder—Follow instructions provided.

When to take:
At the same times each day.

If you forget a dose:
Take as soon as you remember. Wait at least 4 hours for next dose. Resume regular schedule.

What drug does:
Facilitates passage of blood sugar through cell membranes so sugar is usable.

Time lapse before drug works:
30 minutes to 8 hours, depending on type of insulin used.

Continued next column

OVERDOSE

SYMPTOMS:
Low blood sugar (hypoglycemia)—Anxiety; chills, cold sweats, pale skin; drowsiness; excessive hunger; headache; nausea; nervousness; fast heartbeat; shakiness; unusual tiredness or weakness.
WHAT TO DO:

- **Eat some type of sugar immediately, such as glucose product, orange juice (add some sugar), nondiet sodas, candy (such as 5 Lifesavers), honey.**
- **If patient loses consciousness, give glucagon if you have it and know how to use it.**
- **Dial 911 (emergency) for medical help or call poison control center 1-800-222-1222 for instructions.**
- **See emergency information on last 3 pages of this book.**

Don't take with:
Any other medicine or any dietary supplement without consulting your doctor or pharmacist.

POSSIBLE ADVERSE REACTIONS OR SIDE EFFECTS

SYMPTOMS	WHAT TO DO
Life-threatening:	
Hives, rash, intense itching, faintness soon after a dose (anaphylaxis).	Seek emergency treatment immediately.
Common:	
None expected.	
Infrequent:	
• Symptoms of low blood sugar—nervousness, hunger (excessive), cold sweats, rapid pulse, anxiety, cold skin, chills, confusion, concentration loss, drowsiness, headache, nausea, weakness, shakiness, vision changes.	Seek treatment (eat some form of quick-acting sugar—glucose tablets, sugar, fruit juice, corn syrup, honey).
• Symptoms of high blood sugar—increased urination, unusual thirst, dry mouth, drowsiness, flushed or dry skin, fruit-like breath odor, appetite loss, stomach pain or vomiting, tiredness, trouble breathing, increased blood sugar level.	Seek emergency treatment immediately.
• Swelling, redness, itch or warmth at injection site.	Continue. Call doctor when convenient.
Rare:	
None expected.	

WARNINGS & PRECAUTIONS

Don't take if:

- Your diagnosis and dose schedule is not established.
- You don't know how to deal with overdose emergencies.
- You are allergic to insulin.

Before you start, consult your doctor if:

- You take MAO inhibitors.
- You have liver or kidney disease or low thyroid function.

Over age 60:
Guard against hypoglycemia. Repeated episodes can cause permanent confusion and abnormal behavior.

Pregnancy:
Adhere rigidly to diabetes treatment program. Risk category B (see page xviii).

Breast-feeding:
No problems expected. Consult doctor.

Infants & children:
Use only under medical supervision.

Prolonged use:
Talk to your doctor about the need for follow-up medical examinations or laboratory studies to check blood sugar, serum potassium, urine.

Skin & sunlight:
No problems expected.

Driving, piloting or hazardous work:
No problems expected after dose is established.

Discontinuing:
Don't discontinue without doctor's advice until you complete prescribed dose, even though symptoms diminish or disappear.

Others:
- Diet and exercise affect how much insulin you need. Work with your doctor to determine accurate dose.
- Notify your doctor if you skip a dose, overeat, have fever or infection.
- Notify doctor if you develop symptoms of high blood sugar: drowsiness, dry skin, orange fruit-like odor to breath, increased urination, appetite loss, unusual thirst.
- Never freeze insulin.
- May interfere with the accuracy of some medical tests.

POSSIBLE INTERACTION WITH OTHER DRUGS

GENERIC NAME OR DRUG CLASS	COMBINED EFFECT
Adrenocorticoids, systemic	Decreased insulin effect.
Anticonvulsants, hydantoin*	Decreased insulin effect.
Antidiabetics, oral*	Increased antidiabetic effect.
Beta-adrenergic blocking agents*	Possible increased difficulty in regulating blood sugar levels.
Bismuth subsalicylate	Increased insulin effect. May require dosage adjustment.
Carteolol	Hypoglycemic effects may be prolonged.
Contraceptives, oral*	Decreased insulin effect.
Dexfenfluramine	May require dosage change as weight loss occurs.
Diuretics, thiazide*	Decreased insulin effect.
Furosemide	Decreased insulin effect.
Insulin analogs	May require dosage adjustment.
Monoamine oxidase (MAO) inhibitors*	Increased insulin effect.
Nicotine	Increased insulin effect.
Oxyphenbutazone	Increased insulin effect.
Phenylbutazone	Increased insulin effect.
Salicylates*	Increased insulin effect.
Smoking deterrents	May require insulin dosage adjustment.
Sulfa drugs*	Increased insulin effect.
Tetracyclines*	Increased insulin effect.
Thyroid hormones*	Decreased insulin effect.

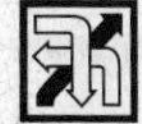

POSSIBLE INTERACTION WITH OTHER SUBSTANCES

INTERACTS WITH	COMBINED EFFECT
Alcohol:	Increased insulin effect. Blood sugar problems. Avoid.
Beverages:	None expected.
Cocaine:	Unknown effect. Avoid.
Foods:	None expected. Follow your diabetic diet instructions.
Marijuana:	Possible increase in blood sugar. Avoid.
Tobacco:	Decreased insulin absorption. Avoid.

*See Glossary

INSULIN ANALOGS

GENERIC AND BRAND NAMES

INSULIN ASPART
- **Novolog**
- **Novolog FlexPen**
- **Novolog Mix 50/50**

INSULIN DETEMIR
- **Levemir**

INSULIN GLARGINE
- **Lantus**
- **Lantus OptiClik**
- **Lantus Solostar Pen**

INSULIN GLULISINE
- **Apidra**
- **Apidra SoloStar**

INSULIN LISPRO
- **Humalog**
- **Humalog Mix 50/50**
- **Humalog Mix 75/25**

BASIC INFORMATION

Habit forming? No
Prescription needed? Yes
Available as generic? No
Drug class: Antidiabetic

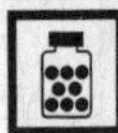

USES

Treats diabetes, a metabolic disorder, in which patients have high levels of sugar in their blood. The drug keeps blood sugar levels from going too high after eating.

DOSAGE & USAGE INFORMATION

How to take:
Taken by injection under the skin. Use disposable, sterile needles, or disposable pen. Rotate injection sites. Follow instructions provided with product.

Continued next column

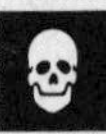

OVERDOSE

SYMPTOMS:
Low blood sugar (hypoglycemia)—Anxiety; chills, cold sweats, pale skin; drowsiness; excessive hunger; headache; nausea; nervousness; fast heartbeat; shakiness; unusual tiredness or weakness.

WHAT TO DO:
- **Eat some type of sugar immediately, such as glucose product, orange juice (add some sugar), nondiet sodas, candy (such as 5 Lifesavers), honey.**
- **If person is unconscious, give glucagon if you have it and know how to use it.**
- **Dial 911 (emergency) for medical help or call poison control center 1-800-222-1222 for instructions.**
- **See emergency information on last 3 pages of this book.**

When to take:
At the same times each day. If taken at mealtime, use it within a 15 minute period prior to the meal. May need to be taken in combination with a long-acting insulin to prevent hyperglycemia.

If you forget a dose:
Follow your doctor's instructions. If unsure, call your doctor or pharmacist.

What drug does:
These drugs are rapid- or fast-acting and work quickly in the body after injection. They are variations (analogs) of human insulin and more closely mimic the time action of natural insulin that comes from the pancreas.

Time lapse before drug works:
30 minutes to 1 hour, which is faster than regular insulin. Insulin aspart and insulin lispro finish acting in 3-4 hours, insulin glargine in 24 hours.

Don't take with:
Any other medicine or any dietary supplement without consulting your doctor or pharmacist.

POSSIBLE ADVERSE REACTIONS OR SIDE EFFECTS

SYMPTOMS	WHAT TO DO
Life-threatening:	
Hives, rash, intense itching, faintness, swelling, breathing difficulty soon after a dose (anaphylaxis).	Seek emergency treatment immediately.
Common:	
None expected.	
Infrequent:	
• Symptoms of low blood sugar—nervousness, hunger (excessive), cold sweats, rapid pulse, anxiety, cold skin, chills, confusion, concentration loss, drowsiness, headache, nausea, weakness, shakiness, vision changes.	Seek treatment (eat some form of quick-acting sugar—glucose tablets, sugar, fruit juice, corn syrup, honey).
• Symptoms of high blood sugar—increased urination, unusual thirst, dry mouth, drowsiness, flushed or dry skin, fruit-like breath odor, appetite loss, stomach pain or vomiting, tiredness, trouble breathing, increased blood sugar level.	Seek emergency treatment immediately.

• Swelling, redness, itch or warmth at injection site; other skin changes at injection site (e.g., thinning or thickened skin).	Continue. Call doctor when convenient.
Rare:	
Dry mouth, excessive thirst, weak or fast pulse, heartbeat irregularities, mental or mood changes, nausea or vomiting, unusual tiredness or weakness, muscle cramps (may be symptoms of hypokalemia).	Continue, but call doctor right away.

WARNINGS & PRECAUTIONS

Don't take if:
If you are allergic to insulin.

Before you start, consult your doctor if:
- Your diagnosis and dose schedule are not established or you don't know how to deal with overdose emergencies.
- You take MAO inhibitors.*
- You have hypoglycemia, liver or kidney disease or low thyroid function.

Over age 60:
Insulin requirements may change. The family should notify the doctor if abnormal behavior or confusion occurs in an older person.

Pregnancy:
Risk category B for aspart, lispro, detemir and category C for glargine, glulisine. See page xviii and consult doctor.

Breast-feeding:
Unknown if drugs pass into milk. May require dosage adjustment. Consult doctor.

Infants & children:
Use only under medical supervision.

Prolonged use:
Talk to your doctor about the need for follow-up medical examinations or laboratory studies to check effectiveness of drug.

Skin & sunlight:
No problems expected.

Driving, piloting or hazardous work:
No problems expected after dose is established. Need to be cautious for signs of hypoglycemia.

Discontinuing:
Don't discontinue without doctor's advice, even though symptoms diminish or disappear.

Others:
- Diet and exercise affect how much insulin you need. Work with your doctor to determine accurate dose. Monitor your glucose levels as directed.
- Notify your doctor if you have a fever, infection, diarrhea, or experience vomiting.
- Advise any doctor or dentist whom you consult that you take this medicine.
- Never freeze insulin.
- Wear medical identification that indicates you have diabetes and take insulin.
- You and your family should educate yourselves about diabetes and learn to recognize hypoglycemia and treat it with sugar or glucagon.
- May interfere with the accuracy of some medical tests.

POSSIBLE INTERACTION WITH OTHER DRUGS

GENERIC NAME OR DRUG CLASS	COMBINED EFFECT
Antidiabetics, oral*	Increased antidiabetic effect.
Hyperglycemia-causing agents*	May need increased dosage of insulin.
Hypoglycemia-causing agents*	May need decreased dosage of insulin.
Insulin	May need dosage adjustment.
Sympatholytics*	Increased insulin effect.
Smoking deterrents	May require insulin dosage adjustment.

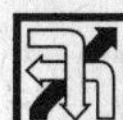

POSSIBLE INTERACTION WITH OTHER SUBSTANCES

INTERACTS WITH	COMBINED EFFECT
Alcohol:	Increased insulin effect. Blood sugar problems. Avoid.
Beverages:	None expected.
Cocaine:	Unknown effect. Avoid.
Foods:	None expected. Follow your diabetic diet instructions.
Marijuana:	Possible increase in blood sugar. Avoid.
Tobacco:	Decreased insulin absorption. Avoid.

***See Glossary**

INTEGRASE INHIBITORS

GENERIC AND BRAND NAMES

ELVITEGRAVIR
Stribild

RALTEGRAVIR
Isentress

BASIC INFORMATION

Habit forming? No
Prescription needed? Yes
Available as generic? No
Drug class: Antiviral agent

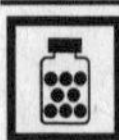

USES

Treatment of human immunodeficiency virus (HIV). HIV is the virus that causes acquired immunodeficiency syndrome (AIDS).

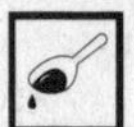

DOSAGE & USAGE INFORMATION

How to take:
Tablet—Swallow with liquid. Raltegravir may be taken with or without food. Take elvitegravir with food.

When to take:
Take raltegravir twice a day at the same times each day. Take elvitegravir once a day at the same time each day.

If you forget a dose:
Take as soon as you remember. If it is almost time for the next dose, wait for next scheduled dose (don't double this dose).

What drug does:
It helps control HIV infection by inhibiting an enzyme that is required for HIV replication. This may reduce the amount of HIV in the blood and may increase immune system cells. The drug does not cure HIV or AIDS.

Time lapse before drug works:
May require several weeks or months before full benefits are apparent.

Don't take with:
Any other medicine or any dietary supplement without consulting your doctor or pharmacist. This is very important with HIV drugs.

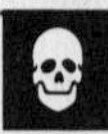

OVERDOSE

SYMPTOMS:
Unknown.
WHAT TO DO:
If person takes much larger amount than prescribed or if accidentally swallowed, call doctor or poison control center 1-800-222-1222 for help.

POSSIBLE ADVERSE REACTIONS OR SIDE EFFECTS

SYMPTOMS	WHAT TO DO
Life-threatening:	
Rare allergic reaction (hives, itching, rash, trouble breathing, tightness in chest, swelling of lips or tongue or throat).	Seek emergency treatment immediately.
Common:	
Diarrhea, nausea, headache, fever.	Continue. Call doctor when convenient.
Infrequent:	
Lightheadedness or dizziness, mild stomach pain, muscle or joint pain, tiredness, vomiting, dark urine, increased hunger or thirst.	Continue. Call doctor when convenient.
Rare:	
• Chest pain, fast heartbeat, shortness of breath.	Discontinue. Call doctor right away.
• Bruising or bleeding, signs of infection, confusion, mood changes, decreased urination, yellow skin or eyes.	Continue, but call doctor right away.
• Body aches, loss of appetite, a feeling of discomfort, body fat increases or fat moves to different areas of body, bloating, weight gain, excessive sweating, swelling, drowsiness, constipation, other unexplained symptoms.	Continue. Call doctor when convenient.

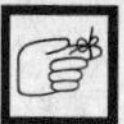

WARNINGS & PRECAUTIONS

Don't take if:
You are allergic to integrase inhibitors.

Before you start, consult your doctor if:
- You are allergic to any medicine, food or other substance, or have a family history of allergies.
- You have a muscle disorder.
- You have kidney or liver disease.

Over age 60:
Use with caution as adverse reactions and side effects may be more frequent and severe than in younger persons.

Pregnancy:
Decide with your doctor if drug benefits justify risk to unborn child. Risk category C (see page xviii). HIV can be passed to the baby if the mother is not properly treated during pregnancy. Talk to your doctor about being included in the Antiretroviral Pregnancy Registry.

Breast-feeding:
It is unknown if drug passes into milk. It is not recommended that HIV-infected mothers breast-feed. Consult your doctor.

Infants & children:
Approved for use in children over age 2.

Prolonged use:
- Long-term effects of using this drug have not been established.
- Talk to your doctor about the need for follow-up blood tests and liver function studies.

Skin & sunlight:
No problems expected.

Driving, piloting or hazardous work:
No problems expected.

Discontinuing:
Don't discontinue without doctor's advice.

Others:
- Advise any doctor or dentist whom you consult that you take this medicine.
- Taking this drug does not prevent you from passing HIV to another person through sexual contact or sharing needles. Avoid sexual contact or practice safe sex (e.g., using condoms) to help prevent the transmission of HIV. Never share or re-use needles. If you have questions, ask your doctor for advice.
- Consult your doctor right away if you develop a new infection (e.g., fever, chills, sore throat or other symptoms).
- Consult your doctor right away if you develop muscle pain, especially if you take HMG CoA reductase inhibitors or fibrates.
- Brand name Stribild contains four drugs. One is cobicistat which is not covered in this book.
- Take drug daily as prescribed. Do not increase or decrease dosage of drug without doctor's approval.

POSSIBLE INTERACTION WITH OTHER DRUGS

GENERIC NAME OR DRUG CLASS	COMBINED EFFECT
Rifampin	Decreased effect of integrase inhibitor.

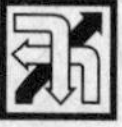

POSSIBLE INTERACTION WITH OTHER SUBSTANCES

INTERACTS WITH	COMBINED EFFECT
Alcohol:	None expected.
Beverages:	None expected.
Cocaine:	Unknown effect. Best to avoid.
Foods:	None expected.
Marijuana:	Unknown effect. Best to avoid.
Tobacco:	None expected.

INTERMITTENT CLAUDICATION AGENTS

GENERIC AND BRAND NAMES

CILOSTAZOL
Pletal

BASIC INFORMATION

Habit forming? No
Prescription needed? Yes
Available as generic? No
Drug class: Vasodilator

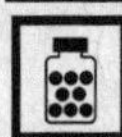

USES

- Treats intermittent claudication (leg pain caused by poor circulation).
- Improves blood vessel function.
- Treatment for other disorders as determined by your doctor.

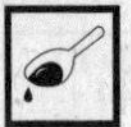

DOSAGE & USAGE INFORMATION

How to take:
Tablet—Swallow with liquid. If you can't swallow tablet whole, ask your pharmacist for advice.

When to take:
Twice a day. Take one half hour before or 2 hours after breakfast and dinner.

If you forget a dose:
Take as soon as you remember. If it is almost time for the next dose, wait for that dose (don't double this dose) and resume regular schedule.

What drug does:
Exact way it works is unknown. It increases blood flow by relaxing and expanding blood vessel walls. It keeps blood from clotting.

Time lapse before drug works:
3-4 weeks, but takes 12 weeks for full benefit.

Don't take with:
Any other medicine, herbal remedy or dietary supplements without consulting your doctor or pharmacist.

OVERDOSE

SYMPTOMS:
Severe headache, severe diarrhea, dizziness, change in heartbeat, nausea or vomiting; flushed, hot face.
WHAT TO DO:
Overdose unlikely to threaten life. If person uses much larger amount than prescribed or if accidentally swallowed, call doctor or poison control center 1-800-222-1222 for help.

POSSIBLE ADVERSE REACTIONS OR SIDE EFFECTS

SYMPTOMS	WHAT TO DO
Life-threatening: None expected.	
Common:	
• Fever, rapid or irregular heartbeat.	Discontinue. Call doctor right away.
• Back pain, gas, dizziness, cough, diarrhea, headache, muscle stiffness or pain, runny or stuffy nose, sore throat.	Continue. Call doctor when convenient.
Infrequent: Fainting, stools are bloody or black or tarry, nausea or indigestion or heartburn (severe or ongoing), tongue swelling, stiff neck, nosebleeds, severe stomach pain or cramping, vomiting blood or material like coffee grounds, unusual bleeding or bruising.	Discontinue. Call doctor right away.
Rare: Burning feeling in throat or chest, bone pain, difficulty in swallowing, ringing or buzzing in the ears, hives, joint pain or stiffness, swelling (face, arms, fingers or lower legs).	Continue. Call doctor when convenient.

INTERMITTENT CLAUDICATION AGENTS

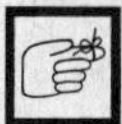

WARNINGS & PRECAUTIONS

Don't take if:
- You are allergic to cilostazol.
- You have congestive heart failure.

Before you start, consult your doctor if:
- You have heart disease, heart rhythm disorder or a bleeding disorder.
- You have liver or kidney disease.
- You suffer from migraines.
- You are a smoker.

Over age 60:
Adverse reactions and side effects may be more frequent and severe than in younger persons.

Pregnancy:
Decide with your doctor if drug benefits justify risk to unborn child. Risk category C (see page xviii).

Breast-feeding:
Drug passes into milk. Avoid drug or discontinue nursing until you finish medicine. Consult doctor about maintaining milk supply.

Infants & children:
Not recommended. Safety and dosage has not been established.

Prolonged use:
No problems expected.

Skin & sunlight:
No problems expected.

Driving, piloting or hazardous work:
Avoid if you feel dizzy or weak. Otherwise, no problems expected.

Discontinuing:
Don't discontinue without doctor's advice until you complete prescribed dose, even though symptoms diminish or disappear.

Others:
- Response to drug varies. If your symptoms don't improve after 3 weeks of use, consult doctor.
- Avoid smoking while taking this medication, as it may worsen your condition.
- Advise any doctor or dentist whom you consult that you take this medicine.

POSSIBLE INTERACTION WITH OTHER DRUGS

GENERIC NAME OR DRUG CLASS	COMBINED EFFECT
Enzyme inhibitors*	Increased effect of intermittent claudication agent.
Sertraline	Increased effect of intermittent claudication agent

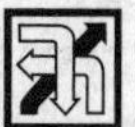

POSSIBLE INTERACTION WITH OTHER SUBSTANCES

INTERACTS WITH	COMBINED EFFECT
Alcohol:	None expected.
Beverages: Grapefruit juice.	Increased effect of intermittent claudication agent.
Cocaine:	Unknown effect. Avoid.
Foods: Grapefruit.	Increased effect of intermittent claudication agent.
Marijuana:	Unknown effect. Avoid.
Tobacco:	Decreased effect of intermittent claudication agent. Also, nicotine narrows your blood vessels. Avoid.

*See Glossary

IODOQUINOL

BRAND NAMES

Diiodohydroxyquin
Diodoquin
Diquinol
Yodoquinol
Yodoxin

BASIC INFORMATION

Habit forming? No
Prescription needed? Yes
Available as generic? Yes
Drug class: Antiprotozoal, antiparasitic

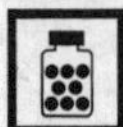

USES

Treatment for intestinal amebiasis and balantidiasis.

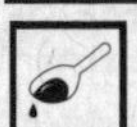

DOSAGE & USAGE INFORMATION

How to take:
Tablet—Mix with applesauce or chocolate syrup if unable to swallow tablets.

When to take:
Three times daily after meals for 20 days. Treatment may be repeated after 2 to 3 weeks.

If you forget a dose:
Take as soon as you remember. If it is almost time for the next dose, wait for that dose (don't double this dose) and resume regular schedule.

What drug does:
Kills amoeba (microscopic parasites) in intestinal tract.

Time lapse before drug works:
May require full course of treatment (20 days) to cure.

Don't take with:
Any other medicine or any dietary supplement without consulting your doctor or pharmacist.

OVERDOSE

SYMPTOMS:
- **Prolonged dosing at high level may produce blurred vision, muscle pain, eye pain, numbness and tingling in hands or feet.**
- **Single overdosage unlikely to threaten life.**

WHAT TO DO:
If person takes much larger amount than prescribed, dial 911 (emergency) for medical help or call poison control center 1-800-222-1222 for instructions.

POSSIBLE ADVERSE REACTIONS OR SIDE EFFECTS

SYMPTOMS	WHAT TO DO
Life-threatening: None expected.	
Common: Diarrhea, nausea, vomiting, abdominal pain.	Continue. Call doctor when convenient.
Infrequent: • Clumsiness, rash, hives, itching, blurred vision, muscle pain, numbness or tingling in hands or feet, chills, fever, weakness.	Discontinue. Call doctor right away.
• Swelling of neck (thyroid gland).	Continue. Call doctor when convenient.
Rare: Dizziness, headache, rectal itching.	Continue. Call doctor when convenient.

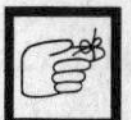

WARNINGS & PRECAUTIONS

Don't take if:
You are allergic to iodoquinol.

Before you start, consult your doctor if:
- You have optic atrophy or thyroid disease.
- You have kidney or liver disease.

Over age 60:
Adverse reactions and side effects may be more frequent and severe than in younger persons.

Pregnancy:
Decide with your doctor if drug benefits justify risk to unborn child. Risk category C (see page xviii).

Breast-feeding:
No proven problems, but avoid if possible. Discontinue nursing until you finish medicine. Consult doctor for advice on maintaining milk supply.

Infants & children:
Not recommended. Safety and dosage has not been established.

Prolonged use:
Not recommended.

Skin & sunlight:
No problems expected.

Driving, piloting or hazardous work:
No problems expected.

Discontinuing:
Don't discontinue without consulting doctor.

Others:
- Thyroid tests may be inaccurate for as long as 6 months after discontinuing iodoquinol treatment.
- May interfere with the accuracy of some medical tests.

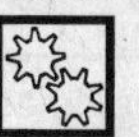

POSSIBLE INTERACTION WITH OTHER DRUGS

GENERIC NAME OR DRUG CLASS	COMBINED EFFECT
None expected.	

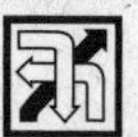

POSSIBLE INTERACTION WITH OTHER SUBSTANCES

INTERACTS WITH	COMBINED EFFECT
Alcohol:	None expected.
Beverages:	None expected.
Cocaine:	None expected.
Foods:	Taking with food may decrease gastrointestinal side effects.
Marijuana:	None expected.
Tobacco:	None expected.

IPRATROPIUM

BRAND NAMES

Apo-Ipravent
Atrovent
Atrovent Inhalation Aerosol
Combivent Respimat
Duoneb
Kendral-Ipratropium

BASIC INFORMATION

Habit forming? No
Prescription needed? Yes
Available as generic? Yes
Drug class: Bronchodilator, anticholinergic

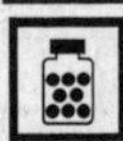

USES

- Treats asthma, bronchitis and emphysema.
- Should not be used alone for acute asthma attacks. May be used with inhalation forms of albuterol or fenoterol.
- May be used to treat rhinorrhea (runny nose).

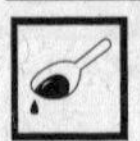

DOSAGE & USAGE INFORMATION

How to use:

- Inhalation aerosol or solution—Carefully follow the printed instructions provided with the inhaler. Avoid contact with eyes.
- Nasal spray—Prime the nasal spray pump as directed, then spray in each nostril. Avoid contact with eyes.

When to take:
Inhalation form may be started at 2 inhalations, 4 times a day and increased by your doctor as needed. Usual dose of nasal form is 2 sprays in each nostril, 2 to 3 times a day.

If you forget a dose:
Use as soon as you remember. If it is almost time for the next dose, wait for next scheduled dose (don't double this dose).

What drug does:
Dilates (opens or widens) bronchial tubes or nasal passages by direct effect on them.

Continued next column

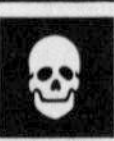

OVERDOSE

SYMPTOMS:
None likely.
WHAT TO DO:
Overdose unlikely to threaten life. If person uses much larger amount than prescribed or if accidentally swallowed, call doctor or poison control center 1-800-222-1222 for help.

Time lapse before drug works:
Inhalation form may take 2 to 3 days for full effectiveness. Effect of nasal form may begin right away or take a few days.

Don't take with:
Any other medicines (including over-the-counter drugs such as cough and cold medicines, laxatives, antacids, diet pills, caffeine, nose drops or vitamins) without consulting your doctor or pharmacist.

POSSIBLE ADVERSE REACTIONS OR SIDE EFFECTS

SYMPTOMS	WHAT TO DO
Life-threatening:	
Rare allergic reaction—Breathing difficulty; closing of the throat; swelling of hands, feet, face, lips or tongue; hives.	Discontinue. Seek emergency treatment.
Common:	
Cough, dry mouth, unpleasant taste.	Continue. Call doctor when convenient.
Infrequent:	
Blurred vision or other vision changes, difficult urination, stuffy nose, sweating, tremors, weakness, dizziness, nervousness, headache.	Continue. Call doctor when convenient.
Rare:	
Skin rash or hives, ongoing constipation, increased wheezing, chest tightness or difficulty in breathing, pounding heartbeat, stomach pain or bloating, severe eye pain.	Discontinue. Call doctor right away.

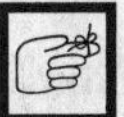

WARNINGS & PRECAUTIONS

Don't take if:
You are sensitive to ipratropium, belladonna, atropine or soybeans, soy lecithin or peanuts.

Before you start, consult your doctor if:
- You have prostate trouble.
- You have glaucoma.
- You have difficulty in urinating.

Over age 60:
Adverse reactions and side effects may be more frequent and severe than in younger persons. You may need smaller doses for shorter periods of time.

Pregnancy:
Decide with your doctor if drug benefits justify risk to unborn child. Risk category B (see page xviii).

Breast-feeding:
It is unknown if drug passes into milk. Avoid drug or discontinue nursing until you finish medicine. Consult doctor for advice on maintaining milk supply.

Infants & children:
Inhalation form may be used in children over age 12. Nasal spray may be used in children over age 6.

Prolonged use:
- For inhalation form, see your doctor to verify drug's effectiveness and for dose adjustment if needed and for eye pressure exams.
- Nasal form should not be used for more than 4 days.

Skin & sunlight:
No problems expected.

Driving, piloting or hazardous work:
Avoid if you feel confused, drowsy or dizzy.

Discontinuing:
No special problems expected.

Others:
- Advise any doctor or dentist whom you consult that you take this medicine.
- Do not increase the drug dosage without your doctor's approval.
- Allow 5-minute intervals between ipratropium inhalations and inhalations of cromolyn, cortisone or other inhalant medicines.

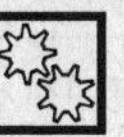

POSSIBLE INTERACTION WITH OTHER DRUGS

GENERIC NAME OR DRUG CLASS	COMBINED EFFECT
Anticholinergics*	Increased anticholinergic effect.
Cromolyn (inhalation form)	Wait 5 minutes after using ipratropium before using cromolyn.

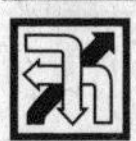

POSSIBLE INTERACTION WITH OTHER SUBSTANCES

INTERACTS WITH	COMBINED EFFECT
Alcohol:	None expected.
Beverages:	None expected.
Cocaine:	Unknown effect. Avoid.
Foods:	None expected.
Marijuana:	Unknown effect. Avoid.
Tobacco:	None expected, but smoking should be avoided.

***See Glossary**

IRON SUPPLEMENTS

GENERIC AND BRAND NAMES

See full list of generic and brand names in the *Generic and Brand Name Directory*, page 886.

BASIC INFORMATION

Habit forming? No
Prescription needed? No
Available as generic? Yes
Drug class: Mineral supplement (iron)

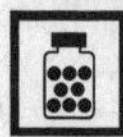

USES

Treatment for dietary iron deficiency or iron-deficiency anemia from other causes.

DOSAGE & USAGE INFORMATION

How to take:
- Tablet, capsule or syrup—Swallow with liquid or food to lessen stomach irritation. If you can't swallow whole, crumble tablet or open capsule and take with liquid or food. Place medicine far back on tongue to avoid staining teeth.
- Extended-release capsule—Swallow whole with liquid. Do not crush.
- Chewable tablet—Chew well before swallowing.
- Liquid—Dilute dose in beverage before swallowing and drink through a straw.

When to take:
1 hour before or 2 hours after eating.

If you forget a dose:
Take as soon as you remember. If it is almost time for the next dose, wait for that dose (don't double this dose) and resume regular schedule.

Continued next column

OVERDOSE

SYMPTOMS:
- **Moderate overdose—Stomach pain, vomiting, diarrhea, black stools, lethargy.**
- **Serious overdose—Weakness and collapse; pallor, weak and rapid heartbeat; shallow breathing; convulsions and coma.**

WHAT TO DO:
- **Dial 911 (emergency) for medical help or call poison control center 1-800-222-1222 for instructions.**
- **See emergency information on last 3 pages of this book.**

What drug does:
Stimulates bone marrow's production of hemoglobin (red blood cell pigment that carries oxygen to body cells).

Time lapse before drug works:
3 to 7 days. May require 3 weeks for maximum benefit.

Don't take with:
Any other medicine or any dietary supplement without consulting your doctor or pharmacist.

POSSIBLE ADVERSE REACTIONS OR SIDE EFFECTS

SYMPTOMS	WHAT TO DO
Life-threatening: In case of overdose, see previous column.	
Common:	
• Stomach pain that is continuing.	Discontinue. Call doctor right away.
• Dark green or black stool, teeth stained with liquid iron, constipation, diarrhea, mild nausea or vomiting.	Continue. Call doctor when convenient.
Infrequent: None expected.	
Rare:	
• Throat pain on swallowing, chest pain, cramps, blood in stool or black stool that has sticky consistency.	Discontinue. Call doctor right away.
• Darkened urine, heartburn.	Continue. Call doctor when convenient.

WARNINGS & PRECAUTIONS

Don't take if:
- You are allergic to any iron supplement or tartrazine dye.
- You take iron injections.
- You have acute hepatitis, hemosiderosis or hemochromatosis (conditions involving excess iron in body).
- You have hemolytic anemia.

Before you start, consult your doctor if:
- You plan to become pregnant while on medication.
- You have had stomach surgery.
- You have had peptic ulcer, enteritis or colitis.

Over age 60:
May cause hemochromatosis (iron storage disease) with bronze skin, liver damage, diabetes, heart problems and impotence.

Pregnancy:
Take only if your doctor advises. Risk category C (see page xviii).

Breast-feeding:
No problems expected. Take only if your doctor confirms you have a dietary deficiency or an iron-deficiency anemia.

Infants & children:
Use only under medical supervision. Overdose common and dangerous. Keep out of children's reach.

Prolonged use:
- May cause hemochromatosis (iron storage disease) with bronze skin, liver damage, diabetes, heart problems and impotence.
- Talk to your doctor about the need for follow-up medical examinations or laboratory studies to check complete blood counts (white blood cell count, platelet count, red blood cell count, hemoglobin, hematocrit), serum iron, total iron-binding capacity.

Skin & sunlight:
No problems expected.

Driving, piloting or hazardous work:
No problems expected.

Discontinuing:
May be unnecessary to finish medicine. Follow doctor's instructions.

Others:
- Liquid form stains teeth. Mix with water or juice to lessen the effect. Brush with baking soda or hydrogen peroxide to help remove stain.
- Some products contain tartrazine dye. Avoid, especially if you are allergic to aspirin.
- May interfere with the accuracy of some medical tests.
- If using extended-release form or coated tablet and your stools don't turn black, consult doctor. The tablet may not be breaking down, and an underdose may result.

POSSIBLE INTERACTION WITH OTHER DRUGS

GENERIC NAME OR DRUG CLASS	COMBINED EFFECT
Acetohydroxamic acid	Decreased effects of both drugs.
Antacids*	Poor iron absorption.
Chloramphenicol	Decreased effect of iron. Interferes with formation of red blood cells and hemoglobin.
Cholestyramine	Decreased iron effect.
Etidronate	Decreased etidronate effect. Take at least 2 hours after iron supplement.
H_2 antagonists*	Decreased iron effect.
Iron supplements, other*	Possible excess iron storage in liver.
Proton pump inhibitors	May decrease effect of iron supplement.
Tetracyclines*	Decreased tetracycline effect. Take iron 3 hours before or 2 hours after taking tetracycline.
Vitamin E	Decreased iron and vitamin E effect.
Zinc supplements	Increased need for zinc.

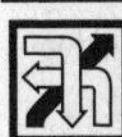

POSSIBLE INTERACTION WITH OTHER SUBSTANCES

INTERACTS WITH	COMBINED EFFECT
Alcohol:	Increased iron absorption. May cause organ damage. Avoid or use in moderation.
Beverages: Milk, tea.	Decreased iron effect.
Cocaine:	None expected.
Foods: Dairy foods, eggs, whole-grain bread and cereal.	Decreased iron effect.
Marijuana:	None expected.
Tobacco:	None expected.

*See Glossary

ISONIAZID

BRAND NAMES

INH
Isotamine
Laniazid
Nydrazid
PMS Isoniazid
Rifamate
Tubizid

BASIC INFORMATION

Habit forming? No
Prescription needed? Yes
Available as generic? Yes
Drug class: Antitubercular

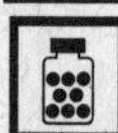

USES

Kills tuberculosis germs.

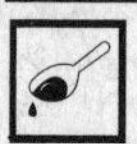

DOSAGE & USAGE INFORMATION

How to take:
- Tablet—Swallow with liquid to lessen stomach irritation.
- Syrup—Follow label directions.

When to take:
At the same time each day.

If you forget a dose:
Take as soon as you remember up to 12 hours late. If more than 12 hours, wait for next scheduled dose (don't double this dose).

What drug does:
Interferes with TB germ metabolism. Eventually destroys the germ.

Time lapse before drug works:
3 to 6 months. You may need to take drug as long as 2 years.

Don't take with:
Any other medicine or any dietary supplement without consulting your doctor or pharmacist.

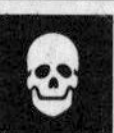

OVERDOSE

SYMPTOMS:
Difficult breathing, convulsions, coma.
WHAT TO DO:
- **Dial 911 (emergency) for medical help or call poison control center 1-800-222-1222 for instructions.**
- **If person is unconscious, check breathing and pulse. If not breathing, begin mouth-to-mouth rescue breathing. If heart is not beating, begin chest compressions.**
- **See emergency information on last 3 pages of this book.**

POSSIBLE ADVERSE REACTIONS OR SIDE EFFECTS

SYMPTOMS	WHAT TO DO
Life-threatening: In case of overdose, see previous column.	
Common:	
• Muscle pain and pain in joints, tingling or numbness in extremities, jaundice.	Discontinue. Call doctor right away.
• Confusion, unsteady walk.	Continue. Call doctor when convenient.
Infrequent:	
• Swollen glands, nausea, indigestion, diarrhea, vomiting.	Discontinue. Call doctor right away.
• Dizziness, appetite loss.	Continue. Call doctor when convenient.
Rare:	
• Rash, fever, impaired vision, anemia with fatigue, weakness, fever, sore throat, unusual bleeding or bruising.	Discontinue. Call doctor right away.
• Breast enlargement or discomfort.	Continue. Tell doctor at next visit.

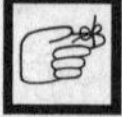

WARNINGS & PRECAUTIONS

Don't take if:
You are allergic to isoniazid.

Before you start, consult your doctor if:
- You plan to become pregnant within medication period.
- You are allergic to ethionamide, pyrazinamide or nicotinic acid.
- You drink alcohol.
- You have liver or kidney disease.
- You have epilepsy, diabetes or lupus.

Over age 60:
Adverse reactions and side effects, especially jaundice, may be more frequent and severe than in younger persons. Kidneys may be less efficient.

Pregnancy:
Decide with your doctor if drug benefits justify risk to unborn child. Risk category C (see page xviii).

Breast-feeding:
Drug passes into milk. Avoid drug or discontinue nursing until you finish medicine. Consult doctor for advice on maintaining milk supply.

Infants & children:
Use only under medical supervision.

Prolonged use:
- Numbness and tingling of hands and feet.
- Talk to your doctor about the need for follow-up medical examinations or laboratory studies to check liver function, eyes.

Skin & sunlight:
No problems expected.

Driving, piloting or hazardous work:
Avoid if you feel dizzy. Otherwise, no problems expected.

Discontinuing:
Don't discontinue without doctor's advice until you complete prescribed dose, even though symptoms diminish or disappear.

Others:
- Diabetic patients may have false blood sugar tests.
- Periodic liver function tests and laboratory blood studies recommended.
- Prescription for vitamin B-6 (pyridoxine) recommended to prevent nerve damage.
- Advise any doctor or dentist whom you consult that you take this medicine.

POSSIBLE INTERACTION WITH OTHER DRUGS

GENERIC NAME OR DRUG CLASS	COMBINED EFFECT
Acetaminophen	Increased risk of liver damage.
Adrenocorticoids, systemic	Decreased isoniazid effect.
Alfentanil	Prolonged duration of alfentanil effect (undesirable).
Antacids* (aluminum-containing)	Decreased absorption of isoniazid.
Anticholinergics*	May increase pressure within eyeball.
Anticoagulants, oral*	Increased anticoagulant effect.
Antidiabetics*	Increased antidiabetic effect.
Antihypertensives*	Increased antihypertensive effect.
Antivirals, HIV/AIDS*	Increased risk of peripheral neuropathy.
Carbamazepine	Increased risk of liver damage.
Cycloserine	Increased risk of central nervous system effects.
Disulfiram	Increased effect of disulfiram.
Laxatives*	Decreased absorption and effect of isoniazid.
Hepatotoxics*	Increased risk of liver damage.
Ketoconazole	Increased risk of liver damage.
Narcotics*	Increased narcotic effect.
Phenytoin	Increased phenytoin effect.
Pyridoxine (Vitamin B-6)	Decreases risk of nerve damage in extremities.
Rifampin	Increased isoniazid toxicity to liver.
Sedatives*	Increased sedative effect.
Stimulants*	Increased stimulant effect.

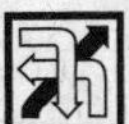

POSSIBLE INTERACTION WITH OTHER SUBSTANCES

INTERACTS WITH	COMBINED EFFECT
Alcohol:	Increased incidence of liver disease and seizures.
Beverages:	None expected.
Cocaine:	None expected.
Foods: Swiss or Cheshire cheese, fish.	Red or itching skin, fast heartbeat. Seek emergency treatment.
Marijuana:	No interactions expected, but marijuana may slow body's recovery.
Tobacco:	No interactions expected, but tobacco may slow body's recovery.

*See Glossary

ISOTRETINOIN

BRAND NAMES

Absorica
Amnesteem
Claravis
Sotret

BASIC INFORMATION

Habit forming? No
Prescription needed? Yes
Available as generic? Yes
Drug classification: Antiacne (systemic)

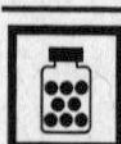

USES

- Decreases cystic acne formation in severe cases.
- Treats certain other skin disorders involving an overabundance of outer skin layer.

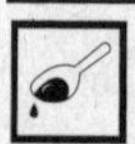

DOSAGE & USAGE INFORMATION

How to take:
Capsule—Swallow whole with a glass of water or liquid (this helps decrease risk of esophagus irritation). Do not chew, crush or open capsule.

When to take:
Twice a day. Follow prescription directions.

If you forget a dose:
Take as soon as you remember. If it is almost time for the next dose, wait for that dose (don't double this dose) and resume regular schedule.

What drug does:
Reduces sebaceous gland activity and size.

Time lapse before drug works:
May require 15 to 20 weeks to experience full benefit.

Don't take with:
- Vitamin A or supplements containing Vitamin A.
- Any other medicine or any dietary supplement without consulting your doctor or pharmacist.

OVERDOSE

SYMPTOMS:
None reported.
WHAT TO DO:
Overdose unlikely to threaten life. If person uses much larger amount than prescribed or if accidentally swallowed, call doctor or poison control center 1-800-222-1222 for help.

POSSIBLE ADVERSE REACTIONS OR SIDE EFFECTS

SYMPTOMS	WHAT TO DO
Life-threatening: None expected.	
Common:	
• Burning, red, itching eyes; lip scaling; burning pain; nosebleeds.	Discontinue. Call doctor right away.
• Itchy skin.	Continue. Call doctor when convenient.
• Dry mouth.	Continue. Tell doctor at next visit. (Suck ice or chew gum).
Infrequent:	
• Rash, infection, nausea, vomiting.	Discontinue. Call doctor right away.
• Pain in muscles, bones, joints; hair thinning; tiredness.	Continue. Call doctor when convenient.
Rare:	
• Severe stomach pain, bleeding gums, blurred vision, severe diarrhea, continuing headache, vomiting, eye pain, rectal bleeding, yellow skin or eyes, serious depression, psychosis, thoughts of suicide.	Discontinue. Call doctor right away.
• Mild headache, increased sensitivity to light, stomach upset, peeling of skin on palms or soles of feet.	Continue. Call doctor when convenient.

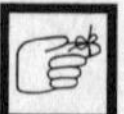

WARNINGS & PRECAUTIONS

Don't take if:
- You are allergic to isotretinoin, etretinate, tretinoin or vitamin A derivatives.
- You are pregnant or plan pregnancy.
- *You are even able to bear children. Read, understand and follow the patient information enclosed with your prescription.*

Before you start, consult your doctor if:
- You have diabetes.
- You or any member of family have high triglyceride levels in blood.
- You or family members have a history of severe depression.

Over age 60:
Adverse reactions and side effects may be more frequent and severe than in younger persons.

Pregnancy:
Causes birth defects in fetus. Don't use. Risk category X (see page xviii).

Breast-feeding:
Effect unknown. Not recommended. Consult doctor.

Infants & children:
Not approved for ages under 12. Use under close medical supervision for ages 13 to 18.

Prolonged use:
- Possible damage to cornea of the eye.
- Talk to your doctor about the need for follow-up medical examinations or laboratory studies to check complete blood counts (white blood cell count, platelet count, red blood cell count, hemoglobin, hematocrit), liver function, blood lipids, blood sugar.

Skin & sunlight:
May cause rash or intensify sunburn in areas exposed to sun or ultraviolet light (photosensitivity reaction). Avoid overexposure. Notify doctor if reaction occurs.

Driving, piloting or hazardous work:
Use caution if there is a decrease in your night vision or you are unable to see well. Consult doctor.

Discontinuing:
Single course of treatment is usually all that's needed. If second course required, wait 8 weeks after completing first course.

Others:
- Use only for severe cases of cystic acne that have not responded to less hazardous forms of acne treatment.
- May interfere with the accuracy of some medical tests.
- May cause bone problems (osteoporosis, fractures, delayed healing).
- Don't donate blood for at least 30 days after discontinuing medicine.
- Acne may worsen at the start of treatment.
- Contact lens wearers may experience discomfort during treatment with this drug.
- Contact doctor right away if a person taking this drug develops symptoms of depression, psychosis (severe mental problems) or has any suicide thoughts or suicide behaviors.
- Advise any doctor or dentist whom you consult that you take this medicine.
- **If you are planning pregnancy or are at risk of pregnancy, don't take this drug.**

POSSIBLE INTERACTION WITH OTHER DRUGS

GENERIC NAME OR DRUG CLASS	COMBINED EFFECT
Antiacne topical preparations* (other), cosmetics (medicated), skin preparations with alcohol, soaps or cleansers (abrasive)	Severe skin irritation.
Etretinate	Increased chance of toxicity of each drug.
Tetracyclines*	Increased risk of developing pseudotumor cerebri.*
Topical drugs or cosmetics	May interact with isotretinoin.
Tretinoin	Increased chance of toxicity.
Vitamin A	Additive toxic effect of each. Avoid.

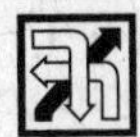

POSSIBLE INTERACTION WITH OTHER SUBSTANCES

INTERACTS WITH	COMBINED EFFECT
Alcohol:	Increase in triglycerides in blood. Avoid.
Beverages:	None expected.
Cocaine:	Increased chance of toxicity of isotretinoin. Avoid.
Foods:	None expected.
Marijuana:	Increased chance of toxicity of isotretinoin. Avoid.
Tobacco:	May decrease absorption of drug. Avoid tobacco during treatment.

***See Glossary**

ISOXSUPRINE

BRAND NAMES

Vasodilan
Vasoprine

BASIC INFORMATION

Habit forming? No
Prescription needed? Yes
Available as generic? Yes
Drug class: Vasodilator

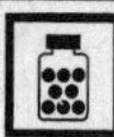

USES

- May improve poor blood circulation.
- Management of premature labor.
- Treatment for painful menstruation.

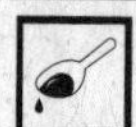

DOSAGE & USAGE INFORMATION

How to take:
Tablet—Swallow with liquid or food to lessen stomach irritation. If you can't swallow whole, crumble tablet and take with liquid or food.

When to take:
At the same times each day.

If you forget a dose:
Take as soon as you remember. If it is almost time for the next dose, wait for that dose (don't double this dose) and resume regular schedule.

What drug does:
Expands blood vessels, increasing flow and permitting distribution of oxygen and nutrients.

Time lapse before drug works:
1 hour.

Don't take with:
Any other medicine or any dietary supplement without consulting your doctor or pharmacist.

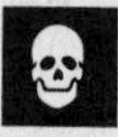

OVERDOSE

SYMPTOMS:
Headache, dizziness, flush, vomiting, weakness, sweating, fainting, shortness of breath, coma.
WHAT TO DO:

- **Dial 911 (emergency) for medical help or call poison control center 1-800-222-1222 for instructions.**
- **If person is unconscious, check breathing and pulse. If not breathing, begin mouth-to-mouth rescue breathing. If heart is not beating, begin chest compressions.**
- **See emergency information on last 3 pages of this book.**

POSSIBLE ADVERSE REACTIONS OR SIDE EFFECTS

SYMPTOMS	WHAT TO DO
Life-threatening: In case of overdose, see previous column.	
Common: None expected.	
Infrequent: Nausea, vomiting.	Continue. Call doctor when convenient.
Rare: Rapid or irregular heartbeat, rash, chest pain, shortness of breath.	Discontinue. Call doctor right away.

WARNINGS & PRECAUTIONS

Don't take if:

- You are allergic to any vasodilator.
- You have any bleeding disease.

Before you start, consult your doctor if:

- You have high blood pressure, hardening of the arteries or heart disease.
- You plan to become pregnant within medication period.
- You have glaucoma.

Over age 60:
Adverse reactions and side effects may be more frequent and severe than in younger persons.

Pregnancy:
Decide with your doctor whether drug benefits justify risk to unborn child. Risk category C (see page xviii).

Breast-feeding:
No problems expected, but consult doctor.

Infants & children:
Not recommended.

Prolonged use:
Talk to your doctor about the need for follow-up medical examinations or laboratory studies.

Skin & sunlight:
No problems expected.

Driving, piloting or hazardous work:
Avoid if you feel dizzy or faint. Otherwise, no problems expected.

Discontinuing:
Don't discontinue without doctor's advice until you complete prescribed dose, even though symptoms diminish or disappear.

Others:

- Be cautious when arising from lying or sitting position, when climbing stairs, or if dizziness occurs.
- May interfere with the accuracy of some medical tests.
- Advise any doctor or dentist whom you consult that you take this medicine.

POSSIBLE INTERACTION WITH OTHER DRUGS

GENERIC NAME OR DRUG CLASS	COMBINED EFFECT
None significant.	

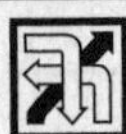

POSSIBLE INTERACTION WITH OTHER SUBSTANCES

INTERACTS WITH	COMBINED EFFECT
Alcohol:	None expected.
Beverages: Milk.	Decreased stomach irritation.
Cocaine:	Decreased blood circulation to extremities. Avoid.
Foods:	None expected.
Marijuana:	Rapid heartbeat.
Tobacco:	Decreased isoxsuprine effect; nicotine constricts blood vessels.

KANAMYCIN

BRAND NAMES

Kantrex

BASIC INFORMATION

Habit forming? No
Prescription needed? Yes
Available as generic? No
Drug class: Bowel preparation

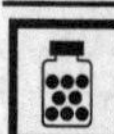

USES

- To cleanse bowel of bacteria prior to intestinal surgery.
- Treats hepatic coma.

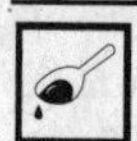

DOSAGE & USAGE INFORMATION

How to take:
Capsule—Swallow with liquid. If you can't swallow whole, open capsule and take with liquid or food. Instructions to take on empty stomach mean 1 hour before or 2 hours after eating.

When to take:
At the same time each day, according to instructions on prescription label.

If you forget a dose:
Take as soon as you remember up to 2 hours late. If more than 2 hours, wait for next scheduled dose (don't double this dose).

What drug does:
Kills susceptible bacteria in the intestines.

Time lapse before drug works:
15 to 30 minutes.

Don't take with:
Any other medicine or any dietary supplement without consulting your doctor or pharmacist.

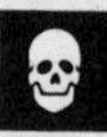

OVERDOSE

SYMPTOMS:
Clumsiness, dizziness, seizures, coma.
WHAT TO DO:

- **Dial 911 (emergency) for medical help or call poison control center 1-800-222-1222 for instructions.**
- **See emergency information on last 3 pages of this book.**

POSSIBLE ADVERSE REACTIONS OR SIDE EFFECTS

SYMPTOMS	WHAT TO DO
Life-threatening: In case of overdose, see previous column.	
Common: Mouth irritation or soreness, nausea.	Continue. Call doctor when convenient.
Infrequent: Vomiting.	Discontinue. Call doctor right away.
Rare: Decreased urine, hearing loss, ringing in ears, clumsiness, unsteadiness, skin rash.	Discontinue. Call doctor right away.

WARNINGS & PRECAUTIONS

Don't take if:
- You are allergic to kanamycin.
- You can't tolerate any aminoglycoside.

Before you start, consult your doctor if:
- You have hearing difficulty.
- You have intestinal obstruction.
- You have severe kidney disease.
- You have ulcerative colitis.

Over age 60:
Adverse reactions and side effects may be more frequent and severe than in younger persons. You may need smaller doses for shorter periods of time.

Pregnancy:
Consult doctor. Risk category D (see page xviii).

Breast-feeding:
No special problems expected. Consult doctor.

Infants & children:
Not recommended for prolonged use.

Prolonged use:
Not recommended for prolonged use.

Skin & sunlight:
No problems expected.

Driving, piloting or hazardous work:
Avoid if you feel confused, drowsy or dizzy.

Discontinuing:
Not recommended for prolonged use.

Others:
No problems expected.

POSSIBLE INTERACTION WITH OTHER DRUGS

GENERIC NAME OR DRUG CLASS	COMBINED EFFECT
None significant.	

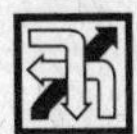

POSSIBLE INTERACTION WITH OTHER SUBSTANCES

INTERACTS WITH	COMBINED EFFECT
Alcohol:	None expected.
Beverages:	None expected.
Cocaine:	None expected.
Foods:	None expected.
Marijuana:	None expected.
Tobacco:	None expected.

KAOLIN & PECTIN

BRAND NAMES

Donnagel-MB
Kao-Con
Kaotin
Kapectolin
Kapectolin with Paregoric
K-C
K-P
K-Pek
Parepectolin

BASIC INFORMATION

Habit forming? No
Prescription needed? No
Available as generic? Yes
Drug class: Antidiarrheal

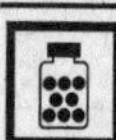

USES

Treats mild to moderate diarrhea. Used in conjunction with fluids, appropriate diet and rest. Treats symptoms only. Does not cure any disorder that causes diarrhea.

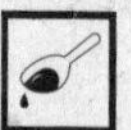

DOSAGE & USAGE INFORMATION

How to take:
Liquid—Swallow prescribed dosage (without diluting) after each loose bowel movement.

When to take:
After each loose bowel movement.

If you forget a dose:
Take when you remember.

What drug does:
Makes loose stools less watery, but may not prevent loss of fluids.

Time lapse before drug works:
15 to 30 minutes.

Don't take with:
Any other medicine or any dietary supplement without consulting your doctor or pharmacist.

OVERDOSE

SYMPTOMS:
Fecal impaction.
WHAT TO DO:
Overdose unlikely to threaten life. If person uses much larger amount than prescribed or if accidentally swallowed, call doctor or poison control center 1-800-222-1222 for help.

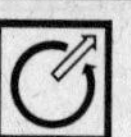

POSSIBLE ADVERSE REACTIONS OR SIDE EFFECTS

SYMPTOMS	WHAT TO DO
Life-threatening: None expected.	
Common: None expected.	
Infrequent: None expected.	
Rare: Constipation (mild).	Continue. Call doctor when convenient.

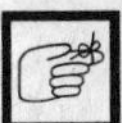

WARNINGS & PRECAUTIONS

Don't take if:
You are allergic to kaolin or pectin.

Before you start, consult your doctor if:
- Patient is child or infant.
- You have any chronic medical problem with heart disease, peptic ulcer, asthma or others.
- You have fever over 101°F.

Over age 60:
Fluid loss caused by diarrhea, especially if taking other medicines, may lead to serious disability. Consult doctor.

Pregnancy:
Consult doctor. Risk category C (see page xviii).

Breast-feeding:
No problems expected.

Infants & children:
Fluid loss caused by diarrhea in infants and children can cause serious dehydration. Consult doctor before giving any medicine for diarrhea.

Prolonged use:
Not recommended.

Skin & sunlight:
No problems expected.

Driving, piloting or hazardous work:
No problems expected.

Discontinuing:
May be unnecessary to finish medicine. Follow doctor's instructions.

Others:
Consult doctor about fluids, diet and rest.

POSSIBLE INTERACTION WITH OTHER DRUGS

GENERIC NAME OR DRUG CLASS	COMBINED EFFECT
Digoxin	Decreases absorption of digoxin. Separate doses by at least 2 hours.
Lincomycins*	Decreases absorption of lincomycin. Separate doses by at least 2 hours.
All other oral medicines	May decrease absorption of other medicines. Separate doses by at least 2 hours.

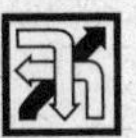

POSSIBLE INTERACTION WITH OTHER SUBSTANCES

INTERACTS WITH	COMBINED EFFECT
Alcohol:	Increased diarrhea. Prevents action of kaolin and pectin.
Beverages:	None expected.
Cocaine:	Aggravates underlying disease. Avoid.
Foods:	None expected.
Marijuana:	Aggravates underlying disease. Avoid.
Tobacco:	Aggravates underlying disease. Avoid.

***See Glossary**

KERATOLYTICS

GENERIC AND BRAND NAMES

See full list of generic and brand names in the *Generic and Brand Name Directory*, page 886.

BASIC INFORMATION

Habit forming? No
Prescription needed? Yes, on some.
Available as generic? Yes
Drug class: Keratolytic, antiacne (topical), antiseborrheic

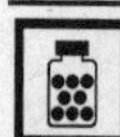

USES

Treatment for skin disorders such as acne, psoriasis, ichthyosis, keratosis, folliculitis, flat warts, eczema, urticaria, calluses, corns, seborrheic dermatitis, dandruff and others.

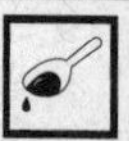

DOSAGE & USAGE INFORMATION

How to use:
Cream, gel, lotion, ointment, pads, plaster, shampoo, soap, topical solution, suspension—Always follow instructions on the label or use as directed by your doctor.

When to use:
At the same time each day or as needed.

If you forget an application:
Use as soon as you remember.

What drug does:
Keratolytics are drugs that soften, loosen and remove keratin (the tough outer layer of the skin).

Time lapse before drug works:
2 to 3 weeks. May require 6 weeks for maximum improvement.

Don't use with:
- Benzoyl peroxide. Apply 12 hours apart.
- Any other topical medicine without consulting your doctor or pharmacist.

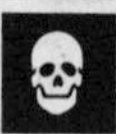

OVERDOSE

SYMPTOMS:
None expected.
WHAT TO DO:
If person swallows drug, dial 911 (emergency) for medical help or call poison control center 1-800-222-1222 for instructions.

POSSIBLE ADVERSE REACTIONS OR SIDE EFFECTS

SYMPTOMS	WHAT TO DO
Life-threatening:	
None expected.	
Common:	
• Pigment change in treated area, warmth or stinging, peeling.	Continue. Tell doctor at next visit.
• Sensitivity to wind or cold.	No action necessary.
Infrequent:	
Blistering, crusting, severe burning, swelling, skin irritation that begins after treatment.	Discontinue. Call doctor right away.
Rare:	
Symptoms of systemic toxicity (diarrhea, nausea, dizziness, headache, breathing difficulty, tiredness, weakness).	Discontinue. Call doctor right away.

WARNINGS & PRECAUTIONS

Don't take if:

- You are allergic to resorcinol or salicylic acid.
- You are sunburned or windburned or have an open skin wound, skin irritation or infection.

Before you start, consult your doctor if:

- You have eczema.
- You have diabetes.
- You have peripheral vascular disease (blood vessel disease).

Over age 60:
No problems expected.

Pregnancy:
Risk factors vary for drugs in this group. See category list on page xviii and consult doctor.

Breast-feeding:
No problems expected. Consult doctor.

Infants & children:
Not recommended. Increased risk of toxicity.

Prolonged use:
No problems expected.

Skin & sunlight:
No special problems expected.

Driving, piloting or hazardous work:
No problems expected.

Discontinuing:
Follow your doctor's instructions or the directions on the label.

Others:

- Acne may get worse before improvement starts in 2 or 3 weeks. Don't wash face more than 2 or 3 times daily.
- Keep medicine away from mouth or eyes. If it accidentally gets into the eyes, flush immediately with clear water.
- Keep medicine away from heat or flame.

POSSIBLE INTERACTION WITH OTHER DRUGS

GENERIC NAME OR DRUG CLASS	COMBINED EFFECT
Antiacne topical preparations (other)	Severe skin irritation.
Cosmetics (medicated)	Severe skin irritation.
Skin preparations with alcohol	Severe skin irritation.
Soaps or cleansers (abrasive)	Severe skin irritation.

POSSIBLE INTERACTION WITH OTHER SUBSTANCES

INTERACTS WITH	COMBINED EFFECT
Alcohol:	None expected.
Beverages:	None expected.
Cocaine:	None expected.
Foods:	None expected.
Marijuana:	None expected.
Tobacco:	None expected.

LACOSAMIDE

BRAND NAMES

Vimpat

BASIC INFORMATION

Habit forming? Possibly
Prescription needed? Yes
Available as generic? No
Drug class: Anticonvulsant; antiepileptic

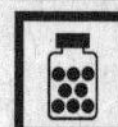

USES

- Treatment of partial-onset seizures in patients with epilepsy. It is used in combination with other antiepileptic drugs.
- Other uses as recommended by your doctor.

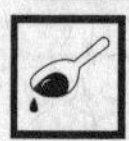

DOSAGE & USAGE INFORMATION

How to take:

- Tablet—Swallow the tablet with a liquid. May be taken with or without food, and on a full or empty stomach.
- Oral solution—Follow instructions on label.
- Injection—Given by medical professional.

When to take:
Tablet is usually taken twice a day at the same times each day. Your doctor will determine the best schedule. Dosages may be increased weekly to achieve maximum benefits.

If you forget a dose:
Take as soon as you remember. If it is almost time for the next dose, skip the missed dose and wait for your next scheduled dose (don't double this dose).

What drug does:
It helps stabilize electrical activity in the brain, but the exact way it controls seizures is unknown.

Time lapse before drug works:
May take several weeks for full effectiveness.

Don't take with:
Any other medicine or any dietary supplement without consulting your doctor or pharmacist.

OVERDOSE

SYMPTOMS:
Unknown (may be similar to side effects).
WHAT TO DO:
Overdose unlikely to threaten life. If person uses much larger amount than prescribed or if accidentally swallowed, call doctor or poison control center 1-800-222-1222 for help.

POSSIBLE ADVERSE REACTIONS OR SIDE EFFECTS

SYMPTOMS	WHAT TO DO
Life-threatening:	
Rare allergic reaction (hives, itching, rash, trouble breathing, tightness in chest, swelling of lips or tongue or face).	Seek emergency treatment immediately.
Common:	
• Dizziness, unsteady walk, shakiness or trembling, unusual drowsiness, lack of coordination.	Continue, but call doctor right away.
• Blurred or double vision, headache, nausea or vomiting.	Continue. Call doctor when convenient.
Infrequent:	
• Mood or mental changes, feeling sad or irritable, forgetfulness, itchy skin, tiredness, trouble sleeping or concentrating, unusual eye movements, depression.	Continue, but call doctor right away.
• Diarrhea, weakness, spinning sensation.	Continue. Call doctor when convenient.
Rare:	
• Tingling or prickling feelings, noises in ears, chills, fever, changes in heartbeat (fast, slow, irregular, pounding), unusual bleeding or bruising, yellow skin or eyes, new or worsening seizures, shortness of breath, fainting, behavior changes, euphoria.	Continue, but call doctor right away.
• Indigestion, heartburn, dry mouth, constipation, muscle spasms.	Continue. Call doctor when convenient.

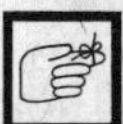

WARNINGS & PRECAUTIONS

Don't take if:
You are allergic to lacosamide.

Before you start, consult your doctor if:
- You have diabetes or kidney or liver problems.
- You have a history of any heart disorder or blood vessel problem.
- You have a history of mental or mood problems (such as depression) or suicidal thoughts or attempts.
- You have a condition that requires you to limit or avoid use of aspartame (oral solution form of drug contains aspartame).
- You are allergic to any medication, food or other substance.

Over age 60:
May be more at risk for side effects or adverse reactions. Use with caution.

Pregnancy:
Decide with your doctor if drug benefits justify risks to unborn child. Risk category C (see page xviii).

Breast-feeding:
It is unknown if drug passes into milk. Avoid drug or discontinue nursing until you finish medicine. Consult doctor for advice on maintaining milk supply.

Infants & children:
Safety and efficacy not established in children younger than age 17.

Prolonged use:
No special problems expected. Follow-up with your doctor on a regular basis to monitor your condition and check for drug side effects.

Skin & sunlight:
No problems expected.

Driving, piloting or hazardous work:
This drug may cause dizziness, coordination problems or blurred or double vision. Don't drive or pilot aircraft until you learn how medicine affects you. Don't work around dangerous machinery. Don't climb ladders or work in high places. The risk of dizziness increases if you drink alcohol.

Discontinuing:
Don't discontinue without doctor's approval due to risk of increased seizure activity. The dosage may need to be gradually decreased before stopping the drug completely.

Others:
- This drug cannot cure epilepsy and will only work to control seizures for as long as you continue to take it.
- Lacosamide is used with other anticonvulsant drugs and additional side effects may occur. If they do, consult your doctor.
- Advise any doctor or dentist whom you consult that you take this medicine.
- Rarely, antiepileptic drugs may lead to suicidal thoughts and behaviors. Call doctor right away if suicidal symptoms or unusual behaviors occur.
- Carry or wear medical identification that lists your seizure disorder and drugs you take.

POSSIBLE INTERACTION WITH OTHER DRUGS

GENERIC NAME OR DRUG CLASS	COMBINED EFFECT
QT interval prolongation-causing drugs*	Increased risk of cardiac (heart) side effects.

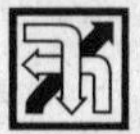

POSSIBLE INTERACTION WITH OTHER SUBSTANCES

INTERACTS WITH	COMBINED EFFECT
Alcohol:	Increased risk of dizziness. Avoid.
Beverages:	None expected.
Cocaine:	Unknown effect. Avoid.
Foods:	None expected.
Marijuana:	Unknown effect. Avoid.
Tobacco:	None expected.

*See Glossary

LAMOTRIGINE

BRAND NAMES

Lamictal
Lamictal Chewable Dispersible Tablet
Lamictal ODT
Lamictal XR

BASIC INFORMATION

Habit forming? No
Prescription needed? Yes
Available as generic? Yes
Drug class: Anticonvulsant, antiepileptic

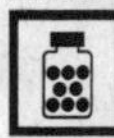

USES

- Treatment for partial (focal) epileptic seizures. May be used in combination with other antiepileptic drugs.
- Treatment of primary generalized tonic-clonic (PGTC) seizures, also known as "grand mal" seizures.
- Maintenance therapy for bipolar disorder.

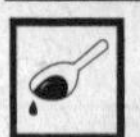

DOSAGE & USAGE INFORMATION

How to take:
- Tablet—Swallow whole with liquid. May be taken with or without food. Do not crush or chew tablet as it can have a bitter taste.
- Chewable dispersible tablet—Swallow whole or chew. If you chew the tablets, drink a small amount of water or diluted fruit juice to aid in swallowing. To mix it in a liquid, follow directions provided with prescription.
- Orally disintegrating tablet—Place tablet on tongue and let it dissolve. Can be taken with or without food or a liquid.
- Extended-release tablet—Swallow whole with liquid. Do not cut, chew or crush tablet.

When to take:
Your doctor will determine the best schedule. Dosages may be increased gradually over the first few weeks of use to achieve maximum benefits.

Continued next column

If you forget a dose:
Take as soon as you remember. If it is almost time for the next dose, then skip the missed dose and wait for your next scheduled dose (don't double this dose).

What drug does:
The exact mechanism is unknown. The anticonvulsant action may result from a decrease in the release of stimulatory neurotransmitters (substances that stimulate nerve cells).

Time lapse before drug works:
May take several weeks for effectiveness.

Don't take with:
Any other medicine or any dietary supplement without consulting your doctor or pharmacist.

OVERDOSE

SYMPTOMS:
Severe drowsiness, severe headache, severe dizziness, coma.
WHAT TO DO:
- **Dial 911 (emergency) for medical help or call poison control center 1-800-222-1222 for instructions.**
- **See emergency information on last 3 pages of this book.**

POSSIBLE ADVERSE REACTIONS OR SIDE EFFECTS

SYMPTOMS	WHAT TO DO
Life-threatening:	
Rare allergic reaction (hives, itching, rash, trouble breathing, tightness in chest, swelling of lips or tongue or face).	Seek emergency treatment immediately.
Common:	
• Skin rash, double vision or blurred vision, clumsiness.	Continue, but call doctor right away.
• Dizziness, nausea or vomiting, headache, drowsiness.	Continue. Call doctor when convenient.
Infrequent:	
Anxiety, depression, confusion, irritability, other mood or mental changes, increase in seizure activity, back-and-forth eye movements (nystagmus).	Continue, but call doctor right away.
Rare:	
• Swelling (hands, face, mouth, feet); breathing difficulty; tiredness or weakness; fever; chills; sore throat; unusual bruising or bleeding; skin peeling, blistering or loosening; muscle cramps or pain; sores on mouth or lips; small red or purple dots on skin; slurred speech; symptoms of aseptic	Continue, but call doctor right away.

meningitis (headache, fever, chills, nausea, vomiting, stiff neck, and sensitivity to light).	
• Indigestion, runny nose, trembling, trouble sleeping, weakness.	Continue. Call doctor when convenient.

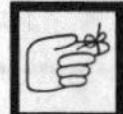

WARNINGS & PRECAUTIONS

Don't take if:
You are allergic to lamotrigine.

Before you start, consult your doctor if:
- You have kidney or liver disease.
- You have any heart disorder.
- You are allergic to any medication, food, or other substance.

Over age 60:
No special problems expected.

Pregnancy:
- Decide with your doctor if drug benefits justify risks to unborn child. Risk category C (see page xviii).
- Use of this drug during the first 3 months of pregnancy may increase chances of baby being born with cleft lip or cleft palate.

Breast-feeding:
Drug passes into milk. Avoid drug or discontinue nursing until you finish medicine. Consult doctor for advice on maintaining milk supply.

Infants & children:
May be used for children age 2 and older. Follow doctor's directions on how to use for your child.

Prolonged use:
Schedule regular visits to your doctor to determine if drug is continuing to be effective in controlling seizures. Follow-up laboratory blood studies may be recommended by your doctor.

Skin & sunlight:
No special problems expected.

Driving, piloting or hazardous work:
Don't drive or pilot aircraft until you learn how medicine affects you. Don't work around dangerous machinery. Don't climb ladders or work in high places. Danger increases if you drink alcohol or take other medicines affecting alertness and reflexes, such as antihistamines, tranquilizers, sedatives, pain medicine, narcotics and mind-altering drugs.

Discontinuing:
Don't discontinue without doctor's approval due to risk of increased seizure activity. Dosage may need to be gradually reduced.

Others:
- Advise any doctor or dentist whom you consult that you take this medicine.
- Use as directed. Don't increase or decrease dosage without doctor's approval.
- A skin rash may indicate a serious, and potentially life-threatening, medical problem. If a skin rash develops, it is usually during the first 4 to 6 weeks after treatment with the drug is started. Call your doctor promptly if you develop any skin rash.
- Rarely, antiepileptic drugs may lead to suicidal thoughts and behaviors. Call doctor right away if suicidal symptoms or unusual behaviors occur.
- Wear or carry medical identification stating your seizure disorder and drugs you take.

POSSIBLE INTERACTION WITH OTHER DRUGS

GENERIC NAME OR DRUG CLASS	COMBINED EFFECT
Carbamazepine	Decreased effect of lamotrigine. Increase in risk of side effects of carbamazepine.
Central nervous system (CNS) depressants*	Increased sedation.
Folate antagonists,* other	Folic acid deficiency.
Phenobarbital	Decreased effect of lamotrigine.
Phenytoin	Decreased effect of lamotrigine.
Primidone	Decreased effect of lamotrigine.
Valproic acid*	Increased effect of lamotrigine.

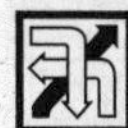

POSSIBLE INTERACTION WITH OTHER SUBSTANCES

INTERACTS WITH	COMBINED EFFECT
Alcohol:	Increased sedation. Avoid.
Beverages:	None expected.
Cocaine:	Problems not known. Best to avoid.
Foods:	None expected.
Marijuana:	Problems not known. Best to avoid.
Tobacco:	None expected.

*See Glossary

LAXATIVES, BULK-FORMING

GENERIC AND BRAND NAMES

See full list of generic and brand names in the *Generic and Brand Name Directory*, page 887.

BASIC INFORMATION

Habit forming? No
Prescription needed? No
Available as generic? Yes
Drug class: Laxative, bulk-forming

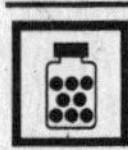

USES

For short-term relief of simple constipation (bowel movements that are abnormally difficult or infrequent). Normal frequency of bowel movements may vary from 2 to 3 times a day to 2 to 3 times a week. Laxatives treat the symptoms of constipation, not the cause.

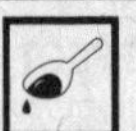

DOSAGE & USAGE INFORMATION

How to take:
Powder, oral solution, tablet, capsule, granules, chewable tablet, caramel, effervescent powder, wafer—Follow package instructions. Swallow with full glass of water or fruit juice. Drink 6 to 8 glasses of water each day in addition to one taken with each dose. Mix all powders thoroughly to avoid any risk of unmixed powder causing intestinal blockage.

When to take:
As directed on the label or according to doctor's instructions.

If you forget a dose:
Take as soon as you remember.

What drug does:
Adds dietary fiber that is not digested. Once in the intestine, it helps to increase fecal bulk, lubricate and soften the intestinal contents and facilitate the passage of stools.

Continued next column

OVERDOSE

SYMPTOMS:
Weakness, increased sweating, confusion, irregular heartbeat, muscle cramps.
WHAT TO DO:
Overdose unlikely to threaten life. If person uses much larger amount than prescribed or if accidentally swallowed, call doctor or poison control center 1-800-222-1222 for help.

Time lapse before drug works:
May work in 12 to 24 hours. Sometimes does not work for 2 to 3 days.

Don't take with:
- Any other medicine or any dietary supplement without consulting your doctor or pharmacist.
- Don't take within 2 hours of taking another medicine. Laxative interferes with absorption of medicine.

POSSIBLE ADVERSE REACTIONS OR SIDE EFFECTS

SYMPTOMS	WHAT TO DO
Life-threatening:	
None expected.	
Common:	
None expected.	
Infrequent:	
Mild stomach cramps, throat irritation with liquid form.	Continue. Call doctor when convenient.
Rare:	
Allergic skin rash or itching, trouble breathing, swallowing difficulty.	Discontinue. Call doctor right away.

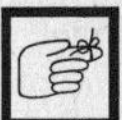

WARNINGS & PRECAUTIONS

Don't take if:
- You have symptoms of appendicitis (abdominal pain, cramping, soreness, bloating, nausea and vomiting). Consult doctor.
- You have dysphagia (swallowing difficulty).
- You are allergic to bulk-forming laxatives.
- You have missed a bowel movement for just 1 or 2 days.

Before you start, consult your doctor if:
- You are allergic to any medicine, food, or other substance or have a family history of allergies.
- You have diabetes or heart or kidney disease.
- You have hypertension (high blood pressure) and the laxative contains sodium.
- You have an intestinal obstruction or undiagnosed rectal bleeding.
- You are taking other laxatives.

Over age 60:
No special problems expected.

Pregnancy:
Most bulk-forming laxatives contain sodium or sugars, which may cause fluid retention. Risk factors vary or may not be designated for these laxatives. Read categories on page xviii and consult doctor.

Breast-feeding:
No special problems expected. Consult doctor.

Infants & children:
- Don't give to children under age 6 without doctor's approval. Young children are not able to describe their symptoms accurately, and a proper diagnosis needs to be made before starting any treatment.
- Don't give to a child who refuses to have a bowel movement (toileting refusal). May force a painful bowel movement and cause the child to hold back even more. Consult doctor.
- For children over age 6, follow package instructions or doctor's directions for correct dosage amount.

Prolonged use:
Don't take for more than 1 week unless under doctor's supervision. Bulk-form laxatives are sometimes used for long-term therapy.

Skin & sunlight:
No special problems expected.

Driving, piloting or hazardous work:
No special problems expected.

Discontinuing:
May be unnecessary to finish medicine. Follow doctor's instructions or instructions on label.

Others:
- Don't give to "flush out" the system or as a "tonic."
- Use as directed. Don't increase or decrease dosage without doctor's approval.
- Excessive use of laxatives in a teenager may indicate an eating disorder such as anorexia nervosa or bulimia nervosa. Consult doctor.
- If there is a sudden change in bowel habits or bowel function that lasts longer than 2 weeks, consult doctor.

POSSIBLE INTERACTION WITH OTHER DRUGS

GENERIC NAME OR DRUG CLASS	COMBINED EFFECT
Antacids*	Irritation of stomach or small intestine.
Anticoagulants*	Decreased anti-coagulant effect. Take 2 hours apart.
Digitalis preparations*	Decreased digitalis effect. Take 2 hours apart.
Diuretics, potassium-sparing*	Decreased potassium effect.
Potassium supplements*	Decreased potassium effect.
Salicylates*	Decreased salicylate effect. Take 2 hours apart.
Tetracyclines*	Decreased tetracycline effect. Take 2 hours apart.

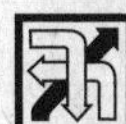

POSSIBLE INTERACTION WITH OTHER SUBSTANCES

INTERACTS WITH	COMBINED EFFECT
Alcohol:	None expected.
Beverages:	None expected.
Cocaine:	None expected.
Foods:	None expected.
Marijuana:	None expected.
Tobacco:	None expected.

*See Glossary

LAXATIVES, OSMOTIC

GENERIC AND BRAND NAMES

See full list of generic and brand names in the *Generic and Brand Name Directory*, page 888.

BASIC INFORMATION

Habit forming? No
Prescription needed? No
Available as generic? Yes
Drug class: Laxative, hyperosmotic

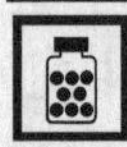

USES

For short-term relief of simple constipation (bowel movements that are abnormally difficult or infrequent). Normal frequency of bowel movements may vary from 2 to 3 times a day to 2 to 3 times a week. Laxatives treat the symptoms of constipation, not the cause.

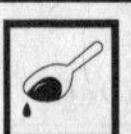

DOSAGE & USAGE INFORMATION

How to take:

- Oral solution, tablet, crystals, effervescent powder, milk of magnesia—Follow package instructions. Swallow with full glass of water or fruit juice. A second glass of liquid is often recommended for best effect. Drink 6 to 8 glasses of water each day, in addition to one taken with each dose.
- Enema or suppository—Read and follow package instructions.

When to take:
Since drug produces stool within 30 minutes to 3 hours following a dose, take it at a time that will not interfere with sleep or other scheduled activities. Don't take late in the day on an empty stomach.

If you forget a dose:
Take as soon as you remember.

Continued next column

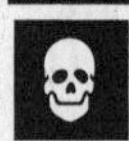

OVERDOSE

SYMPTOMS:
Weakness, increased sweating, confusion, irregular heartbeat, muscle cramps.
WHAT TO DO:
Overdose unlikely to threaten life. If person uses much larger amount than prescribed or if accidentally swallowed, call doctor or poison control center 1-800-222-1222 for help.

What drug does:
Draws water into the bowel from surrounding tissue to help loosen and soften the stool and increases bowel action.

Time lapse before drug works:

- Oral forms—30 minutes to 3 hours. May take longer if taken with a meal.
- Rectal forms—2 to 15 minutes.

Don't take with:

- Any other medicine or any dietary supplement without consulting your doctor or pharmacist.
- Don't take within 2 hours of taking another medicine. Laxative interferes with absorption of medicine.

POSSIBLE ADVERSE REACTIONS OR SIDE EFFECTS

SYMPTOMS	WHAT TO DO
Life-threatening: None expected.	
Common: None expected.	
Infrequent:	
• Belching, cramps, nausea, diarrhea, increased thirst.	Continue. Call doctor when convenient.
• Rectal bleeding, burning, itching or pain (with rectal forms).	Discontinue. Call doctor right away.
Rare: When used too often or dose is too high—Confusion, irregular heartbeat, muscle cramps, unusual tiredness or weakness, dehydration.	Discontinue. Call doctor right away.

WARNINGS & PRECAUTIONS

Don't take if:

- You are having symptoms of appendicitis (abdominal pain, cramping, soreness, bloating, nausea and vomiting). Consult doctor.
- You are allergic to osmotic laxatives.
- You have missed a bowel movement for just 1 or 2 days.

Before you start, consult your doctor if:

- You are allergic to any medicine, food or other substance or have a family history of allergies.
- You have hypertension (high blood pressure) and the laxative contains sodium.
- You have an intestinal obstruction, undiagnosed rectal bleeding or a colostomy or ileostomy.
- You have diabetes or heart or kidney disease.
- You are taking other laxatives.

Over age 60:
- Rectal solutions could cause excess fluid in the body. Consult doctor before using.
- No special problems expected with laxatives taken by mouth.

Pregnancy:
Risk factors vary or may not be designated for these laxatives. Read categories on page xviii and consult doctor.

Breast-feeding:
No special problems expected. Consult doctor.

Infants & children:
- Don't give to children under age 6 without doctor's approval. Young children are not able to describe their symptoms accurately, and a proper diagnosis needs to be made before starting any treatment.
- Don't give to a child who refuses to have a bowel movement (toileting refusal). May force a painful bowel movement and cause the child to hold back even more. Consult doctor.
- For children over age 6, follow package instructions or doctor's directions for correct dosage amount.

Prolonged use:
Don't take for more than 1 week unless under doctor's supervision. May cause laxative dependence in which normal bowel function depends on the laxative to produce a bowel movement.

Skin & sunlight:
No special problems expected.

Driving, piloting or hazardous work:
No special problems expected.

Discontinuing:
May be unnecessary to finish medicine. Follow doctor's instructions or instructions on label.

Others:
- Don't give to "flush out" the system or as a "tonic."
- Use as directed. Don't increase or decrease dosage without doctor's approval.
- Excessive use of laxatives in a teenager may indicate an eating disorder such as anorexia nervosa or bulimia nervosa. Consult doctor.
- If there is a sudden change in bowel habits or bowel function that lasts longer than 2 weeks, consult doctor.

POSSIBLE INTERACTION WITH OTHER DRUGS

GENERIC NAME OR DRUG CLASS	COMBINED EFFECT
Antacids*	Irritation of stomach or small intestine.
Anticoagulants*	Decreased anti-coagulant effect with aluminum- or magnesium-containing laxatives. Avoid.
Ciprofloxacin	Decreased ciprofloxacin effect with magnesium-containing laxatives. Avoid.
Digitalis preparations*	Decreased digitalis effect with aluminum- or magnesium-containing laxatives. Avoid.
Diuretics, potassium-sparing*	Decreased potassium effect.
Etidronate	Decreased etidronate effect if taken with magnesium-containing laxatives. Take 2 hours apart.
Phenothiazines*	Decreased phenothiazine effect with aluminum- or magnesium-containing laxatives. Avoid.
Potassium supplements*	Decreased potassium effect.
Sodium polystyrene	Fluid imbalance in body with magnesium-containing laxatives. Avoid.
Tetracyclines*	Decreased tetracycline effect. Take 2 hours apart.

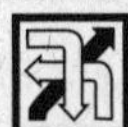

POSSIBLE INTERACTION WITH OTHER SUBSTANCES

INTERACTS WITH	COMBINED EFFECT
Alcohol:	None expected.
Beverages:	None expected.
Cocaine:	None expected.
Foods:	None expected.
Marijuana:	None expected.
Tobacco:	None expected.

*See Glossary

LAXATIVES, SOFTENER/LUBRICANT

GENERIC AND BRAND NAMES

See full list of generic and brand names in the *Generic and Brand Name Directory,* page 888.

BASIC INFORMATION

Habit forming? No
Prescription needed? No
Available as generic? Yes
Drug class: Laxative (stool softener-emollient), lubricant

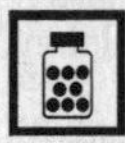

USES

For short-term relief of simple constipation (bowel movements that are abnormally difficult or infrequent). Normal frequency of bowel movements may vary from 2 to 3 times a day to 2 to 3 times a week. Laxatives treat the symptoms of constipation, not the cause.

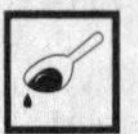

DOSAGE & USAGE INFORMATION

How to take:

- Tablet, capsule, syrup, chewable tablet, oral solution—Follow package instructions. Swallow with full glass of water, fruit juice or milk. Drink 6 to 8 glasses of water each day in addition to one taken with each dose.
- Enema or suppository—Read and follow package instructions.

When to take:
Produces stool within 30 minutes to 3 hours following a dose. Take drug at a time that will not interfere with sleep or scheduled activities. Don't take late in the day on an empty stomach.

If you forget a dose:
Take as soon as you remember.

Continued next column

OVERDOSE

SYMPTOMS:
Weakness, increased sweating, confusion, irregular heartbeat, muscle cramps.
WHAT TO DO:
Overdose unlikely to threaten life. If person uses much larger amount than prescribed or if accidentally swallowed, call doctor or poison control center 1-800-222-1222 for help.

What drug does:
Softener laxatives help liquids mix into the stool to help prevent hard stool masses. Lubricant laxatives coat the stool surface with a thin film that helps ease the passage of the stool through the intestines.

Time lapse before drug works:

- When taken by mouth, usually works within 1 to 2 days after first dose, but may take 3 to 5 days for full effectiveness.
- Rectal dosage forms work in 2 to 15 minutes.

Don't take with:

- Any other medicine or any dietary supplement without consulting your doctor or pharmacist.
- Other stool softener laxatives or mineral oil.
- Don't take within 2 hours of taking another medicine. Laxative interferes with absorption of medicine.

POSSIBLE ADVERSE REACTIONS OR SIDE EFFECTS

SYMPTOMS	WHAT TO DO
Life-threatening:	
None expected.	
Common:	
None expected.	
Infrequent:	
• Mild stomach cramps, throat irritation with liquid forms, diarrhea.	Continue. Call doctor when convenient.
• Rectal bleeding, burning, itching or pain (with rectal forms).	Discontinue. Call doctor right away.
Rare:	
Skin rash.	Discontinue. Call doctor right away.

WARNINGS & PRECAUTIONS

Don't take if:

- You have symptoms of appendicitis (abdominal pain, cramping, soreness, bloating, nausea and vomiting). Consult doctor.
- You are allergic to a softener-emollient or lubricant laxative.
- You have missed a bowel movement for just 1 or 2 days.

Before you start, consult your doctor if:

- You are allergic to any medicine, food or other substance or have a family history of allergies.
- You have hypertension (high blood pressure) and the laxative contains sodium.
- You have an intestinal obstruction, undiagnosed rectal bleeding or a colostomy or ileostomy.
- You are taking other laxatives.
- You have diabetes or heart or kidney disease.
- You have dysphagia (swallowing difficulty) and want to take mineral oil.

Over age 60:
Oral mineral oil is not recommended for bedridden elderly patients; otherwise, no special problems expected.

Pregnancy:
Risk factors vary or may not be designated for these laxatives. Read categories on page xviii and consult doctor.

Breast-feeding:
No special problems expected. Consult doctor.

Infants & children:

- Don't give to children under age 6 without doctor's approval. Young children are not able to describe their symptoms accurately, and a proper diagnosis needs to be made before starting any treatment.
- Don't give to a child who refuses to have a bowel movement (toileting refusal). May force a painful bowel movement and cause the child to hold back even more. Consult doctor.
- For children over age 6, follow package instructions or doctor's directions for correct dosage amount.

Prolonged use:
Don't take for more than 1 week unless under doctor's supervision.

Skin & sunlight:
No special problems expected.

Driving, piloting or hazardous work:
No special problems expected.

Discontinuing:
May be unnecessary to finish medicine. Follow doctor's instructions or instructions on label.

Others:

- Don't give to "flush out" the system or as a "tonic."
- Use as directed. Don't increase or decrease dosage without doctor's approval.
- Excessive use of laxatives in a teenager may indicate an eating disorder such as anorexia nervosa or bulimia nervosa. Consult doctor.
- If there is a sudden change in bowel habits or bowel function that lasts longer than 2 weeks, consult doctor.

POSSIBLE INTERACTION WITH OTHER DRUGS

GENERIC NAME OR DRUG CLASS	COMBINED EFFECT
Antacids*	Irritation of stomach or small intestine.
Anticoagulants*	Decreased anticoagulant effect with mineral oil.
Contraceptives, oral*	Decreased contraceptive effect with mineral oil.
Danthron	Increased danthron effect.
Digitalis preparations*	Decreased digitalis effect with mineral oil.
Diuretics, potassium-sparing*	Decreased potassium effect.
Phenolphthalein	Increased phenolphthalein effect.
Potassium supplements*	Decreased potassium effect.
Vitamins A, D, E, K	Decreased vitamin effect with mineral oil.

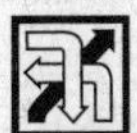

POSSIBLE INTERACTION WITH OTHER SUBSTANCES

INTERACTS WITH	COMBINED EFFECT
Alcohol:	None expected.
Beverages:	None expected.
Cocaine:	None expected.
Foods:	None expected.
Marijuana:	None expected.
Tobacco:	None expected.

*See Glossary

LAXATIVES, STIMULANT

GENERIC AND BRAND NAMES

See full list of generic and brand names in the *Generic and Brand Name Directory*, page 888.

BASIC INFORMATION

Habit forming? Potentially
Prescription needed? No
Available as generic? Yes
Drug class: Laxative (stimulant)

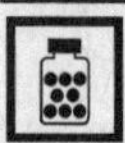

USES

For short-term relief of simple constipation (bowel movements that are abnormally difficult or infrequent). Normal frequency of bowel movements may vary from 2 to 3 times a day to 2 to 3 times a week. Laxatives treat the symptoms of constipation, not the cause.

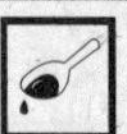

DOSAGE & USAGE INFORMATION

How to take:

- Tablet, chewable tablet, syrup, chewing gum, oral solution, granules, fluidextract, emulsion, wafer—Follow package instructions. Swallow with full glass of water, fruit juice or milk. Give child 6 to 8 glasses of fluid each day in addition to the one taken with each dose to keep stool soft. Give on an empty stomach. Results may be delayed if given with food.
- Enema—Lubricate rectal area with petroleum jelly before inserting enema applicator. Insert carefully to avoid damage to rectal wall. To mix powder for rectal solution, follow instructions on package.
- Suppository—Remove wrapper and moisten suppository with water. Gently insert tapered end into rectum. Push well into rectum with finger. Retain in rectum 20 to 30 minutes.

Continued next column

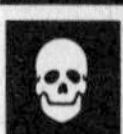

OVERDOSE

SYMPTOMS:
Weakness, increased sweating, confusion, irregular heartbeat, muscle cramps.
WHAT TO DO:
Overdose unlikely to threaten life. If person uses much larger amount than prescribed or if accidentally swallowed, call doctor or poison control center 1-800-222-1222 for help.

When to take:
Usually at bedtime on an empty stomach, unless directed otherwise. Castor oil is usually taken late in the day, as it works within 2 to 6 hours.

If you forget a dose:
Take as soon as you remember.

What drug does:
Acts on smooth muscles of intestinal wall to cause vigorous bowel movement.

Time lapse before drug works:
Oral form within 6 to 10 hours (castor oil 2 to 6 hours). Rectal form within 15 minutes to 1 hour.

Don't take with:

- Any other medicine or any dietary supplement without consulting your doctor or pharmacist.
- Don't take within 2 hours of another medicine. Laxative interferes with absorption of medicine.

POSSIBLE ADVERSE REACTIONS OR SIDE EFFECTS

SYMPTOMS	WHAT TO DO
Life-threatening: None expected.	
Common: None expected.	
Infrequent:	
• Belching, cramps, nausea, diarrhea, throat irritation.	Continue. Call doctor when convenient.
• Rectal bleeding, burning, itching or pain (with rectal forms).	Discontinue. Call doctor right away.
Rare: Confusion, irregular heartbeat, muscle cramps, unusual tiredness or weakness; pink to red color of urine and stools (with phenolphthalein); pink, red or violet to brown urine color (with cascara, danthron or senna); yellow to brown color of urine (with cascara, phenolphthalein or senna); skin rash (allergy).	Discontinue. Call doctor right away.

WARNINGS & PRECAUTIONS

Don't take if:

- You have symptoms of appendicitis (abdominal pain, cramping, soreness, bloating, nausea and vomiting). Consult doctor.
- You are allergic to a stimulant laxative.
- You have missed a bowel movement for just 1 or 2 days.

Before you start, consult your doctor if:

- You are a allergic to any medicine, food or other substance or have a family history of allergies.
- You have hypertension (high blood pressure) and the laxative contains sodium.
- You have an intestinal obstruction or undiagnosed rectal bleeding.
- You have diabetes or heart or kidney disease.
- You are taking other laxatives.

Over age 60:
Excessive use of stimulant laxatives may cause excess loss of body fluid, resulting in weakness and lack of coordination.

Pregnancy:
Risk factors vary or may not be designated for these laxatives. Read categories on page xviii and consult doctor.

Breast-feeding:
Some of the stimulant laxatives may pass into breast milk. Consult doctor.

Infants & children:

- Don't give to children under age 6 without doctor's approval. Young children are not able to describe their symptoms accurately, and a proper diagnosis needs to be made before starting any treatment.
- Don't give to a child who refuses to have a bowel movement (toileting refusal). May force a painful bowel movement and cause the child to hold back even more. Consult doctor.
- For children over age 6, follow package instructions or doctor's directions for correct dosage amount.

Prolonged use:
Don't take for more than 1 week unless under doctor's supervision.

Skin & sunlight:
No special problems expected.

Driving, piloting or hazardous work:
No special problems expected.

Discontinuing:
May be unnecessary to finish medicine. Follow doctor's instructions or instructions on label.

Others:

- Don't give to "flush out" the system or as a "tonic."
- Use as directed. Don't increase or decrease dosage without doctor's approval.
- Excessive use of laxatives in a teenager may indicate an eating disorder such as anorexia nervosa or bulimia nervosa. Consult doctor.
- If there is a sudden change in bowel habits or bowel function that lasts longer than 2 weeks, consult doctor.

POSSIBLE INTERACTION WITH OTHER DRUGS

GENERIC NAME OR DRUG CLASS	COMBINED EFFECT
Antacids*	Irritation of stomach or small intestine.
Diuretics, potassium-sparing*	Decreased potassium effect.
Histamine H_2 receptor antagonists*	Stomach irritation with bisacodyl. Take 1 hour apart.
Potassium supplements*	Decreased potassium effect.

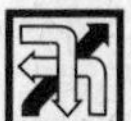

POSSIBLE INTERACTION WITH OTHER SUBSTANCES

INTERACTS WITH	COMBINED EFFECT
Alcohol:	None expected.
Beverages: Milk.	Stomach irritation with bisacodyl. Take 1 hour apart.
Cocaine:	None expected.
Foods:	None expected.
Marijuana:	None expected.
Tobacco:	None expected.

*See Glossary

LEFLUNOMIDE

BRAND NAMES

Arava

BASIC INFORMATION

Habit forming? No
Prescription needed? Yes
Available as generic? Yes
Drug class: Antirheumatic

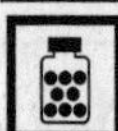

USES

Treats symptoms caused by rheumatoid arthritis, such as inflammation, swelling, stiffness and joint pain. Slows deterioration of joint.

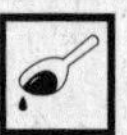

DOSAGE & USAGE INFORMATION

How to take:
Tablet—Take with full glass of water. If you can't swallow whole, crumble tablet and take with liquid or food.

When to take:
At the same time each day.

If you forget a dose:
Take as soon as you remember. However, if it is almost time for your next dose, skip the missed dose and go back to your regular dosing schedule (don't double this dose).

What drug does:
Stops the body from producing too many of the immune cells that are responsible for the swelling and inflammation (immunosuppressive and antiinflammatory).

Time lapse before drug works:
6 to 12 hours.

Don't take with:
Any other medicine or any dietary supplement without consulting your doctor or pharmacist.

OVERDOSE

SYMPTOMS:
None expected.
WHAT TO DO:
Overdose unlikely to threaten life. If person uses much larger amount than prescribed or if accidentally swallowed, call doctor or poison control center 1-800-222-1222 for help.

POSSIBLE ADVERSE REACTIONS OR SIDE EFFECTS

SYMPTOMS	WHAT TO DO
Life-threatening: None expected.	
Common:	
• Chest congestion, cough, difficulty in breathing, loss of appetite, nausea, vomiting, yellow eyes or skin, dizziness, fever, sneezing, sore throat, pain or burning while urinating, frequent urge to urinate.	Continue. Call doctor right away.
• Abdominal pain, hair loss, back pain, diarrhea, heartburn, rash, unexplained weight loss.	Continue. Call doctor if symptoms persist.
Infrequent:	
• Unusual tiredness or weakness, shortness of breath, indigestion, pounding heartbeat, burning or tingling sensation in fingers and toes, joint or muscle pain, rapid heartbeat.	Continue. Call doctor right away.
• Acne, loss of appetite, anxiety, red or irritated eyes, constipation, dry mouth, gas, mouth ulcer, pain or burning in throat, itching, runny nose.	Continue. Call doctor when convenient.
Rare: None expected.	

WARNINGS & PRECAUTIONS

Don't take if:
You are allergic to leflunomide.

Before you start, consult your doctor if:
- You have immune system problems.
- You have severe or uncontrolled infections.
- You have a liver disease or you have elevated liver enzymes (per medical tests).
- You have kidney disease.

Over age 60:
Side effects or problems experienced with this medication appear to be the same in older people as in younger adults.

Pregnancy:
Risk to unborn child outweighs drug benefits. Don't use. Risk category X (see page xviii).

Breast-feeding:
Drug may pass into milk. Avoid drug or discontinue nursing until you finish medicine. Consult doctor for advice on maintaining milk supply.

Infants & children:
Studies on this medicine have been done only in adult patients. Consult doctor before giving this medicine to persons under age 18.

Prolonged use:
Follow-up with your doctor on a regular basis to monitor your condition and check for drug side effects.

Skin & sunlight:
None expected.

Driving, piloting or hazardous work:
None expected.

Discontinuing:
Don't discontinue without consulting doctor or before completing prescribed dosage.

Others:
- May affect accuracy of some laboratory tests.
- Women of childbearing age are advised to use reliable contraception before receiving leflunomide. If you become pregnant while taking this drug, notify your doctor immediately.
- Use of leflunomide by men during time of conception may cause birth defects in their children. Therefore, men taking leflunomide should use condoms as a form of birth control.
- Severe liver injury may occur while taking this drug. Blood tests to check liver enzymes should be done at least monthly for 3 months after starting the drug and every 3 months thereafter.
- Don't have any immunizations during or after treatment with this drug without doctor's approval.
- Advise any doctor or dentist whom you consult that you take this medicine.

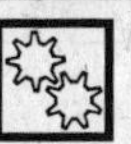

POSSIBLE INTERACTION WITH OTHER DRUGS

GENERIC NAME OR DRUG CLASS	COMBINED EFFECT
Charcoal, activated	Decreased leflunomide effect.
Cholestyramine	Decreased leflunomide effect.
Hepatotoxics*	Increased risk of liver injury.
Methotrexate	Increased risk of side effects.
Rifampin	May increase risk of leflunomide toxicity.

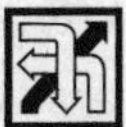

POSSIBLE INTERACTION WITH OTHER SUBSTANCES

INTERACTS WITH	COMBINED EFFECT
Alcohol:	Increases the chance of liver problems. Avoid.
Beverages:	None expected.
Cocaine:	Effect unknown. Avoid.
Foods:	None expected.
Marijuana:	Effect unknown. Avoid
Tobacco:	None expected.

***See Glossary**

LEUCOVORIN

BRAND NAMES

Citrocovorin Calcium
Citrovorum Factor
Folinic Acid
Wellcovorin

BASIC INFORMATION

Habit forming? No
Prescription needed? Yes
Available as generic? Yes
Drug class: Antianemic

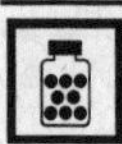

USES

- Antidote to folic acid antagonists.
- Treats anemia.

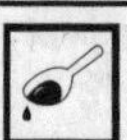

DOSAGE & USAGE INFORMATION

How to take:
Tablet—Swallow with liquid or food to lessen stomach irritation. If you can't swallow whole, crumble tablet and take with liquid or food.

When to take:
At the same time each day, according to instructions on prescription label.

If you forget a dose:
Take as soon as you remember. If it is almost time for the next dose, wait for that dose (don't double this dose) and resume regular schedule.

What drug does:
Favors development of DNA, RNA and protein synthesis.

Time lapse before drug works:
20 to 30 minutes.

Don't take with:
Any other medicine or any dietary supplement without consulting your doctor or pharmacist.

OVERDOSE

SYMPTOMS:
Unlikely to threaten life. If overdose is suspected, follow instructions below.
WHAT TO DO:
- **Dial 911 (emergency) for medical help or call poison control center 1-800-222-1222 for instructions.**
- **See emergency information on last 3 pages of this book.**

POSSIBLE ADVERSE REACTIONS OR SIDE EFFECTS

SYMPTOMS	WHAT TO DO
Life-threatening:	
Wheezing.	Seek emergency treatment immediately.
Common:	
None expected.	
Infrequent:	
None expected.	
Rare:	
Skin rash, hives.	Discontinue. Call doctor right away.

WARNINGS & PRECAUTIONS

Don't take if:
You are allergic to leucovorin.

Before you start, consult your doctor if:
- You have acid urine, ascites, dehydration.
- You have kidney function impairment.
- You have pernicious anemia.
- You have vitamin B-12 deficiency.

Over age 60:
Adverse reactions and side effects may be more frequent and severe than in younger persons. You may need smaller doses for shorter periods of time.

Pregnancy:
Recommended for the treatment of megaloblastic anemia caused by pregnancy. Decide with your doctor if drug benefits justify risk to unborn child. Risk category C (see page xviii).

Breast-feeding:
It is unknown if drug passes into milk. Avoid drug or discontinue nursing until you finish medicine. Consult doctor for advice on maintaining milk supply.

Infants & children:
May increase frequency of seizures. Avoid if possible.

Prolonged use:
No problems expected.

Skin & sunlight:
No problems expected.

Driving, piloting or hazardous work:
Don't drive or pilot aircraft until you learn how medicine affects you. Don't work around dangerous machinery. Don't climb ladders or work in high places. Danger increases if you drink alcohol or take medicine affecting alertness and reflexes.

Discontinuing:
Don't discontinue without consulting doctor. Dose may require gradual reduction if you have taken drug for a long time. Doses of other drugs may also require adjustment.

Others:
Advise any doctor or dentist whom you consult that you take this medicine.

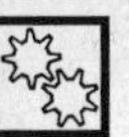

POSSIBLE INTERACTION WITH OTHER DRUGS

GENERIC NAME OR DRUG CLASS	COMBINED EFFECT
Anticonvulsants, barbiturate and hydantoin*	Large doses of leucovorin may counteract the effects of these medicines.
Central nervous system (CNS) depressants*	High alcohol content of leucovorin may cause adverse effects.
Fluorouracil	Increased levels of fluorouracil.
Primidone	Large doses of leucovorin may counteract the effects of both drugs.

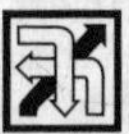

POSSIBLE INTERACTION WITH OTHER SUBSTANCES

INTERACTS WITH	COMBINED EFFECT
Alcohol:	Increased adverse reactions of both.
Beverages:	None expected.
Cocaine:	Increased adverse reactions of both drugs.
Foods:	None expected.
Marijuana:	Increased adverse reactions of both drugs.
Tobacco:	Increased adverse reactions of both.

LEUKOTRIENE MODIFIERS

GENERIC AND BRAND NAMES

MONTELUKAST
Singulair
ZAFIRLUKAST
Accolate
ZILEUTON
Zyflo CR

BASIC INFORMATION

Habit forming? No
Prescription needed? Yes
Available as generic? Yes, for some
Drug class: Antiasthmatic

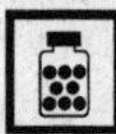

USES

- Treatment of mild to moderate asthma. Not used to treat an active asthma attack. May be used with other asthma medications as directed by your doctor. Montelukast is used for prophylaxis (preventive) and chronic treatment of asthma.
- Prevention of exercise-induced bronchoconstriction (EIB) in patients age 15 and older.
- Montelukast is used for treatment of seasonal allergies (hay fever) and perennial allergic rhinitis (PAR), also known as indoor allergies.

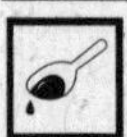

DOSAGE & USAGE INFORMATION

How to take:
- Tablet—Swallow with water, with or without food, except for zafirlukast which must be taken on an empty stomach 1 hour before or 2 hours after a meal.
- Chewable tablet—Chew tablet before you swallow it.
- Extended-release tablet—Swallow whole with liquid. Do not cut, chew or crush tablet.
- Oral granules—Take granules directly in the mouth or mix with a spoonful of cold or room temperature soft food.

Continued next column

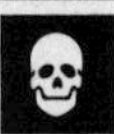

OVERDOSE

SYMPTOMS:
It is unknown what symptoms may occur.
WHAT TO DO:
If person uses much larger amount than prescribed, dial 911 (emergency) for medical help or call poison control center 1-800-222-1222 for instructions.

When to take:
- Montelukast—At the same time each day.
- Zafirlukast—Twice a day at the same times.
- Zileuton—Four times a day at the same times. Take extended-release zileuton within one hour after morning and evening meals.

If you forget a dose:
Take as soon as you remember. If it is almost time for the next dose, wait for that dose (don't double this dose) and resume regular schedule.

What drug does:
Inhibits inflammatory cells associated with asthma. Inhibits reflex reactions to irritants, exercise and cold.

Time lapse before drug works:
30 minutes to 4 hours.

Don't take with:
Any other medicine or any dietary supplement without consulting your doctor or pharmacist.

POSSIBLE ADVERSE REACTIONS OR SIDE EFFECTS

SYMPTOMS	WHAT TO DO
Life-threatening:	
None expected.	
Common:	
Headache, stomach upset, nausea.	Continue. Call doctor when convenient.
Infrequent:	
Weak feeling, pain in abdomen, headache, unusual tiredness, cough, dental pain, dizziness, heartburn, fever, stuffy nose, skin rash.	Continue. Call doctor when convenient.
Rare:	
Liver problems (yellow eyes or skin, fatigue, symptoms of flu, itching, pain in upper right abdominal area); mental and nervous problems (agitation, aggression, abnormal dreams, being anxious, hallucinations, irritable, depression, insomnia, restlessness, tremor, suicidal thinking and behavior [including suicide]).	Discontinue. Call doctor right away.

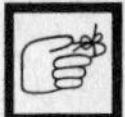

WARNINGS & PRECAUTIONS

Don't take if:
You are allergic to leukotriene modifiers.

Before you start, consult your doctor if:
- You have any other medical problem.
- You have a liver or kidney disease.
- You have a history of alcoholism.

Over age 60:
In some cases older patients taking zafirlukast experienced more infections; otherwise, no problems expected.

Pregnancy:
Decide with your doctor whether drug benefits justify risk to unborn child. Montelukast and zafirlukast are risk category B; zileuton is risk category C (see page xviii).

Breast-feeding:
- Montelukast and zileuton—It is unknown if drug passes into milk. Avoid drug or discontinue nursing until you finish medicine. Consult doctor for advice on maintaining milk supply.
- Zafirlukast—Drug passes into milk. Avoid drug or discontinue nursing until you finish medicine.

Infants & children:
- Montelukast is approved for children 12 months and older.
- Zafirlukast is approved for children over 6 years.
- Zileuton should only be given under close supervision, especially to children under 12 years old.

Prolonged use:
Schedule regular visits with your doctor to determine if the drug continues its effectiveness in controlling asthma symptoms.

Skin & sunlight:
No problems expected.

Driving, piloting or hazardous work:
No problems expected.

Discontinuing:
Don't discontinue without consulting doctor.

Others:
- In a few rare instances, patients taking zafirlukast while having their oral steroid dosage reduced developed Churg-Strauss syndrome (a rare and sometimes fatal condition). It is not known if the problem is caused by zafirlukast. Symptoms of Churg-Strauss syndrome are similar to those caused by flu. Before starting zafirlukast and reducing oral steroids, discuss the benefits and risk factors with your doctor.
- Advise any doctor or dentist you consult that you take this medicine.
- Talk to your doctor if your asthma attacks are not being controlled by the usual dosage of your fast-acting bronchodilator.
- This drug may affect results in some medical tests.
- This drug should be taken every day, even if you are not having asthma symptoms.

POSSIBLE INTERACTION WITH OTHER DRUGS

GENERIC NAME OR DRUG CLASS	COMBINED EFFECT
Beta adrenergic blocking agents	Increased beta blocker effect.
Calcium channel blockers	Increased effect of calcium channel blocker.
Carbamazepine	Increased effect of carbamazepine.
Cisapride	Increased effect of cisapride.
Cyclosporine	Increased effect of cyclosporine.
Dofetilide	Increased dofetilide effect.
Erythromycin	Decreased effect of zafirlukast.
Phenobarbital	Decreased effect of montelukast.
Phenytoin	Increased effect of phenytoin.
Tolbutamide	Increased effect of tolbutamide.
Warfarin	Increased effect of warfarin.

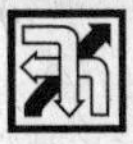

POSSIBLE INTERACTION WITH OTHER SUBSTANCES

INTERACTS WITH	COMBINED EFFECT
Alcohol:	None expected.
Beverages:	None expected.
Cocaine:	Effects unknown. Avoid.
Foods:	None expected.
Marijuana:	Effects unknown. Avoid.
Tobacco:	None expected.

LEVAMISOLE

BRAND NAMES

Ergamisol

BASIC INFORMATION

Habit forming? No
Prescription needed? Yes
Available as generic? No
Drug class: Anticancer treatment adjunct

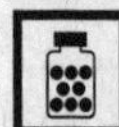

USES

- Treats colorectal cancer when used in combination with fluorouracil.
- Treats malignant melanoma after surgical removal when there is no evidence of spread to organs other than the skin.

DOSAGE & USAGE INFORMATION

How to take:
Tablet—Swallow with liquid or food to lessen stomach irritation. If you can't swallow whole, crumble tablet and take with liquid or food.

When to take:
At the same time each day, according to instructions on prescription label.

If you forget a dose:
Don't take until you notify your doctor.

What drug does:
Acts to help restore the immune system. May activate T-cell lymphocytes and other white cells. Also elevates mood.

Time lapse before drug works:
1-1/2 to 2 hours.

Don't take with:
Any other medicine or any dietary supplement without consulting your doctor or pharmacist.

OVERDOSE

SYMPTOMS:
None expected.
WHAT TO DO:
Overdose unlikely to threaten life. If person uses much larger amount than prescribed or if accidentally swallowed, call doctor or poison control center 1-800-222-1222 for help.

POSSIBLE ADVERSE REACTIONS OR SIDE EFFECTS

SYMPTOMS	WHAT TO DO
Life-threatening:	
Fever, muscle aches, headache, cough, hoarseness, sore throat, painful or difficult urination, low back or side pain.	Seek emergency treatment.
Common:	
• Diarrhea, metallic taste, nausea, joint or muscle pain, skin rash, insomnia, mental depression, nightmares, sleepiness or tiredness, increased dental problems.	Continue. Call doctor when convenient.
• Hair loss.	No action necessary.
Infrequent:	
Mouth, tongue and lip sores.	Call doctor right away.
Rare:	
Unsteady gait while walking; blurred vision; confusion; tremors; tingling or numbness in hands, feet or face; seizures; smacking and puckering of lips; uncontrolled tongue movements.	Call doctor right away.

WARNINGS & PRECAUTIONS

Don't take if:
You are allergic to levamisole.

Before you start, consult your doctor if:
- You take other drugs for cancer.
- You have an active infection.
- You have a seizure disorder.
- You have allergies to other medications.

Over age 60:
No special problems expected.

Pregnancy:
Adequate studies not yet done. Consult your doctor. Risk category C (see page xviii).

Breast-feeding:
Effect unknown. Consult doctor.

Infants & children:
Effect not documented. Consult your doctor.

Prolonged use:
No special problems expected.

Skin & sunlight:
No special problems expected.

Driving, piloting or hazardous work:
No special problems expected.

Discontinuing:
Don't discontinue without consulting doctor. Dose may require gradual reduction if you have taken drug for a long time. Doses of other drugs may also require adjustment.

Others:
- Advise any doctor or dentist whom you consult that you take this medicine.
- Defer dental treatments until your blood count is normal. Pay particular attention to dental hygiene. You may be subject to additional risk of oral infection, delayed healing and bleeding.
- Avoid aspirin. May increase risk of internal bleeding.
- Avoid constipation. May increase risk of internal bleeding.

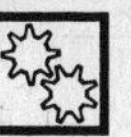

POSSIBLE INTERACTION WITH OTHER DRUGS

GENERIC NAME OR DRUG CLASS	COMBINED EFFECT
Anticoagulants*	Increased risk of bleeding.
Aspirin	Increased risk of bleeding.
Bone marrow depressants*	Increased risk of bone marrow depression.

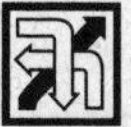

POSSIBLE INTERACTION WITH OTHER SUBSTANCES

INTERACTS WITH	COMBINED EFFECT
Alcohol:	Increased risk of gastritis and internal bleeding.
Beverages:	None expected.
Cocaine:	Increased risk of mental disturbances. Avoid.
Foods:	None expected.
Marijuana:	None expected.
Tobacco:	None expected.

***See Glossary**

LEVETIRACETAM

BRAND NAMES

Keppra
Keppra XR

BASIC INFORMATION

Habit forming? No
Prescription needed? Yes
Available as generic? Yes
Drug class: Anticonvulsant; antiepileptic

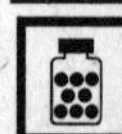

USES

Used to help control some types of seizures in the treatment of epilepsy. This medicine cannot cure epilepsy and will only work to control seizures for as long as you continue to take it.

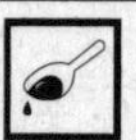

DOSAGE & USAGE INFORMATION

How to take:

- Tablet or extended-release tablet—Swallow whole with a liquid. Do not crush, chew or break tablet. May be taken with or without food, and on a full or empty stomach.
- Oral solution—Follow instructions on prescription.

When to take:
At the same time(s) each day. Your doctor will determine the schedule. Dose may be increased every two weeks to achieve maximum benefits.

If you forget a dose:
Take as soon as you remember. If it is almost time for the next dose, wait for that dose (don't double this dose) and resume regular schedule.

What drug does:
The exact mechanism of the anticonvulsant activity of levetiracetam is unknown.

Time lapse before drug works:
May take several weeks for effectiveness.

Don't take with:
Any other medicine or any dietary supplement without consulting your doctor or pharmacist.

OVERDOSE

SYMPTOMS:
Possibly drowsiness or other symptoms.
WHAT TO DO:
Overdose unlikely to threaten life. If person uses much larger amount than prescribed or if accidentally swallowed, call doctor or poison control center 1-800-222-1222 for help.

POSSIBLE ADVERSE REACTIONS OR SIDE EFFECTS

SYMPTOMS	WHAT TO DO
Life-threatening: None expected.	
Common:	
Cough; dizziness; dry or sore throat; hoarseness; loss of strength or energy; muscle pain or weakness; runny nose; sleepiness; tender, swollen glands in neck; trouble in swallowing; unusual tiredness or weakness; voice changes.	Continue. Call doctor when convenient.
Infrequent:	
• Clumsiness or unsteadiness, crying, depression, double vision, fever or chills, headache, loss of memory or problems with memory, lower back or side pain, mood or mental changes, suicidal thoughts or feelings, nervousness, angry outbursts, pain or tenderness around eyes and cheekbones, painful or difficult urination, paranoia, muscle control problems, overreacting, shortness of breath or trouble breathing, chest tightness, wheezing.	Continue, but call doctor right away. Seek emergency care for severe symptoms.
• Burning, crawling, itching, numbness, prickling, or tingling feelings; feeling of constant movement of self or surroundings; loss of appetite; spinning sensation; weight loss.	Continue. Call doctor when convenient.
Rare:	
Other symptoms.	Continue. Call doctor when convenient.

WARNINGS & PRECAUTIONS

Don't take if:
You are allergic to levetiracetam.

Before you start, consult your doctor if:
- You have kidney disease.
- You are allergic to any medication, food or other substance.
- You have any other medical problems.

Over age 60:
No special problems expected.

Pregnancy:
Decide with your doctor if drug benefits justify risks to unborn child. Risk category C (see page xviii).

Breast-feeding:
It is unknown if drug passes into milk. Avoid drug or discontinue nursing until you finish medicine. Consult doctor for advice on maintaining milk supply.

Infants & children:
Approved for children one month of age and older. Carefully follow prescription instructions.

Prolonged use:
No special problems expected. Follow-up laboratory blood studies may be recommended by your doctor.

Skin & sunlight:
No problems expected.

Driving, piloting or hazardous work:
Don't drive or pilot aircraft until you learn how medicine affects you. Don't work around dangerous machinery. Don't climb ladders or work in high places. Danger increases if you drink alcohol or take other medicines affecting alertness and reflexes such as antihistamines, tranquilizers, sedatives, pain medicine, narcotics and mind-altering drugs.

Discontinuing:
Don't discontinue without doctor's approval due to risk of increased seizure activity. The dosage may need to be gradually decreased before stopping the drug completely.

Others:
- Advise any doctor or dentist whom you consult that you take this medicine.
- Levetiracetam may be used with other anticonvulsant drugs and additional side effects may also occur. If they do, discuss them with your doctor.
- Rarely, antiepileptic drugs may lead to suicidal thoughts and behaviors. Call doctor right away if suicidal symptoms or unusual behaviors occur.
- Wear or carry medical identification to show your seizure disorder and the drugs you take.

POSSIBLE INTERACTION WITH OTHER DRUGS

GENERIC NAME OR DRUG CLASS	COMBINED EFFECT
Anticonvulsants,* other	May decrease or increase effect of both drugs.
CNS Depressants*	Increased sedative effect.

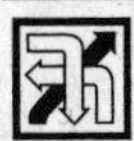

POSSIBLE INTERACTION WITH OTHER SUBSTANCES

INTERACTS WITH	COMBINED EFFECT
Alcohol:	Increased sedative effect. Avoid.
Beverages:	None expected.
Cocaine:	Unknown effect. Avoid.
Foods:	None expected.
Marijuana:	Unknown effect. Avoid.
Tobacco:	None expected.

*See Glossary

LEVOCARNITINE

BRAND NAMES

Carnitor
Carnitor Sugar-free Oral Solution
L-Carnitine
VitaCarn

BASIC INFORMATION

Habit forming? No
Prescription needed? Yes
Available as generic? Yes
Drug class: Nutritional supplement

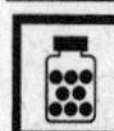

USES

Treats carnitine deficiency, a genetic impairment preventing normal utilization from diet.

DOSAGE & USAGE INFORMATION

How to take:

- Oral solution—Take after meals with liquid to decrease stomach irritation.
- Tablet—Swallow with liquid or food to lessen stomach irritation. If you can't swallow whole, crumble tablet and take with liquid or food.
- Injection—Given by medical professional.

When to take:
Immediately following or during meals to reduce stomach irritation.

If you forget a dose:
Take as soon as you remember. If it is almost time for the next dose, wait for that dose (don't double this dose) and resume regular schedule.

What drug does:
Facilitates normal use of fat to produce energy. Dietary source is meat and milk.

Time lapse before drug works:
Immediate action.

Don't take with:
Any other medicine or any dietary supplement without consulting your doctor or pharmacist.

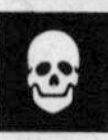

OVERDOSE

SYMPTOMS:
Severe muscle weakness.
WHAT TO DO:

- **Dial 911 (emergency) for medical help or call poison control center 1-800-222-1222 for instructions.**
- **See emergency information on last 3 pages of this book.**

POSSIBLE ADVERSE REACTIONS OR SIDE EFFECTS

SYMPTOMS	WHAT TO DO
Life-threatening: None expected.	
Common: Changed body odor.	Continue. Call doctor when convenient.
Infrequent: Diarrhea, abdominal pain, nausea, vomiting.	Continue, but call doctor right away.
Rare: None expected.	

WARNINGS & PRECAUTIONS

Don't take if:
You are allergic to levocarnitine.

Before you start, consult your doctor if:
- You have a seizure disorder.
- You have severe kidney disorder.

Over age 60:
No problems expected.

Pregnancy:
No proven harm to unborn child, but avoid if possible. Consult doctor. Risk category B (see page xviii).

Breast-feeding:
No problems expected. Consult doctor.

Infants & children:
No problems expected. Deficiency can cause impaired growth and development.

Prolonged use:
Talk to your doctor about the need for follow-up medical examinations or laboratory studies to check triglycerides.

Skin & sunlight:
No problems expected.

Driving, piloting or hazardous work:
No problems expected.

Discontinuing:
Don't discontinue without consulting doctor. Dose may require gradual reduction if you have taken drug for a long time. Doses of other drugs may also require adjustment.

Others:
- Advise any doctor or dentist whom you consult that you take this medicine.
- Do not use a product named "vitamin B-T" sold in health food stores. It contains dextro- and levo- carnitine. This product completely negates the effectiveness of levocarnitine (L-carnitine). Only the L-carnitine form is effective in treating carnitine deficiency.

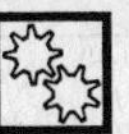

POSSIBLE INTERACTION WITH OTHER DRUGS

GENERIC NAME OR DRUG CLASS	COMBINED EFFECT
None expected.	

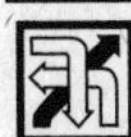

POSSIBLE INTERACTION WITH OTHER SUBSTANCES

INTERACTS WITH	COMBINED EFFECT
Alcohol:	None expected.
Beverages:	None expected.
Cocaine:	None expected.
Foods:	None expected.
Marijuana:	None expected.
Tobacco:	None expected.

LEVODOPA

BRAND NAMES

Dopar
Larodopa

BASIC INFORMATION

Habit forming? No
Prescription needed? Yes
Available as generic? Yes
Drug class: Antiparkinsonism

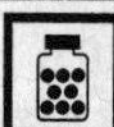

USES

Controls Parkinson's disease symptoms such as rigidity, tremor and unsteady gait.

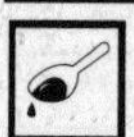

DOSAGE & USAGE INFORMATION

How to take:
Tablet or capsule—Swallow with liquid or food to lessen stomach irritation. If you can't swallow whole, crumble tablet or open capsule and take with liquid or food.

When to take:
At the same times each day.

If you forget a dose:
Take as soon as you remember. If it is almost time for the next dose, wait for that dose (don't double this dose) and resume regular schedule.

What drug does:
Restores chemical balance necessary for normal nerve impulses.

Time lapse before drug works:
2 to 3 weeks to improve; 6 weeks or longer for maximum benefit.

Don't take with:
Any other medicine or any dietary supplement without consulting your doctor or pharmacist.

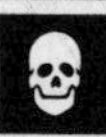

OVERDOSE

SYMPTOMS:
Muscle twitch, spastic eyelid closure, nausea, vomiting, diarrhea, irregular and rapid pulse, weakness, fainting, confusion, agitation, hallucination, coma.
WHAT TO DO:
- **Dial 911 (emergency) for medical help or call poison control center 1-800-222-1222 for instructions.**
- **If person is unconscious, check breathing and pulse. If not breathing, begin mouth-to-mouth rescue breathing. If heart is not beating, begin chest compressions.**
- **See emergency information on last 3 pages of this book.**

POSSIBLE ADVERSE REACTIONS OR SIDE EFFECTS

SYMPTOMS	WHAT TO DO
Life-threatening: In case of overdose, see previous column.	
Common:	
• Uncontrollable body movements.	Discontinue. Call doctor right away.
• Mood change, diarrhea, depression, anxiety.	Continue. Call doctor when convenient.
• Dry mouth, body odor.	No action necessary.
Infrequent:	
• Fainting, severe dizziness, headache, insomnia, nightmares, itchy skin, rash, nausea, vomiting, irregular heartbeat, eyelid spasm.	Discontinue. Call doctor right away.
• Flushed face, muscle twitching, discolored or dark urine, difficult urination, blurred vision, appetite loss.	Continue. Call doctor when convenient.
• Constipation, tiredness.	Continue. Tell doctor at next visit.
Rare:	
• High blood pressure.	Discontinue. Call doctor right away.
• Upper abdominal pain, anemia, increased sex drive.	Continue. Call doctor when convenient.

WARNINGS & PRECAUTIONS

Don't take if:
- You are allergic to levodopa or carbidopa.
- You have taken a monoamine oxidase (MAO) inhibitor* in past 2 weeks.
- You have glaucoma (narrow-angle type).

Before you start, consult your doctor if:
- You have diabetes or epilepsy.
- You have had high blood pressure, heart or lung disease.
- You have had liver or kidney disease.
- You have a peptic ulcer.
- You have malignant melanoma.
- You will have surgery within 2 months, including dental surgery, requiring general or spinal anesthesia.

Over age 60:
Adverse reactions and side effects may be more frequent and severe than in younger persons.

Pregnancy:
Decide with your doctor if drug benefits justify risk to unborn child. Risk category C (see page xviii).

Breast-feeding:
Drug filters into milk. May harm child. Avoid.

Infants & children:
Not recommended.

Prolonged use:
- May lead to uncontrolled movements of head, face, mouth, tongue, arms or legs.
- Talk to your doctor about the need for follow-up medical examinations or laboratory studies to check complete blood counts (white blood cell count, platelet count, red blood cell count, hemoglobin, hematocrit), kidney function, liver function.

Skin & sunlight:
No problems expected.

Driving, piloting or hazardous work:
Don't drive or pilot aircraft until you learn how medicine affects you. Don't work around dangerous machinery. Don't climb ladders or work in high places. Danger increases if you drink alcohol or take medicine affecting alertness and reflexes, such as antihistamines, tranquilizers, sedatives, pain medicine, narcotics and mind-altering drugs.

Discontinuing:
Don't discontinue without doctor's advice until you complete prescribed dose, even though symptoms diminish or disappear.

Others:
- Expect to start with small dose and increase gradually to lessen frequency and severity of adverse reactions.
- Advise any doctor or dentist whom you consult that you take this medicine.

POSSIBLE INTERACTION WITH OTHER DRUGS

GENERIC NAME OR DRUG CLASS	COMBINED EFFECT
Antidepressants, tricyclic (TCA)*	Decreased blood pressure. Weakness and faintness when arising from bed or chair.
Antiparkinsonism drugs, other*	Increased levodopa effect.
Bupropion	Increased levodopa effect.
Haloperidol	Decreased levodopa effect.
Loxapine	Decreased levodopa effect.
MAO inhibitors*	Dangerous rise in blood pressure.
Methyldopa	Decreased levodopa effect.
Molindone	Decreased levodopa effect.
Olanzapine	May decrease levodopa effect.
Papaverine	Decreased levodopa effect.
Phenothiazines*	Decreased levodopa effect.
Phenytoin	Decreased levodopa effect.
Pyridoxine (Vitamin B-6)	Decreased levodopa effect.
Quetiapine	Decreased levodopa effect.
Rauwolfia alkaloids*	Decreased levodopa effect.
Selegiline	May require reduced dosage of levodopa.
Thioxanthenes*	Decreased levodopa effect.
Ziprasidone	Decreased levodopa effect.

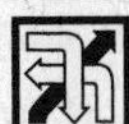

POSSIBLE INTERACTION WITH OTHER SUBSTANCES

INTERACTS WITH	COMBINED EFFECT
Alcohol:	None expected.
Beverages:	None expected.
Cocaine:	Increased risk of heartbeat irregularity.
Foods: High-protein diet.	Decreased levodopa effect.
Marijuana:	Increased fatigue, lethargy, fainting.
Tobacco:	None expected.

LINACLOTIDE

BRAND NAMES

Linzess

BASIC INFORMATION

Habit forming? No
Prescription needed? Yes
Available as generic? No
Drug class: Guanylate cyclase-C agonist

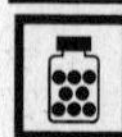

USES

- Relieves symptoms of irritable bowel syndrome (IBS) with constipation.
- Treats chronic constipation of unknown cause (idiopathic constipation).

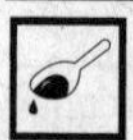

DOSAGE & USAGE INFORMATION

How to take:
Capsule—Swallow whole with a glass of water. Do not break, chew or crush capsule.

When to take:
Drug is taken once a day (at the same time each day) on an empty stomach and at least 30 minutes before your first meal of the day.

If you forget a dose:
Take as soon as you remember. If it is almost time for the next dose, wait for the next scheduled dose (don't double this dose).

What drug does:
It works in the intestine (it is not absorbed in the body) by increasing intestinal fluid secretion which eases the passage of stool and relieves the symptoms associated with constipation.

Time lapse before drug works:
A few days to a week.

Don't take with:
Any other medicine or any dietary supplement without consulting your doctor or pharmacist.

OVERDOSE

SYMPTOMS:
Diarrhea and possibly other symptoms.
WHAT TO DO:
Overdose unlikely to threaten life. If person takes much larger amount than prescribed or if accidentally swallowed, call doctor or poison control center 1-800-222-1222 for help.

POSSIBLE ADVERSE REACTIONS OR SIDE EFFECTS

SYMPTOMS	WHAT TO DO
Life-threatening: None expected.	
Common:	
• Diarrhea (may be severe), pain in abdomen or stomach.	Discontinue. Call doctor right away.
• Passing gas, feeling bloated.	Continue. Call doctor when convenient.
Infrequent: Upset stomach, vomiting, heartburn, unable to control bowel movements, gastrointestinal infections, headache.	Continue. Call doctor when convenient.
Rare:	
• Bleeding from the rectum, black or tarry stool.	Discontinue. Call doctor right away.
• Unusual symptoms that cause concern.	Continue. Call doctor when convenient.

WARNINGS & PRECAUTIONS

Don't take if:
- You are allergic to linaclotide.
- Patient is under age 6.

Before you start, consult your doctor if:
- You have or have had any problem with bowel or stomach blockage (may be referred to as mechanical gastrointestinal obstruction).
- You have severe diarrhea.

Over age 60:
No problems expected.

Pregnancy:
Decide with your doctor whether drug benefits justify risk to unborn child. Risk category C (see page xviii).

Breast-feeding:
It is unknown if drug passes into breast milk. Consult your doctor for advice.

Infants & children:
Do not give to children under age 6. Safety and efficacy for children ages 6 to 17 has not been established.

Prolonged use:
See your doctor for regular visits to make sure the drug is working properly and to check for unwanted effects.

Skin & sunlight:
No problems expected.

Driving, piloting or hazardous work:
No problems expected.

Discontinuing:
No problems expected, but consult your doctor before discontinuing.

Others:
- Advise any doctor, dentist or pharmacist whom you consult that you take this drug.
- Keep drug in its original container. Do not remove the drying agent in the container.

POSSIBLE INTERACTION WITH OTHER DRUGS

GENERIC NAME OR DRUG CLASS	COMBINED EFFECT
None expected	

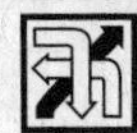

POSSIBLE INTERACTION WITH OTHER SUBSTANCES

INTERACTS WITH	COMBINED EFFECT
Alcohol:	None expected.
Beverages:	None expected.
Cocaine:	None expected.
Foods:	None expected.
Marijuana:	None expected.
Tobacco:	None expected.

LINCOMYCIN

BRAND NAMES

Lincocin

BASIC INFORMATION

Habit forming? No
Prescription needed? Yes
Available as generic? Yes
Drug class: Antibacterial

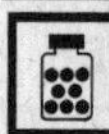

USES

Treatment of bacterial infections that are susceptible to lincomycin.

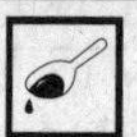

DOSAGE & USAGE INFORMATION

How to take:
Capsule—Swallow with liquid 1 hour before or 2 hours after eating. Drink 8 ounces of water with each dose.

When to take:
At the same times each day.

If you forget a dose:
Take as soon as you remember. If it is almost time for the next dose, wait for that dose (don't double this dose) and resume regular schedule.

What drug does:
Destroys susceptible bacteria. Does not kill viruses.

Time lapse before drug works:
3 to 5 days.

Don't take with:
Any other medicine or any dietary supplement without consulting your doctor or pharmacist.

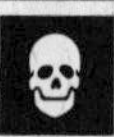

OVERDOSE

SYMPTOMS:
Severe nausea, vomiting, diarrhea.
WHAT TO DO:
Overdose unlikely to threaten life. If person uses much larger amount than prescribed or if accidentally swallowed, call doctor or poison control center 1-800-222-1222 for help.

POSSIBLE ADVERSE REACTIONS OR SIDE EFFECTS

SYMPTOMS	WHAT TO DO
Life-threatening:	
Hives, wheezing, faintness, itching, coma.	Seek emergency treatment.
Common:	
Mild diarrhea, mild stomach cramps, nausea.	Continue. Call doctor when convenient.
Infrequent:	
• Unusual thirst; vomiting; stomach cramps; severe and watery diarrhea with blood or mucus; painful, swollen joints; jaundice; fever; tiredness; weakness; weight loss.	Discontinue. Call doctor right away.
• Itch around groin, rectum or armpits; white patches in mouth; vaginal discharge, itching.	Continue. Call doctor when convenient.
Rare:	
Skin rash.	Discontinue. Call doctor right away.

WARNINGS & PRECAUTIONS

Don't take if:
- You are allergic to lincomycins.
- You have had ulcerative colitis.
- Prescribed for infant under 1 month old.

Before you start, consult your doctor if:
- You have had yeast infections of mouth, skin or vagina.
- You will have surgery within 2 months, including dental surgery, requiring general or spinal anesthesia.
- You have kidney or liver disease.
- You have allergies of any kind.

Over age 60:
Adverse reactions and side effects may be more frequent and severe than in younger persons.

Pregnancy:
Decide with your doctor if drug benefits justify risk to unborn child. Risk category C (see page xviii).

Breast-feeding:
Drug passes into milk. Avoid drug or discontinue nursing until you finish medicine. Consult doctor for advice on maintaining milk supply.

Infants & children:
Don't give to infants younger than 1 month. Use for children only under medical supervision.

Prolonged use:
- Severe colitis with diarrhea and bleeding.
- You may become more susceptible to infections caused by germs not responsive to lincomycin.
- Talk to your doctor about the need for follow-up medical examinations or laboratory studies or proctosigmoidoscopy.

Skin & sunlight:
No problems expected.

Driving, piloting or hazardous work:
No problems expected.

Discontinuing:
Don't discontinue without doctor's advice until you complete prescribed dose, even though symptoms diminish or disappear.

Others:
- May interfere with the accuracy of some medical tests.
- Advise any doctor or dentist whom you consult that you take use medicine.

POSSIBLE INTERACTION WITH OTHER DRUGS

GENERIC NAME OR DRUG CLASS	COMBINED EFFECT
Antidiarrheal preparations*	Decreased lincomycin effect.
Attapulgite	May decrease effectiveness of lincomycin.
Chloramphenicol	Decreased lincomycin effect.
Erythromycins*	Decreased lincomycin effect.
Narcotics*	Increased risk of respiratory problems.

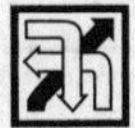

POSSIBLE INTERACTION WITH OTHER SUBSTANCES

INTERACTS WITH	COMBINED EFFECT
Alcohol:	None expected.
Beverages:	None expected.
Cocaine:	None expected.
Foods:	None expected.
Marijuana:	None expected.
Tobacco:	None expected.

***See Glossary**

LINEZOLID

BRAND NAMES

Zyvox

BASIC INFORMATION

Habit forming? No
Prescription needed? Yes
Available as generic? No
Drug class: Antibacterial, antibiotic (oxazolidinone)

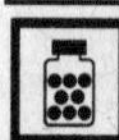

USES

Treats bacterial infections of the blood, lungs and skin. It may also be used for other conditions as determined by your doctor.

DOSAGE & USAGE INFORMATION

How to take:

- Tablet—Take with full glass of water. If you can't swallow whole, crumble tablet and take with liquid or food.
- Oral suspension—Take as directed on label. The medicine should be gently mixed by inverting the bottle 3 to 5 times before each dose. Do not shake the bottle.

When to take:
As directed by your doctor. Usually every 12 hours.

If you forget a dose:
Take as soon as you remember. If it is almost time for the next dose, wait for that dose (don't double this dose) and resume regular schedule.

What drug does:
Destroys bacteria in the body, probably by blocking protein production inside bacteria.

Time lapse before drug works:
10 to 14 days for most infections, but some infections may take longer. Continue taking this medicine for the full time of treatment even if you begin to feel better after a few days.

Continued next column

OVERDOSE

SYMPTOMS:
Unknown.
WHAT TO DO:
Overdose unlikely to threaten life. If person uses much larger amount than prescribed or if accidentally swallowed, call doctor or poison control center 1-800-222-1222 for help.

Don't take with:
Any other medicine or any dietary supplement without consulting your doctor or pharmacist.

POSSIBLE ADVERSE REACTIONS OR SIDE EFFECTS

SYMPTOMS	WHAT TO DO
Life-threatening: None expected.	
Common:	
• Diarrhea, headache.	Continue. Call doctor when convenient.
• Nausea.	Continue. Call doctor if symptoms persist.
Infrequent:	
• Fever, sore mouth or tongue, rash, black tarry stools, chest pain, chills, cough, painful or difficult urination, unusual bleeding or bruising, unusual tiredness or weakness, vomiting.	Discontinue. Call doctor right away.
• Constipation, change in taste, sleeplessness, vaginal yeast infection.	Continue. Call doctor when convenient.
Rare: None expected.	

WARNINGS & PRECAUTIONS

Don't take if:
You are allergic to linezolid.

Before you start, consult your doctor if:
- You are using any other medication.
- You have a history of bleeding problems, diarrhea, high blood pressure or any other medical problems.

Over age 60:
Side effects or problems experienced with this medication appear to be the same in older people as in younger adults.

Pregnancy:
Decide with your doctor if drug benefits justify risk to unborn child. Risk category C (see page xviii).

Breast-feeding:
It is unknown if drug passes into milk. Avoid drug or discontinue nursing until you finish medicine. Consult doctor for advice on maintaining milk supply.

Infants & children:
Studies on this medicine have been done only in adult patients. Consult doctor before giving this medicine to persons under age 18.

Prolonged use:
Usually not prescribed for long-term use.

Skin & sunlight:
None expected.

Driving, piloting or hazardous work:
None expected.

Discontinuing:
Don't discontinue without consulting doctor or completing prescribed dosage.

Others:
- May affect accuracy of some laboratory test values.
- Do not store in the bathroom, near the kitchen sink or in other damp places. Heat or moisture may cause the medicine to break down.
- Advise any doctor or dentist whom you consult that you take this medicine.

POSSIBLE INTERACTION WITH OTHER DRUGS

GENERIC NAME OR DRUG CLASS	COMBINED EFFECT
Pseudoephedrine	May increase blood pressure.
Serotonergics*	Serotonin syndrome.*

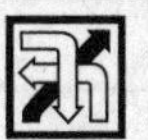

POSSIBLE INTERACTION WITH OTHER SUBSTANCES

INTERACTS WITH	COMBINED EFFECT
Alcohol:	None expected.
Beverages:	None expected.
Cocaine:	Effect unknown. Avoid.
Foods:	None expected.
Marijuana:	Effect unknown. Avoid
Tobacco:	None expected.

***See Glossary**

LITHIUM

BRAND NAMES

Carbolith
Cibalith-S
Duralith
Eskalith
Eskalith CR
Lithane
Lithizine
Lithobid
Lithonate
Lithotabs

BASIC INFORMATION

Habit forming? No
Prescription needed? Yes
Available as generic? Yes
Drug class: Mood stabilizer

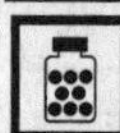

USES

- Normalizes mood and behavior in bipolar (manic-depressive) disorder.
- Treats alcohol toxicity and addiction.
- Treats schizoid personality disorders.

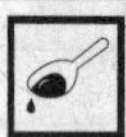

DOSAGE & USAGE INFORMATION

How to take:
- Tablet or capsule—Swallow with liquid or food to lessen stomach irritation. If you can't swallow whole, crumble tablet or open capsule and take with liquid or food. Drink plenty of liquids each day, especially in hot weather.
- Extended-release tablet—Swallow each dose whole. Do not crush.
- Syrup—Take at mealtime. Follow with 8 oz. water.

When to take:
At the same times each day, preferably at mealtime.

If you forget a dose:
Take as soon as you remember. If it is almost time for the next dose, wait for that dose (don't double this dose) and resume regular schedule.

Continued next column

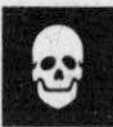

OVERDOSE

SYMPTOMS:
Moderate overdose increases some side effects and may cause diarrhea, nausea. Large overdose may cause vomiting, muscle weakness, convulsions, stupor and coma.

WHAT TO DO:
- **Dial 911 (emergency) for medical help or call poison control center 1-800-222-1222 for instructions.**
- **See emergency information on last 3 pages of this book.**

What drug does:
May correct chemical imbalance in brain's transmission of nerve impulses that influence mood and behavior.

Time lapse before drug works:
1 to 3 weeks. May require 3 months before depressive phase of illness improves.

Don't take with:
Any other medicine or any dietary supplement without consulting your doctor or pharmacist.

POSSIBLE ADVERSE REACTIONS OR SIDE EFFECTS

SYMPTOMS	WHAT TO DO
Life-threatening: In case of overdose, see previous column.	
Common:	
• Dizziness, diarrhea, nausea, vomiting, shakiness, tremor.	Continue. Call doctor when convenient.
• Dry mouth, thirst, decreased sexual ability, increased urination, anorexia.	Continue. Tell doctor at next visit.
Infrequent:	
• Rash, stomach pain, fainting, heartbeat irregularities, shortness of breath, ear noises, swollen hands or feet, slurred speech.	Discontinue. Call doctor right away.
• Thyroid impairment (coldness; dry, puffy skin), muscle aches, headache, weight gain, fatigue, menstrual irregularities, acnelike breakouts, drowsiness, confusion, weakness.	Continue. Call doctor when convenient.
Rare:	
• Blurred vision, eye pain.	Discontinue. Call doctor right away.
• Jerking of arms and legs, worsening of psoriasis, hair loss.	Continue. Call doctor when convenient.

WARNINGS & PRECAUTIONS

Don't take if:
- You are allergic to lithium or tartrazine dye.
- You have kidney or heart disease.
- Patient is younger than 12.

Before you start, consult your doctor if:
- You plan to become pregnant within medication period.

- You have diabetes, thyroid disorder, epilepsy, brain disease, schizophrenia, difficult urination, heart disease, kidney disorder, Parkinson's or history of leukemia.
- You are on a low-salt diet or drink more than 4 cups of coffee per day.
- You plan surgery within 2 months.

Over age 60:
Adverse reactions and side effects may be more frequent and severe than in younger persons.

Pregnancy:
Some fetal risk, but benefits may outweigh risks. Risk category D (see page xviii).

Breast-feeding:
Drug passes into milk. Avoid drug or discontinue nursing until you finish medicine. Consult doctor for advice on maintaining milk supply.

Infants & children:
Don't give to children younger than 12.

Prolonged use:
- Enlarged thyroid with possible impaired function.
- Talk to your doctor about the need for follow-up medical examinations or laboratory studies to check lithium levels, ECG,* kidney function, thyroid, complete blood counts (white blood cell count, platelet count, red blood cell count, hemoglobin, hematocrit).

Skin & sunlight:
No problems expected.

Driving, piloting or hazardous work:
Don't drive or pilot aircraft until you learn how medicine affects you. Don't work around dangerous machinery. Don't climb ladders or work in high places. Danger increases if you drink alcohol or take medicine affecting alertness and reflexes.

Discontinuing:
Don't discontinue without consulting doctor. Dose may require gradual reduction if you have taken drug for a long time. Doses of other drugs may also require adjustment. Quitting this medication when feeling well creates risk of relapse which may not respond to restarting the medication.

Others:
- Regular checkups, periodic blood tests, and tests of lithium levels and thyroid function recommended.
- Avoid exercise in hot weather and other activities that cause heavy sweating. This contributes to lithium poisoning. It is essential to take adequate fluids during hot weather to avoid toxicity.
- Call your doctor if you have an illness that causes heavy sweating, vomiting, or diarrhea. The loss of too much salt and water from your body could cause lithium toxicity.
- Advise any doctor or dentist whom you consult that you take this medicine.
- Some products contain tartrazine dye. Avoid, especially if allergic to aspirin.

POSSIBLE INTERACTION WITH OTHER DRUGS

GENERIC NAME OR DRUG CLASS	COMBINED EFFECT
Acetazolamide	Decreased lithium effect.
Antihistamines*	Possible excessive sedation.
Anti-inflammatory drugs, nonsteroidal (NSAIDs)*	Increased toxic effect of lithium.
Bupropion	Increased risk of seizures.
Carbamazepine	Increased lithium effect.
Desmopressin	Possible decreased desmopressin effect.
Diazepam	Possible hypothermia.
Diclofenac	Possible increase in effect and toxicity.
Didanosine	Increased risk of peripheral neuropathy.

Continued on page 918

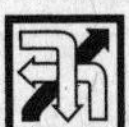

POSSIBLE INTERACTION WITH OTHER SUBSTANCES

INTERACTS WITH	COMBINED EFFECT
Alcohol:	Possible lithium poisoning.
Beverages: Caffeine drinks.	Decreased lithium effect.
Cocaine:	Possible psychosis.
Foods: Salt.	High intake could decrease lithium effect. Low intake could increase lithium effect. *Don't* restrict intake.
Marijuana:	Increased tremor and possible psychosis.
Tobacco:	None expected.

***See Glossary**

LOMUSTINE

BRAND NAMES

CCNU CeeNU

BASIC INFORMATION

Habit forming? No
Prescription needed? Yes
Available as generic? No
Drug class: Antineoplastic

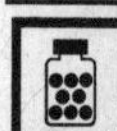

USES

- Treats brain cancer and Hodgkin's lymphoma.
- Sometimes used to treat breast, lung, skin and gastrointestinal cancer.

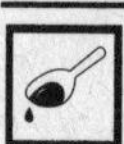

DOSAGE & USAGE INFORMATION

How to take:
Capsule—Swallow with liquid. If you can't swallow whole, open capsule and take with liquid or food. Instructions to take on empty stomach mean 1 hour before or 2 hours after eating. Note: There may be two or more different types of capsules in the container. This is not an error.

When to take:
According to doctor's instructions. Usual course of treatment requires single dosage repeated every 6 weeks.

If you forget a dose:
Take as soon as you remember. Don't ever double doses.

What drug does:
Interferes with growth of cancer cells.

Time lapse before drug works:
None. Works immediately.

Don't take with:
Any other medicine or any dietary supplement without consulting your doctor or pharmacist.

OVERDOSE

SYMPTOMS:
Decreased urine (kidney failure); high fever, chills (infection); bloody or black stools (bleeding).
WHAT TO DO:
- **Dial 911 (emergency) for medical help or call poison control center 1-800-222-1222 for instructions.**
- **See emergency information on last 3 pages of this book.**

POSSIBLE ADVERSE REACTIONS OR SIDE EFFECTS

SYMPTOMS	WHAT TO DO
Life-threatening: In case of overdose, see previous column.	
Common:	
• Fever, chills, difficult urination, unusual bleeding.	Continue. Call doctor when convenient.
• Appetite loss, nausea, hair loss.	No action necessary.
Infrequent:	
• Anemia, confusion, slurred speech, mouth sores, skin rash.	Continue. Call doctor when convenient.
• Darkened skin.	No action necessary.
Rare:	
• Shortness of breath.	Discontinue. Call doctor right away.
• Jaundice (yellow skin and eyes), cough.	Continue. Call doctor when convenient.

WARNINGS & PRECAUTIONS

Don't take if:
- You have chicken pox.
- You have shingles (herpes zoster).

Before you start, consult your doctor if:
- You have an infection.
- You have kidney or lung disease.
- You have had previous cancer chemotherapy or radiation treatment.

Over age 60:
Adverse reactions and side effects may be more frequent and severe than in younger persons. You may need smaller doses for shorter periods of time.

Pregnancy:
Risk to unborn child outweighs drug benefits. Don't use. Risk category D (see page xviii).

Breast-feeding:
Drug passes into milk. Avoid drug or discontinue nursing until you finish medicine. Consult doctor for advice on maintaining milk supply.

Infants & children:
Effect not documented. Consult your doctor.

Prolonged use:
Talk to your doctor about the need for follow-up medical examinations or laboratory studies to check kidney function, liver function and complete blood counts (white blood cell count, platelet count, red blood cell count, hemoglobin, hematocrit).

Skin & sunlight:
No problems expected.

Driving, piloting or hazardous work:
Don't drive or pilot aircraft until you learn how medicine affects you. Don't work around dangerous machinery. Don't climb ladders or work in high places. Danger increases if you drink alcohol or take medicine affecting alertness and reflexes.

Discontinuing:
Call doctor if any of these occur after discontinuing: black or tarry stools, bloody urine, hoarseness, bleeding or bruising, fever or chills.

Others:
- Advise any doctor or dentist whom you consult that you take this medicine.
- May affect results in some medical tests.
- Most adverse reactions and side effects are unavoidable.
- Avoid immunizations, if possible.
- Avoid persons with infections.
- Check with doctor about brushing or flossing teeth.
- Avoid contact sports.

POSSIBLE INTERACTION WITH OTHER DRUGS

GENERIC NAME OR DRUG CLASS	COMBINED EFFECT
Antineoplastic drugs, other*	Increased chance of drug toxicity.
Blood dyscrasia-causing medicines*	Adverse effect on bone marrow, causing decreased white cells and platelets.
Bone marrow depressants,* other	Increased risk of bone marrow depression.
Clozapine	Toxic effect on bone marrow.
Levamisole	Increased risk of bone marrow depression.
Tiopronin	Increased risk of toxicity to bone marrow.
Vaccines, live or killed virus	Increased chance of toxicity or reduced effectiveness of vaccine. Wait 3 to 12 months after lomustine treatment before getting vaccination.

POSSIBLE INTERACTION WITH OTHER SUBSTANCES

INTERACTS WITH	COMBINED EFFECT
Alcohol:	Increased chance of liver damage.
Beverages:	None expected.
Cocaine:	Increased chance of central nervous system toxicity.
Foods:	None expected.
Marijuana:	None expected.
Tobacco:	None expected.

***See Glossary**

LOPERAMIDE

BRAND NAMES

Apo-Loperamide Caplets
Imodium
Imodium A-D
Imodium Advanced
Imodium Multi Symptom Relief
Kaopectate II Caplets
Pepto Diarrhea Control

BASIC INFORMATION

Habit forming? No, unless taken in high doses for long periods.
Prescription needed? Yes, for some
Available as generic? Yes
Drug class: Antidiarrheal

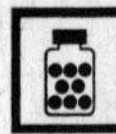

USES

- Treats mild to moderate diarrhea. Used in conjunction with fluids, appropriate diet and rest. Treats symptoms only. Does not cure any disorder that causes diarrhea.
- Treats chronic diarrhea associated with inflammatory bowel disease.

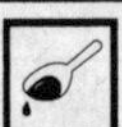

DOSAGE & USAGE INFORMATION

How to take:
- Tablet or capsule—Swallow with food to lessen stomach irritation.
- Liquid—Follow label instructions and use marked dropper.

When to take:
No more often than directed on label.

If you forget a dose:
Take as soon as you remember. If it is almost time for the next dose, wait for that dose (don't double this dose) and resume regular schedule.

What drug does:
Blocks digestive tract's nerve supply, which reduces irritability and contractions in intestinal tract.

Continued next column

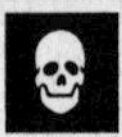

OVERDOSE

SYMPTOMS:
Constipation, lethargy, drowsiness or unconsciousness.
WHAT TO DO:
Overdose unlikely to threaten life. If person uses much larger amount than prescribed or if accidentally swallowed, call doctor or poison control center 1-800-222-1222 for help.

Time lapse before drug works:
1 to 2 hours.

Don't take with:
Any other medicine or any dietary supplement without consulting your doctor or pharmacist.

POSSIBLE ADVERSE REACTIONS OR SIDE EFFECTS

SYMPTOMS	WHAT TO DO
Life-threatening: None expected.	
Common: None expected.	
Infrequent: None expected.	
Rare:	
• Drowsiness, dizziness, dry mouth.	Continue. Call doctor when convenient.
• Nausea, vomiting, bloating, constipation, appetite loss, rash, abdominal pain.	Discontinue. Call doctor right away.

WARNINGS & PRECAUTIONS

Don't take if:
- You have severe colitis.
- You have colitis resulting from antibiotic treatment or infection.
- You are allergic to loperamide.

Before you start, consult your doctor if:
- You are dehydrated from fluid loss caused by diarrhea.
- You have liver disease.

Over age 60:
Adverse reactions and side effects may be more frequent and severe than in younger persons.

Pregnancy:
No proven harm. Avoid if possible. Consult doctor. Risk category B (see page xviii).

Breast-feeding:
No proven problems, but avoid if possible or discontinue nursing until you finish medicine. Consult doctor for advice on maintaining milk supply.

Infants & children:
Don't give to infants or toddlers. Use only under doctor's supervision for children older than 2.

Prolonged use:
Habit forming at high dose.

Skin & sunlight:
No problems expected.

Driving, piloting or hazardous work:
Don't drive or pilot aircraft until you learn how medicine affects you. Don't work around dangerous machinery. Don't climb ladders or work in high places. Danger increases if you drink alcohol or take medicine affecting alertness and reflexes.

Discontinuing:
- May be unnecessary to finish medicine. Follow doctor's instructions.
- After discontinuing, consult doctor if you experience muscle cramps, nausea, vomiting, trembling, stomach cramps or unusual sweating.

Others:
If acute diarrhea lasts longer than 48 hours, discontinue and call doctor. In chronic diarrhea, loperamide is unlikely to be effective if diarrhea doesn't improve in 10 days.

POSSIBLE INTERACTION WITH OTHER DRUGS

GENERIC NAME OR DRUG CLASS	COMBINED EFFECT
Antibiotics*	Increased risk of diarrhea.
Narcotic analgesics	Increased risk of severe constipation.

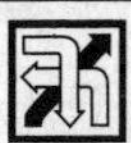

POSSIBLE INTERACTION WITH OTHER SUBSTANCES

INTERACTS WITH	COMBINED EFFECT
Alcohol:	Depressed brain function. Avoid.
Beverages:	None expected.
Cocaine:	Decreased loperamide effect.
Foods:	None expected.
Marijuana:	None expected.
Tobacco:	None expected.

*See Glossary

LORCASERIN

BRAND NAMES

Belviq

BASIC INFORMATION

Habit forming? May be habit forming
Prescription needed? Yes
Available as generic? No
Drug class: Central nervous systemic stimulant; anorexiant

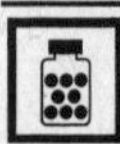

USES

It is used along with a reduced-calorie diet and exercise program to treat obesity in adults who have a BMI (body mass index) over 30. It is also used in adults with a BMI over 27 who have high blood pressure, high cholesterol or diabetes.

DOSAGE & USAGE INFORMATION

How to take:
Tablet—Swallow whole with water. It may be taken with or without food.

When to take:
Twice a day at the same times each day (in the morning and evening).

If you forget a dose:
Take as soon as you remember. If it is almost time for the next dose, wait for the next scheduled dose (don't double this dose).

What drug does:
It works by activating an area of the brain called the serotonin 2C receptor. This action helps a person feel full faster so they eat less than usual.

Time lapse before drug works:
It starts working within hours, but its weight loss effectiveness is determined after taking the drug for 12 weeks.

Don't take with:
Any other medicine or any dietary supplement without consulting your doctor or pharmacist.

OVERDOSE

SYMPTOMS:
Specific symptoms are unclear; may have more severe side effects (e.g., nausea, headache, dizziness, euphoria, hallucinations).
WHAT TO DO:
Overdose unlikely to threaten life. If person takes much larger amount than prescribed or if accidentally swallowed, call doctor or poison control center 1-800-222-1222 for help.

POSSIBLE ADVERSE REACTIONS OR SIDE EFFECTS

SYMPTOMS	WHAT TO DO
Life-threatening:	
Rare allergic reaction (hives, itching, rash, wheezing, tightness in chest, swelling of lips or tongue or throat).	Seek emergency treatment immediately.
Common:	
Headache, dizziness, fatigue, nausea, cold symptoms, back pain, dry mouth, cough, constipation, low blood sugar in diabetic patients.	Continue, but call doctor right away.
Infrequent:	
Diarrhea, urinary tract infection, tooth or throat pain, upset stomach, sinus infection; patients with diabetes may have high blood pressure or swelling of feet and ankles or worsening of diabetes.	Continue, but call doctor right away.
Rare:	
• Confusion, difficulty with concentration or memory, mood changes, depression, hallucinations, feeling euphoric, thoughts of suicide, priapism in males (an erection lasts over 4 hours), enlarged breasts in males, breast milk without childbirth, slow heart rate, serotonin syndrome or neuroleptic malignant syndrome (see Glossary for list of symptoms of each), heart valve problem (shortness of breath, swelling of feet or ankles, chest pain).	Discontinue. Call doctor right away or seek emergency help.
• Feeling anxious or stressed, insomnia, rash, dry eyes or blurred vision or other eye symptoms, muscle pain or spasms.	Continue, but call doctor right away.

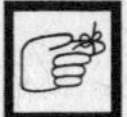

WARNINGS & PRECAUTIONS

Don't take if:
You are allergic to lorcaserin or you are pregnant or plan to become pregnant.

Before you start, consult your doctor if:
- You have liver or kidney problems.
- You have or have had slow heartbeat, heart block, congestive heart failure or heart valvular disease.
- You suffer from depression or mental illness.
- You have pulmonary hypertension.
- You have diabetes or low blood sugar.
- You have cancer or a blood disorder.
- You have a physical abnormality of the penis.

Over age 60:
No problems expected, but dosage may need to be adjusted depending on health status.

Pregnancy:
This drug should not be used in women who are or may become pregnant due to the risk of harm to the baby. Risk category X (see page xviii).

Breast-feeding:
It is unknown if drug passes into breast milk. Consult your doctor for advice.

Infants & children:
Safety and efficacy have not been established for ages under 18.

Prolonged use:
Effects of long term use are unknown. Talk to your doctor about the need for follow-up medical exams or laboratory studies to check the effectiveness of the treatment.

Skin & sunlight:
No problems expected.

Driving, piloting or hazardous work:
Don't drive or pilot aircraft until you learn how medicine affects you. Don't work around dangerous machinery. Don't climb ladders or work in high places. Danger increases if you drink alcohol or take medicine affecting alertness and reflexes.

Discontinuing:
No problems expected, but consult your doctor before stopping the drug.

Others:
- Advise any doctor, dentist or pharmacist whom you consult that you take this drug.
- In addition to taking the drug, be sure to follow the diet and exercise plan your doctor has recommended for you.
- If you have not lost 5% of your body weight by 12 weeks of use, your doctor will likely have you stop the drug. Further use of this drug is unlikely to be of benefit in weight loss.

POSSIBLE INTERACTION WITH OTHER DRUGS

GENERIC NAME OR DRUG CLASS	COMBINED EFFECT
Antidiabetic agents*	Increased risk of low blood sugar.
Erectile dysfunction agents*	Increased risk of side effects.
Serotonergics*	Increased risk of serotonin syndrome* or neuroleptic malignant syndrome.*
Thioridazine	Increased effect of thioridazine. Avoid.
Weight loss products, other	Unknown effect. Consult doctor.

POSSIBLE INTERACTION WITH OTHER SUBSTANCES

INTERACTS WITH	COMBINED EFFECT
Alcohol:	None expected.
Beverages:	None expected.
Cocaine:	Effect unknown. Avoid.
Foods:	None expected.
Marijuana:	Effect unknown. Avoid.
Tobacco:	None expected.

*See Glossary

LOXAPINE

BRAND NAMES

Loxapac
Loxitane
Loxitane C

BASIC INFORMATION

Habit forming? No
Prescription needed? Yes
Available as generic? Yes
Drug class: Tranquilizer, antidepressant

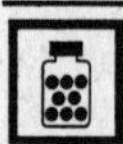

USES

- Treats serious mental illness.
- Treats anxiety and depression.

DOSAGE & USAGE INFORMATION

How to take:
- Oral solution—Take after meals with liquid to decrease stomach irritation.
- Tablet—Swallow with liquid or food to lessen stomach irritation. If you can't swallow whole, crumble tablet and take with liquid or food.
- Capsule—Swallow with liquid or food to lessen stomach irritation. If you can't swallow whole, open capsule and take with liquid or food.

When to take:
At the same times each day, according to instructions on prescription label.

If you forget a dose:
Take as soon as you remember. If it is almost time for the next dose, wait for that dose (don't double this dose) and resume regular schedule.

What drug does:
Blocks the effects of dopamine* in the brain.

Time lapse before drug works:
1/2 to 3 hours.

Don't take with:
Any other medicine or any dietary supplement without consulting your doctor or pharmacist.

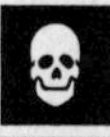

OVERDOSE

SYMPTOMS:
Dizziness, drowsiness, severe shortness of breath, muscle spasms, coma.
WHAT TO DO:
- **Dial 911 (emergency) for medical help or call poison control center 1-800-222-1222 for instructions.**
- **See emergency information on last 3 pages of this book.**

POSSIBLE ADVERSE REACTIONS OR SIDE EFFECTS

SYMPTOMS	WHAT TO DO
Life-threatening:	
Severe shortness of breath, skin rash, heartbeat irregularities, profuse sweating, fever, convulsions (rare).	Seek emergency treatment immediately.
Common:	
• Increased dental problems because of dry mouth and less salivation.	Consult your dentist about a prevention program.
• Swallowing difficulty, expressionless face, stiff arms and legs, dizziness.	Discontinue. Call doctor right away.
Infrequent:	
• Chewing movements with lip smacking, loss of balance, shuffling walk, tremor of fingers and hands, uncontrolled tongue movements.	Discontinue. Call doctor right away.
• Constipation, difficult urination, blurred vision, confusion, loss of sex drive, headache, insomnia, menstrual irregularities, weight gain, light sensitivity, nausea.	Continue. Call doctor when convenient.
Rare:	
Rapid heartbeat, fever, sore throat, jaundice, unusual bleeding.	Discontinue. Call doctor right away.

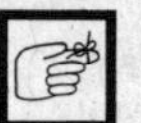

WARNINGS & PRECAUTIONS

Don't take if:
You are allergic to loxapine.

Before you start, consult your doctor if:
- You have a seizure disorder.
- You have an enlarged prostate, glaucoma, Parkinson's disease, heart disease, asthma, emphysema, bronchitis, urinary tract problem, blood pressure problem, blood or blood vessel disorder, kidney or liver disorder or abuse alcohol.

Over age 60:
- Adverse reactions and side effects may be more severe. You may need smaller doses.
- Use of antipsychotic drugs in elderly patients with dementia-related psychosis may increase risk of death. Consult doctor.

Pregnancy:
Decide with your doctor if drug benefits justify risk to unborn child. Risk category C (see page xviii).

Breast-feeding:
Drug may pass into milk. Avoid drug or discontinue nursing until you finish medicine. Consult doctor for advice on maintaining milk supply.

Infants & children:
Not recommended.

Prolonged use:
Talk to your doctor about the need for follow-up medical examinations or laboratory studies.

Skin & sunlight:
May cause rash or intensify sunburn in areas exposed to sun or ultraviolet light (photosensitivity reaction). Avoid overexposure and use sunscreen. Notify doctor if reaction occurs.

Driving, piloting or hazardous work:
Don't drive or pilot aircraft until you learn how medicine affects you. Don't work around dangerous machinery. Don't climb ladders or work in high places. Danger increases if you drink alcohol or take medicine affecting alertness and reflexes.

Discontinuing:
- Don't discontinue without consulting doctor. Dose may require gradual reduction if you have taken drug for a long time. Doses of other drugs may also require adjustment.
- These symptoms may occur after medicine has been discontinued: dizziness; nausea; abdominal pain; uncontrolled movements of mouth, tongue and jaw.

Others:
- Use careful oral hygiene.
- Advise any doctor or dentist whom you consult that you take this medicine.

POSSIBLE INTERACTION WITH OTHER DRUGS

GENERIC NAME OR DRUG CLASS	COMBINED EFFECT
Anticonvulsants*	Decreased effect of anticonvulsant.
Antidepressants, tricyclic*	May increase toxic effects of both drugs.
Bupropion	Increased risk of seizures.
Central nervous system (CNS) depressants*	Increased sedative effects of both drugs.
Epinephrine	Rapid heart rate and severe drop in blood pressure.
Extrapyramidal reaction*-causing drugs	Increased risk of side effects.
Fluoxetine	Increased depressant effects of both drugs.
Guanadrel	Decreased effect of guanadrel.
Guanethidine	Decreased effect of guanethidine.
Guanfacine	Increased effects of both drugs.
Haloperidol	May increase toxic effects of both drugs.
Leucovorin	High alcohol content of leucovorin may cause adverse effects.
Methyldopa	May increase toxic effects of both drugs.
Metoclopramide	May increase toxic effects of both drugs.
Molindone	May increase toxic effects of both drugs.
Pemoline	Increased central nervous stimulation.
Pergolide	Decreased pergolide effect.
Phenothiazines*	May increase toxic effects of both drugs.
Pimozide	May increase toxic effects of both drugs.

Continued on page 918

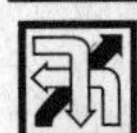

POSSIBLE INTERACTION WITH OTHER SUBSTANCES

INTERACTS WITH	COMBINED EFFECT
Alcohol:	May decrease effect of loxapine. Avoid.
Beverages:	None expected.
Cocaine:	May increase toxicity of both drugs. Avoid.
Foods:	None expected.
Marijuana:	May increase toxicity of both drugs. Avoid.
Tobacco:	May increase toxicity.

*See Glossary

LUBIPROSTONE

BRAND NAMES

Amitiza

BASIC INFORMATION

Habit forming? No
Prescription needed? Yes
Available as generic? No
Drug class: Laxative

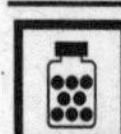

USES

- Treatment for chronic idiopathic constipation and its associated symptoms. Idiopathic means the cause of the constipation is unknown or unapparent. The constipation is not caused by a disease or medications.
- Treatment for irritable bowel syndrome with constipation in adult women.
- May be used for treatment of other disorders as determined by your doctor.

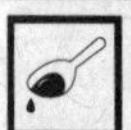

DOSAGE & USAGE INFORMATION

How to take:
Capsule—Swallow with liquid and take with food to help reduce any nausea symptoms.

When to take:
At the same time each day, usually twice a day with a meal or snack.

If you forget a dose:
Take as soon as you remember. If it is almost time for the next dose, wait for next scheduled dose (don't double this dose).

What drug does:
It works in the gastrointestinal system to increase fluid secretion. The increased fluid softens the stool and stimulates bowel activity which helps produce bowel movements. The constipation symptoms of bloating, straining and abdominal discomfort are reduced.

Continued next column

OVERDOSE

SYMPTOMS:
Nausea, vomiting, diarrhea, dizziness, loose or watery stools, headache, retching, hot flush or flushing, abdominal pain and possibly other symptoms.
WHAT TO DO:
Overdose unlikely to threaten life. If person uses much larger amount than prescribed or if accidentally swallowed, call doctor or poison control center 1-800-222-1222 for help.

Time lapse before drug works:
Spontaneous bowel movements may occur within 24 hours of taking the first dose. Several spontaneous bowel movements should occur within the first week.

Don't take with:
Any other medicine or any dietary supplement without consulting your doctor or pharmacist.

POSSIBLE ADVERSE REACTIONS OR SIDE EFFECTS

SYMPTOMS	WHAT TO DO
Life-threatening: None expected.	
Common: Nausea, headache, diarrhea, abdominal pain and distension, flatulence.	Continue. Call doctor when convenient.
Infrequent: Severe diarrhea.	Discontinue. Call doctor right away.
Rare: Other symptoms that cause concern (they may or may not be caused by the drug).	Continue. Call doctor when convenient.

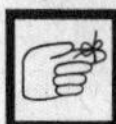

WARNINGS & PRECAUTIONS

Don't take if:
You are allergic to lubiprostone.

Before you start, consult your doctor if:
You have a mechanical gastrointestinal obstruction (this can include problems such as adhesions, carcinomas [cancers] or hernias).

Over age 60:
No problems expected.

Pregnancy:
Decide with your doctor whether drug benefits justify risk to unborn child. Risk category C (see page xviii).

Breast-feeding:
It is unknown if drug passes into milk. Avoid drug or discontinue nursing until you finish medicine. Consult doctor for advice on maintaining milk supply.

Infants & children:
It is not approved for use in those under age 18.

Prolonged use:
Talk to your doctor periodically to determine if continued use of the drug is necessary.

Skin & sunlight:
No problems expected.

Driving, piloting or hazardous work:
No problems expected.

Discontinuing:
No problems expected.

Others:
- Advise any doctor or dentist whom you consult that you take this medicine.
- Consult your doctor if severe diarrhea occurs.

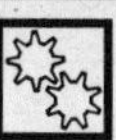

POSSIBLE INTERACTION WITH OTHER DRUGS

GENERIC NAME OR DRUG CLASS	COMBINED EFFECT
None expected.	

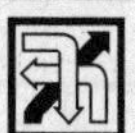

POSSIBLE INTERACTION WITH OTHER SUBSTANCES

INTERACTS WITH	COMBINED EFFECT
Alcohol:	None expected.
Beverages:	None expected.
Cocaine:	Unknown. Best to avoid.
Foods:	None expected.
Marijuana:	Unknown. Best to avoid.
Tobacco:	None expected.

LURASIDONE

BRAND NAMES

Latuda

BASIC INFORMATION

Habit forming? No
Prescription needed? Yes
Available as generic? No
Drug class: Antipsychotic

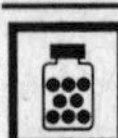

USES

- Treatment for schizophrenia.
- Other uses as recommended by your doctor.

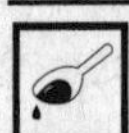

DOSAGE & USAGE INFORMATION

How to take:
Tablet—Swallow with liquid. It should be taken with a meal to help your body absorb the drug. If you can't swallow tablet whole, ask your doctor or pharmacist for advice.

When to take:
Usually once a day at the same time each day.

If you forget a dose:
Take as soon as you remember. If it is almost time for the next dose, wait for the next scheduled dose (don't double this dose).

What drug does:
The exact way it works is unknown. It appears to suppress levels of certain brain chemicals (e.g., dopamine and serotonin) that may be elevated in people with schizophrenia.

Time lapse before drug works:
Starts working within hours, but can take up to several weeks for full effect.

Don't take with:
Any other medicine or any dietary supplement without consulting your doctor or pharmacist.

OVERDOSE

SYMPTOMS:
May include fast heart rate, drowsiness, lightheadedness, faintness, or uncontrolled muscle movements.
WHAT TO DO:
Dial 911 (emergency) for medical help or call poison control center 1-800-222-1222 for instructions.

POSSIBLE ADVERSE REACTIONS OR SIDE EFFECTS

SYMPTOMS	WHAT TO DO
Life-threatening:	
Rare allergic reaction (hives, itching, rash, wheezing, tightness in chest, swelling of lips or tongue or throat).	Seek emergency treatment immediately.
Common:	
Drowsiness, jittery feeling, restlessness, nausea or vomiting, insomnia, indigestion, heartburn, tremor, slow movement, muscle stiffness, fast heartbeat.	Continue. Call doctor when convenient.
Infrequent:	
Fatigue, excess saliva, back pain, agitation, dizziness, anxiety, rash, blurred vision, abdominal pain, diarrhea, decreased appetite, itching, drooling.	Continue. Call doctor when convenient.
Rare:	
• Trouble swallowing, neuroleptic malignant syndrome (high fever; stiff muscles; confusion; blood pressure changes, sweating; muscle pain; weakness), tardive dyskinesia (uncontrolled movements of the face, tongue and other body parts), seizures, thoughts of suicide.	Discontinue. Call doctor right away.
• Weight gain, high blood sugar (frequent urination, feeling unusually thirsty or weak or hungry), lack of menstrual periods, leaking or enlarged breasts, impotence, symptoms of infection or other unexplained symptoms.	Continue. Call doctor when convenient.

WARNINGS & PRECAUTIONS

Don't take if:
You are allergic to lurasidone.

Before you start, consult your doctor if:
- You have or have had liver or kidney disease.
- You have heart disease, low blood pressure, congestive heart failure, other heart problems.
- You take certain drugs classified as enzyme inducers* or enzyme inhibitors.*
- You have cerebrovascular disease or history of stroke.
- You have a history of breast cancer.
- You have seizures or epilepsy.
- You have Parkinson's disease.
- You have high cholesterol or triglycerides.
- You have or have had low white blood cell counts.
- You have trouble swallowing.
- You have or have had suicidal thoughts or attempts or alcohol abuse or dependence.
- Patient has Alzheimer's or dementia.
- You have a family history of, or have diabetes.
- You have tardive dyskinesia.
- You have had neuroleptic malignant syndrome (serious or fatal problems may occur).

Over age 60:
- Adverse reactions and side effects may be more severe than in younger persons.
- Use of antipsychotic drugs in elderly patients with dementia-related psychosis may increase risk of death. Consult doctor.

Pregnancy:
Decide with your doctor if drug benefits justify any possible risk to unborn child. Risk category B (see page xviii).

Breast-feeding:
It is unknown if drug passes into milk. Consult doctor for advice.

Infants & children:
Safety and efficacy have not been established. Use only under close medical supervision.

Prolonged use:
Consult with your doctor on a regular basis while taking this drug to monitor your progress, check for side effects and for recommended lab tests.

Skin & sunlight:
No problems expected.

Driving, piloting or hazardous work:
Don't drive or pilot aircraft until you learn how medicine affects you. Don't work around dangerous machinery. Don't climb ladders or work in high places. Danger increases if you drink alcohol or take medicine affecting alertness and reflexes.

Discontinuing:
Don't discontinue this drug without consulting doctor. Dosage may require a gradual reduction before stopping.

Others:
- Get up slowly from a sitting or lying position to avoid dizziness, faintness or lightheadedness.
- Advise any doctor or dentist whom you consult that you take this medicine.
- Drug can affect body's ability to maintain normal temperature. You may be more sensitive to temperature extremes such as very hot or cold conditions. Avoid getting too cold or becoming overheated or dehydrated. Drink plenty of fluids.
- Drug is not approved for the treatment of patients with dementia-related psychosis.
- Take medicine only as directed. Do not change the dosage without doctor's approval.

POSSIBLE INTERACTION WITH OTHER DRUGS

GENERIC NAME OR DRUG CLASS	COMBINED EFFECT
Antihypertensives*	Increased risk of low blood pressure.
Central nervous system (CNS) depressants*	Increased sedative effect.
Dopamine agonists*	Decreased dopamine agonist effect.
Enzyme inhibitors*	May increase lurasidone effect.
Enzyme inducers*	May decrease lurasidone effect.

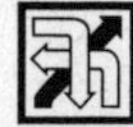

POSSIBLE INTERACTION WITH OTHER SUBSTANCES

INTERACTS WITH	COMBINED EFFECT
Alcohol:	Increased sedative affect. Avoid.
Beverages: Grapefruit juice.	May increase effect of drug.
Cocaine:	Unknown. Avoid.
Foods: Grapefruit.	May increase effect of drug.
Marijuana:	Sedation. Avoid.
Tobacco:	None expected.

*See Glossary

MACROLIDE ANTIBIOTICS

GENERIC AND BRAND NAMES

AZITHROMYCIN
Zithromax
Zmax
CLARITHROMYCIN
Biaxin
Omeclamox-Pak
DIRITHROMYCIN
Dynabac
FIDAXOMICIN
Dificid

BASIC INFORMATION

Habit forming? No
Prescription needed? Yes
Available as generic? Yes, for some
Drug class: Antibiotic (macrolide),

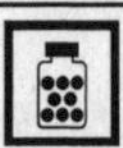

USES

Treatment for mild to moderate bacterial infections responsive to macrolide antibiotics. These include bronchitis, tonsillitis, some pneumonias, ear infections, skin infections (e.g., acne), sinusitis, streptococcal sore throat, urethritis, *Clostridium difficile*-associated diarrhea and others. (Note: Erythromycin is also a macrolide antibiotic and has its own chart.)

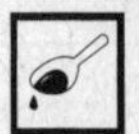

DOSAGE & USAGE INFORMATION

How to take:
- Enteric-coated tablet or delayed-release tablet—Swallow with liquid. Do not crush or chew tablet.
- Tablet or capsule—Swallow with liquid. If you can't swallow whole, ask your doctor or pharmacist for advice.
- Oral suspension or extended-release oral suspension—Follow directions on your prescription label.

When to take:
At the same time each day. Follow directions on your prescription label about taking the drug with food or on an empty stomach or if it makes no difference.

Continued next column

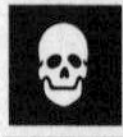

OVERDOSE

SYMPTOMS:
Possibly diarrhea, nausea, vomiting, abdominal pain.
WHAT TO DO:
Overdose unlikely to threaten life. If person uses much larger amount than prescribed or if accidentally swallowed, call doctor or poison control center 1-800-222-1222 for help.

If you forget a dose:
Take as soon as you remember. If it is almost time for the next dose, wait for that dose (don't double this dose) and resume regular schedule.

What drug does:
Prevents growth and reproduction of susceptible bacteria.

Time lapse before drug works:
Usually 2 to 5 days. Some infections may take 10 days or longer to resolve.

Don't take with:
Any other medicine or any dietary supplement without consulting your doctor or pharmacist.

POSSIBLE ADVERSE REACTIONS OR SIDE EFFECTS

SYMPTOMS	WHAT TO DO
Life-threatening:	
Rare allergic reaction (hives, itching, rash, trouble breathing, tightness in chest, swelling of lips or tongue or face).	Seek emergency treatment immediately.
Common:	
None expected.	
Infrequent:	
Nausea, vomiting, abdominal discomfort, diarrhea.	Continue. Call doctor when convenient.
Rare:	
• Allergic reaction (skin rash, itching), liver damage (yellow skin or eyes, nausea, abdominal pain, unusual bleeding or bruising, severe fatigue).	Discontinue. Call doctor right away.
• Headache, dizziness.	Continue. Call doctor when convenient.

WARNINGS & PRECAUTIONS

Don't take if:
You are allergic to macrolide antibiotics.

Before you start, consult your doctor if:
- You have any liver or kidney disorder.
- You have had jaundice.
- You have QT prolongation (a heart disorder) or cardiac arrhythmia.
- You have any muscle disorder, immune system problem or blood disorder.
- You are allergic to any medication, food or other substance.

Over age 60:
May be more at risk of adverse effects.

Pregnancy:
Risk factors vary for drugs in this group. See page xviii and consult doctor.

Breast-feeding:
One or more of these drugs may pass into milk. Avoid drug or discontinue nursing until you finish drug schedule. Consult doctor for advice on maintaining milk supply.

Infants & children:
Give only under close medical supervision to those under age 12. Young children may not complain or recognize adverse effects of drug. Observe child closely for any reactions.

Prolonged use:
Not recommended. The drug is discontinued once the infection is cured.

Skin & sunlight:
No special problems expected.

Driving, piloting or hazardous work:
Avoid if you experience dizziness. Otherwise, no problems expected.

Discontinuing:
Don't discontinue without doctor's advice until you complete prescribed dose, even though symptoms diminish or disappear.

Others:
- Advise any doctor or dentist whom you consult that you take this medicine.
- Some macrolide antibiotics may cause QT interval prolongation and heart arrhythmia (very rarely can be fatal). Consult doctor about your risks.
- May affect the results of some medical tests.

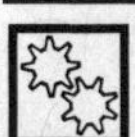

POSSIBLE INTERACTION WITH OTHER DRUGS

GENERIC NAME OR DRUG CLASS	COMBINED EFFECT
Antacids,* aluminum- or magnesium-containing	Take one hour apart.
Bromocriptine	Increased effect of bromocriptine.
Carbamazepine	Increased effect of carbamazepine.
Cisapride	May increase toxic effects. Avoid.
Cyclosporine	Increased effect of cyclosporine.
Digoxin	Increased effect of digoxin.
Disopyramide	Unknown effect. Use with caution.
Enzyme inhibitors*	Increased effect of enzyme inhibitor (with clarithromycin).
Ergot preparations*	Can cause serious or life-threatening problems with blood circulation. Avoid.
HMG-CoA reductase inhibitors	Increased effect of HMG-CoA reductase inhibitor and risk of serious muscle injury. Avoid.
Iron supplements	Decreased effect of dirithromycin. Take 1 hour apart.
Phenytoin	Decreased effect of phenytoin.
Pimozide	May increase toxic effects. Avoid.
Rifabutin	Decreased effect of antibiotic.
Rifampin	Decreased effect of antibiotic.
Tacrolimus	Increased effect of tacrolimus.
Theophylline	Increased effect of theophylline.
Triazolam	Increased risk of triazolam.
Warfarin	Increased risk of bleeding.
Zidovudine	Decreased effect of zidovudine.

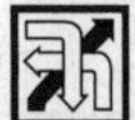

POSSIBLE INTERACTION WITH OTHER SUBSTANCES

INTERACTS WITH	COMBINED EFFECT
Alcohol:	None expected.
Beverages:	None expected.
Cocaine:	None expected.
Foods:	None expected
Marijuana:	None expected.
Tobacco:	None expected.

***See Glossary**

MAPROTILINE

BRAND NAMES

Ludiomil

BASIC INFORMATION

Habit forming? No
Prescription needed? Yes
Available as generic? Yes
Drug class: Antidepressant

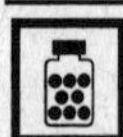

USES

Treatment for depression or anxiety associated with depression.

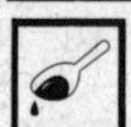

DOSAGE & USAGE INFORMATION

How to take:
Tablet—Swallow with liquid.

When to take:
At the same time each day, usually bedtime.

If you forget a dose:
Bedtime dose—If you forget your once-a-day bedtime dose, don't take it more than 3 hours late. If more than 3 hours, wait for next scheduled dose. Don't double this dose.

What drug does:
Probably affects part of brain that controls messages between nerve cells.

Time lapse before drug works:
Begins in 1 to 2 weeks. May require 4 to 6 weeks for maximum benefit.

Don't take with:
Any other medicine or any dietary supplement without consulting your doctor or pharmacist.

OVERDOSE

SYMPTOMS:
Respiratory failure, fever, cardiac arrhythmia, muscle stiffness, drowsiness, hallucinations, convulsions, coma.
WHAT TO DO:

- **Dial 911 (emergency) for medical help or call poison control center 1-800-222-1222 for instructions.**
- **If person is unconscious, check breathing and pulse. If not breathing, begin mouth-to-mouth rescue breathing. If heart is not beating, begin chest compressions.**
- **See emergency information on last 3 pages of this book.**

POSSIBLE ADVERSE REACTIONS OR SIDE EFFECTS

SYMPTOMS	WHAT TO DO
Life-threatening:	
Seizures.	Seek emergency treatment immediately.
Common:	
• Tremor.	Discontinue. Call doctor right away.
• Headache, dry mouth or unpleasant taste, constipation, diarrhea, indigestion, fatigue, weakness, nausea, drowsiness, nervousness, anxiety, excessive sweating.	Continue. Call doctor when convenient.
• Insomnia, craving sweets.	Continue. Tell doctor at next visit.
Infrequent:	
• Hallucinations, shakiness, dizziness, fainting, blurred vision, eye pain, vomiting, irregular heartbeat or slow pulse, inflamed tongue, abdominal pain, jaundice, hair loss, rash, chills, joint pain, vision changes, hiccups, palpitations.	Discontinue. Call doctor right away.
• Painful or difficult urination; fatigue; decreased sex drive; abnormal dreams; nasal congestion; back pain; muscle aches; frequent urination; painful, absent or irregular menstruation.	Continue. Call doctor when convenient.
Rare:	
Itchy skin; sore throat; fever; involuntary movements of jaw, lips and tongue; nightmares; confusion; swollen breasts in men.	Discontinue. Call doctor right away.

WARNINGS & PRECAUTIONS

Don't take if:
- You are allergic to maprotiline.
- You have had a heart attack within 6 weeks.
- You have taken a monoamine oxidase (MAO) inhibitor* within 2 weeks.

Before you start, consult your doctor if:
- You will have surgery within 2 months, including dental surgery, requiring anesthesia.
- You have a history of drug or alcohol abuse.
- You have an enlarged prostate, heart disease or high blood pressure, stomach or intestinal problems, overactive thyroid, asthma, liver disease, schizophrenia, urinary retention, glaucoma, respiratory disorder, seizure disorders, diabetes, or kidney disease.

Over age 60:
More likely to develop urination difficulty and side effects such as hallucinations, shakiness, dizziness, fainting, headache or insomnia.

Pregnancy:
Consult doctor. Risk category B (see page xviii).

Breast-feeding:
Drug passes into milk. Avoid drug or discontinue nursing until you finish medicine. Consult doctor for advice on maintaining milk supply.

Infants & children:
Not approved in ages under 18. If prescribed, carefully read information provided with prescription. Contact doctor right away if symptoms get worse or any there is any talk of suicide or suicide behaviors. Read information under Others.

Prolonged use:
Request blood cell counts, liver function studies; monitor blood pressure closely.

Skin & sunlight:
May cause rash or intensify sunburn in areas exposed to sun or ultraviolet light (photosensitivity reaction). Avoid overexposure and use sunscreen. Notify doctor if reaction occurs.

Driving, piloting or hazardous work:
Don't drive or pilot aircraft until you learn how medicine affects you. Don't work around dangerous machinery. Don't climb ladders or work in high places. Danger increases if you drink alcohol or take medicine affecting alertness and reflexes.

Discontinuing:
Don't discontinue without consulting doctor. Dose may require gradual reduction if you have taken drug for a long time. Doses of other drugs may also require adjustment.

Others:
- Advise any doctor or dentist whom you consult that you take this drug.
- Adults and children taking antidepressants may experience a worsening of the depression symptoms and may have increased suicidal thoughts or behaviors. Call doctor right away if these symptoms or behaviors occur.
- For dry mouth, suck sugarless hard candy or chew sugarless gum. If dry mouth persists, consult your dentist.

POSSIBLE INTERACTION WITH OTHER DRUGS

GENERIC NAME OR DRUG CLASS	COMBINED EFFECT
Anticholinergics*	Increased sedation.
Antiglaucoma agents	Heart rhythm problems, high blood pressure.
Antihistamines*	Increased antihistamine effect.
Barbiturates*	Decreased antidepressant effect.
Benzodiazepines*	Increased sedation.
Bupropion	Increased risk of seizures.
Central nervous system (CNS) depressants*	Increased sedation.
Cimetidine	Possible increased antidepressant effect and toxicity.

Continued on page 918

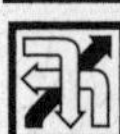

POSSIBLE INTERACTION WITH OTHER SUBSTANCES

INTERACTS WITH	COMBINED EFFECT
Alcohol: Beverages or medicines with alcohol.	Excessive intoxication. Avoid.
Beverages:	None expected.
Cocaine:	Excessive intoxication. Avoid.
Foods:	None expected.
Marijuana:	Excessive drowsiness. Avoid.
Tobacco:	May decrease absorption of maprotiline. Avoid.

***See Glossary**

MARAVIROC

BRAND NAMES

Selzentry

BASIC INFORMATION

Habit forming? No
Prescription needed? Yes
Available as generic? No
Drug class: Antiviral agent

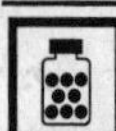

USES

Treatment of adults infected with human immunodeficiency virus (HIV) who have failed other antiviral drug therapy. This drug specifically treats patients with CCR5-tropic HIV-1. The drug is used in combination with other antiviral drugs. HIV is the virus that causes acquired immunodeficiency syndrome (AIDS).

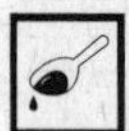

DOSAGE & USAGE INFORMATION

How to take:
Tablet—Swallow with liquid. May be taken with or without food.

When to take:
Take twice a day at the same times each day.

If you forget a dose:
Take as soon as you remember. If it is almost time for the next dose, wait for next scheduled dose (don't double this dose).

What drug does:
It helps control HIV infection by blocking the virus from entering your immune system cells. This helps your immune system stay healthy so it can fight the infection. The drug does not cure HIV or AIDS.

Time lapse before drug works:
May require several weeks or months before full benefits are apparent.

Don't take with:
Any other medicine or any dietary supplement without consulting your doctor or pharmacist. This is very important with HIV drugs.

OVERDOSE

SYMPTOMS:
Feeling faint or lightheaded, cold sweats.
WHAT TO DO:

- **Call doctor or poison control center 1-800-222-1222 for instructions.**
- **See emergency information on last 3 pages of this book.**

POSSIBLE ADVERSE REACTIONS OR SIDE EFFECTS

SYMPTOMS	WHAT TO DO
Life-threatening:	
Rare allergic reaction (hives, itching, rash, trouble breathing, tightness in chest, swelling of lips or tongue or throat).	Seek emergency treatment immediately.
Common:	
Diarrhea, dizziness, fatigue, nausea, cough, fever, other mild cold symptoms, abdominal pain.	Continue. Call doctor when convenient.
Infrequent:	
Swelling, stomach pain, muscle or joint pain, white patches or sores inside mouth or on lips, constipation, urination problems, changes in body fat, sleeping problems, dizziness when getting up from a sitting or lying down position, cold sores or sores on genital or anal area, itching.	Continue. Call doctor when convenient.
Rare:	
• Skin rash, liver problem (symptoms may include nausea, stomach pain, loss of appetite, skin rash, dark urine, clay-colored stools, yellow skin or eyes), chest pain, new infection (fever, chills, cough, flu-like symptoms), light-headedness or near fainting, breathing difficulty.	Discontinue. Call doctor right away.
• Other unexplained symptoms.	Continue. Call doctor when convenient.

WARNINGS & PRECAUTIONS

Don't take if:
You are allergic to maraviroc.

Before you start, consult your doctor if:
- You are allergic to any medicine, food or other substance, or have a family history of allergies.
- You have kidney or liver disease (especially hepatitis B or C), or diabetes.
- You have heart disease, low blood pressure, circulation problems, or a history of heart attack or stroke.

Over age 60:
Use with caution as adverse reactions and side effects may be more frequent and severe than in younger persons.

Pregnancy:
Decide with your doctor if drug benefits justify risk to unborn child. Risk category B (see page xviii). HIV can be passed to the baby if the mother is not properly treated during pregnancy. Talk to your doctor about being included in the Antiretroviral Pregnancy Registry.

Breast-feeding:
It is unknown if drug passes into milk. It is not recommended that HIV-infected mothers breast-feed. Consult your doctor.

Infants & children:
Safety and efficacy have not been established for children under age 16. Consult doctor.

Prolonged use:
- Long-term effects of using this drug have not been established.
- Talk to your doctor about the need for follow up blood tests and liver function studies.

Skin & sunlight:
No problems expected.

Driving, piloting or hazardous work:
Don't drive or pilot aircraft until you learn how medicine affects you. Don't work around dangerous machinery. Don't climb ladders or work in high places. Danger increases if you drink alcohol or take medicine affecting alertness and reflexes, such as antihistamines, tranquilizers, sedatives, pain medicine, narcotics and mind-altering drugs.

Discontinuing:
Don't discontinue (even for a short time) without doctor's advice.

Others:
- Advise any doctor or dentist whom you consult that you take this medicine.
- Taking this drug does not prevent you from passing HIV to another person through sexual contact or sharing needles. Avoid sexual contact or practice safe sex (e.g., using condoms) to help prevent the transmission of HIV. Never share or re-use needles. If you have questions, ask your doctor for advice.
- Liver damage may develop with use of this drug. See symptoms in Possible Adverse Reactions or Side Effects—Rare.
- Consult your doctor right away if you develop symptoms of a new infection.
- Take drug daily as prescribed. Do not increase or decrease dosage of drug without doctor's approval.

POSSIBLE INTERACTION WITH OTHER DRUGS

GENERIC NAME OR DRUG CLASS	COMBINED EFFECT
Antihypertensives*	Increased risk of dizziness. Use with caution.
Enzyme inducers*	Decreased effect of maraviroc.
Enzyme inhibitors*	Increased effect of maraviroc.
St. John's wort	Decreased effect of maraviroc. Avoid.

POSSIBLE INTERACTION WITH OTHER SUBSTANCES

INTERACTS WITH	COMBINED EFFECT
Alcohol:	None expected.
Beverages:	None expected.
Cocaine:	Unknown effect. Best to avoid.
Foods:	None expected.
Marijuana:	Unknown effect. Best to avoid.
Tobacco:	None expected.

*See Glossary

MASOPROCOL

BRAND NAMES

Actinex

BASIC INFORMATION

Habit forming? No
Prescription needed? Yes
Available as generic? No
Drug class: Antineoplastic (topical)

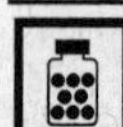

USES

Treats actinic keratoses (scaly, flat or slightly raised skin lesions).

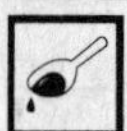

DOSAGE & USAGE INFORMATION

How to take:
Cream—Wash and dry the skin where lesions are located. Massage cream into affected area. Wash hands immediately after use.

When to take:
Use at the same times each day.

If you forget a dose:
Apply as soon as you remember, then resume regular schedule.

What drug does:
Selectively destroys actively proliferating cells.

Time lapse before drug works:
1 to 2 months.

Don't take with:
Any other medicine or any dietary supplement without consulting your doctor or pharmacist.

OVERDOSE

SYMPTOMS:
None reported.
WHAT TO DO:
Not for internal use. If child accidentally swallows, call poison control center 1-800-222-1222 for help.

POSSIBLE ADVERSE REACTIONS OR SIDE EFFECTS

SYMPTOMS	WHAT TO DO
Life-threatening: None expected.	
Common:	
• Redness and swelling of otherwise normal skin.	Discontinue. Call doctor right away.
• Skin reactions including itching, redness, dryness, flaking where medicine applied.	Continue. Call doctor when convenient.
• Temporary burning sensation right after application.	No action necessary.
Infrequent:	
• Allergic reaction to sulfites—bluish skin, severe dizziness, faintness, wheezing, breathing difficulty.	Discontinue. Seek emergency help.
• Swelling, soreness, persistent burning in treated area.	Continue. Call doctor when convenient.
Rare:	
Bleeding, oozing, blistering skin.	Discontinue. Call doctor right away.

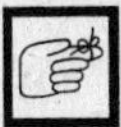

WARNINGS & PRECAUTIONS

Don't take if:
You are allergic to masoprocol.

Before you start, consult your doctor if:
You have a sulfite sensitivity.

Over age 60:
No problems expected.

Pregnancy:
Consult doctor. Risk category B (see page xviii).

Breast-feeding:
Effect not documented. Consult your doctor.

Infants & children:
Not used in this age group.

Prolonged use:
Effects of long-term use unknown. Visit doctor on a regular basis to determine effectiveness of treatment.

Skin & sunlight:
Drug does not cause sensitivity to sunlight. However, keratoses are related to sun exposure, so avoid sunlight when possible.

Driving, piloting or hazardous work:
No problems expected.

Discontinuing:
No problems expected.

Others:
- If you accidentally get masoprocol in your eye, promptly wash the eye with water.
- The cream may stain your clothing.
- Get doctor's approval before using cosmetics or make-up on the skin area you are treating.
- Leave the treated skin areas exposed. Don't cover them with a bandage or a dressing.

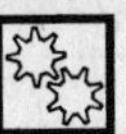

POSSIBLE INTERACTION WITH OTHER DRUGS

GENERIC NAME OR DRUG CLASS	COMBINED EFFECT
None significant.	

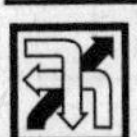

POSSIBLE INTERACTION WITH OTHER SUBSTANCES

INTERACTS WITH	COMBINED EFFECT
Alcohol:	None expected.
Beverages:	None expected.
Cocaine:	None expected.
Foods:	None expected.
Marijuana:	None expected.
Tobacco:	None expected.

MECHLORETHAMINE (Topical)

BRAND NAMES

Mustargen

BASIC INFORMATION

Habit forming? No
Prescription needed? Yes
Available as generic? No
Drug class: Antineoplastic (topical)

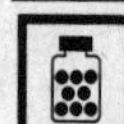

USES

- Treats mycosis fungoides.
- Treats other malignancies (by injection).

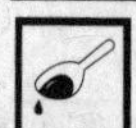

DOSAGE & USAGE INFORMATION

How to use:

- Solution—It is mixed according to doctor's instructions. Don't inhale vapors or powder. Shower and rinse before treatment. Use rubber gloves to apply over entire body. Avoid contact with eyes, nose and mouth.
- Ointment—Use according to doctor's instructions.

When to use:
Usually once a day.

If you forget a dose:
Apply as soon as you remember. If it is almost time for the next scheduled dose, wait and apply that dose at regular time (don't double this dose).

What drug does:
Destroys cells that produce mycosis fungoides.

Time lapse before drug works:
Starts to work right away, but response to treatment may take 3 to 6 months.

Don't use with:
Any other topical or oral medicines (including over-the-counter drugs such as cough and cold medicines, laxatives, antacids, diet pills, caffeine, nose drops or vitamins) without consulting your doctor or pharmacist.

OVERDOSE

SYMPTOMS:
None expected for topical solutions.
WHAT TO DO:
Not intended for internal use. If child accidentally swallows, call doctor or poison control center 1-800-222-1222 for help.

POSSIBLE ADVERSE REACTIONS OR SIDE EFFECTS

SYMPTOMS	WHAT TO DO
Life-threatening: Immediate hives, shortness of breath.	Seek emergency treatment immediately.
Common: Darkening, dry skin.	Continue. Tell doctor at next visit.
Infrequent: Allergic reaction with rash, itching, hives.	Seek emergency treatment immediately.
Rare: None expected.	

WARNINGS & PRECAUTIONS

Don't use if:
You are allergic to mechlorethamine.

Before you start, consult your doctor if:
- You have chicken pox.
- You have shingles (herpes zoster).
- You have skin infection.

Over age 60:
No special problems expected.

Pregnancy:
Risk to unborn child outweighs drug benefits. Don't use. Risk category D (see page xviii).

Breast-feeding:
Drug may be absorbed and pass into milk. Avoid drug or discontinue nursing until you finish medicine. Consult doctor for advice on maintaining milk supply.

Infants & children:
Effect unknown. Consult doctor.

Prolonged use:
- Allergic or hypersensitive reactions more likely. The ointment form is less likely to cause a reaction.
- Talk to your doctor about the need for follow-up medical examinations or laboratory studies to check liver function, complete blood counts (white blood cell count, platelet count, red blood cell count, hemoglobin, hematocrit) and hearing tests.

Skin & sunlight:
No problems expected.

Driving, piloting or hazardous work:
Don't drive or pilot aircraft until you learn how medicine affects you. Don't work around dangerous machinery. Don't climb ladders or work in high places. Danger increases if you drink alcohol or take medicine affecting alertness and reflexes.

Discontinuing:
No special problems expected.

Others:
- Advise any doctor or dentist whom you consult that you take this medicine.
- May affect results in some medical tests.
- Don't use if solution is discolored.

POSSIBLE INTERACTION WITH OTHER DRUGS

GENERIC NAME OR DRUG CLASS	COMBINED EFFECT
None significant.	

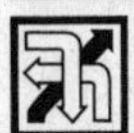

POSSIBLE INTERACTION WITH OTHER SUBSTANCES

INTERACTS WITH	COMBINED EFFECT
Alcohol:	None expected.
Beverages:	None expected.
Cocaine:	None expected.
Foods:	None expected.
Marijuana:	None expected.
Tobacco:	None expected.

MEGLITINIDES

GENERIC AND BRAND NAMES

NATEGLINIDE
Starlix

REPAGLINIDE
PrandiMet
Prandin

BASIC INFORMATION

Habit forming? No
Prescription needed? Yes
Available as generic? No
Drug class: Antidiabetic

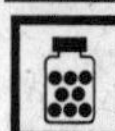

USES

Helps control, but does not cure type 2 (non-insulin dependent) diabetes. Used alone or in combination with other antidiabetic drugs, along with diet and exercise.

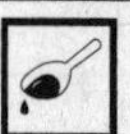

DOSAGE & USAGE INFORMATION

How to take:
Tablet—Take with water between 15-30 minutes before a meal. If you skip the meal, also skip the dose of medicine. If you have an extra meal, take an extra dose.

When to use:
15-30 minutes before each meal or as directed by doctor.

If you forget a dose:
If it is almost time for your next dose, take only that dose. Do not double doses.

What drug does:
Increases amount of insulin secreted from the pancreas, which helps to control blood sugar.

Continued next column

OVERDOSE

SYMPTOMS:
Cold sweats, confusion, cool pale skin, difficulty in concentrating, drowsiness, excessive hunger, rapid heartbeat, nausea, nervousness, nightmares, restless sleep, seizures, shakiness, slurred speech, unusual tiredness or weakness, coma.

WHAT TO DO:

- **For mild low blood sugar symptoms, eat or drink something with sugar in it right away.**
- **For more severe symptoms, dial 911 (emergency) for medical help or call poison control center 1-800-222-1222 for instructions.**
- **See emergency information on last 3 pages of this book.**

Time lapse before drug works:
10-30 minutes; peaks in 1 hour.

Don't take with:
Any other medicine or any dietary supplement without consulting your doctor or pharmacist.

POSSIBLE ADVERSE REACTIONS OR SIDE EFFECTS

SYMPTOMS	WHAT TO DO
Life-threatening: In case of overdose or low blood sugar, see previous column.	
Common:	
Symptoms of a cold (sore throat, runny or stuffy nose, cough), back pain, diarrhea, joint pain.	Continue. Call doctor when convenient.
Frequent:	
Low blood sugar symptoms: anxiety, cold sweats, shakiness, rapid heartbeat, blurred vision, pale skin, behavior changes similar to being drunk, confusion or difficulty thinking, drowsiness, excessive hunger, headache, nausea, nightmares, restless sleep, unusual tiredness or weakness.	Treat the low blood sugar. If symptoms are severe, seek emergency treatment.
Infrequent	
Bloody or cloudy urine, urination problems (burning, painful, difficult, frequent, urge to urinate), wheezing, chills, skin rash or itching or hives, eyes tearing, vomiting.	Discontinue. Call doctor right away.
Rare:	
• Unusual bleeding or bruising, red spots on skin, black or tarry stools, hoarseness, lower back or side pain, other side effects not listed occur.	Continue, but call doctor right away.
• Indigestion, feeling of warmth or heat or burning, stomach pain, constipation, dizziness.	Continue. Call doctor when convenient.

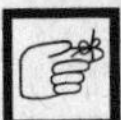

WARNINGS & PRECAUTIONS

Don't use if:
You are allergic to meglitinides.

Before you start, consult your doctor if:

- You have type 1 diabetes or diabetic ketoacidosis (ketones in the blood).
- You have an infection, fever, an injury or trauma, high stress levels or are planning surgery.
- You have a nervous system disorder.
- You have kidney or liver disease or underactive adrenal or pituitary gland.
- You are weak or undernourished.

Over age 60:
Increased risk of developing low blood sugar.

Pregnancy:
Decide with your doctor if drug benefits justify risk to unborn child. Risk category C (see page xviii).

Breast-feeding:
It is not known if drug passes into milk. Avoid drugs or discontinue nursing until you finish medicine. Consult doctor for advice on maintaining milk supply.

Infants & children:
Not recommended. Safety and dosage have not been established.

Prolonged use:
Talk to your doctor about the need for follow up medical examinations or laboratory studies to check blood glucose levels and glycosylated hemoglobin (HbA1c) values.

Skin & sunlight:
No problems expected.

Driving, piloting or hazardous work:
Don't drive or pilot aircraft until you learn how medicine affects you. Don't work around dangerous machinery. Don't climb ladders or work in high places. Danger increases if you drink alcohol or take medicine affecting alertness and reflexes.

Discontinuing:
Don't discontinue without consulting your doctor even if you feel well. You can have diabetes without feeling any symptoms. Untreated diabetes can cause serious problems.

Others:

- Advise any doctor or dentist whom you consult that you take this medicine. It may interfere with the accuracy of some medical tests.
- Follow any special diet your doctor may prescribe. It can help control diabetes.
- Consult doctor if you become ill with vomiting or diarrhea while taking this drug.
- Use caution when exercising. Ask your doctor about an appropriate exercise program.
- Wear medical identification stating that you have diabetes and take this medication.
- Learn to recognize the symptoms of low and high blood sugar. You and your family need to know what to do if these symptoms occur and when to call the doctor for help.
- Have a glucagon kit and syringe in the event severe low blood sugar occurs.

POSSIBLE INTERACTION WITH OTHER DRUGS

GENERIC NAME OR DRUG CLASS	COMBINED EFFECT
Anti-inflammatory drugs nonsteroidal (NSAIDs)	Increased risk of low blood sugar.
Barbiturates	Blood sugar problems.
Beta adrenergic blocking agents	Blood sugar control problems.
Carbamazepine	Blood sugar problems.
Corticosteroids*	Decreased effect of meglitinide.
Diuretics, thiazide	Decreased effect of repaglinide.
Gemfibrozil	Increased effect of meglitinide.
Hyperglycemia-causing medications*	Increased risk of loss of glycemic control.
Monoamine oxidase (MAO) inhibitors*	Increased risk of low blood sugar.
Salicylates	Increased risk of low blood sugar.
Sympathomimetics*	Decreased effect of meglitinide.
Thyroid hormones	Decreased effect of meglitinide.

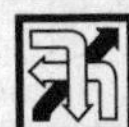

POSSIBLE INTERACTION WITH OTHER SUBSTANCES

INTERACTS WITH	COMBINED EFFECT
Alcohol:	Low blood sugar. Avoid.
Beverages:	None expected.
Cocaine:	None expected.
Foods:	None expected.
Marijuana:	None expected.
Tobacco:	None expected.

***See Glossary**

MELATONIN

BRAND NAMES

Numerous brand names are available.

BASIC INFORMATION

Habit forming? No
Prescription needed? No
Available as generic? Yes
Drug class: Hormone

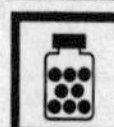

USES

- Melatonin is a hormone produced in the human body by the pineal gland and secreted at night. In most people, the melatonin levels are highest during the normal hours of sleep. The levels increase rapidly in the late evening, peaking after midnight and decreasing toward morning.
- Jet lag: Some research studies have shown that taking melatonin before a flight and continuing for a few days after arrival at the destination helped control jet lag symptoms of fatigue and sleep disturbances. Appears to work best after plane trips that crossed more than six time zones. Timing of doses very important for effectiveness.
- Insomnia and restless leg syndrome: Some research studies have shown that taking melatonin about 2 hours before bedtime decreased the time needed to fall asleep and improved quality of sleep (less wakefulness).
- Other claims that it can slow aging, fight disease, and enhance one's sex life have been less studied and more difficult to prove.

OVERDOSE

SYMPTOMS:
It is unknown what symptoms may occur.
WHAT TO DO:
If person takes much larger amount than prescribed, dial 911 (emergency) for medical help or call poison control center 1-800-222-1222 for instructions.

DOSAGE & USAGE INFORMATION

How to take:
For tablet or capsule—Follow instructions on the label or consult your doctor or pharmacist. Different brands supply different doses. Melatonin, as a product, is marketed as a dietary supplement and is not reviewed by the U.S. Food & Drug Administration (FDA) for effectiveness and safety. The melatonin products being sold are made from animal pineal glands or synthesized. The best dosage amounts are unknown. Use with caution.

When to take:
At the same time each day according to label directions. It is recommended that melatonin be taken at night before bedtime.

If you forget a dose:
Follow label instructions for your particular brand of melatonin. Usually you can take as soon as you remember. If it is almost time for the next dose, wait for that dose (don't double this dose) and resume regular schedule.

What drug does:
- Glands in the body make chemicals called hormones and release them into the bloodstream. Hormones taken as supplements also end up in the bloodstream. In either case, the blood then carries hormones to different parts of the body. There, hormones influence the way organs and tissues work.
- Hormone supplements may not have the same effects on the body as naturally produced hormones have, because the body processes them differently. Higher doses of supplements may result in higher amounts of hormones in the blood than are healthy.

Time lapse before drug works:
Effectiveness will vary from person to person and will also depend on the reason for taking melatonin.

Don't take with:
Any other medicine or any dietary supplement without consulting your doctor or pharmacist.

POSSIBLE ADVERSE REACTIONS OR SIDE EFFECTS

SYMPTOMS	WHAT TO DO
Life-threatening: None expected.	
Common: Unknown.	
Infrequent: Drowsiness, confusion, headache or grogginess may occur the following morning.	Reduce dosage or discontinue taking.
Rare: Unknown. If symptoms occur that you are concerned about, talk to your doctor or pharmacist. Further research may uncover other side effects.	

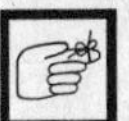

WARNINGS & PRECAUTIONS

Don't use if:
You are allergic to melatonin.

Before you start, consult your doctor if:
- You have any chronic health problem.
- You have high blood pressure (hypertension) or cardiovascular disease. Some studies in animals suggest that melatonin may constrict blood vessels (a problem that could be dangerous for people with these conditions).
- You are allergic to any medication, food or other substance.

Over age 60:
A lower starting dosage is often recommended until a response is determined.

Pregnancy:
Melatonin is not recommended for pregnant women. Decide with your doctor if drug benefits justify risk to unborn child. Risk category is unknown since melatonin is not regulated by the FDA (see page xviii).

Breast-feeding:
It is unknown if drug passes into milk. Avoid drug or discontinue nursing until you finish medicine. Consult doctor for advice on maintaining milk supply.

Infants & children:
Not recommended for children.

Prolonged use:
Effects are unknown. More research is needed to determine long-term effects of melatonin use.

Skin & sunlight:
No problems expected.

Driving, piloting or hazardous work:
Since it causes drowsiness, don't drive or pilot aircraft until you learn how medicine affects you. Don't work around dangerous machinery. Don't climb ladders or work in high places. Danger increases if you drink alcohol or take medicine affecting alertness and reflexes.

Discontinuing:
No problems expected.

Others:
- Advise any doctor or dentist whom you consult that you take melatonin.
- Melatonin is not researched carefully as yet, but there does not appear to be any particular problem. Some studies are promising as to its effect on health.
- Before starting melatonin, talk to your doctor about your sleep problems or try other things that can help sleep, such as avoidance of caffeine, chocolate, and especially alcohol in any amount.

POSSIBLE INTERACTION WITH OTHER DRUGS

GENERIC NAME OR DRUG CLASS	COMBINED EFFECT
All medications	Effects are unknown. Talk to your doctor or pharmacist.

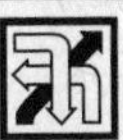

POSSIBLE INTERACTION WITH OTHER SUBSTANCES

INTERACTS WITH	COMBINED EFFECT
Alcohol:	Disrupts the nighttime melatonin effect. Avoid.
Beverages:	None expected.
Cocaine:	Problems not known. Best to avoid.
Foods:	None expected.
Marijuana:	Problems not known. Best to avoid.
Tobacco:	Smoking can disrupt your normal melatonin cycle. Avoid.

MELOXICAM

BRAND NAMES

Mobic

BASIC INFORMATION

Habit forming? No
Prescription needed? Yes
Available as generic? Yes
Drug class: Nonsteroidal anti-inflammatory, antirheumatic

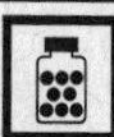

USES

Treatment for joint pain, stiffness, inflammation and swelling of rheumatoid arthritis, osteoarthritis and gout.

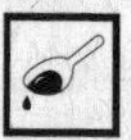

DOSAGE & USAGE INFORMATION

How to take:
Tablet—Swallow whole with liquid. May be taken with or without food.

When to take:
At the same time each day.

If you forget a dose:
Take as soon as you remember; however, if it is the next day, skip the missed dose and return to your normal schedule (don't double this dose).

What drug does:
Reduces tissue concentration of prostaglandins (hormones which produce inflammation and pain).

Continued next column

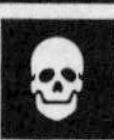

OVERDOSE

SYMPTOMS:
Bloody or black tarry stools; blue lips, fingernails or skin; blurred vision; confusion; changes in urine color or output; difficulty swallowing or breathing; dizziness; fever; chest pain; slow or fast heartbeat; swelling; stomach pain; unusual tiredness or weakness; vomiting of blood or material that looks like coffee grounds; wheezing; yellow eyes or skin.
WHAT TO DO:
- **Dial 911 (emergency) for medical help or call poison control center 1-800-222-1222 for instructions.**
- **See emergency information on last 3 pages of this book.**

Time lapse before drug works:
Begins in 2 to 3 hours. May require 3 weeks of regular use for maximum benefit.

Don't take with:
Any other medicine or any dietary supplement without consulting your doctor or pharmacist.

POSSIBLE ADVERSE REACTIONS OR SIDE EFFECTS

SYMPTOMS	WHAT TO DO
Life-threatening:	
Hives, rash, intense itching, faintness soon after a dose, breathing difficulties (anaphylaxis).	Seek emergency treatment immediately.
Common:	
Diarrhea, heartburn, indigestion, gas.	Continue. Call doctor when convenient.
Infrequent:	
Abdominal pain, anxiety, confusion, constipation, nausea, nervousness, sleepiness.	Continue. Call doctor when convenient.
Rare:	
Difficulty swallowing, swelling around the face, shortness of breath, tightness in chest, unusual tiredness or weakness, bloody or black tarry stools, vomiting, stomach pain.	Discontinue. Seek emergency treatment.

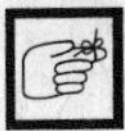

WARNINGS & PRECAUTIONS

Don't take if:
- You are allergic to aspirin or any other nonsteroidal anti-inflammatory drug (NSAIDs).
- You have nasal polyps.

Before you start, consult your doctor if:
- You have a history of alcohol abuse.
- You have bleeding problems or ulcers.
- You have any condition that causes fluid retention (heart problems or high blood pressure) or dehydration.
- You have used tobacco recently.
- You have impaired kidney or liver function.
- You have asthma.

Over age 60:
No problems expected.

Pregnancy:
Decide with your doctor whether drug benefits justify risk to unborn child. Risk category C (see page xviii).

Breast-feeding:
Animal studies show the drug passes into milk. Avoid drug or discontinue nursing until you finish medicine. Consult doctor for advice on maintaining milk supply.

Infants & children:
Not recommended for anyone younger than 18.

Prolonged use:
Talk to your doctor about the need for follow-up medical exams or laboratory studies to check complete blood counts, liver function, stools for blood, and eyes.

Skin & sunlight:
No problems expected.

Driving, piloting or hazardous work:
Don't drive or pilot aircraft until you learn how medicine affects you. Don't work around dangerous machinery. Don't climb ladders or work in high places. Danger increases if you drink alcohol or take medicine affecting alertness and reflexes, such as antihistamines, tranquilizers, sedatives, pain medicine, narcotics and mind-altering drugs.

Discontinuing:
No problems expected. If drug has been taken for a long time, consult doctor before discontinuing.

Others:
- May affect results in some medical tests.
- Advise any doctor or dentist whom you consult that you take this medicine.
- Do not refrigerate.
- Do not store in the bathroom, near the kitchen sink or in other damp places.

POSSIBLE INTERACTION WITH OTHER DRUGS

GENERIC NAME OR DRUG CLASS	COMBINED EFFECT
Angiotensin-converting enzyme (ACE) inhibitors*	May decrease ACE inhibitor effect.
Anti-inflammatory drugs, nonsteroidal (NSAIDs)* other	Increased risk of side effects.
Aspirin	Increased risk of stomach ulcer.
Furosemide	Decreased effect of furosemide.
Lithium	Increased lithium effect.
Warfarin	Increased risk of bleeding problems.

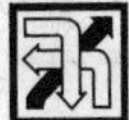

POSSIBLE INTERACTION WITH OTHER SUBSTANCES

INTERACTS WITH	COMBINED EFFECT
Alcohol:	Possible stomach ulcer or bleeding. Avoid.
Beverages:	None expected.
Cocaine:	None expected. Best to avoid.
Foods:	None expected.
Marijuana:	Increased pain relief from NSAIDs.
Tobacco:	Possible stomach ulcer or bleeding.

*See Glossary

MELPHALAN

BRAND NAMES

Alkeran
L-PAM
Phenylalanine Mustard

BASIC INFORMATION

Habit forming? No
Prescription needed? Yes
Available as generic? No
Drug class: Antineoplastic

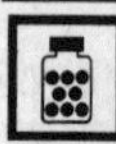

USES

Treatment for certain types of cancer.

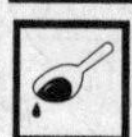

DOSAGE & USAGE INFORMATION

How to take:

- Tablet—Swallow with a full glass of water to help prevent vomiting. Take on an empty stomach, 1 hour before or 2 hours after a meal. If vomiting occurs shortly after taking a dose, consult your doctor for advice.
- IV form—Is given by medical professional.

When to take:
As directed by your doctor. The dosage regimen is individualized. The drug is usually taken for several weeks to start and then followed by a drug rest period for up to 4 weeks.

If you forget a dose:
Skip the missed dose and return to your regular schedule. Don't ever double doses. Consult doctor if you have questions.

What drug does:
It interferes with the growth of cancer cells and causes them to die.

Time lapse before drug works:
May be gradual over weeks or months before your response to the drug can be determined.

Don't take with:
Any other medicine or any dietary supplement without consulting your doctor or pharmacist.

OVERDOSE

SYMPTOMS:
Nausea, vomiting, diarrhea, intestinal bleeding.
WHAT TO DO:
Dial 911 (emergency) for medical help or call poison control center 1-800-222-1222 for instructions.

POSSIBLE ADVERSE REACTIONS OR SIDE EFFECTS

SYMPTOMS	WHAT TO DO
Life-threatening:	
None expected.	
Common:	
Nausea and vomiting.	Continue. Call doctor when convenient.
Infrequent:	
Fever or chills occur with other symptoms (e.g., back or side pain; painful or difficult urination; cough or hoarseness), stools are bloody or tarry or black, bloody urine, fast or irregular heartbeat, small-red spots on skin, shortness of breath, sudden skin rash or itching, troubled breathing, unusual bleeding or bruising, ongoing nausea or vomiting.	Continue, but call doctor right away. Seek emergency care if symptoms are more severe.
Rare:	
• Mouth or lip sores, difficulty swallowing, joint pain, diarrhea, arms or legs become sore or red, feet or lower legs are swollen, unusual lumps or masses, yellow skin or eyes.	Continue, but call doctor right away.
• Menstrual periods stop, weight loss, other side effects not listed.	Continue. Call doctor when convenient.

WARNINGS & PRECAUTIONS

Don't take if:
- You are allergic to melphalan or prior use of the drug has been ineffective.
- Your doctor has not explained the benefits and risks of taking this medicine.

Before you start, consult your doctor if:
- You have gout.
- You have had kidney stones.
- You have impaired kidney or liver function.
- You have taken other anticancer drugs or had radiation treatment in last 3 weeks.
- You have herpes zoster (shingles) or chicken pox (or been exposed).
- You have heart disease, congestive heart failure or other forms of cancer.
- You have bone marrow depression.
- You have an active infection.

Over age 60:
Adverse reactions and side effects may be more frequent and severe than in younger persons.

Pregnancy:
- Consult doctor. Risk category D (see page xviii).
- This drug may cause birth defects if either the male or female is taking it at the time of conception or if it is taken during pregnancy.

Breast-feeding:
It is unknown if drug passes into milk. Breast-feeding is not recommended while you are taking this drug. Consult doctor.

Infants & children:
Safety and effectiveness in this age group have not been established.

Prolonged use:
- Adverse reactions may be more likely the longer drug is required.
- Talk to your doctor about the need for follow-up medical examinations or laboratory studies to check complete blood counts, kidney function and drug's effectiveness.

Skin & sunlight:
No problems expected.

Driving, piloting or hazardous work:
Use caution until you determine how drug affects you.

Discontinuing:
- Don't discontinue without doctor's advice until you complete prescribed dose.
- Some side effects may follow discontinuing. Report to doctor blurred vision, convulsions, confusion, persistent headache, fever or chills, blood in urine, unusual bleeding or other unexpected symptoms.

Others:
- Can cause sterility which could be permanent.
- Your doctor may advise you to drink extra fluids so that you pass more urine (helps prevent kidney problems).
- The drug increases risk for infections and other malignancies. Consult doctor if you develop new or unexpected symptoms.
- Do not have any immunizations (vaccinations) without doctor's approval. Avoid persons who have taken oral polio vaccine within the last several months.
- Advise any doctor or dentist whom you consult that you take this medicine.

POSSIBLE INTERACTION WITH OTHER DRUGS

GENERIC NAME OR DRUG CLASS	COMBINED EFFECT
None expected	With use of tablet (oral) form of melphalan, but do consult your doctor about any other drugs you take.

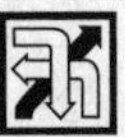

POSSIBLE INTERACTION WITH OTHER SUBSTANCES

INTERACTS WITH	COMBINED EFFECT
Alcohol:	None expected.
Beverages:	None expected.
Cocaine:	Unknown. Avoid.
Foods:	None expected.
Marijuana:	Unknown. Avoid.
Tobacco:	Unknown. Avoid.

MEMANTINE

BRAND NAMES

Namenda
Namenda Oral Solution
Namenda XR

BASIC INFORMATION

Habit forming? No
Prescription needed? Yes
Available as generic? Yes
Drug class: N-methyl-D-aspartate (NMDA) receptor antagonist

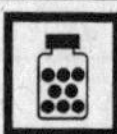

USES

Treats the symptoms of moderate to severe Alzheimer's disease. Alzheimer's is a progressive disease of the brain. Memantine may be used alone or in combination with other drugs for Alzheimer's.

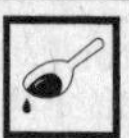

DOSAGE & USAGE INFORMATION

How to take:

- Tablet—Swallow with liquid. It may be taken with or without food.
- Oral solution—Follow the detailed directions provided with the prescription.
- Extended-release capsule—Swallow with liquid. It may be taken with or without food. Do not crush, chew or divide capsule. The capsule may be opened and sprinkled on applesauce and then swallowed.

When to take:
Once or twice daily at the same times each day. A caregiver should monitor usage.

Continued next column

OVERDOSE

SYMPTOMS:
May include agitation, confusion, slow movements, loss of consciousness, restlessness, stupor, unsteady gait, vomiting, vertigo, sleepiness, visual hallucinations.
WHAT TO DO:

- **Dial 911 (emergency) for medical help or call poison control center 1-800-222-1222 for instructions.**
- **See emergency information on last 3 pages of this book.**

If you forget a dose:
Take as soon as possible. If it is almost time for your next dose, skip the missed dose and go back to the regular dosing schedule. Do not double doses.

What drug does:
Blocks excess amounts of a brain chemical called glutamate that can damage or kill nerve cells. It does not cure Alzheimer's disease or treat the underlying cause.

Time lapse before drug works:
Improvement may be seen in weeks, but may take months for maximum benefits. Dosage of the drug may be increased in one-week time periods for the first few weeks.

Don't take with:
Any other medicine or any dietary supplement without consulting your doctor or pharmacist.

POSSIBLE ADVERSE REACTIONS OR SIDE EFFECTS

SYMPTOMS	WHAT TO DO
Life-threatening:	
None expected.	
Common:	
None expected.	
Infrequent:	
Dizziness, headache, constipation, confusion.	Continue. Call doctor when convenient.
Rare:	
Fatigue, back pain, vomiting, sleepiness, high blood pressure. Other symptoms may occur. They may be due to progression of the disease or may be due to the drug.	Continue. Call doctor when convenient.

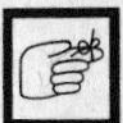

WARNINGS & PRECAUTIONS

Don't take if:
You are allergic to memantine or its components.

Before you start, consult your doctor if:
- You have kidney, liver or heart problems.
- You have a seizure disorder.
- You are allergic to any medication, food or other substance.

Over age 60:
No special problems expected.

Pregnancy:
Decide with your doctor if drug benefits justify risks to unborn child. Risk category B (see page xviii).

Breast-feeding:
This drug is usually not prescribed for reproductive-age women. It is unknown if drug passes into milk. Consult your doctor.

Infants & children:
Not recommended for this age group.

Prolonged use:
Visit the doctor regularly to determine if the drug is continuing to be effective.

Skin & sunlight:
No special problems expected.

Driving, piloting or hazardous work:
Avoid if you feel dizzy, drowsy or confused.

Discontinuing:
No problems expected. Consult doctor.

Others:
- Advise any doctor or dentist whom the patient consults about the use of this medicine.
- The effects of the drug will differ for different patients. Some patients will improve, others may stay the same, and others continue to deteriorate (get worse).

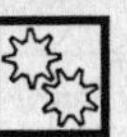

POSSIBLE INTERACTION WITH OTHER DRUGS

GENERIC NAME OR DRUG CLASS	COMBINED EFFECT
Amantadine	May lead to adverse effects of either drug.
Carbonic anhydrase inhibitors	Increased effect of memantine.
Dextromethorphan	May lead to adverse effects of either drug.
Histamine H_2 receptor antagonists	Increased effect of either drug.
Hydrochlorothiazide	Increased effect of both drugs.
Sodium bicarbonate	Increased effect of memantine.
Triamterene	Increased effect of either drug.

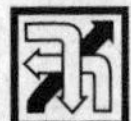

POSSIBLE INTERACTION WITH OTHER SUBSTANCES

INTERACTS WITH	COMBINED EFFECT
Alcohol:	None expected. Best to avoid.
Beverages:	None expected.
Cocaine:	Unknown. Best to avoid.
Foods:	None expected.
Marijuana:	Unknown. Best to avoid.
Tobacco:	None expected.

MEPROBAMATE

BRAND NAMES

See full list of brand names in the *Generic and Brand Name Directory*, page 889.

BASIC INFORMATION

Habit forming? Yes
Prescription needed? Yes
Available as generic? Yes
Drug class: Tranquilizer, antianxiety agent

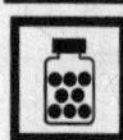

USES

Reduces mild anxiety, tension and insomnia.

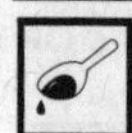

DOSAGE & USAGE INFORMATION

How to take:
- Tablet—Swallow with liquid.
- Extended-release capsule—Swallow each dose whole.

When to take:
At the same times each day.

If you forget a dose:
Take as soon as you remember. If it is almost time for the next dose, wait for that dose (don't double this dose) and resume regular schedule.

What drug does:
Sedates brain centers that control behavior and emotions.

Time lapse before drug works:
1 to 2 hours.

Don't take with:
- Nonprescription drugs containing alcohol or caffeine without consulting doctor.
- Any other medicine or any dietary supplement without consulting your doctor or pharmacist.

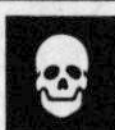

OVERDOSE

SYMPTOMS:
Dizziness, slurred speech, stagger, confusion, depressed breathing and heart function, stupor, coma.
WHAT TO DO:
- **Dial 911 (emergency) for medical help or call poison control center 1-800-222-1222 for instructions.**
- **See emergency information on last 3 pages of this book.**

POSSIBLE ADVERSE REACTIONS OR SIDE EFFECTS

SYMPTOMS	WHAT TO DO
Life-threatening:	
Hives, rash, intense itching, faintness soon after a dose, wheezing (anaphylaxis).	Seek emergency treatment immediately.
Common:	
Dizziness, confusion, agitation, drowsiness, unsteadiness, fatigue, weakness.	Continue. Tell doctor at next visit.
Infrequent:	
• Rash, hives, itchy skin; change in vision; diarrhea, nausea or vomiting, slurred speech, blurred vision.	Discontinue. Call doctor right away.
• False sense of well-being, headache.	Continue. Call doctor when convenient.
Rare:	
Sore throat; fever; rapid, pounding, unusually slow or irregular heartbeat; difficult breathing; unusual bleeding or bruising.	Discontinue. Call doctor right away.

WARNINGS & PRECAUTIONS

Don't take if:
You are allergic to meprobamate, tybamate, carbromal or carisoprodol.

Before you start, consult your doctor if:
- You have epilepsy.
- You have impaired liver or kidney function.
- You have tartrazine dye allergy.
- You suffer from drug abuse or alcoholism, active or in remission.
- You have porphyria.

Over age 60:
Adverse reactions and side effects may be more frequent and severe than in younger persons.

Pregnancy:
Risk to unborn child outweighs drug benefits. Don't use. Risk category D (see page xviii).

Breast-feeding:
Drug passes into milk. May cause sedation in child. Avoid drug or discontinue nursing until you finish medicine. Consult doctor for advice on maintaining milk supply.

Infants & children:
Not recommended.

Prolonged use:
- Habit forming.
- May impair blood cell production.

Skin & sunlight:
No problems expected.

Driving, piloting or hazardous work:
Don't drive or pilot aircraft until you learn how medicine affects you. Don't work around dangerous machinery. Don't climb ladders or work in high places. Danger increases if you drink alcohol or take medicine affecting alertness and reflexes, such as antihistamines, tranquilizers, sedatives, pain medicine, narcotics and mind-altering drugs.

Discontinuing:
Don't discontinue without consulting doctor. Dose may require gradual reduction if you have taken drug for a long time. Doses of other drugs may also require adjustment. Report to your doctor any unusual symptom that begins in the first week you discontinue this medicine. These symptoms may include convulsions, confusion, nightmares, insomnia.

Others:
- Advise any doctor or dentist whom you consult that you take this drug.
- For dry mouth, suck sugarless hard candy or chew sugarless gum. If dry mouth persists, consult your dentist.

POSSIBLE INTERACTION WITH OTHER DRUGS

GENERIC NAME OR DRUG CLASS	COMBINED EFFECT
Addictive drugs*	Increased risk of addictive effect.
Antidepressants, tricyclic*	Increased anti-depressant effect.
Antihistamines*	Possible excessive sedation.
Central nervous system (CNS) depressants*	Increased depressive effects of both drugs.
Monoamine oxidase (MAO) inhibitors*	Increased meprobamate effect.
Narcotics*	Increased narcotic effect.
Sertraline	Increased depressive effects of both drugs.

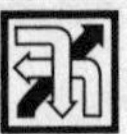

POSSIBLE INTERACTION WITH OTHER SUBSTANCES

INTERACTS WITH	COMBINED EFFECT
Alcohol:	Dangerous increased effect of meprobamate.
Beverages: Caffeine drinks.	Decreased calming effect of meprobamate.
Cocaine:	Decreased meprobamate effect.
Foods:	None expected.
Marijuana:	Increased sedative effect of meprobamate.
Tobacco:	None expected.

*See Glossary

MERCAPTOPURINE

BRAND NAMES

6-MP
Purinethol

BASIC INFORMATION

Habit forming? No
Prescription needed? Yes
Available as generic? Yes
Drug class: Antineoplastic, immunosuppressant

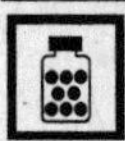

USES

- Treatment for some kinds of cancer.
- Treatment for regional enteritis and ulcerative colitis and other immune disorders.

DOSAGE & USAGE INFORMATION

How to take:
Tablet—Swallow with liquid.

When to take:
At the same time each day.

If you forget a dose:
Skip the missed dose. Don't double the next dose.

What drug does:
Inhibits abnormal cell reproduction.

Time lapse before drug works:
May require 6 weeks for maximum effect.

Don't take with:
Any other medicine or any dietary supplement without consulting your doctor or pharmacist.

OVERDOSE

SYMPTOMS:
Headache, stupor, seizures.
WHAT TO DO:

- **Dial 911 (emergency) for medical help or call poison control center 1-800-222-1222 for instructions.**
- **If person is unconscious, check breathing and pulse. If not breathing, begin mouth-to-mouth rescue breathing. If heart is not beating, begin chest compressions.**
- **See emergency information on last 3 pages of this book.**

POSSIBLE ADVERSE REACTIONS OR SIDE EFFECTS

SYMPTOMS	WHAT TO DO
Life-threatening:	
In case of overdose, see previous column.	
Common:	
• Black stools or bloody vomit.	Discontinue. Seek emergency treatment.
• Mouth sores, sore throat, unusual bleeding or bruising.	Discontinue. Call doctor right away.
• Abdominal pain, nausea, vomiting, weakness, tiredness.	Continue. Call doctor when convenient.
Infrequent:	
• Seizures.	Discontinue. Seek emergency treatment.
• Diarrhea, headache, confusion, blurred vision, shortness of breath, joint pain, blood in urine, jaundice, back pain, appetite loss, feet and leg swelling.	Discontinue. Call doctor right away.
• Cough.	Continue. Call doctor when convenient.
• Acne, boils, hair loss, itchy skin.	Continue. Tell doctor at next visit.
Rare:	
Fever and chills.	Discontinue. Call doctor right away.

WARNINGS & PRECAUTIONS

Don't take if:
You are allergic to any antineoplastic.

Before you start, consult your doctor if:

- You are an alcoholic.
- You have blood, liver or kidney disease.
- You have colitis or peptic ulcer.
- You have gout.
- You have an infection.
- You plan to become pregnant within 3 months.

Over age 60:
Adverse reactions and side effects may be more frequent and severe than in younger persons.

Pregnancy:
Risk to unborn child outweighs drug benefits. Don't use. Risk category D (see page xviii).

Breast-feeding:
Avoid drug or discontinue nursing.

Infants & children:
Use only under special medical supervision.

Prolonged use:
- Adverse reactions more likely the longer drug is required.
- Talk to your doctor about the need for follow-up medical examinations or laboratory studies to check complete blood counts (white blood cell count, platelet count, red blood cell count, hemoglobin, hematocrit), liver function, kidney function, uric acid.

Skin & sunlight:
No problems expected.

Driving, piloting or hazardous work:
Avoid if you feel dizzy, drowsy or confused. Otherwise, no problems expected.

Discontinuing:
Don't discontinue without doctor's advice until you complete prescribed dose, even though symptoms diminish or disappear. Some side effects may follow discontinuing. Report to doctor blurred vision, convulsions, confusion, persistent headache, chills or fever, bloody urine or stools, back pain, jaundice.

Others:
- Drink more fluid than usual so you will have more frequent urination.
- Don't give this medicine to anyone else for any purpose. It is a strong drug that requires close medical supervision.
- Advise any doctor or dentist whom you consult that you take this medicine.
- Report for frequent medical follow-up and laboratory studies.

POSSIBLE INTERACTION WITH OTHER DRUGS

GENERIC NAME OR DRUG CLASS	COMBINED EFFECT
Acetaminophen	Increased likelihood of liver toxicity.
Anticoagulants,* oral	May increase or decrease anticoagulant effect.
Antineoplastic drugs,* other	Increased effect of both (may be desirable) or increased toxicity of each.
Chloramphenicol	Increased toxicity of each.
Clozapine	Toxic effect on bone marrow.
Cyclosporine	May increase risk of infection.
Hepatotoxic drugs*	Increased risk of liver toxicity.
Immunosuppressants,* other	Increased risk of infections and neoplasms.*
Isoniazid	Increased risk of liver damage.
Levamisole	Increased risk of bone marrow depression.
Lovastatin	Increased heart and kidney damage.
Probenecid	Increased toxic effect of mercaptopurine.
Sulfinpyrazone	Increased toxic effect of mercaptopurine.
Tiopronin	Increased risk of toxicity to bone marrow.
Vaccines, live or killed	Increased risk of toxicity or reduced effectiveness of vaccine.

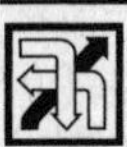

POSSIBLE INTERACTION WITH OTHER SUBSTANCES

INTERACTS WITH	COMBINED EFFECT
Alcohol:	May increase chance of intestinal bleeding.
Beverages:	None expected.
Cocaine:	Increased chance of toxicity.
Foods:	Reduced irritation in stomach.
Marijuana:	None expected.
Tobacco:	Increased lung toxicity.

*See Glossary

MESALAMINE

BRAND NAMES

5-ASA	Lialda
Apriso	Mesalazine
Asacol	Pentasa
Asacol HD	Rowasa
Canasa	Salofalk
Delzicol	sfRowasa

BASIC INFORMATION

Habit forming? No
Prescription needed? Yes
Available as generic? Yes
Drug class: Anti-inflammatory (nonsteroidal)

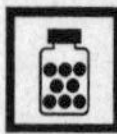

USES

- Treats ulcerative colitis.
- Reduces inflammatory conditions of the lower colon and rectum.

DOSAGE & USAGE INFORMATION

How to use:

- Rectal—Use as an enema. Insert the tip of the pre-packaged medicine container into the rectum. Squeeze container to empty contents. Retain in rectum all night or as long as possible.
- Rectal suppository—Follow instructions on package.
- Delayed-release tablet or capsule; extended-release capsule—Swallow with liquid. Do not crush or chew tablet or open capsule. Take Lialda brand with food.

Continued next column

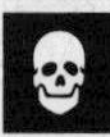

OVERDOSE

SYMPTOMS:
Confusion, severe diarrhea, lightheadedness or dizziness, severe sleepiness, severe headache, ringing or buzzing in ears, hearing loss, nausea and vomiting, sweating, fast or deep breathing.
WHAT TO DO:

- **Dial 911 (emergency) for medical help or call poison control center 1-800-222-1222 for instructions.**
- **See emergency information on last 3 pages of this book.**

When to use:

- Rectal—Each night, preferably after a bowel movement. Continue for 3 to 6 weeks according to your doctor's instructions.
- Rectal suppository—Use 1-3 times a day according to doctor's instructions.
- Oral forms—Follow instructions on label. It may be once-a-day dose or 3 to 4 times a day as directed by doctor.

If you forget a dose:
Take or use as soon as you remember. If it is almost time for the next dose, wait for next scheduled dose (don't double this dose).

What drug does:
It works in the intestinal tract to reduce inflammation and also helps keep the disorder in remission and prevent relapses.

Time lapse before drug works:
3 to 21 days.

Don't take with:

- Oral sulfasalazine concurrently. To do so may increase chances of kidney damage.
- Any other medicine or any dietary supplement without consulting your doctor or pharmacist.

POSSIBLE ADVERSE REACTIONS OR SIDE EFFECTS

SYMPTOMS	WHAT TO DO
Life-threatening: None expected.	
Common: None expected.	
Infrequent: None expected.	
Rare:	
• Abdominal pain, bloody diarrhea, fever, skin rash, anal irritation, chest pain, shortness of breath.	Discontinue. Call doctor right away.
• Gaseousness, nausea, headache, mild hair loss, diarrhea.	Continue. Call doctor when convenient.

WARNINGS & PRECAUTIONS

Don't take if:
You are allergic to mesalamine, salicylates* or any medication containing sulfasalazine (such as Azulfidine).

Before you start, consult your doctor if:
- You have had chronic kidney disease.
- You have pancreatitis.
- You have heart inflammation (pericarditis).

Over age 60:
More sensitive to drug. Aggravates symptoms of enlarged prostate. Causes impaired thinking, hallucinations, nightmares. Consult doctor about any of these.

Pregnancy:
Consult doctor. Risk category B (see page xviii).

Breast-feeding:
It is unknown if drug passes into milk. Avoid nursing until you finish medicine. Consult doctor for advice on maintaining milk supply.

Infants & children:
Use for children only under doctor's supervision.

Prolonged use:
Talk to your doctor about the need for follow-up medical examinations or laboratory studies to check urine.

Skin & sunlight:
No problems expected.

Driving, piloting or hazardous work:
Don't drive or pilot aircraft until you learn how medicine affects you. Don't work around dangerous machinery. Don't climb ladders or work in high places. Danger increases if you drink alcohol or take medicine affecting alertness and reflexes.

Discontinuing:
Don't discontinue without consulting doctor. Dose may require gradual reduction if you have taken drug for a long time. Doses of other drugs may also require adjustment.

Others:
- Internal eye pressure should be measured regularly.
- Canasa may stain things it touches.

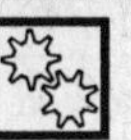

POSSIBLE INTERACTION WITH OTHER DRUGS

GENERIC NAME OR DRUG CLASS	COMBINED EFFECT
Antacids*	Affects the dosage of brand name Apriso. Avoid.

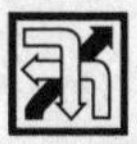

POSSIBLE INTERACTION WITH OTHER SUBSTANCES

INTERACTS WITH	COMBINED EFFECT
Alcohol:	None expected.
Beverages:	None expected.
Cocaine:	None expected.
Foods:	None expected.
Marijuana:	None expected.
Tobacco:	None expected.

METFORMIN

BRAND NAMES

See full list of brand names in the *Generic and Brand Name Directory*, page 889.

BASIC INFORMATION

Habit forming? No
Prescription needed? Yes
Available as generic? Yes
Drug class: Antihyperglycemic, antidiabetic

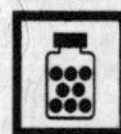

USES

Treatment for hyperglycemia (excess sugar in the blood) that cannot be controlled by diet alone in patients with diabetes type 2.

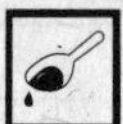

DOSAGE & USAGE INFORMATION

How to take:

- Tablet—Swallow with liquid. Take with food.
- Extended release tablet—Swallow whole. Take with food. Do not break, crush or chew before swallowing.
- Chewable tablet—Follow product instructions.
- Oral solution—Follow product instructions.

Continued next column

When to take:
Usually 1 to 3 times a day as directed by doctor. Take with meals to lessen stomach irritation. Dosage may be increased on a weekly basis until maximum benefits are achieved.

If you forget a dose:
Take as soon as you remember. If it is almost time for the next dose, skip the missed dose and wait for your next scheduled dose (don't double this dose).

What drug does:
Helps to lower blood sugar when it is too high. Treats the symptoms of diabetes, but does not cure it.

Time lapse before drug works:
May take several weeks for full effectiveness.

Don't take with:
Any other medicine or any dietary supplement without consulting your doctor or pharmacist.

OVERDOSE

SYMPTOMS:

- **Symptoms of lactic acidosis (acid in the blood)—chills, diarrhea, fatigue, muscle pain, sleepiness, slow heartbeat, breathing difficulty, unusual weakness.**
- **Hypoglycemia symptoms (low blood sugar) —stomach pain, nervousness, shakiness anxious feeling, confusion, cold sweats, chills, convulsions, cool pale skin, excess hunger, unsteady walk, nausea or vomiting, rapid heartbeat, unusual weakness or tiredness, vision changes, unconsciousness.**

WHAT TO DO:

- **For symptoms of lactic acidosis, call doctor immediately.**
- **For mild low blood sugar symptoms, drink or eat something containing sugar right away.**
- **For more severe symptoms, dial 911 (emergency) for medical help or call poison control center 1-800-222-1222 for instructions.**
- **See emergency information on last 3 pages of this book.**

POSSIBLE ADVERSE REACTIONS OR SIDE EFFECTS

SYMPTOMS	WHAT TO DO
Life-threatening: In case of overdose or low blood sugar, see previous column.	
Common:	
• Stomach pain, diarrhea, vomiting.	Continue, but call doctor right away.
• Decreased appetite, changes in taste, gas, headache, weight loss, feeling of fullness or stomach discomfort, nausea.	Continue. Call doctor when convenient.
Infrequent: None expected.	
Rare:	
Lactic acidosis or severe low blood sugar (see symptoms under Overdose).	Discontinue. Call doctor right away or seek emergency help.

WARNINGS & PRECAUTIONS

Don't take if:
You are allergic to metformin.

Before you start, consult your doctor if:

- You have any kidney or liver disease or any heart or blood vessel disorder.
- You have any chronic health problem.
- You have an infection, illness or any condition that can cause low blood sugar.
- You have a history of acid in the blood (metabolic acidosis or ketoacidosis).

- You are allergic to any medication, food or other substance.

Over age 60:
No special problems expected. A lower starting dosage may be recommended by your doctor.

Pregnancy:
Decide with your doctor if drug benefits justify risks to unborn child. Risk category B (see page xviii).

Breast-feeding:
Drug passes into milk. Avoid drug or discontinue nursing until you finish medicine. Consult doctor for advice on maintaining milk supply.

Infants & children:
Most forms of metformin are approved for children age 10 and over. Use only under close medical supervision.

Prolonged use:
- Schedule regular doctor visits to determine if the drug is continuing to be effective in controlling the diabetes and to check for any problems in kidney function.
- You will most likely require an antidiabetic medicine for the rest of your life.
- You will need to test your blood glucose levels several times a day or, for some, once to several times a week.

Skin & sunlight:
No special problems expected.

Driving, piloting or hazardous work:
No special problems expected.

Discontinuing:
Don't discontinue without consulting your doctor, even if you feel well. You can have diabetes without feeling any symptoms. Untreated diabetes can cause serious problems.

Others:
- Advise any doctor or dentist whom you consult that you take this medicine. Drug may interfere with the accuracy of some medical tests.
- Follow any special diet your doctor may prescribe. It can help control diabetes.
- Consult doctor if you become ill with vomiting or diarrhea.
- Use caution when exercising. Ask your doctor about an appropriate exercise program.
- Wear medical identification stating that you have diabetes and take this medication.
- Learn to recognize the symptoms of low blood sugar. You and your family need to know what to do if these symptoms occur.
- Have a glucagon kit and syringe in the event severe low blood sugar occurs. Carry a quick-acting sugar to treat symptoms of mild low blood sugar.
- High blood sugar (hyperglycemia) may occur with diabetes. Ask your doctor about symptoms to watch for and treatment steps to take.
- This drug may be discontinued temporarily prior to x-ray studies or some surgeries.
- Educate yourself about diabetes.

POSSIBLE INTERACTION WITH OTHER DRUGS

GENERIC NAME OR DRUG CLASS	COMBINED EFFECT
Amiloride	Increased metformin effect.
Calcium channel blockers*	Increased metformin effect.
Cimetidine	Increased metformin effect.
Dexfenfluramine	May require dosage change as weight loss occurs.
Digoxin	Increased metformin effect.
Dofetilide	Increased dofetilide effect.
Furosemide	Increased metformin effect.
Hyperglycemia-causing medications*	Increased risk of hyperglycemia.
Hypoglycemia-causing medications*	Increased risk of hypoglycemia.
Morphine	Increased metformin effect.
Penicillins*	Increased risk of methotrexate toxicity.
Procainamide	Increased metformin effect.
Quinidine	Increased metformin effect.

Continued on page 919

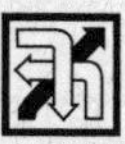

POSSIBLE INTERACTION WITH OTHER SUBSTANCES

INTERACTS WITH	COMBINED EFFECT
Alcohol:	Increased risk of hypoglycemia. Avoid excessive amounts.
Beverages:	None expected.
Cocaine:	None expected.
Foods:	None expected.
Marijuana:	None expected.
Tobacco:	None expected.

***See Glossary**

METHENAMINE

BRAND NAMES

Hiprex
Mandelamine
Urex

BASIC INFORMATION

Habit forming? No
Prescription needed? Yes
Available as generic? Yes
Drug class: Anti-infective (urinary)

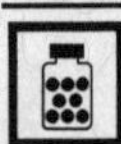

USES

Suppresses chronic urinary tract infections.

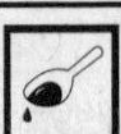

DOSAGE & USAGE INFORMATION

How to take:

- Tablet—Swallow with liquid or food to lessen stomach irritation. If you can't swallow whole, crumble tablet and take with liquid or food. If enteric-coated tablet, swallow whole.
- Liquid form—Use a measuring spoon to ensure correct dose.
- Granules—Dissolve dose in 4 oz. of water. Drink all the liquid.

When to take:
At the same times each day.

If you forget a dose:
Take as soon as you remember. If it is almost time for the next dose, wait for that dose (don't double this dose) and resume regular schedule.

What drug does:
A chemical reaction in the urine changes methenamine into formaldehyde, which destroys certain bacteria.

Time lapse before drug works:
Continual use for 3 to 6 months.

Continued next column

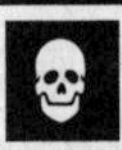

OVERDOSE

SYMPTOMS:
Bloody urine, weakness, deep breathing, stupor, coma.
WHAT TO DO:

- **Dial 911 (emergency) for medical help or call poison control center 1-800-222-1222 for instructions.**
- **See emergency information on last 3 pages of this book.**

Don't take with:
Any other medicine or any dietary supplement without consulting your doctor or pharmacist.

POSSIBLE ADVERSE REACTIONS OR SIDE EFFECTS

SYMPTOMS	WHAT TO DO
Life-threatening:	
In case of overdose, see previous column.	
Common:	
• Rash.	Discontinue. Call doctor right away.
• Nausea, difficult urination.	Continue. Call doctor when convenient.
Infrequent:	
• Blood in urine.	Discontinue. Call doctor right away.
• Burning on urination, lower back pain.	Continue. Call doctor when convenient.
Rare:	
None expected.	

WARNINGS & PRECAUTIONS

Don't take if:
- You are allergic to methenamine.
- You have a severe impairment of kidney or liver function.
- Your urine cannot or should not be acidified (check with your doctor).

Before you start, consult your doctor if:
- You have had kidney or liver disease.
- You plan to become pregnant within medication period.
- You have had gout.

Over age 60:
Don't exceed recommended dose.

Pregnancy:
Decide with your doctor if drug benefits justify risk to unborn child. Risk category C (see page xviii).

Breast-feeding:
Drug passes into milk in small amounts. Consult doctor.

Infants & children:
Use only under medical supervision.

Prolonged use:
No problems expected.

Skin & sunlight:
No problems expected.

Driving, piloting or hazardous work:
No problems expected.

Discontinuing:
Don't discontinue without doctor's advice until you complete prescribed dose, even though symptoms diminish or disappear.

Others:
- Requires an acid urine to be effective. Eat more protein foods, cranberries, cranberry juice with vitamin C, plums, prunes.
- Advise any doctor or dentist whom you consult that you take this medicine.

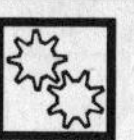

POSSIBLE INTERACTION WITH OTHER DRUGS

GENERIC NAME OR DRUG CLASS	COMBINED EFFECT
Antacids*	Decreased methenamine effect.
Carbonic anhydrase inhibitors*	Decreased methenamine effect.
Citrates*	Decreases effects of methenamine.
Diuretics, thiazide*	Decreased urine acidity.
Sodium bicarbonate	Decreased methenamine effect.
Sulfadoxine and pyrimethamine	Increased risk of kidney toxicity.
Sulfa drugs*	Possible kidney damage.

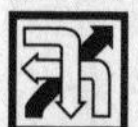

POSSIBLE INTERACTION WITH OTHER SUBSTANCES

INTERACTS WITH	COMBINED EFFECT
Alcohol:	Possible brain depression. Avoid or use with caution.
Beverages: Milk and other dairy products.	Decreased methenamine effect.
Cocaine:	None expected.
Foods: Citrus, cranberries, plums, prunes.	Increased methenamine effect.
Marijuana:	Drowsiness, muscle weakness or blood pressure drop.
Tobacco:	None expected.

***See Glossary**

METHOTREXATE

BRAND NAMES

Amethopterin
Folex
Folex PFS
Mexate
Mexate AQ
Rheumatrex
Trexall

BASIC INFORMATION

Habit forming? No
Prescription needed? Yes
Available as generic? Yes
Drug class: Antimetabolite, antipsoriatic

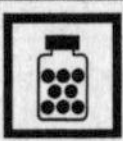

USES

- Treatment for certain types of cancer.
- Treatment for psoriasis in patients with severe problems.
- Treatment for severe rheumatoid arthritis.

DOSAGE & USAGE INFORMATION

How to take:
- Tablet—Swallow with liquid.
- Injectable form—Is sometimes self-injected or used as an oral dose; consult doctor.

When to take:
At the same time each day.

If you forget a dose:
Skip the missed dose. Don't double the next dose.

What drug does:
Inhibits abnormal cell reproduction.

Time lapse before drug works:
May require 6 weeks for maximum effect.

Don't take with:
Any other medicine or any dietary supplement without consulting your doctor or pharmacist.

OVERDOSE

SYMPTOMS:
Headache, stupor, seizures.
WHAT TO DO:
- **Dial 911 (emergency) for medical help or call poison control center 1-800-222-1222 for instructions.**
- **If person is unconscious, check breathing and pulse. If not breathing, begin mouth-to-mouth rescue breathing. If heart is not beating, begin chest compressions.**
- **See emergency information on last 3 pages of this book.**

POSSIBLE ADVERSE REACTIONS OR SIDE EFFECTS

SYMPTOMS	WHAT TO DO
Life-threatening:	
Hives, rash, intense itching, faintness soon after a dose (anaphylaxis).	Seek emergency treatment immediately.
Common:	
• Black stools or bloody vomit.	Discontinue. Seek emergency treatment.
• Sore throat, fever, mouth sores; chills; unusual bleeding or bruising.	Discontinue. Call doctor right away.
• Abdominal pain, nausea, vomiting.	Continue. Call doctor when convenient.
Infrequent:	
• Seizures.	Discontinue. Seek emergency treatment.
• Dizziness when standing after sitting or lying, drowsiness, headache, confusion, blurred vision, shortness of breath, joint pain, blood in urine, jaundice, diarrhea, red skin, back pain.	Discontinue. Call doctor right away.
• Cough, rash, sexual difficulties in males.	Continue. Call doctor when convenient.
• Acne, boils, hair loss, itchy skin.	Continue. Tell doctor at next visit.
Rare:	
Painful urination.	Discontinue. Call doctor right away.

WARNINGS & PRECAUTIONS

Don't take if:
You are allergic to any antimetabolite.

Before you start, consult your doctor if:
- You are an alcoholic.
- You have blood, liver or kidney disease.
- You have colitis or peptic ulcer.
- You have gout.
- You have an infection.
- You plan to become pregnant within 3 months.

Over age 60:
Adverse reactions and side effects may be more frequent and severe than in younger persons.

Pregnancy:
- Psoriasis—Risk to unborn child outweighs drug benefits. Don't use.
- Cancer—Consult doctor.
- Risk category X (see page xviii).

Breast-feeding:
Drug passes into milk. Avoid drug or discontinue nursing.

Infants & children:
Use only under special medical supervision.

Prolonged use:
- Adverse reactions more likely the longer drug is required.
- Talk to your doctor about the need for follow-up medical examinations or laboratory studies to check liver function, kidney function, complete blood counts (white blood cell count, platelet count, red blood cell count, hemoglobin, hematocrit).

Skin & sunlight:
May cause rash or intensify sunburn in areas exposed to sun or ultraviolet light (photosensitivity reaction). Avoid overexposure. Notify doctor if reaction occurs.

Driving, piloting or hazardous work:
Avoid if you feel dizzy, drowsy or confused. Otherwise, no problems expected.

Discontinuing:
Don't discontinue without doctor's advice until you complete prescribed dose, even though symptoms diminish or disappear. Some side effects may follow discontinuing. Consult doctor if blurred vision, convulsions, confusion, or persistent headache occur.

Others:
- Drink more water than usual to cause frequent urination.
- Don't give this medicine to anyone else for any purpose. It is a strong drug that requires close medical supervision.
- Report for frequent medical follow-up and laboratory studies.
- Advise any doctor or dentist whom you consult that you take this medicine.

POSSIBLE INTERACTION WITH OTHER DRUGS

GENERIC NAME OR DRUG CLASS	COMBINED EFFECT
Anticoagulants,* oral	Increased anticoagulant effect.
Anticonvulsants,* hydantoin	Possible methotrexate toxicity.
Antigout drugs*	Decreased antigout effect. Toxic levels of methotrexate.
Anti-inflammatory drugs, nonsteroidal (NSAIDs)*	Possible increased methotrexate toxicity.
Asparaginase	Decreased methotrexate effect.
Bone marrow depressants,* other	Increased risk of bone marrow depression.
Clozapine	Toxic effect on bone marrow.
Diclofenac	May increase toxicity.
Etretinate	Increased chance of toxicity to liver.
Fluorouracil	Decreased methotrexate effect.
Folic acid	Possible decreased methotrexate effect.
Isoniazid	Increased risk of liver damage.
Leflunomide	Increased risk of side effects.
Leucovorin calcium	Decreased methotrexate toxicity.
Levamisole	Increased risk of bone marrow depression.
Oxyphenbutazone	Possible methotrexate toxicity.
Penicillins*	Increased risk of methotrexate toxicity.
Phenylbutazone	Possible methotrexate toxicity.

Continued on page 919

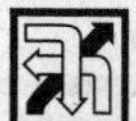

POSSIBLE INTERACTION WITH OTHER SUBSTANCES

INTERACTS WITH	COMBINED EFFECT
Alcohol:	Likely liver damage. Avoid.
Beverages:	Extra fluid intake decreases chance of methotrexate toxicity.
Cocaine:	Increased chance of methotrexate adverse reactions. Avoid.
Foods:	None expected.
Marijuana:	None expected.
Tobacco:	None expected.

***See Glossary**

METOCLOPRAMIDE

BRAND NAMES

Apo-Metoclop
Clopra
Emex
Maxeran
Metozolv ODT
Octamide
Octamide PFS
Reclomide
Reglan

BASIC INFORMATION

Habit forming? No
Prescription needed? Yes
Available as generic? Yes
Drug class: Antiemetic; dopaminergic blocker

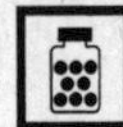

USES

Treatment for gastroesophageal reflux disease (GERD) and for diabetic gastroparesis.

DOSAGE & USAGE INFORMATION

How to take:

- Tablet or syrup—Swallow with liquid or food to lessen stomach irritation.
- Oral disintegrating tablet—Let tablet dissolve on tongue. Don't swallow with water.

When to take:
30 minutes before each meal and at bedtime or take before symptoms expected, up to 4 times a day.

If you forget a dose:
Take as soon as you remember. If it is almost time for the next dose, wait for the next scheduled dose (don't double this dose).

What drug does:
Prevents smooth muscle in stomach from relaxing, thereby helping to empty stomach more quickly.

Continued next column

OVERDOSE

SYMPTOMS:
Severe drowsiness, muscle spasms, mental confusion, trembling, seizure, coma.
WHAT TO DO:

- **Dial 911 (emergency) for medical help or call poison control center 1-800-222-1222 for instructions.**
- **If person is unconscious, check breathing and pulse. If not breathing, begin mouth-to-mouth rescue breathing. If heart is not beating, begin chest compressions.**
- **See emergency information on last 3 pages of this book.**

Time lapse before drug works:
30 to 60 minutes.

Don't take with:
Any other medicine or any dietary supplement without consulting your doctor or pharmacist.

POSSIBLE ADVERSE REACTIONS OR SIDE EFFECTS

SYMPTOMS	WHAT TO DO
Life-threatening:	
In case of overdose, see previous column.	
Common:	
Drowsiness, restlessness, rash.	Continue. Call doctor when convenient.
Infrequent:	
• Wheezing, shortness of breath.	Discontinue. Call doctor right away.
• Dizziness; headache; insomnia; tender, swollen breasts; increased milk flow; menstrual changes; decreased sex drive.	Continue. Call doctor when convenient.
Rare:	
• Abnormal, involuntary movements of jaw, lips and tongue; depression; Parkinson's syndrome.*	Discontinue. Call doctor right away.
• Constipation, nausea, diarrhea, dry mouth.	Continue. Call doctor when convenient.

WARNINGS & PRECAUTIONS

Don't take if:
You are allergic to procaine, procainamide or metoclopramide.

Before you start, consult your doctor if:

- You have Parkinson's disease.
- You have liver or kidney disease.
- You have epilepsy.
- You have bleeding from gastrointestinal tract or intestinal obstruction.
- You will have surgery within 2 months, including dental surgery, requiring general or spinal anesthesia.

Over age 60:
Adverse reactions and side effects may be more frequent and severe than in younger persons.

Pregnancy:
No proven harm to unborn child. Avoid if possible. Consult doctor. Risk category B (see page xviii).

Breast-feeding:
Unknown effect. Consult doctor.

Infants & children:
Adverse reactions more likely to occur than in adults.

Prolonged use:
Adverse reactions including muscle spasms and trembling hands more likely to occur.

Skin & sunlight:
No problems expected.

Driving, piloting or hazardous work:
Don't drive or pilot aircraft until you learn how medicine affects you. Don't work around dangerous machinery. Don't climb ladders or work in high places. Danger increases if you drink alcohol or take medicine affecting alertness and reflexes, such as antihistamines, tranquilizers, sedatives, pain medicine, narcotics and mind-altering drugs.

Discontinuing:
May be unnecessary to finish medicine. Follow doctor's instructions.

Others:
Advise any doctor or dentist whom you consult that you take this medicine.

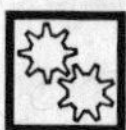

POSSIBLE INTERACTION WITH OTHER DRUGS

GENERIC NAME OR DRUG CLASS	COMBINED EFFECT
Acetaminophen	Increased absorption of acetaminophen.
Anticholinergics*	Decreased metoclopramide effect.
Aspirin	Increased absorption of aspirin.
Bromocriptine	Decreased bromocriptine effect.
Butyrophenone	Increased chance of muscle spasm and trembling.
Central nervous system (CNS) depressants*	Excess sedation.
Clozapine	Toxic effect on the central nervous system.
Digitalis preparations*	Decreased absorption of digitalis.
Ethinamate	Dangerous increased effects of ethinamate. Avoid combining.
Fluoxetine	Increased depressant effects of both drugs.
Guanfacine	May increase depressant effects of either drug.
Insulin	Unpredictable changes in blood glucose. Dosages may require adjustment.
Leucovorin	High alcohol content of leucovorin may cause adverse effects.
Levodopa	Increased absorption of levodopa.
Lithium	Increased absorption of lithium.
Loxapine	May increase toxic effects of both drugs.
Methyprylon	Increased sedative effect, perhaps to dangerous level. Avoid.
Nabilone	Greater depression of central nervous system.
Narcotics*	Decreased metoclopramide effect.
Nizatidine	Decreased nizatidine absorption.
Pergolide	Decreased pergolide effect.

Continued on page 919

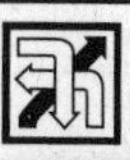

POSSIBLE INTERACTION WITH OTHER SUBSTANCES

INTERACTS WITH	COMBINED EFFECT
Alcohol:	Excess sedation. Avoid.
Beverages: Coffee.	Decreased metoclopramide effect.
Cocaine:	Decreased metoclopramide effect.
Foods:	None expected.
Marijuana:	Decreased metoclopramide effect.
Tobacco:	Decreased metoclopramide effect.

***See Glossary**

METYRAPONE

BRAND NAMES

Metopirone

BASIC INFORMATION

Habit forming? No
Prescription needed? Yes
Available as generic? No
Drug class: Antiadrenal

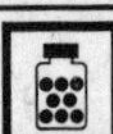

USES

- To diagnose the function of the pituitary gland.
- Treats Cushing's syndrome, a disorder characterized by higher than normal concentrations of cortisol (one of the hormones secreted by the adrenal glands) in the blood.

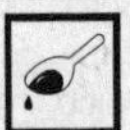

DOSAGE & USAGE INFORMATION

How to take:
- For medical testing purposes—Take the prescribed number of tablets with milk or food on the day before the scheduled test. On the day of the test, blood and urine studies will show the amount of hormones in your blood. Results of the test will help establish your diagnosis.
- For treatment of Cushing's syndrome—Swallow tablet with liquid. If you can't swallow whole, crumble tablet and take with liquid or food.

When to take:
- For medical testing—Take the prescribed number of tablets on the day before the scheduled test.
- For treatment of Cushing's syndrome—Take total daily amount in divided doses. Follow prescription directions carefully.

Continued next column

OVERDOSE

SYMPTOMS:
Nausea (severe), vomiting, diarrhea, abdominal pain, sudden weakness, irregular heartbeat.
WHAT TO DO:
- **Dial 911 (emergency) for medical help or call poison control center 1-800-222-1222 for instructions.**
- **See emergency information on last 3 pages of this book.**

If you forget a dose:
Take as soon as you remember. If it is almost time for the next dose, wait for that dose (don't double this dose) and resume regular schedule.

What drug does:
Prevents one of the chemical reactions in the production of cortisol by the adrenal glands.

Time lapse before drug works:
Approximately 1 hour.

Don't take with:
- Cortisone*-like medicines for 48 hours prior to testing.
- Any other medicine or any dietary supplement without consulting your doctor or pharmacist.

POSSIBLE ADVERSE REACTIONS OR SIDE EFFECTS

SYMPTOMS	WHAT TO DO
Life-threatening: In case of overdose, see previous column.	
Common:	
Dizziness, headache, nausea.	Continue. Call doctor when convenient.
Infrequent:	
Drowsiness.	Continue. Call doctor when convenient.
Rare:	
Hair loss or excess growth, decreased appetite, confusion, acne (may begin or may worsen if already present).	Continue. Call doctor when convenient.

WARNINGS & PRECAUTIONS

Don't take if:
You are allergic to metyrapone.

Before you start, consult your doctor if:
- You have porphyria.
- You have adrenal insufficiency (Addison's disease).
- You have decreased pituitary function.

Over age 60:
No special problems expected.

Pregnancy:
Safety not established. Take only under careful supervision of medical professional. Risk category C (see page xviii).

Breast-feeding:
Drug may pass into milk, although controlled studies in humans have not been performed. Since the possibility exists, avoid nursing until you finish the medicine.

Infants & children:
No special problems expected.

Prolonged use:
No special problems expected.

Skin & sunlight:
No special problems expected.

Driving, piloting or hazardous work:
Don't drive or pilot aircraft until you learn how medicine affects you. Don't work around dangerous machinery. Don't climb ladders or work in high places. Danger increases if you drink alcohol or take medicine affecting alertness and reflexes.

Discontinuing:
No special problems expected.

Others:
Advise any doctor or dentist whom you consult that you take this medicine.

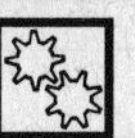

POSSIBLE INTERACTION WITH OTHER DRUGS

GENERIC NAME OR DRUG CLASS	COMBINED EFFECT
Antidiabetics, oral*	Increased risk of adverse reactions.
Contraceptives, oral*	Possible inaccurate test results.
Estrogens*	Possible inaccurate test results.
Insulin	Increased risk of adverse reactions.
Phenytoin	Possible inaccurate test results.

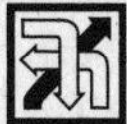

POSSIBLE INTERACTION WITH OTHER SUBSTANCES

INTERACTS WITH	COMBINED EFFECT
Alcohol:	None expected.
Beverages:	None expected.
Cocaine:	None expected.
Foods:	Increased appetite and absorption of nutrients, causing difficulty with weight control.
Marijuana:	None expected.
Tobacco:	None expected.

*See Glossary

MEXILETINE

BRAND NAMES

Mexitil

BASIC INFORMATION

Habit forming? No
Prescription needed? Yes
Available as generic? Yes
Drug class: Antiarrhythmic

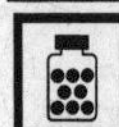

USES

Stabilizes irregular heartbeat.

DOSAGE & USAGE INFORMATION

How to take:
Capsule—Swallow whole with food, milk or antacid to lessen stomach irritation.

When to take:
At the same times each day as directed by your doctor.

If you forget a dose:
Take as soon as you remember. If it is almost time for the next dose, wait for that dose (don't double this dose) and resume regular schedule.

What drug does:
Blocks the fast sodium channel in heart tissue.

Time lapse before drug works:
30 minutes to 2 hours.

Don't take with:
Any other medicine or any dietary supplement without consulting your doctor or pharmacist.

OVERDOSE

SYMPTOMS:
Nausea, vomiting, seizures, convulsions, cardiac arrest.
WHAT TO DO:
- **Dial 911 (emergency) for medical help or call poison control center 1-800-222-1222 for instructions.**
- **See emergency information on last 3 pages of this book.**

POSSIBLE ADVERSE REACTIONS OR SIDE EFFECTS

SYMPTOMS	WHAT TO DO
Life-threatening:	
Chest pain, shortness of breath, irregular or fast heartbeat.	Discontinue. Seek emergency treatment.
Common:	
Dizziness, anxiety, shakiness, unsteadiness when walking, heartburn, nausea, vomiting.	Discontinue. Call doctor right away.
Infrequent:	
• Sore throat, fever, mouth sores, blurred vision, confusion, constipation, diarrhea, headache, numbness or tingling in hands or feet, ringing in ears, unexplained bleeding or bruising, rash, slurred speech, insomnia, weakness, difficult swallowing.	Discontinue. Call doctor right away.
• Loss of taste.	Continue. Call doctor when convenient.
Rare:	
• Seizures.	Discontinue. Seek emergency treatment.
• Hallucinations, psychosis, memory loss, difficult breathing, swollen feet and ankles, hiccups, jaundice.	Discontinue. Call doctor right away.
• Hair loss, impotence.	Continue. Call doctor when convenient.

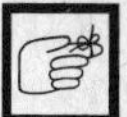

WARNINGS & PRECAUTIONS

Don't take if:
You are allergic to mexiletine, lidocaine or tocainide.

Before you start, consult your doctor if:
- You have had liver or kidney disease or impaired kidney function.
- You have had lupus.
- You have a history of seizures.
- You will have surgery within 2 months, including dental surgery, requiring general or spinal anesthesia.
- You have heart disease or low blood pressure.

Over age 60:
Adverse reactions and side effects may be more frequent and severe than in younger persons. Ask doctor about smaller doses.

Pregnancy:
Decide with your doctor if drug benefits justify risk to unborn child. Risk category C (see page xviii).

Breast-feeding:
Drug passes into milk. Avoid drug or discontinue nursing until you finish medicine. Consult doctor for advice on maintaining milk supply.

Infants & children:
Use only under close medical supervision.

Prolonged use:
- May cause lupus*-like illness.
- Talk to your doctor about the need for follow-up medical examinations or laboratory studies to check ECG,* liver function.

Skin & sunlight:
No problems expected.

Driving, piloting or hazardous work:
Use caution if you feel dizzy or weak. Otherwise, no problems expected.

Discontinuing:
Don't discontinue without consulting doctor. Dose may require gradual reduction if you have taken drug for a long time. Doses of other drugs may also require adjustment.

Others:
Advise any doctor or dentist whom you consult that you take this medicine.

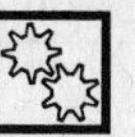

POSSIBLE INTERACTION WITH OTHER DRUGS

GENERIC NAME OR DRUG CLASS	COMBINED EFFECT
Cimetidine	Increased mexiletine effect and toxicity.
Encainide	Increased effect of toxicity on the heart muscle.
Nicardipine	Possible increased effect and toxicity of each drug.
Phenobarbital	Decreased mexiletine effect.
Phenytoin	Decreased mexiletine effect.
Propafenone	Increased effect of both drugs and increased risk of toxicity.
Rifampin	Decreased mexiletine effect.
Urinary acidifiers*	May decrease effectiveness of medicine.
Urinary alkalizers*	May slow elimination of mexiletine and cause need to adjust dosage.

POSSIBLE INTERACTION WITH OTHER SUBSTANCES

INTERACTS WITH	COMBINED EFFECT
Alcohol:	Causes irregular effectiveness of mexiletine. Avoid.
Beverages: Caffeine drinks, iced drinks.	Irregular heartbeat.
Cocaine:	Decreased mexiletine effect.
Foods:	None expected.
Marijuana:	Irregular heartbeat. Avoid.
Tobacco:	Dangerous combination. May lead to liver problems and reduce excretion of mexiletine.

MIFEPRISTONE (RU-486)

BRAND NAMES

Mifeprex

BASIC INFORMATION

Habit forming? No
Prescription needed? Yes
Available as generic? No
Drug class: Abortifacient

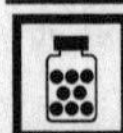

USES

- Terminates pregnancy in the early stages (up to 7 weeks or 49 days since the beginning of the last menstrual period). Mifepristone is not approved for ending later pregnancies. Requires three trips to your doctor's office: day one for administration, day three for a second medication (if you are still pregnant) and day fourteen for follow-up and determination of the status of your pregnancy.
- Note: The brand name drug Korlym is used to treat Cushing's syndrome and is not covered in this drug chart. Consult your doctor or pharmacist if you have questions.

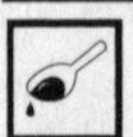

DOSAGE & USAGE INFORMATION

How to take:
Tablet—Taken on day one under strict compliance in the presence of your doctor. On day three misoprostol is taken in your doctor's office (if you are still pregnant).

When to take:
At your doctor's office.

What drug does:
Mifepristone blocks a hormone (progesterone) needed for your pregnancy to continue.

If you forget a dose:
Medication is taken at your doctor's office.

Continued next column

OVERDOSE

SYMPTOMS:
Symptoms are unknown. Drug is taken in medical office so overdose is not likely to occur.
WHAT TO DO:
Overdose unlikely to threaten life. If person uses much larger amount than prescribed or if accidentally swallowed, call doctor or poison control center 1-800-222-1222 for help.

Time lapse before drug works:
A few days to two weeks. If you are still pregnant after two weeks, your doctor will discuss other options you have including a surgical alternative to terminate your pregnancy.

Don't take with:
Any other medicine or any dietary supplement without consulting your doctor or pharmacist.

POSSIBLE ADVERSE REACTIONS OR SIDE EFFECTS

SYMPTOMS	WHAT TO DO
Life-threatening: None expected.	
Common: Nausea or vomiting, diarrhea, abdominal pain, back pain, dizziness, unusual tiredness or weakness, headache.	Call doctor if symptoms persist.
Infrequent:	
• Excessive and heavy vaginal bleeding.	Call doctor right away.
• Pale skin, troubled breathing, unusual bleeding or bruising, anxiety, upset stomach, acid indigestion, fever, insomnia, leg pain, increased clear or white vaginal discharge, shaking, stuffy nose, cough, fainting, genital itching or pain, chills or flu-like symptoms, sinusitis.	Call doctor if symptoms persist.
Rare: None expected.	

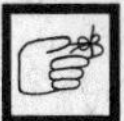

WARNINGS & PRECAUTIONS

Don't take if:
You are allergic to mifepristone or misoprostol.

Before you start, consult your doctor if:
- You have a history of adrenal failure.
- You have a history of hemorrhagic (bleeding) disorders.
- You have an ectopic pregnancy (a pregnancy outside the uterus).
- You have any other medical problems.
- You have anemia.
- You have an in-place intra-uterine device (IUD).
- You cannot easily get emergency medical help during the two weeks after you take the drug.
- You have a family history of porphyria.

Over age 60:
Not used in this age group.

Pregnancy:
Mifepristone is used to terminate pregnancy.

Breast-feeding:
It is unknown if mifepristone is distributed into breast milk. Avoid drug or discontinue nursing until you finish medicine. Consult doctor for advice on maintaining milk supply.

Infants & children:
Safety and efficacy not established. Not used in this age group.

Prolonged use:
Not intended for prolonged use.

Skin & sunlight:
No problems expected.

Driving, piloting or hazardous work:
No problems expected.

Discontinuing:
Drug is administered in the presence of a licensed medical professional who has registered with the manufacturer.

Others:
- Prior to using this medication, you will be required to sign a statement that you have decided to end your pregnancy.
- Advise any doctor or dentist whom you consult that you take this medicine.
- The follow-up doctor visits are very important. Don't miss them.
- May affect the results in some medical tests.
- An ultrasonographic scan may be scheduled 14 days after mifepristone administration to confirm termination of pregnancy and assess bleeding.
- If you do not want to become pregnant again, start using a birth control method as soon as your pregnancy ends.
- Serious bacterial infection and sepsis (blood infection) may occur without the usual signs of infection, such as fever and pelvic tenderness.
- If you are still pregnant after the two weeks, there may be birth defects if the pregnancy continues. Your doctor will discuss other options to end your pregnancy.

POSSIBLE INTERACTION WITH OTHER DRUGS

GENERIC NAME OR DRUG CLASS	COMBINED EFFECT
Anticoagulants*	Excessive bleeding.
Corticosteroids* (long term use)	Effects unknown. Avoid.
Dabigatran	Increased risk of vaginal bleeding.
Enzyme inducers*	May decrease effect of mifepristone.
Enzyme inhibitors*	May increase effect of mifepristone.

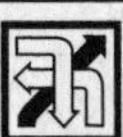

POSSIBLE INTERACTION WITH OTHER SUBSTANCES

INTERACTS WITH	COMBINED EFFECT
Alcohol:	None expected. Best to avoid.
Beverages: Grapefruit juice.	May increase effect of mifepristone.
Cocaine:	Unknown. Avoid.
Foods:	None expected.
Marijuana:	None expected.
Tobacco:	None expected.

*See Glossary

MIGLITOL

BRAND NAMES

Glyset

BASIC INFORMATION

Habit forming? No
Prescription needed? Yes
Available as generic? No
Drug class: Antidiabetic

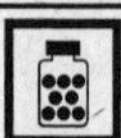

USES

Treatment for hyperglycemia (excess sugar in the blood) that cannot be controlled by diet alone in patients with type 2 diabetes. The drug may be used alone or in combination with other antidiabetic drugs.

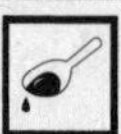

DOSAGE & USAGE INFORMATION

How to take:
Tablet—Swallow with liquid. Take at the very beginning of a meal.

When to take:
Usually 3 times a day or as directed by doctor. Dosage may be increased at 4 to 8 week intervals until maximum benefits are achieved.

If you forget a dose:
And your meal is finished, then skip the missed dose and wait for your next meal and next scheduled dose (don't double this dose).

What drug does:
Impedes the digestion and absorption of carbohydrates and their subsequent conversion into glucose. This improves control of blood glucose and may reduce the complications of diabetes. However, miglitol does not cure diabetes.

Continued next column

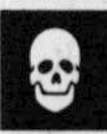

OVERDOSE

SYMPTOMS:
An overdose may cause flatulence, diarrhea and abdominal pain. It is unlikely to produce serious side effects. The drug itself will not produce low blood sugar (hypoglycemia).
WHAT TO DO:
Overdose unlikely to threaten life. If person uses much larger amount than prescribed or if accidentally swallowed, call doctor or poison control center 1-800-222-1222 for help.

Time lapse before drug works:
May take several weeks for full effectiveness.

Don't take with:
Any other medicine or any dietary supplement without consulting your doctor or pharmacist.

POSSIBLE ADVERSE REACTIONS OR SIDE EFFECTS

SYMPTOMS	WHAT TO DO
Life-threatening: None expected from the drug by itself.	
Common: Diarrhea, stomach cramps, gas, bloating feeling.	Continue. Call doctor when convenient.
Infrequent: Skin rash.	Continue. Call doctor when convenient.
Rare: Low blood sugar (hypoglycemia) may occur if you are taking other drugs for diabetes and you do not consume enough calories. Symptoms may include stomach pain, anxious feeling, cold sweats, chills, confusion, convulsions, cool pale skin, excessive hunger, nausea or vomiting, rapid heartbeat, nervousness, shakiness, unsteady walk, unusual weakness or tiredness, vision changes,	For low blood sugar, take glucose or eat honey or drink orange juice. For more severe symptoms, call doctor right away or seek emergency help.

WARNINGS & PRECAUTIONS

Don't take if:
You are allergic to miglitol.

Before you start, consult your doctor if:
- You have any kidney or liver disease or any heart or blood vessel disorder.
- You have any chronic health problem.
- You have an infection, illness or any condition that can cause low blood sugar.
- You have a history of acid in the blood (metabolic acidosis or ketoacidosis).
- You have inflammatory bowel disease or any other intestinal disorder.
- You are allergic to any medication, food or other substance.

Over age 60:
No special problems expected.

Pregnancy:
Decide with your doctor if drug benefits justify risks to unborn child. Risk category B (see page xviii).

Breast-feeding:
Drug passes into milk. It is not recommended for use in nursing mothers.

Infants & children:
Safety and efficacy have not been established. Use only under close medical supervision.

Prolonged use:
- Schedule regular doctor visits to determine if the drug is continuing to be effective in controlling the diabetes and to check for any problems in kidney function.
- You will most likely require an antidiabetic medicine for the rest of your life.
- You will need to test your blood glucose levels several times a day, or for some, once to several times a week.

Skin & sunlight:
No special problems expected.

Driving, piloting or hazardous work:
No special problems expected.

Discontinuing:
Don't discontinue without consulting your doctor even if you feel well. You can have diabetes without feeling any symptoms. Untreated diabetes can cause serious problems.

Others:
- Advise any doctor or dentist whom you consult that you take this medicine.
- It may interfere with the accuracy of some medical tests.
- Follow any special diet your doctor may prescribe. It can help control diabetes.
- Consult doctor if you become ill with vomiting or diarrhea while taking this drug.
- Use caution when exercising. Ask your doctor about an appropriate exercise program.
- Wear medical identification stating that you have diabetes and take this medication.
- Learn to recognize the symptoms of low blood sugar. You and your family need to know what to do if these symptoms occur.
- Have a glucagon kit and syringe in the event severe low blood sugar occurs.
- High blood sugar (hyperglycemia) may occur with diabetes. Ask your doctor about symptoms to watch for and treatment steps to take.
- Educate yourself about diabetes.

POSSIBLE INTERACTION WITH OTHER DRUGS

GENERIC NAME OR DRUG CLASS	COMBINED EFFECT
Amylase (Pancreatic enzyme)	Decreased miglitol effect.
Antidiabetic agents, sulfonylurea	May cause hypoglycemia.
Charcoal, activated	Decreased miglitol effect.
Pancreatin (Pancreatic enzyme)	Decreased miglitol effect.
Pramlintide	Decreased absorption of nutrients.
Propranolol	Decreased effect of propranolol.
Ranitidine	Decreased effect of ranitidine.

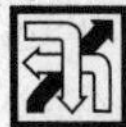

POSSIBLE INTERACTION WITH OTHER SUBSTANCES

INTERACTS WITH	COMBINED EFFECT
Alcohol:	May increase effect of miglitol. Avoid excessive amounts.
Beverages:	None expected.
Cocaine:	None expected. Best to avoid.
Foods:	None expected.
Marijuana:	None expected. Best to avoid.
Tobacco:	People with diabetes should not smoke.

MINOXIDIL

BRAND NAMES

Loniten

BASIC INFORMATION

Habit forming? No
Prescription needed? Yes
Available as generic? Yes
Drug class: Antihypertensive

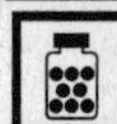

USES

- Treatment for high blood pressure in conjunction with other drugs, such as beta-adrenergic blockers and diuretics.
- Treatment for congestive heart failure.
- Can stimulate hair growth.

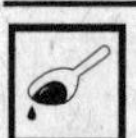

DOSAGE & USAGE INFORMATION

How to take:
Tablet—Swallow with liquid. If you can't swallow whole, crumble tablet and take with liquid or food.

When to take:
At the same time each day, according to instructions on prescription label.

If you forget a dose:
Take as soon as you remember. If it is almost time for the next dose, wait for that dose (don't double this dose) and resume regular schedule.

What drug does:
Relaxes small blood vessels (arterioles) so blood can pass through more easily.

Time lapse before drug works:
2 to 3 hours for effect to begin; 3 to 7 days of continuous use may be necessary for maximum blood pressure response.

Don't take with:
Any other medicine or any dietary supplement without consulting your doctor or pharmacist.

OVERDOSE

SYMPTOMS:
Low blood pressure, fainting, chest pain, shortness of breath, coma.
WHAT TO DO:

- **Dial 911 (emergency) for medical help or call poison control center 1-800-222-1222 for instructions.**
- **See emergency information on last 3 pages of this book.**

POSSIBLE ADVERSE REACTIONS OR SIDE EFFECTS

SYMPTOMS	WHAT TO DO
Life-threatening: In case of overdose, see previous column.	
Common:	
• Excessive hair growth, flushed skin or redness.	Continue. Call doctor when convenient.
• Bloating.	Discontinue. Call doctor right away.
Infrequent:	
• Chest pain, irregular or slow heartbeat, shortness of breath, swollen feet or legs, rapid weight gain.	Discontinue. Call doctor right away.
• Numbness of hands, feet or face; headache; tender breasts; darkening of skin.	Continue. Call doctor when convenient.
Rare:	
Rash.	Discontinue. Call doctor right away.

WARNINGS & PRECAUTIONS

Don't take if:
You are allergic to minoxidil.

Before you start, consult your doctor if:
- You have had a recent stroke or heart attack or angina pectoris in past 3 weeks.
- You have impaired kidney function.
- You have pheochromocytoma.*

Over age 60:
Adverse reactions and side effects may be more frequent and severe than in younger persons.

Pregnancy:
Decide with your doctor if drug benefits justify risk to unborn child. Risk category C (see page xviii).

Breast-feeding:
Drug may pass into milk. Avoid drug or discontinue nursing until you finish medicine. Consult doctor about maintaining milk supply.

Infants & children:
Not recommended. Safety and dosage have not been established.

Prolonged use:
Request periodic blood examinations that include potassium levels.

Skin & sunlight:
May cause rash or intensify sunburn in areas exposed to sun or ultraviolet light (photosensitivity reaction). Avoid overexposure. Notify doctor if reaction occurs.

Driving, piloting or hazardous work:
Avoid if you become dizzy or faint. Otherwise, no problems expected.

Discontinuing:
Don't discontinue without consulting doctor. Dose may require gradual reduction if you have taken drug for a long time. Doses of other drugs may also require adjustment.

Others:
- Advise any doctor or dentist whom you consult that you take this medicine.
- Check blood pressure frequently.

POSSIBLE INTERACTION WITH OTHER DRUGS

GENERIC NAME OR DRUG CLASS	COMBINED EFFECT
Anesthesia	Drastic blood pressure drop.
Antihypertensives,* other	Dosage adjustments may be necessary to keep blood pressure at desired level.
Carteolol	Increased anti-hypertensive effect.
Diuretics*	Dosage adjustments may be necessary to keep blood pressure at desired level.
Estrogens*	May increase blood pressure.
Guanadrel	Weakness and faintness when arising from bed or chair.
Guanethidine	Weakness and faintness when arising from bed or chair.
Lisinopril	Increased anti-hypertensive effect. Dosage of each may require adjustment.
Nicardipine	Blood pressure drop. Dosages may require adjustment.
Nimodipine	Dangerous blood pressure drop.
Nitrates*	Drastic blood pressure drop.
Sotalol	Increased anti-hypertensive effect.
Sympathomimetics*	Possible decreased minoxidil effect.
Terazosin	Decreased effectiveness of terazosin.

POSSIBLE INTERACTION WITH OTHER SUBSTANCES

INTERACTS WITH	COMBINED EFFECT
Alcohol:	Possible excessive blood pressure drop.
Beverages:	None expected.
Cocaine:	Increased risk of heart block and high blood pressure.
Foods: Salt substitutes.	Possible excessive potassium levels in blood.
Marijuana:	Increased dizziness.
Tobacco:	May decrease minoxidil effect. Avoid.

MINOXIDIL (Topical)

BRAND NAMES

Dermal
Men's Rogaine Topical Foam
Rogaine
Rogaine Extra Strength for Men
Rogaine for Men
Rogaine for Women

BASIC INFORMATION

Habit forming? No
Prescription needed? No
Available as generic? Yes
Drug class: Hair growth stimulant

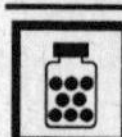

USES

Treats hair loss on scalp from male and female pattern baldness (alopecia androgenetica).

DOSAGE & USAGE INFORMATION

How to use:
Topical solution

- Apply only to dry hair and scalp. With the provided applicator, apply the amount prescribed to the scalp area being treated. Begin in center of the treated area.
- Wash hands immediately after use.
- Don't use a blow dryer.
- If you are using at bedtime, wait 30 minutes after applying before retiring.

When to use:
Twice a day or as directed.

If you forget a dose:
Use as soon as you remember. No need to ever double the dose.

What drug does:
Stimulates hair growth by possibly dilating small blood capillaries, thereby providing more blood to hair follicles.

Time lapse before drug works:
Varies with individuals.

Don't use with:
Other hair-growth products without consulting your doctor or pharmacist.

OVERDOSE

SYMPTOMS:
None expected.
WHAT TO DO:
Not for internal use. If child accidentally swallows, dial 911 (emergency) for medical help or call poison control center 1-800-222-1222 for instructions.

POSSIBLE ADVERSE REACTIONS OR SIDE EFFECTS

SYMPTOMS	WHAT TO DO
Life-threatening:	
Fast, irregular heartbeat (rare; represents too much absorbed into body).	Discontinue. Seek emergency treatment.
Common:	
None expected.	
Infrequent:	
Itching scalp; flaking, reddened skin.	Continue. Call doctor when convenient.
Rare:	
Burning scalp, skin rash, swollen face, headache, dizziness or fainting, hands and feet numb or tingling, rapid weight gain.	Discontinue. Call doctor right away.

WARNINGS & PRECAUTIONS

Don't use if:
You are allergic to minoxidil.

Before you start, consult your doctor if:
- You are allergic to anything.
- You have heart disease or high blood pressure.
- You have skin irritation or abrasion or severe sunburn (systemic absorption may be increased).

Over age 60:
No problems expected.

Pregnancy:
Decide with your doctor if drug benefits justify risk to unborn child. Risk category C (see page xviii).

Breast-feeding:
Drug may pass into milk. Avoid drug or discontinue nursing until you finish medicine. Consult doctor about maintaining milk supply.

Infants & children:
Don't use.

Prolonged use:
No problems expected.

Skin & sunlight:
No problems expected.

Driving, piloting or hazardous work:
No problems expected.

Discontinuing:
No problems expected.

Others:
- Keep away from eyes, nose and mouth. Flush with plain water if accident occurs.
- New hair will drop out when you stop using minoxidil.
- Keep solution cool, but don't freeze.

POSSIBLE INTERACTION WITH OTHER DRUGS

GENERIC NAME OR DRUG CLASS	COMBINED EFFECT
Adrenocorticoids,* topical	May cause undesirable absorption of minoxidil.
Minoxidil, oral	Increased risk of toxicity.
Petrolatum, topical	May cause undesirable absorption of minoxidil.
Retinoids,* topical	May cause undesirable absorption of minoxidil.

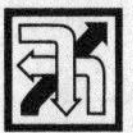

POSSIBLE INTERACTION WITH OTHER SUBSTANCES

INTERACTS WITH	COMBINED EFFECT
Alcohol:	None expected.
Beverages:	None expected.
Cocaine:	None expected.
Foods:	None expected.
Marijuana:	None expected.
Tobacco:	None expected.

*See Glossary

MIRABEGRON

BRAND NAMES

Myrbetriq

BASIC INFORMATION

Habit forming? No
Prescription needed? Yes
Available as generic? No
Drug class: Antispasmodic (urinary tract)

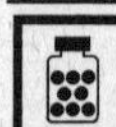

USES

It is used to treat overactive bladder (symptoms include an urgent need to urinate, a need to urinate often or leakage of urine).

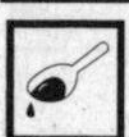

DOSAGE & USAGE INFORMATION

How to take:
Extended-release tablet—Swallow whole with liquid. Do not break, crush or chew tablet. It may be taken with or without food

When to take:
The drug is taken once a day at the same time each day.

If you forget a dose:
Take as soon as you remember. If it is almost time for the next dose, wait for the next scheduled dose (don't double this dose).

What drug does:
It works by relaxing the detrusor (bladder muscle) which helps the bladder hold more urine. This helps reduce the symptoms of an overactive bladder.

Time lapse before drug works:
It can take up to 8 weeks for symptoms to improve. The starting dosage may be increased after 8 weeks to achieve full effectiveness.

Don't take with:
Any other medicine or any dietary supplement without consulting your doctor or pharmacist.

OVERDOSE

SYMPTOMS:
Heart palpitations, fast pulse rate.
WHAT TO DO:
If person takes much larger amount than prescribed or if accidentally swallowed, call doctor or poison control center 1-800-222-1222 for help.

POSSIBLE ADVERSE REACTIONS OR SIDE EFFECTS

SYMPTOMS	WHAT TO DO
Life-threatening:	
Rare allergic reaction (hives, itching, rash, wheezing, tightness in chest, swelling of lips or tongue or throat).	Seek emergency treatment immediately.
Common:	
• Urinary tract infection, high blood pressure,	Continue, but call doctor right away.
• Cold symptoms, mild headache, nausea.	Continue. Call doctor when convenient.
Infrequent:	
• Heartbeat is fast or slow or irregular, unable to completely empty bladder (urinary retention), weak urine stream.	Continue, but call doctor right away.
• Constipation or diarrhea, dizziness, symptoms of flu or sinus infection, back pain, blurred vision, muscle aches, dry mouth.	Continue. Call doctor when convenient.
Rare:	
• New, severe and unusual symptoms.	Discontinue. Call doctor right away.
• Abdominal pain, fatigue, rash or itching.	Continue. Call doctor when convenient.

WARNINGS & PRECAUTIONS

Don't take if:
You are allergic to mirabegron.

Before you start, consult your doctor if:
- You have bladder problems (such as blockage) or an enlarged prostate.
- You have high blood pressure.
- You have liver or kidney problems.

Over age 60:
No problems expected.

Pregnancy:
Decide with your doctor whether drug benefits justify risk to unborn child. Risk category C (see page xviii).

Breast-feeding:
It is unknown if drug passes into breast milk. Consult your doctor for advice.

Infants & children:
Safety and efficacy for children under age 18 has not been established.

Prolonged use:
See your doctor for regular visits to make sure the drug is working properly and to check for unwanted effects (such as high blood pressure).

Skin & sunlight:
No problems expected.

Driving, piloting or hazardous work:
Don't drive or pilot aircraft until you learn how medicine affects you. Don't work around dangerous machinery. Don't climb ladders or work in high places. Danger increases if you drink alcohol or take medicine affecting alertness and reflexes.

Discontinuing:
No problems expected, but consult your doctor before stopping the drug.

Others:
- Advise any doctor, dentist or pharmacist whom you consult that you take this drug.
- Follow your doctor's recommendations for other treatment steps, such as diet changes, bladder training and/or pelvic floor exercises.

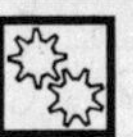

POSSIBLE INTERACTION WITH OTHER DRUGS

GENERIC NAME OR DRUG CLASS	COMBINED EFFECT
Digoxin	Increased effect of digoxin.
Desipramine	Increased effect of desipramine.
Flecainide	Increased effect of flecainide.
Metoprolol	Increased effect of metoprolol.
Muscarinic receptor antagonists	Increased risk of urinary retention. Use caution.
Propafenone	Increased effect of propafenone.
Thioridazine	Increased effect of thioridazine. Avoid.
Warfarin	May increase w arfarin effect.

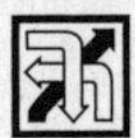

POSSIBLE INTERACTION WITH OTHER SUBSTANCES

INTERACTS WITH	COMBINED EFFECT
Alcohol:	None expected.
Beverages:	None expected.
Cocaine:	Effect unknown. Avoid.
Foods:	None expected.
Marijuana:	Effect unknown. Avoid.
Tobacco:	None expected.

MIRTAZAPINE

BRAND NAMES

Remeron | Remeron SolTab

BASIC INFORMATION

Habit forming? Not expected
Prescription needed? Yes
Available as generic? Yes
Drug class: Antidepressant

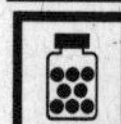

USES

Treats symptoms of mental depression.

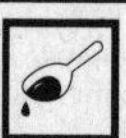

DOSAGE & USAGE INFORMATION

How to take:

- Tablet—Swallow with liquid. May be taken with or without food.
- Oral disintegrating tablet—Let tablet dissolve in your mouth.

When to take:
At the same time each day, usually in the evening before bedtime.

If you forget a dose:
Take as soon as you remember up to 12 hours late. If more than 12 hours, wait for the next scheduled dose (don't double this dose).

What drug does:
The exact mechanism is unknown. It appears to block certain chemicals in the brain, which in turn helps production of other brain chemicals that play a role in helping to relieve symptoms of depression.

Time lapse before drug works:
Will take up to several weeks to show improvement of the depression symptoms.

Don't take with:
Any other medicine or any dietary supplement without consulting your doctor or pharmacist.

OVERDOSE

SYMPTOMS:
Drowsiness, disorientation, memory impairment, rapid heartbeat.
WHAT TO DO:

- **Dial 911 (emergency) for medical help or call poison control center 1-800-222-1222 for instructions.**
- **See emergency information on last 3 pages of this book.**

POSSIBLE ADVERSE REACTIONS OR SIDE EFFECTS

SYMPTOMS	WHAT TO DO
Life-threatening: None expected.	
Common:	
• Abdominal pain, vomiting, joint pain, increased cough, rash, itching, agitation, anxiety, twitching, apathy.	Discontinue. Call doctor right away.
• Sleepiness, increased appetite, weight gain, dizziness, dry mouth, constipation, tiredness, increased thirst.	Continue. Call doctor when convenient.
Infrequent:	
• Slow heartbeat, migraine, dehydration, weight loss, unusual weakness, pain in any part of the body, changes in menstrual periods, changes in vision or hearing, mouth sores, mood or mental changes, breathing difficulty, lack of coordination.	Discontinue. Call doctor right away.
• Forgetfulness, lightheadedness.	Continue. Call doctor when convenient.
Rare:	
• Swelling of hands, feet or legs; infection (fever, chills, aches or pains, sore throat); swollen or discolored tongue; changes in urinary function; hives.	Discontinue. Call doctor right away.
• Muscle aches, strange dreams, headache.	Continue. Call doctor when convenient.

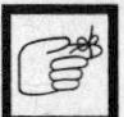

WARNINGS & PRECAUTIONS

Don't take if:
You are allergic to mirtazapine.

Before you start, consult your doctor if:
- You have seizure disorder, heart disease, blood circulation problem or had a stroke.
- You are dehydrated.
- You have a history of drug dependence or drug abuse.
- You have kidney or liver disease.
- You have a history of mood disorders, such as mania, or thoughts of suicide.
- You are allergic to any other medication, food or other substances.

Over age 60:
A lower starting dosage is usually recommended until a response is determined.

Pregnancy:
Decide with your doctor if drug benefits justify risk to unborn child. Risk category C (see page xviii).

Breast-feeding:
It is unknown if drug passes into milk. Avoid drug or discontinue nursing until you finish medicine. Consult doctor for advice on maintaining milk supply.

Infants & children:
Not approved for ages under 18. If prescribed, carefully read information provided with prescription. Contact doctor right away if depression symptoms get worse or there is any talk of suicide or suicide behaviors. Also, read information under Others.

Prolonged use:
Consult with your doctor on a regular basis while taking this drug to check your progress, to discuss any increase or changes in side effects and the need for continued treatment.

Skin & sunlight:
May cause a rash or intensify sunburn in areas exposed to sun or ultraviolet light (photosensitivity reaction). Avoid excessive sun exposure. Consult doctor if reaction occurs.

Driving, piloting or hazardous work:
Don't drive or pilot aircraft until you learn how medicine affects you. Don't climb ladders or work in high places. Danger increases if you drink alcohol or take medicine affecting alertness and reflexes.

Discontinuing:
Consult doctor before discontinuing this drug.

Others:
- Get up slowly from a sitting or lying position to avoid dizziness, faintness or lightheadedness.
- Advise any doctor or dentist whom you consult that you take this medicine.
- Adults and children taking antidepressants may experience a worsening of the depression symptoms and may have increased suicidal thoughts or behaviors. Call doctor right away if these symptoms or behaviors occur.
- Do not increase or reduce dosage without doctor's approval.

POSSIBLE INTERACTION WITH OTHER DRUGS

GENERIC NAME OR DRUG CLASS	COMBINED EFFECT
Benzodiazepines	Increased sedative effect. Avoid.
Monoamine oxidase, (MAO) inhibitors	Potentially life-threatening. Allow 14 days between use of 2 drugs.
Other medications	Complete studies have not been done to evaluate interactions with other drugs, but the potential exists for a variety of possible interactions. Consult doctor or pharmacist.

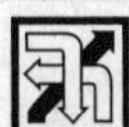

POSSIBLE INTERACTION WITH OTHER SUBSTANCES

INTERACTS WITH	COMBINED EFFECT
Alcohol:	Increased sedative affect. Avoid.
Beverages:	None expected.
Cocaine:	Unknown effect. Best to avoid.
Foods:	None expected.
Marijuana:	Unknown effect. Best to avoid.
Tobacco:	None expected.

MISOPROSTOL

BRAND NAMES

Arthrotec
Cytotec

BASIC INFORMATION

Habit forming? No
Prescription needed? Yes
Available as generic? Yes
Drug class: Antiulcer agent

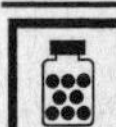

USES

Prevents development of stomach ulcers in persons taking nonsteroidal anti-inflammatory drugs (NSAIDs), including aspirin.

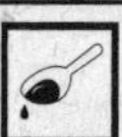

DOSAGE & USAGE INFORMATION

How to take:
Tablet—Swallow with liquid. Swallow Arthrotec brand whole. If you can't swallow Cytotec brand whole, crumble tablet and take with liquid or food. Instructions to take on empty stomach mean 1 hour before or 2 hours after eating.

When to take:
Usually 4 times a day while awake, with or after meals and at bedtime.

If you forget a dose:
Take as soon as you remember. If it is almost time for the next dose, wait for that dose (don't double this dose) and resume regular schedule.

What drug does:
- Improves defense against peptic ulcers by strengthening natural defenses of the stomach lining.
- Decreases stomach acid production.

Time lapse before drug works:
10 to 15 minutes.

Don't take with:
Any other medicines (including over-the-counter drugs such as cough and cold medicines, laxatives, antacids, diet pills, caffeine, nose drops or vitamins) without consulting your doctor or pharmacist.

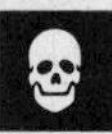

OVERDOSE

SYMPTOMS:
None expected.
WHAT TO DO:
Overdose unlikely to threaten life. If person uses much larger amount than prescribed or if accidentally swallowed, call doctor or poison control center 1-800-222-1222 for help.

POSSIBLE ADVERSE REACTIONS OR SIDE EFFECTS

SYMPTOMS	WHAT TO DO
Life-threatening: None expected.	
Common: Abdominal pain, diarrhea.	Discontinue. Call doctor right away.
Infrequent:	
• Nausea or vomiting.	Continue. Call doctor when convenient.
• Constipation, headache.	Continue. Tell doctor at next visit.
Rare:	
• Gaseousness.	Continue. Tell doctor at next visit.
• Vaginal bleeding.	Discontinue. Call doctor right away.

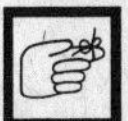

WARNINGS & PRECAUTIONS

Don't take if:
- You are allergic to any prostaglandin.*
- You are pregnant or of child-bearing age.

Before you start, consult your doctor if:
- You have epilepsy.
- You have heart disease.
- You have blood vessel disease of any kind.

Over age 60:
No special problems expected.

Pregnancy:
- Risk to unborn child outweighs drug benefits. Don't use.
- May also lead to serious complications in pregnant women, including excessive bleeding and future infertility.
- Risk category X (see page xviii).

Breast-feeding:
Drug passes into milk. Avoid drug or discontinue nursing until you finish medicine. Consult doctor for advice on maintaining milk supply.

Infants & children:
Not recommended for children under 18.

Prolonged use:
Talk to your doctor about the need for follow-up medical examinations or laboratory studies to check gastric analysis.

Skin & sunlight:
No problems expected.

Driving, piloting or hazardous work:
Avoid if you feel confused, drowsy or dizzy.

Discontinuing:
No special problems expected.

Others:
Advise any doctor or dentist whom you consult that you take this medicine.

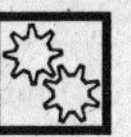

POSSIBLE INTERACTION WITH OTHER DRUGS

GENERIC NAME OR DRUG CLASS	COMBINED EFFECT
Antacids,* magnesium-containing	Severe diarrhea.

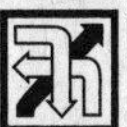

POSSIBLE INTERACTION WITH OTHER SUBSTANCES

INTERACTS WITH	COMBINED EFFECT
Alcohol:	Decreases misoprostol effect. Avoid.
Beverages: Caffeine-containing.	Decreases misoprostol effect. Avoid.
Cocaine:	Decreases misoprostol effect. Avoid.
Foods:	None expected.
Marijuana:	Decreases misoprostol effect. Avoid.
Tobacco:	Decreases misoprostol effect. Avoid.

MONOAMINE OXIDASE (MAO) INHIBITORS

GENERIC AND BRAND NAMES

ISOCARBOXAZID
Marplan
PHENELZINE
Nardil
TRANYLCYPROMINE
Parnate

BASIC INFORMATION

Habit forming? No
Prescription needed? Yes
Available as generic? No
Drug class: MAO (monoamine oxidase) inhibitor, antidepressant

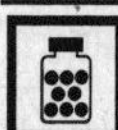

USES

- Treatment for depression and panic disorder.
- Prevention of vascular or tension headaches.

DOSAGE & USAGE INFORMATION

How to take:
Tablet—Swallow with liquid. If you can't swallow whole, crumble tablet and take with liquid or food.

When to take:
At the same times each day.

If you forget a dose:
Take as soon as you remember. If it is almost time for the next dose, wait for that dose (don't double this dose) and resume regular schedule.

What drug does:
Inhibits nerve transmissions in brain that may cause depression.

Time lapse before drug works:
4 to 6 weeks for maximum effect.

Don't take with:
- Foods containing tyramine.* Life-threatening elevation of blood pressure may result.
- Any other medicine or any dietary supplement without consulting your doctor or pharmacist.

OVERDOSE

SYMPTOMS:
Restlessness, agitation, excitement, fever, confusion, dizziness, heartbeat irregularities, hallucinations, sweating, breathing difficulties, insomnia, irritability, convulsions, coma.
WHAT TO DO:
- **Dial 911 (emergency) for medical help or call poison control center 1-800-222-1222 for instructions.**
- **See emergency information on last 3 pages of this book.**

POSSIBLE ADVERSE REACTIONS OR SIDE EFFECTS

SYMPTOMS	WHAT TO DO
Life-threatening: In case of overdose, see previous column. Also read information about dangers associated with tyramine.	
Common:	
• Fatigue, weakness.	Continue. Call doctor when convenient.
• Dizziness when changing position, restlessness, tremors, dry mouth, constipation, difficult urination, blurred vision, "sweet tooth."	Continue. Tell doctor at next visit.
Infrequent:	
• Fainting, enlarged pupils, severe headache, chest pain, rapid or pounding heartbeat.	Discontinue. Seek emergency treatment.
• Hallucinations, insomnia, nightmares, diarrhea, swollen feet or legs, joint pain.	Continue. Call doctor when convenient.
• Diminished sex drive.	Continue. Tell doctor at next visit.
Rare:	
Rash, nausea, vomiting, stiff neck, jaundice, fever, increased sweating, dark urine, slurred speech, staggering gait.	Discontinue. Call doctor right away.

WARNINGS & PRECAUTIONS

Don't take if:
- You are allergic to any MAO inhibitor.
- You have heart disease, congestive heart failure, heart rhythm irregularities or high blood pressure.
- You have liver or kidney disease.

Before you start, consult your doctor if:
- You are an alcoholic.
- You have had a stroke.
- You have diabetes, epilepsy, asthma, overactive thyroid, schizophrenia, Parkinson's disease, adrenal gland tumor.
- You will have surgery within 2 months, including dental surgery, requiring anesthesia.

Over age 60:
Adverse effects more likely.

Pregnancy:
Decide with your doctor if drug benefits justify risk to unborn child. Risk category C (see page xviii).

Breast-feeding:
Safety not established. Consult doctor.

Infants & children:
Not approved for ages under 16. If prescribed, carefully read information provided with prescription. Contact doctor right away if depression symptoms get worse or there is any talk of suicide or suicide behaviors. Also, read information under Others.

Prolonged use:
- May be toxic to liver.
- Talk to your doctor about the need for follow-up medical examinations or laboratory studies to check blood pressure, liver function.

Skin & sunlight:
No special problems expected.

Driving, piloting or hazardous work:
Don't drive or pilot aircraft until you learn how medicine affects you. Don't work around dangerous machinery. Don't climb ladders or work in high places. Danger increases if you drink alcohol or take medicine affecting alertness and reflexes.

Discontinuing:
- Don't discontinue without doctor's advice until you complete prescribed dose, even though symptoms diminish or disappear.
- Follow precautions regarding foods, drinks and other medicines for 2 weeks after discontinuing.
- Adverse symptoms caused by this medicine may occur even after discontinuation. If you develop any of the symptoms listed under Overdose, notify your doctor immediately.

Others:
- May affect blood sugar levels in patients with diabetes.
- Advise any doctor or dentist whom you consult about the use of this medicine.
- Adults and children taking antidepressants may experience a worsening of the depression symptoms and may have increased suicidal thoughts or behaviors. Call doctor right away if these symptoms or behaviors occur.
- Fever may indicate that MAO inhibitor dose requires adjustment.

POSSIBLE INTERACTION WITH OTHER DRUGS

GENERIC NAME OR DRUG CLASS	COMBINED EFFECT
Amphetamines*	Blood pressure rise to life-threatening level.
Anticholinergics*	Increased anticholinergic effect.
Anticonvulsants*	Changed seizure pattern.
Antidepressants, tricyclic*	Blood pressure rise to life-threatening level. Possible fever, convulsions, delirium.
Antidiabetic agents, oral* and insulin	Excessively low blood sugar.
Antihypertensives*	Excessively low blood pressure.
Beta-adrenergic blocking agents*	Possible blood pressure rise if MAO inhibitor is discontinued after simultaneous use with acebutolol.
Bupropion	Increased risk of side effects.
Buspirone	Very high blood pressure.
Caffeine	Irregular heartbeat or high blood pressure.
Carbamazepine	Fever, seizures. Avoid.

Continued on page 920

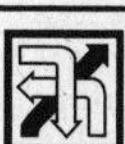

POSSIBLE INTERACTION WITH OTHER SUBSTANCES

INTERACTS WITH	COMBINED EFFECT
Alcohol:	Increased sedation to dangerous level.
Beverages:	
Caffeine drinks.	Irregular heartbeat or high blood pressure.
Drinks containing tyramine.*	Blood pressure rise to life-threatening level.
Cocaine:	Overstimulation. Possibly fatal.
Foods:	
Foods containing tyramine.*	Blood pressure rise to life-threatening level.
Marijuana:	Overstimulation. Avoid.
Tobacco:	None expected.

***See Glossary**

MONOAMINE OXIDASE TYPE B (MAO-B) INHIBITORS

GENERIC AND BRAND NAMES

RASAGILINE
Azilect
SELEGILINE
Apo-Selegiline
Atapryl
Carbex
Eldepryl
Emsam
SELEGILINE (con't)
Gen-Selegiline
Movergan
Novo-Selegiline
Nu-Selegiline
Selpak
Zelepar

BASIC INFORMATION

Habit forming? No
Prescription needed? Yes
Available as generic? Yes, for some
Drug class: Antiparkinsonism; antidyskinetic

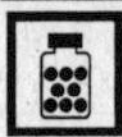

USES

- Treats symptoms of Parkinson's disease.
- Treats major depressive disorder (MDD).
- Treats other disorders per doctor's advice.

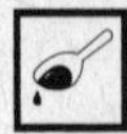

DOSAGE & USAGE INFORMATION

How to take:
- Tablet or capsule—Swallow whole with liquid.
- Oral disintegrating tablet—Let it dissolve on tongue. Do not swallow tablet whole.
- Skin patch—Follow prescription instructions.

When to take:
Take as directed. The oral form is usually taken at breakfast and lunch to help avoid interfering with sleep. Change patch daily at same time.

If you forget a dose:
Take as soon as you remember. If it is almost time for the next dose, wait for that dose (don't double this dose) and resume regular schedule.

Continued next column

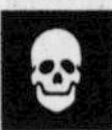

OVERDOSE

SYMPTOMS:
Unknown; may cause sweating, dizziness, insomnia, severe headache, hallucinations, excitement, nervousness, irritability, weakness, seizures, high or low blood pressure, muscle spasm, coma.
WHAT TO DO:
- **Dial 911 (emergency) for medical help or call poison control center 1-800-222-1222 for instructions.**
- **See emergency information on last 3 pages of this book.**

What drug does:
It helps prevent breakdown of dopamine levels in the brain. Dopamine is a brain chemical having to do with control of movement and coordination.

Time lapse before drug works:
Starts working in 1-2 hours, but may take 4-6 weeks to determine drug's full effectiveness.

Don't take with:
- Foods containing tyramine.* Rarely may cause severe high blood pressure (hypertension).
- Any other medicine or diet supplement without consulting your doctor or pharmacist.

POSSIBLE ADVERSE REACTIONS OR SIDE EFFECTS

SYMPTOMS	WHAT TO DO
Life-threatening:	
Rare hypertensive crisis (chest pain, large pupils, heartbeat fast or slow, severe headache, light sensitivity, fever, cold skin, stiff or sore neck, severe nausea/vomiting). Rare allergic reaction (trouble breathing; closing of throat; hives; swelling of lips, tongue or face).	Discontinue. Seek emergency care.
Common:	
• Mood or mental changes, increase in uncontrolled body movements.	Discontinue. Call doctor right away.
• Stomach pain, dry mouth, dizziness, insomnia, feeling faint, mild nausea or vomiting, patch causes mild skin reaction.	Continue. Call doctor when convenient.
Infrequent:	
Bloody or tarry stools, urination difficult or frequent, trouble with breathing or speaking, dizziness or lightheaded when getting up from sitting or lying down, lip smacking, hallucinations, lack of balance, unusual tongue or chewing movements, stomach pain, restlessness, swollen feet or legs, new or odd movements of arms or legs or other body parts, vomiting blood or coffee-ground-like material, wheezing.	Discontinue. Call doctor right away.

MONOAMINE OXIDASE TYPE B (MAO-B) INHIBITORS

Rare:

Constipation, anxiety, tiredness, eyelid spasm, changes in taste, blurred or double vision, leg pain, ringing in ears, diarrhea, burning of lips or mouth or throat, drowsiness, sensitivity to light, sweating, loss of appetite, memory problems, muscle cramps, nervousness, numbness in fingers or toes, red or raised or itchy skin, taste changes, unusual weight loss, heartburn, jaw clenching or teeth gnashing, excess feeling of well-being.	Continue. Call doctor when convenient.

WARNINGS & PRECAUTIONS

Don't take if:
You are allergic to selegiline or rasagiline.

Before you start, consult your doctor if:
- You have a history of ulcers.
- You have tardive dyskinesia or a tremor.
- Patient has profound dementia or severe psychosis.

Over age 60:
No problems expected.

Pregnancy:
Decide with your doctor if drug benefits justify risk to unborn child. Risk category C (see page xviii).

Breast-feeding:
It is unknown if drug passes into milk. Consult doctor for advice.

Infants & children:
Not recommended.

Prolonged use:
Follow up with your doctor on a regular basis to verify the continued effectiveness of the drug.

Skin & sunlight:
May cause rash or intensify sunburn in areas exposed to sun or ultraviolet light (photosensitivity reaction). Avoid overexposure. Notify doctor if reaction occurs.

Driving, piloting or hazardous work:
Don't drive or pilot aircraft until you learn how medicine affects you. Don't work around dangerous machinery. Don't climb ladders or work in high places. Danger increases if you drink alcohol or take medicine affecting alertness and reflexes.

Discontinuing:
Don't discontinue without your doctor's approval as symptoms may worsen. A gradual reduction in dosage may be required.

Others:
- Avoid sudden rises from lying-down or sitting positions.
- Advise any doctor or dentist whom you consult that you take this medicine.

POSSIBLE INTERACTION WITH OTHER DRUGS

GENERIC NAME OR DRUG CLASS	COMBINED EFFECT
Antidepressants, tricyclic	Serious reactions. Avoid or take at least 14 days apart.
Enzyme inducers*	May decrease effect of rasagiline.
Enzyme inhibitors*	May increase effect of rasagiline.
Levodopa	Increased risk of adverse reactions.
Meperidine	Life-threatening. reactions. Avoid.
Narcotics*	Serious reactions. Avoid.
Serotonergic agents,* other	May cause a serotonin syndrome* type reaction. Avoid.

POSSIBLE INTERACTION WITH OTHER SUBSTANCES

INTERACTS WITH	COMBINED EFFECT
Alcohol:	Increased sedation. Avoid.
Beverages:	
Caffeine	Increased effect of caffeine. Limit use.
Cocaine:	High blood pressure, rapid heartbeat. Avoid.
Foods:	
Tyramine-containing*	Severe hypertension. Avoid.
Marijuana:	Excess drowsiness. Avoid.
Tobacco:	None expected.

***See Glossary**

MUSCARINIC RECEPTOR ANTAGONISTS

GENERIC AND BRAND NAMES

DARIFENACIN
- Enablex

FESOTERODINE
- Toviaz

OXYBUTYNIN
- Anturol
- Ditropan
- Ditropan XL
- Gelnique
- Oxytrol
- Oxytrol for Women

SOLIFENACIN
- Vesicare

TOLTERODINE
- Detrol
- Detrol LA

TROSPIUM
- Sanctura
- Sanctura XR

BASIC INFORMATION

Habit forming? No
Prescription needed? Yes, for most
Available as generic? Yes, for some
Drug class: Antispasmodic; anticholinergic

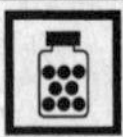

USES

Used to treat an overactive bladder in men and women.

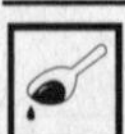

DOSAGE & USAGE INFORMATION

How to take:
- Tablet—Swallow whole with liquid. May be taken with or without food. Take trospium 1 hour before eating or on an empty stomach.
- Extended-release capsule or tablet—Swallow whole with liquid. Take with or without food.
- Syrup, skin patch, or gel (oxybutynin)—Follow instructions on prescription.

When to take:
Take one or more times (as directed) a day at the same time each day. The patch should be applied twice a week. The gel is applied daily.

Continued next column

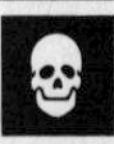

OVERDOSE

SYMPTOMS:
Unsteadiness, confusion, dizziness, severe drowsiness, fast heartbeat, fever, red face, hallucinations, difficult breathing, enlarged pupils, unusual nervousness or excitement.
WHAT TO DO:
- **Dial 911 (emergency) for medical help or call poison control center 1-800-222-1222 for instructions.**
- **See emergency information on last 3 pages of this book.**

If you forget a dose:
Take as soon as you remember. If it is almost time for the next dose, wait for that dose (don't double this dose) and resume regular schedule.

What drug does:
The drugs increase the amount of urine the bladder can hold and also decrease the pressure involved with the urge to urinate.

Time lapse before drug works:
Symptoms should start to improve in about a week. It may take 4 to 6 weeks for full benefits.

Don't take with:
Any other medicine or any dietary supplement without consulting your doctor or pharmacist.

POSSIBLE ADVERSE REACTIONS OR SIDE EFFECTS

SYMPTOMS	WHAT TO DO
Life-threatening:	
Rare allergic reaction—Breathing difficulty; closing of the throat; swelling of hands, feet, face, lips or tongue; hives.	Discontinue. Seek emergency treatment.
Common:	
Constipation, dry mouth, dry eyes or throat, blurred vision, sweating decreased, urinary retention, drowsiness, skin patch causes itching at application site.	Continue. Call doctor if symptoms persist.
Infrequent:	
Flu-like symptoms, decreased sexual ability, difficulty in urinating, headache, sensitivity to light, nausea, vomiting, abdominal pain, insomnia, dizziness, fatigue, depression, diarrhea, gas.	Continue. Call doctor when convenient.
Rare:	
• Eye pain, fast heart rate, urinary tract infection, swelling of arms or legs, changes in mental status, confusion, fainting, skin changes (blistering, peeling or loosening), dark color urine, chest pain, high blood pressure.	Discontinue. Call doctor right away.
• Back or muscle pain, dry skin, skin rash.	Continue. Call doctor when convenient.

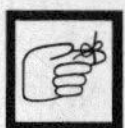

WARNINGS & PRECAUTIONS

Don't take if:
You are allergic to muscarinic receptor antagonists or anticholinergic drugs.

Before you start, consult your doctor if:
- You have heart disease, bleeding disorder or high blood pressure.
- You have hiatal hernia; liver, kidney or thyroid disease; enlarged prostate or myasthenia gravis.
- You have any gastrointestinal disorder or intestinal or urinary tract blockage.
- You have a bladder emptying problem.
- You have glaucoma.
- You have severe ulcerative colitis.
- Patient has Alzheimer's or dementia.

Over age 60:
Adverse reactions and side effects may be more frequent and severe than in younger persons.

Pregnancy:
Decide with your doctor if drug benefits justify any possible risk to unborn child. Risk category for oxybutynin is B, others are C (see page xviii).

Breast-feeding:
It is unknown if these drugs pass into milk. Avoid drug or discontinue nursing until you finish medicine. Consult doctor for advice on maintaining milk supply.

Infants & children:
Oxybutynin is approved for use in children over age 5. Safety and effectiveness of other drugs in this group for use in children under age 18 has not been established.

Prolonged use:
No special problems expected.

Skin & sunlight:
No special problems expected.

Driving, piloting or hazardous work:
Don't drive or pilot aircraft until you learn how drug affects you. Don't work around dangerous machinery. Don't climb ladders or work in high places. Danger increases if you drink alcohol or take drugs affecting alertness and reflexes.

Discontinuing:
No special problems expected. Follow doctor's instructions.

Others:
- Advise any doctor or dentist whom you consult that you take this drug.
- Be careful in hot weather, hot tubs or saunas. The drug can increase your risk of heat stroke (due to decreased sweating).
- Chew sugarless gum or suck on ice chips to relieve a dry mouth. Call your doctor or dentist if the dry mouth lasts longer than 2 weeks.

POSSIBLE INTERACTION WITH OTHER DRUGS

GENERIC NAME OR DRUG CLASS	COMBINED EFFECT
Anticholinergics,* other	Increased risk of side effects from either drug.
Antidepressants, tricyclic*	Increased effect of antidepressant.
Cationic drugs*	May increase effect of trospium.
Central nervous system (CNS) depressants*	Increased sedative effect.
Enzyme inducers*	Decreased effect of darifenacin or solifenacin.
Enzyme inhibitors*	Increased effect of darifenacin, solifenacin or tolterodine.
Flecainide	Increased effect of flecainide. Use caution.
Ketoconazole	Increased effect of solifenacin.
QT prolongation-causing drugs*	Increased risk of heart problems.
Thioridazine	Increased effect of thioridazine.

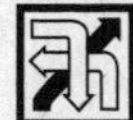

POSSIBLE INTERACTION WITH OTHER SUBSTANCES

INTERACTS WITH	COMBINED EFFECT
Alcohol:	Increased sedative effect. Avoid.
Beverages: Grapefruit juice.	May increase effect. of darifenacin, solifenacin or tolterodine.
Cocaine:	Unknown effect. Avoid.
Foods:	None expected.
Marijuana:	Drowsiness and dry mouth. Avoid.
Tobacco:	None expected.

***See Glossary**

MUSCLE RELAXANTS, SKELETAL

GENERIC AND BRAND NAMES

CARISOPRODOL
- Rela
- Sodol
- Soma
- Soma Compound with Codeine
- Sopridol
- Soridol

CHLORPHENESIN
- Maolate

CHLORZOXAZONE
- Paraflex
- Parafon Forte

METAXALONE
- Skelaxin

METHOCARBAMOL
- Carbacot
- Delaxin
- Marbaxin
- Robamol
- Robaxin
- Robaxisal
- Robomol
- Skelex

BASIC INFORMATION

Habit forming? Possibly
Prescription needed? Yes
Available as generic? Yes, for some.
Drug class: Muscle relaxant

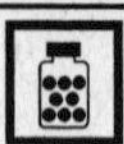

USES

Adjunctive treatment to rest, analgesics and physical therapy for muscle spasms.

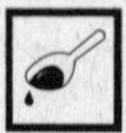

DOSAGE & USAGE INFORMATION

How to take:
- Tablet—Swallow with liquid. If you can't swallow whole, crumble tablet and take with liquid or food. Instructions to take on empty stomach mean 1 hour before or 2 hours after eating.
- Extended-release tablet—Swallow whole with liquid. Don't crumble tablet.

When to take:
As needed, no more often than every 4 hours.

Continued next column

OVERDOSE

SYMPTOMS:
Nausea, vomiting, diarrhea, convulsions, headache. May progress to severe weakness, difficult breathing, sensation of paralysis, coma.

WHAT TO DO:
- **Dial 911 (emergency) for medical help or call poison control center 1-800-222-1222 for instructions.**
- **See emergency information on last 3 pages of this book.**

If you forget a dose:
Take as soon as you remember. If it is almost time for the next dose, wait for that dose (don't double this dose) and resume regular schedule.

What drug does:
Blocks body's pain messages to brain. Also causes sedation.

Time lapse before drug works:
30 to 60 minutes.

Don't take with:
Any other medicine or any dietary supplement without consulting your doctor or pharmacist.

POSSIBLE ADVERSE REACTIONS OR SIDE EFFECTS

SYMPTOMS	WHAT TO DO
Life-threatening:	
Hives, rash, intense itching, faintness soon after a dose (anaphylaxis); extreme weakness, transient paralysis, temporary vision loss.	Seek emergency treatment immediately.
Common:	
• Drowsiness, dizziness.	Continue. Call doctor when convenient.
• Orange or red-purple urine.	No action necessary.
Infrequent:	
• Agitation, constipation or diarrhea, nausea, cramps, vomiting, wheezing, shortness of breath, headache, depression, muscle weakness, trembling, insomnia, uncontrolled eye movements, fainting.	Discontinue. Call doctor right away.
• Blurred vision.	Continue. Call Doctor when convenient.
Rare:	
• Black, tarry or bloody stool; convulsions.	Discontinue. Seek emergency treatment.
• Rash, hives, itching, fever, yellow skin or eyes, sore throat, tiredness, hiccups.	Discontinue. Call doctor right away.

WARNINGS & PRECAUTIONS

Don't take if:

- You are allergic to any skeletal muscle relaxant.
- You have porphyria.

Before you start, consult your doctor if:

- You have had liver or kidney disease.
- You plan pregnancy within medication period.
- You are allergic to tartrazine dye.
- You suffer from depression.

Over age 60:
Adverse reactions and side effects may be more frequent and severe than in younger persons.

Pregnancy:
Safety not proven. Avoid if possible. Consult doctor. Risk category C (see page xviii).

Breast-feeding:
Drug may pass into milk. Avoid drug or discontinue nursing until you finish medicine. Consult doctor for advice on maintaining milk supply.

Infants & children:
Not recommended.

Prolonged use:
Talk to your doctor about the need for follow-up medical examinations or laboratory studies to check liver function, kidney function, complete blood counts (white blood cell count, platelet count, red blood cell count, hemoglobin, hematocrit).

Skin & sunlight:
No problems expected.

Driving, piloting or hazardous work:
Don't drive or pilot aircraft until you learn how medicine affects you. Don't work around dangerous machinery. Don't climb ladders or work in high places. Danger increases if you drink alcohol or take medicine affecting alertness and reflexes, such as antihistamines, tranquilizers, sedatives, pain medicine, narcotics and mind-altering drugs.

Discontinuing:
Don't discontinue without doctor's advice until you complete prescribed dose, even though symptoms diminish or disappear.

Others:

- May affect results in some medical tests.
- Advise any doctor or dentist whom you consult that you take this medicine.

POSSIBLE INTERACTION WITH OTHER DRUGS

GENERIC NAME OR DRUG CLASS	COMBINED EFFECT
Antidepressants*	Increased sedation.
Antihistamines*	Increased sedation.
Central nervous system (CNS) depressants*	Increased depressive effects of both drugs.
Clozapine	Toxic effect on the central nervous system.
Dronabinol	Increased effect of dronabinol on central nervous system. Avoid combination.
Mind-altering drugs*	Increased sedation.
Muscle relaxants,* others	Increased sedation.
Narcotics*	Increased sedation.
Sedatives*	Increased sedation.
Sertraline	Increased depressive effects of both drugs.
Sleep inducers*	Increased sedation.
Tranquilizers*	Increased sedation.

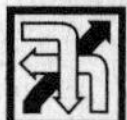

POSSIBLE INTERACTION WITH OTHER SUBSTANCES

INTERACTS WITH	COMBINED EFFECT
Alcohol:	Increased sedation.
Beverages:	None expected.
Cocaine:	Lack of coordination, increased sedation.
Foods:	None expected.
Marijuana:	Lack of coordination, drowsiness, fainting.
Tobacco:	None expected.

NABILONE

BRAND NAMES

Cesamet

BASIC INFORMATION

Habit forming? No
Prescription needed? Yes
Available as generic? No
Drug class: Antiemetic

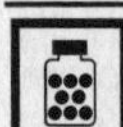

USES

- Treats nausea and vomiting.
- Prevents nausea and vomiting in patients receiving cancer chemotherapy.

DOSAGE & USAGE INFORMATION

How to take:
Capsule—Swallow with liquid. If you can't swallow whole, open capsule and take with liquid or food.

When to take:
At the same times each day, according to instructions on prescription label.

If you forget a dose:
Take as soon as you remember. If it is almost time for the next dose, wait for that dose (don't double this dose) and resume regular schedule.

What drug does:
Chemically related to marijuana, it probably regulates the vomiting control center in the brain.

Time lapse before drug works:
2 hours.

Continued next column

OVERDOSE

SYMPTOMS:
Mood changes; confusion and delusions; hallucinations; mental depression; nervousness; breathing difficulty; fast, slow or pounding heartbeat; fainting.
WHAT TO DO:
- **Dial 911 (emergency) for medical help or call poison control center 1-800-222-1222 for instructions.**
- **If person is unconscious, check breathing and pulse. If not breathing, begin mouth-to-mouth rescue breathing. If heart is not beating, begin chest compressions.**
- **See emergency information on last 3 pages of this book.**

Don't take with:
- Alcohol or any drug that depresses the central nervous system. See Central Nervous System (CNS) Depressants in the Glossary.
- Any other medicine or any dietary supplement without consulting your doctor or pharmacist.

POSSIBLE ADVERSE REACTIONS OR SIDE EFFECTS

SYMPTOMS	WHAT TO DO
Life-threatening:	
Mood changes; fainting; hallucinations; fast, slow or pounding heartbeat; confusion and delusions; mental depression; nervousness; breathing difficulty.	Seek emergency treatment.
Common:	
Dry mouth.	Continue. Call doctor when convenient.
Infrequent:	
Clumsiness, mental changes, drowsiness, headache, false sense of well-being.	Discontinue. Call doctor right away.
Rare:	
Blurred vision, dizziness on standing, appetite loss, muscle pain.	Discontinue. Call doctor right away.

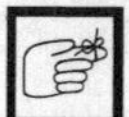

WARNINGS & PRECAUTIONS

Don't take if:
- You are allergic to nabilone or marijuana.
- You have schizophrenic, manic or depressive states.

Before you start, consult your doctor if:
- You have abused drugs or are dependent on them, including alcohol.
- You have had high blood pressure or heart disease.
- You have had impaired liver function.

Over age 60:
Adverse reactions and side effects may be more frequent and severe than in younger persons. You may need smaller doses for shorter periods of time.

Pregnancy:
Decide with your doctor whether drug benefits justify risk to unborn child. Risk category C (see page xviii).

Breast-feeding:
Drug passes into milk. Avoid drug or discontinue nursing until you finish medicine. Consult doctor for advice on maintaining milk supply.

Infants & children:
Not recommended for children 18 and younger. Use only under doctor's supervision.

Prolonged use:
- Avoid prolonged use. This medicine is intended to be used only during a cycle of cancer chemotherapy.
- Talk to your doctor about the need for follow-up medical examinations or laboratory studies to check blood pressure, heart function.

Skin & sunlight:
No problems expected.

Driving, piloting or hazardous work:
Don't drive or pilot aircraft until you learn how medicine affects you. Don't work around dangerous machinery. Don't climb ladders or work in high places. Danger increases if you drink alcohol or take medicine affecting alertness and reflexes.

Discontinuing:
No problems expected.

Others:
- Blood pressure should be measured regularly.
- Learn to count and recognize changes in your pulse.
- Get up from bed or chair slowly to avoid fainting.

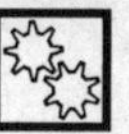

POSSIBLE INTERACTION WITH OTHER DRUGS

GENERIC NAME OR DRUG CLASS	COMBINED EFFECT
Apomorphine	Decreased effect of apomorphine.
Central nervous system (CNS) depressants,* other	Greater depression of the central nervous system.

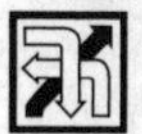

POSSIBLE INTERACTION WITH OTHER SUBSTANCES

INTERACTS WITH	COMBINED EFFECT
Alcohol:	Dangerous depression of the central nervous system. Avoid.
Beverages:	None expected.
Cocaine:	Decreased nabilone effect. Avoid.
Foods:	None expected.
Marijuana:	None expected.
Tobacco:	None expected.

***See Glossary**

NAFARELIN

BRAND NAMES

Synarel

BASIC INFORMATION

Habit forming? No
Prescription needed? Yes
Available as generic? No
Drug class: Gonadotropin inhibitor

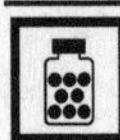

USES

- Treatment for endometriosis to relieve pain and reduce scattered implants of endometrial tissue.
- Treatment for central precocious puberty.

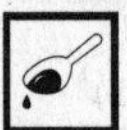

DOSAGE & USAGE INFORMATION

How to take:
Nasal spray—Follow instructions on package insert provided with your medicine.

When to take:
As directed by your doctor. Usually two times a day.

If you forget a dose:
Take as soon as you remember. Don't double this dose.

What drug does:
Reduces estrogen production by ovaries.

Time lapse before drug works:
May require 6 months for full effect.

Don't take with:
- Birth control pills.
- Nasal sprays to decongest the membranes in the nose.
- Any other medicine or any dietary supplement without consulting your doctor or pharmacist.

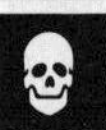

OVERDOSE

SYMPTOMS:
None expected.
WHAT TO DO:
Overdose unlikely to threaten life. If person uses much larger amount than prescribed or if accidentally swallowed, call doctor or poison control center 1-800-222-1222 for help.

POSSIBLE ADVERSE REACTIONS OR SIDE EFFECTS

SYMPTOMS	WHAT TO DO
Life-threatening: None expected.	
Common: Hot flashes.	No action necessary.
Infrequent: Decreased sexual desire, vaginal dryness, headache, acne, swelling of hands and feet, reduction of breast size, weight gain, itchy scalp with flaking, muscle ache, nasal irritation.	Continue. Call doctor when convenient.
Rare: Insomnia, depression, weight loss.	Continue. Call doctor when convenient.

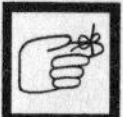

WARNINGS & PRECAUTIONS

Don't take if:
- You become pregnant.
- You have breast cancer.
- You are allergic to any of the ingredients in nafarelin.
- You have undiagnosed abnormal vaginal bleeding.

Before you start, consult your doctor if:
- You take birth control pills.
- You have diabetes.
- You have heart disease.
- You have epilepsy.
- You have kidney disease.
- You have liver disease.
- You have migraine headaches.
- You need to use topical nasal decongestants.

Over age 60:
Not used in this age group.

Pregnancy:
Risk to unborn child outweighs drug benefits. Don't use. Stop if you get pregnant. Consult doctor. Risk category X (see page xviii).

Breast-feeding:
Unknown whether medicine filters into milk. Consult doctor.

Infants & children:
Use only with medical supervision.

Prolonged use:
- Full effect requires prolonged use. Don't discontinue without consulting doctor.
- Talk to your doctor about the need for mammogram, follow-up medical examinations or laboratory studies to check liver function.

Skin & sunlight:
No special problems expected.

Driving, piloting or hazardous work:
No special problems expected.

Discontinuing:
Don't discontinue without consulting doctor. Menstrual periods may be absent for 2 to 3 months after discontinuation.

Others:
- May alter blood sugar levels in diabetic persons.
- Interferes with accuracy of laboratory tests to study pituitary gonadotropic and gonadal functions.
- Bone density decreases during treatment phase, but recovers following treatment.

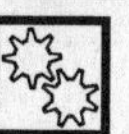

POSSIBLE INTERACTION WITH OTHER DRUGS

GENERIC NAME OR DRUG CLASS	COMBINED EFFECT
Decongestant nasal sprays*	Decreased absorption of nafarelin.

POSSIBLE INTERACTION WITH OTHER SUBSTANCES

INTERACTS WITH	COMBINED EFFECT
Alcohol:	Excessive nervous system depression. Avoid.
Beverages: Caffeine drinks.	Rapid, irregular heartbeat. Avoid.
Cocaine:	May interfere with expected action of nafarelin. Avoid.
Foods:	None expected.
Marijuana:	May interfere with expected action of nafarelin. Avoid.
Tobacco:	Rapid, irregular heartbeat; increased leg cramps. Avoid.

***See Glossary**

NALTREXONE

BRAND NAMES

Barr
Embeda
ReVia
Vivitrol

BASIC INFORMATION

Habit forming? No
Prescription needed? Yes
Available as generic? Yes
Drug class: Narcotic antagonist

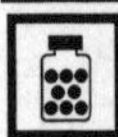

USES

- Treats detoxified former opioid (narcotics) addicts (along with a counseling program). It helps you maintain a drug-free life.
- May be used to treat alcoholism (along with a counseling program).
- The brand name Embeda treats moderate to severe chronic pain (when treatment is needed for an extended period of time).

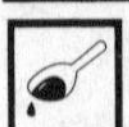

DOSAGE & USAGE INFORMATION

How to take:
- For former addicts—*Don't take drug until detoxification has been accomplished.*
- Tablet—Swallow with liquid or food to lessen stomach irritation. If you can't swallow whole, crumble tablet and take with liquid or food.
- Extended-release injectable—Given by a health care provider.
- Extended-release capsule (Embeda)—Swallow whole or open capsule and sprinkle contents on applesauce. Do not crush, chew or dissolve contents (pellets) as this can lead to potentially fatal dose.

When to take:
- Dosing can be flexible with oral form. You and your doctor will determine a routine.
- Extended-release injectable is given monthly.

Continued next column

OVERDOSE

SYMPTOMS:
Seizures, nausea, stomach pain, dizziness, coma.
WHAT TO DO:
- **Dial 911 (emergency) for medical help or call poison control center 1-800-222-1222 for instructions.**
- **See emergency information on last 3 pages of this book.**

If you forget a dose:
Follow detailed instructions provided with the prescription.

What drug does:
- It works in the brain to block the pleasurable effects or high feeling you get when you use narcotics and decreases craving for alcohol.
- It is unknown how it works for pain relief.

Time lapse before drug works:
1 hour.

Don't take with:
Narcotics, any other medicine, any dietary supplement, especially those that contain alcohol without consulting your doctor or pharmacist.

POSSIBLE ADVERSE REACTIONS OR SIDE EFFECTS

SYMPTOMS	WHAT TO DO
Life-threatening:	
Rare allergic reaction (hives, itching, rash, wheezing, tightness in chest, swelling of lips or tongue or throat).	Seek emergency treatment immediately.
Common:	
Stomach cramps or mild pain, anxiety, nervousness, joint or muscle pain, restlessness, headache, trouble sleeping, unusual tiredness, nausea or vomiting, depression.	Continue. Call doctor when convenient.
Infrequent:	
• Skin rash.	Continue, but call doctor right away.
• Constipation or diarrhea, dizziness, increased thirst, cough, hoarseness, runny or stuffy nose, chills, sneezing, sore throat, irritability, appetite loss, male sexual problems, injection site reaction (pain, tender, itching or hard lump).	Continue. Call doctor when convenient.
Rare:	
• Severe stomach pain, eye symptoms (blurred vision, aching, burning, swollen), chest pain, shortness of breath, frequent or painful urination, swelling (face, feet or	Continue, but call doctor right away.

lower legs), fever, confusion, mood or mental changes, hallucinations, itching, ringing in ears, weight gain.	
• Other symptoms that cause concern.	Continue. Call doctor when convenient.

WARNINGS & PRECAUTIONS

Don't take if:

- You are allergic to naltrexone.
- You are still using opioids or are in opioid withdrawal or have failed naloxone challenge test.
- You are actively drinking alcohol.
- You have liver disease.

Before you start, consult your doctor if:

- You have milder liver disease, kidney disease or bleeding disorder such as hemophilia.
- You have a history of depression or suicidal thoughts or attempts.

Over age 60:
May require dose adjustment.

Pregnancy:
Decide with your doctor whether drug benefits justify risk to unborn child. Risk category C (see page xviii).

Breast-feeding:
It is unknown if drug passes into milk. Avoid drug or discontinue nursing until you finish medicine. Consult doctor for advice on maintaining milk supply.

Infants & children:
Safety and efficacy not established.

Prolonged use:
Consult your doctor about long-term use.

Skin & sunlight:
No problems expected.

Driving, piloting or hazardous work:
Don't drive or pilot aircraft until you learn how medicine affects you. Don't work around dangerous machinery. Don't climb ladders or work in high places. Danger increases if you drink alcohol or take medicine affecting alertness and reflexes.

Discontinuing:
Don't discontinue without consulting doctor. Dose may require gradual reduction if you have taken drug for a long time. Doses of other drugs may also require adjustment.

Others:

- Must be given under close supervision by people experienced in using naltrexone to treat addicts.
- See your doctor on a regular basis to check treatment progress and for recommended medical exams and lab tests.
- Excessive doses of this drug can cause liver injury.
- Attempting to use narcotics to overcome effects of naltrexone may lead to coma and death.
- The drug does not treat narcotic or alcohol withdrawal symptoms.
- Advise any doctor or dentist whom you consult that you take this drug.
- Wear or carry medical ID that indicates you are taking this drug.
- Consult doctor about stopping this drug several days prior to an expected surgery.

POSSIBLE INTERACTION WITH OTHER DRUGS

GENERIC NAME OR DRUG CLASS	COMBINED EFFECT
Hepatotoxics,* other	Increased risk of liver damage.
Narcotic medicines*	1. Can cause withdrawal symptoms. May lead to cardiac arrest, coma and death (if naltrexone taken while person is dependent on these drugs). 2. If these drugs are taken while person is taking naltrexone, opioid effect (pain relief) will be blocked.

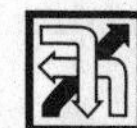

POSSIBLE INTERACTION WITH OTHER SUBSTANCES

INTERACTS WITH	COMBINED EFFECT
Alcohol:	Severe side effects. Must avoid.
Beverages:	None expected.
Cocaine:	Severe side effects. Must avoid.
Foods:	None expected.
Marijuana:	Unpredictable effects. Avoid.
Tobacco:	None expected.

*See Glossary

NARCOTIC ANALGESICS

GENERIC AND BRAND NAMES

See full list of generic and brand names in the *Generic and Brand Name Directory*, page 889.

BASIC INFORMATION

Habit forming? Yes
Prescription needed? Yes
Available as generic? Yes
Drug class: Narcotic

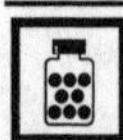

USES

Relieves pain and diarrhea; suppresses cough.

DOSAGE & USAGE INFORMATION

How to take:

- Tablet, capsule or extended-release tablet—Swallow with liquid. Do not crush, crumble or open extended release forms, especially the Palladone brand (could lead to a fatal dose).
- Liquid form of morphine—Mix with fruit juice just before taking to improve taste.
- Syrup—Mix with one-half glass of water (4 oz.) before swallowing.
- Dispersible tablets—Stir into water or fruit juice just before taking each dose.
- Liquid form—May need to be diluted with water before taking. Follow directions on label.
- Suppositories—Remove wrapper and moisten suppository with water. Gently insert into rectum, small end first.
- Nasal, transmucosal, lozenge form, transdermal or the brand name Embeda—Follow prescription instructions carefully.
- Buccal tablet—Let tablet dissolve in mouth per instructions. Do not chew or swallow whole.

Continued next column

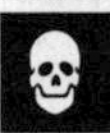

OVERDOSE

SYMPTOMS:
Deep sleep, slow breathing; slow pulse; respiratory arrest; flushed, warm skin; seizures; constricted pupils.
WHAT TO DO:

- **Dial 911 (emergency) for medical help or call poison control center 1-800-222-1222 for instructions.**
- **If person is unconscious, check breathing and pulse. If not breathing, begin mouth-to-mouth rescue breathing. If heart is not beating, begin chest compressions.**
- **See emergency information on last 3 pages of this book.**

When to take:
When needed. No more often than every 4 hours.

If you forget a dose:
Take as soon as you remember. Wait 4 hours for next dose.

What drug does:

- Blocks pain messages to brain and spinal cord.
- Reduces sensitivity of brain's cough control center.

Time lapse before drug works:
30 minutes.

Don't take with:
Any other medicine or any dietary supplement without consulting your doctor or pharmacist.

POSSIBLE ADVERSE REACTIONS OR SIDE EFFECTS

SYMPTOMS	WHAT TO DO
Life-threatening:	
Irregular or slow heartbeat, difficult breathing, wheezing.	Discontinue. Seek emergency treatment.
Common:	
Dizziness, drowsiness, tiredness, headache, lightheadedness, nausea or vomiting, stomach cramps, overexcitement.	Continue. Call doctor when convenient.
Infrequent:	
• Black, tarry stools; bloody or cloudy urine; painful or frequent urination; fast, slow or pounding heartbeat; hallucinations; breathing problems, wheezing; back or side pain; red dots on skin; red or flushed face; ringing or buzzing in ears; skin rash, hives or itching; sore throat; fever; face swelling; decreased urine; trembling; uncontrolled muscle movements; unusual bleeding or bruising; yellow skin or eyes.	Discontinue. Call doctor right away.
• Feeling depressed, pale stools.	Continue. Call doctor when convenient.
Rare:	
Changes in vision, constipation, dry mouth, loss of appetite, restlessness, night-mares, trouble sleeping.	Discontinue. Call doctor when convenient.

WARNINGS & PRECAUTIONS

Don't take if:
- You are allergic to any narcotic.
- You have acute breathing problem or diarrhea that is due to effect of drugs or poison.

Before you start, consult your doctor if:
You have asthma or any lung disorder, liver or kidney problems, heart disorder, seizure disorder, drug abuse or dependence, emotional instability, suicidal thoughts or attempts, gall bladder problems, recent renal or gastrointestinal surgery, head injury or other brain disorder, low thyroid, severe inflammatory bowel disease, high or low blood pressure, prostate problems.

Over age 60:
Increased risk of drug's adverse effects.

Pregnancy:
Risk factors vary for drugs in this group. See category list on page xviii and consult doctor.

Breast-feeding:
One or more of these drugs can pass into milk. Consult doctor.

Infants & children:
Use only with doctor's advice.

Prolonged use:
- High doses and long-term use can be habit forming. Consult doctor on a regular basis.
- May cause chronic constipation.

Skin & sunlight:
No special problems expected.

Driving, piloting or hazardous work:
Don't drive or pilot aircraft until you learn how medicine affects you. Don't work around dangerous machinery. Don't climb ladders or work in high places. Danger increases if you drink alcohol or take drugs affecting alertness.

Discontinuing:
If used for several weeks or more, consult doctor before discontinuing. Report to the doctor any symptoms that develop after discontinuing, such as gooseflesh, irritability, insomnia, yawning, weakness, large eye pupils.

Others:
- Some products contain tartrazine dye. Avoid, especially if you are allergic to aspirin.
- Advise any doctor or dentist whom you consult that you take this medicine.
- Follow directions exactly for using the fentanyl skin patch to avoid an overdose that could lead to severe side effects (including death). Follow all other safety precautions carefully.
- Lying down after the first few doses may decrease unwanted effects of nausea, vomiting, lightheadedness or dizziness.
- Use propoxyphene only as directed to avoid overdose (which can be fatal).

POSSIBLE INTERACTION WITH OTHER DRUGS

GENERIC NAME OR DRUG CLASS	COMBINED EFFECT
Analgesics,* other	Increased analgesic effect.
Anticoagulants,* oral	Possible increased anticoagulant effect.
Anticholinergics*	Increased anticholinergic effect.
Antidepressants*	Increased sedative effect.
Antihistamines*	Increased sedative effect.
Anti-inflammatory drugs, nonsteroidal (NSAIDs)*	Increased narcotic effect.
Butorphanol	Possibly precipitates withdrawal with chronic narcotic use.
Carbamazepine	Increased carbamazepine effect possible with propoxyphene.
Carteolol	Increased narcotic effect. Dangerous sedation.

Continued on page 921

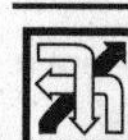

POSSIBLE INTERACTION WITH OTHER SUBSTANCES

INTERACTS WITH	COMBINED EFFECT
Alcohol:	Increased intoxicating effect of alcohol (especially with Avinza brand). Do not drink alcohol or take alcohol-containing drugs.
Beverages:	None expected.
Cocaine:	Increased toxic effects of cocaine. Avoid.
Foods:	None expected.
Marijuana:	Impaired physical and mental performance. Avoid.
Tobacco:	None expected.

***See Glossary**

NARCOTIC ANALGESICS & ACETAMINOPHEN

GENERIC AND BRAND NAMES

See full list of generic and brand names in the *Generic and Brand Name Directory*, page 890.

BASIC INFORMATION

Habit forming? Yes
Prescription needed? Yes
Available as generic? Yes
Drug class: Narcotic, analgesic, fever reducer

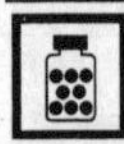

USES

Relieves pain, reduces fever.

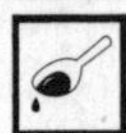

DOSAGE & USAGE INFORMATION

How to take:

- Tablet or capsule—Swallow with liquid. If you can't swallow whole, crumble tablet or open capsule and take with liquid or food.
- Syrup—Mix with one-half glass of water (4 oz.) before swallowing.
- Liquid form—May need to be diluted with water before taking. Follow directions on label.

When to take:
When needed. No more often than every 4 hours or as directed.

If you forget a dose:
Take as soon as you remember. If it is almost time for the next dose, wait for the next scheduled dose (don't double this dose).

What drug does:

- May affect hypothalamus—the part of the brain that helps regulate body heat and receives body's pain messages.

Continued next column

OVERDOSE

SYMPTOMS:
Stomach upset; irritability; sweating, convulsions; deep sleep; slow breathing; slow pulse; flushed, warm skin; constricted pupils; coma.
WHAT TO DO:

- **Dial 911 (emergency) for medical help or call poison control center 1-800-222-1222 for instructions.**
- **If person is unconscious, check breathing and pulse. If not breathing, begin mouth-to-mouth rescue breathing. If heart is not beating, begin chest compressions.**
- **See emergency information on last 3 pages of this book.**

- Blocks pain messages to brain and spinal cord.
- Reduces sensitivity of brain's cough control center.

Time lapse before drug works:
15 to 30 minutes. May last 4 hours.

Don't take with:

- Other drugs containing acetaminophen. Too much acetaminophen can damage liver and kidneys.
- Any other medicine or any dietary supplement without consulting your doctor or pharmacist.

POSSIBLE ADVERSE REACTIONS OR SIDE EFFECTS

SYMPTOMS	WHAT TO DO
Life-threatening:	
Rare allergic reaction (hives, itching, rash, trouble breathing, tightness in chest, swelling of lips or tongue or face).	Seek emergency treatment immediately.
Common:	
Dizziness, drowsiness, tiredness, headache, lightheadedness, nausea or vomiting, stomach cramps, overexcitement.	Continue. Call doctor when convenient.
Infrequent:	
• Black, tarry stools; bloody or cloudy urine; painful or frequent urination; fast, slow or pounding heartbeat; hallucinations; breathing problems, wheezing; back or side pain; red dots on skin; red or flushed face; ringing or buzzing in ears; skin rash, hives or itching; sore throat; fever; face swelling; decreased urine; trembling; uncontrolled muscle movements; unusual bleeding or bruising; yellow skin or eyes.	Discontinue. Call doctor right away.
• Feeling depressed, pale stools.	Continue. Call doctor when convenient.
Rare:	
Changes in vision, constipation, dry mouth, loss of appetite, restlessness, nightmares, trouble sleeping.	Discontinue. Call doctor when convenient.

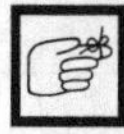

WARNINGS & PRECAUTIONS

Don't take if:

- You are allergic to narcotics or acetaminophen.
- You have acute breathing problem or diarrhea that is due to effect of drugs or poison.

Before you start, consult your doctor if:
You have asthma or any lung disorder, liver or kidney problems, heart disorder, seizure disorder, drug abuse or dependence, emotional instability, suicidal thoughts or attempts, gall bladder problems, recent renal or gastrointestinal surgery, head injury or other brain disorder, low thyroid, severe inflammatory bowel disease, high or low blood pressure, prostate problems.

Over age 60:
Increased risk of drug's adverse effects.

Pregnancy:
Risk factors vary for drugs in this group. See category list on page xviii and consult doctor.

Breast-feeding:
One or more of these drugs can pass into milk. Consult doctor.

Infants & children:
Use only with doctor's advice.

Prolonged use:

- High doses and long-term use can be habit forming or cause liver problems. Consult doctor on a regular basis.
- May cause chronic constipation.

Skin & sunlight:
No special problems expected.

Driving, piloting or hazardous work:
Don't drive or pilot aircraft until you learn how drug affects you. Don't work around dangerous machinery. Don't climb ladders or work in high places. Danger increases if you drink alcohol or take drugs affecting alertness and reflexes.

Discontinuing:
If used for several weeks or more, consult doctor before discontinuing. Report to the doctor any symptoms that develop after discontinuing, such as gooseflesh, irritability, insomnia, yawning, weakness, large eye pupils.

Others:

- Some products contain tartrazine dye. Avoid, especially if you are allergic to aspirin.
- Advise any doctor or dentist whom you consult that you take this medicine.
- Follow directions exactly for using the fentanyl skin patch to avoid an overdose that could lead to severe side effects (including death).
- Lying down after the first few doses may decrease unwanted effects of nausea, vomiting, lightheadedness or dizziness.
- Use propoxyphene only as directed to avoid overdose (which can be fatal).
- There is a risk for severe liver injury if person takes more than recommended dose, takes high doses on regular basis or takes with other drug containing acetaminophen.

POSSIBLE INTERACTION WITH OTHER DRUGS

GENERIC NAME OR DRUG CLASS	COMBINED EFFECT
Analgesics,* other	Increased analgesic effect.
Anticoagulants,* other	May increase anticoagulant effect. Prothrombin times should be monitored.
Anticholinergics*	Increased anticholinergic effect.
Antidepressants*	Increased sedative effect.
Antihistamines*	Increased sedative effect.
Carteolol	Increased narcotic effect. Dangerous sedation.
Mind-altering drugs*	Increased sedative effect.
Narcotics,* other	Increased narcotic effect.
Nitrates*	Excessive blood pressure drop.

Continued on page 921

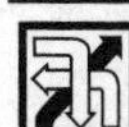

POSSIBLE INTERACTION WITH OTHER SUBSTANCES

INTERACTS WITH	COMBINED EFFECT
Alcohol:	Increased toxic effect of alcohol or liver damage. Don't drink alcohol or take drugs containing alcohol.
Beverages:	None expected.
Cocaine:	Increased toxic effects. Avoid.
Foods:	None expected.
Marijuana:	Physical and mental. problems. Avoid.
Tobacco:	None expected.

***See Glossary**

NARCOTIC ANALGESICS & ASPIRIN

GENERIC AND BRAND NAMES

See full list of generic and brand names in the *Generic and Brand Name Directory*, page 891.

BASIC INFORMATION

Habit forming? Yes
Prescription needed? Yes
Available as generic? Yes
Drug class: Narcotic, analgesic, anti-inflammatory (nonsteroidal)

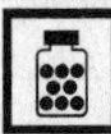

USES

Reduces pain, fever and inflammation.

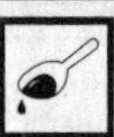

DOSAGE & USAGE INFORMATION

How to take:
Tablet or capsule—Swallow with liquid. If you can't swallow whole, crumble tablet or open capsule and take with liquid or food.

When to take:
As needed. No more often than every 4 hours.

If you forget a dose:
Take as soon as you remember. Wait 4 hours for next dose.

What drug does:
- Affects hypothalamus, the part of the brain which regulates temperature, by dilating small blood vessels in skin.
- Prevents clumping of platelets (small blood cells) so blood vessels remain open.
- Decreases prostaglandin effect.
- Suppresses body's pain messages.
- Suppresses cough reflex.

Continued next column

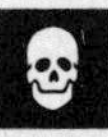

OVERDOSE

SYMPTOMS:
Ringing in ears; nausea; vomiting; dizziness; fever; deep sleep; slow breathing; slow pulse; flushed, warm skin; constricted pupils; hallucinations; convulsions; coma.
WHAT TO DO:
- **Dial 911 (emergency) for medical help or call poison control center 1-800-222-1222 for instructions.**
- **If person is unconscious, check breathing and pulse. If not breathing, begin mouth-to-mouth rescue breathing. If heart is not beating, begin chest compressions.**
- **See emergency information on last 3 pages of this book.**

Time lapse before drug works:
30 minutes.

Don't take with:
- Tetracyclines. Space doses 1 hour apart.
- Any other medicine or any dietary supplement without consulting your doctor or pharmacist.

POSSIBLE ADVERSE REACTIONS OR SIDE EFFECTS

SYMPTOMS	WHAT TO DO
Life-threatening:	
Irregular or slow heartbeat, difficult breathing, wheezing.	Discontinue. Seek emergency treatment.
Common:	
Dizziness, drowsiness, tiredness, headache, lightheadedness, nausea or vomiting, stomach cramps, overexcitement.	Continue. Call doctor when convenient.
Infrequent:	
• Black, tarry stools; bloody or cloudy urine; painful or frequent urination; fast, slow or pounding heartbeat; hallucinations; breathing problems, wheezing; back or side pain; red dots on skin; red or flushed face; ringing or buzzing in ears; skin rash, hives or itching; sore throat; fever; face swelling; decreased urine; trembling; uncontrolled muscle movements; unusual bleeding or bruising; yellow skin or eyes.	Discontinue. Call doctor right away.
• Feeling depressed, pale stools.	Continue. Call doctor when convenient.
Rare:	
• Stomach pain that doesn't go away, vomiting blood.	Discontinue. Call doctor right away.
• Changes in vision, constipation, dry mouth, loss of appetite, restlessness, nightmares, trouble sleeping.	Discontinue. Call doctor when convenient.

WARNINGS & PRECAUTIONS

Don't take if:
- You are allergic to narcotics, aspirin or NSAIDs.
- You have acute breathing problem or diarrhea that is due to effect of drugs or poison.

Before you start, consult your doctor if:
You have ulcers, asthma or any lung disorder, liver or kidney problems, heart disorder, seizure disorder, drug abuse or dependence, emotional instability, suicidal thoughts or attempts, gallbladder problems, recent gastrointestinal or renal surgery, head injury or other brain disorder, low thyroid, severe inflammatory bowel disease, high or low blood pressure, prostate problems, or you have increased risk for stomach bleeding problems.

Over age 60:
Increased risk of drug's adverse effects.

Pregnancy:
Risk factors vary for drugs in this group. See category list on page xviii and consult doctor.

Breast-feeding:
One or more of these drugs can pass into milk. Consult doctor.

Infants & children:
Use only with doctor's advice.

Prolonged use:
- High doses and long-term use can be habit forming. Consult doctor on a regular basis.
- May cause chronic constipation.

Skin & sunlight:
No special problems expected.

Driving, piloting or hazardous work:
Don't drive or pilot aircraft until you learn how medicine affects you. Don't work around dangerous machinery. Don't climb ladders or work in high places. Danger increases if you drink alcohol or take medicine affecting alertness and reflexes.

Discontinuing:
If used for several weeks or more, consult doctor before discontinuing. Report to the doctor any symptoms that develop after discontinuing, such as gooseflesh, irritability, insomnia, yawning, weakness, large eye pupils.

Others:
- Aspirin can complicate surgery; illness; pregnancy, labor and delivery.
- Urine tests for blood sugar may be inaccurate.
- Advise any doctor or dentist whom you consult that you take this medicine.
- Lying down after the first few doses may decrease unwanted effects of nausea, vomiting, lightheadedness or dizziness.
- Don't use if medicine has a strong vinegar-like odor. This means the aspirin is breaking down.
- Use propoxyphene only as directed to avoid overdose (which can be fatal).

POSSIBLE INTERACTION WITH OTHER DRUGS

GENERIC NAME OR DRUG CLASS	COMBINED EFFECT
Acebutolol	Decreased anti-hypertensive effect of acebutolol.
Adrenocorticoids, systemic	Increased risk of ulcers. Increased adrenocorticoid effect.
Alendronate	Increased risk of stomach irritation.
Allopurinol	Decreased allopurinol effect.
Angiotensin-converting enzyme (ACE) inhibitors*	Decreased effect of ACE inhibitor.
Antacids*	Decreased aspirin effect.
Anticoagulants,* oral	Increased anticoagulant effect. Abnormal bleeding.
Antidepressants*	Increased sedative effect.

Continued on page 922

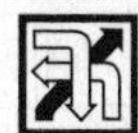

POSSIBLE INTERACTION WITH OTHER SUBSTANCES

INTERACTS WITH	COMBINED EFFECT
Alcohol:	Increased intoxicating effect of alcohol. Do not drink alcohol or take alcohol-containing drugs.
Beverages:	None expected.
Cocaine:	Unknown. Avoid.
Foods:	None expected.
Marijuana:	Impaired physical and mental performance. Avoid.
Tobacco:	None expected.

***See Glossary**

NEFAZODONE

BRAND NAMES

Serzone

BASIC INFORMATION

Habit forming? No
Prescription needed? Yes
Available as generic? Yes
Drug class: Antidepressant (phenylpiperazine)

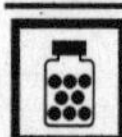

USES

Treats symptoms of mental depression.

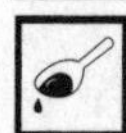

DOSAGE & USAGE INFORMATION

How to take:
Tablet—Swallow with liquid. May be taken with or without food.

When to take:
At the same times each day. The prescribed dosage may be increased weekly until maximum benefits are achieved.

If you forget a dose:
Take as soon as you remember. If it is almost time for the next dose, wait for that dose (don't double this dose) and resume regular schedule.

What drug does:
The exact mechanism is unknown. It appears to block reuptake of serotonin and norepinephrine (stimulating chemicals in the brain that play a role in emotions and psychological disturbances).

Time lapse before drug works:
Will take up to several weeks to relieve the depression.

Don't take with:
Any other medicine or any dietary supplement without consulting your doctor or pharmacist.

OVERDOSE

SYMPTOMS:
Drowsiness, nausea, vomiting, low blood pressure (faintness, weakness, dizziness, lightheadedness) or increased severity of adverse reactions.
WHAT TO DO:
- **Dial 911 (emergency) for medical help or call poison control center 1-800-222-1222 for instructions.**
- **See emergency information on last 3 pages of this book.**

POSSIBLE ADVERSE REACTIONS OR SIDE EFFECTS

SYMPTOMS	WHAT TO DO
Life-threatening: In case of overdose, see previous column.	
Common:	
• Clumsiness or unsteadiness, blurred vision or other vision changes, fainting, lightheadedness, ringing in the ears, skin rash or itching.	Discontinue. Call doctor right away.
• Strange dreams, constipation or diarrhea, dry mouth, heartburn, fever, chills, flushing or feeling warm, headache, increased appetite, insomnia, coughing, tingling or prickly sensations, sore throat, trembling, drowsiness, confusion or agitation, memory lapses.	Continue. Call doctor when convenient.
Infrequent:	
• Tightness in chest; trouble breathing; wheezing; eye pain; combination of nausea, vomiting, diarrhea and stomach pain.	Discontinue. Call doctor right away.
• Joint pain, breast pain, increased thirst.	Continue. Call doctor when convenient.
Rare:	
• Face swelling, hives, muscle pain or stiffness, chest pain, fast heartbeat, mood or mental changes, difficulty speaking, hallucinations, uncontrolled excited behavior, twitching, ear pain, increased hearing sensitivity, bleeding or bruising, irritated red eyes, eyes sensitive to light, pain in back or side, swollen glands, problems with urination.	Discontinue. Call doctor right away.
• Unusual tiredness or weakness, false sense of well-being, menstrual changes, change in sexual desire or function.	Continue. Call doctor when convenient.

WARNINGS & PRECAUTIONS

Don't use if:
You are allergic to nefazodone or trazodone (phenylpiperazine antidepressants).

Before you start, consult your doctor if:
- You have or have had liver disease.
- You have a seizure disorder, heart disease or blood circulation problem or have had a stroke.
- You are dehydrated.
- You have a history of drug abuse.
- You have a history of mood disorders (such as mania) or thoughts of suicide.
- You are allergic to any medication.

Over age 60:
A lower starting dosage is usually recommended until a response is determined.

Pregnancy:
Decide with your doctor if drug benefits justify risk to unborn child. Risk category C (see page xviii).

Breast-feeding:
It is unknown if drug passes into milk. Avoid drug or discontinue nursing until you finish medicine. Consult doctor for advice on maintaining milk supply.

Infants & children:
Not approved for ages under 18. If prescribed, carefully read information provided with prescription. Contact doctor right away if depression symptoms get worse or there is any talk of suicide or suicide behaviors. Also, read information under Others.

Prolonged use:
Consult with your doctor on a regular basis while taking this drug to check your progress and to discuss any increase or changes in side effects and the need for continued treatment.

Skin & sunlight:
May cause a rash or intensify sunburn in areas exposed to sun or ultraviolet light (photosensitivity reaction). Avoid excess sun exposure and use sunscreen. Call doctor if reaction occurs.

Driving, piloting or hazardous work:
Don't drive or pilot aircraft until you learn how medicine affects you. Don't work around dangerous machinery. Don't climb ladders or work in high places. Danger increases if you drink alcohol or take medicine affecting alertness and reflexes.

Discontinuing:
Don't discontinue this drug without consulting doctor. Dosage may require a gradual reduction before stopping.

Others:
- Get up slowly from a sitting or lying position to avoid dizziness, faintness or lightheadedness.
- Advise any doctor or dentist whom you consult that you take this medicine.
- Take drug only as directed. Do not increase or reduce dosage without doctor's approval.
- Adults and children taking antidepressants may experience a worsening of the depression symptoms and may have increased suicidal thoughts or behaviors. Call doctor right away if these symptoms or behaviors occur.
- Use of this drug may result in hepatic (liver) problems that can be life-threatening. Call doctor right away if yellow skin or eyes, stomach problems, appetite loss or fatigue occur.

POSSIBLE INTERACTION WITH OTHER DRUGS

GENERIC NAME OR DRUG CLASS	COMBINED EFFECT
Alprazolam	Increased effect of alprazolam.
Antihypertensives*	Possible too-low blood pressure.
Carbamazepine	Decreased effect of nefazodone. Avoid.
Central nervous system (CNS) depressants*	Increased sedation.
Cisapride	Increased effect of cisapride. Avoid.
Digoxin	Increased digoxin effect.
Fluoxetine	Increased risk of side effects.

Continued on page 922

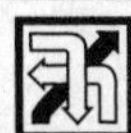

POSSIBLE INTERACTION WITH OTHER SUBSTANCES

INTERACTS WITH	COMBINED EFFECT
Alcohol:	Increased sedative affect. Avoid.
Beverages:	None expected.
Cocaine:	Unknown. Avoid.
Foods:	None expected.
Marijuana:	Unknown. Best to avoid.
Tobacco:	None expected.

NEOMYCIN (Oral)

BRAND NAMES

Mycifradin

BASIC INFORMATION

Habit forming? No
Prescription needed? Yes
Available as generic? Yes
Drug class: Antibacterial

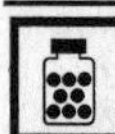

USES

- Clears intestinal tract of germs prior to surgery.
- Treats some causes of diarrhea.
- Lowers blood cholesterol.
- Lessens symptoms of hepatic coma.

DOSAGE & USAGE INFORMATION

How to take:
Tablet—Swallow with liquid or food to lessen stomach irritation. If you can't swallow whole, crumble tablet and take with liquid or food.

When to take:
According to directions on prescription.

If you forget a dose:
Take as soon as you remember. If it is almost time for the next dose, wait for that dose (don't double this dose) and resume regular schedule.

What drug does:
Kills germs susceptible to neomycin.

Time lapse before drug works:
2 to 3 days.

Don't take with:
Any other medicine or any dietary supplement without consulting your doctor or pharmacist.

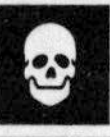

OVERDOSE

SYMPTOMS:
Loss of hearing, difficulty breathing, respiratory paralysis.
WHAT TO DO:

- **Dial 911 (emergency) for medical help or call poison control center 1-800-222-1222 for instructions.**
- **If person is unconscious, check breathing and pulse. If not breathing, begin mouth-to-mouth rescue breathing. If heart is not beating, begin chest compressions.**
- **See emergency information on last 3 pages of this book.**

POSSIBLE ADVERSE REACTIONS OR SIDE EFFECTS

SYMPTOMS	WHAT TO DO
Life-threatening: In case of overdose, see previous column.	
Common: Sore mouth or rectum, nausea, vomiting.	Continue. Call doctor when convenient.
Infrequent: None expected.	
Rare: Clumsiness, dizziness, rash, hearing loss, ringing or noises in ear, frothy stools, gaseousness, decreased frequency of urination, diarrhea.	Discontinue. Call doctor right away.

WARNINGS & PRECAUTIONS

Don't take if:
You are allergic to neomycin or any aminoglycoside.*

Before you start, consult your doctor if:
- You will have surgery within 2 months, including dental surgery, requiring general or spinal anesthesia.
- You have hearing loss or loss of balance secondary to 8th cranial nerve disease.
- You have intestinal obstruction.
- You have myasthenia gravis, Parkinson's disease, kidney disease, ulcers in intestines.

Over age 60:
Adverse reactions and side effects may be more frequent and severe than in younger persons.

Pregnancy:
Risk to unborn child outweighs drug benefits. Don't use. Risk category D (see page xviii).

Breast-feeding:
Avoid if possible. Effect unknown. Consult doctor.

Infants & children:
Give only under close medical supervision.

Prolonged use:
- Adverse effects more likely.
- Talk to your doctor about the need for follow-up medical examinations or laboratory studies to check hearing, kidney function.

Skin & sunlight:
No problems expected.

Driving, piloting or hazardous work:
No problems expected.

Discontinuing:
May be unnecessary to finish medicine. Follow doctor's instructions.

Others:
Advise any doctor or dentist whom you consult that you take this medicine.

POSSIBLE INTERACTION WITH OTHER DRUGS

GENERIC NAME OR DRUG CLASS	COMBINED EFFECT
Aminoglycosides*	Increased chance of toxic effect on hearing, kidneys, muscles.
Beta carotene	Decreased absorption of beta carotene.
Capreomycin	Increased chance of toxic effects on hearing, kidneys.
Cephalothin	Increased chance of toxic effect on kidneys.
Cisplatin	Increased chance of toxic effects on hearing, kidneys.
Ethacrynic acid	Increased chance of toxic effects on hearing, kidneys.
Furosemide	Increased chance of toxic effects on hearing, kidneys.
Mercaptomerin	Increased chance of toxic effects on hearing, kidneys.
Penicillins*	Decreased antibiotic effect.
Tiopronin	Increased risk of toxicity to kidneys.
Vancomycin	Increased chance of toxic effects on hearing, kidneys.

POSSIBLE INTERACTION WITH OTHER SUBSTANCES

INTERACTS WITH	COMBINED EFFECT
Alcohol:	Increased chance of toxicity. Avoid.
Beverages:	None expected.
Cocaine:	Increased chance of toxicity. Avoid.
Foods:	None expected.
Marijuana:	Increased chance of toxicity. Avoid.
Tobacco:	None expected.

***See Glossary**

NEOMYCIN (Topical)

BRAND NAMES

Myciguent

BASIC INFORMATION

Habit forming? No
Prescription needed? No
Available as generic? Yes
Drug class: Antibacterial (topical)

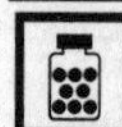

USES

Treats skin infections that may accompany burns, superficial boils, insect bites or stings, skin ulcers, minor surgical wounds.

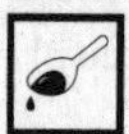

DOSAGE & USAGE INFORMATION

How to take:
Cream, lotion, ointment—Bathe and dry area before use. Apply small amount and rub gently. May cover with gauze or bandage if desired.

When to take:
3 or 4 times daily or as directed by doctor.

If you forget a dose:
Use as soon as you remember.

What drug does:
Kills susceptible bacteria by interfering with bacterial DNA and RNA.

Time lapse before drug works:
Begins first day. May require treatment for a week or longer to cure infection.

Don't take with:
Any other topical medicine without consulting your doctor or pharmacist.

OVERDOSE

SYMPTOMS:
None expected.
WHAT TO DO:
Dial 911 (emergency) for medical help or call poison control center 1-800-222-1222 for instructions.

POSSIBLE ADVERSE REACTIONS OR SIDE EFFECTS

SYMPTOMS	WHAT TO DO
Life-threatening: None expected.	
Common: None expected.	
Infrequent: Itching, swollen, red skin.	Discontinue. Call doctor right away.
Rare: None expected.	

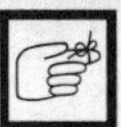

WARNINGS & PRECAUTIONS

Don't take if:
You are allergic to neomycin or any topical medicine.

Before you start, consult your doctor if:
Any lesions on the skin are open sores.

Over age 60:
No problems expected.

Pregnancy:
Consult doctor. Risk category C (see page xviii).

Breast-feeding:
No problems expected, but check with doctor.

Infants & children:
No problems expected, but check with doctor.

Prolonged use:
No problems expected, but check with doctor.

Skin & sunlight:
No special problems expected.

Driving, piloting or hazardous work:
No problems expected, but check with doctor.

Discontinuing:
No problems expected, but check with doctor.

Others:
- Heat and moisture in bathroom medicine cabinet can cause breakdown of medicine. Store someplace else.
- Keep medicine cool, but don't freeze.

POSSIBLE INTERACTION WITH OTHER DRUGS

GENERIC NAME OR DRUG CLASS	COMBINED EFFECT
Any other topical medication	Hypersensitivity reactions more likely to occur.

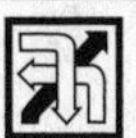

POSSIBLE INTERACTION WITH OTHER SUBSTANCES

INTERACTS WITH	COMBINED EFFECT
Alcohol:	None expected.
Beverages:	None expected.
Cocaine:	None expected.
Foods:	None expected.
Marijuana:	None expected.
Tobacco:	None expected.

NIACIN
(Vitamin B-3, Nicotinic Acid, Nicotinamide)

BRAND NAMES

Advicor
Endur-Acin
Nia-Bid
Niac
Niacels
Niacin
Niacor
Niaspan
Nico-400
Nicobid
Nicolar
Nicotinex
Nicotinyl alcohol
Papulex
Roniacol
Ronigen
Rycotin
Simcor
Slo-Niacin
Span-Niacin
Tega-Span
Tri-B3

Numerous brands of single vitamin and multivitamin combinations are available.

BASIC INFORMATION

Habit forming? No
Prescription needed? Yes, for some
Available as generic? Yes
Drug class: Vitamin supplement, vasodilator, antihyperlipidemic

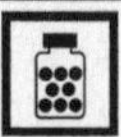

USES

- Replacement for niacin lost due to inadequate diet.
- Treatment for vertigo (dizziness) and ringing in ears.
- Prevention of premenstrual headache.
- Reduction of blood levels of cholesterol and triglycerides.
- Treatment for pellagra.

OVERDOSE

SYMPTOMS:
Body flush, nausea, vomiting, abdominal cramps, diarrhea, weakness, lightheadedness, fainting, sweating.
WHAT TO DO:
Overdose unlikely to threaten life. If person uses much larger amount than prescribed or if accidentally swallowed, call doctor or poison control center 1-800-222-1222 for help.

DOSAGE & USAGE INFORMATION

How to take:
- Tablet, capsule or liquid—Swallow with liquid or food to lessen stomach irritation.
- Extended-release tablets or capsules—Swallow each dose whole.

When to take:
At the same times each day.

If you forget a dose:
Take as soon as you remember. If it is almost time for the next dose, wait for that dose (don't double this dose) and resume regular schedule.

What drug does:
- Corrects niacin deficiency.
- Dilates blood vessels.
- In large doses, decreases cholesterol production.

Time lapse before drug works:
15 to 20 minutes.

Don't take with:
Any other medicine or any dietary supplement without consulting your doctor or pharmacist.

POSSIBLE ADVERSE REACTIONS OR SIDE EFFECTS

SYMPTOMS	WHAT TO DO
Life-threatening:	
None expected.	
Common:	
Dry skin.	Continue. Call doctor when convenient.
Infrequent:	
• Upper abdominal pain, diarrhea.	Discontinue. Call doctor right away.
• Headache, dizziness, faintness, temporary numbness and tingling in hands and feet.	Continue. Call doctor when convenient.
• "Hot" feeling, flush.	No action necessary.
Rare:	
Rash, itching, jaundice, double vision, weakness and faintness when arising from bed or chair.	Discontinue. Call doctor right away.

NIACIN (Vitamin B-3, Nicotinic Acid, Nicotinamide)

WARNINGS & PRECAUTIONS

Don't take if:
You are allergic to niacin or any niacin-containing vitamin mixtures.

Before you start, consult your doctor if:
- You have sensitivity to tartrazine dye.
- You have diabetes.
- You have gout.
- You have gallbladder or liver disease.
- You have impaired liver function.
- You have active peptic ulcer.

Over age 60:
Response to drug cannot be predicted. Dose must be individualized.

Pregnancy:
Consult doctor. Risk category C (see page xviii).

Breast-feeding:
Studies inconclusive. Consult doctor.

Infants & children:
- Use only under medical supervision.
- Keep vitamin-mineral supplements out of children's reach.

Prolonged use:
- May cause impaired liver function.
- Talk to your doctor about the need for follow-up medical examinations or laboratory studies to check liver function, blood sugar.

Skin & sunlight:
No problems expected.

Driving, piloting or hazardous work:
Avoid if you feel dizzy or faint. Otherwise, no problems expected.

Discontinuing:
May be unnecessary to finish medicine. Follow doctor's instructions.

Others:
- A balanced diet should provide all the niacin a healthy person needs and make supplements unnecessary. Best sources are meat, eggs and dairy products.
- Store in original container in cool, dry, dark place.
- Obesity reduces effectiveness.
- Some nicotinic acid products contain tartrazine dye. Read labels carefully if sensitive to tartrazine.

POSSIBLE INTERACTION WITH OTHER DRUGS

GENERIC NAME OR DRUG CLASS	COMBINED EFFECT
Antidiabetics*	Decreased antidiabetic effect.
Beta-adrenergic blocking agents*	Excessively low blood pressure.
Dexfenfluramine	May require dosage change as weight loss occurs.
HMG-CoA reductase inhibitors*	Increased risk of muscle or kidney problems.
Mecamylamine	Excessively low blood pressure.
Methyldopa	Excessively low blood pressure.
Probenecid	Decreased effect of probenecid.
Sulfinpyrazone	Decreased effect of sulfinpyrazone.

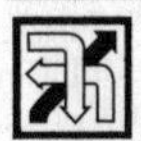

POSSIBLE INTERACTION WITH OTHER SUBSTANCES

INTERACTS WITH	COMBINED EFFECT
Alcohol:	Excessively low blood pressure. Use caution.
Beverages:	None expected.
Cocaine:	Increased flushing.
Foods:	None expected.
Marijuana:	None expected.
Tobacco:	Decreased niacin effect.

***See Glossary**

NICOTINE

BRAND NAMES

Commit
Habitrol
Nicoderm
Nicoderm CQ
Nicoderm CQ Thin
 Flex patch
Nicorette
Nicorette DS
Nicorette Fresh Mint
Nicorette Lozenge
Nicotrol
Nicotrol NS
Prostep
Thrive Gum
Thrive Lozenge

BASIC INFORMATION

Habit Forming? Yes
Prescription needed? No
Available as generic? Yes, for some
Drug class: Antismoking agent

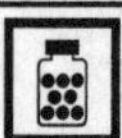

USES

Treatment aid to giving up smoking. Nicotine replacement is to be used in conjunction with a medically supervised behavioral modification program for smoking cessation.

DOSAGE & USAGE INFORMATION

How to use:

- Skin patch—Apply to clean, nonhairy site on the trunk or upper outer arm. Fold old patch in half (sticky sides together) and dispose of where children and pets cannot get to it.
- Chewing gum—Chew gum pieces slowly and intermittently (chew several times, then place between cheek and gum) for best effect.
- Nasal spray—Use 2-3 sprays in each nostril.
- Lozenge—Use as directed on package.

Continued next column

OVERDOSE

SYMPTOMS:
Early symptoms—Nausea, vomiting, severe diarrhea, increased mouth watering, abdominal pain, cold sweat, severe headache, dizziness, confusion, vision and hearing changes.
Late symptoms—Irregular or fast pulse, fainting, breathing difficulty, convulsions.
WHAT TO DO:

- **Dial 911 (emergency) for medical help or call poison control center 1-800-222-1222 for instructions.**
- **See emergency information on last 3 pages of this book.**

When to use:

- Skin patch—Daily. Remove old patch and apply new patch to new location on the skin.
- Chewing gum—When there is an urge to smoke, chew the gum for about 30 minutes. For the brand name Thrive Gum, follow instructions on label.
- Nasal spray—Hourly, or as directed. Dosage adjustments should be made as needed.
- Lozenge—Follow label instructions.
- For all—Always follow product's directions.

If you forget a dose:

- Skin patch—Remove old patch and apply new patch as soon as you remember, then return to regular schedule.
- Chewing gum or nasal spray—Use as soon as you remember (don't double dosages).

What drug does:
Delivers a supply of nicotine to the body for relief of smoking withdrawal symptoms (irritability, headache, nervousness, drowsiness, fatigue). Reduces craving for cigarettes.

Time lapse before drug works:
Minutes to hours depending on type of product.

Don't take with:
Any other medicine or any dietary supplement without consulting your doctor or pharmacist.

POSSIBLE ADVERSE REACTIONS OR SIDE EFFECTS

SYMPTOMS	WHAT TO DO
Life-threatening: In case of overdose, see previous column.	
Common:	
• Skin patch—itching, redness, burning or skin rash at site of patch.	Continue. Call doctor when convenient.
• Chewing gum—dental problems, sore mouth or throat, belching, mouth watering.	Continue. Call doctor when convenient.
• Nasal spray—runny nose, watering eyes, throat irritation, sneezing and cough.	Continue. Call doctor when convenient.
Infrequent:	
Diarrhea, dizziness, indigestion, nervousness, strange dreams, muscle aches, nausea, constipation, increased cough, tiredness, irritability, changes in menstruation, insomnia, headache, increase in sweating.	Continue. Call doctor when convenient.

Rare:

• Allergic reaction (swelling, hives, rash, itching, vomiting, irregular or fast heartbeat); symptoms of overdose occur (high doses of nicotine can cause toxic effects, even in people who are nicotine tolerant).	Discontinue. Call doctor right away.
• Hiccups or hoarseness with chewing gum.	Continue. Call doctor when convenient.

WARNINGS & PRECAUTIONS

Don't take if:
You are allergic to nicotine or any of the components in the skin patch.

Before you start, consult your doctor if:
- You are pregnant.
- You have a skin disorder; mouth, throat, dental or TMJ disorder; long-term nasal disorder (allergy, hay fever, sinusitis, polyps) or asthma.
- You have cardiovascular or peripheral vascular disease or high blood pressure.
- You have liver or kidney disease.
- You have hyperthyroidism, insulin-dependent diabetes, pheochromocytoma, peptic ulcer disease or endocrine disorder.

Over age 60:
Adverse reactions and side effects may be more frequent and severe than in younger persons.

Pregnancy:
Tobacco smoke and nicotine are harmful to the fetus. The specific effects of nicotine from these drugs are unknown. Discuss the risks of both with your doctor. Risk category varies for drugs in this group (see page xviii).

Breast-feeding:
Drug passes into breast milk. Avoid drug or discontinue nursing until you finish medicine. Consult doctor for advice on maintaining milk supply.

Infants & children:
Not recommended.

Prolonged use:
Treatment may take several months. Nicotine replacement therapy is not intended for long-term use.

Skin & sunlight:
No problems expected.

Driving, piloting or hazardous work:
Avoid if you feel dizzy or lightheaded. Otherwise, no problems expected.

Discontinuing:
Adverse reactions and side effects related to nicotine withdrawal may continue for some time after discontinuing.

Others:
- Advise any doctor or dentist whom you consult that you take this medicine.
- May affect results of some medical tests.
- Keep both the used and unused skin patches out of the reach of children and pets. Dispose of old patches according to directions.
- For full benefit from this treatment and to decrease risk of side effects, stop cigarette smoking as soon as you begin treatment.

POSSIBLE INTERACTION WITH OTHER DRUGS

GENERIC NAME OR DRUG CLASS	COMBINED EFFECT
Acetaminophen	Increased effect of acetaminophen.
Beta-adrenergic blocking agents*	Increased effect of beta blocker.
Bronchodilators, xanthine* (except dyphylline)	Increased bronchodilator effect.
Imipramine	Increased effect of imipramine.
Insulin & insulin lispro	May require insulin dosage adjustment.
Isoproterenol	Decreased effect of isoproterenol.
Oxazepam	Increased effect of oxazepam.

Continued on page 923

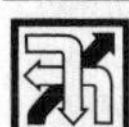

POSSIBLE INTERACTION WITH OTHER SUBSTANCES

INTERACTS WITH	COMBINED EFFECT
Alcohol:	Increased cardiac irritability. Avoid.
Beverages:	None expected.
Cocaine:	Increased cardiac irritability. Avoid.
Foods:	None expected.
Marijuana:	Increased toxic effects. Avoid.
Tobacco:	Increased adverse effects of nicotine. Must avoid.

***See Glossary**

NITAZOXANIDE

BRAND NAMES

Alinia

BASIC INFORMATION

Habit forming? No
Prescription needed? Yes
Available as generic? No
Drug class: Antiprotozoal; antidiarrheal

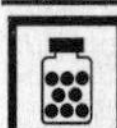

USES

- Treatment of diarrhea and other symptoms caused by two parasitic infections (*Cryptosporidium parvum* and *Giardia lamblia*). These two types of parasites are common causes of persistent diarrhea in children and adults. Outbreaks have been associated with day care centers, swimming pools, water parks and public water supplies.
- May be used for treatment of other disorders as determined by your doctor.

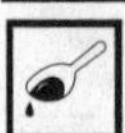

DOSAGE & USAGE INFORMATION

How to take:
- Oral suspension—Follow label instructions and take with food.
- Tablet—Swallow with liquid and take with food.

When to take:
Usual dose is twice a day for 3 days.

If you forget a dose:
Take as soon as you remember. If it is almost time for your next dose, skip the missed dose and go back to your regular dosing schedule. Do not double doses.

What drug does:
Prevents enzyme reactions that are needed for the parasites to survive. Thousands of enzymes are present in the body with a range of functions including food digestion and toxin elimination.

Continued next column

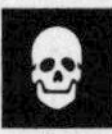

OVERDOSE

SYMPTOMS:
Unknown symptoms.
WHAT TO DO:
Overdose unlikely to threaten life. If person uses much larger amount than prescribed or if accidentally swallowed, call doctor or poison control center 1-800-222-1222 for help.

Time lapse before drug works:
Starts working in a few hours, but takes 3 days for effective treatment.

Don't take with:
Any other medicine or any dietary supplement without consulting your doctor or pharmacist.

POSSIBLE ADVERSE REACTIONS OR SIDE EFFECTS

SYMPTOMS	WHAT TO DO
Life-threatening: None expected.	
Common: None expected.	
Infrequent: None expected.	
Rare: Abdominal pain, diarrhea, vomiting, headache.	Continue. Call doctor if symptoms persist or are severe.

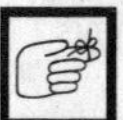

WARNINGS & PRECAUTIONS

Don't take if:
You are allergic to nitazoxanide.

Before you start, consult your doctor if:
- You have liver or kidney disease.
- You have bile or gallbladder problems.
- You have diabetes (the drug contains sucrose).
- You are immunosuppressed due to illness or drugs.

Over age 60:
No problems expected.

Pregnancy:
Decide with your doctor if drug benefits justify risk to unborn child. Risk category B. (See page xviii).

Breast-feeding:
It is unknown if drug passes into milk. Avoid drug or discontinue nursing until you finish medicine. Consult doctor for advice on maintaining milk supply.

Infants & children:
Approved for children over age one.

Prolonged use:
Not used for more than 3 days.

Skin & sunlight:
No problems expected.

Driving, piloting or hazardous work:
No problems expected.

Discontinuing:
No problems expected.

Others:
- Safety and effectiveness of nitazoxanide for HIV positive patients and immunodeficient patients have not been established.
- Advise any doctor or dentist whom you consult that you take this drug.

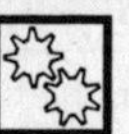

POSSIBLE INTERACTION WITH OTHER DRUGS

GENERIC NAME OR DRUG CLASS	COMBINED EFFECT
Protein bound drugs*	May increase effect of nitazoxanide.

Note: Specific studies on interactions of nitazoxanide with other drugs have not been conducted. If you have a concern about an interaction between drugs, consult your doctor or pharmacist.

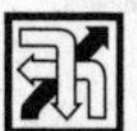

POSSIBLE INTERACTION WITH OTHER SUBSTANCES

INTERACTS WITH	COMBINED EFFECT
Alcohol:	None expected.
Beverages:	None expected.
Cocaine:	None expected.
Foods:	None expected.
Marijuana:	None expected.
Tobacco:	None expected.

*See Glossary

NITRATES

GENERIC AND BRAND NAMES

See full list of generic and brand names in the *Generic and Brand Name Directory*, page 891.

BASIC INFORMATION

Habit forming? No
Prescription needed? Yes
Available as generic? Yes
Drug class: Antianginal (nitrate)

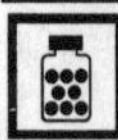

USES

- Reduces frequency and severity of angina attacks.
- Treats congestive heart failure.
- The brand name BiDil is approved to treat heart failure specifically in African Americans.

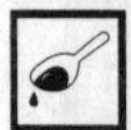

DOSAGE & USAGE INFORMATION

How to take:

- Extended-release tablet or capsule—Swallow each dose whole with liquid.
- Chewable tablet—Chew tablet at earliest sign of angina, and hold in mouth for 2 minutes.
- Regular tablet or capsule—Swallow whole with liquid. Don't crush, chew or open.
- Buccal tablet—Allow to dissolve inside of mouth.
- Lingual spray—Spray under tongue according to instructions enclosed with prescription.
- Ointment—Apply as directed.
- Patch—Apply to skin according to package instructions.
- Sublingual tablet—Place under tongue every 3 to 5 minutes at earliest sign of angina. If you don't have complete relief with 3 or 4 tablets, call doctor.

Continued next column

When to take:

- Swallowed tablet—Take at the same times each day, 1 or 2 hours after meals.
- Sublingual tablet or spray—At onset of angina.
- Ointment—Follow prescription directions.
- Patch—According to physician's instructions.

If you forget a dose:
Take as soon as you remember. If it is almost time for the next dose, wait for that dose (don't double this dose) and resume regular schedule.

What drug does:
Relaxes blood vessels, increasing blood flow to heart muscle.

Time lapse before drug works:

- Sublingual tablets and spray—1 to 3 minutes.
- Other forms—15 to 30 minutes. Will not stop an attack, but may prevent attacks.

Don't take with:
Any other medicine or any dietary supplement without consulting your doctor or pharmacist.

OVERDOSE

SYMPTOMS:
Dizziness; blue fingernails and lips; feeling of pressure in head; fever; fainting; shortness of breath; weak, fast heartbeat; convulsions.
WHAT TO DO:

- **Dial 911 (emergency) for medical help or call poison control center 1-800-222-1222 for instructions.**
- **See emergency information on last 3 pages of this book.**

POSSIBLE ADVERSE REACTIONS OR SIDE EFFECTS

SYMPTOMS	WHAT TO DO
Life-threatening:	
In case of overdose, see previous column.	
Common:	
Headache, flushed face and neck, dry mouth, nausea, vomiting.	Continue. Tell doctor at next visit.
Infrequent:	
• Fainting, rapid heartbeat.	Discontinue. Call doctor right away.
• Restlessness, blurred vision, dizziness.	Continue. Call doctor when convenient.
Rare:	
• Rash.	Discontinue. Call doctor right away.
• Severe irritation, peeling skin.	Continue. Call doctor when convenient.

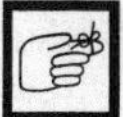

WARNINGS & PRECAUTIONS

Don't take if:
You are allergic to nitrates, including nitroglycerin.

Before you start, consult your doctor if:
- You are taking nonprescription drugs.
- You plan to become pregnant within medication period.
- You have glaucoma.
- You have reacted badly to any vasodilator drug.
- You drink alcoholic beverages or smoke marijuana.

Over age 60:
Adverse reactions and side effects may be more frequent and severe than in younger persons.

Pregnancy:
Decide with your doctor if drug benefits justify risk to unborn child. Risk category C (see page xviii).

Breast-feeding:
Effect unknown. Consult your doctor.

Infants & children:
Not recommended.

Prolonged use:
- Drug may become less effective and require higher doses.
- Talk to your doctor about the need for follow-up medical examinations or laboratory studies to check blood pressure, heart rate.

Skin & sunlight:
No problems expected.

Driving, piloting or hazardous work:
Don't drive or pilot aircraft until you learn how medicine affects you. Don't work around dangerous machinery. Don't climb ladders or work in high places. Danger increases if you drink alcohol or take medicine affecting alertness and reflexes.

Discontinuing:
Except for sublingual tablets, don't discontinue without doctor's advice until you complete prescribed dose, even though symptoms diminish or disappear.

Others:
- If discomfort is not caused by angina, nitrate medication will not bring relief. Call doctor if discomfort persists.
- Periodic urine and laboratory blood studies of white cell counts recommended if you take nitrates.
- Keep sublingual tablets in original container. Always carry them with you, but keep from body heat if possible.
- Sublingual tablets produce a burning, stinging sensation when placed under the tongue. Replace supply if no burning or stinging is noted.
- To avoid development of tolerance, drug-free intervals of 10 hours are sufficient.

POSSIBLE INTERACTION WITH OTHER DRUGS

GENERIC NAME OR DRUG CLASS	COMBINED EFFECT
Anticholinergics*	Increased internal eye pressure.
Antihypertensives*	Excessive blood pressure drop.
Beta-adrenergic blocking agents*	Excessive blood pressure drop.
Calcium channel blockers*	Decreased blood pressure.
Carteolol	Possible excessive blood pressure drop.
Guanfacine	Increased effects of both drugs.
Narcotics*	Excessive blood pressure drop.
Phenothiazines*	May decrease blood pressure.
Sildenafil	Increased effect of nitrates.
Sympathomimetics*	Possible reduced effects of both medicines.

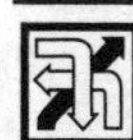

POSSIBLE INTERACTION WITH OTHER SUBSTANCES

INTERACTS WITH	COMBINED EFFECT
Alcohol:	Excessive blood pressure drop.
Beverages:	None expected.
Cocaine:	Reduced effectiveness of nitrates.
Foods:	None expected.
Marijuana:	Decreased nitrate effect.
Tobacco:	Decreased nitrate effect.

***See Glossary**

NITROFURANTOIN

BRAND NAMES

Apo-Nitrofurantoin
Cyantin
Furadantin
Furalan
Furaloid
Furan
Furanite
Furantoin
Furatine
Furaton
Macrobid
Macrodantin
Nephronex
Nifuran
Nitrex
Nitrofan
Nitrofor
Nitrofuracot
Novofuran
Ro-Antoin
Sarodant
Trantoin
Urotoin

BASIC INFORMATION

Habit forming? No
Prescription needed? Yes
Available as generic? Yes
Drug class: Antimicrobial, antibacterial (antibiotic)

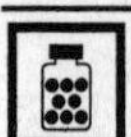

USES

Treatment for urinary tract infections.

DOSAGE & USAGE INFORMATION

How to take:

- Tablet or capsule—Swallow with food or milk to lessen stomach irritation. If you can't swallow whole, crumble tablet or open capsule and take with liquid or food.
- Extended-release capsule—Swallow with liquid. Do not open capsule.
- Liquid—Shake well and take with food. Use a measuring spoon to ensure accuracy.

When to take:
At the same times each day.

If you forget a dose:
Take as soon as you remember. If it is almost time for the next dose, wait for that dose (don't double this dose) and resume regular schedule.

Continued next column

OVERDOSE

SYMPTOMS:
Nausea, vomiting, abdominal pain, diarrhea.
WHAT TO DO:
Overdose unlikely to threaten life. If person uses much larger amount than prescribed or if accidentally swallowed, call doctor or poison control center 1-800-222-1222 for help.

What drug does:
Prevents susceptible bacteria in the urinary tract from growing and multiplying.

Time lapse before drug works:
1 to 2 weeks.

Don't take with:
Any other medicine or any dietary supplement without consulting your doctor or pharmacist.

POSSIBLE ADVERSE REACTIONS OR SIDE EFFECTS

SYMPTOMS	WHAT TO DO
Life-threatening:	
Hives, rash, intense itching, faintness soon after a dose (anaphylaxis).	Seek emergency treatment immediately.
Common:	
• Diarrhea, appetite loss, nausea, vomiting, chest pain, cough, difficult breathing, chills or unexplained fever, abdominal pain.	Discontinue. Call doctor right away.
• Rusty-colored or brown urine.	No action necessary.
Infrequent:	
• Rash, itchy skin, numbness, tingling or burning of face or mouth, fatigue, weakness.	Discontinue. Call doctor right away.
• Dizziness, headache, drowsiness, paleness (in children), discolored teeth (from liquid form).	Continue. Call doctor when convenient.
Rare:	
Jaundice.	Discontinue. Call doctor right away.

WARNINGS & PRECAUTIONS

Don't take if:

- You are allergic to nitrofurantoin.
- You have impaired kidney function.
- You drink alcohol.

Before you start, consult your doctor if:

- You are prone to allergic reactions.
- You are pregnant and within 2 weeks of delivery.
- You have had kidney disease, lung disease, anemia, nerve damage, or G6PD* deficiency (a metabolic deficiency).
- You have diabetes. Drug may affect urine sugar tests.

Over age 60:
Adverse reactions and side effects may be more frequent and severe than in younger persons.

Pregnancy:
Consult doctor. Risk category B (see page xviii).

Breast-feeding:
Drug passes into milk. Avoid drug or discontinue nursing until you finish medicine. Consult doctor for advice on maintaining milk supply.

Infants & children:
Don't give to infants younger than 1 month. Use only under medical supervision for older children.

Prolonged use:

- Chest pain, cough, shortness of breath.
- Talk to your doctor about the need for follow-up medical examinations or laboratory studies to check liver function, lung function.

Skin & sunlight:
No problems expected.

Driving, piloting or hazardous work:
Avoid if you feel dizzy or drowsy. Otherwise, no problems expected.

Discontinuing:
Don't discontinue without consulting doctor. Dose may require gradual reduction if you have taken drug for a long time. Doses of other drugs may also require adjustment.

Others:

- Periodic blood counts, liver function tests, and chest x-rays recommended.
- Advise any doctor or dentist whom you consult that you take this drug.

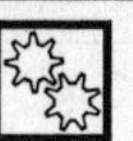

POSSIBLE INTERACTION WITH OTHER DRUGS

GENERIC NAME OR DRUG CLASS	COMBINED EFFECT
Antivirals, HIV/AIDS*	Increased risk of pancreatitis and peripheral neuropathy.
Hemolytics,* other	Increased risk of toxicity.
Nalidixic acid	Decreased nitrofurantoin effect.
Neurotoxic medicines*	Increased risk of damage to nerve cells.
Probenecid	Increased nitrofurantoin effect.
Sulfinpyrazone	Possible nitrofurantoin toxicity.

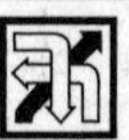

POSSIBLE INTERACTION WITH OTHER SUBSTANCES

INTERACTS WITH	COMBINED EFFECT
Alcohol:	Possible disulfiram reaction.* Avoid.
Beverages:	None expected.
Cocaine:	None expected.
Foods:	None expected.
Marijuana:	None expected.
Tobacco:	None expected.

***See Glossary**

NITROIMIDAZOLES

GENERIC AND BRAND NAMES

METRONIDAZOLE
- **Apo-Metronidazole**
- **Flagyl**
- **Helidac**
- **Metizol**
- **Metric 21**
- **Metro Cream**
- **MetroGel**
- **MetroGel-Vaginal**
- **Neo-Metric**
- **Noritate**

METRONIDAZOLE (con't)
- **Novonidazol**
- **PMS Metronidazole**
- **Protostat**
- **Pylera**
- **Satric**
- **Trikacide**
- **Vandazole**

TINIDAZOLE
- **Tindamax**

BASIC INFORMATION

Habit forming? No
Prescription needed? Yes
Available as generic? Yes, for some
Drug class: Antiprotozoal; antibacterial

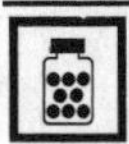

USES

- Treatment for parasitic infections (such as amebiasis, trichomoniasis or giardiasis).
- Treatment for certain bacterial infections.
- Treatment (combined with other drugs) for ulcer caused by *Helicobacter pylori* infection.
- Topical form treats acne rosacea.
- Vaginal forms treats vaginal infections.
- Other uses as determined by your doctor.

DOSAGE & USAGE INFORMATION

How to take:
- Tablet or capsule—Swallow with liquid. Take with food to lessen stomach irritation. The metronidazole tablet may be crushed and taken with food. Ask your pharmacist about crushing tinidazole tablet.
- Extended-release tablet—Swallow with liquid. Take with food to lessen stomach irritation. Do not crush or crumble tablet.
- Cream—Apply to affected area.
- Vaginal form—Follow instructions provided.

Continued next column

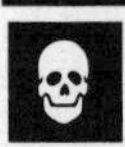

OVERDOSE

SYMPTOMS:
Weakness, nausea, vomiting, diarrhea, confusion, dizziness, numbness, seizures.
WHAT TO DO:
Overdose unlikely to threaten life. If person uses much larger amount than prescribed or if accidentally swallowed, call doctor or poison control center 1-800-222-1222 for help.

When to take:
- Oral form—At the same times each day.
- Topical cream—Apply twice a day.
- Vaginal cream, gel or tablet—Use as directed.

If you forget a dose:
Take as soon as you remember. If it is almost time for the next dose, wait for that dose (don't double this dose) and resume regular schedule.

What drug does:
Kills or stops the growth of protozoa or bacteria.

Time lapse before drug works:
Depends on the infection. May take one day or up to 14 days or longer for a complete cure.

Don't take with:
- Drugs (such as some cough remedies) or supplements containing alcohol.
- Any other medicine or any dietary supplement without consulting your doctor or pharmacist.

POSSIBLE ADVERSE REACTIONS OR SIDE EFFECTS

SYMPTOMS	WHAT TO DO
Life-threatening:	
Rare allergic reaction—Breathing difficulty; closing of the throat; swelling of hands, feet, face, lips or tongue; hives.	Discontinue. Seek emergency treatment.
Common:	
Appetite loss, nausea, stomach pain or cramps, diarrhea, vomiting, lightheaded, mild dizziness.	Continue. Call doctor when convenient.
Infrequent:	
• Metallic or bitter taste, dry mouth, headache.	Continue. Call doctor when convenient.
• Numbness, tingling, weakness or pain in hands or feet (peripheral neuropathy).	Discontinue. Call doctor right away.
• Dark urine (will go away after treatment).	No action necessary.
Rare:	
Unsteadiness or clumsiness, mood or mental changes, skin symptoms (rash, hives, redness, itching), sore throat and fever, seizures, severe stomach or back pain, unusual bleeding or bruising, vaginal irritation or dryness or discharge, changes in urination (painful, frequent, unable to control or decreased).	Discontinue. Call doctor right away.

WARNINGS & PRECAUTIONS

Don't take if:
You are allergic to nitroimidazoles or in the first trimester of pregnancy.

Before you start, consult your doctor if:
- You have seizure, nervous system, or brain disorder.
- You have a stomach or intestinal disorder.
- You have a blood disorder.
- You have liver, kidney or heart disease.
- You have a history of alcoholism.

Over age 60:
No special problems expected.

Pregnancy:
Decide with your doctor if drug benefits justify any possible risk to unborn child. The drugs are not recommended during the first trimester of pregnancy. Metronidazole is risk category B and tinidazole is category C (see page xviii).

Breast-feeding:
Drugs pass into milk. Avoid drug or discontinue nursing until you finish medicine. Consult doctor for advice on maintaining milk supply.

Infants & children:
May be used in children, but always under close medical supervision.

Prolonged use:
These drugs are not intended for long-term use.

Skin & sunlight:
No problems expected.

Driving, piloting or hazardous work:
Don't drive or pilot aircraft until you learn how medicine affects you. Don't work around dangerous machinery. Don't climb ladders or work in high places. Danger increases if you drink alcohol or take other medicines affecting alertness and reflexes.

Discontinuing:
Don't discontinue without doctor's advice until you complete prescribed dose, even though symptoms diminish or disappear.

Others:
- Advise any doctor or dentist whom you consult that you take this medicine. May affect results in some medical tests.
- Contact your doctor if symptoms do not improve in 24 to 48 hours.
- If you are being treated for trichomoniasis, your doctor may want your sexual partner treated at the same time (even if the person has no symptoms).
- These drugs may cause a yeast infection (oral or vaginal) to worsen. Contact your doctor if this occurs.

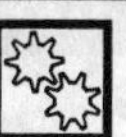

POSSIBLE INTERACTION WITH OTHER DRUGS

GENERIC NAME OR DRUG CLASS	COMBINED EFFECT
Anticoagulants,* oral	Increased anti-coagulant effect. (bleeding or bruising).
Antivirals, HIV/AIDS*	Increased risk of peripheral neuropathy.*
Cholestyramine	Decreased effect of nitroimidazole. Take several hours apart.
Cyclosporine	Increased cyclosporine effect.
Disulfiram	Disulfiram reaction.* Take 2 weeks apart.
Enzyme inducers*	Decreased effect of nitroimidazole.
Enzyme inhibitors*	Increased effect of nitroimidazole.
Fluorouracil	Increased risk of side effects.
Lithium	Increased lithium effect.
Neurotoxic medications*	Increased risk of side effects.
Oxytetracycline	Decreased metronidazole effect.
Phenytoin	Increased phenytoin effect. Decreased nitroimidazole effect.
Tacrolimus	Increased tacrolimus effect.

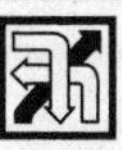

POSSIBLE INTERACTION WITH OTHER SUBSTANCES

INTERACTS WITH	COMBINED EFFECT
Alcohol:	Possible disulfiram reaction.* Avoid alcohol while taking drug and for 3 days after finishing.
Beverages:	None expected.
Cocaine:	Unknown. Avoid.
Foods:	None expected.
Marijuana:	Unknown. Avoid.
Tobacco:	None expected.

***See Glossary**

NON-NUCLEOSIDE REVERSE TRANSCRIPTASE INHIBITORS

GENERIC AND BRAND NAMES

DELAVIRDINE
Rescriptor
EFAVIRENZ
Sustiva
Atripla
ETRAVIRINE
Intelence
NEVIRAPINE
Viramune
Viramune XR
RILPIVIRINE
Complera
Edurant

BASIC INFORMATION

Habit forming? No
Prescription needed? Yes
Available as generic? No
Drug class: Antiviral, HIV and AIDS

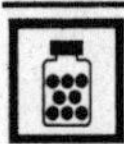

USES

For treatment of HIV and AIDS patients. Used in combination with one or more of the other AIDS drugs. May be used to prevent HIV transmission.

DOSAGE & USAGE INFORMATION

How to take:

- Oral suspension—Swallow with liquid.
- Tablet—Swallow with liquid. May be taken with or without food. Efavirenz should not be taken with a high fat meal.
- Extended-release tablet—Swallow whole with liquid. Do not crush, chew or divide tablet. May be taken with or without food.

When to take:
At the same time each day. At the start of treatment, one tablet is taken daily for 2 weeks and then increased to 2 tablets daily. This helps to decrease risk of side effects.

Continued next column

If you forget a dose:
Take as soon as you remember. If it is almost time for the next dose, wait for that dose (don't double this dose) and resume regular schedule.

What drug does:
Interferes with HIV replication. It helps slow the progress of HIV disease, but does not cure it.

Time lapse before drug works:
May require several weeks or months before full benefits are apparent.

Don't take with:
Any other medicine or any dietary supplement without consulting your doctor or pharmacist. This is very important with these antiviral drugs.

OVERDOSE

SYMPTOMS:
Swelling, extreme tiredness, fever, insomnia, rash, dizziness, vomiting, feeling of movement.
WHAT TO DO:
Overdose unlikely to threaten life. If person uses much larger amount than prescribed or if accidentally swallowed, call doctor or poison control center 1-800-222-1222 for help.

POSSIBLE ADVERSE REACTIONS OR SIDE EFFECTS

SYMPTOMS	WHAT TO DO
Life-threatening:	
Severe skin rash.	Discontinue. Call doctor right away or get emergency help.
Common:	
Mild to moderate skin rash, chills, fever, sore throat.	Discontinue. Call doctor right away.
Infrequent:	
• Fever, blistering skin, mouth sores, aching joints or muscles, eye inflammation, unusual tiredness.	Continue, but call doctor right away.
• Headache, nausea, diarrhea burning or tingling feeling, numbness, sleepiness, loss of appetite, constipation, mood or mental changes, intense dreams, anxiety, difficulty concentrating.	Continue. Call doctor when convenient.
Rare:	
• Yellow skin or eyes, dark urine, heart palpitations, thoughts of suicide.	Discontinue. Call doctor right away.
• Any other unusual symptoms that occur (may be due to the illness, this drug or other drugs being taken).	Continue, but call doctor right away.

NON-NUCLEOSIDE REVERSE TRANSCRIPTASE INHIBITORS

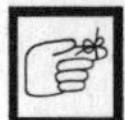

WARNINGS & PRECAUTIONS

Don't take if:
You are allergic to non-nucleoside reverse transcriptase inhibitors.

Before you start, consult your doctor if:
- You are allergic to any medicine, food or other substance, or have a family history of allergies.
- You have kidney or liver disease.

Over age 60:
Adverse reactions and side effects may be more frequent and severe than in younger persons.

Pregnancy:
- Decide with your doctor if drug benefits justify risk to unborn child. Risk category C (see page xviii).
- Efavirenz may cause fetal harm when used during the first trimester. Talk to your doctor about this risk.

Breast-feeding:
Drug passes into milk. Avoid drug or discontinue nursing until you finish medicine. Consult doctor for advice on maintaining milk supply.

Infants & children:
Safety and efficacy have not been established. Use only under close medical supervision.

Prolonged use:
Talk to your doctor about frequent blood counts and liver function studies.

Skin & sunlight:
No problems expected.

Driving, piloting or hazardous work:
Don't drive or pilot aircraft until you learn how medicine affects you. Don't work around dangerous machinery. Don't climb ladders or work in high places. Danger increases if you drink alcohol or take medicine affecting alertness and reflexes.

Discontinuing:
Don't discontinue without doctor's advice until you complete prescribed dose, even though symptoms diminish or disappear.

Others:
- Advise any doctor or dentist whom you consult that you take this medicine.
- Taking this drug does not prevent you from passing HIV to another person through sexual contact or sharing needles. Avoid sexual contact or practice safe sex (e.g., using condoms) to help prevent the transmission of HIV. Never share or re-use needles. If you have questions, ask your doctor for advice.
- Consult your doctor right away if you develop a new infection (e.g., fever, chills, sore throat or other symptoms).
- Do not increase or decrease dosage of drug without doctor's approval.

POSSIBLE INTERACTION WITH OTHER DRUGS

GENERIC NAME OR DRUG CLASS	COMBINED EFFECT
Amphetamines	May require dosage adjustment of amphetamine.
Antacids	Take 1-2 hours apart.
Benzodiazepines	May require dosage adjustment of benzodiazepine.
Calcium channel blockers	May require dosage adjustment of calcium channel blocker.
Carbamazepine	Decreased antiviral drug effect.
Clarithromycin	Interaction effects vary.
Contraceptives, oral*	Decreased contraceptive effect. Use alternative birth control method.
Didanosine	Take at least 1 hour apart.
Ergot preparations*	May require dosage adjustment of ergot drug.
Fluoxetine	Increased antiviral effect.
Histamine H_2 receptor antagonists	May require dosage adjustment of antiviral drug.

POSSIBLE INTERACTION WITH OTHER SUBSTANCES

INTERACTS WITH	COMBINED EFFECT
Alcohol:	None expected.
Beverages:	None expected.
Cocaine:	Unknown effect. Best to avoid.
Foods:	None expected.
Marijuana:	Unknown effect. Best to avoid.
Tobacco:	None expected.

***See Glossary**

NUCLEOSIDE REVERSE TRANSCRIPTASE INHIBITORS

GENERIC AND BRAND NAMES

ABACAVIR
- Epzicom
- Trizivir
- Ziagen

DIDANOSINE
- Videx
- Videx EC

EMTRICITABINE
- Atripla
- Complera
- Emtriva
- Stribild

LAMIVUDINE
- Combivir
- Epivir
- Epzicom
- Trizivir

STAVUDINE
- d4T
- Zerit

ZIDOVUDINE
- Apo-Zidovudine
- AZT
- Combivir
- Novo-AZT
- Retrovir
- Trizivir

BASIC INFORMATION

Habit forming? No
Prescription needed? Yes
Available as generic? Yes, for some
Drug class: Antiviral

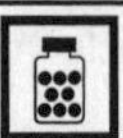

USES

Treats human immunodeficiency virus (HIV) and acquired immunodeficiency syndrome (AIDS).

DOSAGE & USAGE INFORMATION

How to take:
- Tablet or capsule—Swallow with water. Take with or without food as directed.
- Didanosine tablet—Chew or manually crumble tablet. If you crumble tablet, mix with at least 1 oz. of water. Swallow right away. Take 1 hour before or 2 hours after meal.

Continued next column

OVERDOSE

SYMPTOMS:
Seizures, severe nausea and vomiting, extreme tiredness or weakness, increase in bruising or bleeding, loss of coordination, involuntary eye movements.
WHAT TO DO:
- **Dial 911 (emergency) for medical help or call poison control center 1-800-222-1222 for instructions.**
- **See emergency information on last 3 pages of this book.**

- Syrup—Measure correct dosage with a specially marked measuring device.
- Buffered didanosine for oral solution—Follow instructions on label. Swallow immediately after mixing.

When to take:
At the same time each day, according to instructions on prescription label. Follow directions on label for taking with or without food.

If you forget a dose:
Take as soon as you remember. If it is almost time for the next dose, wait for that dose (don't double this dose) and resume regular schedule.

What drug does:
Suppresses replication of human immunodeficiency virus.

Time lapse before drug works:
Depends on the progress of the disease.

Don't take with:
Any other medicine or any dietary supplement without consulting your doctor or pharmacist.

POSSIBLE ADVERSE REACTIONS OR SIDE EFFECTS

SYMPTOMS	WHAT TO DO
Life-threatening:	
In case of overdose, see previous column.	
Common:	
• Tingling, numbness and burning in the feet and ankles (peripheral neuropathy).	Discontinue. Call doctor right away.
• Headache, anxiety, restlessness, digestive disturbances, diarrhea.	Continue. Call doctor when convenient.
Infrequent:	
• Unusual tiredness and weakness, fever, chills, sore throat, unusual bleeding or bruising, yellow skin and eyes, skin rash, pale skin, muscle or joint pain, mouth or throat sores, stomach pain, nausea and vomiting.	Discontinue. Call doctor right away.
• Lack of strength or energy, difficulty sleeping, discolored nails.	Continue. Call doctor when convenient.
Rare:	
Seizures, mood or mental changes, confusion.	Discontinue. Call doctor right away.

NUCLEOSIDE REVERSE TRANSCRIPTASE INHIBITORS

WARNINGS & PRECAUTIONS

Don't take if:
You are allergic to antivirals for HIV and AIDS.

Before you start, consult your doctor if:
- You have a history of alcoholism.
- You have hypertriglyceridemia, anemia, liver or kidney disease, gout, phenylketonuria, peripheral neuropathy or pancreatitis.
- You have a condition that limits sodium intake.
- A gene test is needed before starting abacavir.

Over age 60:
No special problems expected.

Pregnancy:
Risk factors vary for drugs in this group. See category list on page xviii and consult doctor.

Breast-feeding:
Unknown effects. Consult doctor.

Infants & children:
May cause depigmentation of the retina. Children should have eye exams every 3 to 6 months to check for vision changes.

Prolonged use:
Talk with your doctor about the need for follow-up medical examination or laboratory studies to check blood serum and uric acid levels.

Skin & sunlight:
No special problems expected.

Driving, piloting or hazardous work:
Don't drive or pilot aircraft until you learn how medicine affects you. Don't work around dangerous machinery. Don't climb ladders or work in high places. Danger increases if you drink alcohol or take medicine affecting alertness and reflexes.

Discontinuing:
Don't discontinue without consulting doctor. Dose may require gradual reduction if you have taken drug for a long time. Doses of other drugs may require adjustment.

Others:
- Advise any doctor or dentist whom you consult that you take this medicine.
- Taking this drug does not prevent you from passing HIV to another person through sexual contact or sharing needles. Avoid sexual contact or practice safe sex (e.g., using condoms) to help prevent the transmission of HIV. Never share or re-use needles. If you have questions, ask your doctor for advice.
- Consult your doctor right away if you develop a new infection (e.g., fever, chills, sore throat or other symptoms).
- Severe liver complications (non-cirrhotic portal hypertension) may occur with didanosine use. Consult doctor about your risks.
- Brand name Stribild contains four drugs. One is cobicistat which is not covered in this book.
- Do not increase or decrease dosage of drug without doctor's approval.

POSSIBLE INTERACTION WITH OTHER DRUGS

GENERIC NAME OR DRUG CLASS	COMBINED EFFECT
Bone marrow depressants,* other	Drugs may need dosage changes.
Cimetidine	Increased effect of zidovudine.
Clarithromycin	Decreased effect of zidovudine.
Dapsone	Increased risk of peripheral neuropathy. Decreased effect of both drugs.
Fluoroquinolones	Decreased fluoroquinolone effect.
Ganciclovir	Increased toxicity of both drugs. Use with caution.
Itraconazole	Decreased absorption of itraconazole.
Ketoconazole	Decreased effect of ketoconazole.
Pancreatitis-associated drugs*	Increased risk of pancreatitis with didanosine.
Peripheral neuropathy-associated drugs*	Increased risk of peripheral neuropathy.

Continued on page 923

POSSIBLE INTERACTION WITH OTHER SUBSTANCES

INTERACTS WITH	COMBINED EFFECT
Alcohol:	Risk of adverse effects. Avoid.
Beverages:	None expected.
Cocaine:	None expected.
Foods:	None expected.
Marijuana:	None expected.
Tobacco:	None expected.

***See Glossary**

NUCLEOTIDE REVERSE TRANSCRIPTASE INHIBITORS

GENERIC AND BRAND NAMES

TENOFOVIR

Atripla	**Truvada**
Complera	**Viread**
Stribild	

BASIC INFORMATION

Habit forming? No
Prescription needed? Yes
Available as generic? No
Drug class: Antiviral

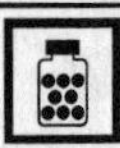

USES

- Treats human immunodeficiency virus (HIV) and acquired immunodeficiency syndrome (AIDS). Used in combination with other antiretroviral agents. Does not cure or prevent HIV or AIDS.
- Treatment of chronic hepatitis B.

DOSAGE & USAGE INFORMATION

How to take:
- Tablets—Swallow with water. Take with or without food as directed.
- Oral powder—Follow instructions for product.

When to take:
At the same time each day, according to instructions on prescription label.

If you forget a dose:
Take as soon as you remember. If it is almost time for the next dose, wait for next scheduled dose (don't double this dose).

What drug does:
Suppresses replication of human immunodeficiency virus.

Time lapse before drug works:
Depends on the progress of the disease.

Don't take with:
Any other medicine or any dietary supplement without consulting your doctor or pharmacist.

OVERDOSE

SYMPTOMS:
Unknown effects.
WHAT TO DO:
If person takes much larger amount than prescribed, dial 911 (emergency) for medical help or call poison control center 1-800-222-1222 for instructions.

POSSIBLE ADVERSE REACTIONS OR SIDE EFFECTS

SYMPTOMS	WHAT TO DO
Life-threatening:	
None expected.	
Common:	
Vomiting, lack or loss of strength.	Continue. Call doctor when convenient.
Infrequent:	
Gaseousness, weight loss, diarrhea.	Continue. Call doctor when convenient.
Rare:	
Breathing fast or shallow, shortness of breath, unusual tiredness, sleepiness, stomach discomfort, loss of appetite, muscle cramping or pain, overall feeling of discomfort, any unusual symptoms.	Continue, but call doctor right away.

NUCLEOTIDE REVERSE TRANSCRIPTASE INHIBITORS

WARNINGS & PRECAUTIONS

Don't take if:
You are allergic to tenofovir.

Before you start, consult your doctor if:
You have liver or kidney disease.

Over age 60:
Studies have not been done in this age group.

Pregnancy:
Consult your doctor. Risk category B (see page xviii).

Breast-feeding:
It is unknown if drug passes into milk. It is not recommended that HIV-infected mothers breast-feed if other options are available. Consult your doctor.

Infants & children:
Approved for use in children over age 2. Use only with close medical supervision.

Prolonged use:

- Talk with your doctor about the need for follow-up medical examination or laboratory studies to check drug's effectiveness.
- Long-term effects of this drug are unknown. Studies are ongoing.

Skin & sunlight:
No special problems expected.

Driving, piloting or hazardous work:
No problems expected.

Discontinuing:
Don't discontinue without consulting doctor.

Others:

- Advise any doctor or dentist whom you consult that you take this medicine.
- Taking this drug does not prevent you from passing HIV to another person through sexual contact or sharing needles. Avoid sexual contact or practice safe sex (e.g., using condoms) to help prevent the transmission of HIV. Never share or re-use needles. If you have questions, ask your doctor for advice.
- Consult your doctor right away if you develop a new infection (e.g., fever, chills, sore throat or other symptoms).
- Brand name Stribild contains four drugs. One is cobicistat which is not covered in this book.
- Do not increase or decrease dosage of drug without doctor's approval.

POSSIBLE INTERACTION WITH OTHER DRUGS

GENERIC NAME OR DRUG CLASS	COMBINED EFFECT
Antivirals for herpes virus	Increased effect of tenofovir.
Didanosine	Increased effect of didanosine. Take tenofovir 2 hours before or 1 hour after didanosine.

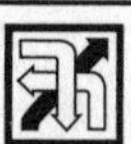

POSSIBLE INTERACTION WITH OTHER SUBSTANCES

INTERACTS WITH	COMBINED EFFECT
Alcohol:	None expected.
Beverages:	None expected.
Cocaine:	None expected. Best to avoid.
Foods:	None expected.
Marijuana:	None expected. Best to avoid.
Tobacco:	None expected.

NYSTATIN

BRAND NAMES

Dermacomb	Mykacet II
Myco II	Mytrex
Mycobiotic II	Nadostine
Mycogen II	Nilstat
Mycolog II	Nystaform
Mycostatin	Nystex
Myco-Triacet II	Tristatin II
Mykacet	

BASIC INFORMATION

Habit forming? No
Prescription needed? Yes
Available as generic? Yes
Drug class: Antifungal

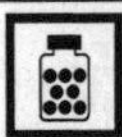

USES

Treatment of fungus infections of the mouth or vagina that are susceptible to nystatin.

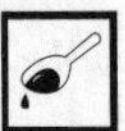

DOSAGE & USAGE INFORMATION

How to take:

- Tablet—Swallow with liquid. May take with or without food.
- Ointment, cream, lotion or powder—Use as directed by doctor and label.
- Liquid or powder for oral suspension—Take as directed. Instruction varies by preparation.
- Lozenge—Take as directed on label.

When to take:
At the same time each day.

If you forget a dose:
Take as soon as you remember. If it is almost time for the next dose, wait for that dose (don't double this dose) and resume regular schedule.

Continued next column

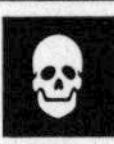

OVERDOSE

SYMPTOMS:
Mild overdose may cause nausea, vomiting, diarrhea.
WHAT TO DO:
Overdose unlikely to threaten life. If person uses much larger amount than prescribed or if accidentally swallowed, call doctor or poison control center 1-800-222-1222 for help.

What drug does:
Prevents growth and reproduction of fungus.

Time lapse before drug works:
Begins immediately. May require 3 weeks for maximum benefit, depending on location and severity of infection.

Don't take with:
Any other medicine or any dietary supplement without consulting your doctor or pharmacist.

POSSIBLE ADVERSE REACTIONS OR SIDE EFFECTS

SYMPTOMS	WHAT TO DO
Life-threatening: None expected.	
Common: (at high doses) Nausea, stomach pain, vomiting, diarrhea.	Discontinue. Call doctor right away.
Infrequent: Mild irritation, itch at application site.	Discontinue. Call doctor right away.
Rare: None expected.	

WARNINGS & PRECAUTIONS

Don't take if:
You are allergic to nystatin.

Before you start, consult your doctor if:
You plan to become pregnant within medication period.

Over age 60:
No problems expected.

Pregnancy:
No proven harm to unborn child. Avoid if possible. Consult doctor. Risk category B (see page xviii).

Breast-feeding:
No proven problems. Consult doctor.

Infants & children:
No problems expected.

Prolonged use:
No problems expected.

Skin & sunlight:
No problems expected.

Driving, piloting or hazardous work:
No problems expected.

Discontinuing:
Don't discontinue without doctor's advice until you complete prescribed dose, even though symptoms diminish or disappear.

Others:
No problems expected.

POSSIBLE INTERACTION WITH OTHER DRUGS

GENERIC NAME OR DRUG CLASS	COMBINED EFFECT
None reported.	

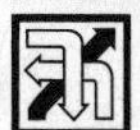

POSSIBLE INTERACTION WITH OTHER SUBSTANCES

INTERACTS WITH	COMBINED EFFECT
Alcohol:	None expected.
Beverages:	None expected.
Cocaine:	None expected.
Foods:	None expected.
Marijuana:	None expected.
Tobacco:	None expected.

OLANZAPINE

BRAND NAMES

Symbyax
Zyprexa
Zyprexa Relprevv
Zyprexa Zydis

BASIC INFORMATION

Habit forming? No
Prescription needed? Yes
Available as generic? Yes
Drug class: Antipsychotic

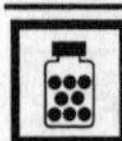

USES

- Treatment for symptoms of schizophrenia, acute mania and other psychotic disorders.
- Treatment for bipolar disorder.

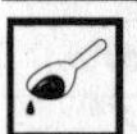

DOSAGE & USAGE INFORMATION

How to take:

- Tablet or capsule—Swallow with liquid. May be taken with or without food.
- Oral disintegrating tablet—Let tablet dissolve in mouth.
- Injection—Given by health care professional.

When to take:

- Oral—once a day at the same time each day.
- Injection—Given every 2 to 4 weeks. Must wait in medical office 3 hours after each dose.

If you forget a dose:
Take as soon as you remember. If it is almost time for the next dose, wait for the next scheduled dose (don't double this dose).

What drug does:
The exact mechanism is unknown. It appears to relieve symptoms by blocking certain nerve impulses between nerve cells.

Time lapse before drug works:
One to 7 days. Further increases in dosage may be needed to relieve symptoms in some patients.

Don't take with:
Any other medicine or any dietary supplement without consulting your doctor or pharmacist.

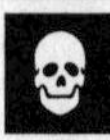

OVERDOSE

SYMPTOMS:
Drowsiness, slurred speech, rapid heartbeat, agitation, severe sweating, rigid muscles, breathing difficulty, stupor, seizures, coma.
WHAT TO DO:
If person takes much larger amount than prescribed, dial 911 (emergency) for medical help or call poison control center 1-800-222-1222 for instructions.

POSSIBLE ADVERSE REACTIONS OR SIDE EFFECTS

SYMPTOMS	WHAT TO DO
Life-threatening:	
High fever, rapid pulse, profuse sweating, muscle rigidity, confusion and irritability, seizures (rare neuroleptic malignant syndrome).	Discontinue. Seek emergency treatment.
Common:	
• Dizziness, difficulty in speaking or swallowing, shaking hands and fingers, trembling, vision problems, weakness, lightheadedness when arising from a sitting or lying position.	Continue. Call doctor right away.
• Drowsiness, constipation, weight gain, agitation, insomnia, headache, nervousness, runny nose, anxiety, dry mouth, arm or leg stiffness, injection site redness or swelling.	Continue. Call doctor when convenient.
Infrequent:	
• Jerky or involuntary movements (in face, lips, jaw, tongue), fast heartbeat, chest pain.	Continue. Call doctor right away.
• Fever, flu-like symptoms, twitching, mood or mental changes, speech unclear, swollen feet or ankles, appetite increased, cough, saliva increased, muscle tightness, muscle spasms (face, neck, back), joint pain, nausea, vomiting, sore throat, incontinence, abdominal pain.	Continue. Call doctor when convenient.
Rare:	
• New symptoms occur after drug injection.	Call doctor right away.
• Breathing difficulty, high blood sugar (thirstiness, frequent urination, increased hunger, weakness).	Discontinue. Call doctor right away.
• Swollen face, rash, confusion, decreased sex drive, menstrual changes, sluggishness.	Continue. Call doctor when convenient.

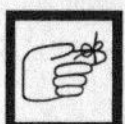

WARNINGS & PRECAUTIONS

Don't take if:
You are allergic to olanzapine.

Before you start, consult your doctor if:
- You have liver disease, heart disease, a blood vessel disorder or history of seizures.
- You have a history of breast cancer.
- You have intestinal blockage.
- You are subject to dehydration or low body temperature.
- You have a history of drug abuse/dependence.
- You have a family history of, are at risk for, or have diabetes.
- You have glaucoma or prostate problems.
- Patient has Alzheimer's.
- You are allergic to any medication, food or other substance.

Over age 60:
- Adverse reactions and side effects may be more severe than in younger persons. A lower starting dosage is usually recommended until a response is determined.
- Use of antipsychotic drugs in elderly patients with dementia-related psychosis may increase risk of death. Consult doctor.

Pregnancy:
Decide with your doctor if drug benefits justify any possible risk to unborn child. Risk category C (see page xviii).

Breast-feeding:
It is unknown if drug passes into milk. It is not recommended for nursing mothers.

Infants & children:
Not approved for ages under 18. If prescribed, carefully read information provided with prescription. Contact doctor right away if depression symptoms get worse or there is any talk of suicide or suicide behaviors. Also, read information under Others.

Prolonged use:
Consult with your doctor on a regular basis while taking this drug to check your progress or to discuss any increase or changes in side effects and the need for continued treatment.

Skin & sunlight:
May cause rash or intensify sunburn in areas exposed to sun or ultraviolet light (photosensitivity reaction). Use sunscreen and avoid over-exposure. Notify doctor if reaction occurs.

Driving, piloting or hazardous work:
Don't drive or pilot aircraft until you learn how medicine affects you. Don't work around dangerous machinery. Don't climb ladders or work in high places. Danger increases if you drink alcohol or take drug affecting alertness and reflexes.

Discontinuing:
Don't discontinue this drug without consulting doctor. Dosage may require a gradual reduction before stopping.

Others:
- Get up slowly from a sitting or lying position to avoid any dizziness or lightheadedness.
- Hot temperatures, exercise, and hot baths can increase risk of heatstroke. Drug may affect body's ability to maintain normal temperature.
- Advise any doctor or dentist whom you consult that you take this medicine.
- Take drug only as directed. Do not increase or reduce dosage without doctor's approval.
- Adults and children taking antidepressants may experience a worsening of the depression symptoms and may have increased suicidal thoughts or behaviors. Call doctor right away if these symptoms or behaviors occur.
- Injected form has risk of PDSS (post-injection delirium/sedation syndrome). Get medical help if severe drowsiness (may be unconscious or in a coma), confusion or disorientation occurs.

POSSIBLE INTERACTION WITH OTHER DRUGS

GENERIC NAME OR DRUG CLASS	COMBINED EFFECT
Anticholinergics,* other	Increased risk of side effects.
Antihypertensives*	Increased effect of antihypertensive.
Carbamazepine	Decreased effect of olanzapine.
Enzyme inducers*	May decrease olanzapine effect.
Enzyme inhibitors*	May increase olanzapine effect.

Continued on page 923

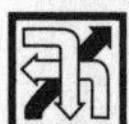

POSSIBLE INTERACTION WITH OTHER SUBSTANCES

INTERACTS WITH	COMBINED EFFECT
Alcohol:	Increased sedation and dizziness. Avoid.
Beverages:	None expected.
Cocaine:	Unknown. Avoid.
Foods:	None expected.
Marijuana:	Unknown. Avoid.
Tobacco:	Decreased olanzapine effect. Avoid.

***See Glossary**

OLSALAZINE

BRAND NAMES

Dipentum

BASIC INFORMATION

Habit forming? No
Prescription needed? Yes
Available as generic? No
Drug class: Inflammatory bowel disease suppressant

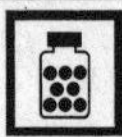

USES

- To maintain remission of ulcerative colitis. Generally prescribed when intolerance to sulfasalazine exists.
- Treatment for Crohn's disease.

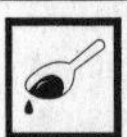

DOSAGE & USAGE INFORMATION

How to take:
Capsule—Swallow with liquid or food to lessen stomach irritation. If you can't swallow whole, open capsule and take with liquid or food.

When to take:
Usually twice a day, or as directed on prescription label.

If you forget a dose:
- Take as soon as possible.
- Skip if it is almost time for next dose.
- Don't double next dose.
- Notify your doctor if there are questions.

What drug does:
Inhibits prostaglandin production in the colon.

Time lapse before drug works:
1 hour.

Don't take with:
Any other medicine or any dietary supplement without consulting your doctor or pharmacist.

OVERDOSE

SYMPTOMS:
None expected.
WHAT TO DO:
Overdose unlikely to threaten life. If person uses much larger amount than prescribed or if accidentally swallowed, call doctor or poison control center 1-800-222-1222 for help.

POSSIBLE ADVERSE REACTIONS OR SIDE EFFECTS

SYMPTOMS	WHAT TO DO
Life-threatening:	
Fever, sore throat, paleness, unusual bleeding (representing effect on blood, a rare complication).	Seek emergency treatment.
Common:	
Diarrhea, appetite loss, nausea, vomiting.	Continue. Call doctor when convenient.
Infrequent:	
Mood changes, sleeplessness, headache.	Continue. Call doctor when convenient.
Rare:	
Skin eruption (acne-like), muscle aches.	Continue. Call doctor when convenient.

WARNINGS & PRECAUTIONS

Don't take if:

- You are allergic to olsalazine, aspirin or any other salicylate.
- You are allergic to mesalamine.

Before you start, consult your doctor if:

- You have kidney disease.
- You are taking any other prescription or nonprescription medicine.

Over age 60:
No special problems expected.

Pregnancy:
Decide with your doctor if drug benefits justify risk to unborn child. Risk category C (see page xviii).

Breast-feeding:
Unknown effects. Consult doctor.

Infants & children:
Effect not documented. Consult your family doctor or pediatrician.

Prolonged use:
Follow through with full prescribed course of treatment.

Skin & sunlight:
No special problems expected.

Driving, piloting or hazardous work:
Don't drive or pilot aircraft until you learn how medicine affects you. Don't work around dangerous machinery. Don't climb ladders or work in high places. Danger increases if you drink alcohol or take medicine affecting alertness and reflexes.

Discontinuing:
Don't discontinue without consulting doctor. Dose may require gradual reduction if you have taken drug for a long time. Doses of other drugs may also require adjustment.

Others:
Request your doctor to check blood counts and kidney function on a regular basis.

POSSIBLE INTERACTION WITH OTHER DRUGS

GENERIC NAME OR DRUG CLASS	COMBINED EFFECT
None expected since olsalazine is not appreciably absorbed from the gastrointestinal tract into the bloodstream.	

POSSIBLE INTERACTION WITH OTHER SUBSTANCES

INTERACTS WITH	COMBINED EFFECT
Alcohol:	Increased risk of gastrointestinal upset and/or bleeding.
Beverages: Highly spiced beverages.	Will irritate underlying condition that olsalazine treats.
Cocaine:	Avoid.
Foods: Highly spiced foods.	Will irritate underlying condition that olsalazine treats.
Marijuana:	Avoid.
Tobacco:	Will irritate underlying condition that olsalazine treats. Avoid.

OMEGA-3-ACID ETHYL ESTERS

BRAND NAMES

Lovaza | Vascepa

BASIC INFORMATION

Habit forming? No
Prescription needed? Yes
Available as generic? No
Drug class: Antihyperlipidemic

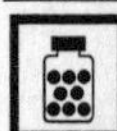

USES

- Helps to lower very high triglyceride (fat-like substance) levels in the blood. Its use is recommended in combination with an appropriate heart-healthy diet and exercise program.
- May be used for treatment of other disorders as determined by your doctor.

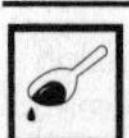

DOSAGE & USAGE INFORMATION

How to take:
Capsule—Swallow whole with liquid. It is advised that it be taken with food.

When to take:
It may be taken 1 to 2 times a day. Follow the instructions on your prescription.

If you forget a dose:
Take as soon as you remember. If it is almost time for the next dose, wait for next scheduled dose (don't double this dose).

What drug does:
Omega-3-acid ethyl esters are derived from fish oil. They help reduce the production of fatty substances (triglycerides) in the liver. The exact way they work is not completely understood. They may also increase the level of low-density lipoprotein (LDL) cholesterol. LDL is considered the "bad" cholesterol.

Time lapse before drug works:
About two months for measurable results as determined by laboratory testing.

Don't take with:
Any other medicine or any dietary supplement without consulting your doctor or pharmacist.

Continued next column

OVERDOSE

SYMPTOMS:
Exact symptoms are unknown.
WHAT TO DO:
Overdose unlikely to threaten life. If person uses much larger amount than prescribed or if accidentally swallowed, call doctor or poison control center 1-800-222-1222 for help.

POSSIBLE ADVERSE REACTIONS OR SIDE EFFECTS

SYMPTOMS	WHAT TO DO
Life-threatening:	
An allergic reaction is unlikely. Symptoms could include itching, difficulty breathing, chest tightness, closing of the throat, swelling of the lips or face or tongue, hives.	Seek emergency treatment immediately.
Common:	
Burping, infection, flu-like symptoms, upset stomach, taste changes, back pain.	Continue. Call doctor when convenient
Infrequent:	
Chest pain.	Discontinue. Call doctor right away.
Rare:	
None expected.	

WARNINGS & PRECAUTIONS

Don't take if:
You are allergic to any omega-3-acid ethyl esters, fish oil or fish.

Before you start, consult your doctor if:
- You have medical problems that may contribute to high triglycerides (e.g., diabetes or hypothyroidism).
- You take drugs such as beta blockers, estrogens or thiazide diuretics. They can be a risk factor for high triglycerides.
- You have liver disease.
- You have a blood clotting problem.
- You are obese.

Over age 60:
No special problems expected.

Pregnancy:
Decide with your doctor if drug benefits justify any possible risk to unborn child. Risk category C (see page xviii).

Breast-feeding:
It is unknown if drug passes into milk. Avoid drug or discontinue nursing until you finish medicine. Consult doctor for advice on maintaining milk supply.

Infants & children:
Safety and effectiveness in children has not been established. Consult your child's doctor.

Prolonged use:
No problems expected. Ask your doctor about routine laboratory studies to verify continued effectiveness of the drug therapy and to check your triglyceride levels.

Skin & sunlight:
No problems expected.

Driving, piloting or hazardous work:
No problems expected.

Discontinuing:
No problems expected.

Others:
- Follow your doctor's advice carefully regarding proper diet and an exercise program. Drugs such as this one are usually prescribed only when more help is needed.
- Consult your doctor about routine monitoring of LDL cholesterol levels to be sure they are not increasing excessively.
- Diabetic patients may experience worsening of blood sugar control.
- Advise any doctor or dentist whom you consult that you take this medicine.
- This drug was previously named Omacor. It was changed to Lovaza.

POSSIBLE INTERACTION WITH OTHER DRUGS

GENERIC NAME OR DRUG CLASS	COMBINED EFFECT
Anticoagulants, oral*	May increase anticoagulant effect. Consult doctor.

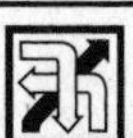

POSSIBLE INTERACTION WITH OTHER SUBSTANCES

INTERACTS WITH	COMBINED EFFECT
Alcohol:	None expected. Decreased alcohol intake is often recommended to help reduce triglyceride levels.
Beverages:	None expected.
Cocaine:	None expected. Best to avoid.
Foods:	None expected.
Marijuana:	None expected. Best to avoid.
Tobacco:	None expected. Smoking can contribute to high triglycerides.

*See Glossary

ORLISTAT

BRAND NAMES

Alli
Xenical

BASIC INFORMATION

Habit forming? No
Prescription needed? Yes, for Xenical
Available as generic? No
Drug class: Antiobesity; lipase inhibitor

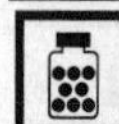

USES

- Treatment for obesity and weight loss. To be used in conjunction with a reduced-calorie diet. Treatment with this drug is not recommended for cosmetic weight loss.
- Used to delay onset of type 2 diabetes.

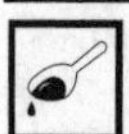

DOSAGE & USAGE INFORMATION

How to take:
Capsule—Swallow with liquid. If you can't swallow whole, open capsule and take with liquid.

When to take:
With or shortly following meals (containing fats) up to three times daily.

If you forget a dose:
Skip the missed dose and return to your regular dosing schedule. Do not double dose.

What drug does:
Blocks some of the normal absorption of fats from the intestines, causing them to be excreted in the feces.

Time lapse before drug works:
Several months or longer for maximum benefit.

Don't take with:
Any other medicine or any dietary supplement without consulting your doctor or pharmacist.

OVERDOSE

SYMPTOMS:
None expected.
WHAT TO DO:
Overdose unlikely to threaten life. If person uses much larger amount than prescribed or if accidentally swallowed, call doctor or poison control center 1-800-222-1222 for help.

POSSIBLE ADVERSE REACTIONS OR SIDE EFFECTS

SYMPTOMS	WHAT TO DO
Life-threatening: None expected.	
Common:	
• Flu-like symptoms, runny nose, congestion, sneezing, sore throat, cough, fever.	Continue. Call doctor when convenient.
• Abdominal pain, oily bowel movements, inability to hold bowel movements, immediate need to have bowel movements, gas with leaky bowel movements, oily spotting of underwear, headaches.	Continue. Call doctor if symptoms persist.
Infrequent:	
• Troubled breathing, tightness in chest, wheezing.	Discontinue. Call doctor right away.
• Anxiety, back pain, menstrual irregularities, rectal pain or discomfort, tooth or gum problems.	Continue. Call doctor if symptoms persist.
Rare:	
• Diarrhea, hearing changes, pain in ear, bloody or cloudy urine, difficult or painful urination, frequent urge to urinate, possible liver damage (itching, yellow skin or eyes, dark urine, appetite loss, light-colored stools).	Discontinue. Call doctor right away.
• Joint pain, dizziness, dry skin, fatigue, insomnia, muscle pain, nausea, skin rash, vomiting.	Continue. Call doctor if symptoms persist.

WARNINGS & PRECAUTIONS

Don't take if:
- You are allergic to orlistat.
- You have been diagnosed with malabsorption.
- You have cholestasis (blocked bile flow).

Before you start, consult your doctor if:
- You are allergic to any foods or dyes.
- You are taking any other medications or dietary supplements for weight loss.
- You have a history of anorexia or bulimia.
- You have any liver disorder, kidney stones or gallbladder problems.
- You are pregnant or are planning to become pregnant.

Over age 60:
Adverse reactions and side effects may be more frequent and severe than in younger persons.

Pregnancy:
Not recommended for use during pregnancy. Risk category B (see page xviii).

Breast-feeding:
It is unknown if orlistat passes into milk. Avoid drug or discontinue nursing until you finish medicine. Consult doctor for advice on maintaining milk supply.

Infants & children:
Not recommended for persons under age 12.

Prolonged use:
Talk to your doctor about the need for follow-up medical examinations or laboratory studies.

Skin & sunlight:
No problems expected.

Driving, piloting or hazardous work:
No special problems expected.

Discontinuing:
Don't discontinue without doctor's advice.

Others:
- Expect to start with small doses and increase gradually to lessen frequency and severity of adverse reactions.
- Orlistat may interfere with your body's absorption of certain vitamins; therefore, you should take a multivitamin supplement daily, two hours before or after taking orlistat.
- During treatment, you should be on a nutritionally balanced reduced-calorie diet that contains no more than 30 percent of calories from fat.
- Drug may affect the results of some medical tests.
- Severe liver injury has been reported rarely with the use of this drug. Discontinue drug and call doctor if you develop signs or symptoms of liver injury (see Rare under Possible Adverse Reactions or Side Effects).
- Patients with diabetes may require a reduced dosage of oral hypoglycemic medicine or insulin due to weight loss.
- Advise any doctor or dentist whom you consult that you take this medicine.

POSSIBLE INTERACTION WITH OTHER DRUGS

GENERIC NAME OR DRUG CLASS	COMBINED EFFECT
Cyclosporine	Unknown effect. Monitor closely.
Hepatotoxics*	Increased risk of liver injury.
Pravastatin	Increased pravastatin effect.
Vitamins A, D, E, K	Decreased vitamin effect.
Warfarin	Increased warfarin effect.

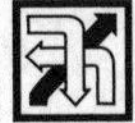

POSSIBLE INTERACTION WITH OTHER SUBSTANCES

INTERACTS WITH	COMBINED EFFECT
Alcohol:	None expected.
Beverages:	None expected.
Cocaine:	Effects unknown. Avoid.
Foods:	None expected.
Marijuana:	Effects unknown. Avoid.
Tobacco:	None expected.

*See Glossary

ORPHENADRINE

BRAND NAMES

Banflex
Blanex
Disipal
Flexagin
Flexain
Flexoject
Flexon
K-Flex
Marflex
Myolin
Myotrol
Neocyten
Noradex
Norflex
O-Flex
Orflagen
Orfro
Orphenate
Tega-Flex

BASIC INFORMATION

Habit forming? Possibly
Prescription needed?
U.S.: Yes
Canada: No
Available as generic? Yes
Drug class: Muscle relaxant, anticholinergic, antihistamine, antiparkinsonism

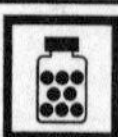

USES

- Reduces discomfort of muscle strain.
- Relieves symptoms of Parkinson's disease.
- Adjunctive treatment to rest, analgesics and physical therapy for muscle spasms.

DOSAGE & USAGE INFORMATION

How to take:
- Tablet—Swallow with liquid. If you can't swallow whole, crumble tablet and take with liquid or food.
- Extended-release tablet—Swallow whole. Do not crumble.

When to take:
At the same times each day.

Continued next column

OVERDOSE

SYMPTOMS:
Fainting, confusion, blurred vision, difficulty swallowing, difficulty breathing, decreased urination, widely dilated pupils, rapid heartbeat, rapid pulse, paralysis, convulsions, coma.
WHAT TO DO:
- **Dial 911 (emergency) for medical help or call poison control center 1-800-222-1222 for instructions.**
- **See emergency information on last 3 pages of this book.**

If you forget a dose:
Take as soon as you remember. If it is almost time for the next dose, wait for that dose (don't double this dose) and resume regular schedule.

What drug does:
Sedative and analgesic effects reduce spasm and pain in skeletal muscles.

Time lapse before drug works:
1 to 2 hours.

Don't take with:
Any other medicine or any dietary supplement without consulting your doctor or pharmacist.

POSSIBLE ADVERSE REACTIONS OR SIDE EFFECTS

SYMPTOMS	WHAT TO DO
Life-threatening:	
Extreme weakness; transient paralysis; temporary loss of vision; hives, rash, intense itching, faintness soon after a dose (anaphylaxis).	Seek emergency treatment immediately.
Common:	
None expected.	
Infrequent:	
• Weakness, headache, dizziness, agitation, drowsiness, tremor, confusion, rapid or pounding heartbeat, depression, hearing loss.	Discontinue. Call doctor right away.
• Dry mouth, nausea, vomiting, constipation, urinary hesitancy or retention, abdominal pain, muscle weakness.	Continue. Call doctor when convenient.
Rare:	
Rash, itchy skin, blurred vision, hallucinations.	Discontinue. Call doctor right away.

WARNINGS & PRECAUTIONS

Don't take if:
- You are allergic to orphenadrine.
- You are allergic to tartrazine dye.

Before you start, consult your doctor if:
- You have glaucoma.
- You have myasthenia gravis.
- You have difficulty emptying bladder.
- You have had heart disease or heart rhythm disturbance.
- You have had a peptic ulcer.
- You have prostate enlargement.

Over age 60:
Adverse reactions and side effects may be more frequent and severe than in younger persons.

Pregnancy:
Decide with your doctor if drug benefits justify risk to unborn child. Risk category C (see page xviii).

Breast-feeding:
It is unknown if drug passes into milk. Avoid drug or discontinue nursing until you finish medicine. Consult doctor for advice on maintaining milk supply.

Infants & children:
Not recommended for children younger than 12.

Prolonged use:

- Increased internal eye pressure.
- Talk to your doctor about the need for follow-up medical examinations or laboratory studies to check complete blood counts (white blood cell count, platelet count, red blood cell count, hemoglobin, hematocrit), liver function, kidney function.

Skin & sunlight:
No problems expected.

Driving, piloting or hazardous work:
Don't drive or pilot aircraft until you learn how medicine affects you. Don't work around dangerous machinery. Don't climb ladders or work in high places. Danger increases if you drink alcohol or take medicine affecting alertness and reflexes, such as antihistamines, tranquilizers, sedatives, pain medicine, narcotics and mind-altering drugs.

Discontinuing:
May be unnecessary to finish medicine. Follow doctor's instructions.

Others:
Advise any doctor or dentist whom you consult that you take this drug.

POSSIBLE INTERACTION WITH OTHER DRUGS

GENERIC NAME OR DRUG CLASS	COMBINED EFFECT
Anticholinergics*	Increased anticholinergic effect.
Antidepressants, tricyclic*	Increased sedation.
Antihistamines*	Increased sedation.
Attapulgite	Decreased orphenadrine effect.
Carteolol	Decreased antihistamine effect.
Chlorpromazine	Hypoglycemia (low blood sugar).
Cisapride	Decreased orphenadrine effect.
Contraceptives, oral*	Decreased contraceptive effect.
Griseofulvin	Decreased griseofulvin effect.
Levodopa	Increased levodopa effect. (Improves effectiveness in treating Parkinson's disease).
Nabilone	Greater depression of central nervous system.
Nitrates*	Increased internal eye pressure.
Nizatidine	Increased nizatidine effect.
Phenylbutazone	Decreased phenylbutazone effect.
Potassium supplements*	Increased possibility of intestinal ulcers with oral potassium tablets.
Propoxyphene	Possible confusion, nervousness, tremors.

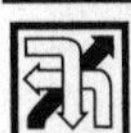

POSSIBLE INTERACTION WITH OTHER SUBSTANCES

INTERACTS WITH	COMBINED EFFECT
Alcohol:	Increased drowsiness. Avoid.
Beverages:	None expected.
Cocaine:	Decreased orphenadrine effect. Avoid.
Foods:	None expected.
Marijuana:	Increased drowsiness, mouth dryness, muscle weakness, fainting.
Tobacco:	None expected.

*See Glossary

ORPHENADRINE, ASPIRIN & CAFFEINE

BRAND NAMES

N3 Gesic
N3 Gesic Forte
Norgesic
Norgesic Forte
Norphadrine
Norphadrine Forte
Orphenagesic
Orphenagesic Forte

BASIC INFORMATION

Habit forming? Yes
Prescription needed? Yes
Available as generic? No
Drug class: Stimulant, vasoconstrictor, muscle relaxant, analgesic, anti-inflammatory (nonsteroidal)

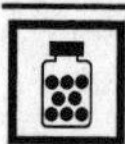

USES

- Reduces discomfort of muscle strain.
- Reduces pain, fever, inflammation.
- Relieves swelling, stiffness, joint pain.
- Treats drowsiness and fatigue.

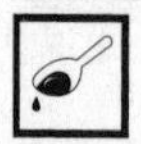

DOSAGE & USAGE INFORMATION

How to take:
Tablet—Swallow with liquid. If you can't swallow whole, crumble and take with liquid or food.

When to take:
At the same times each day.

If you forget a dose:
Take as soon as you remember. If it is almost time for the next dose, wait for that dose (don't double this dose) and resume regular schedule.

What drug does:
- Sedative and analgesic effects reduce spasm and pain in skeletal muscles.
- Affects hypothalamus, the part of the brain which regulates temperature by dilating small blood vessels in skin.

Continued next column

- Prevents clumping of platelets (small blood cells) so blood vessels remain open.
- Decreases prostaglandin effect.
- Suppresses body's pain messages.
- Constricts blood vessel walls.
- Stimulates central nervous system.

Time lapse before drug works:
1 hour.

Don't take with:
- Tetracyclines. Space doses 1 hour apart.
- Any other medicine or any dietary supplement without consulting your doctor or pharmacist.

OVERDOSE

SYMPTOMS:
Fainting, confusion, widely dilated pupils, rapid pulse, ringing in ears, nausea, vomiting, dizziness, fever, deep and rapid breathing, excitement, rapid heartbeat, hallucinations, coma.
WHAT TO DO:
- **Dial 911 (emergency) for medical help or call poison control center 1-800-222-1222 for instructions.**
- **See emergency information on last 3 pages of this book.**

POSSIBLE ADVERSE REACTIONS OR SIDE EFFECTS

SYMPTOMS	WHAT TO DO
Life-threatening:	
Hives, rash, intense itching, wheezing, faintness soon after a dose (anaphylaxis), convulsions, fever.	Seek emergency treatment immediately.
Common:	
• Nausea, vomiting, abdominal cramps, nervousness, urgent urination, low blood sugar (hunger, anxiety, cold sweats, rapid pulse).	Discontinue. Call doctor right away.
• Ringing in ears, indigestion, heart-burn, insomnia.	Continue. Call doctor when convenient.
Infrequent:	
• Weakness, headache, dizziness, drowsiness, agitation, tremor, confusion, irregular heartbeat, hearing loss, diarrhea, hallucinations.	Discontinue. Call doctor right away.
• Dry mouth, constipation.	Continue. Call doctor when convenient.
Rare:	
• Black or bloody vomit.	Discontinue. Seek emergency treatment.
• Change in vision; blurred vision; black, bloody or tarry stool; bloody urine; dilated pupils; uncontrolled movement of hands; sore throat; fever.	Discontinue. Call doctor right away.

WARNINGS & PRECAUTIONS

Don't take if:

- You need to restrict sodium in your diet. Buffered effervescent tablets and sodium salicylate are high in sodium.
- Aspirin has a strong vinegar-like odor, which means it has decomposed.
- You have a peptic ulcer of stomach or duodenum, a bleeding disorder, heart disease.
- You are allergic to any stimulant, aspirin or orphenadrine.

Before you start, consult your doctor if:

- You have had stomach or duodenal ulcers, gout, heart disease or heart rhythm disturbance, peptic ulcer.
- You have asthma, nasal polyps, irregular heartbeat, hypoglycemia (low blood sugar), epilepsy, glaucoma, myasthenia gravis, difficulty emptying bladder, prostate enlargement.

Over age 60:

- More likely to cause hidden bleeding in stomach or intestines. Watch for dark stools.
- Adverse reactions and side effects may be more frequent and severe than in younger persons.

Pregnancy:
Risk to unborn child outweighs drug benefits. Don't use. Risk category D (see page xviii).

Breast-feeding:
Drug passes into milk. Avoid drug or discontinue nursing until you finish medicine. Consult doctor for advice on maintaining milk supply.

Infants & children:

- Overdose frequent and severe. Keep bottles out of children's reach.
- Consult doctor before giving to persons under age 18 who have fever and discomfort of viral illness, especially chicken pox and influenza. Probably increases risk of Reye's syndrome.
- Not recommended for children under 12.

Prolonged use:

- Kidney damage. Periodic kidney function test recommended.
- Stomach ulcers more likely.
- Increased internal eye pressure.
- Talk to your doctor about the need for follow-up medical examinations or laboratory studies to check liver function, complete blood counts (white blood cell count, platelet count, red blood cell count, hemoglobin, hematocrit).

Skin & sunlight:
No special problems expected.

Driving, piloting or hazardous work:
Don't drive or pilot aircraft until you learn how medicine affects you. Don't work around dangerous machinery. Don't climb ladders or work in high places. Danger increases if you drink alcohol or take medicine affecting alertness and reflexes, such as antihistamines, tranquilizers, sedatives, pain medicine, narcotics and mind-altering drugs.

Discontinuing:

- For chronic illness—Don't discontinue without doctor's advice until you complete prescribed dose, even though symptoms diminish or disappear.
- May be unnecessary to finish medicine if you take it for a short-term illness. Follow doctor's instructions.

Others:

- Aspirin can complicate surgery, illness, pregnancy, labor and delivery.
- For arthritis, don't change dose without consulting doctor.
- May produce or aggravate fibrocystic breast disease in women.

POSSIBLE INTERACTION WITH OTHER DRUGS

GENERIC NAME OR DRUG CLASS	COMBINED EFFECT
Acebutolol	Decreased antihypertensive effect of acebutolol.

Continued on page 923

POSSIBLE INTERACTION WITH OTHER SUBSTANCES

INTERACTS WITH	COMBINED EFFECT
Alcohol:	Possible stomach irritation and bleeding, increased drowsiness. Avoid.
Beverages: Caffeine drinks.	Increased caffeine effect.
Cocaine:	Decreased orphenadrine effect. Overstimulation. Avoid.
Foods:	None expected.
Marijuana:	Increased effect of drugs. May lead to dangerous, rapid heartbeat. Increased dry mouth. Avoid.
Tobacco:	Increased heartbeat. Avoid.

OXCARBAZEPINE

BRAND NAMES

Oxtellar XR
Trileptal

BASIC INFORMATION

Habit forming? No
Prescription needed? Yes
Available as generic? Yes
Drug class: Anticonvulsant, antiepileptic

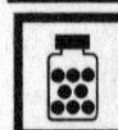

USES

- Treatment for partial (focal) epileptic seizures. May be used alone or in combination with other antiepileptic drugs.
- Other uses as determined by your doctor.

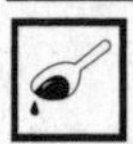

DOSAGE & USAGE INFORMATION

How to take:
- Tablet—Swallow with liquid. May be taken with or without food.
- Oral suspension—Follow product instructions.
- Extended-release tablet—Swallow whole with liquid. Take on an empty stomach. Do not chew, crush or split tablet.

When to take:
Your doctor will determine the best schedule. Dosages will be increased rapidly over the first few days of use. Further increases may be necessary to achieve maximum benefits.

If you forget a dose:
Take as soon as you remember. If it is almost time for the next dose, wait for that dose (don't double this dose) and resume regular schedule.

What drug does:
The exact mechanism is unknown, but it helps decrease abnormal electrical activity in the brain.

Time lapse before drug works:
May take several weeks for effectiveness.

Don't take with:
Any other medicine or any dietary supplement without consulting your doctor or pharmacist.

OVERDOSE

SYMPTOMS:
Double vision, slurred speech, drowsiness, tiredness, diarrhea.
WHAT TO DO:
Overdose unlikely to threaten life. If person uses much larger amount than prescribed or if accidentally swallowed, call doctor or poison control center 1-800-222-1222 for help.

POSSIBLE ADVERSE REACTIONS OR SIDE EFFECTS

SYMPTOMS	WHAT TO DO
Life-threatening:	
Severe skin reaction.	Seek emergency help.
Common:	
• Cough with fever and sneezing and sore throat, clumsiness, vision changes, dizziness, crying, depression, false sense of well-being, spinning sensation, uncontrolled eye movement, feeling of constant movement of self or surroundings.	Continue, but call doctor right away.
• Runny or stuffy nose, nausea or vomiting, sleepiness.	Continue. Call doctor when convenient.
Infrequent:	
• Blurred vision, cloudy or bloody urine, urination changes (decreased or increased, painful, urgent), confusion, falling, bruising, ill feeling, thirstiness, hoarseness, vaginal itching, heartbeat irregularities, facial pain, memory loss, coordination problems, trembling, shortness of breath, unusual tiredness or weakness.	Continue, but call doctor right away.
• Sour stomach, acne, changes in taste, dry mouth, constipation or diarrhea, heartburn, sweating, feeling of warmth in face or chest, back pain, belching, bloody nose.	Continue. Call doctor when convenient.
Rare:	
Sore or bleeding lips, chills, chest pain, irritability, hives or itching, muscle or joint pain, nervousness, rectal bleeding, peeling or blistering skin, sores in mouth, swollen legs, purple spots on skin, burning feeling in chest or stomach.	Continue, but call, doctor right away.

WARNINGS & PRECAUTIONS

Don't take if:
You are allergic to oxcarbazepine or carbamazepine.

Before you start, consult your doctor if:
- You have a history of kidney or liver disease.
- You have hyponatremia (too little sodium in the body).
- You are allergic to any medication, food or other substance.
- You have any other medical problems.

Over age 60:
No special problems expected.

Pregnancy:
Decide with your doctor if drug benefits justify risks to unborn child. Risk category C (see page xviii).

Breast-feeding:
Drug passes into milk. Avoid drug or discontinue nursing until you finish medicine. Consult doctor for advice on maintaining milk supply.

Infants & children:
Approved for children over age two (when drug used with other anticonvulsants) and over age four (drug may be used alone).

Prolonged use:
No special problems expected. Follow-up laboratory blood studies may be recommended by your doctor.

Skin & sunlight:
No problems expected.

Driving, piloting or hazardous work:
Don't drive or pilot aircraft until you learn how medicine affects you. Don't work around dangerous machinery. Don't climb ladders or work in high places. Danger increases if you drink alcohol or take other medicines affecting alertness and reflexes such as antihistamines, tranquilizers, sedatives, pain medicine, narcotics and mind-altering drugs.

Discontinuing:
Don't discontinue without doctor's approval due to risk of increased seizure activity. The dosage may need to be gradually decreased before stopping the drug completely.

Others:
- Advise any doctor or dentist whom you consult that you take this medicine.
- The effectiveness of oral contraceptives that contain estrogen may be reduced. Talk to your doctor about other forms of birth control.
- Oxcarbazepine may be used with other anticonvulsant drugs and additional side effects may occur. If they do, discuss them with your doctor.
- There is a small risk of life threatening skin reactions while taking this drug. If you develop an allergic reaction or a skin rash, contact your doctor right away.
- This medicine alone may cause drowsiness, dizziness, or lightheadedness, especially when getting up from a sitting or lying position.
- Rarely, antiepileptic drugs may lead to suicidal thoughts and behaviors. Call doctor right away if suicidal symptoms or unusual behaviors occur.
- Wear or carry medical identification to show your seizure disorder and the drugs you take.

POSSIBLE INTERACTION WITH OTHER DRUGS

GENERIC NAME OR DRUG CLASS	COMBINED EFFECT
Anticonvulsants,* other	Increased risk of side effects.
CNS Depressants*	Increased sedative effect.
Contraceptives, oral*	Decreased effect of contraceptive.
Felodipine	Decreased effect of felodipine.
Verapamil	Decreased effect of oxcarbazepine.

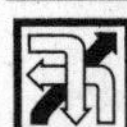

POSSIBLE INTERACTION WITH OTHER SUBSTANCES

INTERACTS WITH	COMBINED EFFECT
Alcohol:	Increased sedative effect. Avoid.
Beverages:	None expected.
Cocaine:	Unknown effect. Avoid.
Foods:	None expected.
Marijuana:	Unknown effect. Avoid.
Tobacco:	None expected.

*See Glossary

OXYMETAZOLINE (Nasal)

BRAND NAMES

See full list of brand names in the *Generic and Brand Name Directory*, page 891.

BASIC INFORMATION

Habit forming? No
Prescription needed? No
Available as generic? Yes
Drug class: Sympathomimetic

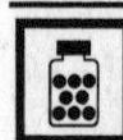

USES

Relieves congestion of nose, sinuses and throat from allergies and infections.

DOSAGE & USAGE INFORMATION

How to take:
Nasal solution, nasal spray—Use as directed on label. Avoid contamination. Don't use same container for more than 1 person.

When to take:
When needed, no more often than every 4 hours.

If you forget a dose:
Use as soon as you remember. Wait 4 hours for next dose.

What drug does:
Constricts walls of small arteries in nose, sinuses and eustachian tubes.

Time lapse before drug works:
5 to 30 minutes. May last 8 to 12 hours.

Continued next column

OVERDOSE

SYMPTOMS:
Headache, sweating, anxiety, agitation, rapid and irregular heartbeat (rare occurrence with systemic absorption) or if child accidentally swallows.
WHAT TO DO:
- **Dial 911 (emergency) for medical help or call poison control center 1-800-222-1222 for instructions.**
- **If person is unconscious, check breathing and pulse. If not breathing, begin mouth-to-mouth rescue breathing. If heart is not beating, begin chest compressions.**
- **See emergency information on last 3 pages of this book.**

Don't take with:
- Nonprescription drugs for allergy, cough or cold without consulting doctor.
- Any other medicine or any dietary supplement without consulting your doctor or pharmacist.

POSSIBLE ADVERSE REACTIONS OR SIDE EFFECTS

SYMPTOMS	WHAT TO DO
Life-threatening: In case of overdose, see previous column.	
Common: None expected.	
Infrequent:	
Burning, dry or stinging nasal passages.	Continue. Call doctor when convenient.
Rare:	
Rebound congestion (increased runny or stuffy nose), headache, insomnia, nervousness (may occur with systemic absorption).	Discontinue. Call doctor right away.

WARNINGS & PRECAUTIONS

Don't take if:
You are allergic to oxymetazoline or other nasal spray.

Before you start, consult your doctor if:
- You have heart disease or high blood pressure.
- You have diabetes.
- You have overactive thyroid.
- You have taken MAO inhibitors in past 2 weeks.
- You have glaucoma.

Over age 60:
Adverse reactions and side effects may be more frequent and severe than in younger persons.

Pregnancy:
Consult doctor. Risk category C (see page xviii).

Breast-feeding:
No proven problems. Consult doctor.

Infants & children:
Don't give to children younger than 2.

Prolonged use:
Drug may lose effectiveness, cause increased congestion (rebound effect*) and irritate nasal membranes.

Skin & sunlight:
No problems expected.

Driving, piloting or hazardous work:
No problems expected.

Discontinuing:
May be unnecessary to finish medicine. Follow doctor's instructions.

Others:
- Don't use for more than 3 days in a row.
- Keep product out of the reach of children.

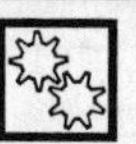

POSSIBLE INTERACTION WITH OTHER DRUGS

GENERIC NAME OR DRUG CLASS	COMBINED EFFECT
Antidepressants, tricyclic*	Possible rise in blood pressure.
Butorphanol	Delays start of butorphanol effect.
Maprotiline	Possible increased blood pressure.

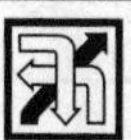

POSSIBLE INTERACTION WITH OTHER SUBSTANCES

INTERACTS WITH	COMBINED EFFECT
Alcohol:	None expected.
Beverages: Caffeine drinks.	Nervousness or insomnia.
Cocaine:	High risk of heartbeat irregularities and high blood pressure.
Foods:	None expected.
Marijuana:	Overstimulation. Avoid.
Tobacco:	None expected.

*See Glossary

PACLITAXEL

BRAND NAMES

Abraxane
Taxol

BASIC INFORMATION

Habit forming? No
Prescription needed? Yes
Available as generic? Yes
Drug class: Antineoplastic

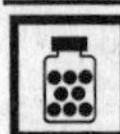

USES

Treats ovarian cancer, breast cancer and some lung cancers.

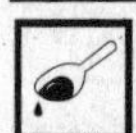

DOSAGE & USAGE INFORMATION

How to take:
Injection—Administered only by a doctor or under the supervision of a doctor.

When to take:
Your doctor will determine the schedule. Usually the drug is infused over a 24-hour period at 21-day intervals. Other drugs may be given prior to paclitaxel injection to help prevent adverse effects.

If you forget a dose:
Not a concern since drug is administered by a doctor.

What drug does:
Interferes with the growth of cancer cells, which are eventually destroyed.

Time lapse before drug works:
Results may not show for several weeks or months.

Don't take with:
Any other medicine or any dietary supplement without consulting your doctor or pharmacist.

OVERDOSE

SYMPTOMS:
None expected.
WHAT TO DO:
Overdose is unlikely. You will be monitored by medical personnel during the time of the infusion.

POSSIBLE ADVERSE REACTIONS OR SIDE EFFECTS

SYMPTOMS	WHAT TO DO
Life-threatening:	
Anaphylactic reaction soon after an injection (hives, rash, intense itching, faintness, breathing difficulty).	Emergency care will be provided.
Common:	
• Paleness, tiredness, flushing of face, skin rash or itching, shortness of breath, fever, chills, cough or hoarseness, back or side pain, difficult or painful urination, unusual bleeding or bruising, black or tarry stools, blood in stool or urine, pinpoint red spots on skin, bleeding gums, delayed wound healing.	Call doctor right away.
• Pain in joints or muscles; diarrhea; nausea and vomiting; numbness, burning or tingling in hands or feet.	Call doctor when convenient.
• Loss of hair (should regrow after treatment completed).	No action necessary.
Infrequent:	
Heart rhythm disturbances, chest pain.	Call doctor right away.
Rare:	
Pain or redness at injection site; mouth or lip sores.	Call doctor right away.

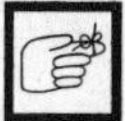

WARNINGS & PRECAUTIONS

Don't take if:
You are allergic to paclitaxel.

Before you start, consult your doctor if:
- You have an infection or any other medical problem.
- You have or recently had chickenpox or herpes zoster (shingles).
- You have heart problems.
- You are pregnant or if you plan to become pregnant.
- You have had radiation therapy or previously taken anticancer drugs.

Over age 60:
No problems expected.

Pregnancy:
Discuss with your doctor whether drug benefits justify risk to unborn child. Risk category D (see page xviii).

Breast-feeding:
Not known if drug passes into milk. Avoid drug or discontinue nursing until you finish medicine. Consult doctor for advice on maintaining milk supply.

Infants & children:
Safety and effectiveness of use in children not established.

Prolonged use:
Not recommended for long-term use.

Skin & sunlight:
No problems expected.

Driving, piloting or hazardous work:
Avoid if you feel side effects such as nausea and vomiting.

Discontinuing:
Your doctor will determine the schedule.

Others:
- Advise any doctor or dentist whom you consult that you take this medicine.
- May affect the results in some medical tests.
- Do not have any immunizations (vaccinations) without doctor's approval. Other household members should not take oral polio vaccine. It could pass the polio virus on to you. Avoid any contact with persons who have taken oral polio vaccine.
- Possible delayed effects (including some types of cancers) may occur months to years after use. Your doctor should discuss with you all risks involving this drug.
- You will have increased risk of infections. Take extra precautions (handwashing), and avoid people with infections. Avoid crowds if possible. Contact your doctor immediately if you develop signs or symptoms of infection.
- Use care in the use of toothbrushes, dental floss and toothpicks. Talk to your medical doctor before you have dental work done.
- Do not touch your eyes or the inside of your nose without carefully washing your hands first.
- Avoid activities (e.g., contact sports) that could cause bruising or injury.
- Avoid cutting yourself when using a safety razor, fingernail or toenail clippers.

POSSIBLE INTERACTION WITH OTHER DRUGS

GENERIC NAME OR DRUG CLASS	COMBINED EFFECT
Blood dyscrasia-causing medicines*	Increased risk of paclitaxel toxicity.
Bone marrow depressants,* (other)	Increased risk of paclitaxel toxicity.

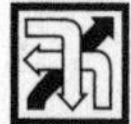

POSSIBLE INTERACTION WITH OTHER SUBSTANCES

INTERACTS WITH	COMBINED EFFECT
Alcohol:	None expected.
Beverages:	None expected.
Cocaine:	None expected.
Foods:	None expected.
Marijuana:	None expected.
Tobacco:	None expected.

***See Glossary**

PANCRELIPASE

BRAND NAMES

Creon
Pancreaze
Pertyze
Ultresa
Viokace
Zenpep

BASIC INFORMATION

Habit forming? No
Prescription needed? Yes
Available as generic? Yes
Drug class: Enzyme (pancreatic)

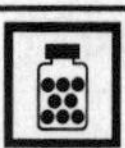

USES

- Replaces pancreatic enzymes lost due to surgery or disease.
- Treats fatty stools (steatorrhea).

DOSAGE & USAGE INFORMATION

How to take:

- Tablet, capsule or delayed-release capsule—Swallow whole. Do not take with milk or milk products.
- Powder—Sprinkle on liquid or soft food.

When to take:
Before meals.

If you forget a dose:
Take as soon as you remember. If it is almost time for the next dose, wait for that dose (don't double this dose) and resume regular schedule.

What drug does:
Enhances digestion of proteins, carbohydrates and fats.

Time lapse before drug works:
30 minutes.

Don't take with:
Any other medicine or any dietary supplement without consulting your doctor or pharmacist.

OVERDOSE

SYMPTOMS:
Shortness of breath, wheezing, diarrhea.
WHAT TO DO:
Overdose unlikely to threaten life. If person uses much larger amount than prescribed or if accidentally swallowed, call doctor or poison control center 1-800-222-1222 for help.

POSSIBLE ADVERSE REACTIONS OR SIDE EFFECTS

SYMPTOMS	WHAT TO DO
Life-threatening: None expected.	
Common: None expected.	
Infrequent: Diarrhea, asthma.	Discontinue. Call doctor right away.
Rare:	
• Rash, hives, blood in urine, swollen feet or legs, abdominal cramps.	Discontinue. Call doctor right away.
• Nausea, joint pain.	Continue. Call doctor when convenient.

WARNINGS & PRECAUTIONS

Don't take if:
You are allergic to pancreatin, pancrelipase, or pork.

Before you start, consult your doctor if:
You take any other medicines.

Over age 60:
Adverse reactions and side effects may be more frequent and severe than in younger persons.

Pregnancy:
Decide with your doctor if drug benefits justify risk to unborn child. Risk category C (see page xviii).

Breast-feeding:
Drug may pass into milk. Avoid drug or discontinue nursing until you finish medicine. Consult doctor for advice on maintaining milk supply.

Infants & children:
Give under close medical supervision only.

Prolonged use:
No additional problems expected.

Skin & sunlight:
No problems expected.

Driving, piloting or hazardous work:
No problems expected.

Discontinuing:
Don't discontinue without consulting doctor. Dose may require gradual reduction if you have taken drug for a long time. Doses of other drugs may also require adjustment.

Others:
- If you take powder form, avoid inhaling.
- Advise any doctor or dentist whom you consult that you take this medicine.

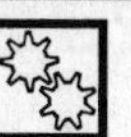

POSSIBLE INTERACTION WITH OTHER DRUGS

GENERIC NAME OR DRUG CLASS	COMBINED EFFECT
Calcium carbonate antacids*	Decreased effect of pancrelipase.
Iron supplements	Decreased iron absorption.
Magnesium hydroxide antacids*	Decreased effect of pancrelipase.

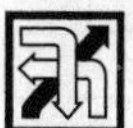

POSSIBLE INTERACTION WITH OTHER SUBSTANCES

INTERACTS WITH	COMBINED EFFECT
Alcohol:	Unknown.
Beverages: Milk.	Decreased effect of pancrelipase.
Cocaine:	Unknown.
Foods: Ice cream, milk products.	Decreased effect of pancrelipase.
Marijuana:	Decreased absorption of pancrelipase.
Tobacco:	Decreased absorption of pancrelipase.

***See Glossary**

PANTOTHENIC ACID (Vitamin B-5)

GENERIC AND BRAND NAMES

CALCIUM PANTOTHENATE — **Dexol T.D.**

Numerous brands of single vitamin and multivitamin combinations may be available.

BASIC INFORMATION

Habit forming? No
Prescription needed? No
Available as generic? Yes
Drug class: Vitamin supplement

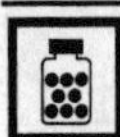

USES

Prevents and treats vitamin B-5 deficiency.

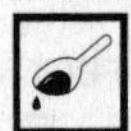

DOSAGE & USAGE INFORMATION

How to take:
Tablet—Swallow with liquid.

When to take:
At the same times each day.

If you forget a dose:
Take as soon as you remember, then resume regular schedule.

What drug does:
Acts as co-enzyme in carbohydrate, protein and fat metabolism.

Time lapse before drug works:
15 to 20 minutes.

Don't take with:
- Levodopa—Small amounts of pantothenic acid will nullify levodopa effect. Carbidopa-levodopa combination not affected by this interaction.
- Any other medicine or any dietary supplement without consulting your doctor or pharmacist.

OVERDOSE

SYMPTOMS:
None expected.
WHAT TO DO:
Overdose unlikely to threaten life. If person uses much larger amount than prescribed or if accidentally swallowed, call doctor or poison control center 1-800-222-1222 for help.

POSSIBLE ADVERSE REACTIONS OR SIDE EFFECTS

SYMPTOMS	WHAT TO DO
Life-threatening: None expected.	
Common: Heartburn.	Discontinue. Call doctor when convenient.
Infrequent: Cramps.	Discontinue. Call doctor when convenient.
Rare: Rash, hives, difficult breathing.	Discontinue. Seek emergency treatment.

PANTOTHENIC ACID (Vitamin B-5)

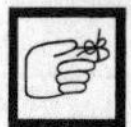

WARNINGS & PRECAUTIONS

Don't take if:
You are allergic to pantothenic acid.

Before you start, consult your doctor if:
You have hemophilia.

Over age 60:
No problems expected.

Pregnancy:
Risk factor not designated. See category list on page xviii and consult doctor.

Breast-feeding:
Don't exceed recommended dose. Consult doctor.

Infants & children:
Don't exceed recommended dose.

Prolonged use:
Large doses for more than 1 month may cause toxicity.

Skin & sunlight:
No problems expected.

Driving, piloting or hazardous work:
No problems expected.

Discontinuing:
No problems expected.

Others:
Regular pantothenic acid supplements are recommended if you take chloramphenicol, cycloserine, ethionamide, hydralazine, immunosuppressants,* isoniazid or penicillamine. These decrease pantothenic acid absorption and can cause anemia or tingling and numbness in hands and feet.

POSSIBLE INTERACTION WITH OTHER DRUGS

GENERIC NAME OR DRUG CLASS	COMBINED EFFECT
None significant.	

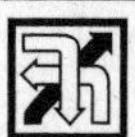

POSSIBLE INTERACTION WITH OTHER SUBSTANCES

INTERACTS WITH	COMBINED EFFECT
Alcohol:	None expected.
Beverages:	None expected.
Cocaine:	None expected.
Foods:	None expected.
Marijuana:	None expected.
Tobacco:	May decrease pantothenic acid absorption. Decreased pantothenic acid effect.

*See Glossary

PAPAVERINE

BRAND NAMES

Cerespan
Genabid
Pavabid
Pavabid Plateau Caps
Pavacot
Pavagen
Pavarine
Pavased
Pavatine
Pavatym
Paverolan

BASIC INFORMATION

Habit forming? No
Prescription needed? Yes
Available as generic? Yes
Drug class: Vasodilator

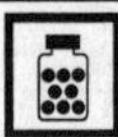

USES

- May improve circulation in the extremities or brain.
- Injected into penis to produce erections.

DOSAGE & USAGE INFORMATION

How to take:
- Tablet—Swallow with liquid or food to lessen stomach irritation. If you can't swallow whole, crumble tablet and take with liquid or food.
- Extended-release capsule—Swallow whole with liquid.
- Injections to penis—Follow doctor's instructions.

When to take:
At the same times each day.

If you forget a dose:
Take as soon as you remember. If it is almost time for the next dose, wait for that dose (don't double this dose) and resume regular schedule.

What drug does:
Relaxes and expands blood vessel walls, allowing better distribution of oxygen and nutrients.

Continued next column

OVERDOSE

SYMPTOMS:
Weakness, fainting, flush, sweating, stupor, irregular heartbeat.
WHAT TO DO:
- **Dial 911 (emergency) for medical help or call poison control center 1-800-222-1222 for instructions.**
- **See emergency information on last 3 pages of this book.**

Time lapse before drug works:
30 to 60 minutes.

Don't take with:
Any other medicine or any dietary supplement without consulting your doctor or pharmacist.

POSSIBLE ADVERSE REACTIONS OR SIDE EFFECTS

SYMPTOMS	WHAT TO DO
Life-threatening:	
None expected.	
Common:	
• Drowsiness, dizziness, headache, flushed face, stomach irritation, indigestion, nausea, mild constipation.	Continue. Call doctor when convenient.
• Dry mouth, throat.	Continue. Tell doctor at next visit.
Infrequent:	
Rash, itchy skin, blurred or double vision, weakness, fast heartbeat.	Discontinue. Call doctor right away.
Rare:	
Jaundice.	Discontinue. Call doctor right away.

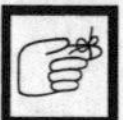

WARNINGS & PRECAUTIONS

Don't take if:
You are allergic to papaverine.

Before you start, consult your doctor if:
- You plan to become pregnant within medication period.
- You have had a heart attack, heart disease, angina or stroke.
- You have Parkinson's disease.

Over age 60:
Adverse reactions and side effects may be more frequent and severe than in younger persons.

Pregnancy:
Decide with your doctor if drug benefits justify risk to unborn child. Risk category C (see page xviii).

Breast-feeding:
Drug may pass into milk. Avoid drug or discontinue nursing until you finish medicine. Consult doctor for advice on maintaining milk supply.

Infants & children:
Not recommended.

Prolonged use:
No problems expected.

Skin & sunlight:
No problems expected.

Driving, piloting or hazardous work:
Don't drive or pilot aircraft until you learn how medicine affects you. Don't work around dangerous machinery. Don't climb ladders or work in high places. Danger increases if you drink alcohol or take medicine affecting alertness and reflexes, such as antihistamines, tranquilizers, sedatives, pain medicine, narcotics and mind-altering drugs.

Discontinuing:
May be unnecessary to finish medicine. If drug does not help in 1 to 2 weeks, consult doctor about discontinuing.

Others:
- Periodic liver function tests recommended.
- Internal eye pressure measurements recommended if you have glaucoma.
- Advise any doctor or dentist whom you consult that you take this medicine.

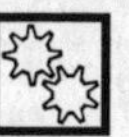

POSSIBLE INTERACTION WITH OTHER DRUGS

GENERIC NAME OR DRUG CLASS	COMBINED EFFECT
Levodopa	Decreased levodopa effect.
Narcotics*	Increased sedation.
Pain relievers*	Increased sedation.
Pergolide	Decreased pergolide effect.
Sedatives*	Increased sedation.
Sympathomimetics*	Reversal of the effect of papaverine.
Tranquilizers*	Increased sedation.

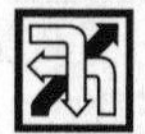

POSSIBLE INTERACTION WITH OTHER SUBSTANCES

INTERACTS WITH	COMBINED EFFECT
Alcohol:	None expected.
Beverages:	None expected.
Cocaine:	Decreased papaverine effect.
Foods:	None expected.
Marijuana:	None expected.
Tobacco:	Decrease in papaverine's dilation of blood vessels.

*See Glossary

PARAGORIC

BRAND NAMES

Brown Mixture
Camphorated Opium Tincture
Kapectolin with Paregoric
Parepectolin

BASIC INFORMATION

Habit forming? Yes
Prescription needed? Yes
Available as generic? Yes
Drug class: Narcotic, antidiarrheal

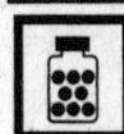

USES

Reduces intestinal cramps and diarrhea.

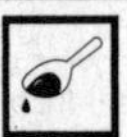

DOSAGE & USAGE INFORMATION

How to take:
Drops or liquid—Dilute dose in beverage before swallowing.

When to take:
As needed for diarrhea, no more often than every 4 hours.

If you forget a dose:
Take as soon as you remember. If it is almost time for the next dose, wait for that dose (don't double this dose) and resume regular schedule.

What drug does:
Anesthetizes surface membranes of intestines and blocks nerve impulses.

Time lapse before drug works:
2 to 6 hours.

Don't take with:
Any other medicine or any dietary supplement without consulting your doctor or pharmacist.

OVERDOSE

SYMPTOMS:
Deep sleep; slow breathing; slow pulse; flushed, warm skin; constricted pupils.
WHAT TO DO:

- **Dial 911 (emergency) for medical help or call poison control center 1-800-222-1222 for instructions.**
- **If person is unconscious, check breathing and pulse. If not breathing, begin mouth-to-mouth rescue breathing. If heart is not beating, begin chest compressions.**
- **See emergency information on last 3 pages of this book.**

POSSIBLE ADVERSE REACTIONS OR SIDE EFFECTS

SYMPTOMS	WHAT TO DO
Life-threatening:	
In case of overdose, see previous column.	
Common:	
Dizziness, flushed face, unusual tiredness, difficult urination.	Continue. Call doctor when convenient.
Infrequent:	
Severe constipation, abdominal pain, vomiting.	Discontinue. Call doctor right away.
Rare:	
• Hives, rash, itchy skin, slow heartbeat, irregular breathing.	Discontinue. Call doctor right away.
• Depression.	Continue. Call doctor when convenient.

WARNINGS & PRECAUTIONS

Don't take if:
You are allergic to any narcotic.*

Before you start, consult your doctor if:
You have impaired liver or kidney function.

Over age 60:
More likely to be drowsy, dizzy, unsteady or constipated.

Pregnancy:
Risk factor varies with length of pregnancy. See category list on page xviii and consult doctor.

Breast-feeding:
Drug filters into milk. May depress infant. Avoid.

Infants & children:
Use only under medical supervision.

Prolonged use:
Causes psychological and physical dependence.

Skin & sunlight:
No problems expected.

Driving, piloting or hazardous work:
Don't drive or pilot aircraft until you learn how medicine affects you. Don't work around dangerous machinery. Don't climb ladders or work in high places. Danger increases if you drink alcohol or take medicine affecting alertness and reflexes, such as antihistamines, tranquilizers, sedatives, pain medicine, narcotics and mind-altering drugs.

Discontinuing:
May be unnecessary to finish medicine. Follow doctor's instructions.

Others:
Great potential for abuse.

POSSIBLE INTERACTION WITH OTHER DRUGS

GENERIC NAME OR DRUG CLASS	COMBINED EFFECT
Analgesics*	Increased analgesic effect.
Anticholinergics*	Increased risk of constipation.
Antidepressants*	Increased sedation.
Antidiarrheal preparations*	Increased sedative effect. Avoid.
Antihistamines*	Increased sedation.
Central nervous system (CNS) depressants*	Increased central nerve system depression.
Naloxone	Decreased paregoric effect.
Naltrexone	Decreased paregoric effect.
Narcotics,* other	Increased narcotic effect.

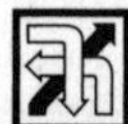

POSSIBLE INTERACTION WITH OTHER SUBSTANCES

INTERACTS WITH	COMBINED EFFECT
Alcohol:	Increases alcohol's intoxicating effect. Avoid.
Beverages:	None expected.
Cocaine:	None expected.
Foods:	None expected.
Marijuana:	Impairs physical and mental performance.
Tobacco:	None expected.

***See Glossary**

PEDICULICIDES (Topical)

GENERIC AND BRAND NAMES

BENZOYL ALCOHOL
Ulesfia
IVERMECTIN (topical)
Sklice Lotion
LINDANE
GBH
G-Well
Kwellada
Kwildane
PMS Lindane
MALATHION
Derbac
Ovide
PERMETHRIN
Acticin
Elimite Cream
Nix Cream Rinse
PYRETHRINS & PIPERONYL BUTOXIDE
A-200 Gel
A-200 Shampoo
Barc
Blue
Lice-Enz Foam and Comb Lice Killing Shampoo Kit
Pyrinyl
R&C
TISIT
TISIT Blue
Triple X
SPINOSAD
Natroba Topical Suspension

BASIC INFORMATION

Habit forming? No
Prescription needed? Yes
Available as generic? Yes, for some
Drug class: Pediculicide, scabicide

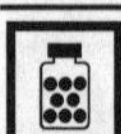

USES

- Treats scabies and lice infections of skin or scalp.
- Cream and lotion treats scabies.
- Shampoo treats lice infections.

OVERDOSE

SYMPTOMS:
Rarely (toxic effects from too much absorbed through skin)—Vomiting, muscle cramps, dizziness, seizure, rapid heartbeat.
WHAT TO DO:
- **Not for internal use. If child accidentally swallows, call poison center 1-800-222-1222 for instructions.**
- **Dial 911 (emergency) for medical help or call poison control center 1-800-222-1222 for help.**
- **See emergency information on last 3 pages of this book.**

DOSAGE & USAGE INFORMATION

How to use:
- All household members should be examined for infestation and treated if infested.
- Read directions on product for proper application technique and length of time to leave on the body.
- Wear plastic gloves when you apply. Use care not to apply more than directed. Avoid contact with eyes, nose and mouth. Flush eyes with water if product gets in the eyes.
- Bathe before applying. Wash hands after applying.
- Use in well-ventilated room.

When to use:
As directed on package.

If you forget a dose:
Use as soon as you remember.

What drug does:
Most types are absorbed into bodies of lice and scabies organisms, killing them. Benzoyl alcohol kills lice by suffocation.

Time lapse before drug works:
Cream or lotion requires 8 to 12 hours contact with skin.

Don't use with:
Other medicines for scabies or lice without consulting your doctor or pharmacist.

POSSIBLE ADVERSE REACTIONS OR SIDE EFFECTS

SYMPTOMS	WHAT TO DO
Life-threatening: None expected.	
Common: None expected.	
Infrequent: None expected.	
Rare:	
• Skin irritation or rash.	Discontinue. Call doctor right away.
• Skin itch that continues 1 week to several weeks after treatment.	Call doctor when convenient.

WARNINGS & PRECAUTIONS

Don't use if:
You are allergic to any pediculicide.

Before you start, consult your doctor if:
- You are allergic to anything that touches your skin.
- You are using any other medicines, creams, lotions or oils.

Over age 60:
Adverse reactions and side effects may be more frequent and severe than in younger persons. Ask doctor about smaller doses.

Pregnancy:
Risk factors vary for drugs in this group. See category list on page xviii and consult doctor.

Breast-feeding:
Effect unknown. Avoid if possible. Consult doctor.

Infants & children:
- More likely to be toxic. Use only under close medical supervision.
- Lindane is not recommended for use in infants. For other children, follow package instructions. Never use more of the product than instructed.

Prolonged use:
Not recommended. Avoid.

Skin & sunlight:
No problems expected, but check with doctor.

Driving, piloting or hazardous work:
No problems expected, but check with doctor.

Discontinuing:
No problems expected, but check with doctor.

Others:
- Don't use on open sores or wounds.
- Even after successful treatment, itching can continue due to remaining inflammation in the skin. This should not be confused with a reinfestation. Consult doctor if you are unsure.

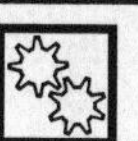

POSSIBLE INTERACTION WITH OTHER DRUGS

GENERIC NAME OR DRUG CLASS	COMBINED EFFECT
Antimyasthenics*	Excessive absorption and chance of toxicity (with malathion only).
Cholinesterase inhibitors*	Excessive absorption and chance of toxicity (with malathion only).

POSSIBLE INTERACTION WITH OTHER SUBSTANCES

INTERACTS WITH	COMBINED EFFECT
Alcohol:	None expected.
Beverages:	None expected.
Cocaine:	None expected.
Foods:	None expected.
Marijuana:	None expected.
Tobacco:	None expected.

***See Glossary**

PENICILLAMINE

BRAND NAMES

Cuprimine Depen

BASIC INFORMATION

Habit forming? No
Prescription needed? Yes
Available as generic? No
Drug class: Chelating agent, antirheumatic, antidote (heavy metal)

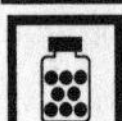

USES

- Treatment for rheumatoid arthritis.
- Prevention of kidney stones.
- Treatment for heavy metal poisoning.

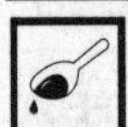

DOSAGE & USAGE INFORMATION

How to take:
Tablet or capsule—Swallow with liquid on an empty stomach 1 hour before or 2 hours after eating.

When to take:
At the same times each day.

If you forget a dose:
- 1 dose a day—Take as soon as you remember up to 12 hours late. If more than 12 hours, wait for next scheduled dose (don't double this dose).
- More than 1 dose a day—Take as soon as you remember. If it is almost time for the next dose, wait for that dose (don't double this dose) and resume regular schedule.

What drug does:
- Combines with heavy metals so kidney can excrete them.
- Combines with cysteine (amino acid found in many foods) to prevent cysteine kidney stones.
- May improve protective function of some white blood cells against rheumatoid arthritis.

Continued next column

OVERDOSE

SYMPTOMS:
Ulcers, sores, convulsions, coughing up blood, coma.
WHAT TO DO:
- **Dial 911 (emergency) for medical help or call poison control center 1-800-222-1222 for instructions.**
- **See emergency information on last 3 pages of this book.**

Time lapse before drug works:
2 to 3 months.

Don't take with:
Any other medicine or any dietary supplement without consulting your doctor or pharmacist.

POSSIBLE ADVERSE REACTIONS OR SIDE EFFECTS

SYMPTOMS	WHAT TO DO
Life-threatening: In case of overdose, see previous column.	
Common: Rash, itchy skin, swollen lymph glands, appetite loss, nausea, diarrhea, vomiting, decreased taste.	Discontinue. Call doctor right away.
Infrequent: Sore throat, fever, unusual bruising, swollen feet or legs, bloody or cloudy urine, weight gain, fatigue, weakness, joint pain.	Discontinue. Call doctor right away.
Rare: Double or blurred vision; pain; ringing in ears; ulcers, sores, white spots in mouth; difficult breathing; coughing up blood; jaundice; abdominal pain; skin blisters; peeling skin.	Discontinue. Call doctor right away.

WARNINGS & PRECAUTIONS

Don't take if:
- You are allergic to penicillamine.
- You have severe anemia.

Before you start, consult your doctor if:
- You have kidney disease.
- You are allergic to any penicillin antibiotic.

Over age 60:
More likely to damage blood cells and kidneys.

Pregnancy:
Decide with your doctor if drug benefits justify risk to unborn child. Risk category C (see page xviii).

Breast-feeding:
Safety not established. Consult doctor.

Infants & children:
Use only under medical supervision.

Prolonged use:
- May damage blood cells, kidney, liver.
- Talk to your doctor about the need for follow-up medical examinations or laboratory studies to check complete blood counts (white blood cell count, platelet count, red blood cell count, hemoglobin, hematocrit), kidney function, liver function.

Skin & sunlight:
No problems expected.

Driving, piloting or hazardous work:
No problems expected.

Discontinuing:
No problems expected.

Others:
- Request laboratory studies on blood and urine every 2 weeks. Kidney and liver function studies recommended every 6 months.
- Advise any doctor or dentist you consult that you use this medicine.

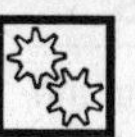

POSSIBLE INTERACTION WITH OTHER DRUGS

GENERIC NAME OR DRUG CLASS	COMBINED EFFECT
Gold compounds*	Damage to blood cells and kidney.
Immuno-suppressants*	Damage to blood cells and kidney.
Iron supplements*	Decreased effect of penicillamine. Wait 2 hours between doses.
Pyridoxine (vitamin B-6)	Increased need for pyridoxine.

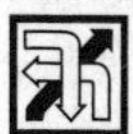

POSSIBLE INTERACTION WITH OTHER SUBSTANCES

INTERACTS WITH	COMBINED EFFECT
Alcohol:	Increased side effects of penicillamine.
Beverages:	None expected.
Cocaine:	Increased side effects of penicillamine.
Foods:	Possible decreased penicillamine effect due to decreased absorption.
Marijuana:	Increased side effects of penicillamine.
Tobacco:	None expected.

***See Glossary**

PENICILLINS

GENERIC AND BRAND NAMES

See full list of generic and brand names in the *Generic and Brand Name Directory*, page 892.

BASIC INFORMATION

Habit forming? No
Prescription needed? Yes
Available as generic? Yes
Drug class: Antibacterial

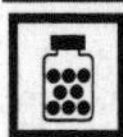

USES

Treatment of bacterial infections that are susceptible to penicillin, including lower respiratory tract infections, otitis media, sinusitis, skin and skin structure infections, urinary tract infections, gastrointestinal disorders, ulcers, endocarditis, pharyngitis. Different penicillins treat different kinds of infections.

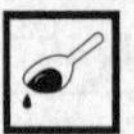

DOSAGE & USAGE INFORMATION

How to take:

- Tablet or capsule—Swallow with liquid on an empty stomach 1 hour before or 2 hours after eating. You may take amoxicillin, penicillin V, pivampicillin or pivmecillinam on a full stomach.
- Chewable tablet—Chew or crush before swallowing.
- Oral suspension—Measure each dose with an accurate measuring device (not a household teaspoon). Store according to instructions.
- Tablets for oral suspension—Mix one tablet in 2 teaspoonfuls of water. Drink right away.

When to take:
Follow instructions on prescription label, or take as directed by doctor. The number of doses, the time between doses and the length of treatment will depend on the problem being treated.

Continued next column

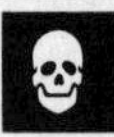

OVERDOSE

SYMPTOMS:
Severe diarrhea, nausea or vomiting.
WHAT TO DO:
Overdose unlikely to threaten life. If person uses much larger amount than prescribed or if accidentally swallowed, call doctor or poison control center 1-800-222-1222 for help.

If you forget a dose:
Take as soon as you remember, then continue regular schedule. If it is almost time for the next dose, wait for that dose (don't double that dose).

What drug does:
Destroys susceptible bacteria. Does not kill viruses (e.g., colds or influenza), fungi or parasites.

Time lapse before drug works:
May be several days before medicine affects infection.

Don't take with:
Any other medicine or any dietary supplement without consulting your doctor or pharmacist.

POSSIBLE ADVERSE REACTIONS OR SIDE EFFECTS

SYMPTOMS	WHAT TO DO
Life-threatening:	
Hives, rash, intense itching, shortness of breath, faintness soon after a dose (anaphylaxis).	Seek emergency treatment immediately.
Common:	
Nausea, vomiting or diarrhea (all mild); sore mouth or tongue; white patches in mouth or on tongue; vaginal itching or discharge; stomach pain.	Continue. Call doctor when convenient.
Infrequent:	
None expected.	
Rare:	
Unexplained bleeding or bruising, weakness, sore throat, fever, severe abdominal cramps, diarrhea (watery and severe), convulsions.	Discontinue. Call doctor right away.

WARNINGS & PRECAUTIONS

Don't take if:
You are allergic to penicillins* or cephalosporins.* A life-threatening reaction may occur.

Before you start, consult your doctor if:
- You are allergic to any substance or drug.
- You have mononucleosis.
- You have congestive heart failure.
- You have high blood pressure or any bleeding disorder.
- You have cystic fibrosis.
- You have kidney disease or a stomach or intestinal disorder.

Over age 60:
No special problems expected.

Pregnancy:
Consult doctor. Risk category B (see page xviii).

Breast-feeding:
Drug passes into milk. Child may become sensitive to penicillins and have allergic reactions to penicillin drugs. Discuss risks and benefits with your doctor.

Infants & children:
No special problems expected.

Prolonged use:
- You may become more susceptible to infections caused by germs not responsive to penicillins.
- Talk to your doctor about the need for follow-up medical examinations or laboratory studies.

Skin & sunlight:
No problems expected.

Driving, piloting or hazardous work:
Usually not dangerous. Most hazardous reactions likely to occur a few minutes after taking penicillin.

Discontinuing:
Don't discontinue without doctor's advice until you complete prescribed dose, even though symptoms diminish or disappear.

Others:
- Urine sugar test for diabetes may show false positive result.
- If your symptoms don't improve within a few days (or if they worsen), call your doctor.
- Don't take medicines for diarrhea without your doctor's approval.
- Birth control pills may not be effective. Use additional birth control methods.

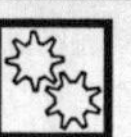

POSSIBLE INTERACTION WITH OTHER DRUGS

GENERIC NAME OR DRUG CLASS	COMBINED EFFECT
Chloramphenicol	Decreased effect of both drugs.
Cholestyramine	May decrease penicillin effect.
Colestipol	May decrease penicillin effect.
Contraceptives, oral*	Impaired contraceptive efficiency.
Erythromycins*	Decreased effect of both drugs.
Methotrexate	Increased risk of methotrexate toxicity.
Probenecid	Increased effect of all penicillins.
Sodium benzoate & sodium phenylacetate	May reduce effect of sodium benzoate & sodium phenylacetate.
Sulfonamides*	Decreased penicillin effect.
Tetracyclines*	Decreased effect of both drugs.

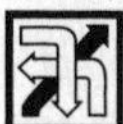

POSSIBLE INTERACTION WITH OTHER SUBSTANCES

INTERACTS WITH	COMBINED EFFECT
Alcohol:	Occasional stomach irritation.
Beverages:	None expected.
Cocaine:	None expected.
Foods: Acidic fruits or juices, aged cheese, wines, syrups (if taken with penicillin G).	Decreased antibiotic effect.
Marijuana:	None expected.
Tobacco:	None expected.

*See Glossary

PENICILLINS & BETA-LACTAMASE INHIBITORS

GENERIC AND BRAND NAMES

AMOXICILLIN & CLAVULANATE
Augmentin
Augmentin ES-600
Augmentin SR
Clavulin

BASIC INFORMATION

Habit forming? No
Prescription needed? Yes
Available as generic? Yes
Drug class: Antibacterial

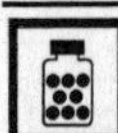

USES

Treatment of bacterial infections that are susceptible to penicillin and beta-lactamase inhibitors, including lower respiratory tract infections, otitis media, sinusitis, skin and skin structure infections, and urinary tract infections.

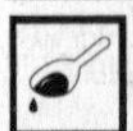

DOSAGE & USAGE INFORMATION

How to take:

- Tablet—Swallow with liquid on a full or empty stomach. Taking with food may lessen any stomach irritation.
- Chewable tablet—Chew or crush before swallowing.
- Oral suspension—Measure each dose with an accurate measuring device (not a household teaspoon).

When to take:
Follow instructions on prescription label, or take as directed by doctor. Normally the drug is taken every 8 hours for 7 to 10 days.

If you forget a dose:
Take as soon as you remember. If it is almost time for the next dose, wait for that dose (don't double this dose) and resume regular schedule.

Continued next column

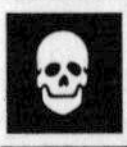

OVERDOSE

SYMPTOMS:
Severe diarrhea, nausea or vomiting.
WHAT TO DO:
Overdose unlikely to threaten life. If person uses much larger amount than prescribed or if accidentally swallowed, call doctor or poison control center 1-800-222-1222 for help.

What drug does:
Destroys susceptible bacteria. Does not kill viruses, fungi or parasites. Beta-lactamase inhibitors increase penicillin's effectiveness by inactivating beta-lactamase (a substance in some bacteria which destroys the penicillin).

Time lapse before drug works:
May be several days before medicine affects infection.

Don't take with:
Any other medicine or any dietary supplement without consulting your doctor or pharmacist.

POSSIBLE ADVERSE REACTIONS OR SIDE EFFECTS

SYMPTOMS	WHAT TO DO
Life-threatening:	
Hives, rash, intense itching, shortness of breath, faintness soon after a dose (anaphylaxis).	Seek emergency treatment immediately.
Common:	
Nausea, vomiting or diarrhea (all mild); sore mouth or tongue; white patches in mouth or on tongue; vaginal itching or discharge; stomach pain.	Continue. Call doctor when convenient.
Infrequent:	
None expected.	
Rare:	
Unexplained bleeding or bruising, weakness, sore throat, fever, severe abdominal cramps, diarrhea (watery and severe), convulsions.	Discontinue. Call doctor right away.

PENICILLINS & BETA-LACTAMASE INHIBITORS

WARNINGS & PRECAUTIONS

Don't take if:
You are allergic to penicillins or cephalosporins. Life-threatening reaction may occur.

Before you start, consult your doctor if:
- You are allergic to any substance or drug.
- You have mononucleosis.
- You have congestive heart failure.
- You have high blood pressure or any bleeding disorder.
- You have cystic fibrosis.
- You have kidney disease or a stomach or intestinal disorder.

Over age 60:
No special problems expected.

Pregnancy:
Consult doctor. Risk category B (see page xviii).

Breast-feeding:
Drug passes into milk. Child may become sensitive to penicillins and have allergic reactions to penicillin drugs. Avoid penicillin or discontinue nursing until you finish medicine. Consult doctor for advice on maintaining milk supply.

Infants & children:
No special problems expected.

Prolonged use:
- You may become more susceptible to infections caused by germs not responsive to penicillins.
- Talk to your doctor about the need for follow-up medical examinations or laboratory studies to check SGPT,* SGOT.*

Skin & sunlight:
No problems expected.

Driving, piloting or hazardous work:
Usually not dangerous. Most hazardous reactions likely to occur a few minutes after taking.

Discontinuing:
Don't discontinue without doctor's advice until you complete prescribed dose, even though symptoms diminish or disappear.

Others:
- Urine sugar test for diabetes may show false positive result.
- If your symptoms don't improve within a few days (or if they worsen), call your doctor.
- Don't take for diarrhea without your doctor's approval.
- Birth control pills may not be effective. Use additional birth control methods.

POSSIBLE INTERACTION WITH OTHER DRUGS

GENERIC NAME OR DRUG CLASS	COMBINED EFFECT
Chloramphenicol	Decreased effect of both drugs.
Cholestyramine	May decrease penicillin effect.
Colestipol	May decrease penicillin effect.
Contraceptives, oral*	Impaired contraceptive efficiency.
Erythromycins*	Decreased effect of both drugs.
Methotrexate	Increased risk of methotrexate toxicity.
Probenecid	Increased effect of all penicillins.
Sodium benzoate & sodium phenylacetate	May reduce effect of sodium benzoate & sodium phenylacetate.
Tetracyclines*	Decreased effect of both drugs.

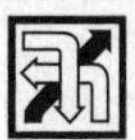

POSSIBLE INTERACTION WITH OTHER SUBSTANCES

INTERACTS WITH	COMBINED EFFECT
Alcohol:	Occasional stomach irritation.
Beverages:	None expected.
Cocaine:	None expected.
Foods:	None expected.
Marijuana:	None expected.
Tobacco:	None expected.

*See Glossary

PENTAMIDINE

BRAND NAMES

NebuPent
Pentacarinat
Pneumopent

BASIC INFORMATION

Habit forming? No
Prescription needed? Yes
Available as generic? No
Drug class: Antiprotozoal

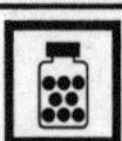

USES

- Treats pneumocystis pneumonia caused by *Pneumocystis jirovecii*.
- Treats some tropical diseases such as leishmaniasis, African sleeping sickness and others.

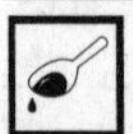

DOSAGE & USAGE INFORMATION

How to take:
Inhalation—Follow package instructions.

When to take:
According to doctor's instructions.

If you forget a dose:
Take as soon as you remember. If it is almost time for the next dose, wait for that dose (don't double this dose) and resume regular schedule.

What drug does:
Interferes with RNA and DNA of infecting organisms.

Time lapse before drug works:
30 minutes to 1 hour.

Don't take with:
Any other medicines (including over-the-counter drugs such as cough and cold medicines, laxatives, antacids, diet pills, caffeine, nose drops or vitamins) without consulting your doctor or pharmacist.

OVERDOSE

SYMPTOMS:
None expected.
WHAT TO DO:
Overdose unlikely to threaten life. If person uses much larger amount than prescribed or if accidentally swallowed, call doctor or poison control center 1-800-222-1222 for help.

POSSIBLE ADVERSE REACTIONS OR SIDE EFFECTS

SYMPTOMS	WHAT TO DO
Life-threatening:	
Unconsciousness, rapid pulse, cold sweats.	Seek emergency treatment immediately.
Common:	
Chest pain or congestion; wheezing; coughing; difficulty in breathing; skin rash; pain, dryness or sensation of lump in throat.	Discontinue. Call doctor right away.
Infrequent:	
• Abdomen or back pain, nausea, vomiting, anxiety, cold sweats, chills, headache, appetite changes, decreased urination, unusual tiredness.	Discontinue. Call doctor right away.
• Bitter or metallic taste.	No action necessary.
Rare:	
None expected.	

WARNINGS & PRECAUTIONS

Don't take if:
You are allergic to pentamidine.

Before you start, consult your doctor if:
You have asthma.

Over age 60:
Adverse reactions and side effects may be more frequent and severe than in younger persons. You may need smaller doses for shorter periods of time.

Pregnancy:
Decide with your doctor if drug benefits justify risk to unborn child. Risk category C (see page xviii).

Breast-feeding:
Unknown effects. Not recommended. Consult doctor.

Infants & children:
Unknown effects. Consult doctor.

Prolonged use:
Talk to your doctor about the need for follow-up medical examinations or laboratory studies to check blood sugar; blood pressure; kidney, liver and heart function; complete blood counts (white blood cell count, platelet count, red blood cell count, hemoglobin, hematocrit); ECG* and serum calcium.

Skin & sunlight:
No problems expected.

Driving, piloting or hazardous work:
Avoid if you feel confused, drowsy or dizzy.

Discontinuing:
No special problems expected.

Others:
- Advise any doctor or dentist whom you consult that you take this medicine.
- May affect results in some medical tests.
- Avoid exposure to people who have infectious diseases.
- To help decrease bitter taste in mouth, suck on a hard candy after taking medicine.
- Consult your doctor for additional information on the injectable form of this drug.

POSSIBLE INTERACTION WITH OTHER DRUGS

GENERIC NAME OR DRUG CLASS	COMBINED EFFECT
None reported with inhalation form of drug.	

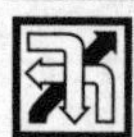

POSSIBLE INTERACTION WITH OTHER SUBSTANCES

INTERACTS WITH	COMBINED EFFECT
Alcohol:	Increased likelihood of adverse reactions. Avoid.
Beverages:	None expected.
Cocaine:	Increased likelihood of adverse reactions. Avoid.
Foods:	None expected.
Marijuana:	Increased likelihood of adverse reactions. Avoid.
Tobacco:	Increased likelihood of adverse reactions. Avoid.

*See Glossary

PENTOXIFYLLINE

BRAND NAMES

Trental

BASIC INFORMATION

Habit forming? No
Prescription needed? Yes
Available as generic? Yes
Drug class: Hemorheologic agent

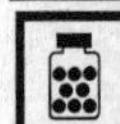

USES

- Reduces pain in legs caused by poor blood circulation (usually due to intermittent claudication).
- May be used for other disorders as determined by your doctor.

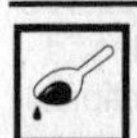

DOSAGE & USAGE INFORMATION

How to take:
Extended-release tablet—Swallow whole with liquid. Do not crush or crumble tablet.

When to take:
At mealtimes. Taking with food decreases the likelihood of irritating the stomach to cause nausea. May take with antacids to help prevent stomach irritation.

If you forget a dose:
Take as soon as you remember. If it is almost time for the next dose, wait for that dose (don't double this dose) and resume regular schedule.

What drug does:
- Reduces "stickiness" of red blood cells and improves flexibility of the red cells.
- Improves blood flow through blood vessels.

Time lapse before drug works:
Several weeks for full effect on circulation.

Don't take with:
Any other medicine or any dietary supplement without consulting your doctor or pharmacist.

OVERDOSE

SYMPTOMS:
Drowsiness, flushed face, fainting, unusual excitement, convulsions.
WHAT TO DO:
- **Dial 911 (emergency) for medical help or call poison control center 1-800-222-1222 for instructions.**
- **See emergency information on last 3 pages of this book.**

POSSIBLE ADVERSE REACTIONS OR SIDE EFFECTS

SYMPTOMS	WHAT TO DO
Life-threatening: None expected.	
Common: None expected.	
Infrequent: Drowsiness, headache, nausea, vomiting, stomach upset.	Continue. Call doctor when convenient.
Rare: Chest pain, irregular heartbeat.	Discontinue. Call doctor right away.

WARNINGS & PRECAUTIONS

Don't take if:
You are allergic to pentoxifylline or other xanthines (caffeine, theophylline, theobromine, aminophylline, dyphylline, or oxtriphylline).

Before you start, consult your doctor if:
- You have coronary artery disease.
- You have active bleeding or any condition where there is a risk of bleeding (e.g., stroke).
- You have cerebrovascular (blood vessels in the brain) disease.
- You have liver or kidney disease.

Over age 60:
Adverse reactions and side effects may be more frequent and severe than in younger persons. Ask doctor about smaller doses.

Pregnancy:
Decide with your doctor if drug benefits justify risk to unborn child. Risk category C (see page xviii).

Breast-feeding:
Drug passes into milk. Avoid drug or discontinue nursing until you finish medicine. Consult doctor for advice on maintaining milk supply.

Infants & children:
Not recommended.

Prolonged use:
No problems expected.

Skin & sunlight:
No problems expected.

Driving, piloting or hazardous work:
Wait to see if drug causes drowsiness. If not, no problems expected.

Discontinuing:
Don't discontinue without doctor's approval.

Others:
- Don't smoke. Nicotine constricts blood vessels and worsens your condition.
- Advise any doctor or dentist you consult that you use this medicine.

POSSIBLE INTERACTION WITH OTHER DRUGS

GENERIC NAME OR DRUG CLASS	COMBINED EFFECT
Anticoagulants,* oral	Possible decreased effect of anticoagulant.
Antihypertensives*	Possible increased effect of hypertensive drug.
Cimetidine	Increased risk of side effects.
Xanthines*	Increased nervous system stimulation.

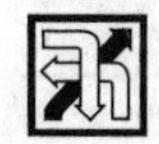

POSSIBLE INTERACTION WITH OTHER SUBSTANCES

INTERACTS WITH	COMBINED EFFECT
Alcohol:	Unknown. Best to avoid.
Beverages: Coffee, tea or other caffeine-containing beverages.	Increased nervous system stimulation.
Cocaine:	Reduced effect of pentoxifylline. Avoid.
Foods:	None expected.
Marijuana:	Decreased effect of pentoxifylline. Avoid.
Tobacco:	Decreased effect of pentoxifylline. Avoid.

*See Glossary

PHENAZOPYRIDINE

BRAND NAMES

Azo-Cheragan
Azo-Gantrisin
Azo-Standard
Baridium
Eridium
Geridium
Phen-Azo
Phenazodine
Pyrazodine
Pyridiate
Pyridium
Pyronium
Urodine
Urogesic
Viridium

BASIC INFORMATION

Habit forming? No
Prescription needed? Yes
Available as generic? Yes
Drug class: Analgesic (urinary)

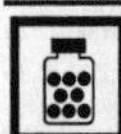

USES

Relieves pain of lower urinary tract irritation, as in cystitis, urethritis or prostatitis. Relieves symptoms only. Phenazopyridine alone does not cure infections.

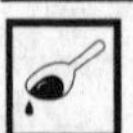

DOSAGE & USAGE INFORMATION

How to take:
Tablet—Swallow with liquid or food to lessen stomach irritation.

When to take:
At the same times each day.

If you forget a dose:
Take as soon as you remember. If it is almost time for the next dose, wait for that dose (don't double this dose) and resume regular schedule.

What drug does:
Anesthetizes lower urinary tract. Relieves pain, burning, pressure and urgency to urinate.

Time lapse before drug works:
1 to 2 hours.

Don't take with:
Any other medicine or any dietary supplement without consulting your doctor or pharmacist.

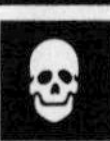

OVERDOSE

SYMPTOMS:
Shortness of breath, weakness.
WHAT TO DO:
Overdose unlikely to threaten life. If person uses much larger amount than prescribed or if accidentally swallowed, call doctor or poison control center 1-800-222-1222 for help.

POSSIBLE ADVERSE REACTIONS OR SIDE EFFECTS

SYMPTOMS	WHAT TO DO
Life-threatening:	
None expected.	
Common:	
Red-orange urine.	No action necessary.
Infrequent:	
Indigestion, fatigue, weakness, dizziness, abdominal pain.	Continue. Call doctor when convenient.
Rare:	
• Rash, jaundice, bluish skin color.	Discontinue. Call doctor right away.
• Headache.	Continue. Call doctor when convenient.

WARNINGS & PRECAUTIONS

Don't take if:

- You have hepatitis.
- You are allergic to any urinary analgesic.

Before you start, consult your doctor if:
You have kidney or liver disease.

Over age 60:
Adverse reactions and side effects may be more frequent and severe than in younger persons.

Pregnancy:
No proven harm to unborn child. Avoid if possible. Consult doctor. Risk category B (see page xviii).

Breast-feeding:
Effect unknown. Consult doctor.

Infants & children:
Not recommended.

Prolonged use:

- Orange or yellow skin.
- Anemia. Occasional blood studies recommended.

Skin & sunlight:
No problems expected.

Driving, piloting or hazardous work:
No problems expected.

Discontinuing:
May be unnecessary to finish medicine. Follow doctor's instructions.

Others:
Advise any doctor or dentist whom you consult that you take this medicine.

POSSIBLE INTERACTION WITH OTHER DRUGS

GENERIC NAME OR DRUG CLASS	COMBINED EFFECT
None significant.	

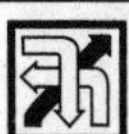

POSSIBLE INTERACTION WITH OTHER SUBSTANCES

INTERACTS WITH	COMBINED EFFECT
Alcohol:	None expected.
Beverages:	None expected.
Cocaine:	None expected.
Foods:	None expected.
Marijuana:	None expected.
Tobacco:	None expected.

PHENOTHIAZINES

GENERIC AND BRAND NAMES

See full list of generic and brand names in the *Generic and Brand Name Directory*, page 892.

BASIC INFORMATION

Habit forming? No
Prescription needed? Yes
Available as generic? Yes, for some.
Drug class: Antipsychotic, antiemetic (phenothiazine)

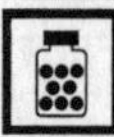

USES

- Treatment for mental and emotional disorders.
- Treats nausea, vomiting, hiccups.
- May be used for other conditions as determined by your doctor.

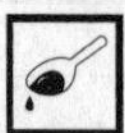

DOSAGE & USAGE INFORMATION

How to take:
- Tablet, sustained release capsule, extended-release capsule—Swallow with liquid or food to lessen stomach irritation.
- Suppository—Remove wrapper and moisten suppository with water. Gently insert into rectum, pointed end first.
- Drops or liquid—Dilute dose in beverage.

When to take:
Times will vary. Take at the same times each day as directed by your doctor.

If you forget a dose:
Take as soon as you remember. If it is almost time for your next dose, skip the missed dose and return to your regular dosing schedule (don't double this dose).

What drug does:
- Suppresses brain centers that control abnormal emotions and behavior.
- Suppresses brain's vomiting center.

Continued next column

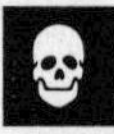

OVERDOSE

SYMPTOMS:
Stupor, convulsions, coma.
WHAT TO DO:
- **Dial 911 (emergency) for medical help or call poison control center 1-800-222-1222 for instructions.**
- **See emergency information on last 3 pages of this book.**

Time lapse before drug works:
Some benefit seen within a week; takes 4 to 6 weeks for full effect.

Don't take with:
- Antacid or medicine for diarrhea at same time.
- Any other medicine or any dietary supplement without consulting your doctor or pharmacist.

POSSIBLE ADVERSE REACTIONS OR SIDE EFFECTS

SYMPTOMS	WHAT TO DO
Life-threatening:	
High fever, rapid pulse, profuse sweating, muscle rigidity, confusion and irritability, seizures.	Discontinue. Seek emergency treatment.
Common:	
Dry mouth, blurred vision, constipation, difficulty urinating; sedation, dizziness, low blood pressure.	Continue. Call doctor when convenient.
Infrequent:	
Continuous jerky or involuntary movements, especially of the face, lips, jaw, tongue; slow-frequency tremor of head or limbs, especially while moving; muscle rigidity, lack of facial expression and slow, inflexible movements. Pacing or restlessness; intermittent spasms of muscles of face, eyes, tongue, jaw, neck, body or limbs; jaundice (yellow skin or eyes).	Discontinue. Call doctor right away.
Rare:	
Other symptoms not listed above.	Continue. Call doctor when convenient.

WARNINGS & PRECAUTIONS

Don't take if:
- You are allergic to any phenothiazine.
- You have a blood or bone marrow disease.

Before you start, consult your doctor if:
- You will have surgery within 2 months, including dental surgery, requiring general or spinal anesthesia.
- You have asthma, emphysema or other lung disorder; glaucoma; or prostate trouble.
- You take nonprescription ulcer medicine, asthma medicine or amphetamines.

Over age 60:
- Adverse reactions and side effects may be more frequent and severe than in younger persons. More likely to develop involuntary movement of jaws, lips, tongue; chewing. Report this to your doctor immediately. Early treatment can help.
- Use of antipsychotic drugs in elderly patients with dementia-related psychosis may increase risk of death. Consult doctor.

Pregnancy:
Risk factors vary for drugs in this group. See category list on page xviii and consult doctor.

Breast-feeding:
Drug passes into milk. Avoid drug or discontinue nursing until you finish medicine. Consult doctor for advice on maintaining milk supply.

Infants & children:
- Don't give to children younger than 2.
- Children more likely than adults to develop adverse reactions from these drugs.

Prolonged use:
May lead to tardive dyskinesia (involuntary movement of jaws, lips, tongue; chewing).

Skin & sunlight:
- One or more drugs in this group may cause rash or intensify sunburn in areas exposed to sun or ultraviolet light (photosensitivity reaction). Use sunscreen and avoid overexposure. Notify doctor if reaction occurs. Sensitivity may remain for 3 months after discontinuing drug.
- Avoid getting overheated or chilled. These drugs affect body temperature and sweating.

Driving, piloting or hazardous work:
Don't drive or pilot aircraft until you learn how medicine affects you. Don't work around dangerous machinery. Don't climb ladders or work in high places. Danger increases if you drink alcohol or take medicine affecting alertness and reflexes.

Discontinuing:
- Nervous and mental disorders—Don't discontinue without doctor's advice until you complete prescribed dose, even though symptoms diminish or disappear.
- Other disorders—Follow doctor's instructions about discontinuing.
- Adverse reactions may occur after drug is discontinued. Consult doctor if new symptoms develop, such as dizziness, nausea, stomach pain, trembling or tardive dyskinesia.*

Others:
- To relieve mouth dryness, chew or suck sugarless gum, candy, or ice.
- Avoid getting the liquid form of the drug on the skin. It may cause a skin rash or irritation.
- Advise any doctor or dentist whom you consult that you take this medicine.

POSSIBLE INTERACTION WITH OTHER DRUGS

GENERIC NAME OR DRUG CLASS	COMBINED EFFECT
Anticholinergics*	Increased phenothiazine effect.
Anticonvulsants*	Increased risk of seizures. May need to increase dosage of anticonvulsant.
Antidepressants, tricyclic*	Increased antidepressant effect.
Antihistamines*	Increased antihistamine effect.
Antihypertensives*	Severe low blood pressure.
Appetite suppressants*	Decreased appetite suppressant effect.
Bupropion	Increased risk of seizures.
Clozapine	Toxic effect on the central nervous system.
Dofetilide	Increased risk of heart problems.

Continued on page 924

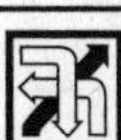

POSSIBLE INTERACTION WITH OTHER SUBSTANCES

INTERACTS WITH	COMBINED EFFECT
Alcohol:	Dangerous oversedation. Avoid.
Beverages:	None expected.
Cocaine:	Decreased phenothiazine effect. Avoid.
Foods:	None expected.
Marijuana:	Drowsiness. May increase antinausea effect.
Tobacco:	None expected.

***See Glossary**

PHENYLEPHRINE

BRAND NAMES

See full list of brand names in the *Generic and Brand Name Directory*, page 892.

BASIC INFORMATION

Habit forming? No
Prescription needed? No
Available as generic? Yes
Drug class: Sympathomimetic, decongestant

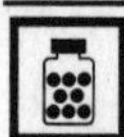

USES

- Temporary relief of congestion of nose and sinuses caused by allergies, colds, hay fever or sinus infection.
- Treats congestion of eustachian tubes caused by middle ear infections.

DOSAGE & USAGE INFORMATION

How to take:

- Nasal drops or spray—Wash hands before use. Blow nose gently, and then use the drops or spray according to instructions on the label.
- Combination drug products—Use according to label directions. Phenylephrine is the decongestant ingredient in many combination cough, cold and hay fever remedies.

When to take:
As needed; no more often than every 4 hours.

If you forget a dose:
Take when you remember. Wait 4 hours or as directed on label for next dose. Never double a dose.

What drug does:
Narrows the blood vessels in the nasal passages or ears which helps relieve the stuffy feeling caused by congestion.

Time lapse before drug works:
5 to 30 minutes.

Continued next column

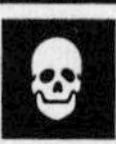

OVERDOSE

SYMPTOMS:
Sweating, dizziness, extreme tiredness, slow heartbeat, coma.
WHAT TO DO:

- **Dial 911 (emergency) for medical help or call poison control center 1-800-222-1222 for instructions.**
- **See emergency information on last 3 pages of this book.**

Don't take with:
Nonprescription drugs for asthma, cough, cold, allergy, appetite suppressants, sleeping pills or drugs containing caffeine without consulting your doctor or pharmacist.

POSSIBLE ADVERSE REACTIONS OR SIDE EFFECTS

SYMPTOMS	WHAT TO DO
Life-threatening:	
Rare allergic reaction (hives, itching, rash, trouble breathing, tightness in chest, swelling of lips or tongue or face).	Seek emergency treatment immediately.
Common:	
Dizziness, insomnia, nervousness, lightheadedness.	Discontinue. Call doctor if symptoms persist.
Infrequent:	
Nasal product may cause burning, dryness, stinging inside nose.	Discontinue. Call doctor if symptoms persist.
Rare:	
• Unusual behavior, fast or pounding heartbeat, seizure, severe shaking.	Discontinue. Call doctor right away.
• Headache, nausea, vomiting, anxiety, mild shaking, sweating.	Discontinue. Call doctor if symptoms persist.

WARNINGS & PRECAUTIONS

Don't take if:
You are allergic to phenylephrine or any sympathomimetic.*

Before you start, consult your doctor if:
- You have high blood pressure.
- You have heart disease.
- You have diabetes.
- You have overactive thyroid.
- You have prostate problems.
- You have urination problems.
- You have glaucoma.
- You have taken MAO inhibitors in past 2 weeks.

Over age 60:
Adverse reactions and side effects may be more frequent and severe than in younger persons.

Pregnancy:
Decide with your doctor if drug benefits justify risk to unborn child. Risk category C (see page xviii).

Breast-feeding:
It is unknown if drug passes into milk. Avoid drug or discontinue nursing until you finish medicine. Consult doctor for advice on maintaining milk supply.

Infants & children:
Read the label on the product to see if it is approved for your child's age. Always follow the directions on product's label about how to use. If unsure, ask your doctor or pharmacist.

Prolonged use:
Do not use product for longer than advised on label or by doctor. Nasal spray may cause rebound congestion* if used longer than recommended on label.

Skin & sunlight:
No problems expected.

Driving, piloting or hazardous work:
Drug may cause dizziness or lightheadedness. Don't drive or pilot aircraft until you learn how medicine affects you. Don't work around dangerous machinery. Don't climb ladders or work in high places.

Discontinuing:
May be unnecessary to finish medicine. Follow label or doctor's instructions.

Others:
- Call the doctor if symptoms worsen or new symptoms develop with use of this medicine.
- Heed all warnings on the product label.
- Advise any doctor or dentist whom you consult that you take this medicine.

POSSIBLE INTERACTION WITH OTHER DRUGS

GENERIC NAME OR DRUG CLASS	COMBINED EFFECT
Antidepressants, tricyclic*	Increased phenylephrine effect.
Antihypertensives*	Increased risk of high blood pressure.
Monoamine oxidase (MAO) inhibitors*	Serious interaction (possibly fatal). Don't use within 14 days.

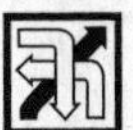

POSSIBLE INTERACTION WITH OTHER SUBSTANCES

INTERACTS WITH	COMBINED EFFECT
Alcohol:	Increased dizziness. Avoid.
Beverages:	None expected.
Cocaine:	Unknown effect. Avoid.
Foods:	None expected.
Marijuana:	Unknown effect. Avoid.
Tobacco:	None expected.

***See Glossary**

PHENYLEPHRINE (Ophthalmic)

BRAND NAMES

Ak-Dilate
Ak-Nefrin
Dilatair
Dionephrine
I-Phrine
Isopto Frin
Minims Phenylephrine
Mydfrin
Neofrin
Ocugestrin
Ocu-Phrin
Phenoptic
Prefrin Liquifilm
Relief Eye Drops for Red Eyes
Spersaphrine

BASIC INFORMATION

Habit forming? No
Prescription needed? Yes, some strengths
Available as generic? No
Drug class: Mydriatic, decongestant (ophthalmic)

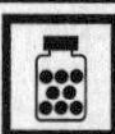

USES

- High-concentration drops—Dilates pupils.
- Low-concentration drops (available without prescription)—Relieves minor eye irritations caused by colds, hay fever, dust, wind, swimming, sun, smog, hard contact lenses, eye strain, smoke.

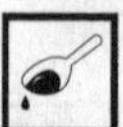

DOSAGE & USAGE INFORMATION

How to use:
Eye drops
- Wash hands.
- Apply pressure to inside corner of eye with middle finger.
- Continue pressure for 1 minute after placing medicine in eye.
- Tilt head backward. Pull lower lid away from eye with index finger of the same hand.
- Drop eye drops into pouch and close eye. Don't blink.
- Keep eyes closed for 1 to 2 minutes.
- Don't touch applicator tip to any surface (including the eye). If you accidentally touch tip, clean with warm water and soap.

Continued next column

- Keep container tightly closed.
- Keep cool, but don't freeze.
- Wash hands immediately after using.

When to use:
As directed on label.

If you forget a dose:
Use as soon as you remember. If it is almost time for the next dose, wait for that dose (don't double this dose) and resume regular schedule.

What drug does:
Acts on small blood vessels to make them constrict.

Time lapse before drug works:
15 to 90 minutes.

Don't use with:
- Other eye drops or ointment without consulting your eye doctor.
- Antidepressants,* guanadrel, guanethidine, maprotiline, pargyline, any monoamine oxidase (MAO) inhibitor.*

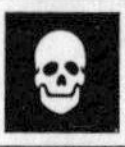

OVERDOSE

SYMPTOMS:
None expected unless too much is absorbed or drops are accidentally swallowed.
WHAT TO DO:
Call poison control center 1-800-222-1222 or doctor for instructions.

POSSIBLE ADVERSE REACTIONS OR SIDE EFFECTS

SYMPTOMS	WHAT TO DO
Life-threatening:	
None expected, unless you use much more than directed.	Discontinue. Call doctor right away.
Common:	
None expected.	
Infrequent:	
Burning or stinging eyes, headache, eyes more sensitive to light, watery eyes, eye irritation not present before.	Continue. Call doctor when convenient.
Rare:	
None expected, unless too much gets absorbed. If so, symptoms will be paleness, dizziness, tremor, increased sweating, irregular or fast heartbeat.	Discontinue. Call doctor right away.

PHENYLEPHRINE (Ophthalmic)

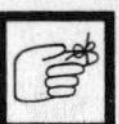

WARNINGS & PRECAUTIONS

Don't use if:

- You are allergic to phenylephrine.
- You have glaucoma.

Before you start, consult your doctor if:

- You have heart disease with irregular heartbeat, high blood pressure, diabetes.
- You take antidepressants,* guanadrel, guanethidine, maprotiline, pargyline, any monoamine oxidase (MAO) inhibitor.*

Over age 60:
Adverse reactions and side effects may be more frequent and severe than in younger persons. Ask doctor about smaller doses.

Pregnancy:
Decide with your doctor if drug benefits justify risk to unborn child. Risk category C (see page xviii).

Breast-feeding:
Safety not established. Consult doctor.

Infants & children:
Use only under close medical supervision.

Prolonged use:
Avoid if possible.

Skin & sunlight:
No special problems expected.

Driving, piloting or hazardous work:
No problems expected.

Discontinuing:
No problems expected.

Others:
Consult doctor if condition doesn't improve in 3 to 4 days.

POSSIBLE INTERACTION WITH OTHER DRUGS

GENERIC NAME OR DRUG CLASS	COMBINED EFFECT

Clinically significant interactions with oral or injected medicines unlikely.

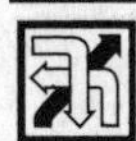

POSSIBLE INTERACTION WITH OTHER SUBSTANCES

INTERACTS WITH	COMBINED EFFECT
Alcohol:	None expected.
Beverages:	None expected.
Cocaine:	None expected.
Foods:	None expected.
Marijuana:	None expected.
Tobacco:	None expected.

***See Glossary**

PILOCARPINE (Oral)

BRAND NAMES

Salagen

BASIC INFORMATION

Habit forming? No
Prescription needed? Yes
Available as generic? Yes
Drug class: Cholinergic

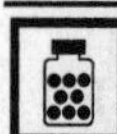

USES

Treatment for dry mouth caused by radiation treatment of patients with cancer (of the head or neck) or patients with Sjogren's syndrome.

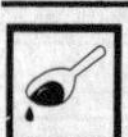

DOSAGE & USAGE INFORMATION

How to take:
Tablet—Follow doctor's directions. May require dosing several times a day.

When to take:
At the same times each day.

If you forget a dose:
Take as soon as you remember. If it is almost time for your next dose, skip the missed dose and return to your regular dosing schedule (don't double this dose).

What drug does:
Stimulates the salivary glands to increase their secretions.

Time lapse before drug works:
20-60 minutes.

Don't take with:
Any other medicine or any dietary supplement without consulting your doctor or pharmacist.

OVERDOSE

SYMPTOMS:
Stomach cramps or pain, diarrhea, severe nausea or vomiting, rapid heartbeat, chest pain, confusion, fainting, bad headache, severe shortness of breath, unusual trembling or shaking, visual problems.
WHAT TO DO:

- **If person takes much larger amount than prescribed, dial 911 (emergency) for medical help or call poison control center 1-800-222-1222 for instructions.**
- **If symptoms are severe or critical, dial 911 (emergency) for medical help or call poison control center 1-800-222-1222 for help.**

POSSIBLE ADVERSE REACTIONS OR SIDE EFFECTS

SYMPTOMS	WHAT TO DO
Life-threatening: In case of overdose, see previous column.	
Common: Runny nose, cough, fever, chills, diarrhea, indigestion, nausea, tiredness or weakness, warm feeling, sweating, skin flushing or red, urinary frequency, joint pain or muscle aches.	Continue. Call doctor when convenient.
Infrequent:	
• Swelling (ankles, feet, face or fingers), rapid heartbeat, visual problems, bloody nose, vomiting.	Discontinue. Call doctor right away.
• Trembling or shaking, trouble with swallowing, voice change, headache.	Continue. Call doctor when convenient.
Rare: None expected.	

WARNINGS & PRECAUTIONS

Don't take if:
You are allergic to pilocarpine (ophthalmic or oral) or have uncontrolled asthma.

Before you start, consult your doctor if:
- You have gallbladder problems.
- You have iritis or glaucoma.
- You have had heart or blood vessel disease.
- You have asthma.
- You have any cognitive or psychiatric problem.
- You have or have had kidney disease.
- You have been told you have a tendency for retinal detachment or have retinal disease.
- You have peptic ulcer disease.

Over age 60:
No problems expected.

Pregnancy:
Decide with your doctor if drug benefits justify risk to unborn child. Risk category C (see page xviii).

Breast-feeding:
It is unknown if pilocarpine passes into breast milk. Avoid drug or discontinue nursing until you finish medicine. Consult doctor for advice on maintaining milk supply.

Infants & children:
Safety and efficacy has not been established in children.

Prolonged use:
If no improvement is seen after twelve weeks of using this medicine, consult doctor.

Skin & sunlight:
No problems expected.

Driving, piloting or hazardous work:
May cause visual disturbances, especially at night. Don't drive or pilot aircraft until you learn how medicine affects you. Don't work around dangerous machinery. Don't climb ladders or work in high places. Danger increases if you drink alcohol or take medicine affecting alertness and reflexes.

Discontinuing:
Consult doctor before discontinuing.

Others:
- Advise any doctor or dentist whom you consult that you take this medicine.
- Since this drug causes sweating, be sure to drink plenty of fluids.

POSSIBLE INTERACTION WITH OTHER DRUGS

GENERIC NAME OR DRUG CLASS	COMBINED EFFECT
Anticholinergics*	Decreased effect of both drugs.
Antiglaucoma agents*	Increased antiglaucoma effect.
Antiglaucoma, beta blockers	Increased risk of side effects.
Beta adrenergic blocking agents	Increased risk of side effects.
Bethanechol	Increased risk of side effects.
Cholinergics,* other	Increased effect of both drugs.

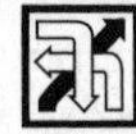

POSSIBLE INTERACTION WITH OTHER SUBSTANCES

INTERACTS WITH	COMBINED EFFECT
Alcohol:	None expected.
Beverages:	None expected.
Cocaine:	None expected. Best to avoid.
Foods:	None expected.
Marijuana:	None expected. Best to avoid.
Tobacco:	None expected.

*See Glossary

PLATELET INHIBITORS

GENERIC AND BRAND NAMES

CLOPIDOGREL
Plavix
PRASUGREL
Effient
TICLOPIDINE
Ticlid

BASIC INFORMATION

Habit forming? No
Prescription needed? Yes
Available as generic? Yes, for some
Drug class: Antithrombotic; platelet aggregation inhibitor

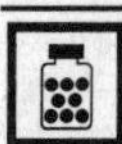

USES

Used for high risk patients to help prevent blood clots and reduce the risk of stroke, heart attack, or other serious problems with the heart or blood vessels. May be used in combination with aspirin therapy.

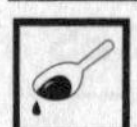

DOSAGE & USAGE INFORMATION

How to take:
Tablet—Swallow with liquid. If you can't swallow tablet whole, ask pharmacist for advice. Take ticlopidine with food. Clopidogrel and prasugrel may be taken with or without food.

When to take:
As directed. Usually twice a day for ticlopidine and once a day for clopidogrel and prasugrel.

If you forget a dose:
Take as soon as you remember. If it is almost time for the next dose, wait for next scheduled dose (don't double this dose).

What drug does:
Prevents certain blood cells from clumping together which reduces the risk of blood clots.

Time lapse before drug works:
1-2 hours. It will take several days for full benefit.

Don't take with:
Any other medicine or any dietary supplement without consulting your doctor or pharmacist.

OVERDOSE

SYMPTOMS:
Bloody vomit or excessive bleeding from gums, nose or rectum, difficult breathing.
WHAT TO DO:
Dial 911 (emergency) for medical help or call poison control center 1-800-222-1222 for instructions.

POSSIBLE ADVERSE REACTIONS OR SIDE EFFECTS

SYMPTOMS	WHAT TO DO
Life-threatening:	
Severe bleeding; rare allergic reaction (hives, itching, rash, trouble breathing, chest tightness, swelling of lips or tongue or face).	Seek emergency treatment immediately.
Common:	
• Chest pain, general body pain, red or purple spots on skin, dizziness, blurred vision.	Continue, but call doctor right away.
• Diarrhea, stomach ache, back pain heartburn, muscle aches, symptoms of a cold.	Continue. Call doctor when convenient.
Infrequent:	
• Unusual bleeding or bruising, slow or fast or irregular heartbeat, shortness of breath, black or tarry stools, bloating or swelling, difficult or painful or decreased urination, swollen glands, chest discomfort, chills, cough, fever, fainting, tingling of hands or feet, unusual weight gain or loss, unusual tiredness or weakness, sore throat, sores on the lips or in mouth, lightheadedness.	Continue, but call doctor right away.
• Mild headache, mild weakness, rash, pain in arms or legs.	Continue. Call doctor when convenient.
Rare:	
• Sudden severe headache or weakness, severe stomach pain, peeling or flaking or blistering skin, being uncoordinated, symptoms of thrombotic thrombocytopenic purpura (mental changes, dark or bloody urine, difficult speaking, pale skin, seizures, yellow eyes or skin, fever, weakness).	Continue, but call doctor right away.

• Loss of appetite, gaseousness, nausea, mild tiredness, constipation, trouble sleeping, anxious or depressed.	Continue. Call doctor when convenient.

WARNINGS & PRECAUTIONS

Don't take if:
- You are allergic to any platelet inhibitor.
- You have active bleeding (e.g., head, bowel or stomach).

Before you start, consult your doctor if:
- You have liver disease, kidney disease, diabetes, stomach ulcers or diverticulitis.
- You have recurrent bleeding (e.g., head, bowel or stomach).
- You have history of stroke, transient ischemic attack (TIA), mini-stroke or heart disorder.
- You weigh under 132 pounds (60 kilograms).
- You have had a recent injury (trauma).
- You have had thrombotic thrombocytopenic purpura.
- You are planning or have had recent surgery or other medical procedure.

Over age 60:
Prasugrel is not recommended for patients 75 years of age and older due to drug's toxicity.

Pregnancy:
Use during pregnancy only if clearly needed. Consult doctor. Risk category B (see page xviii).

Breast-feeding:
It is not known if drug passes into milk. Avoid drug or discontinue nursing until you finish medicine. Consult doctor for advice on maintaining milk supply.

Infants & children:
Not recommended. Safety has not been established.

Prolonged use:
Regular follow up visits to your doctor are important to monitor the effects of the drug.

Skin & sunlight:
No special problems expected.

Driving, piloting or hazardous work:
Don't drive or pilot aircraft until you learn how the medicine affects you. Don't work around dangerous machinery. Don't climb ladders or work in high places. Danger increases if you drink alcohol or take medicine affecting alertness and reflexes.

Discontinuing:
Don't discontinue without medical advice. It can increase your risk for heart attack or stroke.

Others:
- Advise any doctor or dentist whom you consult that you take this medicine. You may be advised to discontinue the drug 1-2 weeks before elective surgery (including dental surgery).
- Wear a medical identification bracelet or tag that indicates you are taking this drug.
- When possible, avoid situations or activities that can increase risk of bleeding or bruising.
- Report any unusual bleeding to your doctor.

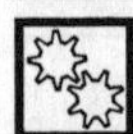

POSSIBLE INTERACTION WITH OTHER DRUGS

GENERIC NAME OR DRUG CLASS	COMBINED EFFECT
Antacids*	Decreased ticlopidine effect.
Anticoagulants	Increased risk of bleeding.
Anti-inflammatory drugs, nonsteroidal (NSAIDs)*	Increased risk of bleeding.
Aspirin	Increased risk of bleeding.
Enzyme inhibitors*	Decreased effect of clopidogrel.
Phenytoin	Increased phenytoin effect with ticlopidine.
Proton pump inhibitors	Decreased effect of clopidogrel.
Thrombolytic agents*	Increased risk of bleeding.
Xanthines*	Increased xanthine effect with ticlopidine.

POSSIBLE INTERACTION WITH OTHER SUBSTANCES

INTERACTS WITH	COMBINED EFFECT
Alcohol:	Increased risk of side effects. Avoid.
Beverages:	None expected.
Cocaine:	Unknown. Avoid.
Foods:	None expected.
Marijuana:	Unknown. Avoid.
Tobacco:	None expected.

***See Glossary**

POTASSIUM SUPPLEMENTS

GENERIC AND BRAND NAMES

See full list of generic and brand names in the *Generic and Brand Name Directory*, page 894.

BASIC INFORMATION

Habit forming? No
Prescription needed? Yes
Available as generic? Yes
Drug class: Mineral supplement (potassium), electrolyte replenisher, antihyperthyroid.

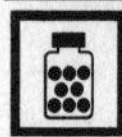

USES

- Treatment for potassium deficiency due to diuretics, cortisone or digitalis medicines.
- Treatment for hypercalcemia due to cancer.
- Treats overactive thyroid disease.
- Treats iodine deficiency.
- Treatment for low potassium associated with some illnesses.

DOSAGE & USAGE INFORMATION

How to take:
- Tablet or capsule—Take as directed on label.
- Effervescent tablets, granules, powder or liquid—Dilute dose in water.

When to take:
At the same time each day, preferably with food or immediately after meals.

If you forget a dose:
Take as soon as you remember. If it is almost time for the next dose, wait for that dose (don't double this dose) and resume regular schedule.

What drug does:
Preserves or restores normal function of nerve cells, thyroid, heart and skeletal muscle cells and kidneys, as well as stomach juice secretions.

Continued next column

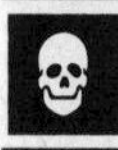

OVERDOSE

SYMPTOMS:
Paralysis of arms and legs, irregular heartbeat, blood pressure drop, convulsions, coma, cardiac arrest.
WHAT TO DO:
- **Dial 911 (emergency) for medical help or call poison control center 1-800-222-1222 for instructions.**
- **See emergency information on last 3 pages of this book.**

Time lapse before drug works:
30 minutes to 2 hours. Full benefit may require 12 to 24 hours.

Don't take with:
Any other medicine or any dietary supplement without consulting your doctor or pharmacist.

POSSIBLE ADVERSE REACTIONS OR SIDE EFFECTS

SYMPTOMS	WHAT TO DO
Life-threatening:	
In case of overdose, see previous column.	
Common:	
• Skin rash, swollen salivary glands.	Discontinue. Call doctor right away.
• Diarrhea, nausea abdominal pain.	Continue. Call doctor when convenient.
Infrequent:	
Bone and joint pain, numbness or tingling in hands or feet, vomiting, dizziness.	Discontinue. Call doctor right away.
Rare:	
Confusion; irregular heartbeat; difficult breathing; unusual fatigue; weakness; heaviness of legs; hemorrhage, perforation with enteric-coated tablets (rarely with wax matrix tablets); esophageal ulceration with tablets; bloody stools.	Discontinue. Call doctor right away.

WARNINGS & PRECAUTIONS

Don't take if:
- You are allergic to any potassium supplement.
- You have acute or chronic kidney disease.

Before you start, consult your doctor if:
- You have Addison's disease or familial periodic paralysis.
- You have heart disease.
- You have intestinal blockage.
- You have a stomach ulcer.
- You use diuretics.
- You have high blood pressure.
- You have kidney disease.
- You have pancreatitis.
- You use heart medicine.
- You use laxatives or have chronic diarrhea.
- You use salt substitutes or low-salt milk.

Over age 60:
Observe dose schedule strictly. Potassium balance is critical.

Pregnancy:
Consult with your doctor before taking potassium supplements, as they may pose a significant risk to your unborn child. Risk category D (see page xviii).

Breast-feeding:
Drug passes into milk. Avoid drug or discontinue nursing until you finish medicine. Consult doctor for advice on maintaining milk supply.

Infants & children:
Use only under doctor's supervision.

Prolonged use:
- Talk to your doctor about the need for follow-up medical examinations or laboratory studies to check serum potassium levels.
- If burning mouth, headache or salivation occur, call doctor.

Skin & sunlight:
No problems expected.

Driving, piloting or hazardous work:
Don't drive or pilot aircraft until you learn how medicine affects you. Don't work around dangerous machinery. Don't climb ladders or work in high places. Danger increases if you drink alcohol or take medicine affecting alertness and reflexes.

Discontinuing:
Don't discontinue without consulting doctor. Dose may require gradual reduction if you have taken drug for a long time. Doses of other drugs may also require adjustment.

Others:
- Overdose or underdose can have serious effect. Frequent EKGs and lab blood studies are recommended to measure serum electrolytes and kidney function.
- Prolonged diarrhea may call for increased dosage of potassium.
- Advise any doctor or dentist you consult that you take this medicine.
- Serious injury may necessitate temporary decrease in potassium.
- Some products contain tartrazine dye. Avoid, especially if you are allergic to aspirin.

POSSIBLE INTERACTION WITH OTHER DRUGS

GENERIC NAME OR DRUG CLASS	COMBINED EFFECT
Adrenocorticoids, systemic	Decreased potassium effect.
Amiloride	Dangerous rise in blood potassium.
Angiotensin-converting enzyme (ACE) inhibitors*	Possible increased potassium effect.
Antacids*	May decrease potassium absorption.
Anticholinergics, other*	Increased possibility of intestinal ulcers, which sometimes occur with oral potassium tablets.
Anti-inflammatory drugs, nonsteroidal (NSAIDs)*	Increased risk of stomach irritation.
Antithyroid drugs*	Excessive effect of antithyroid drugs.
Beta-adrenergic blocking agents*	Increased potassium levels.
Calcium	Decreased potassium effect.
Cortisone drugs*	Increased fluid retention.
Digitalis preparations*	Possible irregular heartbeat.
Diuretics, thiazide or loop*	Decreased potassium effect.
Laxatives*	Possible decreased potassium effect.
Lithium	Increased chance of producing a thyroid goiter.
Losartan	Increased potassium levels.

Continued on page 925

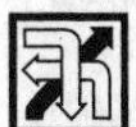

POSSIBLE INTERACTION WITH OTHER SUBSTANCES

INTERACTS WITH	COMBINED EFFECT
Alcohol:	None expected.
Beverages:	
• Salty drinks such as tomato juice, commercial thirst quenchers.	Increased fluid retention.
• Low-salt milk or salt substitutes.	Increased potassium levels.
Cocaine:	May cause irregular heartbeat.
Foods: Salty foods.	Increased fluid retention.
Marijuana:	May cause irregular heartbeat.
Tobacco:	None expected.

*See Glossary

PRAMLINTIDE

BRAND NAMES

Symlin SymlinPen

BASIC INFORMATION

Habit forming? No
Prescription needed? Yes
Available as generic? No
Drug class: Antidiabetic; amylinomimetic

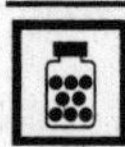

USES

Treatment for certain patients with type 1 or type 2 diabetes who already use insulin, but still need better blood sugar control.

DOSAGE & USAGE INFORMATION

How to take:
Self-injection—Injected under the skin (subcutaneous) of the upper leg (thigh) or stomach area (abdomen). Inject pramlintide at a site that is more than 2 inches away from your insulin injection. Read and carefully follow the instructions provided with the prescription. Your doctor will advise you of any necessary changes in your insulin dosages. Never mix insulin and pramlintide. Use different syringes. Rotate injection sites.

When to take:
Inject it just before major meals. A major meal must have at least 250 calories or 30 grams of carbohydrate. Adjust your pre-meal insulin dose and check blood sugar before and after every meal and at bedtime (or as advised by doctor).

If you forget a dose:
If you forget to inject the dose before you start eating a meal, skip that dose and then inject the next dose as scheduled. Don't double that dose.

Continued next column

OVERDOSE

SYMPTOMS:
Severe nausea, vomiting, diarrhea, dizziness.
WHAT TO DO:

- **Overdose unlikely to threaten life. If person uses much larger amount than prescribed or if accidentally swallowed, call doctor or poison control center 1-800-222-1222 for help.**
- **Be alert to hypoglycemia (low blood sugar) symptoms listed in next column under Infrequent. Pramlintide alone dose not cause hypoglycemia, but it is used with insulin and insulin can induce hypoglycemia.**

What drug does:

- Slows down movement of food through the stomach. This affects how fast sugar enters the blood after eating. It reduces blood sugar output by the liver.
- It reduces appetite by creating a feeling of fulness resulting in potential weight loss.

Time lapse before drug works:
Within the 3 hours after a meal.

Don't take with:
Any other medicine or any dietary supplement without consulting your doctor or pharmacist.

POSSIBLE ADVERSE REACTIONS OR SIDE EFFECTS

SYMPTOMS	WHAT TO DO
Life-threatening:	
Allergic reaction (difficulty breathing, closing of the throat, swelling of the lips or face or tongue, hives).	Seek emergency treatment immediately.
Common:	
Nausea.	Continue. Call doctor if symptom persists.
Infrequent:	
• Indigestion, loss of appetite, vomiting, stomach pain, tiredness, dizziness, injection site reaction (redness, bruising, pain), joint pain, cough, sore throat, headache.	Continue. Call doctor when convenient.
• Symptoms of low blood sugar—nervousness, hunger (excessive), cold sweats, rapid pulse, anxiety, cold skin, chills, confusion, loss of concentration, drowsiness, headache, nausea, weakness, shakiness, vision changes.	Seek treatment (eat some form of quick-acting sugar—glucose tablets, sugar, fruit juice, corn syrup, honey).
• Symptoms of high blood sugar—increased urination, unusual thirst, dry mouth, drowsiness, flushed or dry skin, fruit-like breath odor, appetite loss, stomach pain or vomiting, tiredness, trouble breathing, increased blood sugar level.	Check your blood sugar immediately. Call doctor right away.

Rare:

Other symptoms that cause concern.	Continue. Call doctor when convenient.

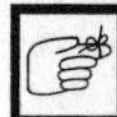

WARNINGS & PRECAUTIONS

Don't take if:
You are allergic to pramlintide.

Before you start, consult your doctor if:
- You suffer from gastroparesis (a condition in which the stomach does not empty properly).
- You have difficulty recognizing symptoms of hypoglycemia (low blood sugar).
- You have poor control of your diabetes (e.g., HbA1c is over 9.0%).
- You have difficulty with your insulin regimen or monitoring your blood sugar levels or have recurrent episodes of hypoglycemia.

Over age 60:
No special problems expected.

Pregnancy:
Decide with your doctor if drug benefits justify risk to unborn child. Risk category C (see page xviii).

Breast-feeding:
It is unknown if drug passes into milk. Consult doctor for advice about the risks and benefits.

Infants & children:
Safety and effectiveness in children has not been established. Consult your child's doctor.

Prolonged use:
Talk to your doctor about the need for follow-up medical examinations and/or laboratory studies to check effectiveness of the drug.

Skin & sunlight:
No problems expected.

Driving, piloting or hazardous work:
No problems expected. You do need to be cautious for symptoms of hypoglycemia (especially at the start of drug treatment).

Discontinuing:
Don't discontinue without doctor's advice.

Others:
- Notify your doctor if you have a fever, infection, diarrhea, or experience vomiting.
- Advise any doctor or dentist whom you consult that you take this medicine.
- Wear or carry medical identification that indicates you have type 1 or type 2 diabetes and the drugs you take.
- You and your family should educate yourselves about diabetes; learn to recognize the symptoms of hypoglycemia and how to treat it. Hypoglycemia may occur in the treatment of diabetes as a result of skipped meals, excessive exercise, or alcohol consumption. Carry non-dietetic candy or glucose tablets to treat episodes of low blood sugar.
- Follow your prescribed diet, drug regimen and exercise routines closely. Changing any of these things can affect blood sugar levels.

POSSIBLE INTERACTION WITH OTHER DRUGS

GENERIC NAME OR DRUG CLASS	COMBINED EFFECT
Acarbose	Decreased absorption of nutrients.
Anticholinergics*	Decreased stomach emptying.
Antidiabetics, oral*	Increased risk of hypoglycemia.
Drugs taken by mouth that need to pass quickly through the stomach (such as oral contraceptives or antibiotics)	May need to take. them 1 hour before or 2 hours after injecting pramlintide.
Drugs that may increase blood sugar lowering or increase risk of hypoglycemia	Increased risk of hypoglycemia.
Insulin	Possible severe hypoglycemia can occur within 3 hours of pramlintide dose.
Miglitol	Decreased absorption of nutrients.

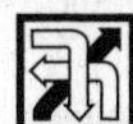

POSSIBLE INTERACTION WITH OTHER SUBSTANCES

INTERACTS WITH	COMBINED EFFECT
Alcohol:	May cause severe low blood sugar. Avoid.
Beverages:	None expected.
Cocaine:	Unknown effect. Avoid.
Foods:	None expected. Follow your diabetic diet instructions.
Marijuana:	Possible increase in blood sugar. Avoid.
Tobacco:	None expected. Best to avoid.

***See Glossary**

PREGABALIN

BRAND NAMES

Lyrica

BASIC INFORMATION

Habit forming? No
Prescription needed? Yes
Available as generic? Yes
Drug class: Antiepileptic

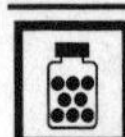

USES

- Treatment for neuropathic (nerve) pain that is associated with disorders such as diabetic peripheral neuropathy, postherpetic neuralgia and spinal cord injuries.
- Treatment for fibromyalgia (a disorder that causes pain, fatigue and sleep problems).
- Used along with other drugs to treat epilepsy.
- Treats other disorders as advised by doctor.

DOSAGE & USAGE INFORMATION

How to take:
- Capsule—Swallow with liquid. Take with or without food.
- Solution—Follow directions on label.

When to take:
2-3 times a day at the same times each day. Dosage may be increased by your doctor after 3-7 days depending on your response.

If you forget a dose:
Take as soon as you remember. If it is almost time for the next dose, wait for that dose (don't double this dose) and resume regular schedule.

What drug does:
The exact mechanism is unclear. It has an affect on certain nerve transmissions in the brain and spinal cord which results in the analgesic (pain relief), anticonvulsant and anti-anxiety activity.

Time lapse before drug works:
Starts working the first day, but may take a week or more to determine full effectiveness.

Continued next column

OVERDOSE

SYMPTOMS:
Unknown (may be similar to side effects).
WHAT TO DO:
Overdose unlikely to threaten life. If person uses much larger amount than prescribed or if accidentally swallowed, call doctor or poison control center 1-800-222-1222 for help.

Don't take with:
Any other medicine or any dietary supplement without consulting your doctor or pharmacist.

POSSIBLE ADVERSE REACTIONS OR SIDE EFFECTS

SYMPTOMS	WHAT TO DO
Life-threatening:	
Rare allergic reaction—Breathing difficulty; closing of the throat; swelling of hands, feet, face, lips or tongue; hives.	Discontinue. Seek emergency treatment.
Common:	
Dizziness, dry mouth, sleepiness, swelling (hands, feet, ankles), blurred or double vision, weight gain, headache, problems with concentration or attention, appetite increased, vomiting, constipation, erectile dysfunction.	Continue. Call doctor when convenient.
Infrequent:	
Emotional changes, diarrhea, unsteady movements (ataxia), euphoric mood, other mood changes, fatigue, sexual function change, hallucinations, unusual dreams, flushing or burning feeling, body symptoms (aches, pain, stiffness, weakness, twitching, tightness), urination changes, dry nose, thirstiness, stomach upset or swollen, eye symptoms (pain, dry, tearing), heartbeat is faster, mild breathing difficulty, rash or hives, insomnia worsens, decreased appetite.	Continue. Call doctor when convenient.
Rare:	
Cold-like symptoms, heartbeat is slower or change in rhythm, changes in blood pressure, menstrual changes, breast pain or discharge, hands or feet feel cold, other new or unexplained symptoms.	Continue. Call doctor when convenient.

WARNINGS & PRECAUTIONS

Don't take if:

- You are allergic to pregabalin.
- You have certain rare hereditary problems (galactose intolerance, the Lapp lactase deficiency or glucose-galactose malabsorption).

Before you start, consult your doctor if:

- You have diabetes.
- You have any kidney disorder.

Over age 60:
If you experience dizziness or sleepiness, take precautions to prevent accidents such as falls.

Pregnancy:
Decide with your doctor if drug benefits justify risk to unborn child. Risk category C (see page xviii).

Breast-feeding:
It is unknown if drug passes into milk. Avoid drug or discontinue nursing until you finish medicine. Consult doctor for advice on maintaining milk supply.

Infants & children:
Safety and effectiveness for children under age 18 has not been established.

Prolonged use:
Talk to your doctor about the need for follow-up examinations to determine continued effectiveness of the drug in treating your disorder.

Skin & sunlight:
No special problems expected.

Driving, piloting or hazardous work:
Don't drive or pilot aircraft until you learn how medicine affects you. Don't work around dangerous machinery. Don't climb ladders or work in high places. Danger increases if you drink alcohol or take other medicines affecting alertness and reflexes.

Discontinuing:
Don't discontinue drug without doctor's advice. Dosage may need to be gradually reduced.

Others:

- Don't increase or decrease drug dosage without doctor's approval.
- Advise any doctor or dentist whom you consult that you take this medicine.
- Rarely, antiepileptic drugs may lead to suicidal thoughts and behaviors. Call doctor right away if suicidal symptoms or unusual behaviors occur.
- Wear or carry medical identification to show your seizure disorder and the drugs you take.

POSSIBLE INTERACTION WITH OTHER DRUGS

GENERIC NAME OR DRUG CLASS	COMBINED EFFECT
Central nervous system (CNS) depressants*	May add to any sedative effect.
Lorazepam	Increased effect of lorazepam.
Oxycodone	Increased risk of side effects.

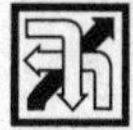

POSSIBLE INTERACTION WITH OTHER SUBSTANCES

INTERACTS WITH	COMBINED EFFECT
Alcohol:	Increased risk of side effects, such as sedation. Avoid.
Beverages:	None expected.
Cocaine:	Effects unknown. Avoid.
Foods:	None expected.
Marijuana:	Effects unknown. Avoid.
Tobacco:	None expected.

*See Glossary

PRIMAQUINE

GENERIC NAMES

PRIMAQUINE

BASIC INFORMATION

Habit forming? No
Prescription needed? Yes
Available as generic? Yes
Drug class: Antiprotozoal (antimalarial)

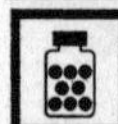

USES

- Treats some forms of malaria.
- Prevents relapses of some forms of malaria.
- Treats *Pneumocystis pneumonia* (used in combination with clindamycin).

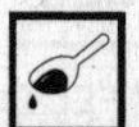

DOSAGE & USAGE INFORMATION

How to take:
Tablet—Take with meals or antacids to minimize stomach irritation.

When to take:
At the same time each day, according to instructions on prescription label.

If you forget a dose:
Take as soon as you remember. If it is almost time for the next dose, wait for that dose (don't double this dose) and resume regular schedule.

What drug does:
Alters the properties of DNA in malaria organisms to prevent them from multiplying.

Time lapse before drug works:
2 to 3 hours.

Don't take with:
Any other medicine or any dietary supplement without consulting your doctor or pharmacist.

OVERDOSE

SYMPTOMS:
None expected.
WHAT TO DO:
Overdose unlikely to threaten life. If person uses much larger amount than prescribed or if accidentally swallowed, call doctor or poison control center 1-800-222-1222 for help.

POSSIBLE ADVERSE REACTIONS OR SIDE EFFECTS

SYMPTOMS	WHAT TO DO
Life-threatening: None expected.	
Common: None expected.	
Infrequent: Dark urine; back, leg or stomach pain; appetite loss; pale skin; fever.	Discontinue. Call doctor right away.
Rare: Blue fingernails, lips and skin; dizziness; difficult breathing; extraordinary tiredness; sore throat.	Discontinue. Call doctor right away.

WARNINGS & PRECAUTIONS

Don't take if:

- You have G6PD* deficiency.
- You are hypersensitive to primaquine.

Before you start, consult your doctor if:
You are Black, Oriental, Asian or of Mediterranean origin.

Over age 60:
No special problems expected.

Pregnancy:
Decide with your doctor if drug benefits justify risk to unborn child. Risk category C (see page xviii).

Breast-feeding:
Effect unknown. Consult doctor.

Infants & children:
No special problems expected.

Prolonged use:
No special problems expected.

Skin & sunlight:
No special problems expected.

Driving, piloting or hazardous work:
No special problems expected.

Discontinuing:
No special problems expected.

Others:

- If you are Black, Asian, Oriental or of Mediterranean origin, insist on a test for G6PD* deficiency before taking this medicine.
- Advise any doctor or dentist whom you consult that you take this medicine.

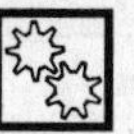

POSSIBLE INTERACTION WITH OTHER DRUGS

GENERIC NAME OR DRUG CLASS	COMBINED EFFECT
Hemolytics,* other	Increased risk of serious side effects affecting the blood.
Quinacrine	Increased toxic effects of primaquine.

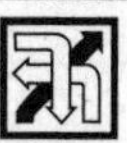

POSSIBLE INTERACTION WITH OTHER SUBSTANCES

INTERACTS WITH	COMBINED EFFECT
Alcohol:	Possible liver toxicity. Avoid.
Beverages:	None expected.
Cocaine:	None expected.
Foods:	None expected.
Marijuana:	None expected.
Tobacco:	None expected.

PRIMIDONE

BRAND NAMES

Apo-Primidone
Myidone
Mysoline
PMS Primidone
Sertan

BASIC INFORMATION

Habit forming? No
Prescription needed? Yes
Available as generic? Yes
Drug class: Anticonvulsant

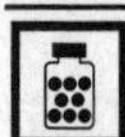

USES

Prevents some forms of epileptic seizures.

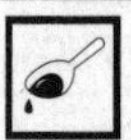

DOSAGE & USAGE INFORMATION

How to take:

- Tablet—Swallow with liquid. If you can't swallow whole, crumble tablet and take with liquid or food.
- Liquid—If desired, dilute dose in beverage before swallowing.

When to take:
Daily in regularly spaced doses, according to doctor's prescription.

If you forget a dose:
Take as soon as you remember. If it is almost time for the next dose, wait for that dose (don't double this dose) and resume regular schedule.

What drug does:
The exact way it works is unknown. It appears to reduce seizures by controlling certain electrical impulses in the brain.

Time lapse before drug works:
2 to 3 weeks for full effectiveness.

Continued next column

OVERDOSE

SYMPTOMS:
Slow, shallow breathing; weak, rapid pulse; confusion, deep sleep, coma.
WHAT TO DO:

- **Dial 911 (emergency) for medical help or call poison control center 1-800-222-1222 for instructions.**
- **If person is unconscious, check breathing and pulse. If not breathing, begin mouth-to-mouth rescue breathing. If heart is not beating, begin chest compressions.**
- **See emergency information on last 3 pages of this book.**

Don't take with:
Any other medicine or any dietary supplement without consulting your doctor or pharmacist.

POSSIBLE ADVERSE REACTIONS OR SIDE EFFECTS

SYMPTOMS	WHAT TO DO
Life-threatening:	
In case of overdose, see previous column.	
Common:	
• Difficult breathing.	Discontinue. Call doctor right away.
• Confusion, change in vision.	Continue. Call doctor when convenient.
• Clumsiness, dizziness, drowsiness.	Continue. Tell doctor at next visit.
Infrequent:	
• Unusual excitement, particularly in children; nausea; vomiting.	Discontinue. Call doctor right away.
• Headache, fatigue, weakness.	Continue. Call doctor when convenient.
Rare:	
• Rash or hives, appetite loss, acute psychosis, hair loss, fever, joint pain.	Discontinue. Call doctor right away.
• Swollen eyelids or legs.	Continue. Call doctor when convenient.
• Decreased sexual ability.	Continue. Tell doctor at next visit.

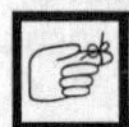

WARNINGS & PRECAUTIONS

Don't take if:

- You are allergic to primidone.
- You have had porphyria.

Before you start, consult your doctor if:

- You have had liver, kidney or lung disease or asthma.
- You have lupus.

Over age 60:
Adverse reactions and side effects may be more frequent and severe than in younger persons.

Pregnancy:
Consult doctor. Risk category D (see page xviii).

Breast-feeding:
Drug filters into milk. May harm child. Avoid. Consult doctor.

Infants & children:
Use only under medical supervision.

Prolonged use:
- Enlarged lymph and thyroid glands.
- Anemia.
- Rickets in children and osteomalacia (insufficient calcium to bones) in adults.
- Talk to your doctor about the need for follow-up medical examinations or laboratory studies.

Skin & sunlight:
No special problems expected.

Driving, piloting or hazardous work:
Don't drive or pilot aircraft until you learn how medicine affects you. Don't work around dangerous machinery. Don't climb ladders or work in high places. Danger increases if you drink alcohol or take medicine affecting alertness and reflexes.

Discontinuing:
Don't discontinue abruptly or without doctor's advice until you complete prescribed dose, even though symptoms diminish or disappear.

Others:
- Tell doctor if you become ill or injured and must interrupt dose schedule.
- Periodic laboratory blood tests of drug level recommended.
- Rarely, antiepileptic drugs may lead to suicidal thoughts and behaviors. Call doctor right away if suicidal symptoms or unusual behaviors occur.
- Wear or carry medical identification to show your seizure disorder and the drugs you take.

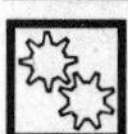

POSSIBLE INTERACTION WITH OTHER DRUGS

GENERIC NAME OR DRUG CLASS	COMBINED EFFECT
Adrenocorticoids, systemic	Decreased adrenocorticoid effect.
Anticoagulants,* oral	Decreased primidone effect.
Anticonvulsants,* other	Changed seizure pattern.
Antidepressants*	Increased antidepressant effect.
Antihistamines*	Increased sedation effect of primidone.
Aspirin	Decreased aspirin effect.
Carbamazepine	Unpredictable increase or decrease of primidone effect.
Carbonic anhydrase inhibitors*	Possible decreased primidone effect.
Central nervous system (CNS) depressants*	Increased CNS depressant effects.
Contraceptives, oral*	Decreased contraceptive effect.
Cyclosporine	Decreased cyclosporine effect.
Digitalis preparations*	Decreased digitalis effect.
Disulfiram	Possible increased primidone effect.
Estrogens*	Decreased estrogen effect.
Griseofulvin	Possible decreased griseofulvin effect.
Isoniazid	Decreased primidone effect.
Lamotrigine	Decreased lamotrigine effect.
Leucovorin (large dose)	May counteract anticonvulsant effect of primidone.
Loxapine	Decreased anticonvulsant effect of primidone.
Metronidazole	Possible decreased metronidazole effect.
Mind-altering drugs*	Increased effect of mind-altering drug.
Monoamine oxidase (MAO) inhibitors*	Increased sedation effect of primidone.
Nabilone	Greater depression of central nervous system.

Continued on page 925

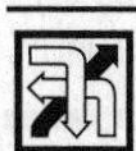

POSSIBLE INTERACTION WITH OTHER SUBSTANCES

INTERACTS WITH	COMBINED EFFECT
Alcohol:	Dangerous sedative effect. Avoid.
Beverages:	None expected.
Cocaine:	Decreased primidone effect.
Foods:	Possible need for more vitamin D.
Marijuana:	Decreased anti-convulsant effect.
Tobacco:	None expected.

*See Glossary

PROBENECID

BRAND NAMES

Benemid
Benuryl
Col-Probenecid
Probalan

BASIC INFORMATION

Habit forming? No
Prescription needed? Yes
Available as generic? Yes
Drug class: Antigout

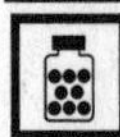

USES

- Treats chronic gout.
- Increases blood levels of penicillins and cephalosporins.

DOSAGE & USAGE INFORMATION

How to take:
Tablet—Swallow with liquid or food to lessen stomach irritation. If you can't swallow whole, crumble tablet and take with liquid or food.

When to take:
At the same time each day.

If you forget a dose:
Take as soon as you remember up to 12 hours late. If more than 12 hours, wait for next scheduled dose (don't double this dose).

What drug does:
- Forces kidneys to excrete uric acid.
- Reduces amount of penicillin excreted in urine.

Time lapse before drug works:
May require several months of regular use to prevent acute gout.

Don't take with:
- Nonprescription drugs containing aspirin or caffeine.
- Any other medicine or any dietary supplement without consulting your doctor or pharmacist.

OVERDOSE

SYMPTOMS:
Breathing difficulty, severe nervous agitation, vomiting, seizures, convulsions, delirium, coma.
WHAT TO DO:
- **Dial 911 (emergency) for medical help or call poison control center 1-800-222-1222 for instructions.**
- **See emergency information on last 3 pages of this book.**

POSSIBLE ADVERSE REACTIONS OR SIDE EFFECTS

SYMPTOMS	WHAT TO DO
Life-threatening: In case of overdose, see previous column.	
Common: Headache, appetite loss, nausea, vomiting.	Continue. Call doctor when convenient.
Infrequent: • Blood in urine, low back pain, worsening gout.	Discontinue. Call doctor right away.
• Dizziness, flushed face, itchy skin.	Continue. Call doctor when convenient.
• Painful or frequent urination, sore gums.	Continue. Tell doctor at next visit.
Rare: Sore throat, fever and chills; difficult breathing; unusual bleeding or bruising; red, painful joint; jaundice; foot, leg or face swelling.	Discontinue. Call doctor right away.

WARNINGS & PRECAUTIONS

Don't take if:
- You are allergic to any uricosuric.*
- You have acute gout.
- Patient is younger than 2.

Before you start, consult your doctor if:
- You have had kidney stones or kidney disease.
- You have a peptic ulcer.
- You have bone marrow or blood cell disease.
- You are undergoing chemotherapy for cancer.

Over age 60:
Adverse reactions and side effects may be more frequent and severe than in younger persons.

Pregnancy:
Consult doctor. Risk category B (see page xviii).

Breast-feeding:
It is unknown if drug passes into milk. Avoid drug or discontinue nursing until you finish medicine. Consult doctor for advice on maintaining milk supply.

Infants & children:
Not recommended.

Prolonged use:
- Possible kidney damage.
- Talk to your doctor about the need for follow-up medical examinations or laboratory studies to check serum uric acid, urine uric acid.

Skin & sunlight:
No problems expected.

Driving, piloting or hazardous work:
Avoid if you feel dizzy. Otherwise, no problems expected.

Discontinuing:
Don't discontinue without consulting doctor. Dose may require gradual reduction if you have taken drug for a long time. Doses of other drugs may also require adjustment.

Others:
- If signs of gout attack develop while taking medicine, consult doctor.
- Advise any doctor or dentist whom you consult that you take this medicine.

POSSIBLE INTERACTION WITH OTHER DRUGS

GENERIC NAME OR DRUG CLASS	COMBINED EFFECT
Allopurinol	Increased effect of each drug.
Anticoagulants,* oral	Increased anticoagulant effect.
Anti-inflammatory drugs, nonsteroidal (NSAIDs)*	Increased toxic risk.
Aspirin	Decreased probenecid effect.
Bismuth subsalicylate	Decreased probenecid effect.
Cephalosporins*	Increased cephalosporin effect.
Ciprofloxacin	May cause kidney dysfunction.
Dapsone	Increased dapsone effect. Increased toxicity.
Diclofenac	Increased diclofenac effect.
Diuretics, thiazide*	Decreased probenecid effect.
Hypoglycemics, oral*	Increased hypoglycemic effect.
Indomethacin	Increased adverse effects of indomethacin.
Ketoprofen	Increased risk of ketoprofen toxicity.
Loracarbef	Increased loracarbef effect.
Methotrexate	Increased methotrexate toxicity.
Nitrofurantoin	Increased effect of nitrofurantoin.
Para-aminosalicylic acid	Increased effect of para-aminosalicylic acid.
Penicillins*	Enhanced penicillin effect.
Pyrazinamide	Decreased probenecid effect.
Salicylates*	Decreased probenecid effect.
Sodium benzoate & sodium phenylacetate	May reduce effect of sodium benzoate & sodium phenylacetate.
Sulfa drugs*	Slows elimination. May cause harmful accumulation of sulfa.
Thioguanine	More likelihood of toxicity of both drugs.
Valacyclovir	Increased valacyclovir effect.
Zidovudine	Increased zidovudine toxicity risk.

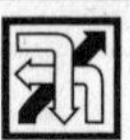

POSSIBLE INTERACTION WITH OTHER SUBSTANCES

INTERACTS WITH	COMBINED EFFECT
Alcohol:	Decreased probenecid effect.
Beverages: Caffeine drinks.	Loss of probenecid effectiveness.
Cocaine:	None expected.
Foods:	None expected.
Marijuana:	Daily use—Decreased probenecid effect.
Tobacco:	None expected.

***See Glossary**

PROCARBAZINE

BRAND NAMES

Matulane
Natulan

BASIC INFORMATION

Habit forming? No
Prescription needed? Yes
Available as generic? No
Drug class: Antineoplastic

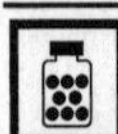

USES

Treatment for certain types of cancer.

DOSAGE & USAGE INFORMATION

How to take:
Capsule—Swallow with liquid after light meal. Don't drink fluids with meals. Drink extra fluids between meals. Avoid sweet or fatty foods.

When to take:
At the same time each day.

If you forget a dose:
Take as soon as you remember. If it is almost time for the next dose, wait for that dose (don't double this dose) and resume regular schedule.

What drug does:
Inhibits abnormal cell reproduction. Procarbazine is an alkylating agent* and an MAO inhibitor.

Time lapse before drug works:
Up to 6 weeks for full effect.

Don't take with:
Any other medicine or any dietary supplement without consulting your doctor or pharmacist.

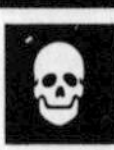

OVERDOSE

SYMPTOMS:
Restlessness, agitation, fever, convulsions, bleeding.
WHAT TO DO:

- **Dial 911 (emergency) for medical help or call poison control center 1-800-222-1222 for instructions.**
- **If person is unconscious, check breathing and pulse. If not breathing, begin mouth-to-mouth rescue breathing. If heart is not beating, begin chest compressions.**
- **See emergency information on last 3 pages of this book.**

POSSIBLE ADVERSE REACTIONS OR SIDE EFFECTS

SYMPTOMS	WHAT TO DO
Life-threatening:	
In case of overdose, see previous column.	
Common:	
• Nausea, vomiting, decreased urination, numbness or tingling in hands or feet, hair loss, rapid or pounding heartbeat, shortness of breath.	Discontinue. Call doctor right away.
• Fatigue, weakness, confusion.	Continue. Call doctor when convenient.
• Dizziness when changing position, dry mouth, inflamed tongue, constipation, difficult urination.	Continue. Tell doctor at next visit.
Infrequent:	
• Fainting.	Discontinue. Seek emergency treatment.
• Severe headache; abnormal bleeding or bruising; muscle, joint or chest pain, enlarged eye pupils; black, tarry stools; bloody urine.	Discontinue. Call doctor right away.
• Hallucinations, insomnia, nightmares, diarrhea, swollen feet or legs, nervousness, eyes sensitive to light, cough or hoarseness, mouth sores, depression.	Continue, but call doctor right away.
• Diminished sex drive.	Continue. Tell doctor at next visit.
Rare:	
Rash, stiff neck, jaundice, fever, sore throat, vomiting blood, wheezing.	Discontinue. Call doctor right away.

WARNINGS & PRECAUTIONS

Don't take if:
You are allergic to any MAO inhibitor.

Before you start, consult your doctor if:

- You are an alcoholic.
- You have asthma.
- You have heart disease, congestive heart failure, heart rhythm irregularities or high blood pressure.

- You have liver or kidney disease.
- You have had a stroke.
- You have diabetes or epilepsy.
- You have overactive thyroid.
- You have schizophrenia.
- You have Parkinson's disease.
- You have adrenal gland tumor.
- You will have surgery within 2 months, including dental surgery, requiring general or spinal anesthesia.

Over age 60:
Adverse reactions and side effects may be more frequent and severe than in younger persons.

Pregnancy:
Consult doctor. Risk category D (see page xviii).

Breast-feeding:
Safety not established. Consult doctor.

Infants & children:
Not recommended.

Prolonged use:
- May be toxic to liver.
- Talk to your doctor about the need for follow-up medical examinations or laboratory studies to check complete blood counts (white blood cell count, platelet count, red blood cell count, hemoglobin, hematocrit), bone marrow, kidney function.

Skin & sunlight:
No special problems expected.

Driving, piloting or hazardous work:
Don't drive or pilot aircraft until you learn how medicine affects you. Don't work around dangerous machinery. Don't climb ladders or work in high places. Danger increases if you drink alcohol or take medicine affecting alertness and reflexes.

Discontinuing:
- Don't discontinue without doctor's advice until you complete prescribed dose, even though symptoms diminish or disappear.
- Follow precautions regarding foods, drinks and other medicines for 2 weeks after discontinuing.

Others:
- May affect blood sugar levels in patients with diabetes.
- Advise any doctor or dentist whom you consult that you take this drug.

POSSIBLE INTERACTION WITH OTHER DRUGS

GENERIC NAME OR DRUG CLASS	COMBINED EFFECT
Amphetamines*	Blood pressure rise to life-threatening level.
Anticonvulsants,* oral	Changed seizure pattern.
Antidepressants, tricyclic*	Blood pressure rise to life-threatening level.
Antidiabetics,* oral and insulin	Excessively low blood sugar.
Antihistamines*	Increased sedation.
Barbiturates*	Increased sedation.
Bone marrow depressants*	Increased toxicity to bone marrow.
Buspirone	Elevated blood pressure.
Caffeine	Irregular heartbeat or high blood pressure.
Carbamazepine	Fever, seizures. Avoid.
Central nervous system (CNS) depressants*	Increased CNS depression.
Clozapine	Toxic effect on bone marrow and central nervous system.
Cyclobenzaprine	Fever, seizures. Avoid.
Dextromethorphan	Fever, hypertension.

Continued on page 925

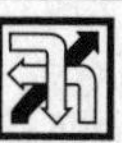

POSSIBLE INTERACTION WITH OTHER SUBSTANCES

INTERACTS WITH	COMBINED EFFECT
Alcohol:	Increased sedation to dangerous level. Disulfiram-like reaction.*
Beverages:	
Caffeine drinks.	Irregular heartbeat or high blood pressure.
Drinks containing tyramine.*	Blood pressure rise to life-threatening level.
Cocaine:	Overstimulation. Possibly fatal.
Foods:	
Foods containing tyramine.*	Blood pressure rise to life-threatening level.
Marijuana:	Overstimulation. Avoid.
Tobacco:	None expected.

***See Glossary**

PROGESTINS

GENERIC AND BRAND NAMES

See full list of generic and brand names in *Generic and Brand Name Directory*, page 894.

BASIC INFORMATION

Habit forming? No
Prescription needed? Yes, for most
Available as generic? Yes, for some.
Drug class: Female sex hormone (progestin)

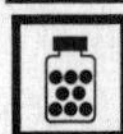

USES

- Treatment for menstrual or uterine disorders.
- Contraceptive (used alone or with estrogen). May be used for emergency contraception.
- Treatment for symptoms of menopause.
- Treatment for several types of cancer.
- Treatment for female hormone imbalance.
- Megestrol is used for treatment of weight loss in AIDS and cancer patients.
- Treatment for female infertility caused by progesterone deficiency.
- Treatment for endometrial hyperplasia.

DOSAGE & USAGE INFORMATION

How to take:

- Capsule—Swallow with liquid. Do not crush, chew or break capsule.
- Tablet—Swallow with liquid or food to lessen stomach irritation. You may crumble tablet.
- Injection—Given by medical provider.
- Transdermal patch—Follow label instructions.
- Implant—Inserted by a health care provider.
- Oral suspension—Follow label instructions.

When to take:

Daily dose at the same time each day. For other forms, follow instructions on label.

If you forget a dose:

- Treatment for menstrual disorders—Take as soon as you remember. If it is almost time for the next dose, wait for that dose (don't double this dose) and resume regular schedule.
- Contraceptive—Consult your doctor or label instructions. You may need to use another birth control method until your next period.

What drug does:

- Progesterone is a female hormone produced in the body. Progestins are synthetic hormones that have progesterone-like actions. They can have multiple effects on the female reproductive system.
- The mechanism that produces weight gain or helps in cancer treatment is unknown.

Time lapse before drug works:

- Menstrual disorders—24 to 48 hours.
- Contraception—3 weeks.
- Cancer—May require 2 to 3 months regular use for maximum benefit.

Don't take with:

Any other medicine or any dietary supplement without consulting your doctor or pharmacist.

OVERDOSE

SYMPTOMS:
Nausea, vomiting, fluid retention, breast discomfort or enlargement, vaginal bleeding.
WHAT TO DO:
Overdose unlikely to threaten life. If person uses much larger amount than prescribed or if accidentally swallowed, call doctor or poison control center 1-800-222-1222 for help.

POSSIBLE ADVERSE REACTIONS OR SIDE EFFECTS

SYMPTOMS	WHAT TO DO
Life-threatening:	
Anaphylaxis (severe allergic reaction).	Seek emergency treatment immediately.
Common:	
• Vaginal bleeding changes (heavy, irregular, spotting, stopped).	Continue, but call doctor right away.
• Abdominal cramping, bloating, swollen feet or ankles, tiredness or weakness, mild headache, nausea, mood changes, skin irritation with injection, skin pain with implant.	Continue. Call doctor when convenient.
Infrequent:	
Depression, acne, tender breasts, changes in facial or body hair, brown spots on skin, loss of sexual desire, insomnia.	Continue. Call doctor when convenient.
Rare:	
• Rash, changes in breast milk.	Continue, but call doctor right away.
• Blood clot with high doses for noncontraceptive use (sudden headache, pain in calf, vision changes, breathing or speech problems).	Discontinue. Seek emergency help.

WARNINGS & PRECAUTIONS

Don't take if:
You are allergic to any progestin hormone.

Before you start, consult your doctor if:
- You have diabetes, heart or kidney disease.
- You have liver or gallbladder disease.
- You have had thrombophlebitis, embolism or stroke, bleeding disorder or high cholesterol.
- You have unexplained vaginal bleeding.
- You have had breast or uterine cancer.
- You have varicose veins.
- You have a seizure disorder.
- You suffer from migraines or depression.
- You have breast disease (lumps, cysts).

Over age 60:
No special problems expected.

Pregnancy:
Risk factors vary for drugs in this group. See category list on page xviii and consult doctor.

Breast-feeding:
Drug passes into milk in small amounts. The low progestin dose used for contraception has not caused problems. Consult doctor for advice about breast-feeding.

Infants & children:
Use only for female children under medical supervision.

Prolonged use:
No problems expected.

Skin & sunlight:
No problems expected.

Driving, piloting or hazardous work:
No problems expected.

Discontinuing:
Consult doctor. This medicine stays in the body and may cause fetal abnormalities. Wait at least 3 months before becoming pregnant. Side effects may also occur (dizziness, nausea, unusual menstrual bleeding).

Others:
- For postmenopausal women, the use of hormone replacement therapy (HRT) which combines estrogen and progestin increases slightly the risk for breast cancer, heart attacks and stroke. HRT does not prevent heart disease. HRT is effective for menopause symptoms (used short term), and helps protect against osteoporosis and colon cancer. Other treatments are available for osteoporosis. Discuss with your doctor if HRT is the right treatment for you.
- Injection form (Depo-Provera) may result in the loss of bone density. The risk increases, the longer the drug is used. The bone loss may not be reversible.
- Patients with diabetes must be monitored closely. Consult doctor if changes in blood glucose levels occur.
- May affect results in some medical tests.
- Advise any doctor or dentist whom you consult that you take this medicine.
- Carefully read the paper called "Information for the Patient" that was given to you with your first prescription or a refill. If you lose it, ask your pharmacist for a copy.

POSSIBLE INTERACTION WITH OTHER DRUGS

GENERIC NAME OR DRUG CLASS	COMBINED EFFECT
Aminoglutethimide	Decreased progestin effect.
Enzyme inducers*	Decreased progestin effect.

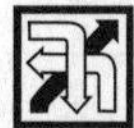

POSSIBLE INTERACTION WITH OTHER SUBSTANCES

INTERACTS WITH	COMBINED EFFECT
Alcohol:	None expected.
Beverages:	None expected.
Cocaine:	Unknown effect. Avoid.
Foods:	None expected.
Marijuana:	Unknown effect. Avoid.
Tobacco: All forms.	Possible blood clots in lung, brain, legs (with high drug doses). Avoid.

***See Glossary**

PROGUANIL

BRAND NAMES

Malarone
Paludrine

BASIC INFORMATION

Habit forming? No
Prescription needed? Yes
Available as generic? No
Drug class: Antimalarial

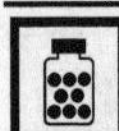

USES

Prevents and treats malaria.

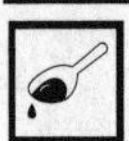

DOSAGE & USAGE INFORMATION

How to take:
Tablet—Swallow whole with liquid after meals.

When to take:
At the same time each day.

If you forget a dose:
Take as soon as you remember. If it is almost time for the next dose, wait for that dose (don't double this dose) and resume regular schedule.

What drug does:
Exact mechanism unknown.

Time lapse before drug works:
1 to 2 weeks.

Don't take with:
Any other medicine or any dietary supplement without consulting your doctor or pharmacist.

OVERDOSE

SYMPTOMS:
Abdominal pain, blood in urine, lower back pain, pain or burning on urination, vomiting.
WHAT TO DO:
If person takes much larger amount than prescribed, dial 911 (emergency) for medical help or call poison control center 1-800-222-1222 for instructions.

POSSIBLE ADVERSE REACTIONS OR SIDE EFFECTS

SYMPTOMS	WHAT TO DO
Life-threatening: None expected.	
Common: Abdominal pain, back pain, coughing, diarrhea, fever, headache, loss of strength, nausea, muscle pain, sore throat, sneezing, vomiting.	Continue. Call doctor if symptoms persist.
Infrequent: Acid or sour stomach, belching, dizziness, flu-like symptoms, heartburn, indigestion, loss of appetite, weight loss, temporary hair loss.	Continue. Call doctor if symptoms persist.
Rare: Skin rash or itching.	Continue. Call doctor when convenient.

WARNINGS & PRECAUTIONS

Don't take if:
You are allergic to proguanil.

Before you start, consult your doctor if:
- You are pregnant or breast-feeding.
- You have kidney problems.

Over age 60:
No problems expected.

Pregnancy:
Decide with your doctor whether drug benefits justify risk to unborn child. Risk category C (see page xviii). Folate supplements should be taken by pregnant women while taking proguanil.

Breast-feeding:
Drug passes into milk. Avoid drug or discontinue nursing until you finish medicine. Consult doctor for advice on maintaining milk supply.

Infants & children:
Not expected to cause different side effects in children than it does in adults.

Prolonged use:
Not intended for long term use.

Skin & sunlight:
No problems expected.

Driving, piloting or hazardous work:
Don't drive or pilot aircraft until you learn how medicine affects you. Don't work around dangerous machinery. Don't climb ladders or work in high places. Danger increases if you drink alcohol or take medicine affecting alertness and reflexes, such as antihistamines, tranquilizers, sedatives, pain medicine, narcotics and mind-altering drugs.

Discontinuing:
Don't discontinue without doctor's advice until you complete the prescribed dosage.

Others:
- Advise any doctor or dentist whom you consult that you take this medicine.
- Persons of Asian or African descent metabolize this drug rapidly, therefore the drug may not reach effective blood levels for protection against malaria.

POSSIBLE INTERACTION WITH OTHER DRUGS

GENERIC NAME OR DRUG CLASS	COMBINED EFFECT
None expected.	

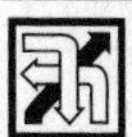

POSSIBLE INTERACTION WITH OTHER SUBSTANCES

INTERACTS WITH	COMBINED EFFECT
Alcohol:	None expected.
Beverages:	None expected.
Cocaine:	None expected.
Foods:	None expected.
Marijuana:	None expected.
Tobacco:	None expected.

PROPAFENONE

BRAND NAMES

Rhythmol

BASIC INFORMATION

Habit forming? No
Prescription needed? Yes
Available as generic? Yes
Drug class: Antiarrhythmic

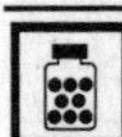

USES

Treats severe heartbeat irregularities (life-threatening ventricular rhythm disturbances).

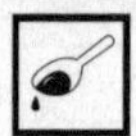

DOSAGE & USAGE INFORMATION

How to take:
Tablet—Swallow with liquid or food to lessen stomach irritation. If you can't swallow whole, crumble tablet and take with liquid or food.

When to take:
At the same time each day, according to instructions on prescription label.

If you forget a dose:
Take as soon as you remember. If it is almost time for the next dose, wait for that dose (don't double this dose) and resume regular schedule.

What drug does:
Slows electrical activity in the heart to decrease the excitability of the heart muscle.

Time lapse before drug works:
3-1/2 hours to 1 week for full effect. Begins working almost immediately.

Don't take with:
Any other medicine (including nonprescription drugs such as cough and cold medicines, nose drops, vitamins, laxatives, antacids, diet pills, or caffeine) without consulting your doctor or pharmacist.

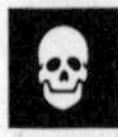

OVERDOSE

SYMPTOMS:
Very rapid heart rate that is also irregular.
WHAT TO DO:
Overdose unlikely to threaten life. If person uses much larger amount than prescribed or if accidentally swallowed, call doctor or poison control center 1-800-222-1222 for help.

POSSIBLE ADVERSE REACTIONS OR SIDE EFFECTS

SYMPTOMS	WHAT TO DO
Life-threatening:	
Severe chest pain, severe shortness of breath.	Seek emergency treatment.
Common:	
• Faster or more irregular heartbeat.	Discontinue. Call doctor right away.
• Taste change, dizziness.	Continue. Call doctor when convenient.
Infrequent:	
• Blurred vision, skin rash.	Discontinue. Call doctor right away.
• Constipation, diarrhea.	Continue. Call doctor when convenient.
• Dry mouth, nausea.	Continue. Tell doctor at next visit.
Rare:	
Fever, chills, trembling, joint pain, slow heartbeat.	Discontinue. Call doctor right away.

WARNINGS & PRECAUTIONS

Don't take if:
You are allergic to propafenone.

Before you start, consult your doctor if:
- You have asthma or bronchospasm.
- You have congestive heart failure.
- You have liver disease or kidney disease.
- You have a recent history of heart attack.
- You have a pacemaker.

Over age 60:
More likely to have decreased kidney function and require dosage modification.

Pregnancy:
Decide with your doctor if drug benefits justify risk to unborn child. Risk category C (see page xviii).

Breast-feeding:
No proven problems. Consult doctor.

Infants & children:
Safety and efficacy not established.

Prolonged use:
Don't discontinue without consulting doctor. Dose may require gradual reduction if you have taken drug for a long time. Dosages of other drugs may also require adjustment.

Skin & sunlight:
No special problems expected.

Driving, piloting or hazardous work:
Don't drive or pilot aircraft until you learn how medicine affects you. Don't work around dangerous machinery. Don't climb ladders or work in high places. Danger increases if you drink alcohol or take medicine affecting alertness and reflexes.

Discontinuing:
Don't discontinue without consulting doctor. Dose may require gradual reduction if you have taken drug for a long time. Doses of other drugs may also require adjustment.

Others:
- Advise any doctor or dentist whom you consult that you take this medicine, especially if you are to be anesthetized.
- Report changes in symptoms to your doctor and return for periodic visits to check progress.
- Carry or wear a medical I.D. card or bracelet that indicate your disorder and the drugs you take.

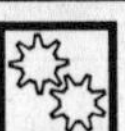

POSSIBLE INTERACTION WITH OTHER DRUGS

GENERIC NAME OR DRUG CLASS	COMBINED EFFECT
Anesthetics, local (e.g., prior to dental procedures)	May increase risk of side effects.
Antiarrhythmics,* other	Increased risk of adverse reactions.
Beta-adrenergic blocking agents*	Increased beta blocker effect.
Digitalis preparations*	Increased digitalis absorption. May require decreased dosage of digitalis preparation.
Doxepin (topical)	Increased risk of toxicity of both drugs.
Enzyme inhibitors*	Increased effect of propafenone.
Warfarin	Increased warfarin effect.

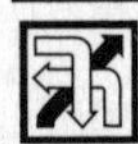

POSSIBLE INTERACTION WITH OTHER SUBSTANCES

INTERACTS WITH	COMBINED EFFECT
Alcohol:	Unpredictable effect on heartbeat. Avoid.
Beverages: Caffeine drinks.	Increased heartbeat irregularity. Avoid.
Cocaine:	Increased heartbeat irregularity. Avoid.
Foods:	None expected.
Marijuana:	Increased heartbeat irregularity. Avoid.
Tobacco:	Increased heartbeat irregularity. Avoid.

***See Glossary**

PROPANTHELINE

BRAND NAMES

Pro-Banthine | Propanthel

BASIC INFORMATION

Habit forming? No
Prescription needed?
High strength: Yes
Low strength: No
Available as generic? Yes
Drug class: Antispasmodic, anticholinergic

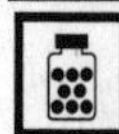

USES

Reduces spasms of digestive system, bladder and urethra.

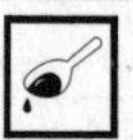

DOSAGE & USAGE INFORMATION

How to take:
Tablet—Swallow with liquid or food to lessen stomach irritation.

When to take:
30 minutes before meals (unless directed otherwise by doctor).

If you forget a dose:
Take as soon as you remember. If it is almost time for the next dose, wait for that dose (don't double this dose) and resume regular schedule.

What drug does:
Blocks nerve impulses at parasympathetic nerve endings, preventing muscle contractions and gland secretions of organs involved.

Time lapse before drug works:
15 to 30 minutes.

Don't take with:
Any other medicine or any dietary supplement without consulting your doctor or pharmacist.

OVERDOSE

SYMPTOMS:
Dilated pupils, blurred vision, rapid pulse and breathing, dizziness, fever, hallucinations, confusion, slurred speech, agitation, flushed face, convulsions, coma.
WHAT TO DO:
- **Dial 911 (emergency) for medical help or call poison control center 1-800-222-1222 for instructions.**
- **See emergency information on last 3 pages of this book.**

POSSIBLE ADVERSE REACTIONS OR SIDE EFFECTS

SYMPTOMS	WHAT TO DO
Life-threatening:	
Hives, rash, intense itching, faintness soon after a dose (anaphylaxis).	Seek emergency treatment immediately.
Common:	
• Confusion, delirium, rapid heartbeat.	Discontinue. Call doctor right away.
• Nausea, vomiting, decreased sweating.	Continue. Call doctor when convenient.
• Constipation, loss of taste.	Continue. Tell doctor at next visit.
• Dry ears, nose, throat, mouth.	No action necessary.
Infrequent:	
• Headache, difficult urination, nasal congestion, altered taste, impotence.	Continue. Call doctor when convenient.
• Lightheadedness.	Discontinue. Call doctor right away.
Rare:	
Rash or hives, eye pain, blurred vision.	Discontinue. Call doctor right away.

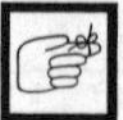

WARNINGS & PRECAUTIONS

Don't take if:
- You are allergic to any anticholinergic.
- You have trouble with stomach bloating.
- You have difficulty emptying your bladder completely.
- You have narrow-angle glaucoma.
- You have severe ulcerative colitis.

Before you start, consult your doctor if:
- You have open-angle glaucoma.
- You have angina.
- You have chronic bronchitis or asthma.
- You have hiatal hernia.
- You have liver, kidney or thyroid disease.
- You have enlarged prostate.
- You have myasthenia gravis.
- You have peptic ulcer.
- You will have surgery within 2 months, including dental surgery, requiring general or spinal anesthesia.

Over age 60:
Adverse reactions and side effects may be more frequent and severe than in younger persons.

Pregnancy:
Decide with your doctor whether drug benefits justify risk to unborn child. Risk category C (see page xviii).

Breast-feeding:
Drug passes into milk and decreases milk flow. Avoid drug or discontinue nursing until you finish medicine. Consult doctor for advice on maintaining milk supply.

Infants & children:
Use only under medical supervision.

Prolonged use:
Chronic constipation, possible fecal impaction. Consult doctor immediately.

Skin & sunlight:
No problems expected.

Driving, piloting or hazardous work:
No problems expected.

Discontinuing:
May be unnecessary to finish medicine. Follow doctor's instructions.

Others:
Advise any doctor or dentist whom you consult that you take this medicine.

POSSIBLE INTERACTION WITH OTHER DRUGS

GENERIC NAME OR DRUG CLASS	COMBINED EFFECT
Adrenocorticoids, systemic	Possible glaucoma.
Amantadine	Increased propantheline effect.
Antacids*	Decreased propantheline effect.
Anticholinergics,* other	Increased propantheline effect.
Antidepressants, tricyclic*	Increased propantheline effect. Increased sedation.
Antidiarrhea preparations*	Reduced propantheline effect.
Antihistamines*	Increased propantheline effect.
Attapulgite	Decreased propantheline effect.
Buclizine	Increased propantheline effect.
Digitalis preparations*	Possible decreased absorption of digitalis.
Haloperidol	Increased internal eye pressure.
Ketoconazole	Decreased ketoconazole effect.
Meperidine	Increased propantheline effect.
Methylphenidate	Increased propantheline effect.
Molindone	Increased anti-cholinergic effect.
Monoamine oxidase (MAO) inhibitors*	Increased propantheline effect.
Nitrates*	Increased internal eye pressure.
Nizatidine	Increased nizatidine effect.
Orphenadrine	Increased propantheline effect.
Phenothiazines*	Increased propantheline effect.
Pilocarpine	Loss of pilocarpine effect in glaucoma treatment.
Potassium supplements*	Increased possibility of intestinal ulcers with oral potassium tablets.
Quinidine	Increased propantheline effect.
Sedatives* or central nervous system (CNS) depressants*	Increased sedative effect of both drugs.
Vitamin C	Decreased propantheline effect. Avoid large doses of vitamin C.

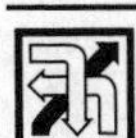

POSSIBLE INTERACTION WITH OTHER SUBSTANCES

INTERACTS WITH	COMBINED EFFECT
Alcohol:	None expected.
Beverages:	None expected.
Cocaine:	Excessively rapid heartbeat. Avoid.
Foods:	None expected.
Marijuana:	Drowsiness and dry mouth.
Tobacco:	None expected.

***See Glossary**

PROTEASE INHIBITORS

GENERIC AND BRAND NAMES

ATAZANAVIR
Reyataz
DARUNAVIR
Prezista
FOSAMPRENAVIR
Lexiva
INDINAVIR
Crixivan
LOPINAVIR
Kaletra
NELFINAVIR
Viracept
RITONAVIR
Kaletra
Norvir
SAQUINAVIR
Invirase
TIPRANAVIR
Aptivus

BASIC INFORMATION

Habit forming? No
Prescription needed? Yes
Available as generic? No
Drug class: Protease inhibitor

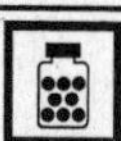

USES

Used in combination with other drugs as a treatment for HIV infection.

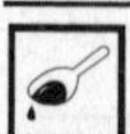

DOSAGE & USAGE INFORMATION

How to take:

- Tablet or capsule—Swallow with liquid. Take with food or meal to enhance drug's absorption. Take tipranavir or darunavir at the same time as ritonavir. Take indinavir 1 hour before or 2 hours after eating. You may take fosamprenavir tablet with or without food. Your doctor may recommend additional methods to help the body absorb the drugs.
- Film-coated tablet (Kaletra)—Can be taken with or without food.
- Liquid ritonavir—Swallow with chocolate milk or liquid nutritional supplement to disguise unpleasant taste.
- Oral solution—Take as directed.

When to take:
At the same times each day, according to instructions on prescription label.

Continued next column

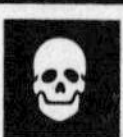

OVERDOSE

SYMPTOMS:
Unknown effect.
WHAT TO DO:
Overdose unlikely to threaten life. If person uses much larger amount than prescribed or if accidentally swallowed, call doctor or poison control center 1-800-222-1222 for help.

If you forget a dose:
Take as soon as you remember. If it is almost time for the next dose, wait for next scheduled dose (don't double this dose).

What drug does:
Blocks an enzyme called protease that is vital to the final stages of HIV replication (reproduction). Blocking protease causes HIV to make copies of itself that can't infect new cells.

Time lapse before drug works:
It will take weeks to months of treatment with the drug to determine the benefits of this therapy.

Don't take with:
Any other medicine or any dietary supplement without consulting your doctor or pharmacist.

POSSIBLE ADVERSE REACTIONS OR SIDE EFFECTS

SYMPTOMS	WHAT TO DO
Life-threatening: None expected.	
Common: Diarrhea, abdominal discomfort, nausea, sores in mouth, dizziness, dry mouth, tiredness, appetite loss.	Continue. Call doctor when convenient.
Infrequent: Rash, muscle or joint pain, headache, abdominal pain, weakness, back pain, numbness or tingling in hands or feet, tingling around mouth.	Continue. Call doctor when convenient.
Rare: • Confusion, yellow skin or eyes, severe skin reaction, lack of coordination, seizures, liver problems (fatigue, loss of appetite, nausea, dark urine, yellow skin or eyes, stomach pain). Watch for warning signs of hyperglycemia or diabetes (increased thirst and hunger, unexplained weight loss, increased urination, fatigue and dry itchy skin).	Continue, but call doctor right away.
• Other symptoms not listed. They may be drug-associated or infection-associated.	Continue. Call doctor when convenient.

WARNINGS & PRECAUTIONS

Don't take if:
You are allergic to protease inhibitors.

Before you start, consult your doctor if:
- You have any liver or kidney disease.
- You have diabetes or hypertension.
- You have peripheral neuropathy.*

Over age 60:
No special problems expected.

Pregnancy:
Risk factors vary for drugs in this group. See category list on page xviii and consult doctor.

Breast-feeding:
Unknown if drug passes into milk. Breast-feeding not recommended in HIV-infected women.

Infants & children:
Some of these drugs are approved for use in infants and children. Consult your child's doctor.

Prolonged use:
Medical studies have shown that HIV can become resistant to the effects of these drugs.

Skin & sunlight:
No special problems expected.

Driving, piloting or hazardous work:
Don't drive or pilot aircraft until you learn how medicine affects you. Don't work around dangerous machinery. Don't climb ladders or work in high places. Danger increases if you drink alcohol or take medicine affecting alertness and reflexes.

Discontinuing:
Don't discontinue without consulting doctor.

Others:
- Advise any doctor or dentist whom you consult that you take this medicine.
- These drugs do not reduce the risk of transmitting HIV to others through sexual contact. Avoid sexual contact or use condoms to help prevent HIV infection. Don't share needles or equipment for injections with other persons.
- These drugs may cause or aggravate diabetes or hypertension.

POSSIBLE INTERACTION WITH OTHER DRUGS

GENERIC NAME OR DRUG CLASS	COMBINED EFFECT
Alfuzosin	Increased alfuzosin effect.
Antacids*	Take 2 hours apart of protease inhibitor.
Anticonvulsants*	Decreased effect of protease inhibitor.
Colchicine	Increased effect of colchicine.
Contraceptives, oral	Less contraceptive effect.
Dexamethasone	Decreased effect of protease inhibitor.
Digoxin	Increased digoxin effect.
Enzyme inducers*	Decreased effect of protease inhibitor.
Enzyme inhibitors*	Increased effect of enzyme inhibitor.
Ergot preparations*	Serious or life-threatening problems. Avoid.
Fluticasone	Increased effect of fluticasone.
Histamine H_2 receptor antagonists	May need dosage adjustment of protease inhibitor.
HMG-CoA reductase inhibitors	Increased risk of muscle damage and kidney failure. Consult doctor.
Methadone	Decreased effect of methadone.
Non-nucleoside reverse transcriptase inhibitors	May need dosage adjustment of protease inhibitor.

Continued on page 926

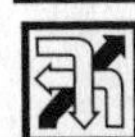

POSSIBLE INTERACTION WITH OTHER SUBSTANCES

INTERACTS WITH	COMBINED EFFECT
Alcohol:	None expected.
Beverages: Grapefruit juice.	May increase effect of protease inhibitor.
Cocaine:	Unknown. Avoid.
Foods: Grapefruit.	May increase effect of protease inhibitor.
Marijuana:	Unknown. Avoid.
Tobacco:	Decreased effect of ritonavir.

***See Glossary**

PROTECTANT (Ophthalmic)

GENERIC AND BRAND NAMES

HYDROXYPROPYL CELLULOSE
Lacrisert

HYDROXYPROPYL METHYLCELLULOSE
Artificial Tears
Bion Tears
Eye Lube
Gonak
Goniosoft
Goniosol
Isopto Alkaline
Isopto Plain
Isopto Tears
Just Tears
Lacril
Methocel
Moisture Drops
Nature's Tears
Ocutears
Tearisol
Tears Naturale
Tears Naturale Free
Tears Naturale II
Tears Renewed
Ultra Tears

BASIC INFORMATION

Habit forming? No
Prescription needed? Yes
Available as generic? Yes, for some
Drug class: Protectant (ophthalmic), artificial tears

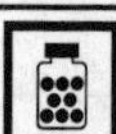

USES

- Relieves eye dryness and irritation caused by inadequate flow of tears.
- Moistens contact lenses and artificial eyes.

OVERDOSE

SYMPTOMS:
None expected.
WHAT TO DO:
Not intended for internal use. If child accidentally swallows, call doctor or poison control center 1-800-222-1222 for help.

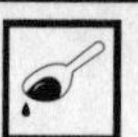

DOSAGE & USAGE INFORMATION

How to use:
Eye drops
- Wash hands.
- Apply pressure to inside corner of eye with middle finger.
- Continue pressure for 1 minute after placing medicine in eye.
- Tilt head backward. Pull lower lid away from eye with index finger of the same hand.
- Drop eye drops into pouch and close eye. Don't blink.
- Keep eyes closed for 1 to 2 minutes.
- Don't touch applicator tip to any surface (including the eye). If you accidentally touch tip, clean with warm water and soap.
- Keep container tightly closed.
- Keep cool, but don't freeze.
- Wash hands immediately after using.

When to use:
As directed. Usually every 3 or 4 hours.

If you forget a dose:
Use as soon as you remember.

What drug does:
- Stabilizes and thickens tear film.
- Lubricates and protects eye.

Time lapse before drug works:
2 to 10 minutes.

Don't use with:
Other eye drops without consulting your doctor or pharmacist.

POSSIBLE ADVERSE REACTIONS OR SIDE EFFECTS

SYMPTOMS	WHAT TO DO
Life-threatening: None expected.	
Common: None expected.	
Infrequent: Eye irritation not present before using artificial tears.	Discontinue. Call doctor right away.
Rare: None expected.	

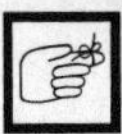

WARNINGS & PRECAUTIONS

Don't use if:
You are allergic to any artificial tears.

Before you start, consult your doctor if:
You use any other eye drops.

Over age 60:
No problems expected.

Pregnancy:
Risk factor not designated. See category list on page xviii and consult doctor.

Breast-feeding:
No problems expected, but check with doctor.

Infants & children:
Don't use.

Prolonged use:
Don't use for more than 3 or 4 days.

Skin & sunlight:
No problems expected.

Driving, piloting or hazardous work:
No problems expected.

Discontinuing:
May not need all the medicine in container. If symptoms disappear, stop using.

Others:
Check with your doctor if eye irritation continues or becomes worse.

POSSIBLE INTERACTION WITH OTHER DRUGS

GENERIC NAME OR DRUG CLASS	COMBINED EFFECT
Clinically significant interactions with oral or injected medicines unlikely.	

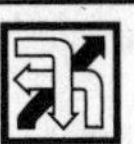

POSSIBLE INTERACTION WITH OTHER SUBSTANCES

INTERACTS WITH	COMBINED EFFECT
Alcohol:	None expected.
Beverages:	None expected.
Cocaine:	None expected.
Foods:	None expected.
Marijuana:	None expected.
Tobacco:	None expected.

PROTON PUMP INHIBITORS

GENERIC AND BRAND NAMES

DEXLANSOPRAZOLE
- Dexilant

ESOMEPRAZOLE
- Nexium Delayed-Release Capsules
- Nexium for Delayed-Release Oral Suspension
- Vimovo

LANSOPRAZOLE
- Prevacid
- Prevacid NapraPAC
- Prevacid Solutab
- Prevacid 24 Hour

OMEPRAZOLE
- Losec
- Omeclamox-Pak
- Prilosec
- Prilosec OTC
- Rapinex Powder for Oral Suspension
- Zegerid Capsules
- Zegerid Chewable Tablets
- Zegerid OTC
- Zegerid Powder

PANTOPRAZOLE
- Pantoloc
- Protonix
- Protonix Delayed Release Oral Suspension

RABEPRAZOLE
- Aciphex

BASIC INFORMATION

Habit forming? No
Prescription needed? Yes, for some
Available as generic? Yes, for some
Drug class: Antiulcer agent; proton pump inhibitor

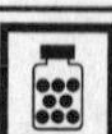

USES

- Treats gastroesophageal reflux disease or GERD (splashing of stomach acid from the stomach up onto the lower end of the esophagus).
- Treats ulcers in the stomach and duodenum.
- Treats any disorder associated with excess production of stomach acid (such as Zollinger-Ellison syndrome).

OVERDOSE

SYMPTOMS:
Severe drowsiness, seizures, breathing difficulty, decreased body temperature.
WHAT TO DO:
- **Dial 911 (emergency) for medical help or call poison control center 1-800-222-1222 for instructions.**
- **See emergency information on last 3 pages of this book.**

DOSAGE & USAGE INFORMATION

How to take:
- Delayed-release and extended-release capsule—Swallow whole with liquid. Do not crush, chew or open (unless allowed on label).
- Delayed-release oral suspension—Follow instructions on prescription.
- Immediate-release capsule—Swallow whole with water (not other liquids). Do not crush, chew or break open.
- Powder—Follow instructions on prescription.
- Tablet (enteric coated)—Swallow whole with liquid. Do not crush, crumble or chew tablet.

When to take:
Once daily, right before a meal (preferably breakfast), unless otherwise directed by your doctor. Dexlansoprazole can be taken without regard to food. With once-a-day dosing, it is important to take the medicine on schedule.

If you forget a dose:
Take as soon as you remember. If it is almost time for the next dose, wait for next scheduled dose (don't double this dose).

What drug does:
Stops the production of stomach acid.

Time lapse before drug works:
Thirty minutes to 3 hours.

Don't take with:
Any other medicine or any dietary supplement without consulting your doctor or pharmacist.

POSSIBLE ADVERSE REACTIONS OR SIDE EFFECTS

SYMPTOMS	WHAT TO DO
Life-threatening: None expected.	
Common: Diarrhea, stomach pain.	Continue. Call doctor when convenient.
Infrequent: Nausea, loss of appetite, headache, heartburn, muscle pain, skin rash, drowsiness.	Continue. Call doctor when convenient.
Rare: Weakness or unusual tiredness, sore throat and fever, sores in mouth, unusual bleeding or bruising, cloudy or bloody urine, urination changes (difficult, frequent or painful).	Discontinue. Call doctor right away.

WARNINGS & PRECAUTIONS

Don't take if:
You are allergic to proton pump inhibitors (PPIs).

Before you start, consult your doctor if:
- You are allergic to any medicines, foods or other substances.
- You have or have had liver disease.
- You have a stomach infection.

Over age 60:
No special problems expected.

Pregnancy:
Risk factors may vary for drugs in this group. See category list on page xviii and consult doctor.

Breast-feeding:
It is unknown if drug passes into milk. Avoid drug or discontinue nursing until you finish medicine. Consult doctor for advice on maintaining milk supply.

Infants & children:
- Lansoprazole is used in children ages 1 to 17.
- Esomeprazole is used in children ages 1 to 17 for the short-term treatment of gastroesophageal reflux disease.
- Rabeprazole is used in children over age 11 for the short-term treatment of gastroesophageal reflux disease.

Prolonged use:
- The length of treatment can run from 4 to 8 weeks or may be indefinite. Symptoms may improve in 1 to 2 weeks, but your doctor will determine when healing is complete.
- Risk of low magnesium blood levels (hypomagnesemia). Symptoms may include muscle spasms, heart rhythm problems or seizures. Consult doctor about your risks.

Skin & sunlight:
No special problems expected.

Driving, piloting or hazardous work:
No special problems expected.

Discontinuing:
Don't discontinue without consulting doctor until you complete prescribed dose, even though symptoms diminish or disappear.

Others:
- Advise any doctor or dentist whom you consult that you take this medicine.
- If directed by your doctor, it is permissible and sometimes helpful to take with antacids* to relieve upper abdominal pain. Antacids may be used more than once daily if needed.
- Brand name Zegerid contains sodium bicarbonate (a form of salt). If you are on a diet that restricts salt or sodium, consult your doctor before using this drug.
- May increase risk of fractures of the hip, wrist, and spine with high doses or long-term use.
- May affect results of some medical tests.
- Drug increases risk of Clostridium difficile diarrhea. Consult doctor if diarrhea persists.

POSSIBLE INTERACTION WITH OTHER DRUGS

GENERIC NAME OR DRUG CLASS	COMBINED EFFECT
Antifungals, azole	Decreased effect of azole antifungal.
Atazanavir	Decreased effect of atazanavir. Avoid.
Clopidogrel	Decreased effect of clopidogrel with some proton pump inhibitors.
Diazepam	Increased effect of diazepam.
Digoxin	Increased effect of digoxin.
Hypomagnesemia-causing drugs,* other	Increased risk of low magnesium.
Iron supplements	Decreased effect of iron supplement.
Phenytoin	Increased effect of phenytoin with omeprazole.
Sucralfate	Decreased effect of some proton pump inhibitors. Take 30 minutes before sucralfate.
Tacrolimus	Increased effect of tacrolimus.
Theophylline	May require dosage adjustment of theophylline with lansoprazole.
Warfarin	May cause abnormal bleeding.

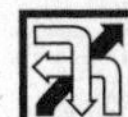

POSSIBLE INTERACTION WITH OTHER SUBSTANCES

INTERACTS WITH	COMBINED EFFECT
Alcohol:	None expected.
Beverages:	None expected.
Cocaine:	None expected.
Foods:	None expected.
Marijuana:	None expected.
Tobacco:	None expected.

***See Glossary**

PSEUDOEPHEDRINE

BRAND NAMES

See full list of brand names in the *Generic and Brand Name Directory*, page 894.

BASIC INFORMATION

Habit forming? No
Prescription needed? Yes, for high strength
Available as generic? Yes
Drug class: Sympathomimetic, decongestant

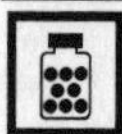

USES

Reduces congestion of nose, sinuses and ears (eustachian tubes) from infections and allergies.

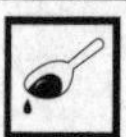

DOSAGE & USAGE INFORMATION

How to take:

- Tablet or capsule—Swallow with liquid. You may chew or crush tablet or open capsule.
- Extended-release tablet or capsule—Swallow whole. Do not crush or chew tablet. The capsule may be opened and the contents mixed with jam or jelly and taken with no chewing.
- Syrup—Take as directed on label.
- Drops—Place directly on tongue and swallow.
- Oral solution—Take as directed on label.
- Combination products—Follow instructions on label.

When to take:

- At the same times each day.
- To prevent insomnia, take last dose of day a few hours before bedtime.

If you forget a dose:
Take as soon as you remember. If it is almost time for the next dose, wait for next scheduled dose (don't double this dose).

Continued next column

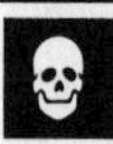

OVERDOSE

SYMPTOMS:
Nervousness, restlessness, headache, rapid or irregular heartbeat, sweating, nausea, vomiting, anxiety, confusion, delirium, muscle tremors, convulsions, hallucinations.
WHAT TO DO:

- **Dial 911 (emergency) for medical help or call poison control center 1-800-222-1222 for instructions.**
- **See emergency information on last 3 pages of this book.**

What drug does:
Decreases blood volume in nasal tissues, shrinking tissues and enlarging airways.

Time lapse before drug works:
15 to 20 minutes.

Don't take with:
Any other medicine or dietary supplement without consulting your doctor or pharmacist.

POSSIBLE ADVERSE REACTIONS OR SIDE EFFECTS

SYMPTOMS	WHAT TO DO
Life-threatening:	
Rare allergic reaction (hives, itching, rash, trouble breathing, tightness in chest, swelling of lips or tongue or throat).	Seek emergency treatment immediately.
Common:	
None expected.	
Infrequent:	
Nervousness, restlessness, trouble sleeping.	Discontinue. Call doctor if symptoms persist.
Rare:	
• Hallucinations, seizures, slow or irregular heart-beat, difficult breathing or shortness of breath.	Discontinue. Seek emergency treatment.
• Dizziness or lightheaded-ness, headache, nausea, vomiting, excess sweating, painful or difficult urination, paleness, weakness, trembling.	Discontinue. Call doctor if symptoms persist.

WARNINGS & PRECAUTIONS

Don't take if:
You are allergic to pseudoephedrine or any sympathomimetic* drug.

Before you start, consult your doctor if:
- You have diabetes or overactive thyroid.
- You have taken any monoamine oxidase (MAO) inhibitor* in past 2 weeks.
- You have high blood pressure or heart or blood vessel disease.
- You have glaucoma.
- You have prostate problems.

Over age 60:
Adverse reactions and side effects may be more frequent and severe than in younger persons.

Pregnancy:
Decide with your doctor if drug benefits justify risk to unborn child. Risk category B (see page xviii).

Breast-feeding:
Drug passes into milk. Avoid drug or discontinue nursing until you finish medicine. Consult doctor for advice on maintaining milk supply.

Infants & children:
Read the label on the product to see if it is approved for your child's age. Always follow the directions on product's label about how to use. If unsure, ask your doctor or pharmacist.

Prolonged use:
Not intended for long-term use. Consult doctor.

Skin & sunlight:
No problems expected.

Driving, piloting or hazardous work:
Avoid if you feel dizzy. Otherwise, no problems expected.

Discontinuing:
May be unnecessary to finish medicine. Follow label directions or doctor's instructions.

Others:
- Call the doctor if symptoms worsen or new symptoms develop with use of this medicine.
- Advise any doctor or dentist whom you consult that you take this medicine.
- Heed all warnings on the product label.
- Most pseudoephedrine-containing products are available without a prescription, but there are restrictions on their sales. This is because pseudoephedrine is a substance often used in the illegal manufacture of methamphetamine or "speed." You will need to ask a pharmacist for the product, show identification, sign a logbook and be limited in the amount you can purchase.

POSSIBLE INTERACTION WITH OTHER DRUGS

GENERIC NAME OR DRUG CLASS	COMBINED EFFECT
Antihypertensives*	Decreased anti-hypertensive effect.
Beta-adrenergic blocking agents*	Decreased effect of beta-blocker.
Citrates	Urinary retention. Increased effect of pseudoephedrine.
Digitalis preparations*	Irregular heartbeat.
Methyldopa	Possible increased blood pressure.
Monoamine oxidase (MAO) inhibitors*	Serious reactions (potentially fatal). Take at least 2 weeks apart.
Nitrates*	Possible decreased nitrate effect.
Rauwolfia alkaloids	Decreased effect of pseudoephedrine.
Sympathomimetics,* other	Increased risk of side effects.
Thyroid hormones	Increased effect of either drug.

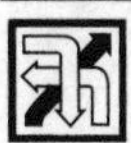

POSSIBLE INTERACTION WITH OTHER SUBSTANCES

INTERACTS WITH	COMBINED EFFECT
Alcohol:	None expected.
Beverages: Caffeine drinks.	Nervousness or insomnia.
Cocaine:	High risk of heartbeat irregularities and high blood pressure. Avoid
Foods:	None expected.
Marijuana:	Rapid heartbeat. Avoid.
Tobacco:	None expected.

*See Glossary

PSORALENS

GENERIC AND BRAND NAMES

METHOXSALEN
- Oxsoralen
- Oxsoralen Topical
- Oxsoralen Ultra
- UltraMOP

TRIOXSALEN
- Trisoralen

BASIC INFORMATION

Habit forming? No
Prescription needed? Yes
Available as generic? No
Drug class: Repigmenting agent (psoralen)

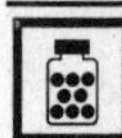

USES

- Repigmenting skin affected with vitiligo (absence of skin pigment).
- Treatment for psoriasis, when other treatments haven't helped.
- Treatment for mycosis fungoides.

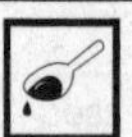

DOSAGE & USAGE INFORMATION

How to take or apply:
- Tablet or capsule—Swallow with liquid or food to lessen stomach irritation.
- Topical—As directed by doctor.

When to take or apply:
2 to 4 hours before exposure to sunlight or sunlamp.

If you forget a dose:
Take as soon as you remember. Delay sun exposure for at least 2 hours after taking.

What drug does:
Helps pigment cells when used in conjunction with ultraviolet light.

Time lapse before drug works:
- For vitiligo, 6 to 9 months.
- For psoriasis, 10 weeks or longer.
- For tanning, 3 to 4 days.

Don't take with:
Any other medicine that causes skin sensitivity to sun. Ask your pharmacist if you have questions.

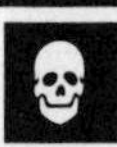

OVERDOSE

SYMPTOMS:
Blistering skin, swelling feet and legs.
WHAT TO DO:
Overdose unlikely to threaten life. If person uses much larger amount than prescribed or if accidentally swallowed, call doctor or poison control center 1-800-222-1222 for help.

POSSIBLE ADVERSE REACTIONS OR SIDE EFFECTS

SYMPTOMS	WHAT TO DO
Life-threatening:	
None expected.	
Common:	
• Increased skin sensitivity to sun.	Always protect from overexposure.
• Increased eye sensitivity to sunlight.	Always protect with wrap-around sunglasses.
• Nausea.	Continue. Call doctor when convenient.
Infrequent:	
• Skin red and sore.	Discontinue. Call doctor right away.
• Dizziness, headache, depression, leg cramps, insomnia.	Continue. Call doctor when convenient.
Rare:	
Hepatitis with jaundice, blistering and peeling.	Discontinue. Call doctor right away.

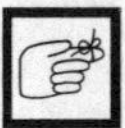

WARNINGS & PRECAUTIONS

Don't take if:
- You are allergic to any psoralen.
- You are unwilling or unable to remain under close medical supervision.

Before you start, consult your doctor if:
- You have heart or liver disease.
- You have allergy to sunlight.
- You have cataracts.
- You have albinism.
- You have lupus erythematosus, porphyria, chronic infection, skin cancer or peptic ulcer.
- You will have surgery within 2 months, including dental surgery, requiring general or spinal anesthesia.
- You have skin cancer.

Over age 60:
Adverse reactions and side effects may be more frequent and severe than in younger persons.

Pregnancy:
Risk factors vary for drugs in this group. See category list on page xviii and consult doctor.

Breast-feeding:
Drug may pass into milk. Avoid drug or discontinue nursing until you finish medicine. Consult doctor for advice on maintaining milk supply.

Infants & children:
Not recommended.

Prolonged use:
- Increased chance of toxic effects.
- Talk to your doctor about the need for follow-up medical examinations or laboratory studies to check ANA titers,* complete blood counts (white blood cell count, platelet count, red blood cell count, hemoglobin, hematocrit), liver function, kidney function, eyes.

Skin & sunlight:
- One or more drugs in this group may cause rash or intensify sunburn in areas exposed to sun or ultraviolet light (photosensitivity reaction). Avoid overexposure. Notify doctor if reaction occurs.
- Too much can burn skin. Cover skin for 24 hours before and 8 hours following treatments.

Driving, piloting or hazardous work:
No problems expected. Protect eyes and skin from bright light.

Discontinuing:
Skin may remain sensitive for some time after treatment stops. Use extra protection from sun.

Others:
- Use sunblock on lips.
- Don't use just to make skin tan.
- Don't use hard gelatin capsules interchangeably with soft gelatin capsules.

POSSIBLE INTERACTION WITH OTHER DRUGS

GENERIC NAME OR DRUG CLASS	COMBINED EFFECT
Photosensitizing medications*	Greatly increased likelihood of extreme sensitivity to sunlight.

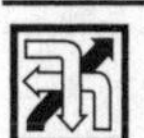

POSSIBLE INTERACTION WITH OTHER SUBSTANCES

INTERACTS WITH	COMBINED EFFECT
Alcohol:	May increase chance of liver toxicity.
Beverages: Lime drinks.	Avoid—toxic.
Cocaine:	Increased chance of toxicity. Avoid.
Foods: Those containing furocoumarin (limes, parsley, figs, parsnips, carrots, celery, mustard).	May cause toxic reaction to psoralens.
Marijuana:	Increased chance of toxicity. Avoid.
Tobacco:	May cause uneven absorption of medicine. Avoid.

*See Glossary

PYRIDOXINE (Vitamin B-6)

BRAND NAMES

Beesix	Rodex
Hexa-Betalin	Vitabec 6
Pyroxine	

Numerous brands of single vitamin and multivitamin combinations may be available.

BASIC INFORMATION

Habit forming? No
Prescription needed?
High strength: Yes
Low strength: No
Available as generic? Yes
Drug class: Vitamin supplement

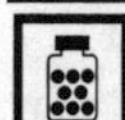

USES

- Prevention and treatment of pyridoxine deficiency.
- Treatment of some forms of anemia.
- Treatment of INH (isonicotinic acid hydrazide), cycloserine poisoning.

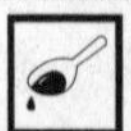

DOSAGE & USAGE INFORMATION

How to take:
- Tablet—Swallow with liquid.
- Extended-release capsule—Swallow each dose whole with liquid.

When to take:
At the same times each day.

If you forget a dose:
Take as soon as you remember, then resume regular schedule.

What drug does:
It is an essential nutrient needed by the body. It acts as co-enzyme in carbohydrate, protein and fat metabolism.

Time lapse before drug works:
15 to 20 minutes.

Don't take with:
Any other medicine or any dietary supplement without consulting your doctor or pharmacist.

OVERDOSE

SYMPTOMS:
None expected.
WHAT TO DO:
Overdose unlikely to threaten life.

POSSIBLE ADVERSE REACTIONS OR SIDE EFFECTS

SYMPTOMS	WHAT TO DO
Life-threatening: None expected.	
Common: None expected.	
Infrequent: Nausea, headache.	Discontinue. Call doctor right away.
Rare: Numbness or tingling in hands or feet (large doses).	Discontinue. Call doctor right away.

WARNINGS & PRECAUTIONS

Don't take if:
You are allergic to pyridoxine.

Before you start, consult your doctor if:
You are pregnant or breast-feeding.

Over age 60:
No problems expected.

Pregnancy:
Don't exceed recommended dose. Consult doctor. Risk category A (see page xviii).

Breast-feeding:
Don't exceed recommended dose. Consult doctor.

Infants & children:
Don't exceed recommended dose.

Prolonged use:
Large doses for more than 1 month may cause toxicity.

Skin & sunlight:
No problems expected.

Driving, piloting or hazardous work:
No problems expected.

Discontinuing:
No problems expected.

Others:
- Advise any doctor or dentist whom you consult that you take this medicine.
- Regular pyridoxine supplements recommended if you take chloramphenicol, cycloserine, ethionamide, hydralazine, immunosuppressants, isoniazid or penicillamine. These decrease pyridoxine absorption and can cause anemia or tingling and numbness in hands and feet.

POSSIBLE INTERACTION WITH OTHER DRUGS

GENERIC NAME OR DRUG CLASS	COMBINED EFFECT
Contraceptives, oral*	Decreased pyridoxine effect.
Cycloserine	Decreased pyridoxine effect.
Estrogens*	Decreased pyridoxine effect.
Ethionamide	Decreased pyridoxine effect.
Hydralazine	Decreased pyridoxine effect.
Hypnotics, barbiturates*	Decreased hypnotic effect.
Immuno-suppressants*	Decreased pyridoxine effect.
Isoniazid	Decreased pyridoxine effect.
Levodopa	Decreased levodopa effect.
Penicillamine	Decreased pyridoxine effect.
Phenobarbital	Possible decreased phenobarbital effect.
Phenytoin	Decreased phenytoin effect.

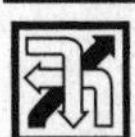

POSSIBLE INTERACTION WITH OTHER SUBSTANCES

INTERACTS WITH	COMBINED EFFECT
Alcohol:	None expected.
Beverages:	None expected.
Cocaine:	None expected.
Foods:	None expected.
Marijuana:	None expected.
Tobacco:	Decreased pyridoxine effect.

***See Glossary**

QUETIAPINE

BRAND NAMES

Seroquel
Seroquel XR

BASIC INFORMATION

Habit forming? No
Prescription needed? Yes
Available as generic? Yes
Drug class: Antipsychotic

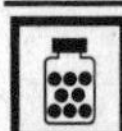

USES

- Treatment for symptoms of schizophrenia.
- Treatment for bipolar disorder and major depressive disorder.

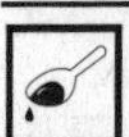

DOSAGE & USAGE INFORMATION

How to take:
- Tablet—Swallow with liquid. May be taken with or without food.
- Extended-release tablet—Swallow each dose whole. Don't crush or chew. Take without food or with a light meal or as advised by doctor.

When to take:
As directed by your doctor—2 to 3 times a day at the same times each day. The dosage may be increased over the first few days of use.

If you forget a dose:
Take as soon as you remember. If it is almost time for the next dose, wait for the next scheduled dose (don't double this dose).

What drug does:
The exact mechanism is unknown. It appears to alleviate symptoms of schizophrenia by blocking certain nerve impulses between nerve cells.

Time lapse before drug works:
One to 7 days. Further increases in the dosage may be needed to relieve symptoms.

Don't take with:
Any other medicine or any dietary supplement without consulting your doctor or pharmacist.

OVERDOSE

SYMPTOMS:
Drowsiness and slurred speech; other symptoms may occur that were not observed in medical studies of the drug.
WHAT TO DO:
If person takes much larger amount than prescribed, dial 911 (emergency) for medical help or call poison control center 1-800-222-1222 for instructions.

POSSIBLE ADVERSE REACTIONS OR SIDE EFFECTS

SYMPTOMS	WHAT TO DO
Life-threatening:	
High fever, rapid pulse, profuse sweating, muscle rigidity, confusion and irritability, seizures (rare neuroleptic malignant syndrome).	Discontinue. Seek emergency treatment.
Common:	
• Dizziness, difficulty in speaking or swallowing, shaking hands and fingers, trembling, vision problems, weakness, lightheadedness when arising from a sitting or lying position.	Continue. Call doctor right away.
• Drowsiness, constipation, weight gain, agitation, insomnia, headache, nervousness, runny nose, anxiety, dry mouth, arm or leg stiffness.	Continue. Call doctor when convenient.
Infrequent:	
• Jerky or involuntary movements (in face, lips, jaw, tongue) chest pain, fast heartbeat.	Continue. Call doctor right away.
• Fever, flu-like symptoms, twitching, mood or mental changes, speech unclear, swollen feet or ankles, appetite increased, cough, saliva increased, muscle tightness, muscle spasms (face, neck, back), joint pain, nausea, vomiting, sore throat, incontinence, abdominal pain.	Continue. Call doctor when convenient.
Rare:	
• Breathing difficulty, high blood sugar (thirstiness, frequent urination, increased hunger, weakness).	Discontinue. Call doctor right away.
• Swollen face, rash, confusion, decreased sex drive, menstrual changes, sluggishness.	Continue. Call doctor when convenient.

WARNINGS & PRECAUTIONS

Don't take if:
You are allergic to quetiapine.

Before you start, consult your doctor if:
- You have a heart problem or disease, high or low blood pressure or blood vessel problem.
- Patient has Alzheimer's or dementia.
- You have a history of breast cancer.
- You are subject to dehydration or low body temperature.
- You have had suicidal thoughts or behaviors.
- You have a history of alcohol or drug abuse.
- You have diabetes or high blood sugar, thyroid problems, liver or kidney disease or high levels of blood fats.
- You have glaucoma or cataracts.
- You have prostate problems.
- You are allergic to any medication, food or other substance.
- You have a history of seizures.

Over age 60:
- Adverse reactions and side effects may be more severe than in younger persons. A lower starting dosage is usually recommended until a response is determined.
- Use of antipsychotic drugs in elderly patients with dementia-related psychosis may increase risk of death. Consult doctor.

Pregnancy:
Decide with your doctor if drug benefits justify any possible risk to unborn child. Risk category C (see page xviii).

Breast-feeding:
It is unknown if drug passes into milk. It is not recommended for nursing mothers.

Infants & children:
Safety in children under age 18 has not been established. Use only under close medical supervision. Contact doctor right away if depression symptoms get worse or there is any talk of suicide or suicide behaviors.

Prolonged use:
- Consult with your doctor on a regular basis to check your progress or to discuss any increase or changes in side effects and the need for continued treatment.
- Get eyes examined every 6 months.

Skin & sunlight:
May cause rash or intensify sunburn in areas exposed to sun or ultraviolet light (photosensitivity reaction). Use sunscreen and avoid overexposure. Notify doctor if reaction occurs.

Driving, piloting or hazardous work:
Don't drive or pilot aircraft until you learn how medicine affects you. Don't work around dangerous machinery. Don't climb ladders or work in high places. Danger increases if you drink alcohol or take drug affecting alertness.

Discontinuing:
Don't discontinue drug without doctor's advice. Dosage may need to be slowly reduced first.

Others:
- Get up slowly from a sitting or lying position to avoid any dizziness or lightheadedness.
- Advise any doctor or dentist whom you consult that you take this medicine.
- Hot temperatures, exercise, and hot baths can increase risk of heatstroke. Drug may affect body's ability to maintain normal temperature.
- Adults and children taking antidepressants may experience a worsening of the depression symptoms and may have increased suicidal thoughts or behaviors. Call doctor right away if these symptoms or behaviors occur.
- Take drug only as directed. Do not increase or reduce dosage without doctor's approval.

POSSIBLE INTERACTION WITH OTHER DRUGS

GENERIC NAME OR DRUG CLASS	COMBINED EFFECT
Antihypertensives*	Increased risk of low blood pressure.
Central nervous system (CNS) depressants,* other	Increased sedative effect.
Enzyme inducers*	May decrease quetiapine effect.
Enzyme inhibitors*	May increase quetiapine effect.

Continued on page 926

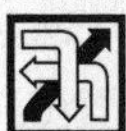

POSSIBLE INTERACTION WITH OTHER SUBSTANCES

INTERACTS WITH	COMBINED EFFECT
Alcohol:	Increased sedation and dizziness. Avoid.
Beverages: Grapefruit juice.	Increased effect of drug. Avoid.
Cocaine:	Unknown. Avoid.
Foods:	None expected.
Marijuana:	Unknown. Avoid.
Tobacco:	None expected.

QUINACRINE

BRAND NAMES

Atabrine

BASIC INFORMATION

Habit forming? No
Prescription needed? Yes
Available as generic? Yes
Drug class: Antiprotozoal

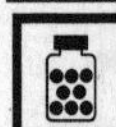

USES

- Treats disease caused by the intestinal parasite *Giardia lamblia.*
- Treats mild to moderate discoid lupus erythematosus.

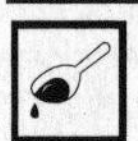

DOSAGE & USAGE INFORMATION

How to take:
Tablet—Swallow with full glass of water, tea or fruit juice. If you can't swallow whole, crumble tablet and mix with jam or chocolate syrup.

When to take:
After meals.

If you forget a dose:
Take as soon as you remember up to 2 hours late. If more than 2 hours, wait for next scheduled dose (don't double this dose).

What drug does:
Destroys *Giardia lamblia* parasites in the gastrointestinal system.

Time lapse before drug works:
1 day.

Continued next column

OVERDOSE

SYMPTOMS:
Severe abdominal cramps, convulsions, severe diarrhea, fainting, irregular heartbeat, restlessness.
WHAT TO DO:
- **Dial 911 (emergency) for medical help or call poison control center 1-800-222-1222 for instructions.**
- **If person is unconscious, check breathing and pulse. If not breathing, begin mouth-to-mouth rescue breathing. If heart is not beating, begin chest compressions.**
- **See emergency information on last 3 pages of this book.**

Don't take with:
Any other medicine or any dietary supplement without consulting your doctor or pharmacist.

POSSIBLE ADVERSE REACTIONS OR SIDE EFFECTS

SYMPTOMS	WHAT TO DO
Life-threatening:	
In case of overdose, see previous column.	
Common:	
• Dizziness, nausea, headache.	Discontinue. Call doctor right away.
• Yellow eyes, skin, urine (due to dye-like characteristics of quinacrine).	Report to doctor, but no action necessary.
Infrequent:	
• Mild abdominal cramps; mild diarrhea; appetite loss; skin rash, itching or peeling.	Discontinue. Call doctor right away.
• Mood changes.	Continue. Call doctor when convenient.
Rare:	
Hallucinations, nightmares.	Discontinue. Call doctor right away.

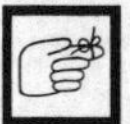

WARNINGS & PRECAUTIONS

Don't take if:
You are allergic to quinacrine.

Before you start, consult your doctor if:
- You have porphyria.
- You have had psoriasis.
- You have a history of severe mental disorders.
- You are on a low-salt, low-sugar or other special diet.

Over age 60:
No special problems.

Pregnancy:
Decide with your doctor whether drug benefits justify risk to unborn child. Treatment best begun after child has been delivered. Risk category C (see page xviii).

Breast-feeding:
Effect unknown. Consult doctor.

Infants & children:
Children tolerate quinacrine poorly. Quinacrine may cause vomiting due to bitter taste. Try crushing tablets in jam, honey or chocolate syrup.

Prolonged use:
- Can cause eye problems, liver disease, aplastic anemia. Don't use for more than 5 days.
- Talk to your doctor about the need for follow-up medical examinations or laboratory studies to check stools for giardiasis.

Skin & sunlight:
No problems expected.

Driving, piloting or hazardous work:
Don't drive or pilot aircraft until you learn how medicine affects you. Don't work around dangerous machinery. Don't climb ladders or work in high places. Danger increases if you drink alcohol or take medicine affecting alertness and reflexes, such as antihistamines, tranquilizers, sedatives, pain medicine, narcotics and mind-altering drugs.

Discontinuing:
Don't discontinue before 5 days without consulting doctor.

Others:
- Advise any doctor or dentist whom you consult that you take this medicine.
- Request 3 stool exams several days apart.

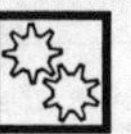

POSSIBLE INTERACTION WITH OTHER DRUGS

GENERIC NAME OR DRUG CLASS	COMBINED EFFECT
Primaquine	Decreased effect of primaquine.

POSSIBLE INTERACTION WITH OTHER SUBSTANCES

INTERACTS WITH	COMBINED EFFECT
Alcohol:	Increased adverse effects of both. Avoid.
Beverages:	None expected.
Cocaine:	None expected.
Foods:	None expected.
Marijuana:	None expected.
Tobacco:	None expected.

QUINIDINE

BRAND NAMES

Apo-Quinidine
Cardioquin
Cin-Quin
Duraquin
Novoquinidin
Quinaglute Dura-Tabs
Quinalan
Quinate
Quinidex Extentabs
Quinora

BASIC INFORMATION

Habit forming? No
Prescription needed?
U.S.: Yes
Canada: No
Available as generic? Yes
Drug class: Antiarrhythmic

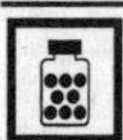

USES

- Corrects heart rhythm disorders.
- May be used in treatment of malaria.

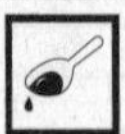

DOSAGE & USAGE INFORMATION

How to take:
- Tablet or capsule—Swallow with liquid or food to lessen stomach irritation. If you can't swallow whole, crush tablet or open capsule and take with small amount of food.
- Extended-release tablet—Swallow each dose whole. Don't crush them.

When to take:
At the same times each day.

If you forget a dose:
Take as soon as you remember up to 2 hours late. If more than 2 hours, wait for next scheduled dose (don't double this dose).

Continued next column

What drug does:
Delays nerve impulses to the heart to regulate heartbeat.

Time lapse before drug works:
2 to 4 hours.

Don't take with:
Any other medicine or any dietary supplement without consulting your doctor or pharmacist.

OVERDOSE

SYMPTOMS:
Confusion, severe blood pressure drop, lethargy, breathing difficulty, fainting, seizures, coma.
WHAT TO DO:
- **Dial 911 (emergency) for medical help or call poison control center 1-800-222-1222 for instructions.**
- **If person is unconscious, check breathing and pulse. If not breathing, begin mouth-to-mouth rescue breathing. If heart is not beating, begin chest compressions.**
- **See emergency information on last 3 pages of this book.**

POSSIBLE ADVERSE REACTIONS OR SIDE EFFECTS

SYMPTOMS	WHAT TO DO
Life-threatening:	
Hives, rash, intense itching, faintness soon after a dose (anaphylaxis); wheezing.	Seek emergency treatment immediately.
Common:	
Bitter taste, diarrhea, nausea, vomiting, appetite loss, abdominal pain.	Discontinue. Call doctor right away.
Infrequent:	
• Dizziness, light-headedness, fainting, headache, confusion, rash, change in vision, difficult breathing, rapid heartbeat.	Discontinue. Call doctor right away.
• Ringing in ears.	Continue. Call doctor when convenient.
Rare:	
• Unusual bleeding or bruising, difficulty or pain on swallowing, fever, joint pain, jaundice, hepatitis.	Discontinue. Call doctor right away.
• Weakness.	Continue. Call doctor when convenient.

WARNINGS & PRECAUTIONS

Don't take if:
- You are allergic to quinidine.
- You have an active infection.

Before you start, consult your doctor if:
- You have an electrolyte disorder.
- You have heart disease or myasthenia gravis.
- You have kidney or liver disease.

Over age 60:
Adverse reactions and side effects may be more frequent and severe than in younger persons.

Pregnancy:
Decide with your doctor if drug benefits justify risk to unborn child. Risk category C (see page xviii).

Breast-feeding:
Drug filters into milk. May harm child. Consult doctor.

Infants & children:
No problems expected.

Prolonged use:
Talk to your doctor about the need for follow-up studies to check complete blood counts (white blood cell count, platelet count, red blood cell count, hemoglobin, hematocrit), liver function, kidney function, serum potassium levels, ECG.*

Skin & sunlight:
May cause rash or intensify sunburn in areas exposed to sun or ultraviolet light (photosensitivity reaction). Avoid overexposure. Notify doctor if reaction occurs.

Driving, piloting or hazardous work:
Don't drive or pilot aircraft until you learn how medicine affects you. Don't work around dangerous machinery. Don't climb ladders or work in high places. Danger increases if you drink alcohol or take medicine affecting alertness and reflexes, such as antihistamines, tranquilizers, sedatives, pain medicine, narcotics and mind-altering drugs.

Discontinuing:
Don't discontinue without doctor's advice until you complete prescribed dose, even though symptoms diminish or disappear.

Others:
Advise any doctor or dentist whom you consult that you take this medicine.

POSSIBLE INTERACTION WITH OTHER DRUGS

GENERIC NAME OR DRUG CLASS	COMBINED EFFECT
Alkalizers, urinary*	Slows quinidine elimination, increasing its effect and toxicity.
Amiodarone	Increased effect of quinidine. Risk of heart rhythm problems.
Antacids	Take at least 2 hours apart.
Anticholinergics	Increased anti-cholinergic effect.
Anticoagulants,* oral	Possible increased anticoagulant effect.
Antidepressants, tricyclic	Increased risk of heart rhythm problems.
Cimetidine	Increased quinidine effect.
Digitalis preparations	May slow heartbeat. Dose adjustments may be needed.
Diltiazem	Increased quinidine effect.
Enzyme inhibitors*	Increased effect of quinidine.
Erythromycin	Possible irregular heartbeat.
Haloperidol	Possible irregular heartbeat.
Mefloquine	Possible irregular heartbeat. Avoid.
Memantine	Increased effect of either drug.
Metformin	Increased metformin effect.
Nifedipine	Possible decreased quinidine effect.
Phenobarbital	Decreased quinidine effect.
Phenothiazines*	Possible increased quinidine effect.
QT interval prolongation-causing drugs*	Heartbeat irregularities.
Verapamil	Increased quinidine effect.

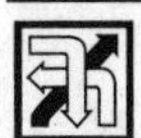

POSSIBLE INTERACTION WITH OTHER SUBSTANCES

INTERACTS WITH	COMBINED EFFECT
Alcohol:	None expected.
Beverages:	
Caffeine drinks.	Causes rapid heartbeat. Use with care.
Grapefruit juice.	Toxicity risk. Avoid.
Cocaine:	Irregular heartbeat. Avoid.
Foods:	None expected.
Marijuana:	Can cause fainting.
Tobacco:	Irregular heartbeat. Avoid.

*See Glossary

QUININE

BRAND NAMES

Qualaquin

BASIC INFORMATION

Habit forming? No
Prescription needed? Yes
Available as generic? Yes
Drug class: Antiprotozoal

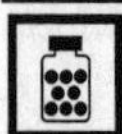

USES

Treatment or prevention of malaria.

DOSAGE & USAGE INFORMATION

How to take:
Tablet or capsule—Swallow with liquid or food to lessen stomach irritation.

When to take:
- Prevention—At the same time each day, usually at bedtime.
- Treatment—At the same times each day in evenly spaced doses.

If you forget a dose:
- Prevention—Take as soon as you remember up to 12 hours late. If more than 12 hours, wait for next scheduled dose (don't double this dose).
- Treatment—Take as soon as you remember up to 2 hours late. If more than 2 hours, wait for next scheduled dose (don't double this dose).

What drug does:
- Reduces contractions of skeletal muscles.
- Increases blood flow.
- Interferes with genes in malaria micro-organisms.

Continued next column

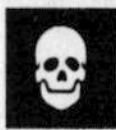

OVERDOSE

SYMPTOMS:
Severe impairment of vision and hearing; severe nausea, vomiting, diarrhea; shallow breathing, fast heartbeat; apprehension, confusion, delirium.
WHAT TO DO:
Dial 911 (emergency) for medical help or call poison control center 1-800-222-1222 for instructions.

Time lapse before drug works:
May require several days or weeks for maximum effect.

Don't take with:
Any other medicine or any dietary supplement without consulting your doctor or pharmacist.

POSSIBLE ADVERSE REACTIONS OR SIDE EFFECTS

SYMPTOMS	WHAT TO DO
Life-threatening:	
In case of overdose, see previous column.	
Common:	
• Blurred vision or change in vision, eyes sensitive to light.	Discontinue. Call doctor right away.
• Dizziness, headache, abdominal discomfort, mild nausea, vomiting, diarrhea.	Continue. Call doctor when convenient.
• Ringing or buzzing in ears, impaired hearing.	Continue. Tell doctor at next visit.
Infrequent:	
Rash, hives, itchy skin, difficult breathing.	Discontinue. Call doctor right away.
Rare:	
Sore throat, fever, unusual bleeding or bruising, unusual tiredness or weakness, angina.	Discontinue. Call doctor right away.

WARNINGS & PRECAUTIONS

Don't take if:
You are allergic to quinine or quinidine.

Before you start, consult your doctor if:
- You plan to become pregnant within medication period.
- You have asthma.
- You have eye disease, hearing problems or ringing in the ears.
- You have heart disease.
- You have myasthenia gravis.

Over age 60:
Adverse reactions and side effects may be more frequent and severe than in younger persons.

Pregnancy:
Risk to unborn child outweighs drug benefits. Don't use. Risk category X (see page xviii).

Breast-feeding:
Drug filters into milk. May harm child. Consult doctor.

Infants & children:
Use only under medical supervision.

Prolonged use:
May develop headache, blurred vision, nausea, temporary hearing loss, but seldom need to discontinue because of these symptoms.

Skin & sunlight:
May cause rash or intensity sunburn in areas exposed to sun or ultraviolet light (photosensitivity reaction). Avoid overexposure. Notify doctor if reaction occurs.

Driving, piloting or hazardous work:
Avoid if you feel dizzy or have blurred vision. Otherwise, no problems expected.

Discontinuing:
Don't discontinue without doctor's advice until you complete prescribed dose, even though symptoms diminish or disappear.

Others:
- Advise any doctor or dentist whom you consult that you take this medicine.
- Quinine is only approved for treating malaria. It is sometimes used as an unapproved treatment for restless leg syndrome or restless leg cramps. This use can lead to serious and life-threatening side effects. Consult your doctor.
- Don't confuse with quinidine, a medicine for heart rhythm problems.

POSSIBLE INTERACTION WITH OTHER DRUGS

GENERIC NAME OR DRUG CLASS	COMBINED EFFECT
Alkalizers,* urinary	Possible toxic effects of quinine.
Antacids* (with aluminum hydroxide)	Decreased quinine effect.
Anticoagulants,* oral	Increased anticoagulant effect.
Dapsone	Increased risk of adverse effect on blood cells.
Digitalis	Possible increased digitalis effect.
Digoxin	Possible increased digoxin effect.
Mefloquine	Increased risk of heartbeat irregularities.
Metformin	Increased metformin effect.
Quinidine	Possible toxic effects of quinine.

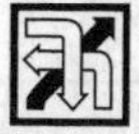

POSSIBLE INTERACTION WITH OTHER SUBSTANCES

INTERACTS WITH	COMBINED EFFECT
Alcohol:	None expected.
Beverages:	None expected.
Cocaine:	None expected.
Foods:	None expected.
Marijuana:	None expected.
Tobacco:	None expected.

***See Glossary**

RALOXIFENE

BRAND NAMES

Evista

BASIC INFORMATION

Habit forming? No
Prescription needed? Yes
Available as generic? No
Drug class: Osteoporosis therapy, prophylactic

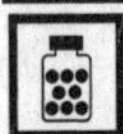

USES

- Prevents and treats osteoporosis in postmenopausal women. Does not treat hot flashes of menopause.
- Lowers low-density lipoprotein (LDL) cholesterol blood levels.
- Used for reduction of breast cancer risk in postmenopausal women.
- Other uses as determined by your doctor.

DOSAGE & USAGE INFORMATION

How to take:
Tablet—Swallow with water, with or without food. If you can't swallow whole, crumble tablet and take with liquid or food.

When to take:
At the same time each day.

If you forget a dose:
Take as soon as you remember up to 12 hours late. If more than 12 hours, wait for next scheduled dose (don't double this dose).

What drug does:
It is a selective estrogen receptor modulator or SERM. These drugs can act both like the hormone estrogen (such as in the bones) or block estrogen (such as in the breast tissue).

Time lapse before drug works:
Up to twelve months.

Don't take with:
Any other medicine or any dietary supplement without consulting your doctor or pharmacist.

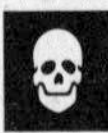

OVERDOSE

SYMPTOMS:
None reported.
WHAT TO DO:
Overdose unlikely to threaten life. If person uses much larger amount than prescribed or if accidentally swallowed, call doctor or poison control center 1-800-222-1222 for help.

POSSIBLE ADVERSE REACTIONS OR SIDE EFFECTS

SYMPTOMS	WHAT TO DO
Life-threatening:	
Blood clot formation.	Discontinue. Seek emergency treatment immediately.
Common:	
• Chest pain; bloody or cloudy urine; burning or painful urination; frequent urge to urinate; infection; cold- or flu-like symptoms; leg cramping; skin rash; swelling of hands, ankles or feet; vaginal itching.	Discontinue. Call doctor right away.
• Joint or muscle pain, swollen joints, gas, upset stomach, vomiting, hot flashes, insomnia, white vaginal discharge, depression, sweating, unexplained weight gain.	Continue. Call doctor if symptoms persist.
Infrequent:	
Abdominal pain, diarrhea, loss of appetite, nausea, weakness, migraine headache, difficulty breathing, fever, congestion.	Discontinue. Call doctor right away.
Rare:	
Blood clot formation (symptoms include swelling in legs, sharp pain in legs, sudden chest pain, coughing up blood, changes in vision).	Discontinue. Seek emergency treatment immediately.

WARNINGS & PRECAUTIONS

Don't take if:
- You are allergic to raloxifene.
- You are scheduled for surgery within 72 hours.

Before you start, consult your doctor if:
- You plan to become pregnant within the medication period.
- You have or have had a history of blood clot (deep vein thrombosis) formation.
- You have a history of stroke, transient ischemic attacks (TIA) or heart disease.
- You have high triglycerides (a blood fat).
- You have or have had cancer or tumors.
- You have liver disease.

Over age 60:
Adverse reactions and side effects in older adults have been similar to those experienced by women who have just undergone menopause.

Pregnancy:
Use of raloxifene is not recommended during pregnancy. Risk category X (see page xviii).

Breast-feeding:
Unknown whether drug passes into milk and is not recommended during breast-feeding. Presently raloxifene is to be used in postmenopausal women only.

Infants & children:
Not recommended for this age group.

Prolonged use:
No problems expected. Your doctor should periodically evaluate your response to the drug and adjust the dose if necessary.

Skin & sunlight:
No problems expected.

Driving, piloting or hazardous work:
No problems expected.

Discontinuing:
Don't discontinue without consulting doctor.

Others:
- Advise any doctor or dentist whom you consult that you take this medicine.
- This drug is associated with an increased risk of developing blood clots in the veins (deep vein thrombosis) or stroke. Consult doctor.
- In addition to taking the drug, weight-bearing exercise and adequate intake of calcium and vitamin D are essential in preventing bone loss. Periods of prolonged inactivity may worsen your condition. Daily dietary supplements of elemental calcium and vitamin D may be recommended by your doctor.
- May help lower low-density lipoprotein (LDL) cholesterol levels.

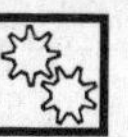

POSSIBLE INTERACTION WITH OTHER DRUGS

GENERIC NAME OR DRUG CLASS	COMBINED EFFECT
Cholestyramine	Lessens the effect of raloxifene.
Estrogens	Not recommended for use with raloxifene.
Protein bound drugs*	Caution is recommended; consult doctor before taking any of these in conjunction with raloxifene.
Warfarin	May lessen the effect of warfarin.

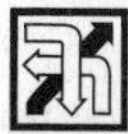

POSSIBLE INTERACTION WITH OTHER SUBSTANCES

INTERACTS WITH	COMBINED EFFECT
Alcohol:	Increased risk of adverse effects. Avoid.
Beverages:	None expected.
Cocaine:	Effects unknown. Avoid.
Foods:	None expected.
Marijuana:	Effects unknown. Avoid.
Tobacco:	Increases risk of blood clot. Avoid.

*See Glossary

RAMELTEON

BRAND NAMES

Rozerem

BASIC INFORMATION

Habit forming? No
Prescription needed? Yes
Available as generic? No
Drug class: Melatonin receptor agonist; nonbenzodiazepine hypnotic

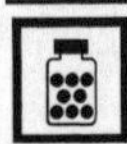

USES

It is used to help you fall asleep faster when you have trouble falling asleep and experience insomnia.

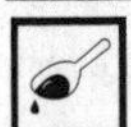

DOSAGE & USAGE INFORMATION

How to take:
Tablet—Swallow whole with liquid. Do not crush or chew the tablet. Take it with or without food. Do not take it with, or immediately after, a high fat meal. Doing so can reduce the effectiveness of the drug.

When to take:
Take within 30 minutes of bedtime. Take the drug only when you know that you will get 8 full hours (or more) of sleep after the dose.

If you forget a dose:
Skip the missed dose. Resume dosage schedule the next night if needed to help you sleep. Do not take more than one dose in a 24 hour period.

What drug does:
It stimulates melatonin receptors (chemicals) in the brain that are responsible for the regulation of the body's 24 hour sleep-wake cycle.

Time lapse before drug works:
Usually within 30 to 90 minutes.

Continued next column

OVERDOSE

SYMPTOMS:
Unknown for sure; may include extreme drowsiness, confusion, dizziness, difficult or slow breathing and unconsciousness.
WHAT TO DO:

- **Dial 911 (emergency) for medical help or call poison control center 1-800-222-1222 for instructions.**
- **See emergency information on last 3 pages of this book.**

Don't take with:
Fluvoxamine or any other medicine or any dietary supplement without consulting your doctor or pharmacist.

POSSIBLE ADVERSE REACTIONS OR SIDE EFFECTS

SYMPTOMS	WHAT TO DO
Life-threatening:	
Allergic reaction (difficulty breathing, closing of the throat, swelling of the lips or face or tongue, hives).	Seek emergency treatment immediately.
Common:	
Dizziness, drowsiness, nausea, headache, fatigue, worsening insomnia.	Discontinue. Call doctor when convenient.
Infrequent:	
Decreased sex drive, menstrual changes, milky discharge from breasts, cold- or flu-like symptoms, muscle or joint or body aches or pain, taste changes, stomach upset.	Discontinue. Call doctor when convenient.
Rare:	
The class of drugs used to treat insomnia are called hypnotics. They can cause a variety of adverse reactions in one's emotions, behavior, cognition (thinking) and mood. Symptoms can include worsening depression, memory problems, confusion, bizarre behaviors, suicidal thoughts, hallucinations, unusual excitement, irritability, aggressiveness, nervousness, sleep-related behaviors,* and possibly others.	Discontinue. Call doctor right away.

WARNINGS & PRECAUTIONS

Don't take if:

- You are allergic to ramelteon.
- You are taking the drug fluvoxamine.

Before you start, consult your doctor if:

- You have or have had liver disease.
- You suffer from depression or a psychiatric disorder or abuse alcohol or drugs.
- You suffer from sleep apnea or emphysema, asthma, bronchitis or other chronic lung disease.

Over age 60:
No special problems expected.

Pregnancy:
Decide with your doctor if drug benefits justify any possible risk to unborn child. Risk category C (see page xviii).

Breast-feeding:
It is unknown if drug passes into milk. It is not recommended during breast-feeding. Consult doctor for advice.

Infants & children:
Safety and effectiveness in children has not been established. Consult your child's doctor.

Prolonged use:
No special problems expected. You and your doctor will decide if there is a need to take the drug for a prolonged period for chronic insomnia (insomnia at least three nights a week for a period of one month or longer).

Skin & sunlight:
No special problems expected.

Driving, piloting or hazardous work:
Don't drive or pilot aircraft until you learn how medicine affects you. Don't work around dangerous machinery. Don't climb ladders or work in high places. Danger increases if you drink alcohol or take other medicines affecting alertness and reflexes.

Discontinuing:
No problems expected. Ramelteon does not appear to produce withdrawal symptoms or lead to physical dependence.

Others:

- Advise any doctor or dentist whom you consult that you take this medicine.
- Consult your doctor if your insomnia symptoms do not improve after taking the drug a few nights.

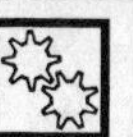

POSSIBLE INTERACTION WITH OTHER DRUGS

GENERIC NAME OR DRUG CLASS	COMBINED EFFECT
Enzyme inducers*	Decreased effect of ramelteon.
Enzyme inhibitors*	Increased effect of ramelteon. Consult your doctor or pharmacist before using.
Fluvoxamine	Increased effect of ramelteon. Avoid.

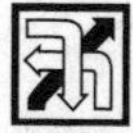

POSSIBLE INTERACTION WITH OTHER SUBSTANCES

INTERACTS WITH	COMBINED EFFECT
Alcohol:	Increased sedation. Avoid.
Beverages:	
Grapefruit juice.	Unknown effect. Consult doctor.
Cocaine:	Unknown. Avoid.
Foods:	
Grapefruit.	Unknown effect. Consult doctor.
High fat meal	Drug effect is decreased if taken with, or right after, the meal.
Marijuana:	Unknown. Avoid.
Tobacco:	None expected.

RANOLAZINE

BRAND NAMES

Ranexa

BASIC INFORMATION

Habit forming? No
Prescription needed? Yes
Available as generic? No
Drug class: Antianginal

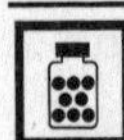

USES

Treatment of chronic angina (chest pain caused by an insufficient supply of oxygen to the heart). It may be used in combination with other drug treatments, such as amlodipine, beta blockers or nitrates.

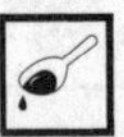

DOSAGE & USAGE INFORMATION

How to take:
Extended-release tablet—Swallow whole with liquid. It may be taken with or without food. Do not crush, crumble or chew tablet.

When to take:
Usually twice a day at the same times each day. Follow the instructions on your prescription.

If you forget a dose:
Take as soon as you remember. If it is almost time for the next dose, wait for next scheduled dose (don't double this dose).

What drug does:
Exact method of action is unknown. It appears to relax contracted heart muscle and return blood flow to normal levels which relieves the pain.

Time lapse before drug works:
Within a few hours. Dosage may be increased by your doctor as needed for pain relief.

Don't take with:
Any other medicine or any dietary supplement without consulting your doctor or pharmacist.

OVERDOSE

SYMPTOMS:
May include dizziness, "pins and needles" feeling, nausea, vomiting, double vision, confusion and fainting.
WHAT TO DO:
Overdose unlikely to threaten life. If person uses much larger amount than prescribed or if accidentally swallowed, call doctor or poison control center 1-800-222-1222 for help.

POSSIBLE ADVERSE REACTIONS OR SIDE EFFECTS

SYMPTOMS	WHAT TO DO
Life-threatening: None expected.	
Common: Dizziness, headache, constipation, nausea, weakness.	Continue. Call doctor when convenient.
Infrequent: Abdominal pain, tinnitus, vomiting, vertigo, dry mouth, tremor, lightheaded or dizzy when arising from sitting or lying position.	Continue. Call doctor when convenient.
Rare: Palpitations, slow heartbeat, blood in urine, blurred vision, fainting.	Discontinue. Call doctor right away.

WARNINGS & PRECAUTIONS

Don't take if:
You are allergic to ranolazine.

Before you start, consult your doctor if:
- You have pre-existing QT interval prolongation (an abnormality of the heart's electrical system as diagnosed by medical testing).
- You have kidney or liver disease.
- You have uncorrected hypokalemia (low potassium level).
- You have a history of ventricular tachycardia.

Over age 60:
Adverse reactions and side effects may be more frequent and severe than in younger persons. You may need smaller doses at start of therapy.

Pregnancy:
Decide with your doctor if drug benefits justify any possible risk to unborn child. Risk category C (see page xviii).

Breast-feeding:
It is unknown if drug passes into milk. Avoid drug or discontinue nursing until you finish medicine. Consult doctor for advice on maintaining milk supply.

Infants & children:
Safety and effectiveness in children has not been established.

Prolonged use:
No problems expected.

Skin & sunlight:
No problems expected.

Driving, piloting or hazardous work:
Don't drive motor vehicles or pilot aircraft until you learn how medicine affects you. Don't work around dangerous machinery. Don't climb ladders or work in high places.

Discontinuing:
No problems expected. Consult your doctor before stopping the drug.

Others:
- Other antianginal drugs should be tried first due to the risk of QT interval prolongation (abnormality of the heart's electrical system).
- An ECG* should be performed prior to starting the drug and periodically during drug therapy.
- It is important to follow your doctor's advice on diet, exercise, smoking and weight control.
- Advise any doctor or dentist whom you consult that you take this medicine.

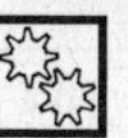

POSSIBLE INTERACTION WITH OTHER DRUGS

GENERIC NAME OR DRUG CLASS	COMBINED EFFECT
Antidepressants, tricyclics	Increased effect of tricyclic antidepressant.
Antipsychotics*	Increased effect of antipsychotic.
Digoxin	Increased effect and blood levels of digoxin.
Enzyme inhibitors*	Risk of abnormal heart rhythm. Avoid.
QT interval prolongation-causing drugs,* other	Risk of abnormal heart rhythm. Avoid.
Simvastatin	Increased effect of simvastatin.

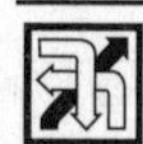

POSSIBLE INTERACTION WITH OTHER SUBSTANCES

INTERACTS WITH	COMBINED EFFECT
Alcohol:	None expected.
Beverages: Grapefruit juice.	Risk of abnormal heart rhythm. Avoid.
Cocaine:	Unknown. Best to avoid.
Foods: Grapefruit.	Risk of abnormal heart rhythm. Avoid.
Marijuana:	Unknown. Best to avoid.
Tobacco:	None expected. Persons with angina should not smoke.

*See Glossary

RAUWOLFIA ALKALOIDS

GENERIC AND BRAND NAMES

See full list of generic and brand names in the *Generic and Brand Name Directory*, page 896.

BASIC INFORMATION

Habit forming? No
Prescription needed? Yes
Available as generic? Yes
Drug class: Antihypertensive, tranquilizer (rauwolfia alkaloid)

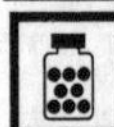

USES

- Treatment for high blood pressure.
- Tranquilizer for mental and emotional disturbances.

DOSAGE & USAGE INFORMATION

How to take:
Tablet—Swallow with liquid or food to lessen stomach irritation. If you can't swallow whole, crumble tablet and take with liquid or food.

When to take:
At the same times each day.

If you forget a dose:
Take as soon as you remember up to 2 hours late. If more than 2 hours, wait for next scheduled dose (don't double this dose).

What drug does:
- Interferes with nerve impulses and relaxes blood vessel muscles, reducing blood pressure.
- Suppresses brain centers that control emotions.

Time lapse before drug works:
3 weeks continual use required to determine effectiveness.

Continued next column

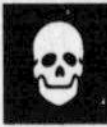

OVERDOSE

SYMPTOMS:
Drowsiness; slow, weak pulse; slow, shallow breathing; diarrhea; coma; flush; low body temperature; pinpoint pupils.
WHAT TO DO:
- **Dial 911 (emergency) for medical help or call poison control center 1-800-222-1222 for instructions.**
- **See emergency information on last 3 pages of this book.**

Don't take with:
Any other medicine or any dietary supplement without consulting your doctor or pharmacist.

POSSIBLE ADVERSE REACTIONS OR SIDE EFFECTS

SYMPTOMS	WHAT TO DO
Life-threatening:	
In case of overdose, see previous column.	
Common:	
• Depression, dizziness.	Continue. Call doctor when convenient.
• Headache, faintness, drowsiness, lethargy, red eyes, stuffy nose, impotence, diminished sex drive, diarrhea, dry mouth.	Continue. Tell doctor at next visit.
Infrequent:	
• Black stool; bloody vomit; chest pain; shortness of breath; irregular or slow heartbeat; stiffness in muscles, bones, joints.	Discontinue. Call doctor right away.
• Trembling hands, foot and leg swelling.	Continue. Call doctor when convenient.
Rare:	
• Rash or itchy skin, sore throat, fever, abdominal pain, nausea, vomiting, unusual bleeding or bruising, jaundice.	Discontinue. Call doctor right away.
• Painful urination, nightmares.	Continue. Call doctor when convenient.

WARNINGS & PRECAUTIONS

Don't take if:
You are allergic to any rauwolfia alkaloid.

Before you start, consult your doctor if:
- You have been depressed.
- You have had peptic ulcer, ulcerative colitis or gallstones.
- You have epilepsy.
- You will have surgery within 2 months, including dental surgery, requiring general or spinal anesthesia.

Over age 60:
Adverse reactions and side effects may be more frequent and severe than in younger persons.

Pregnancy:
Decide with your doctor whether drug benefits justify risk to unborn child. Risk category C (see page xviii).

Breast-feeding:
Drug passes into milk. Avoid drug or discontinue nursing until you finish medicine. Consult doctor for advice on maintaining milk supply.

Infants & children:
Not recommended.

Prolonged use:
- May rarely increase risk of certain cancers. Consult your doctor if you have a family or personal history of cancer.
- Talk to your doctor about the need for follow-up medical examinations or laboratory studies.

Skin & sunlight:
No problems expected.

Driving, piloting or hazardous work:
Avoid if you feel drowsy, dizzy or faint. Otherwise, no problems expected.

Discontinuing:
Don't discontinue without consulting doctor. Dose may require gradual reduction if you have taken drug for a long time. Doses of other drugs may also require adjustment.

Others:
- Advise any doctor or dentist whom you consult that you take this medicine.
- Consult your doctor if you do isometric exercises. These raise blood pressure. Drug may intensify blood pressure rise.

POSSIBLE INTERACTION WITH OTHER DRUGS

GENERIC NAME OR DRUG CLASS	COMBINED EFFECT
Anticoagulants,* oral	Unpredictable increased or decreased effect of anticoagulant.
Anticonvulsants*	Serious change in seizure pattern.
Antidepressants*	Increased anti-depressant effect.
Antihistamines*	Increased anti-histamine effect.
Antihypertensives,* other	Increased rauwolfia effect.
Aspirin	Decreased aspirin effect.
Beta-adrenergic blocking agents*	Increased rauwolfia alkaloid effect. Excessive sedation.
Carteolol	Increased anti-hypertensive effect.
Central nervous system (CNS) depressants*	Increased CNS depression.
Clozapine	Toxic effect on the central nervous system.
Digitalis preparations*	Possible irregular heartbeat.
Dronabinol	Increased effects of both drugs. Avoid.
Ethinamate	Dangerous increased effects of ethinamate. Avoid combining.
Fluoxetine	Increased depressant effects of both drugs.
Guanfacine	May increase depressant effects of either medicine.
Leucovorin	High alcohol content of leucovorin may cause adverse effects.
Levodopa	Decreased levodopa effect.

Continued on page 926

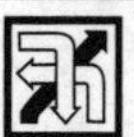

POSSIBLE INTERACTION WITH OTHER SUBSTANCES

INTERACTS WITH	COMBINED EFFECT
Alcohol:	Increased intoxication. Use with extreme caution.
Beverages: Carbonated drinks.	Decreased rauwolfia alkaloid effect.
Cocaine:	Increased risk of heart block and high blood pressure.
Foods: Spicy foods.	Possible digestive upset.
Marijuana:	Occasional use—Mild drowsiness. Daily use—Moderate drowsiness, low blood pressure, depression.
Tobacco:	None expected.

RENIN INHIBITORS

GENERIC AND BRAND NAMES

ALISKIREN
Amturnide
Tekamlo
Tekturna
Tekturna HCT
Valturna

BASIC INFORMATION

Habit forming? No
Prescription needed? Yes
Available as generic? No
Drug class: Antihypertensive; renin inhibitor

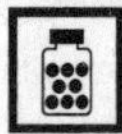

USES

Treatment for hypertension (high blood pressure). May be used alone or along with other antihypertensive medications.

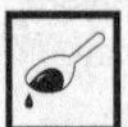

DOSAGE & USAGE INFORMATION

How to take:
Tablet—Swallow with liquid. May be taken with or without food. Do not remove the special drying agent from the bottle.

When to take:
Once daily at the same time each day, or as directed by your doctor.

If you forget a dose:
Take as soon as you remember. If it is almost time for the next dose, then skip the missed dose and wait for your next scheduled dose (don't double this dose).

What drug does:
It inhibits renin, a kidney enzyme associated with the regulation of blood pressure. This helps the blood vessels to relax and widen so blood pressure is lowered.

Continued next column

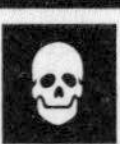

OVERDOSE

SYMPTOMS:
Unknown. Could cause very low blood pressure (hypotension).
WHAT TO DO:
Overdose unlikely to threaten life. If person uses much larger amount than prescribed or if accidentally swallowed, call doctor or poison control center 1-800-222-1222 for help.

Time lapse before drug works:
It starts working within a few hours, but may take several weeks for full effectiveness.

Don't take with:
Any other medicine or any dietary supplement without consulting your doctor or pharmacist.

POSSIBLE ADVERSE REACTIONS OR SIDE EFFECTS

SYMPTOMS	WHAT TO DO
Life-threatening:	
Rare allergic reaction (hives, itching, rash, trouble breathing, tightness in chest, swelling of lips or tongue or throat).	Seek emergency treatment immediately.
Common:	
Diarrhea, headache.	Continue. Call doctor when convenient.
Infrequent:	
Cough, rash.	Continue. Call doctor when convenient.
Rare:	
• Low blood pressure (feeling faint, dizzy or lightheaded), seizure.	Discontinue. Call doctor right away.
• Abdominal pain, bloating, heartburn, nausea, burping, reflux, fatigue, upper respiratory tract infection, back pain, runny or stuffy nose.	Continue. Call doctor when convenient.

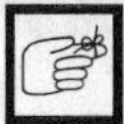

WARNINGS & PRECAUTIONS

Don't take if:
- You are allergic to aliskiren.
- You are pregnant.

Before you start, consult your doctor if:
- You have kidney (renal) disease or disorder.
- You have a history of dialysis, nephrotic syndrome, or renovascular hypertension (high blood pressure caused by narrowing of the arteries that carry blood to the kidneys).
- You have hyperkalemia (high level of potassium in the blood).
- You plan to become pregnant.
- You are allergic to any medication, food or other substance.

Over age 60:
No special problems expected.

Pregnancy:
Decide with your doctor if drug benefits justify any possible risk to unborn child. When used in the second and third trimesters, the drug can cause injury and even death to the developing fetus. Risk category C—first trimester and D—second and third trimesters (see page xviii).

Breast-feeding:
It is unknown if drug passes into milk. Avoid drug or discontinue nursing. Consult doctor for advice.

Infants & children:
Not approved for children under age 18.

Prolonged use:
- No special problems expected. Hypertension usually requires life-long treatment.
- Schedule regular doctor visits to determine if drug is continuing to be effective in controlling the hypertension and to check your potassium levels and kidney function.

Skin & sunlight:
No special problems expected.

Driving, piloting or hazardous work:
Use caution if you feel dizzy or are experiencing other side effects.

Discontinuing:
Don't discontinue without consulting your doctor, even if you feel well. You can have hypertension without feeling any symptoms. Untreated high blood pressure can cause serious problems.

Others:
- Advise any doctor or dentist whom you consult that you take this medicine. May interfere with the accuracy of some medical tests.
- Follow any diet or exercise plan your doctor prescribes. It can help control hypertension.
- Get up slowly from a sitting or lying position to avoid any dizziness, faintness or lightheadedness.

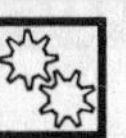

POSSIBLE INTERACTION WITH OTHER DRUGS

GENERIC NAME OR DRUG CLASS	COMBINED EFFECT
Antihypertensives,* other	Increased antihypertensive effect.
Furosemide	May decrease furosemide effect.

POSSIBLE INTERACTION WITH OTHER SUBSTANCES

INTERACTS WITH	COMBINED EFFECT
Alcohol:	None expected.
Beverages:	None expected.
Cocaine:	Unknown effect. Avoid.
Foods:	None expected.
Marijuana:	Unknown effect. Avoid.
Tobacco:	None expected. Best to avoid.

RESERPINE, HYDRALAZINE & HYDROCHLOROTHIAZIDE

BRAND NAMES

Cam-Ap-Es
Cherapas
Ser-A-Gen
Seralazide
Serpazide
Tri-Hydroserpine
Unipres

BASIC INFORMATION

Habit forming? No
Prescription needed? Yes
Available as generic? Yes
Drug class: Antihypertensive

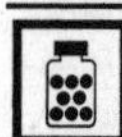

USES

- Treatment for high blood pressure and congestive heart failure.
- Reduces fluid retention (edema).

DOSAGE & USAGE INFORMATION

How to take:
Tablet—Swallow with liquid. If you can't swallow whole, crumble and take with liquid or food.

When to take:
At the same times each day.

If you forget a dose:
Take as soon as you remember up to 2 hours late. If more than 2 hours, wait for next scheduled dose (don't double this dose).

What drug does:
- Relaxes blood vessels, reducing blood pressure.
- Suppresses brain centers that control emotions.
- Reduces body fluid and relaxes arteries, lowering blood pressure.

Time lapse before drug works:
Regular use for several weeks may be necessary to determine drug's effectiveness.

Continued next column

OVERDOSE

SYMPTOMS:
Drowsiness; slow, shallow breathing; pinpoint pupils; diarrhea; flush; low body temperature; rapid, weak heartbeat; fainting; extreme weakness; cold, sweaty skin; cramps, coma.
WHAT TO DO:
- **Dial 911 (emergency) for medical help or call poison control center 1-800-222-1222 for instructions.**
- **See emergency information on last 3 pages of this book.**

Don't take with:
- Nonprescription drugs containing alcohol without consulting doctor.
- Any other medicine or any dietary supplement without consulting your doctor or pharmacist.

POSSIBLE ADVERSE REACTIONS OR SIDE EFFECTS

SYMPTOMS	WHAT TO DO
Life-threatening:	
Rapid or irregular heartbeat, weak pulse, fainting, black stool, black or bloody vomit, chest pain.	Discontinue. Seek emergency treatment.
Common:	
• Nausea, vomiting.	Discontinue. Call doctor right away.
• Headache, diarrhea, drowsiness, runny nose, appetite loss.	Continue. Call doctor when convenient.
Infrequent:	
• Blurred vision, chest pain, abdominal pain, rash, hives, joint pain.	Discontinue. Call doctor right away.
• Dizziness; mood change; headache; dry mouth; weakness; tiredness; weight gain or loss; eyes red, watery, irritated; confusion; constipation; red or flushed face; joint stiffness; depression; anxiety; foot and leg swelling.	Continue. Call doctor when convenient.
Rare:	
• Jaundice; unexplained bleeding or bruising; sore throat, fever, mouth sores; weakness and faintness when arising from bed or chair.	Discontinue. Call doctor right away.
• Numbness, tingling, burning feeling in feet and hands; nasal congestion; impotence; nightmares.	Continue. Call doctor when convenient.

WARNINGS & PRECAUTIONS

Don't take if:
You are allergic to any rauwolfia alkaloid, hydralazine, any thiazide diuretic drug,* or tartrazine dye.

RESERPINE, HYDRALAZINE & HYDROCHLOROTHIAZIDE

Before you start, consult your doctor if:
- You have been depressed.
- You have had peptic ulcer, ulcerative colitis, gallstones, kidney disease or impaired kidney function, lupus or a stroke.
- You have epilepsy, gout, liver, pancreas or kidney disorder.
- You feel pain in chest, neck or arms on physical exertion.
- You are allergic to any sulfa drug.*
- You will have surgery within 2 months, including dental surgery, requiring general or spinal anesthesia.

Over age 60:
Adverse reactions and side effects may be more frequent and severe than in younger persons, especially dizziness and excessive potassium loss.

Pregnancy:
Decide with your doctor if drug benefits justify risk to unborn child. Risk category C (see page xviii).

Breast-feeding:
Drug passes into milk. Avoid drug or discontinue nursing until you finish medicine. Consult doctor.

Infants & children:
Not recommended.

Prolonged use:
- Causes cancer in laboratory animals. Consult your doctor if you have a family or personal history of cancer.
- Possible psychosis.
- May cause lupus; numbness, tingling in hands or feet.
- Talk to your doctor about the need for follow-up medical examinations or laboratory studies.

Skin & sunlight:
One or more drugs in this group may cause rash or intensify sunburn in areas exposed to sun or ultraviolet light (photosensitivity reaction). Avoid overexposure. Notify doctor if reaction occurs.

Driving, piloting or hazardous work:
Don't drive or pilot aircraft until you learn how medicine affects you. Don't work around dangerous machinery. Don't climb ladders or work in high places. Danger increases if you drink alcohol or take medicine affecting alertness and reflexes.

Discontinuing:
Don't discontinue without consulting doctor. Dose may require gradual reduction if you have taken drug for a long time. Doses of other drugs may also require adjustment.

Others:
- Consult your doctor if you do isometric exercises. These raise blood pressure. Drug may intensify blood pressure rise.
- Vitamin B-6 supplement may be advisable. Consult doctor.
- Hot weather and fever may cause dehydration and drop in blood pressure. Dose may require temporary adjustment. Weigh daily and report any unexpected weight decreases to your doctor.
- Advise any doctor or dentist whom you consult that you take this medicine.
- May cause rise in uric acid, leading to gout.
- May cause blood sugar rise in diabetics.
- Some products contain tartrazine dye. Avoid, especially if you are allergic to aspirin.

POSSIBLE INTERACTION WITH OTHER DRUGS

GENERIC NAME OR DRUG CLASS	COMBINED EFFECT
Acebutolol	Possible increased effects of drugs.
Allopurinol	Decreased allopurinol effect.

Continued on page 927

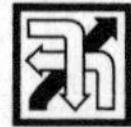

POSSIBLE INTERACTION WITH OTHER SUBSTANCES

INTERACTS WITH	COMBINED EFFECT
Alcohol:	Increased intoxication. Avoid.
Beverages: Carbonated drinks.	Decreased reserpine effect.
Cocaine:	Dangerous blood pressure rise. Avoid.
Foods: Spicy foods.	Possible digestive upset.
Licorice.	Excessive potassium loss that causes dangerous heart rhythms.
Marijuana:	Weakness on standing. May increase blood pressure. Occasional use—Mild drowsiness. Daily use—Moderate drowsiness, low blood pressure, depression.
Tobacco:	Possible angina attacks.

***See Glossary**

RETINOIDS (Oral)

GENERIC AND BRAND NAMES

ACITRETIN
Soriatane

BASIC INFORMATION

Habit forming? No
Prescription needed? Yes
Available as generic? No
Drug class: Antipsoriatic

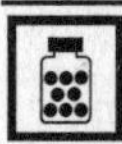

USES

- Treats psoriasis in patients who don't respond well to standard or usual treatment. It may be combined with phototherapy or other antipsoriatic drugs.
- It may be used to improve arthritis symptoms that accompany psoriasis.
- Treatment for certain other skin disorders.

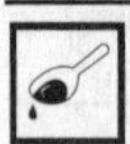

DOSAGE & USAGE INFORMATION

How to take:
Capsule—Swallow with liquid and take with food to lessen stomach irritation.

When to take:
At the same time each day, usually once a day.

If you forget a dose:
Take as soon as you remember. If it is almost time for the next dose, wait for next scheduled dose (don't double this dose).

What drug does:
The exact mechanism of action is unknown. The drug appears to help growth of normal skin cells. It also has anti-inflammatory action.

Time lapse before drug works:
The skin may show improvement in 2 weeks, but full benefit can take 2 to 3 months.

Don't take with:
Any other medicine or any dietary supplement without consulting your doctor or pharmacist.

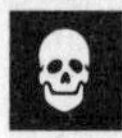

OVERDOSE

SYMPTOMS:
May include nausea, vomiting, severe headache, drowsiness, loss of balance, itching, irritability.
WHAT TO DO:
Overdose unlikely to threaten life. If person takes much larger amount than prescribed, call doctor or poison control center 1-800-222-1222 for help.

POSSIBLE ADVERSE REACTIONS OR SIDE EFFECTS

SYMPTOMS	WHAT TO DO
Life-threatening: None expected.	
Common:	
• Severe headache, severe nausea or vomiting.	Discontinue. Call doctor right away.
• Stiffness or pain in bones or joints or muscles, mild headaches, lip symptoms (chapped, redness, sore, cracking, swollen), dryness of nose or eyes, hair loss, skin sensitivity to sunlight, sore mouth, nose-bleeds, peeling or scaling (eyelids, palms, fingertips, and soles of feet), runny nose, sore or swollen gums, thirstiness.	Continue. Call doctor when convenient.
Infrequent:	
• Blurred vision, eye pain.	Discontinue. Call doctor right away.
• Fingernails loose or skin around them is sore or red, loss of eyebrows or eye lashes, redness of eye or inside eyelid, eyes watery or sensitive to light, swollen eyelids, problem with contact lens use, psoriasis gets worse in early drug use.	Continue. Call doctor when convenient.
Rare:	
• Double vision, decreased night vision, yellow skin or eyes, stomach pain, dark urine, unusual bruising.	Discontinue. Call doctor right away.
• Skin symptoms (spots, infection, sores, stinging, odd odor, burning, rash), ear pain or itching, flu-like symptoms, stye, cough or hoarseness, trouble in speaking, vaginal discharge or itching or irritation.	Continue. Call doctor when convenient.

WARNINGS & PRECAUTIONS

Don't take if:
- You are female and pregnant or may get pregnant in the next 3 years. Severe birth defects have occurred while using and after discontinuing this drug. Don't start drug until you have 2 negative pregnancy tests. Read all the prescribing information carefully.
- If you are allergic to retinoids or parabens (used as preservative in gelatin capsule).

Before you start, consult your doctor if:
- You have high cholesterol or triglycerides.
- You have diabetes or are an alcoholic.
- You have had problems with too much vitamin A in the body (hypervitaminosis).
- You are a female of reproductive age.
- You have kidney, liver or pancreas disease.

Over age 60:
Adverse reactions and side effects may be more frequent and severe than in younger persons. You may need smaller doses for shorter periods of time.

Pregnancy:
- Risk to unborn child outweighs drug benefits. The drug may cause severe birth defects. Don't use. Risk category X (see page xviii).
- Stop taking the drug and consult your doctor right away if you become pregnant while taking the drug or within 3 years after stopping.

Breast-feeding:
The drug may pass into milk. Avoid drug or discontinue nursing until you finish medicine. Consult doctor for advice on maintaining milk supply.

Infants & children:
It may prevent normal bone growth in children. Use only under close medical supervision.

Prolonged use:
Talk to your doctor about follow-up medical exams or laboratory studies to check blood lipids, liver function, eyes or pregnancy tests.

Skin & sunlight:
May cause rash or intensify sunburn in areas exposed to sun or ultraviolet light (photosensitivity reaction). Use sunscreen with SPF of 15 or higher. Avoid overexposure. Notify doctor if reaction occurs.

Driving, piloting or hazardous work:
Don't drive motor vehicles or pilot aircraft until you learn how medicine affects you. Don't work around dangerous machinery. Don't climb ladders or work in high places.

Discontinuing:
Drug use is discontinued once skin has healed sufficiently. Your psoriasis may recur after stopping the drug. Consult doctor for advice. Don't use leftover drug without doctor's approval.

Others:
- Certain methods of birth control may fail while using this drug, including tubal ligation and progestin (minipill) preparations. Other birth control methods may be affected also. Use two different methods of birth control.
- Don't donate blood during drug treatment or for 3 years thereafter.
- Advise any doctor or dentist whom you consult that you take this medicine.
- May cause liver damage or problems in controlling blood sugar.
- Laboratory blood studies for cholesterol and triglyceride levels should be obtained prior to and during treatment.
- Avoid skin products that cause skin dryness or sensitivity. Consult your doctor for advice.

POSSIBLE INTERACTION WITH OTHER DRUGS

GENERIC NAME OR DRUG CLASS	COMBINED EFFECT
Acne preparations*	Excessive drying effect on skin.
Contraceptives, oral* (progestin-only type)	Decreased effect of oral contraceptive.
Isotretinoin	Increased risk of adverse reactions.
Methotrexate	Risk of hepatitis.
Phenytoin	Increased effect of phenytoin.
Tetracyclines*	Risk of pseudotumor cerebri (pressure in the brain).
Tretinoin	Increased risk of adverse reactions.
Vitamin A	Increased risk of adverse reactions.

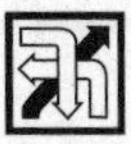

POSSIBLE INTERACTION WITH OTHER SUBSTANCES

INTERACTS WITH	COMBINED EFFECT
Alcohol:	Risk of severe side effects during drug use and after stopping. Avoid alcohol.
Beverages:	None expected.
Cocaine:	Unknown. Avoid.
Foods:	None expected.
Marijuana:	Unknown. Avoid.
Tobacco:	None expected.

RETINOIDS (Topical)

GENERIC AND BRAND NAMES

ADAPALENE
- **Differin**
- **Epiduo**

BEXAROTENE
- **Targretin**

TAZAROTENE
- **Avage**
- **Fabior**
- **Tazorac**

TRETINOIN
- **Atralin Gel**
- **Avita**
- **Renova**
- **Retin-A Cream**
- **Retin-A Cream Regimen Kit**
- **Retin-A Gel**
- **Retin-A Gel Regimen Kit**

TRETINOIN (Con't)
- **Retin-A Solution**
- **Retinoic Acid**
- **Solage**
- **Stieva-A Cream**
- **Stieva-A Cream Forte**
- **Stieva-A Gel**
- **Stieva-A Solutionl**
- **Tretin-X**
- **Tri-Luma**
- **Veltin Gel**
- **Vitamin A Acid Cream**
- **Vitamin A Acid Gel**
- **Ziana Gel**

BASIC INFORMATION

Habit forming? No
Prescription needed? Yes
Available as generic? Yes, for some
Drug class: Antiacne (topical), antipsoriatic

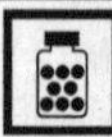

USES

- Treatment for acne, psoriasis, ichthyosis, keratosis, folliculitis, flat warts.
- Treatment for sun-damaged skin (wrinkles), mottled skin, rough skin and pigmented skin.
- Bexarotene treats skin cancer (cutaneous T cell lymphoma).
- Tri-Luma is a combination drug—tretinoin and fluocinolone and hydroquinone (not covered in this book).
- Solage is a combination drug—tretinoin plus mequinol (which is not covered in this book).

OVERDOSE

SYMPTOMS:
None expected.
WHAT TO DO:
- **If person accidentally swallows drug, dial 911 (emergency) for medical help or call poison control center 1-800-222-1222 for instructions.**
- **See emergency information on last 3 pages of this book.**

DOSAGE & USAGE INFORMATION

How to use:
Wash skin with nonmedicated soap, pat dry, wait 20 minutes before applying or as directed.
- Cream, gel or foam—Apply to affected areas with fingertips and rub in gently.
- Solution—Apply to affected areas with gauze pad or cotton swab.
- Avoid getting product into eyes or mouth, onto lips, inside nose or on vagina.

When to use:
Apply once daily, usually in the evening before going to bed.

If you forget a dose:
Use as soon as you remember if it is still the same day. If more than 12 hours late, wait for the next dose (don't double this dose).

What drug does:
Helps control acne inflammation and prevent new acne outbreaks. Increases skin cell turnover so skin layer peels off more easily.

Time lapse before drug works:
May require 2 to 6 weeks for minimum benefit and 3 to 12 months for full benefit.

Don't use with:
Any other topical medicine without consulting your doctor or pharmacist.

POSSIBLE ADVERSE REACTIONS OR SIDE EFFECTS

SYMPTOMS	WHAT TO DO
Life-threatening:	
None expected.	
Common:	
• Mild redness, itching, chapping, dryness of skin during first few weeks of use.	Depending on severity, may reduce frequency of use.
• Worsening of acne or psoriasis during first few weeks of use (due to action of the drug on previous unseen skin breakouts).	Expected effect. No action necessary.
Infrequent:	
Painful skin irritation, darkening or lightening of skin where treated.	Discontinue. Call doctor when convenient.
Rare:	
None expected.	

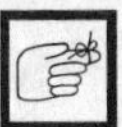

WARNINGS & PRECAUTIONS

Don't take if:
You are allergic to topical retinoids or any of the components of the gel product.

Before you start, consult your doctor if:
- You are using any other prescription or nonprescription medicine for the skin.
- You are using abrasive skin cleansers or medicated cosmetics.

Over age 60:
No problems expected.

Pregnancy:
- Adapalene and tretinoin—Discuss with your doctor if benefits outweigh risks to unborn child. Risk category C (see page xviii).
- Bexarotene and tazarotene—Risk to unborn child outweighs drug's benefits. Don't use. Risk category X (see page xviii).

Breast-feeding:
Effect unknown. Consult doctor.

Infants & children:
Use only as directed by your child's doctor.

Prolonged use:
No problems expected.

Skin & sunlight:
- May cause rash or intensify sunburn in areas exposed to sun or ultraviolet light. Avoid overexposure. Notify doctor if reaction occurs.
- If you are normally exposed to considerable sunlight, use extra caution. Use broad spectrum of sunscreen on treated areas and wear protective clothing (e.g., hat).

Driving, piloting or hazardous work:
No problems expected.

Discontinuing:
- May be unnecessary to finish medicine. Discontinue when acne improves. For some patients, this medicine may be used indefinitely to control acne.
- If skin problem doesn't improve after first few weeks of use, consult doctor.

Others:
- Cold or windy weather may further irritate the skin. Avoid if possible.
- Products with a drying effect on the skin may cause irritation when used with retinoids. These include cosmetics, abrasive soaps and cleansers, astringents, and topical products that contain alcohol, spices or lime.
- Advise any doctor or dentist whom you consult that you use this medicine.
- Brand name Solage also contains the drug mequinol.
- Don't apply drug to skin area that has cuts, abrasions, a rash or is sunburned.

POSSIBLE INTERACTION WITH OTHER DRUGS

GENERIC NAME OR DRUG CLASS	COMBINED EFFECT
Antiacne topical preparations, other	Excessive skin irritation.
Cosmetics (medicated)	Severe skin irritation.
Insect repellents containing DEET	Repellent can be absorbed into skin.
Skin-peeling agents (salicylic acid, sulfur, resorcinol)	Excessive skin irritation.
Skin preparations with alcohol	Severe skin irritation.
Soaps or cleansers (abrasive)	Severe skin irritation.

POSSIBLE INTERACTION WITH OTHER SUBSTANCES

INTERACTS WITH	COMBINED EFFECT
Alcohol:	None expected.
Beverages:	None expected.
Cocaine:	None expected.
Foods:	None expected.
Marijuana:	None expected.
Tobacco:	None expected.

***See Glossary**

RIBAVIRIN

BRAND NAMES

Tribavirin
Virazid
Virazole

BASIC INFORMATION

Habit forming? No
Prescription needed? Yes
Available as generic? Yes
Drug class: Antiviral

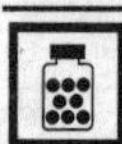

USES

- Treats severe viral pneumonia.
- Treats respiratory syncytial virus (RSV) infections in hospitalized infants or children.
- Treats influenza A and B with some success.
- Does not treat other viruses such as the common cold.
- Brand names Rebetol and Ribasphere are used to treat chronic hepatitis C when combined with another drug. The information in this chart does not include any facts about these two brands. Your doctor will provide you the information and instructions and will follow your therapy carefully.

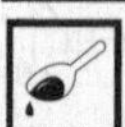

DOSAGE & USAGE INFORMATION

How to take:
By inhalation of a fine mist through mouth. Requires a special sprayer attached to oxygen mask; face mask for infants or hood.

When to take:
As ordered by your doctor.

If you forget a dose:
Use as soon as you remember.

What drug does:
Kills virus or prevents its growth.

Time lapse before drug works:
Begins working in 1 hour. May require treatment for 12 to 18 hours per day for 3 to 7 days.

Don't take with:
Any other medicine or any dietary supplement without consulting your doctor or pharmacist.

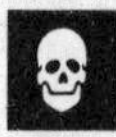

OVERDOSE

SYMPTOMS:
None expected.
WHAT TO DO:
Overdose unlikely to threaten life. If person uses much larger amount than prescribed or if accidentally swallowed, call doctor or poison control center 1-800-222-1222 for help.

POSSIBLE ADVERSE REACTIONS OR SIDE EFFECTS

SYMPTOMS	WHAT TO DO
Life-threatening: None expected.	
Common: None expected.	
Infrequent:	
• Unusual tiredness or weakness.	Discontinue. Call doctor right away.
• Headache, insomnia, appetite loss, nausea.	Continue. Call doctor when convenient.
Rare:	
Skin irritation or rash.	Continue. Call doctor when convenient.

WARNINGS & PRECAUTIONS

Don't take if:
You are allergic to ribavirin.

Before you start, consult your doctor if:
- You are now on low-salt, low-sugar or other special diet.
- You have severe anemia.

Over age 60:
Adverse reactions and side effects may be more frequent and severe than in younger persons. Ask doctor about smaller doses.

Pregnancy:
Risk to unborn child outweighs drug benefits. Don't use. Risk category X (see page xviii).

Breast-feeding:
Drug may pass into milk. Avoid drug or discontinue nursing until you finish medicine. Consult doctor for advice on maintaining milk supply.

Infants & children:
Use only under close medical supervision.

Prolonged use:
No problems expected.

Skin & sunlight:
No special problems expected.

Driving, piloting or hazardous work:
Don't drive or pilot aircraft until you learn how medicine affects you. Don't work around dangerous machinery. Don't climb ladders or work in high places. Danger increases if you drink alcohol or take medicine affecting alertness and reflexes, such as antihistamines, tranquilizers, sedatives, pain medicine, narcotics and mind-altering drugs.

Discontinuing:
Don't discontinue without consulting doctor. Dose may require gradual reduction if you have taken drug for a long time. Doses of other drugs may also require adjustment.

Others:
- Health care workers exposed to ribavirin may experience headache; eye itching, redness or swelling.
- Female health care workers who are pregnant or may become pregnant should avoid exposure to drug.
- The information in this chart does not cover or include the brand names Rebetol or Ribasphere. Your doctor must provide that information for you.

POSSIBLE INTERACTION WITH OTHER DRUGS

GENERIC NAME OR DRUG CLASS	COMBINED EFFECT
Zidovudine	Decreased effect of ribavirin and zidovudine.

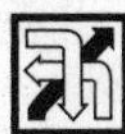

POSSIBLE INTERACTION WITH OTHER SUBSTANCES

INTERACTS WITH	COMBINED EFFECT
Alcohol:	None expected.
Beverages:	None expected.
Cocaine:	None expected.
Foods:	None expected.
Marijuana:	None expected.
Tobacco:	None expected.

RIBOFLAVIN (Vitamin B-2)

BRAND NAMES

Numerous brands of single vitamin and multivitamin combinations are available.

BASIC INFORMATION

Habit forming? No
Prescription needed? No
Available as generic? Yes
Drug class: Vitamin supplement

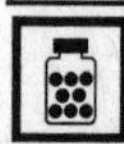

USES

- Dietary supplement to ensure normal growth and health.
- Dietary supplement to treat symptoms caused by deficiency of B-2: sores in mouth, eyes sensitive to light, itching and peeling skin.

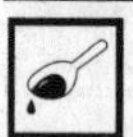

DOSAGE & USAGE INFORMATION

How to take:
Tablet—Swallow with liquid or food to lessen stomach irritation. If you can't swallow whole, crumble tablet and take with liquid or food.

When to take:
At the same times each day.

If you forget a dose:
Take as soon as you remember. If it is almost time for the next dose, wait for that dose (don't double this dose) and resume regular schedule.

What drug does:
Promotes normal growth and health.

Time lapse before drug works:
Requires continual intake.

Don't take with:
Any other medicine or any dietary supplement without consulting your doctor or pharmacist.

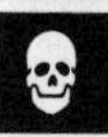

OVERDOSE

SYMPTOMS:
Dark urine, nausea, vomiting.
WHAT TO DO:
Overdose unlikely to threaten life. If person uses much larger amount than prescribed or if accidentally swallowed, call doctor or poison control center 1-800-222-1222 for help.

POSSIBLE ADVERSE REACTIONS OR SIDE EFFECTS

SYMPTOMS	WHAT TO DO
Life-threatening: None expected.	
Common: Urine yellow in color.	No action necessary.
Infrequent: None expected.	
Rare: None expected.	

RIBOFLAVIN (Vitamin B-2)

WARNINGS & PRECAUTIONS

Don't take if:
- You are allergic to any B vitamin.
- You have chronic kidney failure.

Before you start, consult your doctor if:
You are pregnant or plan pregnancy.

Over age 60:
No problems expected.

Pregnancy:
Take within recommended guidelines. Consult doctor. Risk category A (see page xviii).

Breast-feeding:
Take within recommended guidelines. Consult doctor.

Infants & children:
Consult doctor.

Prolonged use:
No problems expected.

Skin & sunlight:
No problems expected.

Driving, piloting or hazardous work:
No problems expected.

Discontinuing:
No problems expected.

Others:
- Advise any doctor or dentist whom you consult that you take this medicine.
- A balanced diet should provide all the vitamin B-2 a healthy person needs and makes supplements unnecessary during periods of good health. Best sources are milk, meats and green leafy vegetables.

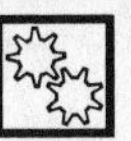

POSSIBLE INTERACTION WITH OTHER DRUGS

GENERIC NAME OR DRUG CLASS	COMBINED EFFECT
Anticholinergics*	Possible increased riboflavin absorption.
Antidepressants, tricyclic*	Decreased riboflavin effect.
Phenothiazines*	Decreased riboflavin effect.
Probenecid	Decreased riboflavin effect.

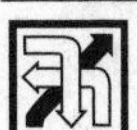

POSSIBLE INTERACTION WITH OTHER SUBSTANCES

INTERACTS WITH	COMBINED EFFECT
Alcohol:	Prevents uptake and absorption of vitamin B-2.
Beverages:	None expected.
Cocaine:	None expected.
Foods:	None expected.
Marijuana:	None expected.
Tobacco:	Prevents absorption of vitamin B-2 and other vitamins and nutrients.

***See Glossary**

RIFAMYCINS

GENERIC AND BRAND NAMES

RIFAMPIN
- Rifadin
- Rifamate
- Rifampicin
- Rimactane

RIFAPENTINE
- Priftin

BASIC INFORMATION

Habit forming? No
Prescription needed? Yes
Available as generic? Yes
Drug class: Antibacterial, antitubercular

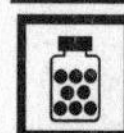

USES

Treatment for tuberculosis and other infections. Used in combination with other antitubercular medications.

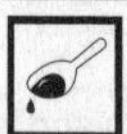

DOSAGE & USAGE INFORMATION

How to take:
Capsule or tablet—Swallow with liquid or food. If you can't swallow whole, open capsule or crumble tablet and take with liquid or small amount of food. For child, mix with small amount of applesauce or jelly.

When to take:
1 hour before or 2 hours after a meal.

If you forget a dose:
Take as soon as you remember. If it is almost time for the next dose, wait for that dose (don't double this dose) and resume regular schedule.

What drug does:
Prevents multiplication of tuberculosis germs.

Continued next column

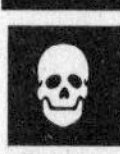

OVERDOSE

SYMPTOMS:
Slow, shallow breathing; weak, rapid pulse; cold, sweaty skin; coma.
WHAT TO DO:
- **Dial 911 (emergency) for medical help or call poison control center 1-800-222-1222 for instructions.**
- **If person is unconscious, check breathing and pulse. If not breathing, begin mouth-to-mouth rescue breathing. If heart is not beating, begin chest compressions.**
- **See emergency information on last 3 pages of this book.**

Time lapse before drug works:
Usually 2 weeks. May require 1 to 2 years without missed doses for maximum benefit.

Don't take with:
Any other medicine or any dietary supplement without consulting your doctor or pharmacist.

POSSIBLE ADVERSE REACTIONS OR SIDE EFFECTS

SYMPTOMS	WHAT TO DO
Life-threatening: In case of overdose, see previous column.	
Common:	
• Diarrhea; reddish urine, stool, saliva, sweat and tears.	Continue. Call doctor when convenient.
• Blood in urine, joint pain, back or side pain, swelling of feet or legs.	Continue, but call doctor right away.
Infrequent:	
• Rash; flushed, itchy skin of face and scalp; blurred vision; difficulty breathing; nausea, vomiting; abdominal cramps; tiredness; bleeding or bruising.	Continue, but call doctor right away.
• Dizziness, unsteady gait, confusion, muscle or bone pain, heartburn, flatulence, chills, headache, fever, mood or behavior changes.	Continue. Call doctor when convenient.
Rare:	
• Sore throat, mouth or tongue; jaundice.	Discontinue. Call doctor right away.
• Appetite loss, less urination.	Continue. Call doctor when convenient.

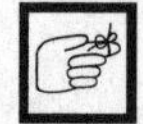

WARNINGS & PRECAUTIONS

Don't take if:
- You are allergic to any of the rifamycins.
- You wear soft contact lenses.

Before you start, consult your doctor if:
You are alcoholic or have liver disease.

Over age 60:
Adverse reactions and side effects may be more frequent and severe than in younger persons.

Pregnancy:
Decide with your doctor if drug benefits justify risk to unborn child. Risk category C (see page xviii).

Breast-feeding:
Effect unknown. Consult doctor.

Infants & children:
Use only under medical supervision.

Prolonged use:
- You may become more susceptible to infections caused by germs not responsive to rifamycins.
- Talk to your doctor about the need for follow-up medical examinations or laboratory studies to check liver function.

Skin & sunlight:
No problems expected.

Driving, piloting or hazardous work:
Don't drive or pilot aircraft until you learn how medicine affects you. Don't work around dangerous machinery. Don't climb ladders or work in high places. Danger increases if you drink alcohol or take medicine affecting alertness and reflexes, such as antihistamines, tranquilizers, sedatives, pain medicine, narcotics and mind-altering drugs.

Discontinuing:
Don't discontinue without doctor's advice until you complete prescribed dose, even though symptoms diminish or disappear.

Others:
- Reddish tears may discolor soft contact lenses.
- Advise any doctor or dentist you consult that you are using this medication.

POSSIBLE INTERACTION WITH OTHER DRUGS

GENERIC NAME OR DRUG CLASS	COMBINED EFFECT
Adrenocorticoids, systemic	Decreased adreno-corticoid effect.
Anticoagulants,* oral	Decreased anticoagulant effect.
Antidepressants,* tricyclic	Decreased anti-depressant effect.
Antidiabetics,* oral	Decreased antidiabetic effect.
Antifungals,* azole	Decreased antifungal effect.
Barbiturates*	Decreased barbiturate effect.
Calcium channel* blockers	Decreased channel blocker effect.
Chloramphenicol	Decreased effect of both drugs.
Clarithromycin	Decreased antibiotic effect.
Clofibrate	Decreased clofibrate effect.
Clozapine	Toxic effect on bone marrow.
Contraceptives, oral*	Decreased contraceptive effect.
Cyclosporine	Decreased effect of both drugs.
Dapsone	Decreased dapsone effect.
Diazepam	Decreased diazepam effect.
Digitalis preparations*	Decreased digitoxin effect.
Disopyramide	Decreased disopyramide effect.
Doxycycline	Decreased antibiotic effect.
Estrogens* (including contraceptive pills)	Decreased effect of both drugs.
Haloperidol	Decreased haloperidol effect.
Hepatotoxics*	Increased risk of liver toxicity.
Isoniazid	Possible toxicity to liver.
Leflunomide	Increased risk of leflunomide toxicity.
Levothyroxine	Decreased levothyroxine effect.
Methadone	Decreased methadone effect.
Mexiletine	Decreased mexiletine effect.
Non-nucleoside reverse transcriptase inhibitors	May require dosage adjustment of rifampin.

Continued on page 928

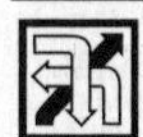

POSSIBLE INTERACTION WITH OTHER SUBSTANCES

INTERACTS WITH	COMBINED EFFECT
Alcohol:	Possible toxicity to liver.
Beverages:	None expected.
Cocaine:	None expected.
Foods:	None expected.
Marijuana:	None expected.
Tobacco:	None expected.

*See Glossary

RIFAXIMIN

BRAND NAMES

Xifaxan

BASIC INFORMATION

Habit forming? No
Prescription needed? Yes
Available as generic? No
Drug class: Antidiarrheal; antibacterial

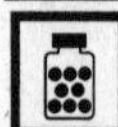

USES

- Treatment for diarrhea (often called travelers' diarrhea) caused by drinking fluids or eating food contaminated by a bacteria (most often *Escherichia coli*). It may not be effective for diarrhea caused by other bacteria or viruses.
- Reduction in risk of overt hepatic encephalopathy recurrence in patients age 18 and older.

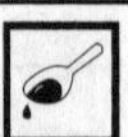

DOSAGE & USAGE INFORMATION

How to take:
Tablet—Swallow with liquid. Take with or without food.

When to take:
Three times a day at the same times each day. It is normally taken for three days.

If you forget a dose:
Take as soon as you remember. If it is almost time for the next dose, wait for that dose (don't double this dose) and resume regular schedule.

What drug does:
It works in the gastrointestinal tract to kill the bacteria causing the diarrhea. It is not absorbed into the bloodstream like most antibiotic drugs.

Continued next column

OVERDOSE

SYMPTOMS:
Unknown, but may include: nausea, vomiting, diarrhea and abdominal discomfort.
WHAT TO DO:
Overdose unlikely to threaten life. If person uses much larger amount than prescribed or if accidentally swallowed, call doctor or poison control center 1-800-222-1222 for help.

Time lapse before drug works:
Starts working in a few hours, but takes three days to cure the infection being treated.

Don't take with:
Any other medicine or any dietary supplement without consulting your doctor or pharmacist.

POSSIBLE ADVERSE REACTIONS OR SIDE EFFECTS

SYMPTOMS	WHAT TO DO
Life-threatening:	
Rare allergic reaction—Breathing difficulty; closing of the throat; swelling of hands, feet, face, lips or tongue; hives.	Discontinue. Seek emergency treatment.
Common:	
Headache.	Continue. Call doctor if symptoms persist.
Infrequent:	
Nausea, vomiting, stomach discomfort, gas, straining with bowel movement, sensitivity reaction including rash.	Continue. Call doctor if symptoms persist.
Rare:	
None expected.	

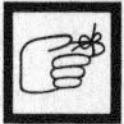

WARNINGS & PRECAUTIONS

Don't take if:
You are allergic to rifaximin or other antibiotics called rifamycins (including rifampin or rifabutin).

Before you start, consult your doctor if:
- You have a fever.
- You have blood in your stool.
- You have dysentery (a severe form of diarrhea).
- You have pseudomembranous colitis.

Over age 60:
No special problems expected.

Pregnancy:
Decide with your doctor if drug benefits justify risk to unborn child. Risk category C (see page xviii).

Breast-feeding:
It is unknown if drug passes into milk. Avoid drug or discontinue nursing until you finish medicine. Consult doctor for advice on maintaining milk supply.

Infants & children:
Safety and effectiveness for children under age 12 has not been established.

Prolonged use:
Not recommended. Medicine is discontinued once the infection is cured.

Skin & sunlight:
No special problems expected.

Driving, piloting or hazardous work:
No problems expected.

Discontinuing:
- Don't discontinue without doctor's advice until you complete prescribed dose, even though symptoms diminish or disappear.
- Do discontinue and call your doctor if diarrhea gets worse, you have bloody diarrhea or develop a fever.

Others:
- Be sure to drink plenty of fluids while you have diarrhea symptoms to prevent dehydration.
- Contact your doctor if symptoms do not improve in 24 to 48 hours.
- Advise any doctor or dentist whom you consult that you take this medicine.

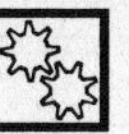

POSSIBLE INTERACTION WITH OTHER DRUGS

GENERIC NAME OR DRUG CLASS	COMBINED EFFECT
None expected.	

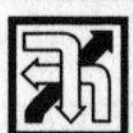

POSSIBLE INTERACTION WITH OTHER SUBSTANCES

INTERACTS WITH	COMBINED EFFECT
Alcohol:	None expected.
Beverages:	None expected.
Cocaine:	Effects unknown. Avoid.
Foods:	None expected.
Marijuana:	Effects unknown. Avoid.
Tobacco:	None expected.

RILUZOLE

BRAND NAMES

Rilutek

BASIC INFORMATION

Habit forming? No
Prescription needed? Yes
Available as generic? Yes
Drug class: Amyotrophic lateral sclerosis therapy agent

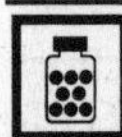

USES

Treatment for amyotrophic lateral sclerosis (ALS or Lou Gehrig's disease), a motor neuron disorder that causes weakness and atrophy of the muscles. Riluzole may extend a patient's survival time and delay the need for surgery for complications. It does not cure the disorder.

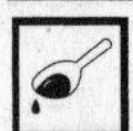

DOSAGE & USAGE INFORMATION

How to take:
Tablet—Swallow with liquid. Instructions to take on an empty stomach mean 1 hour before or 2 hours after eating.

When to take:
Usually every 12 hours.

If you forget a dose:
Take as soon as you remember. If it is almost time for the next dose, wait for that dose (don't double this dose) and resume regular schedule.

What drug does:
The cause of ALS is unknown and the exact mechanism of how the drug works is also unknown. It appears to decrease production of certain chemicals in the body and may affect some cellular activity that leads to the progressive weakness caused by the disorder.

Time lapse before drug works:
6 to 18 months for maximum benefits.

Don't take with:
Any other medicine or any dietary supplement without consulting your doctor or pharmacist.

OVERDOSE

SYMPTOMS:
Unknown.
WHAT TO DO:
If person takes much larger amount than prescribed, dial 911 (emergency) for medical help or call poison control center 1-800-222-1222 for instructions.

POSSIBLE ADVERSE REACTIONS OR SIDE EFFECTS

SYMPTOMS	WHAT TO DO
Life-threatening: None expected.	
Common:	
• Difficulty breathing, abdominal pain, increased coughing, blood pressure increased.	Discontinue. Call doctor right away.
• Mouth has a burning, or tingling feeling, constipation, nausea, vomiting, dizziness, mild weakness, headache, diarrhea.	Continue. Call doctor when convenient.
Infrequent:	
Skin symptoms (redness, itching, scaling, bruising, oozing or thickening), fever, sore feet or legs, sores in mouth or on lips, fast heartbeat.	Discontinue. Call doctor right away.
Rare:	
Changes in vision, tightness in chest, wheezing, memory loss, mood changes, severe drowsiness, hallucinations, mental changes, swelling (face, hands, fingers, feet or legs), nosebleed, blood in urine, unusual bleeding, unusual tiredness or weakness, severe headache, pain in various parts of the body, eyes red or irritated, continued or painful penile erection, noisy breathing, loss of bladder control, hives.	Discontinue. Call doctor right away.

WARNINGS & PRECAUTIONS

Don't take if:
You are sensitive to riluzole.

Before you start, consult your doctor if:
- You are allergic to any medicine, food or other substance, or have a family history of allergies.
- You have liver or kidney disease.

Over age 60:
No problems expected.

Pregnancy:
Decide with your doctor if drug benefits justify risk to unborn child. Risk category C (see page xviii).

Breast-feeding:
Not recommended. Consult doctor.

Infants & children:
Not recommended for this age group.

Prolonged use:
Talk to your doctor about the need for follow-up medical examinations or laboratory studies to check liver function.

Skin & sunlight:
No problems expected.

Driving, piloting or hazardous work:
Don't drive or pilot aircraft until you learn how medicine affects you. Don't work around dangerous machinery. Don't climb ladders or work in high places. Danger increases if you drink alcohol or take other medicines affecting alertness and reflexes.

Discontinuing:
No problems expected.

Others:
- May affect the results of some medical tests.
- Use as directed. Don't increase or decrease dosage without doctor's approval.
- Advise any doctor or dentist whom you consult that you take this medicine.
- Call your doctor if you develop a fever.

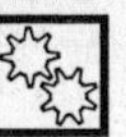

POSSIBLE INTERACTION WITH OTHER DRUGS

GENERIC NAME OR DRUG CLASS	COMBINED EFFECT
Hepatotoxics*	Increased risk of adverse effects.
Other medications	Complete studies have not been done to evaluate interactions with other drugs, but the potential exists for a variety of possible interactions. Consult doctor.

POSSIBLE INTERACTION WITH OTHER SUBSTANCES

INTERACTS WITH	COMBINED EFFECT
Alcohol:	Increased risk of adverse effects.
Beverages:	None expected.
Cocaine:	Problems not known. Best to avoid.
Foods:	None expected.
Marijuana:	Problems not known. Best to avoid.
Tobacco:	May decrease riluzole effect.

*See Glossary

ROFLUMILAST

BRAND NAMES

Daliresp

BASIC INFORMATION

Habit forming? No
Prescription needed? Yes
Available as generic? No
Drug class: Phosphodiesterase-4 (PDE4) inhibitor

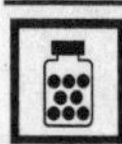

USES

Reduces frequency of flare-ups (exacerbations) in patients with severe chronic obstructive pulmonary disease (COPD) that is linked to chronic bronchitis. This drug is an add-on to bronchodilator treatment. It is not to be taken for the relief of acute bronchospasms.

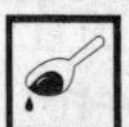

DOSAGE & USAGE INFORMATION

How to take:
Tablet—Swallow whole with liquid. May be taken with or without food.

When to take:
Once a day at the same time each day.

If you forget a dose:
Take as soon as you remember. If it is almost time for the next dose, wait for the next scheduled dose (don't double this dose).

What drug does:
It helps block the inflammatory process in COPD thereby reducing inflammation in the lungs that typically leads to symptoms (e.g., coughing and excess mucus).

Time lapse before drug works:
Starts working within hours, but noticeable improvements in lung function may take 4 to 8 weeks.

Don't take with:
Any other medicine or any dietary supplement without consulting your doctor or pharmacist.

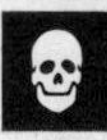

OVERDOSE

SYMPTOMS:
May have headache, dizziness, palpitations, gastrointestinal problem, light-headedness, clamminess and low blood pressure.
WHAT TO DO:
Dial 911 (emergency) for medical help or call poison control center 1-800-222-1222 for instructions.

POSSIBLE ADVERSE REACTIONS OR SIDE EFFECTS

SYMPTOMS	WHAT TO DO
Life-threatening:	
Rare allergic reaction (hives, itching, rash, wheezing, tightness in chest, swelling of lips or tongue or throat).	Seek emergency treatment immediately.
Common:	
Weight loss, nausea, headache, diarrhea, back pain.	Continue. Call doctor when convenient.
Infrequent:	
Dizziness or vertigo, insomnia, appetite loss, flu or cold-like symptoms.	Continue. Call doctor when convenient.
Rare:	
• Unusual changes in behavior or mood, depression or anxiety symptoms worsen, talk or thoughts of suicide.	Discontinue. Call doctor right away.
• Feeling nervous, stomach pain, indigestion, vomiting, muscle spasms, tremors.	Continue. Call doctor when convenient.

WARNINGS & PRECAUTIONS

Don't take if:
You are allergic to roflumilast.

Before you start, consult your doctor if:
- You have any liver disorder.
- You have a history of anxiety, depression or psychiatric disorders.
- You have a history of suicidal thoughts or behavior.

Over age 60:
No special problems expected.

Pregnancy:
Decide with your doctor if drug benefits justify risk to unborn child. Risk category C (see page xviii).

Breast-feeding:
Drug may pass into milk. Avoid drug or discontinue nursing until you finish medicine. Consult doctor for advice on maintaining milk supply.

Infants & children:
Not recommended for ages under 18. COPD does not normally occur in children.

Prolonged use:
- Consult with your doctor on a regular basis while taking this drug to monitor your progress, to check for side effects and to get recommended lab tests.
- The drug may cause weight loss in some patients. If excess weight loss occurs, consult your doctor.

Skin & sunlight:
No problems expected.

Driving, piloting or hazardous work:
No problems expected.

Discontinuing:
No problems expected, but do consult your doctor before stopping the drug.

Others:
- Advise any doctor or dentist whom you consult that you take this medicine.
- Caregivers and families should be alert to unusual changes in the patient's mood or behavior. If new symptoms occur or milder symptoms worsen, consult doctor.

POSSIBLE INTERACTION WITH OTHER DRUGS

GENERIC NAME OR DRUG CLASS	COMBINED EFFECT
Enzyme inhibitors*	Increased effect of roflumilast.
Enzyme inducers*	Decreased effect of roflumilast.
Oral contraceptives* containing ethinyl estradiol or gestodyne	Increased effect of roflumilast.

POSSIBLE INTERACTION WITH OTHER SUBSTANCES

INTERACTS WITH	COMBINED EFFECT
Alcohol:	None expected.
Beverages: Grapefruit juice.	May increase effect of roflumilast.
Cocaine:	Unknown effect. Best to avoid.
Foods: Grapefruit.	May increase effect of roflumilast.
Marijuana:	Unknown effect. Best to avoid.
Tobacco:	None expected. People with COPD should not smoke.

***See Glossary**

SALICYLATES

GENERIC AND BRAND NAMES

See full list of generic and brand names in the *Generic and Brand Name Directory*, page 896.

BASIC INFORMATION

Habit forming? No
Prescription needed? For some
Available as generic? Yes
Drug class: Analgesic, anti-inflammatory (nonsteroidal)

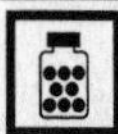

USES

- Reduces pain, fever, inflammation.
- Relieves swelling, stiffness, joint pain of arthritis or rheumatism.
- Decreases risk of myocardial infarction (aspirin only).

DOSAGE & USAGE INFORMATION

How to take:
- Tablet or capsule—Swallow with liquid.
- Extended-release tablet—Swallow each dose whole.
- Suppository—Remove wrapper and moisten suppository with water. Gently insert into rectum, large end first.

When to take:
Pain, fever, inflammation—As needed, no more often than every 4 hours.

If you forget a dose:
- Pain, fever—Take as soon as you remember. Wait 4 hours for next dose.
- Arthritis—Take as soon as you remember up to 2 hours late. Return to regular schedule.

What drug does:
- Affects hypothalamus, the part of the brain that regulates temperature by dilating small blood vessels in skin.

Continued next column

OVERDOSE

SYMPTOMS:
Ringing in ears; nausea; vomiting; dizziness; fever; deep, rapid breathing; hallucinations; convulsions; coma.
WHAT TO DO:
- **Dial 911 (emergency) for medical help or call poison control center 1-800-222-1222 for instructions.**
- **See emergency information on last 3 pages of this book.**

- Prevents clumping of platelets (small blood cells) so blood vessels remain open.
- Decreases prostaglandin effect.
- Suppresses body's pain messages.

Time lapse before drug works:
30 minutes for pain, fever, arthritis.

Don't take with:
- Tetracyclines. Space doses 1 hour apart.
- Any other medicine or any dietary supplement without consulting your doctor or pharmacist.

POSSIBLE ADVERSE REACTIONS OR SIDE EFFECTS

SYMPTOMS	WHAT TO DO
Life-threatening:	
Hives, rash, intense itching, faintness soon after a dose (anaphylaxis); black or bloody vomit; blood in urine.	Seek emergency treatment immediately.
Common:	
• Nausea, vomiting, abdominal pain.	Discontinue. Seek emergency treatment.
• Heartburn, indigestion.	Continue. Call doctor when convenient.
• Ringing in ears.	Continue. Tell doctor at next visit.
Infrequent:	
None expected.	
Rare:	
• Black stools, unexplained fever.	Discontinue. Seek emergency treatment.
• Rash, hives, itchy skin, diminished vision, shortness of breath, wheezing, jaundice.	Discontinue. Call doctor right away.
• Drowsiness, headache.	Continue. Call doctor when convenient.

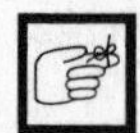

WARNINGS & PRECAUTIONS

Don't take if:
- You are allergic to salicylates.
- You need to restrict sodium in your diet. Buffered effervescent tablets and sodium salicylate are high in sodium.
- Salicylates have a strong vinegar-like odor, which means they have decomposed.
- You have a bleeding disorder.

Before you start, consult your doctor if:
- You have had stomach or duodenal ulcers.
- You have had gout.
- You have asthma or nasal polyps.

ELECTIVE PROGESTERONE RECEPTOR IODULATORS

NERIC AND BRAND NAMES

PRISTAL
lla

ASIC INFORMATION

abit forming? No
rescription needed? Yes
Available as generic? No
Drug class: Contraceptive

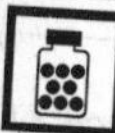

USES

Emergency contraceptive that is used to prevent pregnancy after unprotected sex or after failure of another birth control method.

DOSAGE & USAGE INFORMATION

How to take:
Tablet—Swallow whole with liquid. May be taken with or without food.

When to use:
As soon as possible within 5 days (120 hours) after unprotected sex or after failure of another birth control method. It may be used any time during the menstrual cycle. Repeated use within the same menstrual cycle is not recommended.

If you forget a dose:
It is a one time dose.

What drug does:
It works primarily by stopping or delaying the release of an egg from the ovary. It may also work by preventing egg fertilization or preventing the implantation of a fertilized egg in the uterus.

Time lapse before drug works:
About 1 to 3 hours.

Don't take with:
Any other medicine or any dietary supplement without consulting your doctor or pharmacist.

OVERDOSE

SYMPTOMS:
Unknown. An overdose is unlikely as each package contains one tablet.
WHAT TO DO:
If tablet is accidentally swallowed, call doctor or poison control center 1-800-222-1222 for help.

POSSIBLE ADVERSE REACTIONS OR SIDE EFFECTS

SYMPTOMS	WHAT TO DO
Life-threatening: None expected.	
Common: Headache, nausea, unusual tiredness or weakness, cramps, dizziness, spotting.	Call doctor if symptoms continue.
Infrequent: • Next menstrual period is early or less than a week late, acne.	No action necessary.
• Next menstrual period is over a week late.	Call doctor right away.
Rare: Abdominal or stomach pain 3 to 5 weeks after taking drug.	Call doctor right away.

Over age 60:
More likely to cause hidden bleeding in stomach or intestines. Watch for dark stools.

Pregnancy:
Risk factors vary for drugs in this group. See category list on page xviii and consult doctor.

Breast-feeding:
Drug passes into milk. Avoid drug or discontinue nursing until you finish medicine. Consult doctor for advice on maintaining milk supply.

Infants & children:
- Overdose frequent and severe. Keep bottles out of children's reach.
- Do not give to persons under age 18 who have fever and discomfort of viral illness, especially chicken pox and influenza. Probably increases risk of Reye's syndrome.

Prolonged use:
- Kidney damage. Periodic kidney function test recommended.
- Talk to your doctor about the need for follow-up medical examinations or laboratory studies to check liver function.

Skin & sunlight:
No special problems expected.

Driving, piloting or hazardous work:
No restrictions unless you feel drowsy.

Discontinuing:
For chronic illness—Don't discontinue without doctor's advice until you complete prescribed dose, even though symptoms diminish or disappear.

Others:
- Salicylates can complicate surgery, pregnancy, labor and delivery, and illness.
- Advise any doctor or dentist whom you consult that you take this medicine.
- For arthritis—Don't change dose without consulting doctor.
- Urine tests for blood sugar may be inaccurate.

POSSIBLE INTERACTION WITH OTHER DRUGS

GENERIC NAME OR DRUG CLASS	COMBINED EFFECT
Acetaminophen	Increased risk of kidney damage (with high, prolonged dose of each).
Adrenocorticoids, systemic	Decreased salicylate effect.
Allopurinol	Decreased allopurinol effect.
Angiotensin-converting enzyme (ACE) inhibitors*	Decreased ACE inhibitor effect.
Antacids*	Decreased salicylate effect.
Anticoagulants,* oral	Increased anticoagulant effect. Abnormal bleeding.
Antidiabetics,* oral	Low blood sugar.
Anti-inflammatory drugs, nonsteroidal (NSAIDs)*	Risk of stomach bleeding and ulcers.
Aspirin, other	Likely salicylate toxicity.
Beta-adrenergic blocking agents*	Decreased anti-hypertensive effect.
Bismuth subsalicylate	Increased risk of salicylate toxicity.
Bumetanide	Decreased diuretic effect.
Calcium supplements*	Increased salicylate effect.
Carteolol	Decreased antihypertensive effect of carteolol.
Ethacrynic acid	Decreased diuretic effect.
Furosemide	Possible salicylate toxicity.
Gold compounds*	Increased likelihood of kidney damage.
Indomethacin	Risk of stomach bleeding and ulcers.
Insulin	Decreased blood sugar.

Continued on page 928

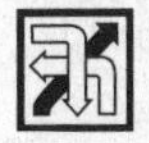

POSSIBLE INTERACTION WITH OTHER SUBSTANCES

INTERACTS WITH	COMBINED EFFECT
Alcohol:	Possible stomach irritation and bleeding. Avoid.
Beverages:	None expected.
Cocaine:	None expected.
Foods:	None expected.
Marijuana:	Possible increased pain relief, but marijuana may slow body's recovery. Avoid.
Tobacco:	None expected.

***See Glossary**

SCOPOLAMINE (Hyoscine)

BRAND NAMES

See full list of brand names in the *Generic and Brand Name Directory*, page 896.

BASIC INFORMATION

Habit forming? No
Prescription needed?
High strength: Yes
Low strength: No
Available as generic? Yes
Drug class: Antispasmodic, anticholinergic

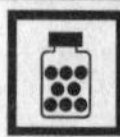

USES

- Reduces spasms of digestive system, bladder and urethra.
- Relieves painful menstruation.
- Prevents motion sickness.

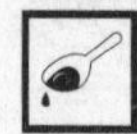

DOSAGE & USAGE INFORMATION

How to take:

- Tablet or capsule—Swallow with liquid or food to lessen stomach irritation.
- Drops—Dilute dose in beverage.
- Skin disc—Clean application site. Change application sites with each dose.

When to take:

- Motion sickness—Apply disc 30 minutes before departure.
- Other uses—Take 30 minutes before meals (unless directed otherwise by doctor).

If you forget a dose:
Take up to 2 hours late. If more than 2 hours, wait for next dose (don't double this dose).

What drug does:
Blocks nerve impulses at parasympathetic nerve endings, preventing muscle contractions and gland secretions of organs involved.

Continued next column

OVERDOSE

SYMPTOMS:
Dilated pupils, blurred vision, rapid pulse and breathing, dizziness, fever, hallucinations, confusion, slurred speech, agitation, flushed face, convulsions, coma.
WHAT TO DO:

- **Dial 911 (emergency) for medical help or call poison control center 1-800-222-1222 for instructions.**
- **See emergency information on last 3 pages of this book.**

Time lapse before drug works:
15 to 30 minutes.

Don't take with:
Any other medicine or any dietary supplement without consulting your doctor or pharmacist.

POSSIBLE ADVERSE REACTIONS OR SIDE EFFECTS

SYMPTOMS	WHAT TO DO
Life-threatening:	
Hives, rash, intense itching, faintness soon after a dose (anaphylaxis).	Seek emergency treatment immediately.
Common:	
• Confusion, delirium, rapid heartbeat.	Discontinue. Call doctor right away.
• Nausea, vomiting, decreased sweating.	Continue. Call doctor when convenient.
• Constipation, changes in taste.	Continue. Tell doctor at next visit.
• Dryness in ears, nose, throat, mouth.	No action necessary.
Infrequent:	
Headache, difficult urination, stuffy nose, feeling lightheaded.	Continue. Call doctor when convenient.
Rare:	
Rash or hives, eye pain, blurred vision.	Discontinue. Call doctor right away.

WARNINGS & PRECAUTIONS

Don't take if:

- You are allergic to any anticholinergic.
- You have trouble with stomach bloating.
- You have difficulty emptying your bladder completely.
- You have narrow-angle glaucoma.
- You have severe ulcerative colitis.

Before you start, consult your doctor if:

- You have open-angle glaucoma, angina, chronic bronchitis or asthma, hiatal hernia, liver disease, enlarged prostate, myasthenia gravis, peptic ulcer, kidney or thyroid disease.
- You will have surgery within 2 months, including dental surgery, requiring general or spinal anesthesia.

Over age 60:
Adverse reactions and side effects may be more frequent and severe than in younger persons.

Pregnancy:
Decide with your doctor whether drug benefits justify risk to unborn child. Risk category C (see page xviii).

Breast-feeding:
Drug passes into milk and decreases milk flow. Avoid drug or discontinue nursing until you finish medicine. Consult doctor for advice on maintaining milk supply.

Infants & children:
Use only under medical supervision.

Prolonged use:
Chronic constipation, possible fecal impaction. Consult doctor immediately.

Skin & sunlight:
No problems expected.

Driving, piloting or hazardous work:
Use disqualifies you for piloting aircraft. Don't drive until you learn how medicine affects you. Don't work around dangerous machinery. Don't climb ladders or work in high places.

Discontinuing:
May be unnecessary to finish medicine. Follow doctor's instructions.

Others:
Advise any doctor or dentist whom you consult that you take this medicine.

POSSIBLE INTERACTION WITH OTHER DRUGS

GENERIC NAME OR DRUG CLASS	COMBINED EFFECT
Adrenocorticoids, systemic	Possible glaucoma.
Amantadine	Increased scopolamine effect.
Antacids*	Decreased scopolamine effect.
Anticholinergics,* other	Increased scopolamine effect.
Antidepressants, tricyclic*	Increased scopolamine effect. Increased sedation.
Antidiarrheals*	Decreased scopolamine effect.
Antihistamines*	Increased scopolamine effect.
Attapulgite	Decreased scopolamine effect.
Buclizine	Increased scopolamine effect.
Clozapine	Toxic effect on the central nervous system.
Digitalis preparations*	s
Encainide	Inc toxi mus
Ethinamate	Dang effects Avoid c
Fluoxetine	Increased depressan both drugs.
Guanfacine	May increase depressant eff either medicine.
Haloperidol	Increased interna eye pressure.
Ketoconazole	Decreased ketoconazole effect.
Leucovorin	High alcohol content of leucovorin may cause adverse effects.
Meperidine	Increased scopolamine effect.
Methylphenidate	Increased scopolamine effect.
Methyprylon	May increase sedative effect to dangerous level. Avoid.
Molindone	Increased anticholinergic effect.
Monoamine oxidase (MAO) inhibitors*	Increased scopolamine effect.

Continued on page 928

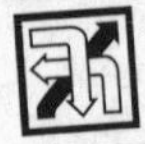

POSSIBLE INTERACTION WITH OTHER SUBSTANCES

INTERACTS WITH	COMBINED EFFECT
Alcohol:	None expected.
Beverages:	None expected.
Cocaine:	Excessively rapid heartbeat. Avoid.
Foods:	None expected.
Marijuana:	Drowsiness, dry mouth.
Tobacco:	None expected.

*See Glossary

SELECTIVE PROGESTERONE RECEPTOR MODULATORS

WARNINGS & PRECAUTIONS

Don't use if:
- You are allergic to ulipristal.
- You are pregnant.

Before you start, consult your doctor if:
- You suspect you are pregnant.
- You are overweight (drug may be less effective).

Over age 60:
Not used in this age group.

Pregnancy:
Consult doctor. Risk category X (see page xviii).

Breast-feeding:
The drug is not recommended in breast-feeding women. Consult doctor.

Infants & children:
May be used by females who have started their menstrual periods.

Prolonged use:
Not used long term.

Skin & sunlight:
No problems expected.

Driving, piloting or hazardous work:
No problems expected.

Discontinuing:
It is a one time dose.

Others:
- Call doctor right away if you have vomiting or diarrhea within three hours of taking this drug. You may need to take another dose.
- The drug will not protect you from getting HIV/AIDS or other sexually transmitted diseases.
- The drug is not intended for routine use as a method of birth control.
- A pregnancy test is recommended if your menstrual period is more than a week late.
- Fertility is likely to return to normal rather quickly after taking this drug. Other methods of birth control should be used as soon as possible after taking ulipristal, as it will not prevent future pregnancies. If you are using hormonal contraceptives,* your doctor may recommend that you also use a barrier method of birth control until your next menstrual period.
- Call doctor right away if you have severe lower abdominal or stomach pain 3 to 5 weeks after taking drug. You may have an ectopic pregnancy (outside of the uterus). This can be serious and life-threatening. It may lead to problems that make it harder for you to become pregnant in the future.

POSSIBLE INTERACTION WITH OTHER DRUGS

GENERIC NAME OR DRUG CLASS	COMBINED EFFECT
Contraceptives, hormonal*	Decreased contraceptive effect.
Enzyme inducers*	May decrease contraceptive effect of ulipristal.
Enzyme inhibitors*	May increase risk of adverse effects of ulipristal.

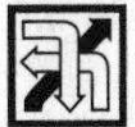

POSSIBLE INTERACTION WITH OTHER SUBSTANCES

INTERACTS WITH	COMBINED EFFECT
Alcohol:	None expected.
Beverages: Grapefruit juice.	May increase risk of side effects.
Cocaine:	None expected.
Food: Grapefruit.	May increase risk of side effects.
Marijuana:	None expected.
Tobacco:	None expected.

SELECTIVE SEROTONIN REUPTAKE INHIBITORS (SSRIs)

GENERIC AND BRAND NAMES

CITALOPRAM
Celexa
ESCITALOPRAM
Lexapro
FLUOXETINE
Prozac
Prozac Weekly
Sarafem
Symbyax
FLUVOXAMINE
Luvox
Luvox CR
PAROXETINE
Paxil
Paxil CR
SERTRALINE
Zoloft

BASIC INFORMATION

Habit forming? No
Prescription needed? Yes
Available as generic? Yes, for some
Drug class: Antidepressant, antiobsessional agent, antianxiety agent.

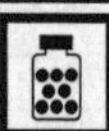

USES

- Treats depression, obsessive compulsive disorder, generalized anxiety disorder, panic disorder, post traumatic stress disorder, social phobia, premenstrual dysphoric disorder and seasonal affective disorder.
- Treats depressive episode of bipolar disorder.

DOSAGE & USAGE INFORMATION

How to take:
- Capsule or tablet—Swallow with water. Take with or without food. If you can't swallow whole, crumble tablet or open capsule and take with liquid or food.
- Oral disintegrating tablet—Dissolve in mouth.
- Oral solution, extended-release capsule or controlled-release tablet—Follow instructions.

When to take:
At the same time each day or weekly, usually in the a.m. Some dosages may be twice daily.

Continued next column

If you forget a dose:
Take as soon as you remember. If it is near the time of your next dose, skip the missed dose and resume normal schedule. Don't double this dose.

What drug does:
Affects serotonin, one of the chemicals in the brain called neurotransmitters, that plays a role in emotions and psychological disturbances.

Time lapse before drug works:
1 to 4 weeks.

Don't take with:
Any other medicine or any dietary supplement without consulting your doctor or pharmacist.

OVERDOSE

SYMPTOMS:
Dizziness, sweating, nausea, vomiting, tremor, heart rhythm disturbances. In rare cases, amnesia, coma and convulsions.
WHAT TO DO:
- **Dial 911 (emergency) for medical help or call poison control center 1-800-222-1222 for instructions.**
- **See emergency information on last 3 pages of this book.**

POSSIBLE ADVERSE REACTIONS OR SIDE EFFECTS

SYMPTOMS	WHAT TO DO
Life-threatening:	
Rash, itchy skin, breathing problems, chest pain (allergic reaction).	Seek emergency treatment immediately.
Common:	
Drowsiness, nausea, cough or hoarseness, lower back or side pain, sores on lips or mouth, constipation or diarrhea, headache, anxiety, changes in sexual desire or function, insomnia, dry mouth, unusual weakness or tiredness.	Continue. Call doctor when convenient.
Infrequent:	
• Vision changes, confusion, apathy (lack of emotion), breathing difficulty, chills, black or tarry stools, fever, enlarged lymph glands, heart rhythm changes, vomiting, skin rash or itching.	Discontinue. Call doctor right away.
• Abdominal pain, loss of appetite, yawning, tingling, skin burning or prickly feeling, stuffy nose, change in sense of taste, tooth grinding, trembling, increased saliva, gas, heartburn, sweating, urinary changes, hair loss, muscle or joint pain, menstrual changes, weight changes.	Continue. Call doctor when convenient.

Rare:

• Seizures (convulsions).	Discontinue. Seek emergency help.
• Abnormal bleeding, breast tenderness or enlargement, red or peeling skin, red or irritated eyes, sore throat, sudden body or facial spasms, dizziness, signs of low blood sugar (anxiety, chills, nervousness, difficulty concentrating), clumsiness.	Discontinue. Call doctor right away.

WARNINGS & PRECAUTIONS

Don't take if:
- You are allergic to any SSRIs.
- You currently take (or took in the last two weeks) a monoamine oxidase (MAO) inhibitor.

Before you start, consult your doctor if:
- You have had kidney or liver problems.
- You have a history of seizure disorders.
- You have a history of drug or alcohol abuse.
- You have a history of mood disorders, mania, or thoughts of suicide.

Over age 60:
Adverse reactions and side effects may be more severe and frequent than in younger patients; dosage may need to be adjusted.

Pregnancy:
Decide with your doctor if drug benefits justify risk to unborn child. Risk category C for drugs in this group except paroxetine. Paroxetine (Paxil) is a risk category D. It may cause birth defects (see page xviii for risk category information).

Breast-feeding:
Drugs pass into milk. Avoid drug or discontinue nursing until you finish medicine. Consult doctor for advice on maintaining milk supply.

Infants & children:
For children under age 18 use only with close medical supervision. Carefully read information provided with prescription. Contact doctor right away if depression symptoms get worse or there is any talk of suicide or suicide behaviors. Read also the information under Others on this page.

Prolonged use:
No problems expected. Your doctor should periodically evaluate your response to the drug and adjust the dose if necessary.

Skin & sunlight:
One or more drugs in this group may cause rash or intensify sunburn in areas exposed to sun or ultraviolet light (photosensitivity reaction). Avoid overexposure. Notify doctor if reaction occurs.

Driving, piloting or hazardous work:
Don't drive or pilot aircraft until you learn how medicine affects you. Don't work around dangerous machinery. Don't climb ladders or work in high places. Danger increases if you drink alcohol or take medicine affecting alertness and reflexes.

Discontinuing:
- Don't discontinue without consulting doctor. You may need to reduce the dose gradually to avoid side effects.
- After discontinuing the drug, call your doctor right away if any new or unusual symptoms develop (emotional or physical).

Others:
- Advise any doctor or dentist whom you consult that you take this medicine.
- Take drug only as directed. Do not increase or reduce dosage without doctor's approval.
- Adults and children taking antidepressants may experience a worsening of the depression symptoms and may have increased suicidal thoughts or behaviors. Call doctor right away if these symptoms or behaviors occur.

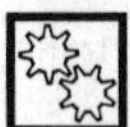

POSSIBLE INTERACTION WITH OTHER DRUGS

GENERIC NAME OR DRUG CLASS	COMBINED EFFECT
Anticoagulants, oral*	Increased risk of side effects of both drugs.
Antidepressants, tricyclic*	Increased risk of side effects.
Anti-inflammatory drugs, nonsteroidal (NSAIDs)*	Risk of stomach bleeding and ulcers.

Continued on page 929

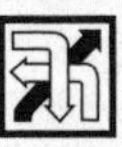

POSSIBLE INTERACTION WITH OTHER SUBSTANCES

INTERACTS WITH	COMBINED EFFECT
Alcohol:	Contributes to depression. Avoid.
Beverages: Grapefruit juice.	Toxicity risk. Avoid.
Cocaine:	Unknown. Avoid.
Foods: Grapefruit.	Toxicity risk. Avoid.
Marijuana:	Unknown. Avoid.
Tobacco:	None expected.

SEROTONIN-DOPAMINE ANTAGONISTS

GENERIC AND BRAND NAMES

ILOPERIDONE
Fanapt
PALIPERIDONE
Invega
Invega Sustenna
RISPERIDONE
Risperdal
Risperdal Consta
Risperdal M-TAB

BASIC INFORMATION

Habit forming? No
Prescription needed? Yes
Available as generic? Yes, for some
Drug class: Antipsychotic

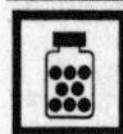

USES

- Treats schizophrenia, schizoaffective disorder and bipolar disorder.
- Treatment of irritability in children with autism.
- Treats other disorders per doctor's advice.

DOSAGE & USAGE INFORMATION

How to take:
- Tablet—Swallow with liquid. May be taken with or without food.
- Injection—Patients will go to a medical office as scheduled for injection.
- Orally disintegrating tablet—Dissolves in the mouth in seconds. Do not chew.
- Oral solution—Dilute in 3 to 4 ounces of water, orange juice, or low fat milk (no cola or tea).
- Extended-release tablet—Swallow whole with liquid.

When to take:
At the same times each day. Take once-a-day dose in morning. Prescribed dosage may be increased gradually over first several days.

If you forget a dose:
Take as soon as you remember. If it is almost time for the next dose, wait for the next scheduled dose (don't double this dose).

Continued next column

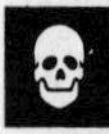

OVERDOSE

SYMPTOMS:
Drowsiness, dizziness, rapid heartbeat, low blood pressure, convulsions, muscle spasms and uncontrolled body movements.
WHAT TO DO:
- **Dial 911 (emergency) for medical help or call poison control center 1-800-222-1222 for instructions.**
- **See emergency information on last 3 pages of this book.**

What drug does:
It appears to act on neurotransmitters (serotonin and dopamine) in the brain to help restore more normal thinking and more normal mood.

Time lapse before drug works:
One to 7 days. A gradual increase in the dosage amount may be necessary to relieve symptoms.

Don't take with:
Any other medicine or diet supplement without consulting your doctor or pharmacist.

POSSIBLE ADVERSE REACTIONS OR SIDE EFFECTS

SYMPTOMS	WHAT TO DO
Life-threatening:	
Neuroleptic malignant syndrome (high fever, fast heart rate, sweating rigid muscles, unstable blood pressure, confusion, seizures, stupor or coma).	Discontinue. Seek emergency treatment.
Common:	
• Difficulty speaking or swallowing, loss of balance, vision changes, mask-like face, shuffling walk, arms or legs are stiff or weak, trembling or twitching, muscle spasms (face, neck, back), unable to move eyes, body twisting.	Discontinue. Call doctor right away.
• Constipation or diarrhea, drowsiness, dry mouth, headache, heartburn, cough, dreaming more, sore throat, nausea, stuffy or runny nose, unusual tiredness or weakness, weight gain, anxiety or nervousness, mood or mental changes, sexual dysfunction, urination problems, restlessness, insomnia, sweating.	Continue. Call doctor when convenient.
Infrequent:	
• Fast or irregular heartbeat, dizziness, lightheadedness, chest pain, trouble breathing.	Discontinue. Call doctor right away.
• Menstrual changes; skin is dry, darker or oily; rash; excess saliva; joint, back or stomach pain; vomiting; appetite loss; weight loss; unexpected breast milk.	Continue. Call doctor when convenient.

Rare:

• High blood sugar (thirstiness, frequent urination, increased hunger, weakness); lip smacking; uncontrolled movements (arms, legs, tongue and chewing); cheek puffing; increased blinking; eyelid spasms; unusual facial or body positions; manic behavior; high or low body temperature; unusual bleeding or bruising.	Discontinue. Call doctor right away.
• Other symptoms that cause concern.	Continue. Call doctor when convenient.

WARNINGS & PRECAUTIONS

Don't take if:
You are allergic to iloperidone, paliperidone or risperidone.

Before you start, consult your doctor if:
- You have or have had liver, kidney, heart or blood vessel disease; stroke; diabetes or pre-diabetes; high or low blood pressure; seizures; Parkinson's disease; breast cancer; electrolyte disorder; Alzheimer's; neuroleptic malignant syndrome; phenylketonuria; suicide thoughts; tardive dyskinesia or trouble swallowing.
- Patient is elderly and has dementia.

Over age 60:
- Adverse reactions and side effects may be more severe than in younger persons. A lower starting dosage is usually recommended.
- Use of antipsychotic drugs in elderly patients with dementia-related psychosis may increase risk of death. Consult doctor.

Pregnancy:
Decide with your doctor if drug benefits justify any possible risk to unborn child. Risk category C (see page xviii).

Breast-feeding:
It is unknown if these drugs pass into milk. Consult your doctor for advice.

Infants & children:
Use only with close medical supervision.

Prolonged use:
See your doctor on a regular basis to monitor drug's effectiveness and any side effects.

Skin & sunlight:
- May cause rash or intensify sunburn in areas exposed to sun or ultraviolet light (photo-sensitivity reaction). Use sunscreen and avoid overexposure. Notify doctor if reaction occurs.
- Hot temperatures and exercise, hot baths can increase risk of heatstroke. Drug may affect body's ability to maintain normal temperature.

Driving, piloting or hazardous work:
Don't drive or pilot aircraft until you learn how drug affects you. Don't work around dangerous machinery. Don't climb ladders or work in high places. Danger increases if you drink alcohol or take drugs affecting alertness and reflexes.

Discontinuing:
- Don't discontinue this drug without doctor's approval. Dosage may require a gradual reduction before stopping.
- Withdrawal effects may occur after stopping drug. Consult doctor if new symptoms develop that cause you concern.

Others:
- Get up slowly from a sitting or lying position to avoid feeling dizzy, faint or lightheaded.
- Advise any doctor or dentist whom you consult that you take this medicine.
- Take drug only as directed. Do not increase or reduce dosage without doctor's approval.

POSSIBLE INTERACTION WITH OTHER DRUGS

GENERIC NAME OR DRUG CLASS	COMBINED EFFECT
Antihypertensives*	Increased risk of low blood pressure.
Carbamazepine	Decreased effect of risperidone.
Central nervous system (CNS) depressants,* other	Increased sedative effect.
Clozapine	Increased effect of risperidone.
Dopamine agonists*	Decreased dopamine agonist effect.
Enzyme Inhibitors*	Increased effect of iloperidone.
QT interval prolongation-causing drugs*	Heartbeat irregularities with iloperidone.

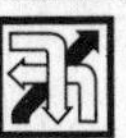

POSSIBLE INTERACTION WITH OTHER SUBSTANCES

INTERACTS WITH	COMBINED EFFECT
Alcohol:	Serious risks. Avoid.
Beverages:	None expected.
Cocaine:	Unknown. Avoid.
Foods:	None expected.
Marijuana:	Unknown. Avoid.
Tobacco:	None expected.

SEROTONIN & NOREPINEPHRINE REUPTAKE INHIBITORS (SNRIs)

GENERIC AND BRAND NAMES

DESVENLAFAXINE
Pristiq
DULOXETINE
Cymbalta
MILNACIPRAN
Savella
VENLAFAXINE
Effexor
Effexor XR

BASIC INFORMATION

Habit forming? No
Prescription needed? Yes
Available as generic? Yes, for some
Drug class: Antidepressant

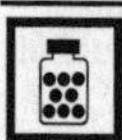

USES

- Treatment for major depressive disorder.
- Treatment for diabetic peripheral neuropathy.
- Treatment for generalized anxiety disorder.
- May be used for chronic pain syndrome, social anxiety disorder, fibromyalgia, hot flashes, stress incontinence or other disorders.

DOSAGE & USAGE INFORMATION

How to take:

- Tablet, extended-release capsule or extended-release tablet—Swallow whole with liquid. Take with food if stomach upset occurs. Capsule may be opened and contents sprinkled into a spoonful of applesauce and swallowed.
- Delayed-release capsule—Swallow with liquid. May be taken with or without food. Do not open, crush or chew capsule.

When to take:
At the same times each day (with meals or with a snack for venlafaxine).

Continued next column

OVERDOSE

SYMPTOMS:
Extreme drowsiness or tiredness or weakness, seizure, fast heartbeat, tingling or burning sensation, tremor, nausea, vomiting, agitation, hyperactive, enlarged pupils. In some cases, may have no symptoms.
WHAT TO DO:

- **Dial 911 (emergency) for medical help or call poison control center 1-800-222-1222 for instructions.**
- **See emergency information on last 3 pages of this book.**

If you forget a dose:
Take as soon as you remember. If it is almost time for the next dose, wait for that dose (don't double this dose) and resume regular schedule.

What drug does:
Increases level of two brain chemicals (serotonin and norepinephrine) that affect behavior and mood and play a role in depression.

Time lapse before drug works:
Begins in 1 to 3 weeks, but may take 4 to 6 weeks for maximum benefit.

Don't take with:
Any other medicine or any dietary supplement without consulting your doctor or pharmacist.

POSSIBLE ADVERSE REACTIONS OR SIDE EFFECTS

SYMPTOMS	WHAT TO DO
Life-threatening:	
Rare allergic reaction—Breathing difficulty; closing of the throat; swelling of hands, feet, face, lips or tongue; hives.	Discontinue. Seek emergency treatment.
Common:	
Nausea, dry mouth, increased sweating, appetite loss, insomnia or drowsiness, fatigue, headache, constipation, diarrhea, rash or itching.	Continue. Call doctor when convenient.
Infrequent:	
Mood or behavior or mental changes, dizziness, impotence, less interest in sex or changes in orgasm, skin flushing, stomach upset or pain, vomiting, weight loss, muscle aches or pain, joint pain or swelling, trembling or shaking, vision changes, abnormal dreams, sore throat, stuffy or runny nose, fever, cough, frequent or hesitant urination, nervousness, weakness, lightheadedness.	Continue. Call doctor when convenient.
Rare:	
Seizures, fainting, irregular heartbeat, abnormal behaviors, severe symptoms such as suicide thoughts or behaviors.	Discontinue. Call doctor right away.

SEROTONIN & NOREPINEPHRINE REUPTAKE INHIBITORS (SNRIs)

WARNINGS & PRECAUTIONS

Don't take if:
You are allergic to serotonin and norepinephrine reuptake inhibitors or take MAO inhibitors.*

Before you start, consult your doctor if:
- You have diabetes; heart, liver, or kidney disease; glaucoma; a blood clotting or bleeding problem or high cholesterol.
- You have high or low blood pressure.
- You have thoughts about suicide.
- You have a brain disorder or brain damage or mental retardation.
- You are losing weight.
- You have bipolar disorder or mania.
- You have a history of seizures or epilepsy.
- You drink excess amounts of alcohol.

Over age 60:
No special problems expected.

Pregnancy:
Decide with your doctor if drug benefits justify any possible risk to unborn child. Risk category C (see page xviii).

Breast-feeding:
Venlafaxine passes into milk. It is unknown if duloxetine passes into milk. Avoid nursing until you finish medicine. Consult doctor for advice on maintaining milk supply.

Infants & children:
Not approved for ages under age 18. If prescribed, carefully read information provided with prescription. Contact doctor right away if depression symptoms get worse or there is any talk of suicide or suicide behaviors. Also, read information under Others.

Prolonged use:
Consult with your doctor on a regular basis while taking this drug to check blood pressure and to determine the need for continued treatment.

Skin & sunlight:
No special problems expected.

Driving, piloting or hazardous work:
Don't drive or pilot aircraft until you learn how medicine affects you. Don't work around dangerous machinery. Don't climb ladders or work in high places. Danger increases if you drink alcohol or take medicine affecting alertness and reflexes.

Discontinuing:
- Don't discontinue without consulting doctor. You may need to reduce the dose gradually.
- If any new or unusual symptoms develop (emotional or physical) after you discontinue the drug, call your doctor right away.

Others:
- Rise slowly from a sitting or lying position to avoid dizziness, faintness or lightheadedness.
- Diabetic patients should consult doctor if blood sugar levels are affected by taking this drug.
- Advise any doctor or dentist whom you consult that you take this drug.
- Adults and children taking antidepressants may experience a worsening of the depression symptoms and may have increased suicidal thoughts or behaviors. Call doctor right away if these symptoms or behaviors occur.
- Take drug as directed. Do not increase or reduce dosage without doctor's approval.

POSSIBLE INTERACTION WITH OTHER DRUGS

GENERIC NAME OR DRUG CLASS	COMBINED EFFECT
Antiarrhythmics*	Increased side effect risk (with duloxetine).
Antidepressants, other	Increased sedative effect.
Antidepressants, tricyclic	Increased side effect risk (with duloxetine).
Central nervous system (CNS) depressants,* other	Increased sedative effect.
Cimetidine	Increased effect of venlafaxine.
Enzyme inhibitors*	Increased effect of either drug.
Monoamine oxidase (MAO) inhibitors*	Severe adverse reactions. Allow 14 days between use.
Phenothiazines	Increased side effect risk (with duloxetine).

Continued on page 929

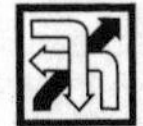

POSSIBLE INTERACTION WITH OTHER SUBSTANCES

INTERACTS WITH	COMBINED EFFECT
Alcohol:	Possible severe liver damage. Avoid.
Beverages:	None expected.
Cocaine:	Unknown. Avoid.
Foods:	None expected.
Marijuana:	Unknown. Avoid.
Tobacco:	None expected.

***See Glossary**

SIMETHICONE

BRAND NAMES

Alka-Seltzer Gas Relief
Degas
Di-Gel
Extra Strength Gas-X
Extra Strength Maalox Anti-Gas
Extra Strength Maalox GRF Gas Relief Formula
Flatulex
Gas Aid
Gas Relief
Gas-X
Gas-X Extra Strength
Gas-X Thin Strips
Gas-X with Maalox
Gelusil
Genasyme
Imodium Advanced
Imodium Multi-Symptom Relief
Maalox Anti-Gas
Maalox GRF Gas Relief Formula
Maximum Strength Mylanta Gas Relief
Maximum Strength Phazyme
Mygel
Mylanta Gas
Mylicon
Mylicon-80
Mylicon-125
Ovol
Ovol 40
Ovol-80
PediaCare Infants' Gas Relief
Phazyme
Phazyme 55
Phazyme 95
Riopan Plus

BASIC INFORMATION

Habit forming? No
Prescription needed? No
Available as generic? Yes, for some
Drug class: Antiflatulent

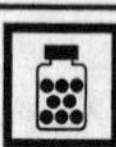

USES

- Treatment for retention of abdominal gas.
- Used prior to x-ray of abdomen.

DOSAGE & USAGE INFORMATION

How to take:
- Tablet or capsule—Swallow with liquid.
- Liquid—Dissolve in water. Drink all of dose.
- Thin strip—Let it dissolve on your tongue.
- Chewable tablet—Chew completely. Don't swallow whole.

Continued next column

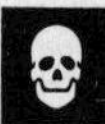

OVERDOSE

SYMPTOMS:
None expected.
WHAT TO DO:
Overdose unlikely to threaten life. If person uses much larger amount than prescribed or if accidentally swallowed, call doctor or poison control center 1-800-222-1222 for help.

When to take:
After meals and at bedtime.

What drug does:
Reduces surface tension of gas bubbles in stomach.

Time lapse before drug works:
10 minutes.

If you forget a dose:
Take when remembered if needed.

Don't take with:
Any other medicine or any dietary supplement without consulting your doctor or pharmacist.

POSSIBLE ADVERSE REACTIONS OR SIDE EFFECTS

SYMPTOMS | **WHAT TO DO**

Life-threatening:
None expected.

Common:
None expected.

Infrequent:
None expected.

Rare:
None expected.

WARNINGS & PRECAUTIONS

Don't take if:
You are allergic to simethicone.

Before you start, consult your doctor if:
You have allergies to other drugs or substances.

Over age 60:
No problems expected.

Pregnancy:
Consult doctor. Risk category C (see page xviii).

Breast-feeding:
No problems expected. Consult doctor.

Infants & children:
Not recommended.

Prolonged use:
No problems expected.

Skin & sunlight:
No problems expected.

Driving, piloting or hazardous work:
No problems expected.

Discontinuing:
May be unnecessary to finish medicine. Discontinue when symptoms disappear.

Others:
No problems expected.

POSSIBLE INTERACTION WITH OTHER DRUGS

GENERIC NAME OR DRUG CLASS	COMBINED EFFECT
None significant.	

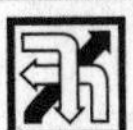

POSSIBLE INTERACTION WITH OTHER SUBSTANCES

INTERACTS WITH	COMBINED EFFECT
Alcohol:	None expected.
Beverages:	None expected.
Cocaine:	None expected.
Foods:	None expected.
Marijuana:	None expected.
Tobacco:	None expected.

SODIUM BICARBONATE

BRAND NAMES

Alka-Seltzer Original
Arm & Hammer Pure Baking Soda
Bell/ans
Bromo-Seltzer
Citrocarbonate Soda Mint
Zegerid Capsules
Zegerid Chewable Tablets
Zegerid OTC
Zegerid Powder

BASIC INFORMATION

Habit forming? No
Prescription needed? No
Available as generic? Yes
Drug class: Alkalizer, antacid

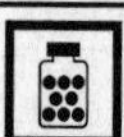

USES

- Treats metabolic acidosis.
- Alkalinizes urine to reduce uric acid kidney stones.
- Treats hyperacidity of the stomach that is present with indigestion, gastroesophageal reflux and peptic ulcer disease.

DOSAGE & USAGE INFORMATION

How to take:
- Tablet—Swallow with liquid. If you can't swallow whole, crumble tablet and take with liquid or food.
- Powder—Mix in a glass of water and drink.
- Effervescent sodium bicarbonate—Mix in a glass of cold water and drink.

When to take:
- For hyperacidity—1 to 3 hours after meals.
- For kidney stones—According to prescription instructions.

If you forget a dose:
Take as soon as you remember. If it is almost time for the next dose, wait for that dose (don't double this dose) and resume regular schedule.

Continued next column

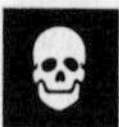

OVERDOSE

SYMPTOMS:
Excessive swelling of feet and lower legs.
WHAT TO DO:
Overdose unlikely to threaten life. If person uses much larger amount than prescribed or if accidentally swallowed, call doctor or poison control center 1-800-222-1222 for help.

What drug does:
- Buffers acid in the stomach.
- Increases excretion of bicarbonate in the urine to help dissolve uric acid stones.

Time lapse before drug works:
Works immediately, but the duration of effect is short.

Don't take with:
Any other medicine or any dietary supplement without consulting your doctor or pharmacist.

POSSIBLE ADVERSE REACTIONS OR SIDE EFFECTS

SYMPTOMS	WHAT TO DO
Life-threatening:	
None expected.	
Common:	
None expected.	
Infrequent:	
• Stomach cramps that continue.	Discontinue. Call doctor right away.
• Nausea, headache, appetite loss (with long-term use).	Continue. Call doctor when convenient.
Rare:	
Muscle pain or twitching, nervousness, breathing difficulty, mild swelling of feet or lower legs (with large doses).	Discontinue. Call doctor right away.

WARNINGS & PRECAUTIONS

Don't take if:
You are allergic to sodium bicarbonate.

Before you start, consult your doctor if:
You have heart disease, kidney disease or toxemia of pregnancy.

Over age 60:
Adverse reactions and side effects may be more frequent and severe than in younger persons.

Pregnancy:
May cause weight gain and swelling of feet and ankles. Avoid if you have high blood pressure. Consult doctor. Risk category C (see page xviii).

Breast-feeding:
No problems expected, but consult doctor.

Infants & children:
Not recommended. Safety and dosage have not been established.

Prolonged use:
Don't use for longer than prescribed or recommended. May cause sodium overload.

Skin & sunlight:
No special problems expected.

Driving, piloting or hazardous work:
No special problems expected.

Discontinuing:
May be unnecessary to finish medicine. Follow doctor's instructions.

Others:
- Heat and moisture in bathroom medicine cabinet can cause breakdown of medicine. Store someplace else.
- May interfere with the accuracy of some medical tests (especially acidosis and urinalysis tests).

POSSIBLE INTERACTION WITH OTHER DRUGS

GENERIC NAME OR DRUG CLASS	COMBINED EFFECT
Adrenocorticoids*	Sodium overload.
Cortisone	Sodium overload.
Ketoconazole	Decreased absorption of ketoconazole.
Mecamylamine	Increased mecamylamine effect.
Memantine	Increased effect of memantine.
Methenamine	Decreased methenamine effect.
Tetracyclines*	Greatly reduced absorption of tetracyclines.
Any other medicine	Decreased absorption of other medicine if taken within 1 to 2 hours of taking sodium bicarbonate.

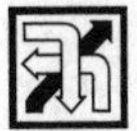

POSSIBLE INTERACTION WITH OTHER SUBSTANCES

INTERACTS WITH	COMBINED EFFECT
Alcohol:	Decreased effectiveness of sodium bicarbonate.
Beverages: Milk and milk products (large amounts).	Increased risk of side effects.
Cocaine:	None expected.
Foods:	None expected.
Marijuana:	None expected.
Tobacco:	Decreased effectiveness of sodium bicarbonate.

*See Glossary

SODIUM FLUORIDE

BRAND NAMES

Fluor-A-Day	Listermint with Fluoride
Fluorident	Luride
Fluoritab	Luride-SF
Fluorodex	Pediaflor
Fluotic	Pedi-Dent
Flura	Solu-Flur
Karidium	

Numerous other multiple vitamin-mineral supplements. Check labels.

BASIC INFORMATION

Habit forming? No
Prescription needed? Yes, for some
Available as generic? Yes
Drug class: Mineral supplement (fluoride)

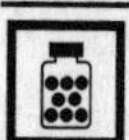

USES

- Reduces tooth cavities.
- Treats osteoporosis.

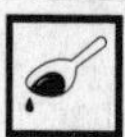

DOSAGE & USAGE INFORMATION

How to take:
- Tablet—Swallow with liquid or crumble tablet and take with liquid (not milk) or food.
- Liquid—Measure with dropper and take directly or with liquid.
- Chewable tablet—Chew slowly and thoroughly before swallowing.

When to take:
Usually at bedtime after teeth are thoroughly brushed.

If you forget a dose:
Take as soon as you remember. If it is almost time for the next dose, wait for that dose (don't double this dose) and resume regular schedule.

Continued next column

OVERDOSE

SYMPTOMS:
Stomach cramps or pain, nausea, faintness, vomiting (possibly bloody), diarrhea, black stools, shallow breathing, muscle spasms, seizures, arrhythmias.
WHAT TO DO:
- **Dial 911 (emergency) for medical help or call poison control center 1-800-222-1222 for instructions.**
- **See emergency information on last 3 pages of this book.**

What drug does:
Provides supplemental fluoride to combat tooth decay.

Time lapse before drug works:
8 weeks to provide maximum effect.

Don't take with:
Any other medicine or any dietary supplement without consulting your doctor or pharmacist.

POSSIBLE ADVERSE REACTIONS OR SIDE EFFECTS

SYMPTOMS	WHAT TO DO
Life-threatening: In case of overdose, see previous column.	
Common:	
Constipation, appetite loss.	Continue. Call doctor when convenient.
Infrequent:	
• Rash.	Discontinue. Call doctor right away.
• Tooth discoloration.	Continue. Call doctor when convenient.
Rare:	
• Severe upsets (digestive) only with overdose.	Discontinue. Seek emergency treatment.
• Mouth and lip sores, aching bones, stiffness.	Discontinue. Call doctor right away.

WARNINGS & PRECAUTIONS

Don't take if:
- Your water supply contains 0.7 parts fluoride per million. Too much fluoride stains teeth permanently.
- You are allergic to any fluoride-containing product.
- You have underactive thyroid.

Before you start, consult your doctor if:
- You have kidney disease.
- You have ulcers.
- You have joint pain.

Over age 60:
No problems expected.

Pregnancy:
Consult doctor. Risk category C (see page xviii).

Breast-feeding:
No problems expected. Consult doctor.

Infants & children:
No problems expected except accidental overdose. Keep vitamin-mineral supplements out of children's reach.

Prolonged use:
Excess may cause discolored teeth and decreased calcium in blood.

Skin & sunlight:
No problems expected.

Driving, piloting or hazardous work:
No problems expected.

Discontinuing:
No problems expected.

Others:
- Store in original plastic container. Fluoride decomposes glass.
- Some products contain tartrazine dye. Avoid, especially if you are allergic to aspirin.

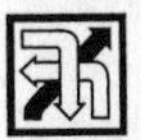

POSSIBLE INTERACTION WITH OTHER DRUGS

GENERIC NAME OR DRUG CLASS	COMBINED EFFECT
Calcium supplements*	Decreased effect of calcium and fluoride.

POSSIBLE INTERACTION WITH OTHER SUBSTANCES

INTERACTS WITH	COMBINED EFFECT
Alcohol:	None expected.
Beverages: Milk.	Prevents absorption of fluoride. Space dose 2 hours before or after milk.
Cocaine:	None expected.
Foods:	None expected.
Marijuana:	None expected.
Tobacco:	None expected.

*See Glossary

STIMULANT MEDICATIONS

GENERIC AND BRAND NAMES

DEXMETHYL PHENIDATE
- Focalin
- Focalin XR

METHYLPHENIDATE
- Concerta
- Daytrana
- Metadate CD
- Metadate ER
- Methylin Chewable

METHYLPHENIDATE (con't)
- Methylin ER
- Methylin Oral Suspension
- PMS Methylpheni date
- Quillivant XR
- Ritalin
- Ritalin LA
- Ritalin SR

BASIC INFORMATION

Habit forming? Yes
Prescription needed? Yes
Available as generic? Yes, for some
Drug class: Central nervous system stimulant, sympathomimetic

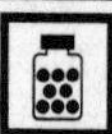

USES

- Decreases overactivity and lengthens attention span in children and adults with attention-deficit hyperactivity disorder (ADHD). A total treatment plan may also include educational, social and psychological therapies.
- Treatment of depression in adults.
- Treatment for narcolepsy and other disorders.

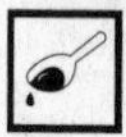

DOSAGE & USAGE INFORMATION

How to take:
- Tablet (short-acting)—Swallow with liquid. Take as directed, usually 30-45 minutes before meals, or with meals if stomach upset occurs. If swallowing is a problem, ask your pharmacist if tablet can be crushed and taken with liquid or small amount of food.

Continued next column

- Skin patch—Follow instructions on label.
- Extended- or sustained-release tablet and capsule—Swallow whole with liquid, usually before breakfast (or as directed). Do not crush tablet. Do not open capsule (unless your label states that the capsule may be opened and sprinkled over cool applesauce and then swallowed right away).
- Oral solution, extended-release oral solution or chewable tablet—Follow instructions on label.

When to take:
At the same times each day. Regular tablets are often taken at breakfast and lunch (best not to take late in day). Extended-release forms are usually taken in the morning.

If you forget a dose:
Take as soon as you remember. If it is almost time for the next dose, wait for next scheduled dose (don't double this dose).

What drug does:
Stimulates brain to improve alertness, concentration and attention span. Calms the hyperactive child and improves ability to focus.

Time lapse before drug works:
May take 2 or more weeks to see effectiveness. Dosage may be increased or decreased depending on the response and side effects.

Don't take with:
Any other medicine or any dietary supplement without consulting your doctor or pharmacist.

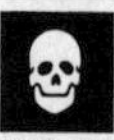

OVERDOSE

SYMPTOMS:
Rapid heartbeat, fever, confusion, vomiting, agitation, hallucinations, convulsions, coma.
WHAT TO DO:
- **Dial 911 (emergency) for medical help or call poison control center 1-800-222-1222 for instructions.**
- **If person is unconscious, check breathing and pulse. If not breathing, begin mouth-to-mouth rescue breathing. If heart is not beating, begin chest compressions.**
- **See emergency information on last 3 pages of this book.**

POSSIBLE ADVERSE REACTIONS OR SIDE EFFECTS

SYMPTOMS	WHAT TO DO
Life-threatening:	
In case of overdose, see previous column.	
Common:	
• Fast heartbeat, blood pressure increased.	Discontinue. Call doctor right away.
• Nervousness, appetite loss, trouble sleeping.	Continue. Call doctor when convenient.
Infrequent:	
• Rash or hives, chest or joint pain, unusual bruising or bleeding, unable to control body movements, fever.	Discontinue. Call doctor right away.
• Nausea, dizziness, headache, stomach pain, drowsiness, muscle cramps.	Continue. Call doctor when convenient.
Rare:	
Changed or blurred vision, unusual vocal outbursts, convulsions, abnormal or manic behavior, trouble breathing, fainting, hallucinations, is suspicious.	Discontinue. Call doctor right away.

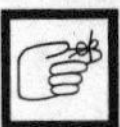

WARNINGS & PRECAUTIONS

Don't take if:
You are allergic to stimulant medications.

Before you start, consult your doctor if:
- You have epilepsy or have seizures.
- You have high blood pressure, any heart or blood vessel disorder or liver problems.
- You have glaucoma.
- You take MAO inhibitors.*
- You suffer from anxiety, agitation, tension, depressive or psychotic problems or have Tourette's syndrome or motor tics.
- You have a history of drug or alcohol abuse.

Over age 60:
Adverse reactions and side effects may be more frequent and severe than in younger persons.

Pregnancy:
Decide with your doctor if drug benefits justify risk to unborn child. Risk category C (see page xviii).

Breast-feeding:
It is unknown if drug passes into milk. Avoid drug or stop nursing until you finish medicine. Consult doctor for advice on maintaining milk supply.

Infants & children:
Use only under medical supervision for children 6 or older. Regular doctor visits are important to monitor drug's effectiveness and side effects.

Prolonged use:
- Increased risk of weight loss and abnormal behaviors. Rare risk of physical growth retardation in children.
- Talk to your doctor about the need for follow up medical examinations or laboratory studies to check drug's effectiveness and monitor any adverse effects.

Skin & sunlight:
No problems expected.

Driving, piloting or hazardous work:
Don't drive, ride a bicycle or pilot aircraft until you learn how drug affects you. Don't work around dangerous machinery. Don't climb ladders or work in high places. Danger increases if you drink alcohol or take drugs affecting alertness and reflexes.

Discontinuing:
- Don't discontinue without doctor's advice even if symptoms diminish or disappear.
- Withdrawal symptoms may occur after you discontinue the drug. Report to your doctor any new physical or emotional symptoms.

Others:
- Drug may cause serious heart and psychiatric (mental) problems, including sudden death. Read warning information provided with prescription. Call doctor right away if symptoms develop (e.g., chest pain, shortness of breath, fainting, or hallucinations).
- Dose must be carefully adjusted by doctor.
- Advise any doctor or dentist whom you consult about the use of this medicine.

POSSIBLE INTERACTION WITH OTHER DRUGS

GENERIC NAME OR DRUG CLASS	COMBINED EFFECT
Anticholinergics*	Increased anticholinergic effect.
Anticoagulants,* oral	Increased anticoagulant effect.
Anticonvulsants*	Increased anticonvulsant effect, or decreased stimulant effect.
Antidepressants, tricyclic*	Increased anti-depressant effect. Decreased stimulant medication effect.
Antihypertensives*	Decreased antihypertensive effect.
Central nervous system (CNS) stimulants*	Overstimulation.
Clonidine	Increased risk of adverse effects.
Dextrothyroxine	Increased stimulant medication effect.
Monoamine oxidase (MAO) inhibitors*	Dangerous rise in blood pressure. Take at least 14 days apart.
Pimozide	May mask the cause of tics.

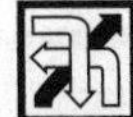

POSSIBLE INTERACTION WITH OTHER SUBSTANCES

INTERACTS WITH	COMBINED EFFECT
Alcohol:	None expected. Best to avoid.
Beverages:	None expected.
Cocaine:	Unknown. Avoid.
Foods:	None expected.
Marijuana:	Unknown. Avoid.
Tobacco:	None expected.

***See Glossary**

STIMULANTS, AMPHETAMINE-RELATED

GENERIC AND BRAND NAMES

ARMODAFINIL	MODAFINIL
Nuvigil	Alertec Provigil Sparlon

BASIC INFORMATION

Habit forming? Possibly
Prescription needed? Yes
Available as generic? Yes, for some
Drug class: Antinarcoleptic; central nervous system stimulant

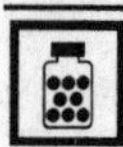

USES

- Treatment to help people who have narcolepsy to stay awake during the day. It does not cure narcolepsy.
- Used to improve wakefulness in patients with excessive sleepiness disorders, improve wakefulness for obstructive sleep apnea and shift work sleep disorder.
- Treatment for attention deficit hyperactivity disorder (ADHD).

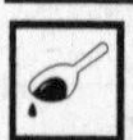

DOSAGE & USAGE INFORMATION

How to take:
Tablet—Swallow whole with liquid. You may take it with or without food.

When to take:
At the same time each day, usually in the morning. Follow instructions on the label.

If you forget a dose:
Take as soon as you remember, until noon of the same day. If you don't remember until later, skip the missed dose to avoid problems getting to sleep. Return to your regular dosing schedule the next day. Do not double doses.

Continued next column

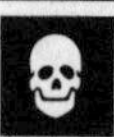

OVERDOSE

SYMPTOMS:
Symptoms may include agitation, increased blood pressure, increased heart rate and insomnia.
WHAT TO DO:
Overdose unlikely to threaten life. If person uses much larger amount than prescribed or if accidentally swallowed, call doctor or poison control center 1-800-222-1222 for help.

What drug does:
Stimulates the central nervous system. The exact way these drugs work is unknown.

Time lapse before drug works:
2 to 4 hours.

Don't take with:
Any other medicine or any dietary supplement without consulting your doctor or pharmacist.

POSSIBLE ADVERSE REACTIONS OR SIDE EFFECTS

SYMPTOMS	WHAT TO DO
Life-threatening:	
Rare allergic reaction—Breathing difficulty; closing of the throat; swelling of hands, feet, face, lips or tongue; hives, any rash.	Discontinue. Seek emergency treatment.
Common:	
Anxiety, headache, nausea, nervousness, trouble sleeping.	Continue. Call doctor when convenient.
Infrequent:	
Appetite changes, diarrhea, dry mouth, skin symptoms (dryness, flushing or tingling), muscle stiffness, stuffy or runny nose, trembling or shaking, vomiting.	Continue. Call doctor when convenient.
Rare:	
Vision changes, chills or fever, confusion, abnormal heart rate, dizziness, fainting, increased thirst or urination, depression, memory or mood changes, shortness of breath, trouble in urinating, uncontrolled movements (face, mouth and tongue).	Discontinue. Call doctor right away.

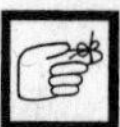

WARNINGS & PRECAUTIONS

Don't take if:
You are allergic to armodafinil or modafinil or other central nervous system stimulants.

Before you start, consult your doctor if:
- You have heart disease or have had a heart attack.
- You have or have had high blood pressure.
- You take oral contraceptives.

- You have liver or kidney disease.
- You have a history of psychosis, depression, mania, or other severe mental illness.

Over age 60:
No special problems expected.

Pregnancy:
Decide with your doctor if drug benefits justify any possible risk to unborn child. Risk category C (see page xviii).

Breast-feeding:
It is unknown if drugs pass into milk. Avoid drug or discontinue nursing until you finish medicine. Consult doctor for advice on maintaining milk supply.

Infants & children:
Not approved for children. One exception—the brand name Sparlon is approved for treatment of attention deficit hyperactivity disorder in children ages 6-17.

Prolonged use:
May lead to physical or mental dependence. Consult your doctor if any of the following signs of dependence occur:
- A strong desire to continue taking this drug.
- A need to increase the dose to receive the effects of the medicine.
- Withdrawal side effects when you stop taking the medicine.

Skin & sunlight:
No problems expected.

Driving, piloting or hazardous work:
Don't drive or pilot aircraft until you learn how medicine affects you. Don't work around dangerous machinery. Don't climb ladders or work in high places. Danger increases if you drink alcohol or take medicine affecting alertness and reflexes such as antihistamines, tranquilizers or sedatives, pain medicine, narcotics and mind-altering drugs.

Discontinuing:
- Consult your doctor if any new or unusual symptoms occur after discontinuing the drug.
- Dose may require gradual reduction if you have taken drug for a long time.

Others:
- If you are using a birth control method, such as pills or implants, they may not be as effective while taking these drugs and for up to one month after stopping them.
- Stop drug and contact your doctor if you experience any sort of unusual rash or mood changes. Rare cases of serious or life-threatening rash and serious psychiatric adverse experiences (including anxiety, mania, hallucinations and thoughts of suicide) have been reported.
- Advise any doctor or dentist whom you consult that you take this medicine.
- May affect the results in some medical tests.

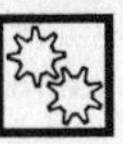

POSSIBLE INTERACTION WITH OTHER DRUGS

GENERIC NAME OR DRUG CLASS	COMBINED EFFECT
Antidepressants, tricyclic*	Increased effect of antidepressant.
CNS stimulants*	Increased stimulant effect.
Contraceptives*	Decreased contraceptive effect.
Diazepam	Decreased diazepam effect.
Enzyme inducers*	Decreased stimulant effect.
Enzyme inhibitors*	Increased stimulant effect.
MAO inhibitors*	Unknown effect. Avoid.
Mephenytoin	Mephenytoin dose may need adjustment.
Theophylline	Decreased theophylline effect.
Warfarin	Increased warfarin effect.

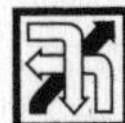

POSSIBLE INTERACTION WITH OTHER SUBSTANCES

INTERACTS WITH	COMBINED EFFECT
Alcohol:	Effects unknown. Avoid.
Beverages: Grapefruit juice.	Unknown effect. Consult doctor.
Cocaine:	Effects unknown. Avoid.
Foods: Grapefruit.	Unknown effect. Consult doctor.
Marijuana:	Effects unknown. Avoid.
Tobacco:	None expected.

***See Glossary**

SUCRALFATE

BRAND NAMES

Carafate
Sulcrate
Sulcrate Suspension Plus

BASIC INFORMATION

Habit forming? No
Prescription needed? Yes
Available as generic? Yes
Drug class: Antiulcer agent

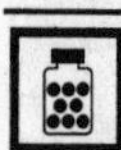

USES

- Treatment for duodenal and gastric ulcers.
- Used to relieve side effects of nonsteroidal anti-inflammatory therapy in rheumatoid arthritis.
- Treatment for gastroesophageal reflux disease (GERD).

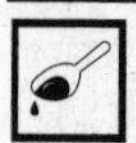

DOSAGE & USAGE INFORMATION

How to take:
- Tablet—Take as directed on an empty stomach.
- Oral suspension—Follow instructions on package.

When to take:
1 hour before meals and at bedtime. Allow 2 hours to elapse before taking other prescription medicines.

If you forget a dose:
Take as soon as you remember. If it is almost time for the next dose, wait for that dose (don't double this dose) and resume regular schedule.

What drug does:
Covers ulcer site and protects from acid, enzymes and bile salts.

Time lapse before drug works:
Begins in 30 minutes. May require several days to relieve pain.

Don't take with:
Any other medicine or any dietary supplement without consulting your doctor or pharmacist.

OVERDOSE

SYMPTOMS:
None expected.
WHAT TO DO:
Overdose unlikely to threaten life. If person uses much larger amount than prescribed or if accidentally swallowed, call doctor or poison control center 1-800-222-1222 for help.

POSSIBLE ADVERSE REACTIONS OR SIDE EFFECTS

SYMPTOMS	WHAT TO DO
Life-threatening: None expected.	
Common: Constipation.	Continue. Call doctor when convenient.
Infrequent: Dizziness, sleepiness, rash, itchy skin, abdominal pain, indigestion, vomiting, nausea, dry mouth, diarrhea.	Continue. Call doctor when convenient.
Rare: Back pain.	Continue. Call doctor when convenient.

WARNINGS & PRECAUTIONS

Don't take if:
You are allergic to sucralfate.

Before you start, consult your doctor if:
- You will have surgery within 2 months, including dental surgery, requiring general or spinal anesthesia.
- You have gastrointestinal or kidney disease.

Over age 60:
Adverse reactions and side effects may be more frequent and severe than in younger persons.

Pregnancy:
No proven harm to unborn child. Avoid if possible. Consult doctor. Risk category B (see page xviii).

Breast-feeding:
Unknown effects. Consult doctor.

Infants & children:
Safety not established.

Prolonged use:
Request blood counts if medicine needed longer than 8 weeks.

Skin & sunlight:
No problems expected.

Driving, piloting or hazardous work:
Don't drive or pilot aircraft until you learn how medicine affects you. Don't work around dangerous machinery. Don't climb ladders or work in high places. Danger increases if you drink alcohol or take medicine affecting alertness and reflexes, such as antihistamines, tranquilizers, sedatives, pain medicine, narcotics and mind-altering drugs.

Discontinuing:
Don't discontinue without consulting doctor. Dose may require gradual reduction if you have taken drug for a long time. Doses of other drugs may also require adjustment.

Others:
Advise any doctor or dentist whom you consult that you take this medicine.

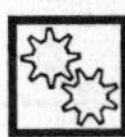

POSSIBLE INTERACTION WITH OTHER DRUGS

GENERIC NAME OR DRUG CLASS	COMBINED EFFECT
Anagrelide	May interfere with anagrelide absorption.
Antacids*	Take 1/2 hour before or after sucralfate.
Cimetidine	Possible decreased absorption of cimetidine if taken simultaneously.
Ciprofloxacin	Decreased absorption of ciprofloxacin. Take 2 hours before sucralfate.
Digoxin	Decreased absorption of digoxin. Take 2 hours before sucralfate.
Fluoroquinolones	Decreased fluoroquinolone effect.
Ketoconazole	Decreased ketoconazole effect.
Norfloxacin	Decreased absorption of norfloxacin. Take 2 hours before sucralfate.
Ofloxacin	Decreased absorption of ofloxacin. Take 2 hours before sucralfate.
Phenytoin	Possible decreased absorption of phenytoin if taken simultaneously.
Proton pump inhibitors	May decrease effect of some proton pump inhibitors. Take 30 minutes before sucralfate.
Theophylline	Decreased absorption of theophylline. Take 2 hours before sucralfate.
Vitamins A, D, E, K	Decreased vitamin absorption.

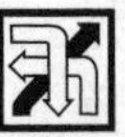

POSSIBLE INTERACTION WITH OTHER SUBSTANCES

INTERACTS WITH	COMBINED EFFECT
Alcohol:	Irritates ulcer. Avoid.
Beverages:	
Caffeine.	Irritates ulcer. Avoid.
Cocaine:	May make ulcer worse. Avoid.
Foods:	No problems expected.
Marijuana:	May make ulcer worse. Avoid.
Tobacco:	May make ulcer worse. Avoid.

*See Glossary

SULFADOXINE & PYRIMETHAMINE

BRAND NAMES

Fansidar

BASIC INFORMATION

Habit forming? No
Prescription needed? Yes
Available as generic? No
Drug class: Antiprotozoal

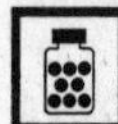

USES

- Treats malaria *(Plasmodium falciparum)*.
- Helps prevent malaria when traveling to areas where it exists.
- Also used to prevent isosporiasis in patients with acquired immunodeficiency disease.

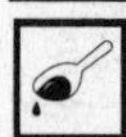

DOSAGE & USAGE INFORMATION

How to take:
Tablet—Swallow with liquid. Instructions to take on empty stomach mean 1 hour before or 2 hours after eating. Drink plenty of fluids while using this drug to help kidneys excrete more urine.

When to take:
Follow doctor's instructions.

If you forget a dose:
Take as soon as you remember. If close to time for next dose, skip this one and wait for next scheduled dose. Don't double dose.

What drug does:
The sulfa component kills bacteria; the pyrimethamine works to kill malaria organisms in red blood cells or human tissue.

Time lapse before drug works:
2 to 6 hours.

Continued next column

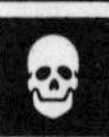

OVERDOSE

SYMPTOMS:
Appetite loss, sore throat and fever, seizure, coma.
WHAT TO DO:
- **Dial 911 (emergency) for medical help or call poison control center 1-800-222-1222 for instructions.**
- **See emergency information on last 3 pages of this book.**

Don't take with:
- Any other medicines (including over-the-counter drugs such as cough and cold medicines, laxatives, antacids, diet pills, caffeine, nose drops or vitamins) without consulting your doctor or pharmacist.
- Mefloquine.

POSSIBLE ADVERSE REACTIONS OR SIDE EFFECTS

SYMPTOMS	WHAT TO DO
Life-threatening:	
Rare allergic reaction (hives, itching, rash, trouble breathing, tightness in chest, swelling of lips or tongue or face).	Seek emergency treatment immediately.
Common:	
Loss or change of taste; diarrhea; skin rash; pale skin; sore throat; sore, red tongue; mouth ulcers; fever; excessive bleeding; tiredness; light sensitivity.	Discontinue. Call doctor right away.
Infrequent:	
Aching joints, fever, skin blisters or peeling, jaundice (yellow skin and eyes).	Discontinue. Call doctor right away.
Rare:	
Bloody urine, burning on urination, back pain, swollen neck.	Discontinue. Call doctor right away.

SULFADOXINE & PYRIMETHAMINE

WARNINGS & PRECAUTIONS

Don't take if:
You are allergic to sulfa drugs, furosemide, thiazide diuretics, or carbonic anhydrase inhibitors.

Before you start, consult your doctor if:
- You have AIDS.
- You have anemia, seizures, G6PD* deficiency, liver disease, porphyria, kidney disease.
- You can't tolerate sulfa drugs.

Over age 60:
Adverse reactions and side effects may be more frequent and severe than in younger persons. You may need smaller doses for shorter periods of time.

Pregnancy:
Use birth control so you won't get pregnant while in an endemic malaria area. Should not be taken during pregnancy if it can possibly be avoided. Consult doctor. Risk category C (see page xviii).

Breast-feeding:
Drug passes into milk. Avoid drug or discontinue nursing until you finish medicine. Consult doctor for advice on maintaining milk supply.

Infants & children:
Don't use in infants under 2 months old.

Prolonged use:
Talk to your doctor about the need for follow-up medical examinations or laboratory studies to check complete blood counts (white blood cell count, platelet count, red blood cell count, hemoglobin, hematocrit) and urinalysis.

Skin & sunlight:
May cause rash or intensify sunburn in areas exposed to sun or ultraviolet light (photosensitivity reaction). Avoid overexposure. Notify doctor if reaction occurs.

Driving, piloting or hazardous work:
Avoid if you feel confused, drowsy or dizzy.

Discontinuing:
Don't discontinue for 4 to 6 weeks after you leave endemic malaria areas.

Others:
- Advise any doctor or dentist whom you consult that you take this medicine.
- May affect results in some medical tests.
- Sleep under mosquito netting while in endemic areas. Wear long-sleeved shirts and long pants.
- Report to your doctor if you develop any symptoms of illness while you take this medicine—even if the symptoms seem minor.

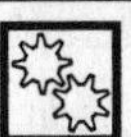

POSSIBLE INTERACTION WITH OTHER DRUGS

GENERIC NAME OR DRUG CLASS	COMBINED EFFECT
Anticoagulants*	Increased risk of toxicity.
Anticonvulsants*	Increased risk of toxicity.
Antidiabetics*	Increased risk of toxicity.
Bone marrow depressants*	Increased risk of bleeding or other toxic symptoms.
Clozapine	Toxic effect on the central nervous system.
Contraceptives, oral*	Reduced reliability of the contraceptive.
Hepatotoxic medicines*	Increased risk of liver toxicity.
Methenamine	Increased risk of kidney toxicity.
Methotrexate	Increased risk of toxicity.
Zidovudine	Increased risk of liver toxicity.

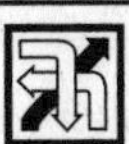

POSSIBLE INTERACTION WITH OTHER SUBSTANCES

INTERACTS WITH	COMBINED EFFECT
Alcohol:	Nausea and vomiting. Avoid.
Beverages:	No special problems expected.
Cocaine:	Increased likelihood of adverse reactions or seizures. Avoid.
Foods:	No special problems expected.
Marijuana:	Increased likelihood of adverse reactions. Avoid.
Tobacco:	No special problems expected.

***See Glossary**

SULFASALAZINE

BRAND NAMES

Azaline
Azulfidine
Azulfidine En-Tabs
PMS Sulfasalazine
PMS Sulfasalazine EC
Salazopyrin
Salazosulfapyridine
Salicylazosulfapyridine
S.A.S. Enteric-500
S.A.S.-500

BASIC INFORMATION

Habit forming? No
Prescription needed? Yes
Available as generic? Yes
Drug class: Sulfa (sulfonamide)

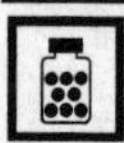

USES

- Treatment for ulceration and bleeding from ulcerative colitis and Crohn's disease.
- Treatment for rheumatoid arthritis for patients not responding to other treatments.

DOSAGE & USAGE INFORMATION

How to take:
Tablet or enteric-coated tablet—Swallow whole with full glass of water. Do not crush or chew tablet. Take after a meal or with food to lessen stomach irritation.

When to take:
At the same times each day, evenly spaced.

If you forget a dose:
Take as soon as you remember. If it is almost time for the next dose, wait for that dose (don't double this dose) and resume regular schedule.

What drug does:
It has an anti-inflammatory action in the body.

Time lapse before drug works:
2 to 5 days.

Don't take with:
Any other medicine or any dietary supplement without consulting your doctor or pharmacist.

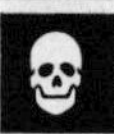

OVERDOSE

SYMPTOMS:
Less urine, bloody urine, coma.
WHAT TO DO:

- **Dial 911 (emergency) for medical help or call poison control center 1-800-222-1222 for instructions.**
- **See emergency information on last 3 pages of this book.**

POSSIBLE ADVERSE REACTIONS OR SIDE EFFECTS

SYMPTOMS	WHAT TO DO
Life-threatening:	
Rare allergic reaction (hives, itching, rash, trouble breathing, tightness in chest, swelling of lips or tongue or face).	Seek emergency treatment immediately.
Common:	
• Itchy skin, rash.	Discontinue. Call doctor right away.
• Headache, nausea, vomiting, diarrhea, appetite loss, skin sensitive to sun.	Continue. Call doctor when convenient.
• Orange urine or skin.	Continue. Tell doctor at next visit.
Infrequent:	
• Red, peeling or blistering skin; sore throat; fever; swallowing difficulty; unusual bruising; aching joints or muscles; jaundice.	Discontinue. Call doctor right away.
• Dizziness, tiredness, weakness, impotence.	Continue. Call doctor when convenient.
Rare:	
Painful urination; low back pain; numbness, tingling, burning feeling in feet and hands; bloody urine; neck swelling.	Discontinue. Call doctor right away.

WARNINGS & PRECAUTIONS

Don't take if:
You are allergic to any sulfa drug.*

Before you start, consult your doctor if:

- You are allergic to carbonic anhydrase inhibitors, oral antidiabetics or thiazide or loop diuretics or other substances.
- You have liver or kidney disease, porphyria, asthma, intestinal blockage or blood problems.

Over age 60:
Adverse reactions and side effects may be more frequent and severe than in younger persons.

Pregnancy:
Consult doctor. Risk category B (see page xviii).

Breast-feeding:
Drug passes into milk. Avoid drug or discontinue nursing until you finish medicine. Consult doctor for advice on maintaining milk supply.

Infants & children:
Don't give to infants younger than 2 years.

Prolonged use:
- May enlarge thyroid gland.
- You may become more susceptible to infections caused by germs not responsive to this drug.
- Request frequent blood counts, liver and kidney function studies.

Skin & sunlight:
May cause rash or intensify sunburn in areas exposed to sun or ultraviolet light (photosensitivity reaction). Avoid overexposure. Notify doctor if reaction occurs.

Driving, piloting or hazardous work:
Avoid if you feel dizzy. Otherwise, no problems expected.

Discontinuing:
Don't discontinue without doctor's advice until you complete prescribed dose, even though symptoms diminish or disappear.

Others:
- Drink plenty of fluids each day to help prevent adverse reactions.
- If you require surgery, tell anesthetist you take sulfa.

POSSIBLE INTERACTION WITH OTHER DRUGS

GENERIC NAME OR DRUG CLASS	COMBINED EFFECT
Aminobenzoates	Possible decreased sulfa effect.
Antibiotics*	Decreased sulfa effect.
Anticoagulants,* oral	Increased anticoagulant effect.
Anticonvulsants, hydantoin*	Toxic effect on brain.
Antidiabetics*	Toxic effect on brain.
Aspirin	Increased sulfa effect.
Calcium supplements*	Decreased sulfa effect.
Clozapine	Toxic effect on the central nervous system.
Digoxin	Decreased digoxin effect.
Hepatotoxic agents*	Increased liver toxicity.
Iron supplements*	Decreased sulfa effect.
Isoniazid	Possible anemia.
Mecamylamine	Decreased antibiotic effect.
Methenamine	Possible kidney blockage.
Methotrexate	Increased methotrexate effect.
Oxyphenbutazone	Increased sulfa effect.
Para-aminosalicylic acid	Decreased sulfa effect.
Penicillins*	Decreased penicillin effect.
Phenylbutazone	Increased sulfa effect.
Probenecid	Increased sulfa effect.
Sulfinpyrazone	Increased sulfa effect.
Sulfonylureas*	May increase hypoglycemic action.
Trimethoprim	Increased sulfa effect.
Vitamin C	Possible kidney damage. Avoid large doses of vitamin C.
Zidovudine	Increased risk of toxic effects of zidovudine.

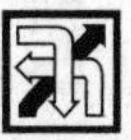

POSSIBLE INTERACTION WITH OTHER SUBSTANCES

INTERACTS WITH	COMBINED EFFECT
Alcohol:	Increased alcohol effect.
Beverages: Less than 2 quarts of fluid daily.	May increase risk of kidney damage.
Cocaine:	None expected.
Foods:	None expected.
Marijuana:	None expected.
Tobacco:	None expected.

***See Glossary**

SULFINPYRAZONE

BRAND NAMES

Anturan
Anturane
Apo-Sulfinpyrazone
Novopyrazone

BASIC INFORMATION

Habit forming? No
Prescription needed? Yes
Available as generic? Yes
Drug class: Antigout

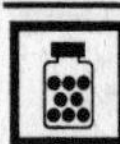

USES

- Treatment for chronic gout.
- May be prescribed to reduce the risk of recurrent heart attack.

DOSAGE & USAGE INFORMATION

How to take:
Tablet or capsule—Swallow with liquid or food to lessen stomach irritation. If you can't swallow whole, crumble tablet or open capsule and take with liquid or food.

When to take:
At the same times each day.

If you forget a dose:
Take as soon as you remember. If it is almost time for the next dose, wait for that dose (don't double this dose) and resume regular schedule.

What drug does:
Reduces uric acid level in blood and tissues by increasing amount of uric acid secreted in urine by kidneys.

Time lapse before drug works:
May require 6 months to prevent gout attacks.

Don't take with:
Any other medicine or any dietary supplement without consulting your doctor or pharmacist.

OVERDOSE

SYMPTOMS:
Breathing difficulty, vomiting, imbalance, seizures, convulsions, coma.
WHAT TO DO:
- **Dial 911 (emergency) for medical help or call poison control center 1-800-222-1222 for instructions.**
- **If person is unconscious, check breathing and pulse. If not breathing, begin mouth-to-mouth rescue breathing. If heart is not beating, begin chest compressions.**
- **See emergency information on last 3 pages of this book.**

POSSIBLE ADVERSE REACTIONS OR SIDE EFFECTS

SYMPTOMS	WHAT TO DO
Life-threatening:	
In case of overdose, see previous column.	
Common:	
None expected.	
Infrequent:	
• Painful or difficult urination, worsening gout.	Discontinue. Call doctor right away.
• Rash, nausea, vomiting, abdominal pain, low back pain.	Continue. Call doctor when convenient.
Rare:	
• Black, bloody or tarry stools.	Discontinue. Seek emergency treatment.
• Sore throat; fever; unusual bleeding or bruising; red, painful joints; blood in urine; fatigue or weakness.	Discontinue. Call doctor right away.

WARNINGS & PRECAUTIONS

Don't take if:
- You are allergic to sulfinpyrazone.
- You have acute gout.
- You have active ulcers (stomach or duodenal), enteritis or ulcerative colitis.
- You have blood cell disorders.
- You are allergic to oxyphenbutazone or phenylbutazone.

Before you start, consult your doctor if:
You have kidney or blood disease.

Over age 60:
Adverse reactions and side effects may be more frequent and severe than in younger persons. You require lower dose because of decreased kidney function.

Pregnancy:
Decide with your doctor whether drug benefits justify risk to unborn child. Risk category C (see page xviii).

Breast-feeding:
Effect unknown. Consult doctor.

Infants & children:
Not recommended.

Prolonged use:
- Possible kidney damage.
- Talk to your doctor about the need for follow-up medical examinations or laboratory studies to check complete blood counts (white blood cell count, platelet count, red blood cell count, hemoglobin, hematocrit), kidney function, serum uric acid and urine uric acid.

Skin & sunlight:
No problems expected.

Driving, piloting or hazardous work:
No problems expected.

Discontinuing:
Don't discontinue without consulting doctor. Dose may require gradual reduction if you have taken drug for a long time. Doses of other drugs may also require adjustment.

Others:
- Drink 10 to 12 glasses of water each day you take this medicine.
- Periodic blood and urine laboratory tests recommended.

POSSIBLE INTERACTION WITH OTHER DRUGS

GENERIC NAME OR DRUG CLASS	COMBINED EFFECT
Allopurinol	Increased effect of each drug.
Anticoagulants,* oral	Increased anticoagulant effect.
Antidiabetics,* oral	Increased antidiabetic effect.
Aspirin	Bleeding tendency. Decreased sulfinpyrazone effect.
Bismuth subsalicylate	Decreased sulfinpyrazone effect.
Cephalosporins*	Increased risk of bleeding.
Cholestyramine	Decreased sulfinpyrazone effect.
Contraceptives, oral*	Increased bleeding between menstrual periods.
Diuretics*	Decreased sulfinpyrazone effect.
Nitrofurantoin	Increased risk of toxicity.
Penicillins*	Increased penicillin effect.
Salicylates*	Bleeding tendency. Decreased sulfinpyrazone effect.
Sulfa drugs*	Increased effect of sulfa drugs.
Thioguanine	May need increased dosage of sulfinpyrazone.

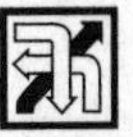

POSSIBLE INTERACTION WITH OTHER SUBSTANCES

INTERACTS WITH	COMBINED EFFECT
Alcohol:	Decreased sulfinpyrazone effect.
Beverages: Caffeine drinks.	Decreased sulfinpyrazone effect.
Cocaine:	None expected.
Foods:	None expected.
Marijuana:	Occasional use—None expected. Daily use—May increase blood level of uric acid.
Tobacco:	None expected.

*See Glossary

SULFONAMIDES

GENERIC AND BRAND NAMES

See full list of generic and brand names in the *Generic and Brand Name Directory*, page 896.

BASIC INFORMATION

Habit forming? No
Prescription needed? Yes
Available as generic? Yes, for some
Drug class: Antibacterial (antibiotic), antiprotozoal, sulfa (sulfonamide)

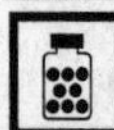

USES

- Treatment of urinary tract and other infections.
- Sulfamethoxazole in combination with trimethoprim may be used to treat bronchitis, certain types of pneumonia, skin infections, middle ear infections, intestinal tract infections and urinary tract infections.

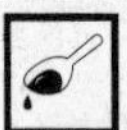

DOSAGE & USAGE INFORMATION

How to take:

- Tablet—Swallow with liquid. Instructions to take on empty stomach mean 1 hour before or 2 hours after eating. Drink an extra amount of water daily so that urine output will be adequate.
- Liquid—Shake carefully before measuring.
- Other forms—Follow label instructions.

When to take:
At the same times each day, evenly spaced.

If you forget a dose:
Take as soon as you remember. If it is almost time for the next dose, wait for that dose (don't double this dose) and resume regular schedule.

What drug does:
Interferes with a nutrient (folic acid) necessary for growth and reproduction of bacteria. Will not attack viruses.

Continued next column

OVERDOSE

SYMPTOMS:
Less urine, bloody urine, stomach pain, lightheadedness, headache, drowsiness, coma.

WHAT TO DO:

- **Dial 911 (emergency) for medical help or call poison control center 1-800-222-1222 for instructions.**
- **See emergency information on last 3 pages of this book.**

Time lapse before drug works:
2 to 5 days to affect infection.

Don't take with:
Any other medicine or any dietary supplement without consulting your doctor or pharmacist.

POSSIBLE ADVERSE REACTIONS OR SIDE EFFECTS

SYMPTOMS	WHAT TO DO
Life-threatening:	
Rare allergic reaction (hives, itching, rash, trouble breathing, tightness in chest, swelling of lips or tongue or face).	Seek emergency treatment immediately.
Common:	
• Itchy skin, rash.	Discontinue. Call doctor right away.
• Headache, nausea, vomiting, diarrhea, appetite loss, skin sensitive to sun, dizziness.	Continue. Call doctor when convenient.
Infrequent:	
• Red, peeling or blistering skin; sore throat; fever; swallowing difficulty; unusual bruising or bleeding; aching joints or muscles; yellow skin or eyes; pale skin.	Discontinue. Call doctor right away.
• Weakness or tiredness.	Continue. Call doctor when convenient.
Rare:	
Painful urination, low back pain, numbness, stomach pain, bloody diarrhea or urine, neck swelling, mood or behavior changes, increased or decreased urine output, thirst.	Discontinue. Call doctor right away.

WARNINGS & PRECAUTIONS

Don't take if:
You are allergic to any sulfa drug.

Before you start, consult your doctor if:
- You are allergic to carbonic anhydrase inhibitors, oral antidiabetics or diuretics (thiazide or loop).
- You are allergic by nature.
- You have liver or kidney disease.
- You have glucose 6-phosphate dehydrogenase (G6PD) disease.
- You have porphyria.
- You have anemia or other blood problems.

Over age 60:
Adverse reactions and side effects may be more frequent and severe than in younger persons.

Pregnancy:
Decide with your doctor if drug benefits justify risk to unborn child. Risk category C (see page xviii).

Breast-feeding:
Drug passes into milk. Avoid drug or discontinue nursing until you finish medicine. Consult doctor for advice on maintaining milk supply.

Infants & children:
Don't give to infants younger than 2 months.

Prolonged use:
- You may become more susceptible to infections caused by germs not responsive to this drug.
- Drug may enlarge thyroid gland (rare).
- Talk to your doctor about the need for frequent blood counts, liver and kidney function studies.

Skin & sunlight:
May cause rash or intensify sunburn in areas exposed to sun or ultraviolet light (photo-sensitivity reaction). Avoid excess exposure. Notify doctor if reaction occurs.

Driving, piloting or hazardous work:
Avoid if you feel dizzy. Otherwise, no problems expected.

Discontinuing:
Don't discontinue without doctor's advice until you complete prescribed dose, even though symptoms diminish or disappear.

Others:
- Drink 2 quarts of liquid each day to prevent side effects or adverse reactions.
- Advise any doctor or dentist whom you consult that you take this medicine.
- If you require surgery, tell anesthetist you take sulfa.

POSSIBLE INTERACTION WITH OTHER DRUGS

GENERIC NAME OR DRUG CLASS	COMBINED EFFECT
Aminobenzoate potassium	Possible decreased sulfonamide effect.
Anticoagulants,* oral	Increased anticoagulant effect.
Anticonvulsants,* hydantoin	Increased anticonvulsant effect.
Antidiabetics,* oral	Increased antidiabetic effect.
Bone marrow depressants*	Increased risk of side effects.
Contraceptives,* oral estrogen	Decreased contraceptive effect.
Cyclosporine	Decreased cyclosporine effect.
Hemolytics,* other	Increased risk of side effects.
Hepatotoxic agents*	Increased liver toxicity.
Mecamylamine	Decreased antibiotic effect.
Methenamine	Possible kidney blockage.
Methotrexate	Increased methotrexate effect.
Penicillins*	Decreased penicillin effect.
Phenylbutazone	Increased sulfonamide effect.
Probenecid	Increased sulfonamide effect.
Sulfinpyrazone	Increased sulfonamide effect.

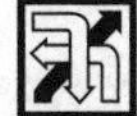

POSSIBLE INTERACTION WITH OTHER SUBSTANCES

INTERACTS WITH	COMBINED EFFECT
Alcohol:	None expected.
Beverages:	
Inadequate fluid intake.	Increased risk of side effects.
Cocaine:	None expected.
Foods:	None expected.
Marijuana:	None expected.
Tobacco:	None expected.

*See Glossary

SULFONAMIDES & PHENAZOPYRIDINE

GENERIC AND BRAND NAMES

SULFAMETHOXAZOLE & PHENAZOPYRIDINE	SULFISOXAZOLE & PHENAZOPYRIDINE
Azo Gantanol	Azo Gantrisin
Azo-Sulfamethoxazole	Azo-Sulfisoxazol
	Azo-Truxazole
	Sul-Azo

BASIC INFORMATION

Habit forming? No
Prescription needed? Yes
Available as generic? Yes
Drug class: Analgesic (urinary), sulfonamide

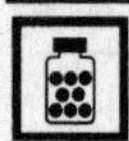

USES

- Treats infections responsive to this drug.
- Relieves pain of lower urinary tract irritation, as in cystitis, urethritis or prostatitis.

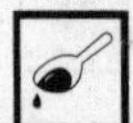

DOSAGE & USAGE INFORMATION

How to take:
Tablet—Swallow with liquid. Instructions to take on empty stomach mean 1 hour before or 2 hours after eating.

When to take:
At the same times each day, after meals.

If you forget a dose:
Take as soon as you remember. If it is almost time for the next dose, wait for that dose (don't double this dose) and resume regular schedule.

What drug does:
- Interferes with a nutrient (folic acid) necessary for growth and reproduction of bacteria. Will not attack viruses.
- Anesthetizes lower urinary tract. Relieves pain, burning, pressure and urgency to urinate.

Time lapse before drug works:
2 to 5 days to affect infection.

Continued next column

OVERDOSE

SYMPTOMS:
Less urine, bloody urine, shortness of breath, weakness, coma.
WHAT TO DO:
- **Dial 911 (emergency) for medical help or call poison control center 1-800-222-1222 for instructions.**
- **See emergency information on last 3 pages of this book.**

Don't take with:
Any other medicine or any dietary supplement without consulting your doctor or pharmacist.

POSSIBLE ADVERSE REACTIONS OR SIDE EFFECTS

SYMPTOMS	WHAT TO DO
Life-threatening:	
Rare allergic reaction (hives, itching, rash, trouble breathing, tightness in chest, swelling of lips or tongue or face).	Seek emergency treatment immediately.
Common:	
• Rash, itchy skin.	Discontinue. Call doctor right away.
• Dizziness, diarrhea, headache, appetite loss, nausea, vomiting, skin sensitive to sun.	Continue. Call doctor when convenient.
Infrequent:	
• Joint pain; swallowing difficulty; pale skin; blistering; peeling of skin; sore throat, fever, mouth sores; unexplained bleeding or bruising; jaundice.	Discontinue. Call doctor right away.
• Abdominal pain, indigestion, weakness, tiredness.	Continue. Call doctor when convenient.
Rare:	
Back pain; neck swelling; numbness, tingling, burning feeling in feet and hands; bloody urine; painful urination.	Discontinue. Call doctor right away.

WARNINGS & PRECAUTIONS

Don't take if:
- You are allergic to any sulfa drug or urinary analgesic.
- You have hepatitis.

Before you start, consult your doctor if:
- You are allergic to carbonic anhydrase inhibitors, oral antidiabetics or thiazide or loop diuretics.
- You are allergic by nature.
- You have liver or kidney disease, porphyria.
- You have developed anemia from use of any drug.
- You have G6PD* deficiency.

Over age 60:
Adverse reactions and side effects may be more frequent and severe than in younger persons.

SULFONAMIDES & PHENAZOPYRIDINE

Pregnancy:
Risk factors vary for drugs in this group. See category list on page xviii and consult doctor.

Breast-feeding:
Drug passes into milk. Avoid drug or discontinue nursing until you finish medicine. Consult doctor for advice on maintaining milk supply.

Infants & children:
Don't give to infants younger than 1 month.

Prolonged use:
- May enlarge thyroid gland.
- You may become more susceptible to infections caused by germs not responsive to this drug.
- Request frequent blood counts, liver and kidney function studies.
- Orange or yellow skin.
- Anemia. Occasional blood studies recommended.

Skin & sunlight:
One or more drugs in this group may cause rash or intensify sunburn in areas exposed to sun or ultraviolet light (photosensitivity reaction). Avoid overexposure. Notify doctor if reaction occurs.

Driving, piloting or hazardous work:
Avoid if you feel dizzy. Otherwise, no problems expected.

Discontinuing:
Don't discontinue without doctor's advice until you complete prescribed dose, even though symptoms diminish or disappear.

Others:
- Drink 2 quarts of liquid each day to prevent adverse reactions.
- If you require surgery, tell anesthetist you take sulfa.
- Will probably cause urine to be reddish orange. Requires no action.
- May stain fabrics.

POSSIBLE INTERACTION WITH OTHER DRUGS

GENERIC NAME OR DRUG CLASS	COMBINED EFFECT
Aminobenzoates	Possible decreased sulfa effect.
Anticoagulants,* oral	Increased anticoagulant effect.
Anticonvulsants, hydantoin*	Toxic effect on brain.
Antidiabetics*	Toxic effect on brain.
Aspirin	Increased sulfa effect.
Clozapine	Toxic effect on the central nervous system.
Didanosine	Increased risk of pancreatitis.
Hepatotoxic agents*	Increased liver toxicity.
Isoniazid	Possible anemia.
Mecamylamine	Decreased antibiotic effect.
Methenamine	Possible kidney blockage.
Methotrexate	Increased methotrexate effect.
Oxyphenbutazone	Increased sulfa effect.
Para-aminosalicylic acid	Decreased sulfa effect.
Penicillins*	Decreased penicillin effect.
Phenylbutazone	Increased sulfa effect.
Probenecid	Increased sulfa effect.
Sulfinpyrazone	Increased sulfa effect.
Sulfonylureas*	May increase hypoglycemic action.
Trimethoprim	Increased sulfa effect.
Zidovudine	Increased risk of toxic effects of zidovudine.

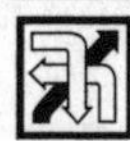

POSSIBLE INTERACTION WITH OTHER SUBSTANCES

INTERACTS WITH	COMBINED EFFECT
Alcohol:	Increased alcohol effect.
Beverages: Inadequate fluid intake.	Increased risk of side effects.
Cocaine:	None expected.
Foods:	None expected.
Marijuana:	None expected.
Tobacco:	None expected.

SULFONYLUREAS

GENERIC AND BRAND NAMES

See full list of generic and brand names in the *Generic and Brand Name Directory*, page 896.

BASIC INFORMATION

Habit forming? No
Prescription needed? Yes
Available as generic? Yes, for some.
Drug class: Antidiabetic (oral), sulfonylurea

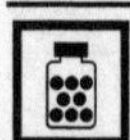

USES

- Treatment for diabetes in adults who can't control blood sugar by diet, weight loss and exercise.
- Treatment for diabetes insipidus (chlorpropamide).

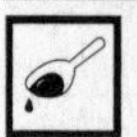

DOSAGE & USAGE INFORMATION

How to take:

- Tablet—Swallow with liquid or food to lessen stomach irritation. If you can't swallow whole, crumble tablet and take with liquid or food.
- Extended-release tablet—Swallow whole with liquid. Do not crush or chew tablet.

When to take:
At the same times each day.

If you forget a dose:
Take as soon as you remember. If it is almost time for the next dose, wait for that dose (don't double this dose) and resume regular schedule.

What drug does:
Stimulates pancreas to produce more insulin. Insulin in blood forces cells to use sugar in blood.

Time lapse before drug works:
3 to 4 hours. May require 2 weeks for maximum benefit.

Don't take with:
Any other medicine or any dietary supplement without consulting your doctor or pharmacist.

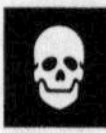

OVERDOSE

SYMPTOMS:
Excessive hunger, nausea, anxiety, cool skin, cold sweats, drowsiness, rapid heartbeat, weakness, unconsciousness, coma.
WHAT TO DO:

- **Dial 911 (emergency) for medical help or call poison control center 1-800-222-1222 for instructions.**
- **See emergency information on last 3 pages of this book.**

POSSIBLE ADVERSE REACTIONS OR SIDE EFFECTS

SYMPTOMS	WHAT TO DO
Life-threatening: In case of overdose, see previous column.	
Common:	
• Dizziness.	Discontinue. Call doctor right away.
• Diarrhea, appetite loss, nausea, stomach pain, heartburn, constipation.	Continue. Call doctor when convenient.
Infrequent:	
• Low blood sugar (hunger, anxiety, cold sweats, rapid pulse), shortness of breath.	Discontinue. Seek emergency treatment.
• Headache.	Continue. Call doctor when convenient.
Rare:	
Fatigue, itchy skin or rash, sore throat, fever, ringing in ears, unusual bleeding or bruising, jaundice, edema, weakness, confusion.	Discontinue. Call doctor when convenient.

WARNINGS & PRECAUTIONS

Don't take if:

- You are allergic to any sulfonylurea.
- You have impaired kidney or liver function.

Before you start, consult your doctor if:

- You have a severe infection.
- You have thyroid disease.
- You take insulin.
- You have heart disease.

Over age 60:
Dose usually smaller than for younger adults. Avoid episodes of low blood sugar because repeated ones can damage brain permanently.

Pregnancy:
Discuss any use of these drugs with your doctor. Risk factors vary for drugs in this group. See category list on page xviii and consult doctor.

Breast-feeding:
Drug filters into milk. May lower baby's blood sugar. Avoid.

Infants & children:
Don't give to infants or children.

Prolonged use:
- Adverse effects more likely.
- Talk to your doctor about the need for follow-up medical examinations or laboratory studies to check blood sugar, complete blood counts (white blood cell count, platelet count, red blood cell count, hemoglobin, hematocrit), eyes.

Skin and sunlight:
One or more drugs in this group may cause rash or intensify sunburn in areas exposed to sun or ultraviolet light (photosensitivity reaction). Avoid overexposure. Notify doctor if reaction occurs.

Driving, piloting or hazardous work:
No problems expected unless you develop hypoglycemia (low blood sugar). If so, avoid driving or hazardous activity.

Discontinuing:
Don't discontinue without consulting doctor. Dose may require gradual reduction if you have taken drug for a long time. Doses of other drugs may also require adjustment.

Others:
- Don't exceed recommended dose. Hypoglycemia (low blood sugar) may occur, even with proper dose schedule. You must balance medicine, diet and exercise.
- May affect results in some medical tests.
- Advise any doctor or dentist whom you consult that you take this medicine.

POSSIBLE INTERACTION WITH OTHER DRUGS

GENERIC NAME OR DRUG CLASS	COMBINED EFFECT
Adrenocorticoids, systemic	Decreased antidiabetic effect.
Androgens*	Increased blood sugar lowering.
Anticoagulants*	Unpredictable prothrombin times.
Anticonvulsants, hydantoin*	Decreased blood sugar lowering.
Antifungals, azoles	Increased blood sugar lowering.
Anti-inflammatory nonsteroidal drugs (NSAIDs)*	Increased blood sugar lowering.
Aspirin	Increased blood sugar lowering.
Beta-adrenergic blocking agents*	Increased blood sugar lowering. Possible increased difficulty in regulating blood sugar levels.
Bismuth subsalicylate	Increased insulin effect. May require dosage adjustment.
Chloramphenicol	Increased blood sugar lowering.
Cimetidine	Increased blood sugar lowering.
Clofibrate	Increased blood sugar lowering.
Contraceptives, oral*	Decreased blood sugar lowering.
Dapsone	Increased risk of adverse effect on blood cells.
Desmopressin	May increase desmopressin effect.
Dexfenfluramine	May require dosage change as weight loss occurs.
Dextrothyroxine	Sulfonylurea may require adjustment.
Digoxin	Possible decreased digoxin effect.
Diuretics* (loop, thiazide)	Decreased blood sugar lowering.
Epinephrine	Increased blood sugar lowering.
Estrogens*	Increased blood sugar lowering.
Guanethidine	Unpredictable blood sugar lowering effect.
Hemolytics*	Increased risk of adverse effect on blood cells.

Continued on page 930

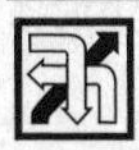

POSSIBLE INTERACTION WITH OTHER SUBSTANCES

INTERACTS WITH	COMBINED EFFECT
Alcohol:	Disulfiram reaction.* Avoid.
Beverages:	None expected.
Cocaine:	None expected.
Foods:	None expected.
Marijuana:	Decreased blood sugar lowering. Avoid.
Tobacco:	None expected.

***See Glossary**

TAMOXIFEN

BRAND NAMES

Alpha-Tamoxifen
Med Tamoxifen
Novo-Tamoxifen
Soltamox
Tamofen
Tamone
Tamoplex

BASIC INFORMATION

Habit forming? No
Prescription needed? Yes
Available as generic? Yes
Drug class: Antineoplastic

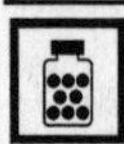

USES

- Treats advanced breast cancer.
- Can help prevent breast cancer in those at risk.

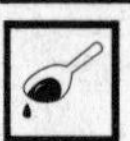

DOSAGE & USAGE INFORMATION

How to take:

- Tablet—Swallow with liquid. If you can't swallow whole, crumble tablet and take with liquid or food. Instructions to take on empty stomach mean 1 hour before or 2 hours after eating.
- Oral solution—Follow the directions provided with the prescription.
- Enteric-coated tablet—Swallow whole. Do not crush or crumble tablet.

When to take:
Follow instructions on prescription.

If you forget a dose:
Take as soon as you remember. If it is almost time for the next dose, wait for that dose (don't double this dose) and resume regular schedule.

What drug does:
Blocks uptake of estradiol and inhibits growth of cancer cells.

Time lapse before drug works:

- 4 to 10 weeks.
- With bone metastases—several months.

Continued next column

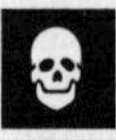

OVERDOSE

SYMPTOMS:
None expected.
WHAT TO DO:
Overdose unlikely to threaten life. If person uses much larger amount than prescribed or if accidentally swallowed, call doctor or poison control center 1-800-222-1222 for help.

Don't take with:
Any other medicines (including over-the-counter drugs such as cough and cold medicines, laxatives, antacids, diet pills, caffeine, nose drops or vitamins) without consulting your doctor or pharmacist.

POSSIBLE ADVERSE REACTIONS OR SIDE EFFECTS

SYMPTOMS	WHAT TO DO
Life-threatening:	
Leg pain, shortness of breath.	Seek emergency treatment immediately.
Common:	
Hot flashes, nausea and vomiting, weight gain.	Continue. Call doctor when convenient.
Infrequent:	
Headache, dry skin, menstrual irregularities, vaginal itching, sleepiness.	Continue. Call doctor when convenient.
Rare:	
Blurred vision, confusion.	Discontinue. Call doctor right away.

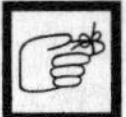

WARNINGS & PRECAUTIONS

Don't take if:
You are allergic to tamoxifen.

Before you start, consult your doctor if:
- You have cataracts.
- You have blood disorders.
- You have high cholesterol.

Over age 60:
Adverse reactions and side effects may be more frequent and severe than in younger persons. You may need smaller doses for shorter periods of time.

Pregnancy:
Consult doctor. Risk category D (see page xviii).

Breast-feeding:
Effect not documented. Consult your doctor.

Infants & children:
Not intended for use in children.

Prolonged use:
Talk to your doctor about the need for follow-up medical examinations (especially pelvic exams) or laboratory studies to check complete blood counts (white blood cell count, platelet count, red blood cell count, hemoglobin, hematocrit) and serum calcium.

Skin & sunlight:
No problems expected.

Driving, piloting or hazardous work:
Avoid if you feel confused, drowsy or dizzy.

Discontinuing:
No special problems expected.

Others:
- Advise any doctor or dentist whom you consult that you take this medicine.
- May affect results in some medical tests.
- Be sure you and your doctor discuss all aspects of using this drug, and read all instructional materials.
- The Nolvadex brand of tamoxifen has been discontinued in the United States.
- May make you more fertile. Talk to your doctor about using some type of birth control.

POSSIBLE INTERACTION WITH OTHER DRUGS

GENERIC NAME OR DRUG CLASS	COMBINED EFFECT
Antacids*	Decreased tamoxifen effect. Take 1 to 2 hours apart.
Cimetidine	Decreased tamoxifen effect.
Estrogens*	Decreased tamoxifen effect.
Famotidine	Decreased tamoxifen effect.
H_2 antagonist antihistamines*	Decreased tamoxifen effect.
Ranitidine	Decreased tamoxifen effect.

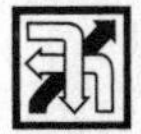

POSSIBLE INTERACTION WITH OTHER SUBSTANCES

INTERACTS WITH	COMBINED EFFECT
Alcohol:	None expected.
Beverages:	None expected.
Cocaine:	None expected.
Foods:	None expected.
Marijuana:	None expected.
Tobacco:	None expected.

***See Glossary**

TAPENTADOL

BRAND NAMES

Nucynta Nucynta ER

BASIC INFORMATION

Habit forming? Yes, with long term use
Prescription needed? Yes
Available as generic? No
Drug class: Analgesic

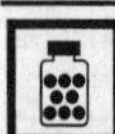

USES

Treatment for moderate to severe pain.

DOSAGE & USAGE INFORMATION

How to take:

- Tablet—Swallow whole with liquid. May be taken with or without food. Do not crush, chew or split tablet. Do not mix tablet into a liquid for snorting or injecting. It is for oral use only.
- Extended-release tablet—Swallow whole. If you can't swallow whole, ask doctor or pharmacist for advice. Do not crush, split, chew, or crumble tablet (could lead to rapid release of drug and side effects that could be fatal).
- Oral solution—Follow doctor's instructions.

When to take:
Immediate-release form—every 4 to 6 hours as needed for pain; extended-release form—every 12 hours (or as directed for either).

If you forget a dose:
If taken on a dosing schedule, take as soon as you remember. If it is almost time for the next dose, wait for next scheduled dose (don't double this dose).

Continued next column

OVERDOSE

SYMPTOMS:
Breathing difficulty, sleepiness, seizures, cold/clammy skin, blurred vision, confusion, vomiting, fainting, weak pulse, slow heartbeat, low blood pressure, stupor, coma. Deaths due to overdose have been reported with abuse and misuse of narcotic drugs, by ingesting, inhaling, or injecting crushed tablets.
WHAT TO DO:

- **Dial 911 (emergency) for medical help or call poison control center 1-800-222-1222 for instructions.**
- **See emergency information on last 3 pages of this book.**

What drug does:
The exact way it works is unknown. It affects certain chemicals in the brain and central nervous system to help reduce both the perception of pain and the emotional response to pain.

Time lapse before drug works:
Usually within 60 minutes.

Don't take with:
Any other medicine or any dietary supplement without consulting your doctor or pharmacist.

POSSIBLE ADVERSE REACTIONS OR SIDE EFFECTS

SYMPTOMS	WHAT TO DO
Life-threatening:	
Rare allergic reaction (hives, itching, rash, trouble breathing, tightness in chest, swelling of lips or tongue or face).	Seek emergency treatment immediately.
Common:	
Constipation, nausea, headache, drowsiness, dizziness, vomiting.	Continue. Call doctor when convenient.
Infrequent:	
• Constant urge to urinate or inability to urinate, blurred vision.	Discontinue. Call doctor right away.
• Loss of appetite, stomach pain, dry mouth, weakness, confusion, sweating, diarrhea, gas, trouble sleeping, changes in mood, nervousness, heartburn, tiredness.	Continue. Call doctor when convenient.
Rare:	
Seizures, balancing difficulty, memory problems, shortness of breath, difficulty performing tasks, skin symptoms (itching, redness or swelling), fainting, lightheadedness when getting up from a sitting or lying position, hallucinations, fast heartbeat, speech problems, agitation, clumsiness, hot flashes, sensations in hands or feet (burning, pain, tingling, weakness, trembling or shaking).	Discontinue. Call doctor right away.

WARNINGS & PRECAUTIONS

Don't take if:
You are allergic to tapentadol, tramadol or narcotic drugs or you are sensitive to any ingredients in the drugs.

Before you start, consult your doctor if:
- You have kidney or liver disease, seizure disorder, stomach disorder, bowel blockage, thyroid disorder, pancreatitis, gallbladder problems, brain tumor or prior head injury.
- You have a history of depression, mental illness or suicidal thoughts or behaviors.
- You have a history of drug abuse or substance abuse, including alcohol abuse.
- You are severely overweight, have sleep apnea or significant curvature of the spine.
- You have any lung or breathing problem.

Over age 60:
Increased risk of side effects. Patients over age 75 usually require a dosage adjustment.

Pregnancy:
Decide with your doctor if drug benefits justify risk to unborn child. Risk category C (see page xviii).

Breast-feeding:
It is unknown if drug passes into milk. Avoid drug or discontinue nursing until you finish medicine. Consult doctor for advice on maintaining milk supply.

Infants & children:
Safety in children under age 18 has not been established.

Prolonged use:
- Consult with your doctor on a regular basis while using this drug.
- Can cause drug dependence, addiction and withdrawal symptoms.

Skin & sunlight:
No special problems expected.

Driving, piloting or hazardous work:
Don't drive or pilot aircraft until you learn how medicine affects you. Don't work around dangerous machinery. Don't climb ladders or work in high places. Danger increases if you drink alcohol or take medicine affecting alertness and reflexes.

Discontinuing:
If you have taken this drug for a long time, consult with your doctor before discontinuing. Withdrawal symptoms may occur if drug is discontinued abruptly. Symptoms include anxiety, sweating, insomnia, pain, nausea, tremors, diarrhea, breathing problems and hallucinations. Call doctor if symptoms occur.

Others:
- Drug can cause constipation. Consult doctor before using a laxative or stool softener to treat or prevent this side effect.
- Don't increase dosage or frequency of use without your doctor's approval.
- Development of a potentially life-threatening serotonin syndrome* or overdose (which can be fatal) may occur with the use of this drug.
- Do not use within 14 days of taking monoamine oxidase (MAO) inhibitors.*
- Advise any doctor or dentist whom you consult that you take this medicine.

POSSIBLE INTERACTION WITH OTHER DRUGS

GENERIC NAME OR DRUG CLASS	COMBINED EFFECT
Central nervous system (CNS) depressants*	Serious adverse events including breathing difficulty.
Monoamine oxidase (MAO) inhibitors*	Serious adverse events including seizures and serotonin syndrome.*
Narcotics*	Breathing difficulty and increased risk of side effects and seizures.
Serotonergics*	Increased risk of seizures and serotonin syndrome.*

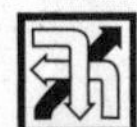

POSSIBLE INTERACTION WITH OTHER SUBSTANCES

INTERACTS WITH	COMBINED EFFECT
Alcohol:	Serious side effects. Avoid.
Beverages:	None expected.
Cocaine:	Unknown. Avoid.
Foods:	None expected.
Marijuana:	Serious side effects. Avoid.
Tobacco:	None expected.

TEGASEROD

BRAND NAMES

Zelnorm

BASIC INFORMATION

Habit forming? No
Prescription needed? Yes
Available as generic? No
Drug class: Gastrointestinal serotonin receptor agonist

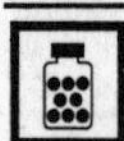

USES

- Treatment for women with constipation-predominant irritable bowel syndrome (IBS or IBS-C). IBS is a common gastrointestinal disorder affecting women more often than men. Symptoms include abdominal pain and discomfort, bloating, constipation or diarrhea.
- Treatment for chronic constipation.
- May be used for treatment of other disorders as determined by your doctor.

Note: This drug is available in the U.S. through a special distribution program. Consult your doctor.

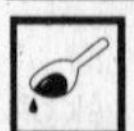

DOSAGE & USAGE INFORMATION

How to take:
Tablet—Take with water on an empty stomach.

When to use:
Twice daily just before a meal (usually morning and evening). Follow prescription instructions.

If you forget a dose:
Take the missed dose just before your next meal (don't double this dose). Then resume your regular schedule.

What drug does:
Helps in the movement of stools through the bowels and prevents constipation by activating certain body nerve cells (5-HT4 receptors) located in the stomach and intestines.

Continued next column

OVERDOSE

SYMPTOMS:
May develop diarrhea, headache and/or abdominal pain.
WHAT TO DO:
Overdose unlikely to threaten life. If person uses much larger amount than prescribed or if accidentally swallowed, call doctor or poison control center 1-800-222-1222 for help.

Time lapse before drug works:
Symptoms may improve within a day to a week, but may take up to 4 weeks to determine if the drug is effective in controlling the IBS symptoms.

Don't take with:
Any other medicine or any dietary supplement without consulting your doctor or pharmacist.

POSSIBLE ADVERSE REACTIONS OR SIDE EFFECTS

SYMPTOMS	WHAT TO DO
Life-threatening: None expected.	
Common: Diarrhea (may stop after one episode), mild abdominal pain, nausea, headache, gaseousness.	Continue. Call doctor when convenient.
Infrequent: Dizziness, flu or cold symptoms, back pain, feeling of fullness.	Continue. Call doctor when convenient.
Rare: Increased severity or worsening of symptoms of abdominal pain or diarrhea (may be bloody), rectal bleeding, dizziness, lightheadedness, fainting.	Discontinue. Call doctor right away.

WARNINGS & PRECAUTIONS

Don't take if:
You are allergic to tegaserod.

Before you start, consult your doctor if:
- You have liver or kidney disease.
- You often have diarrhea.
- You have bowel disease, bowel obstruction, gallbladder disease with symptoms, sphincter disorder, or abdominal adhesions.

Over age 60:
No problems expected.

Pregnancy:
Decide with your doctor if drug benefits justify any possible risk to unborn child. Risk category B (see page xviii).

Breast-feeding:
It is unknown if drug passes into milk. Avoid nursing until you finish medicine. Consult doctor for advice on maintaining milk supply.

Infants & children:
Not approved for children under age 18.

Prolonged use:
The drug is indicated for short term use. Caution is advised for its use longer than 3 months since safety has not been established.

Skin & sunlight:
No problems expected.

Driving, piloting or hazardous work:
No problems expected.

Discontinuing:
No problems expected, but consult your doctor before discontinuing the drug.

Others:
- There has been a small increase in abdominal surgeries in patients taking this drug. It is not known if the drug is involved in the increase. There is some concern that the drug may cause or worsen ovarian cysts. Be sure to discuss any questions with your doctor.
- Advise any doctor or dentist whom you consult that you take this medicine.
- The drug's effectiveness for men with IBS has not been established.
- Follow your doctor's advice and recommendations for any additional treatment steps for IBS. They may involve stress reduction, relaxation techniques, dietary changes and others.
- Take medicine only as directed. Do not increase or reduce dosage without doctor's approval. Have regular medical follow-up while taking this drug.
- Recommended therapy is 4-6 weeks with an additional 4-6 weeks if patient has good response.

POSSIBLE INTERACTION WITH OTHER DRUGS

GENERIC NAME OR DRUG CLASS	COMBINED EFFECT
None expected.	

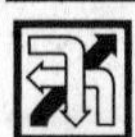

POSSIBLE INTERACTION WITH OTHER SUBSTANCES

INTERACTS WITH	COMBINED EFFECT
Alcohol:	None expected.
Beverages:	None expected.
Cocaine:	None expected.
Foods:	None expected.
Marijuana:	None expected.
Tobacco:	None expected.

TELITHROMYCIN

BRAND NAMES

Ketek

BASIC INFORMATION

Habit forming? No
Prescription needed? Yes
Available as generic? No
Drug class: Antibacterial; antibiotic (ketolide)

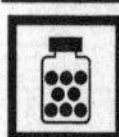

USES

Treatment for pneumonia of mild to moderate severity.

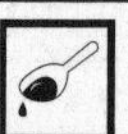

DOSAGE & USAGE INFORMATION

How to take:
Tablet—Swallow with a full glass of water. It may be taken with or without food. Do not crush or chew tablet.

When to take:
Once a day at the same time each day.

If you forget a dose:
Take as soon as you remember. If it is almost time for the next dose, wait for that dose (don't double this dose) and resume regular schedule.

What drug does:
Prevents growth and reproduction of susceptible bacteria.

Time lapse before drug works:
Starts working in a few hours, but takes 5 to 10 days to cure the infection being treated.

Don't take with:
Any other medicine or any dietary supplement without consulting your doctor or pharmacist.

OVERDOSE

SYMPTOMS:
Unknown effects.
WHAT TO DO:
Overdose unlikely to threaten life. If person uses much larger amount than prescribed or if accidentally swallowed, call doctor or poison control center 1-800-222-1222 for help.

POSSIBLE ADVERSE REACTIONS OR SIDE EFFECTS

SYMPTOMS	WHAT TO DO
Life-threatening:	
Rare allergic reaction—Breathing difficulty; closing of the throat; swelling of hands, feet, face, lips or tongue; hives.	Discontinue. Seek emergency treatment.
Common:	
Diarrhea, nausea.	Continue. Call doctor when convenient.
Infrequent:	
• Vision changes (blurred or difficulty in focusing or double vision).	Continue, but call doctor right away.
• Abdominal discomfort, belching, heartburn, vomiting, tingling or numbness or prickling sensations, changes in vaginal discharge, headache, dry lips or skin, flushing or red or warm skin, pale urine, urination increased or more frequent, genital itching, appetite loss, changes in sense of smell or taste, facial pain or tenderness or swelling, insomnia, mood changes, confusion, dizziness or feeling lightheaded.	Continue. Call doctor when convenient.
Rare:	
Stomach or chest, pain, breathing or swallowing difficulty, fainting, fever or chills, heartbeat is irregular or fast or slow, urine is dark or decreased, diarrhea is bloody or watery, yellow skin or eyes, unusual weakness or tiredness, unusual bleeding or bruising, joint or muscle pain, sores or patches on mouth or tongue or throat, skin symptoms (rash, peeling, blistering, itching).	Discontinue. Call doctor right away.

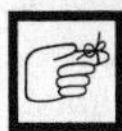

WARNINGS & PRECAUTIONS

Don't take if:
You are allergic to ketolide or macrolide antibiotics or take cisapride or pimozide.

Before you start, consult your doctor if:
- You have kidney or liver problems.
- You have hepatitis or jaundice.
- You have heart rhythm problems or a slow heartbeat (bradycardia).
- You have low potassium or low magnesium levels in your blood.
- You have myasthenia gravis.
- You are allergic to any medication, food or other substance.

Over age 60:
No special problems expected.

Pregnancy:
Decide with your doctor whether drug benefits justify risk to unborn child. Risk category C (see page xviii).

Breast-feeding:
Unknown if drug passes into milk. Avoid drug or discontinue nursing until you finish drug. Consult doctor for advice on maintaining milk supply.

Infants & children:
Safety and effectiveness for children under age 18 has not been established.

Prolonged use:
Drug is discontinued once the infection is cured.

Skin & sunlight:
No special problems expected.

Driving, piloting or hazardous work:
Avoid if you experience vision problems or dizziness. Otherwise, no problems expected.

Discontinuing:
Don't discontinue without doctor's advice until you complete prescribed dose, even though symptoms diminish or disappear.

Others:
- Advise any doctor or dentist whom you consult that you take this medicine.
- May affect the results of some medical tests.

POSSIBLE INTERACTION WITH OTHER DRUGS

GENERIC NAME OR DRUG CLASS	COMBINED EFFECT
Antiarrhythmics	Risk of heart rhythm problems.
Antifungals, azoles	Increased effect of telithromycin.
Benzodiazepines*	Increased effect of benzodiazepine.
Cisapride (this drug has limited availability)	Heart problem risk. Avoid.
Digoxin	Increased effect of digoxin.
Enzyme inducers*	Decreased effect of enzyme inducer or telithromycin.
Enzyme inhibitors*	Increased effect of enzyme inhibitor or telithromycin.
Ergot preparations*	Toxicity risk of ergot preparation. Avoid.
HMG-CoA reductase inhibitors	Increased effect of HMG-CoA reductase inhibitor.
Metoprolol	Increased risk of side effects.
Pimozide	Heart problem risk. Avoid.
QT interval prolongation-causing drugs*	Effects not clear. Use with caution.
Rifampin	Decreased effect of rifampin. Avoid.
Ritonavir	Increased effect of ritonavir.
Sirolimus	Increased effect of sirolimus.
Sotalol	Decreased effect of sotalol.
Tacrolimus	Increased effect of tacrolimus.
Theophylline	Increased risk of side effects. Take one hour apart.
Warfarin	Risk of side effects—bleeding or bruising.

POSSIBLE INTERACTION WITH OTHER SUBSTANCES

INTERACTS WITH	COMBINED EFFECT
Alcohol:	None expected.
Beverages:	None expected.
Cocaine:	Unknown. Avoid.
Foods:	None expected
Marijuana:	Unknown. Avoid.
Tobacco:	None expected, but you shouldn't smoke.

*See Glossary

TERBINAFINE (Oral)

BRAND NAMES

Lamisil Oral Granules
Lamisil Tablets

BASIC INFORMATION

Habit forming? No
Prescription needed? Yes
Available as generic? Yes
Drug class: Antifungal

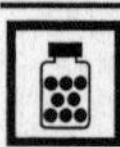

USES

- Treats fungal infection (called onychomycosis) of the toenails or fingernails.
- May be used for other fungal infections as determined by your doctor.
- Note: Another form of this drug is applied topically to the skin. For information, see the drug chart for Antifungals (Topical).

DOSAGE & USAGE INFORMATION

How to take:

- Tablet—Swallow with liquid. May be taken with or without food. If you can't swallow whole, crush tablet and take with liquid or food.
- Oral granules—Sprinkle on food. Follow instructions on prescription on what foods to use.

When to take:

- It is usually taken once a day at the same time each day for a period of weeks to months.
- It may be taken daily for one week per month for 2, 3 or 4 months (called pulse therapy).

If you forget a dose:
Take tablet as soon as you remember. If it is almost time for the next dose, wait for the next scheduled dose (don't double this dose).

Continued next column

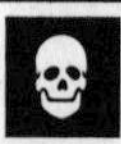

OVERDOSE

SYMPTOMS:
May include nausea, vomiting, abdominal pain, dizziness, rash, frequent urination and headache.
WHAT TO DO:

- **Dial 911 (emergency) for medical help or call poison control center 1-800-222-1222 for instructions.**
- **See emergency information on last 3 pages of this book.**

What drug does:
During the weeks of treatment, the drug will slowly kill the fungus infecting the nail. In many cases, the nail will then grow out normally.

Time lapse before drug works:
Improvement in symptoms may be seen in days or weeks, but fungus infections can be very slow to clear up. The drug is usually prescribed for 6 weeks for fingernail infections and 12 weeks or longer for toenail infections.

Don't take with:
Any other medicine or diet supplement without consulting your doctor or pharmacist.

POSSIBLE ADVERSE REACTIONS OR SIDE EFFECTS

SYMPTOMS	WHAT TO DO
Life-threatening:	
Rare allergic reaction (hives, itching, rash, trouble breathing, tightness in chest, swelling of lips or tongue or throat).	Seek emergency treatment immediately.
Common:	
Nausea, vomiting, mild stomach pain, diarrhea, feeling of fullness, mild appetite loss, headache.	Continue. Call doctor when convenient.
Infrequent:	
• Skin rash, itching.	Discontinue. Call doctor right away.
• Taste changes or loss of taste.	Continue. Call doctor when convenient.
Rare:	
• Nausea or vomiting that is persistent, unusual tiredness or weakness, stomach pain or appetite loss that is more severe, yellow eyes or skin, dark urine, pale stools, fever, chills, sore throat, aching muscles, skin symptoms (redness, blistering, peeling, loosening), unusual bleeding or bruising.	Discontinue. Call doctor right away.
• Hair loss.	Continue. Call doctor when convenient.

WARNINGS & PRECAUTIONS

Don't take if:
You are allergic to terbinafine.

Before you start, consult your doctor if:
- You have chronic or active liver disease or kidney disease.
- You have lupus erythematosus.
- You are an alcoholic.

Over age 60:
No special problems expected.

Pregnancy:
Decide with your doctor if drug should be taken during pregnancy. Treatment of nail fungal infections can usually be postponed until after delivery. Risk category B (see page xviii).

Breast-feeding:
Drug passes into milk. Avoid drug or discontinue nursing until you finish dosage. Consult doctor for advice on maintaining milk supply.

Infants & children:
The safety and effectiveness in this age group has not been established. Use only with doctor's approval and close medical supervision.

Prolonged use:
Use of the drug is usually limited to weeks or months of treatment.

Skin & sunlight:
No problems expected.

Driving, piloting or hazardous work:
No problems expected.

Discontinuing:
Don't discontinue the drug without doctor's advice until you complete prescribed dose, even though symptoms diminish or disappear.

Others:
- Periodic laboratory blood studies and liver and kidney function tests may be recommended.
- Be patient and persistent in following the treatment regimen for nail care. Consult your doctor if symptoms do not improve within a few weeks (or months for onychomycosis), or if they become worse.
- Taste changes caused by the drug usually improve within several weeks after stopping the drug, but a few cases may last a year or more.
- Very rarely, severe complications may occur with use of this drug. They include serious (and possibly fatal) liver disease, an abnormal blood disorder and Stevens Johnson syndrome (a severe allergic skin reaction).
- Advise any doctor or dentist whom you consult that you take this medicine.

POSSIBLE INTERACTION WITH OTHER DRUGS

GENERIC NAME OR DRUG CLASS	COMBINED EFFECT
Caffeine	Increased effect of caffeine.
Enzyme inducers*	May decrease effect of terbinafine or enzyme inducer.
Enzyme inhibitors*	May increase effect of terbinafine or enzyme inhibitor.
Warfarin	May affect blood clotting ability.

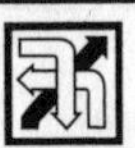

POSSIBLE INTERACTION WITH OTHER SUBSTANCES

INTERACTS WITH	COMBINED EFFECT
Alcohol:	Increased risk of side effects. Avoid.
Beverages:	None expected.
Cocaine:	Unknown. Avoid.
Foods:	None expected.
Marijuana:	Unknown. Avoid.
Tobacco:	None expected.

***See Glossary**

TETRACYCLINES

GENERIC AND BRAND NAMES

See full list of generic and brand names in the *Generic and Brand Name Directory*, page 896

BASIC INFORMATION

Habit forming? No
Prescription needed? Yes
Available as generic? Yes
Drug class: Antibacterial, antiacne

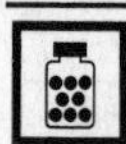

USES

- Treatment for bacterial infections susceptible to any tetracycline. Not used for viruses.
- Treatment for acne, ulcers and used as diuretic.
- Treatment for dental bacterial infections.

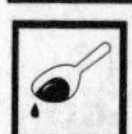

DOSAGE & USAGE INFORMATION

How to take:
- Tablet or capsule—Take on empty stomach 1 hour before or 2 hours after eating. If you can't swallow whole, crumble tablet or open capsule and take with liquid or food.
- Delayed-release capsule or extended-release tablet or capsule—Swallow whole with liquid. Do not open, crush or chew.
- Dental product—Follow package instructions.
- Liquid—Shake well. Take with measuring spoon.

When to take:
At the same times each day, evenly spaced.

If you forget a dose:
Take as soon as you remember. If it is almost time for the next dose, wait for that dose (don't double this dose) and resume regular schedule.

What drug does:
Prevents bacteria growth and reproduction.

Time lapse before drug works:
- Infections—May require 5 days to affect infection.
- Acne—May require 4 weeks to affect acne.

Don't take with:
Any other medicine or any dietary supplement without consulting your doctor or pharmacist.

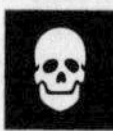

OVERDOSE

SYMPTOMS:
Severe nausea, vomiting, diarrhea.
WHAT TO DO:
Overdose unlikely to threaten life. If person uses much larger amount than prescribed or if accidentally swallowed, call doctor or poison control center 1-800-222-1222 for help.

POSSIBLE ADVERSE REACTIONS OR SIDE EFFECTS

SYMPTOMS	WHAT TO DO
Life-threatening:	
Hives, rash, intense itching, faintness soon after a dose (anaphylaxis).	Seek emergency treatment immediately.
Common:	
• Mild stomach cramps, diarrhea, nausea or vomiting, dizziness, lightheadedness or unsteadiness (with minocycline).	Continue. Call doctor when convenient.
• Increased sensitivity to sunlight, tooth discoloration (in children age 8 and under).	Discontinue. Call doctor right away.
Infrequent:	
• Frequent or increased urination, excessive thirst, unusual tiredness or weakness (with demeclocycline); darker color or discoloration of skin and mucous membranes (with minocycline).	Discontinue. Call doctor right away.
• Sore mouth or tongue, rectal or genital itch.	Continue. Call doctor when convenient.
• Darkened tongue (will go away when drug is discontinued).	No action necessary.
Rare:	
Changes in vision, yellow skin or eyes, continued vomiting, severe stomach cramps, loss of appetite, ongoing headache, bulging fontanel (soft spot on head of infant).	Discontinue. Call doctor right away.

WARNINGS & PRECAUTIONS

Don't take if:
You are allergic to any tetracycline antibiotic.

Before you start, consult your doctor if:
- You have kidney or liver disease.
- You have lupus.
- You have myasthenia gravis.

Over age 60:
Dosage usually less than in younger adults. More likely to cause itching around rectum. Ask your doctor how to prevent it.

Pregnancy:
Risk to unborn child outweighs drug benefits. Don't use. Risk category D (see page xviii).

Breast-feeding:
Drug passes into milk. Avoid drug or discontinue nursing until you finish medicine. Consult doctor for advice on maintaining milk supply.

Infants & children:
May cause permanent teeth malformation or discoloration in children less than 8 years old. Don't use.

Prolonged use:
- You may become more susceptible to infections caused by germs not responsive to tetracycline.
- May cause rare problems in liver, kidney or bone marrow. Periodic laboratory blood studies, liver and kidney function tests recommended if you use drug a long time.

Skin & sunlight:
May cause rash or intensify sunburn in areas exposed to sun or ultraviolet light (photosensitivity reaction). Avoid overexposure. Notify doctor if reaction occurs.

Driving, piloting or hazardous work:
No problems expected.

Discontinuing:
Don't discontinue without doctor's advice until you complete prescribed dose, even though symptoms diminish or disappear.

Others:
- Avoid using outdated drug.
- May affect results in some medical tests.
- Birth control pills may not be effective. Use additional birth control method.
- Advise any doctor or dentist whom you consult that you take this medicine.

POSSIBLE INTERACTION WITH OTHER DRUGS

GENERIC NAME OR DRUG CLASS	COMBINED EFFECT
Antacids*	Decreased tetracycline effect.
Anticoagulants,* oral	Increased anticoagulant effect.
Antivirals, HIV/AIDS*	Decreased antibiotic effect.
Bismuth subsalicylate	Decreased tetracycline absorption.
Calcium supplements*	Decreased tetracycline effect.
Cefixime	Decreased antibiotic effect of cefixime.
Cholestyramine or colestipol	Decreased tetracycline effect.
Contraceptives, oral*	Decreased contraceptive effect.
Desmopressin	Possible decreased desmopressin effect.
Digitalis preparations*	Increased digitalis effect.
Etretinate	Increased chance of adverse reactions of etretinate.
Lithium	Increased lithium effect.
Mineral supplements* (iron, calcium, magnesium, zinc)	Decreased tetracycline absorption. Separate doses by 1 to 2 hours.
Penicillins*	Decreased penicillin effect.
Sodium bicarbonate	Greatly reduced tetracycline absorption.

Continued on page 930

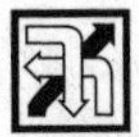

POSSIBLE INTERACTION WITH OTHER SUBSTANCES

INTERACTS WITH	COMBINED EFFECT
Alcohol:	Possible liver damage. Avoid.
Beverages: Milk.	Decreased tetracycline absorption. Take dose 2 hours after or 1 hour before drinking.
Cocaine:	None expected.
Foods: Dairy products.	Decreased tetracycline absorption. Take dose 2 hours after or 1 hour before eating.
Marijuana:	No interactions expected, but marijuana may slow body's recovery. Avoid.
Tobacco:	None expected.

***See Glossary**

THIAMINE (Vitamin B-1)

BRAND NAMES

Betalin S	Bewon
Betaxin	Biamine

Numerous brands of single vitamin and multivitamin combinations may be available.

BASIC INFORMATION

Habit forming? No
Prescription needed? No
Available as generic? Yes
Drug class: Vitamin supplement

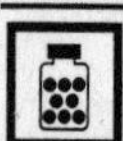

USES

- Dietary supplement to promote normal growth, development and health.
- Treatment for beri-beri (a thiamine-deficiency disease).
- Dietary supplement for alcoholism, cirrhosis, overactive thyroid, infection, breast-feeding, absorption diseases, pregnancy, prolonged diarrhea, burns.

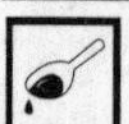

DOSAGE & USAGE INFORMATION

How to take:
Tablet or liquid—Swallow with beverage or food to lessen stomach irritation.

When to take:
At the same time each day.

If you forget a dose:
Take when remembered, then return to regular schedule.

What drug does:
- Promotes normal growth and development.
- Combines with an enzyme to metabolize carbohydrates.

Time lapse before drug works:
15 minutes.

Don't take with:
Any other medicine or any dietary supplement without consulting your doctor or pharmacist.

OVERDOSE

SYMPTOMS:
Increased severity of adverse reactions and side effects.
WHAT TO DO:
Overdose unlikely to threaten life. If person uses much larger amount than prescribed or if accidentally swallowed, call doctor or poison center 1-800-222-1222 for help.

POSSIBLE ADVERSE REACTIONS OR SIDE EFFECTS

SYMPTOMS	WHAT TO DO
Life-threatening: None expected.	
Common: None expected.	
Infrequent: None expected.	
Rare:	
• Wheezing.	Discontinue. Seek emergency treatment.
• Rash or itchy skin.	Discontinue. Call doctor right away.

WARNINGS & PRECAUTIONS

Don't take if:
You are allergic to any B vitamin.

Before you start, consult your doctor if:
You have liver or kidney disease.

Over age 60:
No problems expected.

Pregnancy:
Consult doctor. Risk category A (see page xviii).

Breast-feeding:
No problems expected in meeting child's normal daily requirements. Consult doctor.

Infants & children:
No problems expected.

Prolonged use:
No problems expected.

Skin & sunlight:
No problems expected.

Driving, piloting or hazardous work:
No problems expected.

Discontinuing:
No problems expected.

Others:
A balanced diet should provide enough thiamine for healthy people to make a supplement unnecessary. Best dietary sources of thiamine are whole-grain cereals and meats.

POSSIBLE INTERACTION WITH OTHER DRUGS

GENERIC NAME OR DRUG CLASS	COMBINED EFFECT
Barbiturates*	Decreased thiamine effect.

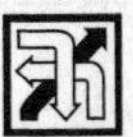

POSSIBLE INTERACTION WITH OTHER SUBSTANCES

INTERACTS WITH	COMBINED EFFECT
Alcohol:	None expected.
Beverages: Carbonates, citrates (additives listed on many beverage labels).	Decreased thiamine effect.
Cocaine:	None expected.
Foods: Carbonates, citrates (additives listed on many food labels).	Decreased thiamine effect.
Marijuana:	None expected.
Tobacco:	None expected.

*See Glossary

THIAZOLIDINEDIONES

GENERIC AND BRAND NAMES

PIOGLITAZONE	ROSIGLITAZONE
Actos	Avandamet
ACTOplus Met	Avandaryl
ACTOplus Met XR	Avandia
Duetact	
Oseni	

BASIC INFORMATION

Habit forming? No
Prescription needed? Yes
Available as generic? Yes, for some
Drug class: Antidiabetic

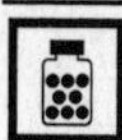

USES

Treatment for type 2 diabetes. Rosiglitazone or pioglitazone may be used alone, with insulin or with other antidiabetic drugs.

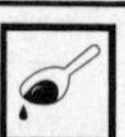

DOSAGE & USAGE INFORMATION

How to take:

- Tablet—Swallow with liquid. Take at mealtime. If you can't swallow whole, crumble tablet and take with liquid or food.
- Extended-release tablet—Swallow whole with liquid. May be taken with or without food. Do not crush, chew or split tablet.

When to take:
Once a day or as directed by doctor. Dosage may be increased after several weeks.

Continued next column

OVERDOSE

SYMPTOMS:
Symptoms of hypoglycemia—stomach pain, anxious feeling, cold sweats, chills, confusion, convulsions, cool pale skin, excessive hunger, nausea or vomiting, rapid heartbeat, nervousness, shakiness, unsteady walk, unusual weakness or tiredness, vision changes, unconsciousness.
WHAT TO DO:

- **For mild hypoglycemia symptoms, drink or eat something with sugar right away.**
- **For more severe symptoms, dial 911 (emergency) for medical help or call poison control center 1-800-222-1222 for instructions.**
- **See emergency information on last 3 pages of this book.**

If you forget a dose:
Wait for your next meal that same day and take dose then. If you forget until the next day, take that day's regular dose on schedule (don't double this dose).

What drug does:
Lowers blood glucose by improving target cell response to insulin. These drugs do not cure diabetes.

Time lapse before drug works:
May take several weeks for full effectiveness.

Don't take with:
Any other medicine or any dietary supplement without consulting your doctor or pharmacist.

POSSIBLE ADVERSE REACTIONS OR SIDE EFFECTS

SYMPTOMS	WHAT TO DO
Life-threatening:	
In case of overdose or low blood sugar, see previous column.	
Common:	
• Pain in back or other body part, infection.	Continue. Call doctor right away.
• Headache, dizziness, nausea, unusual tiredness or weakness.	Continue. Call doctor when convenient.
Infrequent:	
Sore throat, runny nose, diarrhea.	Continue. Call doctor when convenient.
Rare:	
• Severe low blood sugar (see symptoms under Overdose).	Discontinue. Call doctor right away or seek emergency help.
• Liver problems including jaundice (yellow skin or eyes) and hepatitis that could lead to liver transplantation or death; symptoms of heart failure (excessive, rapid weight gain, shortness of breath and swelling of legs or feet) after starting drug.	Discontinue. Call doctor right away.

WARNINGS & PRECAUTIONS

Don't take if:
You are allergic to any of the thiazolidinediones.

Before you start, consult your doctor if:

- You have liver disease or any heart disorder.
- You have any chronic health problem.

- You have a history of acid in the blood (metabolic acidosis or ketoacidosis).
- You are allergic to any medication, food or other substance.

Over age 60:
No special problems expected.

Pregnancy:
Decide with your doctor if drug benefits justify risks to unborn child. Risk category C for pioglitazone and rosiglitazone (see page xviii).

Breast-feeding:
It is unknown if drug passes into milk. It is not recommended for use in nursing mothers.

Infants & children:
Safety and efficacy have not been established. Use only under close medical supervision.

Prolonged use:
- Schedule regular doctor visits to determine if the drug is continuing to be effective in controlling the diabetes and to check for any liver function problems.
- You will most likely require an antidiabetic medicine for the rest of your life.
- You will need to test your blood glucose levels several times a day, or for some, once to several times a week.

Skin & sunlight:
No special problems expected.

Driving, piloting or hazardous work:
No special problems expected.

Discontinuing:
Don't discontinue without consulting your doctor even if you feel well. You can have diabetes without feeling any symptoms. Untreated diabetes can cause serious problems.

Others:
- Use of these drugs may lead to liver problems. Currently, it is necessary to get liver function studies prior to starting the drug, then every other month for 6 months and periodically thereafter while on the drug.
- Rosiglitazone may increase risk of heart attack and heart-related death in certain patients. Consult doctor.
- Use of these drugs can cause fluid retention which may lead to or worsen chronic heart failure.
- Advise any doctor or dentist whom you consult that you take this medicine. It may interfere with the accuracy of some medical tests.
- May cause ovulation to resume in some women with ovarian disorders. Discuss the need for nonhormonal contraception with your doctor.
- Follow any special diet your doctor may prescribe. It can help control diabetes.
- Consult doctor if you become ill with vomiting or diarrhea while taking this drug.
- Use caution when exercising. Ask your doctor about an appropriate exercise program.
- Wear medical identification stating that you have diabetes and take this medication.
- Learn to recognize the symptoms of low blood sugar. You and your family need to know what to do if these symptoms occur.
- Have a glucagon kit and syringe in the event severe low blood sugar occurs.
- Use of these drugs may raise both HDL and LDL cholesterol levels.
- High blood sugar (hyperglycemia) may occur with diabetes. Ask your doctor about symptoms to watch for and treatment steps to take.
- Educate yourself about diabetes.

POSSIBLE INTERACTION WITH OTHER DRUGS

GENERIC NAME OR DRUG CLASS	COMBINED EFFECT
Antidiabetic agents, sulfonylurea	May decrease fasting plasma glucose concentrations.
Contraceptives, oral*	Decreased effect of contraceptive.
Cyclosporine	Decreased effect of cyclosporine.
HMG-CoA reductase inhibitors	Decreased effect of HMG-CoA reductase inhibitor.
Tacrolimus	Decreased effect of tacrolimus.

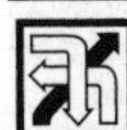

POSSIBLE INTERACTION WITH OTHER SUBSTANCES

INTERACTS WITH	COMBINED EFFECT
Alcohol:	No special problems. Avoid excessive amounts of alcohol.
Beverages:	None expected.
Cocaine:	No special problems. Best to avoid.
Foods:	None expected.
Marijuana:	No special problems. Best to avoid.
Tobacco:	People with diabetes should not smoke.

***See Glossary**

THIOGUANINE

BRAND NAMES

Lanvis

BASIC INFORMATION

Habit forming? No
Prescription needed? Yes
Available as generic? Yes
Drug class: Antineoplastic

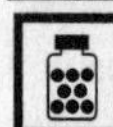

USES

Treats some forms of leukemia.

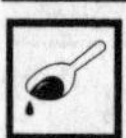

DOSAGE & USAGE INFORMATION

How to take:
Tablet—Swallow with liquid. If you can't swallow whole, crumble tablet and take with liquid or food. Instructions to take on empty stomach mean 1 hour before or 2 hours after eating.

When to take:
According to doctor's instructions.

If you forget a dose:
Skip the missed dose and return to regular schedule. Don't double dose.

What drug does:
Interferes with growth of cancer cells.

Time lapse before drug works:
Varies greatly among patients.

Don't take with:
Any other medicines (including over-the-counter drugs such as cough and cold medicines, laxatives, antacids, diet pills, caffeine, nose drops or vitamins) without consulting your doctor or pharmacist.

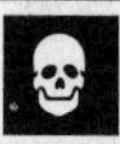

OVERDOSE

SYMPTOMS:
None expected.
WHAT TO DO:
Overdose unlikely to threaten life. If person uses much larger amount than prescribed or if accidentally swallowed, call doctor or poison control center 1-800-222-1222 for help.

POSSIBLE ADVERSE REACTIONS OR SIDE EFFECTS

SYMPTOMS	WHAT TO DO
Life-threatening: None expected.	
Common:	
• Appetite loss, diarrhea, skin rash.	Continue. Call doctor when convenient.
• Nausea.	No action necessary.
Infrequent: Bloody urine, hoarseness or cough; fever or chills, lower back or side pain, painful or difficult urination, red spots on skin, unusual bleeding or bruising, joint pain, swollen feet and legs, unsteady gait, black or tarry stools.	Discontinue. Call doctor right away.
Rare: Mouth and lip sores, jaundice (yellow skin and eyes).	Discontinue. Call doctor right away.

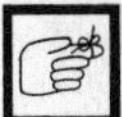

WARNINGS & PRECAUTIONS

Don't take if:
- You are allergic to thioguanine.
- You have chicken pox or shingles.

Before you start, consult your doctor if:
- You have gout.
- You have an infection.
- You have kidney or liver disease.
- You have had radiation or cancer chemotherapy within 6 weeks.

Over age 60:
Adverse reactions and side effects may be more frequent and severe than in younger persons. You may need smaller doses for shorter periods of time.

Pregnancy:
Risk to unborn child outweighs drug benefits. Don't use. Risk category D (see page xviii).

Breast-feeding:
Drug may pass into milk. Avoid drug or discontinue nursing until you finish medicine. Consult doctor for advice on maintaining milk supply.

Infants & children:
No special problems expected.

Prolonged use:
- Increased likelihood of side effects.
- Talk to your doctor about the need for follow-up medical examinations or laboratory studies to check kidney and liver function, serum uric acid, and complete blood counts (white blood cell count, platelet count, red blood cell count, hemoglobin, hematocrit).

Skin & sunlight:
No problems expected.

Driving, piloting or hazardous work:
No problems expected.

Discontinuing:
Report to your doctor any of these symptoms that occur after discontinuing: black, tarry stools; bloody urine; hoarseness or cough; fever or chills; lower back or side pain; painful or difficult urination; red spots on skin; unusual bleeding or bruising.

Others:
- Advise any doctor or dentist whom you consult that you take this medicine.
- May affect results in some medical tests.
- Use an effective form of birth control. Consult doctor for advice.

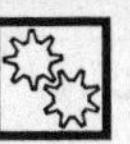

POSSIBLE INTERACTION WITH OTHER DRUGS

GENERIC NAME OR DRUG CLASS	COMBINED EFFECT
Antigout drugs*	May need increased antigout dosage.
Bone marrow depressants,* other	Increased risk of bone marrow depression.
Vaccines, live or killed	Increased risk of toxicity or reduced effectiveness of vaccine.
Zidovudine	More likelihood of toxicity of both drugs.

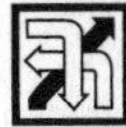

POSSIBLE INTERACTION WITH OTHER SUBSTANCES

INTERACTS WITH	COMBINED EFFECT
Alcohol:	Increased side effects.
Beverages:	None expected.
Cocaine:	Increased side effects.
Foods:	None expected.
Marijuana:	None expected.
Tobacco:	None expected.

*See Glossary

THIOTHIXENE

BRAND NAMES

Navane	Thiothixene HCl Intensol

BASIC INFORMATION

Habit forming? No
Prescription needed? Yes
Available as generic? Yes
Drug class: Antipsychotic (thioxanthene)

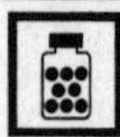

USES

Reduces anxiety, agitation, psychosis.

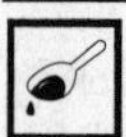

DOSAGE & USAGE INFORMATION

How to take:

- Capsule—Swallow with liquid. If you can't swallow whole, open capsule and take with liquid or food.
- Syrup—Dilute dose in beverage before swallowing.

When to take:
At the same times each day.

If you forget a dose:
Take as soon as you remember. If it is almost time for the next dose, wait for that dose (don't double this dose) and resume regular schedule.

What drug does:
Corrects imbalance of nerve impulses.

Time lapse before drug works:
3 weeks.

Continued next column

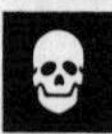

OVERDOSE

SYMPTOMS:
Drowsiness, dizziness, weakness, muscle rigidity, twitching, tremors, confusion, dry mouth, blurred vision, rapid pulse, shallow breathing, low blood pressure, convulsions, coma.
WHAT TO DO:

- **Dial 911 (emergency) for medical help or call poison control center 1-800-222-1222 for instructions.**
- **If person is unconscious, check breathing and pulse. If not breathing, begin mouth-to-mouth rescue breathing. If heart is not beating, begin chest compressions.**
- **See emergency information on last 3 pages of this book.**

Don't take with:
Any other medicine or any dietary supplement without consulting your doctor or pharmacist.

POSSIBLE ADVERSE REACTIONS OR SIDE EFFECTS

SYMPTOMS	WHAT TO DO
Life-threatening:	
High fever, rapid pulse, profuse sweating, muscle rigidity, confusion and irritability, seizures.	Discontinue. Seek emergency treatment.
Common:	
• Jerky or involuntary movements, especially of the face, lips, jaw, tongue; slow-frequency tremor of head or limbs, especially while moving; muscle rigidity, lack of facial expression and slow, inflexible movements.	Discontinue. Call doctor right away.
• Pacing or restlessness; intermittent spasms of muscles of face, eyes, tongue, jaw, neck, body or limbs; dry mouth; blurred vision; constipation; difficulty urinating.	Continue. Call doctor when convenient.
Infrequent:	
• Sedation, low blood pressure and dizziness.	Continue. Call doctor when convenient.
• Other symptoms not listed above.	Continue. Call doctor when convenient.

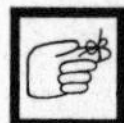

WARNINGS & PRECAUTIONS

Don't take if:

- You are allergic to any thioxanthene or phenothiazine tranquilizer.
- You have serious blood disorder.
- You have Parkinson's disease.
- Patient is younger than 12.

Before you start, consult your doctor if:

- You have had liver or kidney disease.
- You have epilepsy, glaucoma, prostate trouble.
- You have high blood pressure or heart disease (especially angina).
- You use alcohol daily.
- You will have surgery within 2 months, including dental surgery, requiring general or spinal anesthesia.

Over age 60:

- Adverse reactions and side effects may be more frequent and severe than in younger persons.
- Use of antipsychotic drugs in elderly patients with dementia-related psychosis may increase risk of death. Consult doctor.

Pregnancy:
Decide with your doctor if drug benefits justify risk to unborn child. Risk category C (see page xviii).

Breast-feeding:
Studies inconclusive. Consult your doctor.

Infants & children:
Not approved for children under age 12.

Prolonged use:

- Pigment deposits in lens and retina of eye.
- Involuntary movements of jaws, lips, tongue (tardive dyskinesia).
- Talk to your doctor about the need for follow-up medical examinations or laboratory studies to check complete blood counts (white blood cell count, platelet count, red blood cell count, hemoglobin, hematocrit), liver function, eyes.

Skin & sunlight:

- May cause rash or intensify sunburn in areas exposed to sun or ultraviolet light (photosensitivity reaction). Use sunscreen and avoid overexposure. Notify doctor if reaction occurs.
- Hot temperatures and exercise or hot baths can increase risk of heatstroke. Drug may affect body's ability to maintain normal temperature.

Driving, piloting or hazardous work:
Don't drive or pilot aircraft until you learn how medicine affects you. Don't work around dangerous machinery. Don't climb ladders or work in high places. Danger increases if you drink alcohol or take medicine affecting alertness and reflexes.

Discontinuing:
Don't discontinue without consulting doctor. Dose may require gradual reduction if you have taken drug for a long time. Doses of other drugs may also require adjustment.

Others:

- Advise any doctor or dentist whom you consult that you take this medicine.
- For dry mouth, suck sugarless hard candy or chew sugarless gum. If dry mouth persists, consult your dentist.

POSSIBLE INTERACTION WITH OTHER DRUGS

GENERIC NAME OR DRUG CLASS	COMBINED EFFECT
Anticonvulsants*	Change in seizure pattern.
Antidepressants, tricyclic*	Increased thiothixene effect. Excessive sedation.
Antihistamines*	Increased thiothixene effect. Excessive sedation.
Antihypertensives*	Excessively low blood pressure.
Barbiturates*	Increased thiothixene effect. Excessive sedation.
Bupropion	Increased risk of seizures.
Epinephrine	Excessively low blood pressure.
Guanethidine	Decreased guanethidine effect.
Levodopa	Decreased levodopa effect.
Mind-altering drugs*	Increased thiothixene effect. Excessive sedation.
Monoamine oxidase (MAO) inhibitors*	Excessive sedation.
Narcotics*	Increased thiothixene effect. Excessive sedation.
Pergolide	Decreased pergolide effect.
Quinidine	Increased risk of heartbeat irregularities.

Continued on page 930

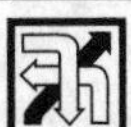

POSSIBLE INTERACTION WITH OTHER SUBSTANCES

INTERACTS WITH	COMBINED EFFECT
Alcohol:	Excessive brain depression. Avoid.
Beverages:	None expected.
Cocaine:	Decreased thiothixene effect. Avoid.
Foods:	None expected.
Marijuana:	Daily use—Fainting likely; possible psychosis.
Tobacco:	None expected.

THYROID HORMONES

GENERIC AND BRAND NAMES

LEVOTHYROXINE	THYROGLOBULIN
Eltroxin	Levoxyl
Levo-T	L-Thyroxine
Levothroid	Proloid
Novothyrox	Synthroid
LIOTHYRONINE	THYROID
Cytomel	Armour Thyroid
LIOTRIX	Thyrar
Euthroid	Thyroid Strong
Thyrolar	Westhroid

BASIC INFORMATION

Habit forming? No
Prescription needed? Yes
Available as generic? Yes, for some
Drug class: Thyroid hormone

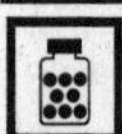

USES

Replacement for thyroid hormones lost due to deficiency.

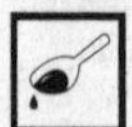

DOSAGE & USAGE INFORMATION

How to take:
Tablet—Swallow with liquid. Levothyroxine tablet should be taken with full glass of water.

When to take:
At the same time each day before a meal or on awakening.

If you forget a dose:
Take as soon as you remember up to 12 hours late. If more than 12 hours, wait for next scheduled dose (don't double this dose).

What drug does:
Increases cell metabolism rate.

Continued next column

OVERDOSE

SYMPTOMS:
"Hot" feeling, heart palpitations, nervousness, sweating, hand tremors, insomnia, rapid and irregular pulse, headache, irritability, diarrhea, weight loss, muscle cramps, angina, congestive heart failure possible.
WHAT TO DO:
Overdose unlikely to threaten life. If person uses much larger amount than prescribed or if accidentally swallowed, call doctor or poison control center 1-800-222-1222 for help.

Time lapse before drug works:
48 hours.

Don't take with:
Any other medicine or any dietary supplement without consulting your doctor or pharmacist.

POSSIBLE ADVERSE REACTIONS OR SIDE EFFECTS

SYMPTOMS	WHAT TO DO
Life-threatening:	
In case of overdose, see previous column.	
Common:	
Tremor, headache, irritability, insomnia, appetite change, diarrhea, leg cramps, menstrual irregularities, fever, heat sensitivity, unusual sweating, weight loss, nervousness.	Continue. Call doctor when convenient.
Infrequent:	
Hives, rash, vomiting, chest pain, rapid and irregular heartbeat, shortness of breath.	Discontinue. Call doctor right away.
Rare:	
None expected.	

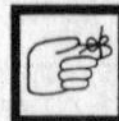

WARNINGS & PRECAUTIONS

Don't take if:
- You have had a heart attack within the past 6 weeks.
- You have no thyroid deficiency, but want to use this to lose weight.

Before you start, consult your doctor if:
- You have heart disease or high blood pressure.
- You have diabetes.
- You have Addison's disease, have had adrenal gland deficiency or use epinephrine, ephedrine or isoproterenol for asthma.

Over age 60:
More sensitive to thyroid hormone. May need smaller doses.

Pregnancy:
Considered safe if for thyroid deficiency only. Consult doctor. Risk category A (see page xviii).

Breast-feeding:
Present in milk. Consult doctor.

Infants & children:
Use only under medical supervision.

Prolonged use:
- No problems expected if dose is correct.
- Talk to your doctor about the need for follow-up medical examinations or laboratory studies to check thyroid, heart.

Skin & sunlight:
No problems expected.

Driving, piloting or hazardous work:
No problems expected.

Discontinuing:
Don't discontinue without consulting doctor. Dose may require gradual reduction if you have taken drug for a long time. Doses of other drugs may also require adjustment.

Others:
- Digestive upsets, tremors, cramps, nervousness, insomnia or diarrhea may indicate need for dose adjustment.
- Different brands can cause different results. Do not change brands without consulting doctor.
- Advise any doctor or dentist whom you consult that you take this medicine.

POSSIBLE INTERACTION WITH OTHER DRUGS

GENERIC NAME OR DRUG CLASS	COMBINED EFFECT
Adrenocorticoids, systemic	May require thyroid hormone dosage change.
Amphetamines*	Increased amphetamine effect.
Anticoagulants,* oral	Increased anticoagulant effect.
Antidepressants, tricyclic*	Increased antidepressant effect. Irregular heartbeat.
Antidiabetics,* oral or insulin	Antidiabetic may require adjustment.
Aspirin (large doses, continuous use)	Increased effect of thyroid hormone.
Barbiturates*	Decreased barbiturate effect.
Beta-adrenergic blocking agents*	Possible decreased effect of beta blocker.
Cholestyramine	Decreased effect of thyroid hormone.
Colestipol	Decreased effect of thyroid hormone.
Contraceptives, oral*	Decreased effect of thyroid hormone.
Digitalis preparations*	Decreased digitalis effect.
Ephedrine	Increased ephedrine effect.
Epinephrine	Increased epinephrine effect.
Estrogens*	Decreased effect of thyroid hormone.
Meglitinides	Increased blood sugar levels.
Methylphenidate	Increased methylphenidate effect.
Phenytoin	Possible decreased effect of thyroid hormone.
Sympathomimetics*	Increased risk of rapid or irregular heartbeat.

POSSIBLE INTERACTION WITH OTHER SUBSTANCES

INTERACTS WITH	COMBINED EFFECT
Alcohol:	None expected.
Beverages:	None expected.
Cocaine:	Excess stimulation. Avoid.
Foods:	None expected.
Marijuana:	None expected.
Tobacco:	None expected.

*See Glossary

TIAGABINE

BRAND NAMES

Gabitril

BASIC INFORMATION

Habit forming? No
Prescription needed? Yes
Available as generic? No
Drug class: Anticonvulsant; antiepileptic

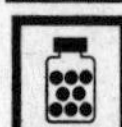

USES

Treatment of partial seizures in patients with epilepsy. It is used in combination with other antiepileptic drugs.

DOSAGE & USAGE INFORMATION

How to take:
Tablet—Swallow whole with a liquid. Take with food or on a full stomach.

When to take:
Usually once a day to start, then taken 2 to 4 times a day at the same times each day. Your doctor will determine the schedule. Dosage may be increased slowly to achieve best results.

If you forget a dose:
Take as soon as you remember. If it is almost time for the next dose, skip the missed dose and wait for your next scheduled dose (don't double this dose).

What drug does:
It is not known exactly how the drug works. It increases the amount of a brain chemical (called GABA) that helps prevent seizure activity.

Continued next column

OVERDOSE

SYMPTOMS:
Seizures including status epilepticus, lack of coordination, confusion, drowsiness, muscle spasms, hostility, impaired speech, agitation, lethargy, stupor, tremors, disorientation, vomiting, temporary paralysis, coma.
WHAT TO DO:
- **Dial 911 (emergency) for medical help or call poison control center 1-800-222-1222 for instructions.**
- **If person is unconscious, check breathing and pulse. If not breathing, begin mouth-to-mouth rescue breathing. If heart is not beating, begin chest compressions.**
- **See emergency information on last 3 pages of this book.**

Time lapse before drug works:
May take several weeks for full effectiveness.

Don't take with:
Any other medicine or any dietary supplement without consulting your doctor or pharmacist.

POSSIBLE ADVERSE REACTIONS OR SIDE EFFECTS

SYMPTOMS	WHAT TO DO
Life-threatening:	
Rare allergic reaction (hives, itching, rash, trouble breathing, tightness in chest, swelling of lips or tongue or face); rare Stevens-Johnson syndrome (mucous membranes and skin have redness, blisters, peeling, looseness).	Seek emergency treatment immediately.
Common:	
Dizziness, weakness, tremor, drowsiness, concentration problems, infection (chills, fever, headache, sore throat), nervousness.	Continue. Call doctor when convenient.
Infrequent:	
• Numbness or burning or tingling sensations, speech problems, agitation, confusion, hostility, memory problems, vision changes, clumsiness.	Continue, but call doctor right away.
• Stomach pain, increased cough, muscle aches or pain or weakness, nausea, sleeping problems, pain, unusual tiredness vomiting, diarrhea.	Continue. Call doctor when convenient.
Rare:	
• Status epilepticus (ongoing seizures), severe weakness, suicidal thoughts.	Seek emergency treatment immediately.
• New or increased, seizures, severe rash, depression, unusual behaviors.	Continue, but call doctor right away.
• Itching, flushing, mild rash, appetite increased, mouth sores, emotional upsets.	Continue. Call doctor when convenient.

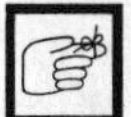

WARNINGS & PRECAUTIONS

Don't take if:
You are allergic to tiagabine.

Before you start, consult your doctor if:
- You do not have seizures or epilepsy.
- You have any type of liver disorder.
- You have a history of mental or mood problems (such as depression) or suicidal thoughts or attempts.
- You are allergic to any medication, food or other substance.

Over age 60:
No problems expected.

Pregnancy:
Decide with your doctor if drug benefits justify risks to unborn child. Risk category C (see page xviii).

Breast-feeding:
It is unknown if drug passes into milk. Avoid drug or discontinue nursing until you finish medicine. Consult doctor for advice on maintaining milk supply.

Infants & children:
Safety and efficacy not established in children younger than age 12.

Prolonged use:
No special problems expected. Follow-up with your doctor on a regular basis to monitor your condition and check for drug side effects.

Skin & sunlight:
No problems expected.

Driving, piloting or hazardous work:
This drug may cause dizziness and drowsiness. Don't drive or pilot aircraft until you learn how medicine affects you. Don't work around dangerous machinery. Don't climb ladders or work in high places. The risk of dizziness increases if you drink alcohol.

Discontinuing:
Don't discontinue without doctor's approval due to risk of increased seizure activity. The dosage may need to be gradually decreased before stopping the drug completely.

Others:
- This drug cannot cure epilepsy and will only work to control seizures for as long as you continue to take it.
- Tiagabine is used with other anticonvulsant drugs and additional side effects may occur. If they do, consult your doctor.
- Advise any doctor or dentist whom you consult that you take this medicine.
- Rarely, antiepileptic drugs may lead to suicidal thoughts and behaviors. Call doctor right away if suicidal symptoms or unusual behaviors occur.
- Carry or wear medical identification that lists your seizure disorder and drugs you take.
- Use of this drug in patients without epilepsy may lead to new onset seizures and status epilepticus. Nonepileptic patients who develop seizures should discontinue the drug. Consult doctor to see if you have a seizure disorder.

POSSIBLE INTERACTION WITH OTHER DRUGS

GENERIC NAME OR DRUG CLASS	COMBINED EFFECT
Enzyme inducing, antiepileptic drugs*	Decreased effect of tiagabine.
Other drugs	Unknown. Consult doctor or pharmacist.
Protein bound drugs*	Increased effect of both drugs.
Seizure threshold lowering drugs*	Increased risk of seizures.
Valproate	May alter affect of either drug. Consult doctor.

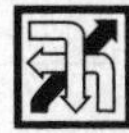

POSSIBLE INTERACTION WITH OTHER SUBSTANCES

INTERACTS WITH	COMBINED EFFECT
Alcohol:	Increased risk of dizziness. Avoid.
Beverages:	Ask your doctor about drinking grapefruit juice.
Cocaine:	Unknown effect. Avoid.
Foods:	None expected.
Marijuana:	Unknown effect. Avoid.
Tobacco:	None expected.

*See Glossary

TICAGRELOR

BRAND NAMES

Brilinta

BASIC INFORMATION

Habit forming? No
Prescription needed? Yes
Available as generic? No
Drug class: Platelet aggregation inhibitor

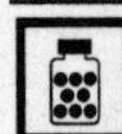

USES

It helps prevent blood clots and reduces the risk of heart attack, stroke or other vascular events. It is used in people who have had a heart attack or have acute coronary syndrome (symptoms include severe chest pain called angina).

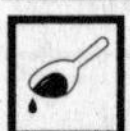

DOSAGE & USAGE INFORMATION

How to take:
Tablet—Swallow whole with water. It may be taken with or without food. Take it with food if the tablet upsets your stomach.

When to take:
Twice a day at the same times each day. This drug is intended to be used in combination with aspirin. Your doctor will advise you of how much aspirin to take each day.

If you forget a dose:
Take as soon as you remember. If it is almost time for the next dose, wait for that dose (don't double this dose) and resume regular schedule.

What drug does:
An antiplatelet drug works by preventing platelets (a type of blood cell) from clumping and forming clots that reduce blood flow and may cause a heart attack or stroke.

Time lapse before drug works:
It starts working within 1 to 2 hours.

Don't take with:
Any other medicine or dietary supplement without consulting your doctor or pharmacist.

OVERDOSE

SYMPTOMS:
Nausea, vomiting, irregular heartbeat, and increased risk of bleeding.
WHAT TO DO:
Overdose unlikely to threaten life. If person takes much larger amount than prescribed or if accidentally swallowed, call doctor or poison control center 1-800-222-1222 for help.

POSSIBLE ADVERSE REACTIONS OR SIDE EFFECTS

SYMPTOMS	WHAT TO DO
Life-threatening:	
Rare allergic reaction (hives, itching, rash, wheezing, tightness in chest, swelling of lips or tongue or throat).	Seek emergency treatment immediately.
Common:	
Difficult breathing or shortness of breath, nosebleeds.	Continue, but call doctor right away.
Infrequent:	
• Unusual bleeding from the gums or vagina or rectum or eyes, black or tarry stools, red or brown urine, coughing up blood or coffee-ground material, unusual bruising, purple or red spots under the skin, fast or slow or irregular heartbeat, chest pain.	Continue, but call doctor right away.
• Dizziness, faintness, headache, diarrhea, upset stomach, unusual tiredness or weakness, back pain, cough, nausea.	Continue. Call doctor when convenient.
Rare:	
• Bleeding in the brain (may have symptoms of sudden numbness or weakness on one side of the body, sudden and severe headache, confusion, balance or vision problems).	Seek emergency help immediately.
• Low or high blood pressure.	Continue. Call doctor when convenient.

WARNINGS & PRECAUTIONS

Don't take if:
You are allergic to ticagrelor.

Before you start, consult your doctor if:

- You have a history of intracranial hemorrhage (bleeding in the brain).
- You have a liver (hepatic) disorder.
- You have a bleeding problem such as a peptic ulcer.
- You have lung disease or breathing problems (e.g., asthma or COPD).
- You plan on having surgery (including dental surgery) in the near future.

Over age 60:
May have increased risk of side effects.

Pregnancy:
Decide with your doctor whether drug benefits justify risk to unborn child. Risk category C (see page xviii).

Breast-feeding:
It is unknown if drug passes into breast milk. Breast-feeding is not recommended while taking this drug. Consult your doctor for advice.

Infants & children:
Safety and efficacy not established for ages under 18.

Prolonged use:
Talk to your doctor about the need for follow-up medical exams or laboratory studies to check the effectiveness of the treatment.

Skin & sunlight:
No problems expected.

Driving, piloting or hazardous work:
Avoid if you experience dizziness or faintness, otherwise no problems expected.

Discontinuing:
Don't discontinue without doctor's approval. Stopping the drug can increase the risk of blood clots and their complications.

Others:

- Advise any doctor, dentist or pharmacist whom you consult that you take this drug.
- While taking this drug you will likely bruise and bleed more easily than usual or bleed for longer than usual. Avoid rough sports or other situations where you could be bruised, cut or injured. Be extra careful when using sharp objects. Bleeding complications can be serious or fatal. Consult doctor if you have any concerns or questions about side effects.
- Drug use may increase risk of serious bleeding during a surgery, other medical procedures or some types of dental work. You may be advised to stop using this drug at least 5 days before a surgery, medical procedure or dental work.

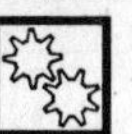

POSSIBLE INTERACTION WITH OTHER DRUGS

GENERIC NAME OR DRUG CLASS	COMBINED EFFECT
Anticoagulants*	Increased risk of bleeding.
Anti-inflammatory drugs, nonsteroidal (NSAIDs)*	Increased risk of bleeding.
Antiplatelet drugs,* other	Increased risk of bleeding.
Aspirin	Decreased effect of ticagrelor if you take more than 100 mg of aspirin daily.
Digoxin	Increased effect of digoxin.
Enzyme inducers*	Decreased effect of ticagrelor.
Enzyme inhibitors*	Increased effect of ticagrelor.
HMG-CoA reductase inhibitors	Increased side effects of certain HMG-CoA inhibitors.

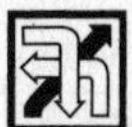

POSSIBLE INTERACTION WITH OTHER SUBSTANCES

INTERACTS WITH	COMBINED EFFECT
Alcohol:	None expected.
Beverages: Grapefruit juice.	May increase effect of ticagrelor.
Cocaine:	Unknown effect. Avoid.
Foods: Grapefruit.	May increase effect of ticagrelor.
Marijuana:	Unknown effect. Avoid.
Tobacco:	None expected, but people with heart disorders should not smoke.

***See Glossary**

TIOPRONIN

BRAND NAMES

Capen
Captimer
Epatiol
Mucolysin
Sutilan
Thiola
Thiosol
Tioglis
Vincol

BASIC INFORMATION

Habit forming? No
Prescription needed? Yes
Available as generic? No
Drug class: Antiurolithic

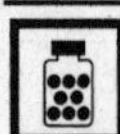

USES

Prevents the formation of kidney stones when there is too much cystine in the urine.

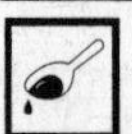

DOSAGE & USAGE INFORMATION

How to take:
Tablet—Swallow with liquid. If you can't swallow whole, crumble tablet and take with liquid or food. Instructions to take on empty stomach mean 1 hour before or 2 hours after eating.

When to take:
3 times daily (once approximately every 8 hours).

If you forget a dose:
Take as soon as you remember. If it is almost time for the next dose, wait for that dose (don't double this dose) and resume regular schedule.

What drug does:
Removes high levels of cystine from the body.

Time lapse before drug works:
It starts working right away, but full benefit may take weeks to months. Laboratory studies are used to measure the cystine in the urine.

Continued next column

OVERDOSE

SYMPTOMS:
None expected. If overdose is suspected, follow instructions below.
WHAT TO DO:
- **Dial 911 (emergency) for medical help or call poison control center 1-800-222-1222 for instructions.**
- **See emergency information on last 3 pages of this book.**

Don't take with:
- Medicines that are known to cause kidney damage or depress bone marrow.
- Any other medicine or any dietary supplement without consulting your doctor or pharmacist.

POSSIBLE ADVERSE REACTIONS OR SIDE EFFECTS

SYMPTOMS	WHAT TO DO
Life-threatening:	
Rare allergic reaction (hives, itching, rash, wheezing, tightness in chest, swelling of lips or tongue or throat).	Seek emergency treatment immediately.
Common:	
• Skin rash, itching skin, mouth sores, mouth ulcers.	Discontinue. Call doctor right away.
• Abdominal pain, gaseousness, diarrhea, nausea or vomiting.	Continue. Call doctor when convenient.
Infrequent:	
• Cloudy urine, chills, breathing difficulty, joint pain.	Discontinue. Call doctor right away.
• Impaired smell or taste.	Continue. Call doctor when convenient.
Rare:	
Coughing up blood, fever, unusual tiredness or weakness, double vision, muscle weakness.	Discontinue. Call doctor right away.

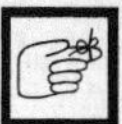

WARNINGS & PRECAUTIONS

Don't take if:
You are allergic to tiopronin or penicillamine.

Before you start, consult your doctor if:
You have had any of the following in the past:
- Agranulocytosis.
- Aplastic anemia.
- Thrombocytopenia.
- Impaired kidney function.

Over age 60:
May require dosage adjustment if kidney function is impaired.

Pregnancy:
Decide with your doctor if drug benefits justify risk to unborn child. Risk category C (see page xviii).

Breast-feeding:
Drug passes into milk. Avoid or discontinue nursing until you finish medicine. Consult doctor for advice on maintaining milk supply.

Infants & children:
Safety not established. Consult doctor.

Prolonged use:
No special problems expected.

Skin & sunlight:
No special problems expected.

Driving, piloting or hazardous work:
Don't drive or pilot aircraft until you learn how medicine affects you. Don't work around dangerous machinery. Don't climb ladders or work in high places. Danger increases if you drink alcohol or take medicine affecting alertness and reflexes.

Discontinuing:
No special problems expected.

Others:
- Advise any doctor or dentist whom you consult that you take this medicine.
- May affect results of some medical tests.

POSSIBLE INTERACTION WITH OTHER DRUGS

GENERIC NAME OR DRUG CLASS	COMBINED EFFECT
Bone marrow depressants*	May increase possibility of toxic effects of tiopronin.
Medications toxic to kidneys (nephrotoxins*)	May increase possibility of toxic effects of tiopronin.

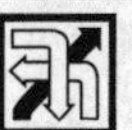

POSSIBLE INTERACTION WITH OTHER SUBSTANCES

INTERACTS WITH	COMBINED EFFECT
Alcohol:	None expected.
Beverages:	
Water.	Enhances effects of tiopronin. Drink 8 to 10 glasses daily.
Cocaine:	None expected.
Foods:	None expected.
Marijuana:	None expected.
Tobacco:	None expected.

***See Glossary**

TIZANIDINE

BRAND NAMES

Zanaflex

BASIC INFORMATION

Habit forming? No
Prescription needed? Yes
Available as generic? Yes
Drug class: Antispastic, muscle relaxant

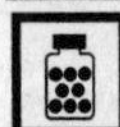

USES

- Relieves muscle spasticity caused by diseases such as multiple sclerosis. It does not appear to improve muscle weakness.
- Relieves muscle spasticity caused by injury to spinal cord.

DOSAGE & USAGE INFORMATION

How to take:
Tablet or capsule—Swallow with liquid. Follow instructions on your prescription about whether to take with food or not. Food can change the amount of the drug absorbed by your body.

When to take:
Up to three times a day or as directed by your doctor.

If you forget a dose:
Take as soon as you remember. If it is almost time for the next dose, wait for that dose (don't double this dose) and resume regular schedule.

What drug does:
Slows nerve impulses that stimulate skeletal muscles, decreasing cramping.

Time lapse before drug works:
Within hours. Dosage may be increased over a several week period to achieve maximum effectiveness.

Don't take with:
Any other medicine or any dietary supplement without consulting your doctor or pharmacist.

OVERDOSE

SYMPTOMS:
Breathing difficulties, heartbeat irregularities, sleepiness, confusion, coma.
WHAT TO DO:
- **Dial 911 (emergency) for medical help or call poison control center 1-800-222-1222 for instructions.**
- **See emergency information on last 3 pages of this book.**

POSSIBLE ADVERSE REACTIONS OR SIDE EFFECTS

SYMPTOMS	WHAT TO DO
Life-threatening:	
In case of overdose, see previous column.	
Common:	
• Nervousness, sensation changes (tingling, burning, prickling), skin sores, anxiety, tiredness or weakness, constipation, back pain, dizziness, dry mouth, depression, drowsiness, heartburn, lightheadedness when getting up from a sitting or lying position, increase in muscle spasm, muscle weakness, sore throat, runny nose, increased sweating.	Continue. Call doctor when convenient.
• Fever, liver problems, (weight loss, nausea, vomiting, yellow skin or eyes), pain or burning when urinating, involuntary movements, diarrhea, vomiting, stomach pain, speech problems.	Discontinue. Call doctor when convenient.
Infrequent:	
• Heartbeat irregularity, black or tarry stools, seizures, bloody vomit, fever and chills, fainting.	Discontinue. Call doctor right away
• Mental changes, mood changes, dry skin, swelling of hands or feet or other areas of the body, difficulty swallowing, migraine, neck pain, trembling or shaking, weight loss, joint or muscle pain, skin rash, feeling of coldness, puffy skin, weight gain, cough, white patches on tongue or in mouth, visual changes or eye pain.	Continue. Call doctor when convenient.
Rare:	
Other symptoms not mentioned above.	Continue. Call doctor when convenient.

WARNINGS & PRECAUTIONS

Don't take if:
You are allergic to tizanidine.

Before you start, consult your doctor if:
- You have liver disease.
- You have kidney disease.
- You are allergic to any medication, food or other substance.
- You are taking an alpha-adrenergic blood pressure medicine.

Over age 60:
Adverse reactions and side effects may be more frequent and severe than in younger persons. Lower dosage may be recommended to start.

Pregnancy:
Decide with your doctor if drug benefits justify risk to unborn child. Risk category C (see page xviii).

Breast-feeding:
It is unknown if drug passes into milk. Avoid nursing or discontinue until you finish drug. Consult doctor.

Infants & children:
Safety and dosage have not been established.

Prolonged use:
Talk to your doctor about the need for liver function studies while using this drug.

Skin & sunlight:
No special problems expected.

Driving, piloting or hazardous work:
Don't drive or pilot aircraft until you learn how medicine affects you. Don't work around dangerous machinery. Don't climb ladders or work in high places. Danger increases if you drink alcohol or take medicine affecting alertness and reflexes, such as antihistamines, tranquilizers, sedatives, pain medicine, narcotics and mind-altering drugs.

Discontinuing:
Don't discontinue without consulting doctor.

Others:
- May interfere with the results in some medical tests.
- Get up slowly from a sitting or lying position to avoid any dizziness, faintness or lightheadedness.
- Advise any doctor or dentist whom you consult that you take this medicine.
- The brand name Zanaflex is available as a tablet and a capsule. The two formulations are not interchangeable. Switching from the capsule to the tablet may increase risk of side effects.
- Take medicine only as directed. Do not increase or reduce dosage without doctor's approval.

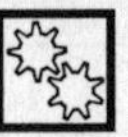

POSSIBLE INTERACTION WITH OTHER DRUGS

GENERIC NAME OR DRUG CLASS	COMBINED EFFECT
Central nervous system (CNS) depressants *	Increased sedation.
Ciprofloxacin	Dangerous increased tizanidine effect. Avoid.
Contraceptives, oral	Increased effect of tizanidine.
Enzyme Inhibitors*	Increased effect of tizanidine.
Fluvoxamine	Dangerous increased tizanidine effect. Avoid.
Hypotension-causing drugs,* other	Increased effect of hypotension.

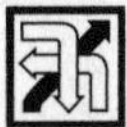

POSSIBLE INTERACTION WITH OTHER SUBSTANCES

INTERACTS WITH	COMBINED EFFECT
Alcohol:	Increased sedation, low blood pressure. Avoid.
Beverages:	None expected.
Cocaine:	Increased spasticity. Avoid.
Foods:	Follow prescription instructions about taking with food.
Marijuana:	Increased spasticity or sedation. Avoid.
Tobacco:	May interfere with absorption of medicine.

***See Glossary**

TOFACITINIB

BRAND NAMES

Xeljanz

BASIC INFORMATION

Habit forming? No
Prescription needed? Yes
Available as generic? No
Drug class: JAK (Janus kinase) inhibitor

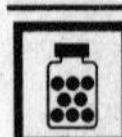

USES

- Treatment of moderate to severe rheumatoid arthritis (RA) in adults. It may be used alone or with other medications.
- May be used to treat other conditions as determined by your doctor.

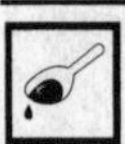

DOSAGE & USAGE INFORMATION

How to take:
Tablet—Swallow whole with liquid. It may be taken with or without food (food may lessen stomach upset).

When to take:
Drug is taken twice a day at the same times each day.

If you forget a dose:
Take as soon as you remember. If it is almost time for the next dose, wait for the next scheduled dose (don't double this dose).

What drug does:
It works by blocking Janus kinase (JAK) a component of the body's cells that plays a role in activating the inflammation involved with RA.

Time lapse before drug works:
One to 2 days, but it takes 2 weeks or longer for symptoms to start improving and may be months to feel full benefits.

Don't take with:
Any other medicine or any dietary supplement without consulting your doctor or pharmacist.

OVERDOSE

SYMPTOMS:
Unknown.
WHAT TO DO:
Overdose unlikely to threaten life. If person takes much larger amount than prescribed or if accidentally swallowed, call doctor or poison control center 1-800-222-1222 for help.

POSSIBLE ADVERSE REACTIONS OR SIDE EFFECTS

SYMPTOMS	WHAT TO DO
Life-threatening:	
Rare allergic reaction (hives, itching, rash, wheezing, tightness in chest, swelling of lips or tongue or throat).	Seek emergency treatment immediately.
Common:	
Cold or flu-like symptoms (stuffy nose, fever, chills, cough, sneezing, sore throat), bloody or cloudy urine, difficult or painful or frequent urination, high blood pressure.	Continue, but call doctor right away.
Infrequent:	
Headache, diarrhea, dizziness, heartburn, indigestion, nausea.	Continue. Call doctor when convenient.
Rare:	
Serious infections may occur and symptoms will vary: unusual weakness or tiredness, yellow eyes or skin, change in stool (lighter color or black or tarry), unusual bruising, painful skin rash or blisters, general ill feeling, abdominal pain, chest pain, persistent cough, loss of appetite, unusual weight loss, night sweats, severe headache or dizziness, shortness of breath, numbness or tingling, swelling (feet, ankles, legs, hands or joints), muscle or joint pain, vomiting or coughing up blood, change in bowel habits, swollen lymph nodes, other symptoms that cause concern.	Discontinue. Call doctor right away.

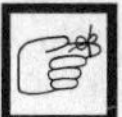

WARNINGS & PRECAUTIONS

Don't take if:
You are allergic to tofacitinib.

Before you start, consult your doctor if:
- You have a history of anemia or low blood cell counts.
- You have an infection or a history of chronic infections (e.g., bacteria, virus or fungus).
- You have stomach or bowel problems (e.g., ulcers, ulcerative colitis, diverticulitis or perforation).
- You have or have had cancer.
- You have or have had kidney or liver disease (including hepatitis).
- You have weakened immune system due to illness (e.g., diabetes or HIV) or drugs.
- You have hyperlipidemia (high cholesterol or fats in the blood).
- You have recently received or are scheduled to receive a vaccine.
- You have or have had or been exposed to tuberculosis (TB). You will need a skin test for TB before taking drug.

Over age 60:
May be more at risk of side effects such as infections.

Pregnancy:
Decide with your doctor whether drug benefits justify risk to unborn child. Risk category C (see page xviii).

Breast-feeding:
It is unknown if drug passes into breast milk. Consult your doctor for advice.

Infants & children:
Safety and efficacy have not been established.

Prolonged use:
- See your doctor for regular visits to make sure the drug is working properly, to obtain recommended blood tests and to check for unwanted effects.
- Long term efficacy of drug is not known.

Skin & sunlight:
No problems expected.

Driving, piloting or hazardous work:
No problems expected.

Discontinuing:
No problems expected, but consult your doctor before discontinuing. Certain lab tests may be required for a period of time after stopping drug.

Others:
- Patients taking this drug are at increased risk for infections that can be serious and possibly fatal. These include bacterial, viral and fungal infections; tuberculosis; cancer; lymphoma; herpes zoster (shingles) and others. Also, gastrointestinal perforations have occurred. Consult doctor about your risks.
- It is important to obtain all recommended laboratory blood tests while taking this drug.
- Advise any doctor, dentist or pharmacist whom you consult that you take this drug.

POSSIBLE INTERACTION WITH OTHER DRUGS

GENERIC NAME OR DRUG CLASS	COMBINED EFFECT
Biologic response modifiers*	Increased risk of infection. Avoid.
Enzyme inducers*	May decrease effect of tofacitinib.
Enzyme inhibitors*	May increase effect of tofacitinib.
Immunosuppressants*	Increased risk of infections. Avoid.
Live vaccines	May decrease vaccine effect. Possible infection. Avoid.

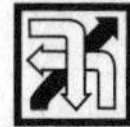

POSSIBLE INTERACTION WITH OTHER SUBSTANCES

INTERACTS WITH	COMBINED EFFECT
Alcohol:	None expected.
Beverages:	None expected.
Cocaine:	Effect unknown. Avoid.
Foods:	None expected.
Marijuana:	Effect unknown. Avoid.
Tobacco:	None expected.

*See Glossary

TOPIRAMATE

BRAND NAMES

Qsymia
Topamax
Topamax Sprinkle Capsules
Trokendi XR

BASIC INFORMATION

Habit forming? No
Prescription needed? Yes
Available as generic? Yes
Drug class: Anticonvulsant, antiepileptic

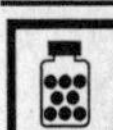

USES

- Treatment for partial (focal) epileptic seizures. May be used alone or in combination with other antiepileptic drugs.
- Treats overweight and obesity in adults.
- Used to prevent migraine headache in adults.

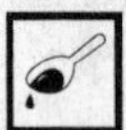

DOSAGE & USAGE INFORMATION

How to take:

- Tablet—Swallow the tablets whole with a drink of water; do not crush or chew (the tablet has a bitter taste). May be taken with or without food and on a full or empty stomach.
- Sprinkle capsules—Can be swallowed whole or opened carefully and the contents sprinkled on a small amount of soft food, such as applesauce, pudding, ice cream, oatmeal or yogurt. Swallow this mixture immediately. Do not chew or store for later use.
- Extended-release capsule—Swallow whole with liquid. Do not crush, chew or open capsule.

When to take:
Your doctor will determine the best schedule. Dosages will be increased rapidly over the first weeks of use. Further increases may be necessary to achieve maximum benefits.

Continued next column

OVERDOSE

SYMPTOMS:
Slow or irregular heartbeat, confusion, dizziness, faintness, unusual tiredness or weakness, blue skin or fingernails, breathing difficulty, coma.
WHAT TO DO:

- **Dial 911 (emergency) for medical help or call poison control center 1-800-222-1222 for instructions.**
- **See emergency information on last 3 pages of this book.**

If you forget a dose:
Take as soon as you remember. If it is almost time for the next dose, skip the missed dose and wait for your next scheduled dose (don't double this dose).

What drug does:
The exact mechanism of the anticonvulsant effect is unknown. It appears to block the spread of seizures rather than raise the seizure threshold like other anticonvulsants. Topiramate's anticonvulsant actions involve several mechanisms.

Time lapse before drug works:
May take several weeks for effectiveness.

Don't take with:
Any other medicine or any dietary supplement without consulting your doctor or pharmacist.

POSSIBLE ADVERSE REACTIONS OR SIDE EFFECTS

SYMPTOMS	WHAT TO DO
Life-threatening:	
In case of overdose, see previous column.	
Common:	
• Burning, prickling, or tingling sensations; clumsiness or unsteadiness; confusion; continuous, uncontrolled back-and-forth or rolling eye movements; dizziness; double vision or other vision problems; drowsiness; generalized slowing of mental and physical activity; memory problems; menstrual changes; menstrual pain; nervousness; speech or language problems; trouble in concentrating or paying attention; unusual tiredness or weakness.	Continue, but call doctor right away.
• Breast pain in women, nausea, tremor.	Continue. Call doctor when convenient.
Infrequent:	
• Abdominal pain; fever, chills; sore throat; lessening of sensations or perception; loss of appetite; mood or mental changes (such as aggression, agitation, apathy, irritability, and depression); red, irritated, or bleeding gums; weight loss.	Continue, but call doctor right away.

• Back pain, chest pain, constipation, heartburn, hot flushes, increased sweating, leg pain.	Continue. Call doctor when convenient.
Rare:	
Eye pain, frequent or difficult urination, bloody urine, hearing loss, itching, unsteadiness, loss of bladder control, lower back or side pain, nosebleeds, pale skin, red or irritated eyes, ringing or buzzing in ears, skin rash, swelling, troubled breathing.	Continue, but call doctor right away.

WARNINGS & PRECAUTIONS

Don't take if:
You are allergic to topiramate.

Before you start, consult your doctor if:
- You have a history of liver disease.
- You have kidney disease or kidney stones (nephrolithiasis).
- You are allergic to any medication, food or other substance.
- You have any other medical problems.

Over age 60:
No special problems expected.

Pregnancy:
Risk of birth defects to unborn child exists. Risk category D (see page xviii).

Breast-feeding:
It is unknown if drug passes into milk. Avoid drug or discontinue nursing until you finish medicine. Consult doctor for advice on maintaining milk supply.

Infants & children:
This medicine is approved for use from age 2 on. Dose is according to body weight. This medicine is not expected to cause different side effects or problems in children than it does in adults.

Prolonged use:
No special problems expected. Follow-up laboratory blood studies may be recommended by your doctor.

Skin & sunlight:
No problems expected.

Driving, piloting or hazardous work:
Don't drive or pilot aircraft until you learn how medicine affects you. Don't work around dangerous machinery. Don't climb ladders or work in high places. Danger increases if you drink alcohol or take other medicines affecting alertness and reflexes.

Discontinuing:
Don't discontinue without doctor's approval due to risk of increased seizure activity. The dosage may need to be gradually decreased before stopping the drug completely.

Others:
- Advise any doctor or dentist whom you consult that you take this medicine.
- Drink plenty of fluids while taking topiramate. If you have had kidney stones in the past, this will help to reduce your chances of forming kidney stones.
- Topiramate may be used with other anticonvulsant drugs and additional side effects may also occur. If they do, discuss them with your doctor.
- Rarely, antiepileptic drugs may lead to suicidal thoughts and behaviors. Call doctor right away if suicidal symptoms or unusual behaviors occur.
- Wear or carry medical identification to show your seizure disorder and the drugs you take.

POSSIBLE INTERACTION WITH OTHER DRUGS

GENERIC NAME OR DRUG CLASS	COMBINED EFFECT
Anticonvulsants,* other	May decrease or increase effect of both drugs.
Carbonic anhydrase inhibitors*	Increased risk of kidney stones.
Central nervous system (CNS) depressants*	Increased sedative effect.
Contraceptives, oral*	Decreased effect of contraceptive.
Digoxin	May decrease effect of digoxin.

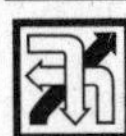

POSSIBLE INTERACTION WITH OTHER SUBSTANCES

INTERACTS WITH	COMBINED EFFECT
Alcohol:	Increased sedative effect. Avoid.
Beverages:	None expected.
Cocaine:	Unknown effect. Avoid.
Foods:	None expected.
Marijuana:	Unknown effect. Avoid.
Tobacco:	None expected.

***See Glossary**

TOREMIFENE

BRAND NAMES

Fareston

BASIC INFORMATION

Habit forming? No
Prescription needed? Yes
Available as generic? No
Drug class: Antineoplastic

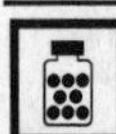

USES

Used to treat breast cancer in postmenopausal women.

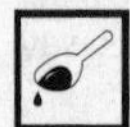

DOSAGE & USAGE INFORMATION

How to take:
Tablet—Swallow with water and take with or without food. If you can't swallow whole, crumble tablet and take with liquid or food.

When to take:
At the same time each day.

If you forget a dose:
Take as soon as possible. If it is almost time for your next dose, skip the missed dose and go back to your regular dosing schedule. Do not double doses.

What drug does:
Exact mechanism unknown. Appears to block growth-stimulating effects of estrogen in the tumor.

Time lapse before drug works:
4 to 6 weeks to determine effectiveness.

Don't take with:
Any other medicine or any dietary supplement without consulting your doctor or pharmacist.

OVERDOSE

SYMPTOMS:
Dizziness, headache, nausea and vomiting.
WHAT TO DO:
Overdose unlikely to threaten life. If person uses much larger amount than prescribed or if accidentally swallowed, call doctor or poison control center 1-800-222-1222 for help.

POSSIBLE ADVERSE REACTIONS OR SIDE EFFECTS

SYMPTOMS	WHAT TO DO
Life-threatening:	
Pain or swelling of feet or lower legs, chest pain, shortness of breath.	Seek emergency treatment immediately.
Common:	
Hot flashes, nausea.	Continue. Call doctor if symptoms persist.
Infrequent:	
• Change in vaginal discharge, pain or feeling of pressure in pelvis, vaginal bleeding, confusion, increased urination, loss of appetite, unusual tiredness, changes in vision.	Continue. Call doctor right away.
• Dizziness, dry eyes, bone pain, vomiting.	Continue. Call doctor if symptoms persist.
Rare:	
None expected.	

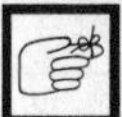

WARNINGS & PRECAUTIONS

Don't take if:
- You are allergic to toremifene.
- You have a history of blood clots or have been diagnosed with thromboembolic disease.

Before you start, consult your doctor if:
- You have any other medical problem.
- You have any blood or bleeding disorder.
- You have ever been diagnosed with endometrial hyperplasia (unusual growth of the lining of the uterus).
- You have a tumor that has spread to your bone.

Over age 60:
No problems expected.

Pregnancy:
Consult doctor. Risk category D (see page xviii).

Breast-feeding:
Drug may pass into milk. Avoid drug or discontinue nursing until you finish medicine. Consult doctor about maintaining milk supply.

Infants & children:
There is no identified potential use of toremifene in children.

Prolonged use:
Talk to your doctor about the need for follow-up laboratory studies to check complete blood count, blood calcium concentrations and liver function.

Skin & sunlight:
Avoid prolonged or extended exposure to direct sunlight and/or artificial sunlight while using this medication.

Driving, piloting or hazardous work:
No problems expected.

Discontinuing:
Don't discontinue without consulting doctor.

Others:
- Advise any doctor or dentist you consult that you are taking this medication.
- May interfere with the accuracy of some medical tests.

POSSIBLE INTERACTION WITH OTHER DRUGS

GENERIC NAME OR DRUG CLASS	COMBINED EFFECT
Anticoagulants	May increase time it takes blood to clot.
Diuretics, thiazide	Possible increased calcium.
Enzyme inducers*	May lessen the effect of toremifene.
Enzyme inhibitors*	May increase the effect of toremifene.

POSSIBLE INTERACTION WITH OTHER SUBSTANCES

INTERACTS WITH	COMBINED EFFECT
Alcohol:	None expected.
Beverages:	None expected.
Cocaine:	Effects unknown. Avoid.
Foods:	None expected.
Marijuana:	Effects unknown. Avoid.
Tobacco:	None expected.

***See Glossary**

TRAMADOL

BRAND NAMES

CIP-Tramadol ER
Ryzolt
Ultracet
Ultram
Ultram ER
Ultram ODT

BASIC INFORMATION

Habit forming? Yes
Prescription needed? Yes
Available as generic? Yes
Drug class: Analgesic

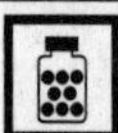

USES

Treatment for moderate to moderately severe pain (used more for chronic than acute pain).

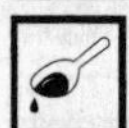

DOSAGE & USAGE INFORMATION

How to take:

- Tablet or extended-release tablet—Swallow whole with liquid. May be taken with or without food. Do not crush, chew or split tablet. It is for oral use only. Read prescription instructions.
- Disintegrating tablet—Let tablet dissolve in mouth. Do not crush, chew or split tablet. It is for oral use only. Read prescription instructions.

When to take:
Every 4 to 6 hours as needed for pain. Extended release form is taken once a day.

If you forget a dose:
Take as soon as you remember. If it is almost time for the next dose, wait for next scheduled dose (don't double this dose).

What drug does:
Exact mechanism unknown. It appears to block pain messages to the brain and spinal cord.

Continued next column

OVERDOSE

SYMPTOMS:
Breathing difficulty, sleepiness, seizures, cold/clammy skin, slow heartbeat, low blood pressure, stupor, coma. Deaths due to overdose have been reported with abuse and misuse of tramadol, by ingesting, inhaling, or injecting the crushed tablets.
WHAT TO DO:

- **Dial 911 (emergency) for medical help or call poison control center 1-800-222-1222 for instructions.**
- **See emergency information on last 3 pages of this book.**

Time lapse before drug works:
Within 60 minutes.

Don't take with:
Any other medicine or any dietary supplement without consulting your doctor or pharmacist.

POSSIBLE ADVERSE REACTIONS OR SIDE EFFECTS

SYMPTOMS	WHAT TO DO
Life-threatening:	
Rare allergic reaction (hives, itching, rash, trouble breathing, tightness in chest, swelling of lips or tongue or face).	Seek emergency treatment immediately.
Common:	
Constipation, nausea, headache, drowsiness, clumsiness, dizziness, itching, flushing or redness of skin, trouble sleeping.	Continue. Call doctor when convenient.
Infrequent:	
• Constant urge to urinate or inability to urinate, blurred vision.	Discontinue. Call doctor right away.
• Loss of appetite, stomach pain, dry mouth, weakness, confusion, sweating, diarrhea, gas, hot flashes, nervousness, heartburn, tiredness.	Continue. Call doctor when convenient.
Rare:	
Seizures, balancing difficulty, skin reaction (itching, redness and swelling), memory problems, shortness of breath, difficulty performing tasks, hallucinations, lightheadedness when getting up from a sitting or lying position, sensations in hands and feet (burning, tingling, pain, weakness, trembling or shaking), faintness, fast heartbeat.	Discontinue. Call doctor right away.

WARNINGS & PRECAUTIONS

Don't take if:
You are allergic to tramadol or narcotic drugs or you are sensitive to any ingredients in the drug.

Before you start, consult your doctor if:
- You have kidney or liver disease, seizure disorder, stomach disorder or prior head injury.
- You have a history of depression, mental illness or suicidal thoughts or behaviors.
- You have a history of drug abuse or substance abuse, including alcohol abuse.
- You have respiratory problems.

Over age 60:
Increased risk of side effects. Patients over age 75 usually require a dosage adjustment.

Pregnancy:
Decide with your doctor if drug benefits justify risk to unborn child. Risk category C (see page xviii).

Breast-feeding:
Drug passes into milk. Avoid drug or discontinue nursing until you finish medicine. Consult doctor for advice on maintaining milk supply.

Infants & children:
Safety in children under age 18 has not been established.

Prolonged use:
- Consult with your doctor on a regular basis while using this drug.
- Can cause drug dependence, addiction and withdrawal symptoms.

Skin & sunlight:
No special problems expected.

Driving, piloting or hazardous work:
Don't drive or pilot aircraft until you learn how medicine affects you. Don't work around dangerous machinery. Don't climb ladders or work in high places. Danger increases if you drink alcohol or take medicine affecting alertness and reflexes.

Discontinuing:
If you have taken this drug for a long time, consult with your doctor before discontinuing. Withdrawal symptoms may occur if drug is discontinued abruptly. Symptoms include: anxiety, sweating, insomnia, pain, nausea, tremors, diarrhea, breathing problems and hallucinations. Call doctor if symptoms occur.

Others:
- Don't increase dosage or frequency of use without your doctor's approval. Development of a potentially life-threatening serotonin syndrome* or overdose (which can be fatal) may occur with the use of tramadol.
- Advise any doctor or dentist whom you consult that you take this medicine.

POSSIBLE INTERACTION WITH OTHER DRUGS

GENERIC NAME OR DRUG CLASS	COMBINED EFFECT
Carbamazepine	Decreased effect of tramadol.
Central nervous system (CNS) depressants*	Serious adverse events including breathing difficulty.
Clozapine	May increase risk of seizures.
Cyclobenzaprine	May increase risk of seizures.
Digoxin	May increase risk of digoxin toxicity.
Enzyme inducers*	May decrease effect of tramadol.
Enzyme inhibitors*	May increase effect of tramadol.
Monoamine oxidase (MAO) inhibitors*	Serious adverse events including seizures and serotonin syndrome.*
Narcotics*	Increased risk of side effects and seizures.
Phenothiazines*	Increased risk of side effects.
Quinidine	Unknown effect. May need to adjust dose.
Serotonergics*	Increased risk of seizures and serotonin syndrome.*
Tranquilizers*	Increased risk of side effects.
Warfarin	May increase risk of bleeding.

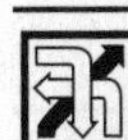

POSSIBLE INTERACTION WITH OTHER SUBSTANCES

INTERACTS WITH	COMBINED EFFECT
Alcohol:	Serious side effects. Avoid.
Beverages:	None expected.
Cocaine:	Unknown. Avoid.
Foods:	None expected.
Marijuana:	Unknown. Avoid.
Tobacco:	None expected.

***See Glossary**

TRAZODONE

BRAND NAMES

Oleptro
Trazon
Trialodine

BASIC INFORMATION

Habit forming? No
Prescription needed? Yes
Available as generic? Yes
Drug class: Antidepressant (nontricyclic)

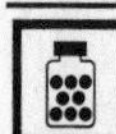

USES

- Treats mental depression.
- Treats anxiety.
- Helps promote sleep.
- Treats some types of chronic pain.

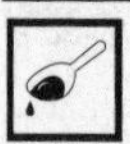

DOSAGE & USAGE INFORMATION

How to take:

- Tablet—Swallow with liquid or food to lessen stomach irritation. If you can't swallow whole, crumble tablet and take with liquid or food.
- Extended release tablet—Swallow whole. Do not crumble or crush tablet.

When to take:
According to prescription directions. Bedtime dose usually higher than other doses.

If you forget a dose:
Take dose as soon as you remember. If it is almost time for the next dose, wait for the next scheduled dose (don't double this dose).

What drug does:
Maintains balance of certain brain chemicals.

Time lapse before drug works:
2 to 4 weeks for full effect.

Continued next column

OVERDOSE

SYMPTOMS:
Fainting, irregular heartbeat, respiratory arrest, chest pain, seizures, coma.
WHAT TO DO:

- **Dial 911 (emergency) for medical help or call poison control center 1-800-222-1222 for instructions.**
- **If person is unconscious, check breathing and pulse. If not breathing, begin mouth-to-mouth rescue breathing. If heart is not beating, begin chest compressions.**
- **See emergency information on last 3 pages of this book.**

Don't take with:
Any other medicine or any dietary supplement without consulting your doctor or pharmacist.

POSSIBLE ADVERSE REACTIONS OR SIDE EFFECTS

SYMPTOMS	WHAT TO DO
Life-threatening:	
In case of overdose, see previous column.	
Common:	
Drowsiness.	Continue. Call doctor when convenient.
Infrequent:	
• Prolonged penile erections that may be very painful (priapism).	Seek emergency treatment immediately.
• Tremor, fainting, incoordination, blood pressure rise or drop, rapid heartbeat, shortness of breath.	Discontinue. Call doctor right away.
• Disorientation, confusion, fatigue, dizziness on standing, headache, nervousness, rash, itchy skin, blurred vision, ringing in ears, dry mouth, bad taste, diarrhea, nausea, vomiting, constipation, aching, menstrual changes, diminished sex drive, nightmares, vivid dreams.	Continue. Call doctor when convenient.
Rare:	
Unusual excitement.	Discontinue. Call doctor right away.

WARNINGS & PRECAUTIONS

Don't take if:

- You are allergic to trazodone.
- You are thinking about suicide.

Before you start, consult your doctor if:

- You have heart rhythm problem.
- You have any heart disease.
- You will have surgery within 2 months, including dental surgery, requiring general or spinal anesthesia.
- You have bipolar (manic-depressive) disorder.
- You have liver or kidney disease.

Over age 60:
Adverse reactions and side effects may be more frequent and severe than in younger persons.

TRILOSTANE

BRAND NAMES

Modrastane

BASIC INFORMATION

Habit forming? No
Prescription needed? Yes
Available as generic? No
Drug class: Antiadrenal

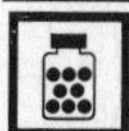

USES

Temporary treatment of Cushing's syndrome until surgery on adrenals or radiation to pituitary gland can be performed.

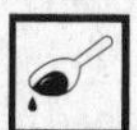

DOSAGE & USAGE INFORMATION

How to take:
Capsule—Swallow with liquid. If you can't swallow whole, open capsule and take with liquid or food. Instructions to take on empty stomach mean 1 hour before or 2 hours after eating.

When to take:
Follow doctor's instructions.

If you forget a dose:
Take as soon as you remember. If it is almost time for the next dose, wait for that dose (don't double this dose) and resume regular schedule.

What drug does:
Decreases function of the adrenal cortex.

Time lapse before drug works:
8 hours.

Don't take with:
Any other medicines (including over-the-counter drugs such as cough and cold medicines, axatives, antacids, diet pills, caffeine, nose drops vitamins) without consulting your doctor or armacist.

OVERDOSE

TOMS:
xpected.
O DO:
e unlikely to threaten life. If person ch larger amount than prescribed or tally swallowed, call doctor or ntrol center 1-800-222-1222 for help.

POSSIBLE ADVERSE REACTIONS OR SIDE EFFECTS

SYMPTOMS	WHAT TO DO
Life-threatening: None expected.	
Common: Diarrhea, abdominal pain.	Discontinue. Call doctor right away.
Infrequent: Muscle ache, bloating, watery eyes, nausea, increased salivation, flushing, burning mouth or nose.	Continue. Call doctor when convenient.
Rare: Darkening skin, tiredness, appetite loss, depression, skin rash, vomiting.	Continue. Call doctor when convenient.

TRAZODONE

Pregnancy:
Decide with your doctor if drug benefits justify risk to unborn child. Risk category C (see page xviii).

Breast-feeding:
Drug passes into milk. Avoid drug or discontinue nursing until you finish medicine. Consult doctor for advice on maintaining milk supply.

Infants & children:
Not approved for ages under 18. If prescribed, carefully read information provided with prescription. Contact doctor right away if depression symptoms get worse or there is any talk of suicide or suicide behaviors. Also, read information under Others.

Prolonged use:
See your doctor for occasional blood counts, especially if you have fever and sore throat.

Skin & sunlight:
May cause rash or intensify sunburn in areas exposed to sun or ultraviolet light (photosensitivity reaction). Use sunscreen and avoid overexposure. Notify doctor if reaction occurs.

Driving, piloting or hazardous work:
Don't drive or pilot aircraft until you learn how medicine affects you. Don't work around dangerous machinery. Don't climb ladders or work in high places. Danger increases if you drink alcohol or take medicine affecting alertness and reflexes, such as antihistamines, tranquilizers, sedatives, pain medicine, narcotics and mind-altering drugs.

Discontinuing:
Don't discontinue without consulting doctor. Dose may require gradual reduction if you have taken drug for a long time. Doses of other drugs may also require adjustment.

Others:
- Advise any doctor or dentist whom you consult that you take this medicine.
- Adults and children taking antidepressants may experience a worsening of the depression symptoms and may have increased suicidal thoughts or behaviors. Call doctor right away if these symptoms or behaviors occur.
- For dry mouth, suck on sugarless hard candy or chew sugarless gum.
- Electroconvulsive therapy* should be avoided. Combined effect is unknown.

POSSIBLE INTERACTION WITH OTHER DRUGS

GENERIC NAME OR DRUG CLASS	COMBINED EFFECT
Antidepressants,* other	Excess drowsiness.
Antihistamines*	Excess drowsiness.
Antihypertensives*	Possible too-low blood pressure. Avoid.
Barbiturates*	Too-low blood pressure and drowsiness. Avoid.
Bupropion	Increased risk of seizures.
Central nervous system (CNS) depressants*	Increased sedation.
Digoxin	Possible increased digitalis effect.
Enzyme Inhibitors*	Increased effect of trazodone.
Guanabenz	Increased effects of both medicines.
Monoamine oxidase (MAO) inhibitors*	May add to toxic effect of each.
Narcotics*	Excess drowsiness.
Phenytoin	Possible increased phenytoin effect.
Ritonavir	Possible increased effect of trazodone.

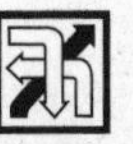

POSSIBLE INTERACTION WITH OTHER SUBSTANCES

INTERACTS WITH	COMBINED EFFECT
Alcohol:	Excess sedation. Avoid.
Beverages: Caffeine.	May add to heartbeat irregularity. Avoid.
Cocaine:	May add to heartbeat irregularity. Avoid.
Foods:	None expected.
Marijuana:	May add to heartbeat irregularity. Avoid.
Tobacco:	May add to heartbeat irregularity. Avoid.

***See Glossary**

BRAND NAMES

Apo-Triazo
Halcion
Novo-Triolam
Nu-Triazo

BASIC INFORMATION

Habit forming? Yes
Prescription needed? Yes
Available as generic? Yes
Drug class: Sedative-hypnotic agent

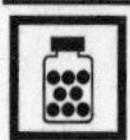

USES

- Treatment for insomnia (short term).
- Prevention or treatment of transient insomnia associated with sudden sleep schedule changes, such as travel across several time zones.

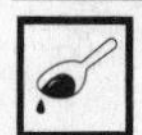

DOSAGE & USAGE INFORMATION

How to take:
Tablet—Swallow with liquid. If you can't swallow whole, crumble tablet and take with liquid or food.

When to take:
At the same time each day, according to instructions on prescription label. You should be in bed when you take your dose.

If you forget a dose:
Take as soon as you remember. If it is almost time for the next dose, wait for that dose (don't double this dose) and resume regular schedule.

What drug does:
Affects limbic system of brain, the part that controls emotions.

Time lapse before drug works:
Within 30 minutes.

Continued next column

OVERDOSE

SYMPTOMS:
Drowsiness, weakness, tremor, stupor, coma.
WHAT TO DO:
- **Dial 911 (emergency) for medical help or call poison control center 1-800-222-1222 for instructions.**
- **If person is unconscious, check breathing and pulse. If not breathing, begin mouth-to-mouth rescue breathing. If heart is not beating, begin chest compressions.**
- **See emergency information on last 3 pages of this book.**

Don't take with:
Any other medicine or any dietary supplement without consulting your doctor or pharmacist.

POSSIBLE ADVERSE REACTIONS OR SIDE EFFECTS

SYMPTOMS	WHAT TO DO
Life-threatening:	
Rare allergic reaction (hives, itching, rash, wheezing, tightness in chest, swelling of lips or tongue or throat).	Seek emergency treatment immediately.
Common:	
Clumsiness, drowsiness, dizziness.	Continue. Call doctor when convenient.
Infrequent:	
• Amnesia, hallucinations, confusion, depression, irritability, rash, itch, vision changes, sore throat, fever, chills, dry mouth.	Discontinue. Call doctor right away.
• Constipation or diarrhea, nausea, vomiting, difficult urination, vivid dreams, behavior changes, abdominal pain, headache.	Continue. Call doctor when convenient.
Rare:	
• Slow heartbeat, breathing difficulty.	Discontinue. Seek emergency treatment.
• Mouth, throat ulcers; jaundice. sleep-related behaviors.*	Discontinue. Call doctor right away.
• Decreased sex drive.	Continue. Call doctor when convenient.

WARNINGS & PRECAUTIONS

Don't take if:
- You are allergic to any benzodiazepine.
- You have myasthenia gravis.
- You are an active or recovering alcoholic.
- Patient is younger than 6 months.

Before you start, consult your doctor if:
- You have liver, kidney or lung disease.
- You have diabetes, epilepsy or porphyria.
- You have glaucoma.

Over age 60:
Adverse reactions and side effects may be more frequent and severe than in younger persons. You may need smaller doses for shorter periods.

Pregnancy:
Risk to unborn child outweighs drug benefits. Don't use. Risk category X (see page xviii).

Breast-feeding:
Drug may pass into milk. Avoid drug or discontinue nursing until you finish medicine. Consult doctor for advice on maintaining milk supply.

Infants & children:
Not recommended.

Prolonged use:
May impair liver function.

Skin & sunlight:
No problems expected.

Driving, piloting or hazardous work:
Don't drive or pilot aircraft until you learn how medicine affects you. Don't work around dangerous machinery. Don't climb ladders or work in high places. Danger increases if you drink alcohol or take medicine affecting alertness and reflexes.

Discontinuing:
Don't discontinue without consulting doctor. Dose may require gradual reduction if you have taken drug for a long time. Doses of other drugs may also require adjustment.

Others:
- Hot weather, heavy exercise and profuse sweating may reduce excretion and cause overdose.
- Blood sugar may rise in diabetics, requiring insulin adjustment.
- Don't use for insomnia more than 4-7 days.
- Advise any doctor or dentist whom you consult that you take this medicine.
- Triazolam has a very short duration of action in the body.

POSSIBLE INTERACTION WITH OTHER DRUGS

GENERIC NAME OR DRUG CLASS	COMBINED EFFECT
Anticonvulsants*	Change in seizure frequency or severity.
Antidepressants*	Increased sedative effects of both drugs.
Antihistamines*	Increased sedative effects of both drugs.
Antihypertensives*	Excessively low blood pressure.
Central nervous system (CNS) depressants,* other	Increased central nervous system depression.
Cimetidine	Increased triazolam effect. May be dangerous.
Clozapine	Toxic effect on the central nervous system.
Contraceptives, oral*	Increased triazolam effect and toxicity.
Disulfiram	Increased triazolam effect and toxicity.
Erythromycins*	Increased triazolam effect and toxicity.
Isoniazid	Increased triazolam effect and toxicity.
Ketoconazole	Increased triazolam effect and toxicity.
Levodopa	Possible decreased levodopa effect.
Molindone	Increased tranquilizer effect.
Monoamine oxidase (MAO) inhibitors*	Convulsions, deep sedation, rage.
Narcotics*	Increased sedative effects of both drugs.
Nefazodone	Increased effects of both drugs.
Omeprazole	Delayed excretion of triazolam causing increased amount of triazolam in blood.
Probenecid	Increased triazola effect.
Zidovudine	Increased tox zidovudine.

*See Glossary

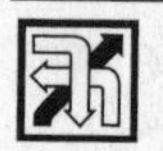

POSSIBLE INTERA WITH OTHER SUB

INTERACTS WITH	CO
Alcohol:	
Beverages: Grapefruit juice.	
Cocaine:	
Foods:	
Marijuana	
Tobac	

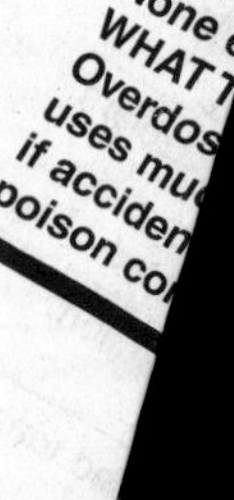

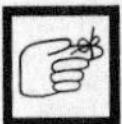

WARNINGS & PRECAUTIONS

Don't take if:
You know you are allergic to trilostane.

Before you start, consult your doctor if:
- You have an infection.
- You will have surgery while taking.
- You have a head injury.
- You have kidney disease.

Over age 60:
Adverse reactions and side effects may be more frequent and severe than in younger persons. You may need smaller doses for shorter periods of time.

Pregnancy:
Risk to unborn child outweighs drug benefits. Don't use. Risk category X (see page xviii).

Breast-feeding:
Safety not established. Consult doctor.

Infants & children:
Effect not documented. Consult your pediatrician.

Prolonged use:
- Not intended for prolonged use.
- Talk to your doctor about the need for follow-up medical examinations or laboratory studies.

Skin & sunlight:
No problems expected.

Driving, piloting or hazardous work:
Avoid if you feel confused, drowsy or dizzy.

Discontinuing:
No special problems expected.

Others:
- Advise any doctor or dentist whom you consult that you take this medicine.
- May affect results in some medical tests.

POSSIBLE INTERACTION WITH OTHER DRUGS

GENERIC NAME OR DRUG CLASS	COMBINED EFFECT
Aminoglutethimide	Too much decrease in adrenal function.
Mitotane	Too much decrease in adrenal function.

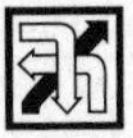

POSSIBLE INTERACTION WITH OTHER SUBSTANCES

INTERACTS WITH	COMBINED EFFECT
Alcohol:	None expected.
Beverages:	None expected.
Cocaine:	None expected.
Foods:	None expected.
Marijuana:	None expected.
Tobacco:	None expected.

TRIMETHOBENZAMIDE

BRAND NAMES

Tigan

BASIC INFORMATION

Habit forming? No
Prescription needed? Yes
Available as generic? Yes
Drug class: Antiemetic

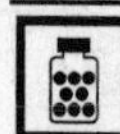

USES

Reduces nausea and vomiting.

DOSAGE & USAGE INFORMATION

How to take:
Capsule—Swallow with liquid. If you can't swallow whole, open capsule and take with liquid or food.

When to take:
When needed, no more often than label directs.

If you forget a dose:
Take when you remember. Wait as long as label directs for next dose.

What drug does:
Exact mechanism unknown. Possibly blocks nerve impulses to brain's vomiting centers.

Time lapse before drug works:
20 to 40 minutes.

Don't take with:
Any other medicine or any dietary supplement without consulting your doctor or pharmacist.

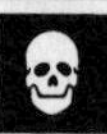

OVERDOSE

SYMPTOMS:
Confusion, convulsions, coma.
WHAT TO DO:

- **Dial 911 (emergency) for medical help or call poison control center 1-800-222-1222 for instructions.**
- **If person is unconscious, check breathing and pulse. If not breathing, begin mouth-to-mouth rescue breathing. If heart is not beating, begin chest compressions.**
- **See emergency information on last 3 pages of this book.**

POSSIBLE ADVERSE REACTIONS OR SIDE EFFECTS

SYMPTOMS	WHAT TO DO
Life-threatening: In case of overdose, see previous column.	
Common: Drowsiness.	Continue. Call doctor when convenient.
Infrequent: Rash, blurred vision, diarrhea, dizziness, headache, muscle cramps, unusual tiredness.	Discontinue. Call doctor right away.
Rare: Seizures, tremor, depression, sore throat, fever, repeated vomiting, back pain, yellow skin or eyes, body spasm (head and heels bent backward and body bowed forward).	Discontinue. Call doctor right away.

WARNINGS & PRECAUTIONS

Don't take if:
You are allergic to trimethobenzamide.

Before you start, consult your doctor if:
You have reacted badly to antihistamines.

Over age 60:
More susceptible to low blood pressure and sedative effects of this drug.

Pregnancy:
Decide with your doctor if drug benefits justify risk to unborn child. Risk category C (see page xviii).

Breast-feeding:
Effect unknown. Avoid if possible. Consult doctor.

Infants & children:
Avoid during viral infections. Drug may contribute to Reye's syndrome.

Prolonged use:

- Damages blood cell production of bone marrow.
- Causes Parkinson's-like symptoms of tremors, rigidity.

Skin & sunlight:
No special problems expected.

Driving, piloting or hazardous work:
Don't drive until you learn how medicine affects you. Don't work around dangerous machinery. Don't climb ladders or work in high places. Danger increases if you drink alcohol or take medicine affecting alertness and reflexes, such as antihistamines, tranquilizers, sedatives, pain medicine, narcotics and mind-altering drugs.

Discontinuing:
May be unnecessary to finish medicine. Follow doctor's instructions.

Others:
Advise any doctor or dentist whom you consult that you take this medicine.

POSSIBLE INTERACTION WITH OTHER DRUGS

GENERIC NAME OR DRUG CLASS	COMBINED EFFECT
Antidepressants*	Increased sedative effect.
Antihistamines*	Increased sedative effect.
Barbiturates*	Increased effect of both drugs.
Belladonna	Increased effect of both drugs.
Cholinergics*	Increased effect of both drugs.
Clozapine	Toxic effect on the central nervous system.
Ethinamate	Dangerous increased effects of ethinamate. Avoid combining.
Fluoxetine	Increased depressant effects of both drugs.
Guanfacine	May increase depressant effects of either medicine.
Leucovorin	High alcohol content of leucovorin may cause adverse effects.
Methyprylon	May increase sedative effect to dangerous level. Avoid.
Mind-altering drugs*	Increased effect of mind-altering drug.
Nabilone	Greater depression of central nervous system.
Narcotics*	Increased sedative effect.
Ototoxic medications*	May mask the symptoms of ototoxicity.
Phenothiazines*	Increased effect of both drugs.
Sedatives*	Increased sedative effect.
Sertraline	Increased depressive effects of both drugs.
Sleep inducers*	Increased effect of sleep inducer.
Tranquilizers*	Increased sedative effect.

POSSIBLE INTERACTION WITH OTHER SUBSTANCES

INTERACTS WITH	COMBINED EFFECT
Alcohol:	Oversedation. Avoid.
Beverages:	None expected.
Cocaine:	None expected.
Foods:	None expected.
Marijuana:	Increased antinausea effect.
Tobacco:	None expected.

*See Glossary

TRIMETHOPRIM

BRAND NAMES

Apo-Sulfatrim
Apo-Sulfatrim DS
Bactrim
Bactrim DS
Bethaprim
Cotrim
Cotrim DS
Co-trimaxizole
Novotrimel
Novotrimel DS
Nu-Cotrimox
Nu-Cotrimox DS
Proloprim
Protrin
Roubac
Septra
Septra DS
SMZ-TMP
Sulfamethoprim
Sulfamethoprim DS
Sulfaprim
Sulfaprim DS
Sulfatrim
Sulfatrim DS
Sulfoxaprim
Sulfoxaprim DS
Sulmeprim
Triazole
Triazole DS
Trimeth-Sulfa
Trimpex
Trisulfam
Uroplus DS
Uroplus SS

BASIC INFORMATION

Habit forming? No
Prescription needed? Yes
Available as generic? Yes
Drug class: Antimicrobial (antibacterial)

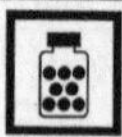

USES

- Treats urinary tract infections susceptible to trimethoprim.
- Helps prevent recurrent urinary tract infections if taken once a day.
- Treats *Pneumocystis pneumonia*.

OVERDOSE

SYMPTOMS:
Nausea, vomiting, diarrhea.
WHAT TO DO:
Overdose unlikely to threaten life. If person uses much larger amount than prescribed or if accidentally swallowed, call doctor or poison control center 1-800-222-1222 for help.

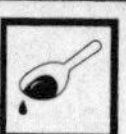

DOSAGE & USAGE INFORMATION

How to take:
- Tablet—Swallow with liquid or food to lessen stomach irritation. If can't swallow whole, crush or crumble tablet and take with food or liquid.
- Oral suspension (in combination with sulfamethoxazole)—Follow directions on label.

When to take:
Space doses evenly in 24 hours to keep constant amount in urine.

If you forget a dose:
Take as soon as you remember. If it is almost time for the next dose, wait for that dose (don't double this dose) and resume regular schedule.

What drug does:
Stops harmful bacterial germs from multiplying. Will not kill viruses.

Time lapse before drug works:
2 to 5 days.

Don't take with:
Any other medicine or any dietary supplement without consulting your doctor or pharmacist.

POSSIBLE ADVERSE REACTIONS OR SIDE EFFECTS

SYMPTOMS	WHAT TO DO
Life-threatening:	
Rare allergic reaction (hives, itching, rash, wheezing, tightness in chest, swelling of lips or tongue or throat).	Seek emergency treatment immediately.
Common:	
None expected.	
Infrequent:	
Diarrhea, nausea, vomiting, stomach cramps, headache.	Continue. Call doctor when convenient.
Rare:	
Blue fingernails, lips and skin; difficult breathing; sore throat; fever; anemia; jaundice; unusual bleeding or bruising; unusual tiredness or weakness; skin changes (rash, itch, redness, blisters, peeling or loosening); aching joints or muscles.	Discontinue. Call doctor right away.

WARNINGS & PRECAUTIONS

Don't take if:
- You are allergic to trimethoprim or any sulfa drug.*
- You are anemic due to folic acid deficiency.

Before you start, consult your doctor if:
You have had liver or kidney disease.

Over age 60:
- Reduced liver and kidney function may require reduced dose.
- More likely to have severe anal and genital itch.
- Increased susceptibility to anemia.

Pregnancy:
Decide with your doctor whether drug benefits justify risk to unborn child. Risk category C (see page xviii).

Breast-feeding:
No proven harm to unborn child. Avoid if possible. Consult doctor.

Infants & children:
Use under medical supervision only.

Prolonged use:
- Anemia.
- Talk to your doctor about the need for follow-up medical examinations or laboratory studies to check complete blood counts (white blood cell count, platelet count, red blood cell count, hemoglobin, hematocrit).

Skin & sunlight:
May cause rash or intensify sunburn in areas exposed to sun or ultraviolet light (photosensitivity reaction). Avoid overexposure. Notify doctor if reaction occurs.

Driving, piloting or hazardous work:
No problems expected.

Discontinuing:
Don't discontinue without doctor's advice until you complete prescribed dose, even though symptoms diminish or disappear.

Others:
Advise any doctor or dentist whom you consult that you take this medicine.

POSSIBLE INTERACTION WITH OTHER DRUGS

GENERIC NAME OR DRUG CLASS	COMBINED EFFECT
Anticonvulsants*	Increased risk of anemia.
Bone marrow depressants*	Increased possibility of bone marrow suppression.
Folate antagonists,* other	Increased risk of anemia.
Metformin	Increased metformin effect.
Phenytoin	Increased phenytoin effect.

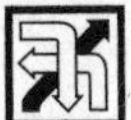

POSSIBLE INTERACTION WITH OTHER SUBSTANCES

INTERACTS WITH	COMBINED EFFECT
Alcohol:	Increased alcohol effect with Bactrim or Septra.
Beverages:	None expected.
Cocaine:	None expected.
Foods:	None expected.
Marijuana:	None expected.
Tobacco:	None expected.

***See Glossary**

TRIPTANS

GENERIC AND BRAND NAMES

ALMOTRIPTAN
Axert
ELETRIPTAN
Relpax
FROVATRIPTAN
Frova
NARATRIPTAN
Amerge
RIZATRIPTAN
Maxalt
Maxalt-MLT
SUMATRIPTAN
Alsuma
Imitrex
Imitrex Nasal Spray
Sumavel DosePro
Treximet
Zecuity
ZOLMITRIPTAN
Zomig
Zomig-Nasal Spray
Zomig-ZMT

BASIC INFORMATION

Habit forming? No
Prescription needed? Yes
Available as generic? Yes, for some
Drug class: Antimigraine

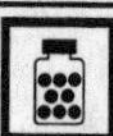

USES

- Treatment for acute migraine headaches not relieved by other medications (e.g., aspirin or acetaminophen). Does not prevent migraines.
- Treatment for cluster headaches.

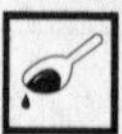

DOSAGE & USAGE INFORMATION

How to take:
- Injection or needle-free system—Follow instructions provided by prescription or doctor for injection technique and how to dispose.
- Tablet—Swallow whole with liquid. Do not crush, break or chew tablet.
- Orally disintegrating tablet—Place on tongue, let it dissolve and swallow with saliva.
- Wafers—Place on tongue to dissolve and be swallowed with saliva.
- Skin patch—Follow prescription instructions.
- Nasal spray—One spray into one nostril as a single dose or as instructed by doctor.

Continued next column

OVERDOSE

SYMPTOMS:
Dizziness, sleepiness, vomiting, slow heartbeat, chest pain, tremor, warm feeling, large pupil, irregular breathing, incoordination.
WHAT TO DO:
- **Dial 911 (emergency) for medical help or call poison control center 1-800-222-1222 for instructions.**
- **See emergency information on last 3 pages of this book.**

When to take:
- At the first sign of a migraine (aura or pain). After using drug, lie down in a quiet, dark room to increase effectiveness of treatment.
- An additional dose may be helpful if the migraine returns. Do not exceed the prescribed quantity or frequency. Do not use additional dose if first dose does not bring substantial relief.
- For treatment of cluster headaches, follow your doctor's instructions.

If you forget a dose:
Triptans are not taken on a routine schedule. They are taken when migraines occur.

What drug does:
Enlarged (dilated) blood vessels in the brain cause migraines. Triptans work by narrowing (constricting) these blood vessels.

Time lapse before drug works:
Relief usually begins within 30 minutes for oral dosage (tablets/wafers), 10 minutes for injection and 15 minutes for nasal spray.

Don't take with:
- Ergotamine-containing drugs. Delay 24 hours.
- Any other medicine or any dietary supplement without consulting your doctor or pharmacist.

POSSIBLE ADVERSE REACTIONS OR SIDE EFFECTS

SYMPTOMS	WHAT TO DO
Life-threatening:	
Rare allergic reaction (hives, itching, rash, wheezing, tightness in chest, swelling of lips or tongue or throat).	Seek emergency treatment immediately.
Common:	
Nausea and/or vomiting (vomiting may be from migraine or from drug), drowsiness or dizziness, migraine recurs.	Continue. Call doctor when convenient.
Infrequent:	
Sensation of burning, warmth, numbness, cold or tingling; lightheadedness; flushing; discomfort of jaw, mouth, throat, nose or sinuses; anxiety; tiredness; vision changes; just feeling ill; muscle weakness, aches, cramps or stiffness; burning, pain, or redness at injection site.	Continue. Call doctor when convenient.

Rare:

Pain, pressure or tightness in the chest; difficulty swallowing; irregular heartbeat; shortness of breath; severe stomach pain.	Discontinue. Call doctor right away or seek emergency help for severe symptoms.

WARNINGS & PRECAUTIONS

Don't take if:
- You are allergic to any triptans.
- You have angina pectoris, a history of myocardial infarction or myocardial ischemia, Prinzmetal's angina, stroke or uncontrolled hypertension (high blood pressure).

Before you start, consult your doctor if:
- You have heart rhythm problems or coronary artery disease.
- You have liver or kidney disease.

Over age 60:
Adverse reactions and side effects may be more frequent and severe than in younger persons. Consult doctor.

Pregnancy:
Decide with your doctor whether drug benefits justify risk to unborn child. Risk category C (see page xviii).

Breast-feeding:
Unknown effects. Decide with your doctor whether drug benefits justify possible risk.

Infants & children:
Some of these drugs are approved for children. Use and dosage will be determined by your child's doctor.

Prolonged use:
No problems expected.

Skin & sunlight:
No problems expected.

Driving, piloting or hazardous work:
Avoid if you feel drowsy or dizzy. Otherwise no problems expected.

Discontinuing:
No problems expected. Talk to your doctor if you have plans to discontinue use of drug.

Others:
- Advise any doctor or dentist whom you consult that you take this medicine.
- Rarely, the drug may affect results in some medical tests.
- Follow your doctor's recommendations for any additional treatments for prevention of migraines.
- Sensitivity to light is a symptom of migraine and is not drug-related.

POSSIBLE INTERACTION WITH OTHER DRUGS

GENERIC NAME OR DRUG CLASS	COMBINED EFFECT
Dihydroergotamine	Increased vasoconstriction. Delay 24 hours between drugs.
Enzyme inhibitors*	Increased effect of eletriptan.
Ergotamine	Increased vasoconstriction. Delay 24 hours between drugs.
Monoamine oxidase (MAO) inhibitors*	Adverse effects unknown. Avoid.
Propranolol	Increased effect of rizatriptan.
Selective serotonin reuptake inhibitors (SSRIs)	Risk of serotonin syndrome.*
Serotonergics*	Risk of serotonin syndrome.*
Serotonin & norepinephrine reuptake inhibitors (SNRIs)	Risk of serotonin syndrome.*
Triptans, other	Increased vasoconstriction. Delay 24 hours between drugs.

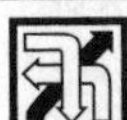

POSSIBLE INTERACTION WITH OTHER SUBSTANCES

INTERACTS WITH	COMBINED EFFECT
Alcohol:	No interaction known, but alcohol aggravates migraines. Avoid.
Beverages: Grapefruit juice.	May increase the effect of eletriptan.
Cocaine:	Unknown. Avoid.
Foods: Grapefruit.	May increase the effect of eletriptan.
Marijuana:	Unknown. avoid.
Tobacco:	None expected.

*See Glossary

TUMOR NECROSIS FACTOR BLOCKERS

GENERIC AND BRAND NAMES

ADALIMUMAB
Humira
CERTOLIZUMAB
Cimzia
ETANERCEPT
Enbrel
GOLIMUMAB
Simponi
INFLIXIMAB
Remicade

BASIC INFORMATION

Habit forming? No
Prescription needed? Yes
Available as generic? No
Drug class: Antirheumatic; biological response modifier

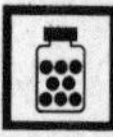

USES

- Treatment of moderately to severely active rheumatoid arthritis. Used for patients who have not responded to one or more disease modifying antirheumatic drugs (DMARDs). May be used alone or in combination with certain other arthritis drugs (e.g., methotrexate).
- Treats Crohn's disease, ulcerative colitis, moderate to severe ankylosing spondylitis, psoriatic arthritis, and moderate to severe plaque psoriasis.
- May be used for other disorders as determined by your doctor.

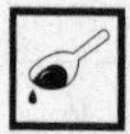

DOSAGE & USAGE INFORMATION

How to take:

- Self injection—The drug may be self-injected under the skin (subcutaneously). Follow your doctor's instructions and the directions provided with the prescription on how and where to inject. Do not use the medication unless you are sure about the proper method for injection. Store medication in the refrigerator (do not freeze) until you plan to use it. After each use, throw away the syringe and any medicine left in it (ask your pharmacist about disposal methods). Never reuse the needles or syringes.

Continued next column

- Infliximab—The drug is given by injection in a medical office. With training, some patients may be able to self-inject the drug.

When to take:
Once or twice a week for etanercept, every other week for adalimumab and certolizumab, monthly for golimumab and infliximab is given several times a year. Read label for specific instructions.

If you forget a dose:
Inject as soon as possible. If it is almost time for your next dose, skip the missed dose and go back to your regular dosing schedule. Do not double doses.

What drug does:
Blocks the damage done to healthy cells by the tumor necrosis factor (TNF), a protein in the body. The drug helps prevent the progressive joint destruction of rheumatoid arthritis.

Time lapse before drug works:
It will take several weeks before full benefits of the drug are noticeable.

Don't use with:
Any other medicine or any dietary supplement without consulting your doctor or pharmacist.

OVERDOSE

SYMPTOMS:
None expected.
WHAT TO DO:
If an overdose is suspected, dial 911 (emergency) for medical help or call poison control center 1-800-222-1222 for instructions.

POSSIBLE ADVERSE REACTIONS OR SIDE EFFECTS

SYMPTOMS	WHAT TO DO
Life-threatening: None expected.	
Common: Chills, fever, chest pain or tightness, hives or itching, flushed face, breathing difficulty, stuffy or runny nose, headache, sneezing, wheezing, sore throat, unusual tiredness or weakness, vomiting, rash (on face, scalp or stomach), reaction at injection site.	Call doctor right away.
Infrequent: Painful or frequent or difficult urination, bloody or colored urine, fast heartbeat, faintness, pain or stiffness in muscles and joints, pain (stomach, back, face, shoulder, rectum), dizziness, diarrhea, sores on mouth or tongue, vaginal itching or burning, sore fingernails or toenails.	Call doctor right away.

Rare:

Allergic reaction (itching, rash hives, swelling of face or lips, wheezing), black or tarry stools, vision problems, constipation, feeling of fullness, yellow skin or eyes, swollen glands, fungal infection (fever, cough, tiredness, weight loss, sweats, shortness of breath).	Call doctor right away.

WARNINGS & PRECAUTIONS

Don't take if:
You are allergic to tumor necrosis factor blockers or their components.

Before you start, consult your doctor if:
- You have congestive heart failure (CHF).
- You have or have had tuberculosis.
- You have a central nervous system disorder or a blood disorder or diabetes.
- You are scheduled for surgery.
- You are allergic to rubber or latex (it is used in the drug product's needle covering).
- You have an active infection.
- You have a chronic disorder or infection, a malignancy, or are immunosuppressed.

Over age 60:
Use with caution in elderly patients, since infections are more common in this age group.

Pregnancy:
Risk factors vary for drugs in this group. See category list on page xviii and consult doctor.

Breast-feeding:
It is unknown if drug passes into milk. Consult doctor for advice on breast-feeding if you use this medication.

Infants & children:
Use only with close medical supervision. Infliximab is used in children 6 and older with certain disorders. Etanercept is used in children ages 4 and older who have juvenile idiopathic arthritis (JIA).

Prolonged use:
- No specific problems expected.
- Talk to your doctor about the need for follow-up medical examinations or laboratory studies to check effectiveness of the drug and to monitor for infections or adverse effects.

Skin & sunlight:
No problems expected.

Driving, piloting or hazardous work:
No problems expected.

Discontinuing:
No problems expected. Consult doctor first.

Others:
- Serious infections (such as bacterial, viral, fungal, and tuberculosis) and death have been reported in patients using these drugs. Consult your doctor if any signs or symptoms of infection occur.
- Infliximab use may lead to liver toxicity and liver failure with symptoms of yellow skin or eyes, vomiting, and abdominal pain. It may also cause blood abnormalities or blood vessel inflammation with symptoms of vision changes, weakness, numbness or tingling, paleness, fever, or easy bruising or bleeding. Call doctor right away if symptoms occur.
- Slight increased risk of cancer and lupus-like syndromes. Ask your doctor about your risks.
- Advise any doctor or dentist whom you consult that you take this medicine.
- See your doctor for regular visits while using this drug.
- Avoid immunizations unless doctor approved.

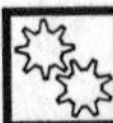

POSSIBLE INTERACTION WITH OTHER DRUGS

GENERIC NAME OR DRUG CLASS	COMBINED EFFECT
Anakinra	Risk of serious infection. Avoid.
Immunosuppressants*	May increase risk of infection.
Live vaccines	May decrease vaccine effect.

Note: Consult your doctor or pharmacist about other possible interactions.

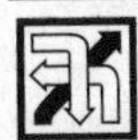

POSSIBLE INTERACTION WITH OTHER SUBSTANCES

INTERACTS WITH	COMBINED EFFECT
Alcohol:	None expected.
Beverages:	None expected.
Cocaine:	None expected. However, cocaine may slow body's recovery. Avoid.
Foods:	None expected.
Marijuana:	None expected. However, marijuana may slow body's recovery. Avoid.
Tobacco:	None expected.

*See Glossary

URSODIOL

BRAND NAMES

Actigall
Urso
Ursofalk

BASIC INFORMATION

Habit forming? No
Prescription needed? Yes
Available as generic? Yes
Drug class: Anticholelithic

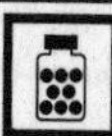

USES

- Dissolves cholesterol gallstones in selected patients who either can't tolerate surgery or don't require surgery for other reasons. Not used when surgery is clearly indicated.
- Prevention of gallstone formation during rapid weight loss.
- Treatment for primary biliary cirrhosis.

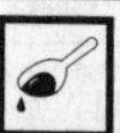

DOSAGE & USAGE INFORMATION

How to take:
Capsule or tablet—Swallow with a full glass of water. You may take with food to lessen stomach irritation. If you can't swallow whole, open capsule and take with liquid or food. Ask pharmacist for information about crushing tablet form.

When to take:
With meals, 2 or 3 times a day according to your doctor's instructions.

If you forget a dose:
Take as soon as you remember. If it is almost time for the next dose, wait for that dose (don't double this dose) and resume regular schedule.

Continued next column

OVERDOSE

SYMPTOMS:
Severe diarrhea.
WHAT TO DO:
Overdose unlikely to threaten life. If person uses much larger amount than prescribed or if accidentally swallowed, call doctor or poison control center 1-800-222-1222 for help.

What drug does:
Decreases secretion of cholesterol into bile by suppressing production and secretion of cholesterol by the liver. Ursodiol will not help gallstone problems unless the gallstones are made of cholesterol. It works best when the stones are small.

Time lapse before drug works:
Unpredictable. Varies among patients. If taken for gallstones, the drug may need to be taken for a long time.

Don't take with:
Any other medicine or any dietary supplement without consulting your doctor or pharmacist.

POSSIBLE ADVERSE REACTIONS OR SIDE EFFECTS

SYMPTOMS	WHAT TO DO
Life-threatening:	
Rare allergic reaction—Breathing difficulty; closing of the throat; swelling of hands, feet, face, lips or tongue; hives.	Discontinue. Seek emergency treatment.
Common:	
None expected.	
Infrequent:	
Diarrhea, nausea, upset stomach, headache.	Continue. Call doctor when convenient.
Rare:	
Any unusual symptoms occur.	Continue. Call doctor when convenient.

WARNINGS & PRECAUTIONS

Don't take if:
You are allergic to any bile acids.

Before you start, consult your doctor if:
- You have complications of gallstones, such as infection, cholecystitis or obstruction of the bile ducts.
- You have had pancreatitis.
- You have heart, liver or kidney disease.

Over age 60:
No special problems expected.

Pregnancy:
Decide with your doctor whether drug benefits justify risk to unborn child. Pregnancy risk category B (see page xviii).

Breast-feeding:
It is unknown if drug passes into milk; however, similar substances appear in breast milk. Consult doctor for advice on breast-feeding if you use this medication.

Infants & children:
Not recommended. Adequate studies have not been performed.

Prolonged use:
- No special problems expected.
- Talk to your doctor about the need for follow-up medical examinations or laboratory studies to check kidney function.

Skin & sunlight:
No problems expected.

Driving, piloting or hazardous work:
Don't pilot aircraft until you learn how medicine affects you. Don't work around dangerous machinery. Don't climb ladders or work in high places. Danger increases if you drink alcohol or take medicine affecting alertness and reflexes, such as antihistamines, tranquilizers, sedatives, pain medicine, narcotics and mind-altering drugs.

Discontinuing:
Don't discontinue without consulting doctor.

Others:
- Plan regular visits to your doctor while you take ursodiol. Have ultrasound and liver function studies done at appropriate intervals. Liver damage is unlikely, but theoretically could happen.
- Advise any doctor or dentist whom you consult that you take this medicine.

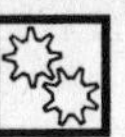

POSSIBLE INTERACTION WITH OTHER DRUGS

GENERIC NAME OR DRUG CLASS	COMBINED EFFECT
Antacids* (aluminum-containing)	Decreased absorption of ursodiol.
Cholestyramine	Decreased absorption of ursodiol.
Clofibrate	Decreased effect of ursodiol.
Colestipol	Decreased absorption of ursodiol.
Estrogens*	Decreased effect of ursodiol.
Progestins	Decreased effect of ursodiol.

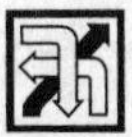

POSSIBLE INTERACTION WITH OTHER SUBSTANCES

INTERACTS WITH	COMBINED EFFECT
Alcohol:	None expected, unless you have impaired liver function from alcohol abuse.
Beverages:	None expected.
Cocaine:	None expected.
Foods:	None expected.
Marijuana:	None expected.
Tobacco:	None reported. However, tobacco may possibly impair absorption from the intestinal tract. Better to avoid.

VALPROIC ACID

BRAND NAMES

Depakene
Stavzor

BASIC INFORMATION

Habit forming? No
Prescription needed? Yes
Available as generic? Yes
Drug class: Anticonvulsant

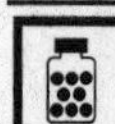

USES

- Treatment of various types of epilepsy.
- Treatment for bipolar (manic-depressive) disorder.
- Prevention of migraine headaches.

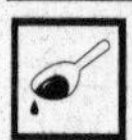

DOSAGE & USAGE INFORMATION

How to take:
- Capsule or syrup—Swallow with liquid or food to lessen stomach irritation. Do not crush or chew capsule.
- Delayed-release capsule—Swallow whole with a glass of water. Do not crush or chew.

When to take:
One to three times a day as directed by doctor.

If you forget a dose:
Take as soon as you remember. If it is almost time for the next dose, wait for the next scheduled dose (don't double this dose).

What drug does:
It helps stabilize electrical and chemical activity in the brain.

Time lapse before drug works:
1 to 4 hours, but full effect may take weeks.

Don't take with:
Any other medicine or any dietary supplement without consulting your doctor or pharmacist.

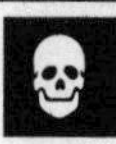

OVERDOSE

SYMPTOMS:
Extreme drowsiness, heart problems, loss of consciousness.
WHAT TO DO:
- **Dial 911 (emergency) for medical help or call poison control center 1-800-222-1222 for instructions.**
- **See emergency information on last 3 pages of this book.**

POSSIBLE ADVERSE REACTIONS OR SIDE EFFECTS

SYMPTOMS	WHAT TO DO
Life-threatening: Rare allergic reaction (hives, itching, rash, wheezing, tightness in chest, swelling lips, or tongue or throat).	Seek emergency treatment immediately.
Common: Mild appetite loss, indigestion, nausea, vomiting, abdominal cramps, diarrhea, tremor, weight gain or loss, menstrual changes in girls, headache.	Continue. Call doctor when convenient.
Infrequent: Clumsiness or unsteadiness, constipation, skin rash, dizziness, drowsiness, irritable or excited, hair loss.	Continue. Call doctor when convenient.
Rare: Mood or behavior changes; continued nausea, vomiting and appetite loss; increase in seizures; swelling (face, feet, legs); clay-color stools; confusion, yellow skin or eyes; tiredness or weakness; back-and-forth eye movements; seeing spots/seeing double; unusual bleeding or bruising; dark urine; low fever; severe stomach cramps.	Continue, but call doctor right away or seek emergency care for severe symptoms.

WARNINGS & PRECAUTIONS

Don't take if:
You are allergic to valproic acid.

Before you start, consult your doctor if:
- You have liver, kidney, blood or brain disorder or pancreatitis or urea cycle disorder.
- Drug is to be used for a young child.
- You have a history of depression or suicide thoughts or suicidal behavior.
- You are a woman of childbearing age.

Over age 60:
Adverse reactions and side effects may be more frequent and severe than in younger persons.

Pregnancy:
Risk of birth defects to unborn child exists. Use only if benefits of drug greatly exceed fetal risk. Risk category D (see page xviii).

Breast-feeding:
Drug passes into milk. Avoid drug or discontinue nursing until you finish medicine. Consult doctor for advice on maintaining milk supply.

Infants & children:
Increased risk for side effects and adverse reactions. Use under close medical supervision only.

Prolonged use:
Request periodic blood tests, liver and kidney function tests. These tests are necessary for safe and effective use.

Skin & sunlight:
No problems expected.

Driving, piloting or hazardous work:
Don't drive or pilot aircraft until you learn how medicine affects you. Don't work around dangerous machinery. Don't climb ladders or work in high places. Danger increases if you drink alcohol or take medicine affecting alertness and reflexes.

Discontinuing:
Don't discontinue without consulting doctor. Dose may require gradual reduction if you have taken drug for a long time. Doses of other drugs may also require adjustment.

Others:

- Read the insert provided with the drug. Follow all instructions and heed all warnings.
- Advise any doctor or dentist whom you consult that you take this drug.
- In rare cases, the drug can cause life-threatening liver failure (especially in children under age 2) or life-threatening pancreatitis (inflammation of the pancreas). Consult your doctor about your risks.
- Rarely, antiepileptic (anticonvulsant) drugs may lead to suicidal thoughts and behaviors. Call doctor right away if suicidal symptoms or unusual behaviors occur.
- Wear or carry medical identification to show your seizure disorder and the drugs you take.

POSSIBLE INTERACTION WITH OTHER DRUGS

GENERIC NAME OR DRUG CLASS	COMBINED EFFECT
Anticoagulants,* oral	Increased risk of bleeding problems.
Anticonvulsants,* other	Each drug may need dosage adjusted.
Anti-inflammatory drugs, nonsteroidal* (NSAIDs)	Increased risk of bleeding problems.
Aspirin	Increased effect of valproic acid.
Carbamazepine	Decreased effect of valproic acid.
Central nervous system (CNS) depressants*	Increased sedative effect.
Clonazepam	May prolong seizure.
Diazepam	Increased effect of diazepam.
Enzyme inducers*	May Increase effect of some enzyme inducers and decrease effect of valproic acid.
Felbamate	Increased effect of valproic acid.
Hepatotoxics*	Increased risk of liver problems.
Lamotrigine	Increased effect of lamotrigine and risk of life-threatening rash.
Phenobarbital	Increased effect of phenobarbital and decreased effect of valproic acid.
Phenytoin	Increased phenytoin effect; decreased valproic acid effect.
Primidone	Increased effect of primidone.
Rifampin	Decreased effect of valproic acid.

Continued on page 930

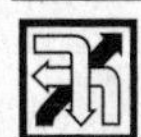

POSSIBLE INTERACTION WITH OTHER SUBSTANCES

INTERACTS WITH	COMBINED EFFECT
Alcohol:	Excess sedation. Avoid.
Beverages:	None expected.
Cocaine:	Unknown. Avoid.
Foods:	None expected.
Marijuana:	Unknown. Avoid.
Tobacco:	None expected.

*See Glossary

VANCOMYCIN

BRAND NAMES

Vancocin

BASIC INFORMATION

Habit forming? No
Prescription needed? Yes
Available as generic? Yes
Drug class: Antibacterial

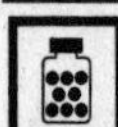

USES

- Treats colitis when caused by *Clostridium* infections.
- Treats some forms of severe diarrhea and other disorders as determined by your doctor.

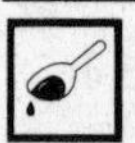

DOSAGE & USAGE INFORMATION

How to take:

- Capsule—Swallow with liquid. If you can't swallow whole, open capsule and take with liquid or food. Instructions to take on empty stomach mean 1 hour before or 2 hours after eating.
- Oral solution—Use the calibrated measuring device. Swallow with other liquid to prevent nausea.
- There is also an injectable form. This information applies to the oral form only.

When to take:
According to doctor's instructions. Usually every 6 hours.

If you forget a dose:
Take as soon as you remember. If it is almost time for the next dose, wait for that dose (don't double this dose) and resume regular schedule.

What drug does:
Kills bacterial cells.

Time lapse before drug works:
None. Works right away. This medicine is not absorbed to a great extent through the intestinal tract.

Continued next column

OVERDOSE

SYMPTOMS:
None expected.
WHAT TO DO:
Overdose unlikely to threaten life. If person uses much larger amount than prescribed or if accidentally swallowed, call doctor or poison control center 1-800-222-1222 for help.

Don't take with:
Any other medicines (including over-the-counter drugs such as cough and cold medicines, laxatives, antacids, diet pills, caffeine, nose drops or vitamins) without consulting your doctor or pharmacist.

POSSIBLE ADVERSE REACTIONS OR SIDE EFFECTS

SYMPTOMS	WHAT TO DO
Life-threatening:	
None expected.	
Common:	
Bitter taste.	Continue. Tell doctor at next visit.
Infrequent:	
Nausea or vomiting.	Continue. Call doctor when convenient.
Rare:	
Hearing loss, ears ringing or buzzing.	Discontinue. Call doctor right away.

WARNINGS & PRECAUTIONS

Don't take if:
You are allergic to vancomycin.

Before you start, consult your doctor if:
- You have hearing problems.
- You have severe kidney disease.
- You have intestinal obstruction.

Over age 60:
Adverse reactions and side effects may be more frequent and severe than in younger persons. You may need smaller doses for shorter periods of time.

Pregnancy:
Consult doctor. Risk category B (see page xviii).

Breast-feeding:
No special problems expected. Consult doctor.

Infants & children:
No special problems expected.

Prolonged use:
Talk to your doctor about the need for follow-up medical examinations or laboratory studies to check hearing acuity, kidney function, vancomycin serum concentration and urinalysis.

Skin & sunlight:
No problems expected.

Driving, piloting or hazardous work:
No problems expected.

Discontinuing:
No special problems expected.

Others:
- Advise any doctor or dentist whom you consult that you take this medicine.
- May affect results in some medical tests.

POSSIBLE INTERACTION WITH OTHER DRUGS

GENERIC NAME OR DRUG CLASS	COMBINED EFFECT
Cholestyramine	Decreased therapeutic effect of vancomycin.
Colestipol	Decreased therapeutic effect of vancomycin.
Metformin	Increased metformin effect.
Nephrotoxics*	Increased risk of kidney problems.

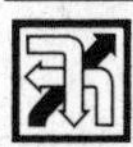

POSSIBLE INTERACTION WITH OTHER SUBSTANCES

INTERACTS WITH	COMBINED EFFECT
Alcohol:	None expected.
Beverages:	None expected.
Cocaine:	None expected.
Foods:	None expected.
Marijuana:	None expected.
Tobacco:	None expected.

***See Glossary**

VARENICLINE

BRAND NAMES

Chantix

BASIC INFORMATION

Habit Forming? No
Prescription needed? Yes
Available as generic? No
Drug class: Antismoking agent

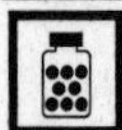

USES

Helps adults quit smoking. It is recommended that patients combine use of this drug with a stop-smoking program (such as counseling, support groups and/or patient education).

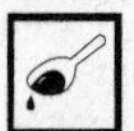

DOSAGE & USAGE INFORMATION

How to take:
Tablet—Swallow whole with a full glass (8 ounces) of water.

When to use:

- The tablet is taken twice a day after eating.
- The first step in treatment is to set a date to quit smoking. Then start taking the drug one week before that date. A lower dose is taken at the start of treatment and increased over the first few days. In most cases, treatment time is 12 weeks. It may be continued for another 12 weeks to improve long-term success in quitting smoking.

If you forget a dose:
Take tablet as soon as you remember. If it is almost time for the next dose, wait for the next scheduled dose (don't double this dose).

Continued next column

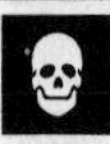

OVERDOSE

SYMPTOMS:
Symptoms of an overdose are unknown.
WHAT TO DO:

- **Dial 911 (emergency) for medical help or call poison control center 1-800-222-1222 for instructions.**
- **See emergency information on last 3 pages of this book.**

What drug does:
It is a nicotine-free drug that acts on the brain to reduce cravings for cigarettes (and other tobacco products). It also blocks the pleasurable effects of smoking. This helps to decrease the desire to smoke and reduces the unpleasant smoking withdrawal symptoms.

Time lapse before drug works:
It may take several days to see the effects. Full benefit may take 12 weeks of treatment.

Don't take with:
Any other medicine or diet supplement without consulting your doctor or pharmacist.

POSSIBLE ADVERSE REACTIONS OR SIDE EFFECTS

SYMPTOMS	WHAT TO DO
Life-threatening:	
Rare allergic reaction (hives, itching, rash, trouble breathing, tightness in chest, swelling of lips or tongue or throat).	Seek emergency treatment immediately.
Common:	
Nausea (may go on for several months), insomnia, headache.	Continue. Call doctor when convenient.
Infrequent:	
Strange dreams, gas, abdominal pain, upset stomach, taste changes, constipation, weak or tired feeling, vomiting.	Continue. Call doctor when convenient.
Rare:	
Chest pain, fast or slow or irregular heartbeat, memory loss, seizures, severe or persistent nausea, suicidal thoughts, unusual mental or mood changes, vision changes, drowsiness, other unusual symptoms.	Discontinue. Call doctor right away.

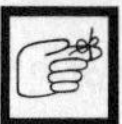

WARNINGS & PRECAUTIONS

Don't take if:
You are allergic to varenicline.

Before you start, consult your doctor if:
- You have kidney disease.
- You have or have had depression or a psychiatric illness.
- You have any chronic medical or health problem.

Over age 60:
Adverse reactions and side effects may be more frequent and severe than in younger persons.

Pregnancy:
Decide with your doctor if drug benefits justify risk to unborn child. Risk category C (see page xviii). (Tobacco smoke and nicotine are known to be harmful to a fetus.)

Breast-feeding:
It is unknown if drug passes into milk. Avoid drug or discontinue nursing until you finish dosage. Consult doctor for advice on maintaining milk supply.

Infants & children:
Safety and effectiveness in children under age 18 has not been established. Consult doctor.

Prolonged use:
It is not intended for long-term use. Usually prescribed for one or two 12-week periods of time.

Skin & sunlight:
No problems expected.

Driving, piloting or hazardous work:
Drug may cause drowsiness. Don't drive or pilot aircraft until you learn how medicine affects you. Don't work around dangerous machinery. Don't climb ladders or work in high places.

Discontinuing:
- Don't discontinue abruptly without doctor's advice. It could increase risk of feeling irritable and cause sleep disturbance.
- Nicotine withdrawal symptoms may occur during and after treatment. These include increased appetite, weight gain, tension, irritability, insomnia, headache and others. Consult doctor if withdrawal symptoms persist.

Others:
- Advise any doctor or dentist whom you consult that you take this medicine.
- For full benefit from a stop-smoking program, follow your doctor's advice.
- Even if you smoke after your quit date, continue to try to quit. Advise your doctor if you do continue to smoke after a few weeks of treatment.
- Patients who are attempting to quit smoking with this drug should be observed for serious mood or behavior changes. Symptoms may include depressed mood, agitation, being aggressive, other emotional changes and thoughts about suicide or possible suicide attempts. Consult doctor about your risks or call doctor right away if any symptoms occur.

POSSIBLE INTERACTION WITH OTHER DRUGS

GENERIC NAME OR DRUG CLASS	COMBINED EFFECT
Cimetidine	May increase effect of varenicline.
Insulin	No interaction, but dosage may need adjustment once you quit smoking.
Nicotine replacement	May increase risk of side effects.
Theophylline	No interaction, but dosage may need adjustment once you quit smoking.
Warfarin	No interaction, but dosage may need adjustment once you quit smoking.

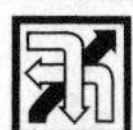

POSSIBLE INTERACTION WITH OTHER SUBSTANCES

INTERACTS WITH	COMBINED EFFECT
Alcohol:	None expected.
Beverages:	None expected.
Cocaine:	Unknown. Avoid.
Foods:	None expected.
Marijuana:	Unknown. Avoid.
Tobacco:	As intended, varenicline blocks the pleasurable effect of nicotine.

VILAZODONE

BRAND NAMES

Viibryd

BASIC INFORMATION

Habit forming? No
Prescription needed? Yes
Available as generic? Yes
Drug class: Antidepressant

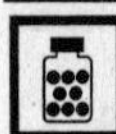

USES

- Treatment for major depressive disorder.
- Other uses as recommended by your doctor.

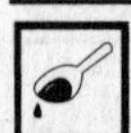

DOSAGE & USAGE INFORMATION

How to take:
Tablet—Swallow with liquid and take with food. The drug may not work as well if you take it on an empty stomach. If you can't swallow tablet whole, ask your doctor or pharmacist for advice.

When to take:
Once a day at the same time each day (usually with a meal).

If you forget a dose:
Take as soon as you remember. If it is almost time for the next dose, wait for the next scheduled dose (don't double this dose).

What drug does:
The exact mechanism is not fully understood. The drug's dual action increases the level and the effects of serotonin (a brain chemical; also called neurotransmitter). Serotonin plays a role in emotions and psychological disturbances.

Time lapse before drug works:
Begins in 1 to 2 weeks. May require 4 to 6 weeks for maximum benefit.

Don't take with:
Any other medicine or any dietary supplement without consulting your doctor or pharmacist.

OVERDOSE

SYMPTOMS:
Restlessness, hallucinations, disorientation, lethargy, serotonin syndrome.*
WHAT TO DO:
- **Dial 911 (emergency) for medical help or call poison control center 1-800-222-1222 for instructions.**
- **See emergency information on last 3 pages of this book.**

POSSIBLE ADVERSE REACTIONS OR SIDE EFFECTS

SYMPTOMS	WHAT TO DO
Life-threatening:	
Rare allergic reaction (hives, itching, rash, wheezing, tightness in chest, swelling of lips or tongue or throat).	Seek emergency treatment immediately.
Common:	
Diarrhea, nausea, trouble sleeping, dizziness, dry mouth, change in sexual desire or function.	Continue. Call doctor when convenient.
Infrequent:	
Vomiting, abnormal dreams, blurred vision, dry eye, migraine, sedation.	Continue. Call doctor when convenient.
Rare:	
New or sudden changes in mood, behavior, actions, thoughts, feelings, speaking, energy (especially if severe); suicidal thinking or behavior; abnormal bleeding; seizures; low sodium levels in your body (weakness, memory problems, headache, mental changes); serotonin syndrome or neuroleptic syndrome (fast heartbeat, muscle twitching or tightness or stiffness, agitation, hallucinations, fever, sweating, confusion, coordination problems).	Discontinue. Call doctor right away.

WARNINGS & PRECAUTIONS

Don't take if:
- You are allergic to vilazodone.
- You have taken a monoamine oxidase (MAO) inhibitor* within 2 weeks.

Before you start, consult your doctor if:
- You have a history or family history of mania or hypomania or bipolar disorder.
- You have or have had seizures or convulsions.
- You have low sodium levels (per lab tests).
- You drink alcohol.
- You have or have had bleeding problems.
- You have liver or kidney problems.

Over age 60:
No special problems expected.

Pregnancy:
Decide with your doctor if drug benefits justify any possible risk to unborn child. Risk category C (see page xviii).

Breast-feeding:
It is unknown if drug passes into milk. Consult doctor for advice.

Infants & children:
Not approved in ages under 18. If prescribed, carefully read information provided with prescription. Contact doctor right away if symptoms get worse or any there is any talk of suicide or suicide behaviors. Read information under Others.

Prolonged use:
Consult with your doctor on a regular basis while taking this drug to monitor your progress, check for side effects and for recommended lab tests.

Skin & sunlight:
No problems expected.

Driving, piloting or hazardous work:
Don't drive or pilot aircraft until you learn how drug affects you. Don't work around dangerous machinery. Don't climb ladders or work in high places. Danger increases if you drink alcohol or take drugs affecting alertness and reflexes.

Discontinuing:
- Don't discontinue without consulting doctor. Dose may require gradual reduction. Doses of other drugs may also require adjustment.
- If new or unexplained symptoms occur after stopping the drug, call doctor right away.

Others:
- Adults and children taking antidepressants may experience a worsening of the depression symptoms, unusual behavior changes and may display increased suicidal thoughts or behavior. Call doctor right away if these symptoms or behaviors occur.
- Advise any doctor or dentist whom you consult that you take this drug.

POSSIBLE INTERACTION WITH OTHER DRUGS

GENERIC NAME OR DRUG CLASS	COMBINED EFFECT
Anticoagulants*	Increased risk of abnormal bleeding.
Anti-inflammatory drugs, nonsteroidal (NSAIDs)*	Increased risk of abnormal bleeding.
Antiplatelet drugs*	Increased risk of abnormal bleeding.
Central nervous system (CNS) depressants*	Increased sedation.
Diuretics*	May increase risk of hyponatremia (low sodium in blood).
Dopamine antagonists*	Risk of neuroleptic malignant syndrome* or serotonin syndrome.*
Enzyme inhibitors*	Increased effect of vilazodone.
Enzyme inducers*	Decrease effect of vilazodone.
Monoamine oxidase (MAO) inhibitors*	Severe adverse reactions. Allow 14 days between use.
Protein bound drugs,* other	Increased effect of protein bound drug.
Serotonergics,* other	Risk of serotonin syndrome.* Avoid.

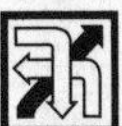

POSSIBLE INTERACTION WITH OTHER SUBSTANCES

INTERACTS WITH	COMBINED EFFECT
Alcohol:	Increased sedation. Avoid.
Beverages: Grapefruit juice.	May increase effect of vilazodone.
Cocaine:	Unknown. Avoid.
Food: Grapefruit.	May increase effect of vilazodone.
Marijuana:	Unknown. Avoid.
Tobacco:	None expected.

***See Glossary**

VITAMIN A

BRAND NAMES

Acon
Afaxin
Alphalin
Aquasol A
Dispatabs
Sust-A

Numerous brands of single vitamin and multivitamin combinations are available.

BASIC INFORMATION

Habit forming? No
Prescription needed? No
Available as generic? Yes
Drug class: Vitamin supplement

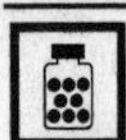

USES

- Dietary supplement to ensure normal growth and health, especially of eyes and skin.
- Beta carotene form decreases severity of sun exposure in patients with porphyria.

DOSAGE & USAGE INFORMATION

How to take:
- Drops or capsule—Swallow with liquid. If you can't swallow whole, open capsule and take with liquid or food.
- Oral solution—Swallow with liquid.
- Tablet—Swallow with liquid.

When to take:
At the same time each day.

If you forget a dose:
Take as soon as you remember. If it is almost time for the next dose, wait for that dose (don't double this dose) and resume regular schedule.

What drug does:
Promotes normal growth and health.

Continued next column

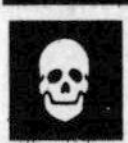

OVERDOSE

SYMPTOMS:
Increased adverse reactions and side effects. Jaundice (rare, but may occur with large doses), malaise, vomiting, irritability, bleeding gums, seizures, double vision, peeling skin.
WHAT TO DO:
If person takes much larger amount than prescribed, dial 911 (emergency) for medical help or call poison control center 1-800-222-1222 for instructions.

Time lapse before drug works:
Requires continual intake.

Don't take with:
Any other medicine or any dietary supplement without consulting your doctor or pharmacist.

POSSIBLE ADVERSE REACTIONS OR SIDE EFFECTS

SYMPTOMS	WHAT TO DO
Life-threatening:	
In case of overdose, see previous column.	
Common:	
None expected.	
Infrequent:	
Confusion; dizziness; drowsiness; headache; irritability; dry, cracked lips; peeling skin; hair loss; sensitivity to light.	Continue. Call doctor when convenient.
Rare:	
• Bulging soft spot on baby's head, double vision, bone or joint pain, abdominal pain, frequent urination, vomiting.	Discontinue. Call doctor right away.
• Diarrhea, appetite loss, nausea.	Continue. Call doctor when convenient.

WARNINGS & PRECAUTIONS

Don't take if:
You have chronic kidney failure.

Before you start, consult your doctor if:
You have any kidney disorder.

Over age 60:
No problems expected.

Pregnancy:
Risk factor determined by length of pregnancy and dosage amount. See category list on page xviii and consult doctor.

Breast-feeding:
No problems expected. Consult doctor.

Infants & children:
- Avoid large doses.
- Keep vitamin-mineral supplements out of children's reach.

Prolonged use:
No problems expected.

Skin & sunlight:
No special problems expected.

Driving, piloting or hazardous work:
No problems expected.

Discontinuing:
Don't discontinue without doctor's advice until you complete prescribed dose, even though symptoms diminish or disappear.

Others:
- Don't exceed recommended dosage. Too much over a long time may be harmful.
- A balanced diet will help provide vitamin A. Best sources are liver; yellow-orange fruits and vegetables; dark-green, leafy vegetables; milk; butter and margarine.

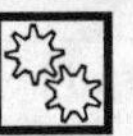

POSSIBLE INTERACTION WITH OTHER DRUGS

GENERIC NAME OR DRUG CLASS	COMBINED EFFECT
Anticoagulants*	Increased anticoagulant effect with large doses (over 10,000 I.U.) of vitamin A.
Calcium supplements*	Decreased vitamin effect.
Cholestyramine	Decreased vitamin A absorption.
Colestipol	Decreased vitamin absorption.
Contraceptives, oral*	Increased vitamin A levels.
Etretinate	Increased risk of toxic effects.
Isotretinoin	Increased risk of toxic effect of each.
Mineral oil (long-term)	Decreased vitamin A absorption.
Neomycin	Decreased vitamin absorption.
Vitamin A derivatives, other	Increased toxicity risk.
Vitamin E (excess dose)	Vitamin A depletion.

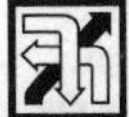

POSSIBLE INTERACTION WITH OTHER SUBSTANCES

INTERACTS WITH	COMBINED EFFECT
Alcohol:	None expected.
Beverages:	None expected.
Cocaine:	None expected.
Foods:	None expected.
Marijuana:	None expected.
Tobacco:	None expected.

*See Glossary

VITAMIN B-12 (Cyanocobalamin)

GENERIC AND BRAND NAMES

CYANOCOBALAMIN
Anocobin
Bedoz
Berubigen
Betalin 12
CaloMist
Cyanabin
Kaybovite
Kaybovite-1000
Nascobal
Redisol
Rubion
Rubramin
Rubramin-PC

HYDROXOCOBALAMIN
Acti-B-12
Alpha Redisol
Alphamin
Codroxomin
Droxomin

Numerous brands of single vitamin and multivitamin combinations may be available.

BASIC INFORMATION

Habit forming? No
Prescription needed? Yes, for some
Available as generic? Yes
Drug class: Vitamin supplement

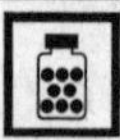

USES

- Dietary supplement for normal growth, development and health.
- Treatment for nerve damage.
- Treatment for pernicious anemia.
- Treatment and prevention of vitamin B-12 deficiencies in people who have had stomach or intestines surgically removed.
- Prevention of vitamin B-12 deficiency in strict vegetarians and persons with absorption diseases.

OVERDOSE

SYMPTOMS:
Increased adverse reactions and side effects.
WHAT TO DO:
Overdose unlikely to threaten life. If person uses much larger amount than prescribed or if accidentally swallowed, call doctor or poison control center 1-800-222-1222 for help.

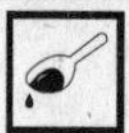

DOSAGE & USAGE INFORMATION

How to take:
- Tablet—Swallow with liquid.
- Extended-release tablet—Swallow whole with liquid. Do not crush or chew.
- Injection—Follow doctor's directions.
- Nasal gel or nasal spray—Follow instructions on product. Use nasal spray 1 hour before or 1 hour after eating hot foods or drinking hot liquids.

When to take:
- Oral—At the same time each day.
- Injection—Follow doctor's directions.
- Nasal gel or spray—Use weekly or as directed on prescription.

If you forget a dose:
Take as soon as you remember. If it is almost time for the next dose, wait for that dose (don't double this dose) and resume regular schedule.

What drug does:
Acts as enzyme to promote normal fat and carbohydrate metabolism and protein synthesis.

Time lapse before drug works:
15 minutes.

Don't take with:
Any other medicine or any dietary supplement without consulting your doctor or pharmacist.

POSSIBLE ADVERSE REACTIONS OR SIDE EFFECTS

SYMPTOMS	WHAT TO DO
Life-threatening:	
Hives, rash, intense itching, faintness soon after a dose (anaphylaxis).	Seek emergency treatment immediately.
Common:	
None expected.	
Infrequent:	
None expected.	
Rare:	
• Itchy skin, wheezing.	Discontinue. Call doctor right away.
• Diarrhea.	Continue. Call doctor when convenient.

VITAMIN B-12 (Cyanocobalamin)

WARNINGS & PRECAUTIONS

Don't take if:
- You are allergic to any B vitamin.
- You have Leber's disease (optic nerve atrophy).

Before you start, consult your doctor if:
- You have gout.
- You have heart disease.

Over age 60:
Don't take more than recommended amount per day unless prescribed by your doctor.

Pregnancy:
Risk factor determined by length of pregnancy and dosage amount. See category list on page xviii and consult doctor.

Breast-feeding:
Effect unknown. Consult doctor.

Infants & children:
No problems expected.

Prolonged use:
No problems expected.

Skin & sunlight:
No problems expected.

Driving, piloting or hazardous work:
No problems expected.

Discontinuing:
Don't discontinue without doctor's advice until you complete prescribed dose, even though symptoms diminish or disappear.

Others:
- A balanced diet should provide all the vitamin B-12 a healthy person needs and make supplements unnecessary. Best sources are meat, fish, egg yolk and cheese.
- Tablets should be used only for diet supplements. All other uses of vitamin B-12 require injections.
- Don't take large doses of vitamin C (1,000 mg or more per day) unless prescribed by your doctor.

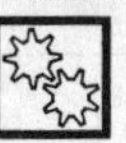

POSSIBLE INTERACTION WITH OTHER DRUGS

GENERIC NAME OR DRUG CLASS	COMBINED EFFECT
Anticonvulsants*	Decreased absorption of vitamin B-12.
Chloramphenicol	Decreased vitamin B-12 effect.
Cholestyramine	Decreased absorption of vitamin B-12.
Cimetidine	Decreased absorption of vitamin B-12.
Colchicine	Decreased absorption of vitamin B-12.
Famotidine	Decreased absorption of vitamin B-12.
H_2 antagonists*	Decreased absorption of vitamin B-12.
Neomycin	Decreased absorption of vitamin B-12.
Para-aminosalicylic acid	Decreased effects of para-aminosalicylic acid.
Potassium (extended-release forms)	Decreased absorption of vitamin B-12.
Ranitidine	Decreased absorption of vitamin B-12.
Vitamin C (ascorbic acid)	Destroys vitamin B-12 if taken at same time. Take 2 hours apart.

POSSIBLE INTERACTION WITH OTHER SUBSTANCES

INTERACTS WITH	COMBINED EFFECT
Alcohol:	Decreased absorption of vitamin B-12.
Beverages:	None expected.
Cocaine:	None expected.
Foods:	None expected.
Marijuana:	None expected.
Tobacco:	None expected.

*See Glossary

VITAMIN C (Ascorbic Acid)

BRAND NAMES

Ascorbicap
Cecon
Cemill
Cenolate
Cetane
Cevalin
Cevi-Bid
Ce-Vi-Sol
Cevita
C-Span
Flavorcee
Redoxon
Sunkist

Numerous brands of single vitamin and multivitamin combinations are available.

BASIC INFORMATION

Habit forming? No
Prescription needed? No
Available as generic? Yes
Drug class: Vitamin supplement

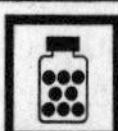

USES

- Prevention and treatment of scurvy and other vitamin C deficiencies.
- Treatment of anemia.
- Maintenance of acid urine.

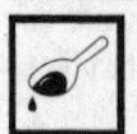

DOSAGE & USAGE INFORMATION

How to take:
- Tablet or capsule—Swallow with liquid.
- Extended-release tablet or extended-release capsule—Swallow whole with liquid. Do not crush or chew.
- Chewable tablet—Chew well, then swallow.
- Effervescent tablet—Follow label instructions. Let tablet dissolve in water and drink entire mixture.
- Suspension, solution or drops—Use a dropper or dose-measuring spoon to measure doses.
- Syrup—Follow label instructions. Use a dose-measuring spoon to measure dosage and then swallow.
- Lozenge—Let dissolve completely in mouth.
- Powder or crystal—Measure and mix as directed. Drink all the mixture right away.

Continued next column

When to take:
1, 2 or 3 times per day, as prescribed on label.

If you forget a dose:
Take as soon as you remember. If it is almost time for the next dose, wait for that dose (don't double this dose) and resume regular schedule.

What drug does:
- May help form collagen.
- Increases iron absorption from intestine.
- Contributes to hemoglobin and red blood cell production in bone marrow.

Time lapse before drug works:
1 week.

Don't take with:
Any other medicine or any dietary supplement without consulting your doctor or pharmacist.

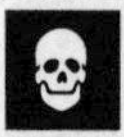

OVERDOSE

SYMPTOMS:
Diarrhea, vomiting, dizziness.
WHAT TO DO:
Overdose unlikely to threaten life. If person uses much larger amount than prescribed or if accidentally swallowed, call doctor or poison control center 1-800-222-1222 for help.

POSSIBLE ADVERSE REACTIONS OR SIDE EFFECTS

SYMPTOMS	WHAT TO DO
Life-threatening:	
None expected.	
Common:	
None expected.	
Infrequent:	
• Mild diarrhea, nausea, vomiting.	Discontinue. Call doctor right away.
• Flushed face.	Continue. Call doctor when convenient.
Rare:	
• Kidney stones with high doses, anemia, abdominal pain.	Discontinue. Call doctor right away.
• Headache.	Continue. Tell doctor at next visit.

VITAMIN C (Ascorbic Acid)

WARNINGS & PRECAUTIONS

Don't take if:
You are allergic to vitamin C.

Before you start, consult your doctor if:
- You have sickle-cell or other anemia.
- You have had kidney stones.
- You have gout.

Over age 60:
Don't take more than recommended amount per day unless prescribed by your doctor.

Pregnancy:
Risk factor determined by length of pregnancy and dosage amount. See category list on page xviii and consult doctor.

Breast-feeding:
Avoid large doses. Consult doctor.

Infants & children:
- Avoid large doses. Follow instructions on label.
- Keep vitamin-mineral supplements out of children's reach.

Prolonged use:
Large doses for longer than 2 months may cause kidney stones.

Skin & sunlight:
No problems expected.

Driving, piloting or hazardous work:
No problems expected.

Discontinuing:
No problems expected.

Others:
- Store in cool, dry place.
- May cause inaccurate tests for sugar in urine or blood in stool.
- May cause crisis in patients with sickle-cell anemia.
- A balanced diet should provide all the vitamin C a healthy person needs and make supplements unnecessary. Best sources are citrus, strawberries, cantaloupe and raw peppers.
- Don't take large doses of vitamin C (1,000 mg or more per day) unless prescribed by your doctor.
- Some products contain tartrazine dye. Avoid, if allergic (especially aspirin hypersensitivity).

POSSIBLE INTERACTION WITH OTHER DRUGS

GENERIC NAME OR DRUG CLASS	COMBINED EFFECT
Amphetamines*	Possible decreased amphetamine effect.
Anticholinergics*	Possible decreased anticholinergic effect.
Anticoagulants,* oral	Possible decreased anticoagulant effect.
Antidepressants, tricyclic (TCA)*	Possible decreased antidepressant effect.
Aspirin	Decreased vitamin C effect and salicylate excretion.
Barbiturates*	Decreased vitamin C effect. Increased barbiturate effect.
Cellulose sodium phosphate	Decreased vitamin C effect.
Contraceptives, oral*	Decreased vitamin C effect.
Estrogens*	Increased likelihood of adverse effects from estrogen with 1 g or more of vitamin C per day.
Iron supplements*	Increased iron absorption.
Mexiletine	Possible decreased effectiveness of mexiletine.
Quinidine	Possible decreased quinidine effect.
Salicylates*	Decreased vitamin C effect and salicylate excretion. May lead to salicylate toxicity.
Tranquilizers* (phenothiazine)	May decrease phenothiazine effect if no vitamin C deficiency exists.

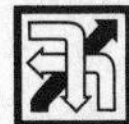

POSSIBLE INTERACTION WITH OTHER SUBSTANCES

INTERACTS WITH	COMBINED EFFECT
Alcohol:	None expected.
Beverages:	None expected.
Cocaine:	None expected.
Foods:	None expected.
Marijuana:	None expected.
Tobacco:	Increased requirement for vitamin C.

VITAMIN D

GENERIC AND BRAND NAMES

ALFACALCIDOL
One-Alpha
CALCIFEDIOL
Calderol
CALCITRIOL
Rocaltrol
CHOLECALCIFEROL
Fosamax Plus D
Fosavance

DIHYDROTACHY-STEROL
DHT
DHT Intensol
Hytakerol
DOXERCALCIFEROL
Hectorol
ERGOCALCIFEROL
Calciferol
Drisdol
Osto Forte
Radiostol
Radiostol Forte

(Many other name brands are available)

BASIC INFORMATION

Habit forming? No
Prescription needed? Only for high strength
Available as generic? Yes
Drug class: Vitamin supplement

USES

- Dietary supplement.
- Prevention of rickets (bone disease).
- Treatment for hypocalcemia (low blood calcium) in kidney disease.
- Supplement in those who use sunscreen daily.

DOSAGE & USAGE INFORMATION

How to take:
- Tablet or capsule—Swallow with liquid.
- Extended-release tablet or extended-release capsule—Swallow whole with liquid. Do not crush or chew.
- Chewable tablet—Chew well, then swallow.
- Effervescent tablet—Follow label instructions. Dissolve tablet in water. Drink entire mixture.

Continued next column

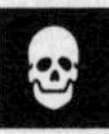

OVERDOSE

SYMPTOMS:
Severe stomach pain, nausea, vomiting, weight loss; bone and muscle pain; increased urination, cloudy urine; mood or mental changes (possible psychosis); high blood pressure, irregular heartbeat; eye irritation or light sensitivity; itchy skin.
WHAT TO DO:
Overdose unlikely to threaten life. If person uses much larger amount than prescribed or if accidentally swallowed, call doctor or poison control center 1-800-222-1222 for help.

- Suspension, solution or drops—Use a dropper or dose-measuring spoon to measure doses.
- Syrup—Follow label instructions. Use a dose-measuring spoon to measure dosage and then swallow.
- Lozenge—Let dissolve completely in mouth.
- Powder or crystal—Measure and mix as directed. Drink all the mixture right away.

When to take:
As directed, usually once a day at the same time each day. Some are taken once a week/month.

If you forget a dose:
Take as soon as you remember. If it is almost time for the next dose, wait for that dose (don't double this dose) and resume regular schedule.

What drug does:
- Maintains growth and health.
- Prevents rickets.
- Essential so body can use calcium and phosphate.

Time lapse before drug works:
2 hours. May require 2 to 3 weeks of continual use for maximum effect.

Don't take with:
Any other medicine or any dietary supplement without consulting your doctor or pharmacist.

POSSIBLE ADVERSE REACTIONS OR SIDE EFFECTS

SYMPTOMS	WHAT TO DO
Life-threatening:	
In case of overdose, see previous column.	
Common:	
None expected.	
Infrequent:	
Headache, metallic taste in mouth, thirst, dry mouth, constipation, appetite loss, nausea, vomiting, weakness, cloudy urine, sensitivity to light.	Continue. Call doctor when convenient.
Rare:	
• Increased urination, pink eye, psychosis, severe abdominal pain, fever.	Discontinue. Call doctor right away.
• Muscle pain, bone pain, diarrhea.	Continue. Tell doctor when convenient.

WARNINGS & PRECAUTIONS

Don't take if:
You are allergic to medicine containing vitamin D.

Before you start, consult your doctor if:
- You plan to become pregnant while taking vitamin D.
- You have epilepsy.
- You have heart or blood-vessel disease.
- You have kidney disease.

Over age 60:
Adverse reactions and side effects may be more frequent and severe than in younger persons.

Pregnancy:
Risk factor determined by length of pregnancy and dosage amount. See category list on page xviii and consult doctor.

Breast-feeding:
No problems expected, but consult doctor.

Infants & children:
- Avoid large doses.
- Keep vitamins out of children's reach.

Prolonged use:
- No problems expected.
- Talk to your doctor about the need for follow-up medical examinations or laboratory studies to check kidney function, liver function, serum calcium.

Skin & sunlight:
No special problems expected.

Driving, piloting or hazardous work:
No problems expected.

Discontinuing:
Don't discontinue without doctor's advice until you complete prescribed dose, even though symptoms diminish or disappear.

Others:
- Don't exceed dose. Too much over a long time may be harmful.
- Some products contain tartrazine dye. Avoid, if allergic (especially aspirin hypersensitivity).
- Sunscreen prevents the body from manufacturing vitamin D from sunshine. Consider supplementary vitamin D if you use sunscreen daily. Ask doctor for advice.

POSSIBLE INTERACTION WITH OTHER DRUGS

GENERIC NAME OR DRUG CLASS	COMBINED EFFECT
Antacids* (magnesium-containing)	Possible excess magnesium.
Anticonvulsants, hydantoin*	Decreased vitamin D effect.
Calcium (high doses)	Excess calcium in blood.
Calcium channel blockers*	Possible decreased effect of calcium channel blockers.
Calcium supplements*	Excessive absorption of vitamin D.
Cholestyramine	Decreased vitamin D effect.
Colestipol	Decreased vitamin D absorption.
Cortisone	Decreased vitamin D effect.
Digitalis preparations*	Heartbeat irregularities.
Diuretics, thiazide*	Possible increased calcium.
Mineral oil	Decreased vitamin D effect.
Neomycin	Decreased vitamin D absorption.
Nicardipine	Decreased nicardipine effect.
Phenobarbital	Decreased vitamin D effect.
Phosphorus preparations*	Accumulation of excess phosphorus.
Rifampin	Possible decreased vitamin D effect.
Vitamin D, other	Possible toxicity.

POSSIBLE INTERACTION WITH OTHER SUBSTANCES

INTERACTS WITH	COMBINED EFFECT
Alcohol:	None expected.
Beverages:	None expected.
Cocaine:	None expected.
Foods:	None expected.
Marijuana:	None expected.
Tobacco:	None expected.

*See Glossary

VITAMIN D (Topical)

GENERIC AND BRAND NAMES

CALCIPOTRIENE
Dovonex
Sorilux
Taclonex

CALCITRIOL (topical)
Vectical

BASIC INFORMATION

Habit forming? No
Prescription needed? Yes
Available as generic? Yes, for some
Drug class: Antipsoriatic

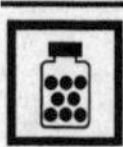

USES

Treats discoid or "plaque" psoriasis, the most common form of the disorder.

DOSAGE & USAGE INFORMATION

How to use:
Cream, ointment, foam or topical solution—Apply a thin layer to the affected skin or scalp as per instructions. Rub in gently and completely. Avoid your eyes, mouth and vagina. Wash hands after use.

When to use:
Twice a day or as advised by your doctor.

If you forget a dose:
Apply as soon as you remember, then return to regular schedule.

What drug does:
It helps slow the growth of abnormal skin cells.

Time lapse before drug works:
2 weeks. May take up to 8 weeks for maximum benefits that can include marked improvement in symptoms for most patients or complete clearing for others.

Continued next column

OVERDOSE

SYMPTOMS:
May be absorbed into the body through excess topical application and increase the levels of calcium and cause nausea, vomiting, loss of appetite, increased thirst and urination, unusual tiredness or weakness.
WHAT TO DO:
Overdose unlikely to threaten life. If person uses much larger amount than prescribed or if accidentally swallowed, call doctor or poison control center 1-800-222-1222 for help.

Don't use with:
Other topical or oral drugs without consulting with your doctor or pharmacist.

POSSIBLE ADVERSE REACTIONS OR SIDE EFFECTS

SYMPTOMS	WHAT TO DO
Life-threatening: None expected.	
Common: Irritation, burning, itching of the skin.	Discontinue. Call doctor when convenient.
Infrequent: Redness, dryness, peeling, rash, worsening of psoriasis.	Discontinue. Call doctor when convenient.
Rare: Darkening of treated areas of skin, pus in hair follicles; very rare symptoms may occur if drug absorbed into body (nausea, vomiting, loss of appetite, increased thirst and urination, unusual tiredness or weakness).	Discontinue. Call doctor when convenient.

WARNINGS & PRECAUTIONS

Don't use if:
- You are allergic to topical vitamin D.
- You have hypercalcemia (excess of calcium in the body).

Before you start, consult your doctor if:
- You have had allergic reaction to other topical drugs, oral drugs, food or other substances.
- You are taking calcium supplements, oral vitamin D or thiazide diuretics.

Over age 60:
Adverse reactions and side effects may be more frequent and severe than in younger persons.

Pregnancy:
Decide with your doctor if drug benefits justify any possible risk to unborn child. Risk category C (see page xviii).

Breast-feeding:
It is unknown if drugs pass into milk. Avoid drug or discontinue nursing until you finish medicine. Consult doctor for advice on maintaining milk supply.

Infants & children:
Approved for use in age 18 and older. Safety in children has not been established. Use only under close medical supervision. Adverse reactions and side effects may be more frequent and severe.

Prolonged use:
Talk to your doctor about the need for follow-up laboratory studies to check calcium levels in your blood or urine.

Skin & sunlight:
Your skin may be more sensitive to sunlight when using this drug. Sunlight exposure (even brief periods) may cause a skin rash, itching, redness, other skin discoloration or a severe sunburn. When you begin using this drug, try to stay out of direct sunlight, especially between the hours of 10:00 a.m. and 3:00 p.m. Apply a sunblock product that has an SPF of 30 or higher. Wear protective clothing, including a hat and sunglasses. Do not use a sun lamp or tanning bed or booth. Consult your doctor if you have any concerns.

Driving, piloting or hazardous work:
No special problems expected.

Discontinuing:
No special problems expected.

Others:
- Wash hands after applying the drug.
- Advise any doctor or dentist whom you consult that you use this medicine.
- One or more of these products is flammable. Read label. Do not use near an open flame.

POSSIBLE INTERACTION WITH OTHER DRUGS

GENERIC NAME OR DRUG CLASS	COMBINED EFFECT
Calcium supplements	Increased calcium in the blood.
Diuretics, thiazide	Increased calcium in the blood.
Vitamin D (oral)	Increased calcium in the blood.

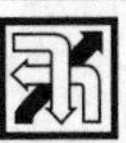

POSSIBLE INTERACTION WITH OTHER SUBSTANCES

INTERACTS WITH	COMBINED EFFECT
Alcohol:	None expected.
Beverages:	None expected.
Cocaine:	None expected.
Foods:	None expected.
Marijuana:	None expected.
Tobacco:	None expected.

*See Glossary

VITAMIN E

BRAND NAMES

Aquasol E
Chew-E
Eprolin
Epsilan-M
Pheryl-E
Viterra E

Numerous brands of single vitamin and multivitamin combinations are available.

BASIC INFORMATION

Habit forming? No
Prescription needed? No
Available as generic? Yes
Drug class: Vitamin supplement

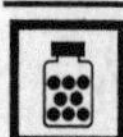

USES

- Dietary supplement to promote normal growth, development and health.
- Treatment and prevention of vitamin E deficiency, especially in premature or low-birth-weight infants.
- Treatment for fibrocystic disease of the breast.
- Treatment for circulatory problems to the lower extremities.
- Treatment for sickle-cell anemia.
- Treatment for lung toxicity from air pollution.

DOSAGE & USAGE INFORMATION

How to take:

- Tablet or capsule—Swallow with liquid.
- Extended-release tablet or extended-release capsule—Swallow whole with liquid. Do not crush or chew.
- Chewable tablet—Chew well, then swallow.
- Effervescent tablet—Follow label instructions. Let tablet dissolve in water and drink entire mixture.
- Suspension, solution or drops—Use a dropper or dose-measuring spoon to measure doses.
- Syrup—Follow label instructions. Use a dose-measuring spoon to measure dosage and then swallow.
- Lozenge—Let dissolve completely in mouth.
- Powder or crystal—Measure and mix as directed. Drink all the mixture right away.

Continued next column

OVERDOSE

SYMPTOMS:
Nausea, vomiting, fatigue.
WHAT TO DO:
Overdose unlikely to threaten life. If person uses much larger amount than prescribed or if accidentally swallowed, call doctor or poison control center 1-800-222-1222 for help.

When to take:
At the same times each day.

If you forget a dose:
Take as soon as you remember. If it is almost time for the next dose, wait for that dose (don't double this dose) and resume regular schedule.

What drug does:

- Promotes normal growth and development.
- Prevents oxidation in body.

Time lapse before drug works:
Will vary depending on the disorder being treated.

Don't take with:
Any other medicine or any dietary supplement without consulting your doctor or pharmacist.

POSSIBLE ADVERSE REACTIONS OR SIDE EFFECTS

SYMPTOMS	WHAT TO DO
Life-threatening: None expected.	
Common: Breast enlargement, dizziness, headache.	Continue. Call doctor when convenient.
Infrequent: Nausea, abdominal pain, muscle aches, pain in lower legs, fever, tiredness, weakness.	Continue. Call doctor when convenient.
Rare: Blurred vision, diarrhea.	Discontinue. Call doctor right away.

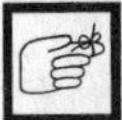

WARNINGS & PRECAUTIONS

Don't take if:
You are allergic to vitamin E.

Before you start, consult your doctor if:
- You have had blood clots in leg veins (thrombophlebitis).
- You have liver disease.

Over age 60:
No problems expected. Avoid excessive doses.

Pregnancy:
No problems expected with normal daily requirements. Don't exceed prescribed dose. Consult doctor.

Breast-feeding:
No problems expected. Consult doctor.

Infants & children:
Use only under medical supervision.

Prolonged use:
Toxic accumulation of vitamin E. Don't exceed recommended dose.

Skin & sunlight:
No problems expected.

Driving, piloting or hazardous work:
No problems expected.

Discontinuing:
No problems expected.

Others:
A balanced diet should provide all the vitamin E a healthy person needs and make supplements unnecessary. Best sources are vegetable oils, whole-grain cereals, liver.

POSSIBLE INTERACTION WITH OTHER DRUGS

GENERIC NAME OR DRUG CLASS	COMBINED EFFECT
Anticoagulants,* oral	Increased anticoagulant effect.
Cholestyramine	Decreased vitamin E absorption.
Colestipol	Decreased vitamin E absorption.
Iron supplements*	Possible decreased effect of iron supplement in patients with iron-deficiency anemia. Decreased vitamin E effect in healthy persons.
Mineral oil	Decreased vitamin E effect.
Neomycin	Decreased vitamin E absorption.
Vitamin A	Recommended dose of vitamin E—Increased benefit and decreased toxicity of vitamin A. Excess dose of vitamin E—Vitamin A depletion.

POSSIBLE INTERACTION WITH OTHER SUBSTANCES

INTERACTS WITH	COMBINED EFFECT
Alcohol:	None expected.
Beverages:	None expected.
Cocaine:	None expected.
Foods:	None expected.
Marijuana:	None expected.
Tobacco:	None expected.

*See Glossary

VITAMIN K

GENERIC AND BRAND NAMES

MENADIOL	PHYTONADIONE
Synkayvite	Mephyton

Numerous brands of single vitamin and multivitamin combinations may be available.

BASIC INFORMATION

Habit forming? No
Prescription needed? No
Available as generic? Yes
Drug class: Vitamin supplement

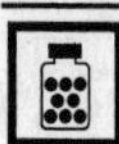

USES

- Dietary supplement.
- Treatment for bleeding disorders and malabsorption diseases due to vitamin K deficiency.
- Treatment for hemorrhagic disease of the newborn.
- Treatment for bleeding due to overdose of oral anticoagulants.

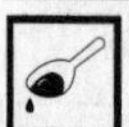

DOSAGE & USAGE INFORMATION

How to take:
- May be given by injection in hospital or doctor's office.
- Tablet or capsule—Swallow with liquid.
- Extended-release tablet or extended-release capsule—Swallow whole with liquid. Do not crush or chew.
- Chewable tablet—Chew well, then swallow.
- Effervescent tablet—Follow label instructions. Let tablet dissolve in water and drink entire mixture.
- Suspension, solution or drops—Use a dropper or dose-measuring spoon to measure doses.
- Syrup—Follow label instructions. Use a dose-measuring spoon to measure dosage and then swallow.
- Lozenge—Let dissolve completely in mouth.
- Powder or crystal—Measure and mix as directed. Drink all the mixture right away.

Continued next column

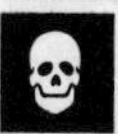

OVERDOSE

SYMPTOMS:
Nausea, vomiting.
WHAT TO DO:
Overdose unlikely to threaten life. If person uses much larger amount than prescribed or if accidentally swallowed, call doctor or poison control center 1-800-222-1222 for help.

When to take:
At the same time each day.

If you forget a dose:
Take as soon as you remember. If it is almost time for the next dose, wait for that dose (don't double this dose) and resume regular schedule.

What drug does:
- Promotes growth, development and good health.
- Supplies a necessary ingredient for blood clotting.

Time lapse before drug works:
15 to 30 minutes to support blood clotting. For some problems, it may take weeks or months.

Don't take with:
Any other medicine or any dietary supplement without consulting your doctor or pharmacist.

POSSIBLE ADVERSE REACTIONS OR SIDE EFFECTS

SYMPTOMS	WHAT TO DO
Life-threatening:	
None expected.	
Common:	
None expected.	
Infrequent:	
Unusual taste, face flushing.	Continue. Call doctor when convenient.
Rare:	
Rash, hives.	Discontinue. Call doctor right away.

WARNINGS & PRECAUTIONS

Don't take if:
- You are allergic to vitamin K.
- You have G6PD* deficiency.
- You have liver disease.

Before you start, consult your doctor if:
You are pregnant.

Over age 60:
No problems expected.

Pregnancy:
Risk factor determined by length of pregnancy and dosage amount. See category list on page xviii and consult doctor.

Breast-feeding:
No problems expected. Consult doctor.

Infants & children:
Phytonadione is the preferred form for hemorrhagic disease of the newborn.

Prolonged use:
Talk to your doctor about the need for follow-up medical examinations or laboratory studies to check prothrombin time.

Skin & sunlight:
No problems expected.

Driving, piloting or hazardous work:
No problems expected.

Discontinuing:
No problems expected.

Others:
- Tell all doctors and dentists you consult that you take this medicine.
- Don't exceed dose. Too much over a long time may be harmful.
- A balanced diet should provide all the vitamin K a healthy person needs and make supplements unnecessary. Best sources are green, leafy vegetables, meat or dairy products.

POSSIBLE INTERACTION WITH OTHER DRUGS

GENERIC NAME OR DRUG CLASS	COMBINED EFFECT
Anticoagulants,* oral	Decreased anticoagulant effect.
Cholestyramine	Decreased vitamin K effect.
Colestipol	Decreased vitamin K absorption.
Dapsone	Increased risk of adverse effect on blood cells.
Mineral oil (long-term)	Vitamin K deficiency.
Neomycin	Decreased vitamin K absorption.
Sulfa drugs*	Vitamin K deficiency.

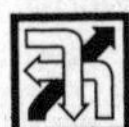

POSSIBLE INTERACTION WITH OTHER SUBSTANCES

INTERACTS WITH	COMBINED EFFECT
Alcohol:	None expected.
Beverages:	None expected.
Cocaine:	None expected.
Foods:	None expected.
Marijuana:	None expected.
Tobacco:	None expected.

*See Glossary

VITAMINS & FLUORIDE

GENERIC AND BRAND NAMES

Adeflor
Cari-Tab
Mulvidren-F
Poly-Vi-Flor
Tri-Vi-Flor
Vi-Daylin/F
Vi-Penta F

Also brands are available in the forms of multiple vitamins & fluoride; vitamins A, D & C & fluoride.

BASIC INFORMATION

Habit forming? No
Prescription needed? Yes
Available as generic? No
Drug class: Vitamins, minerals

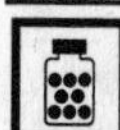

USES

- Reduces incidence of tooth cavities (fluoride). Children who need supplements should take until age 16.
- Prevents deficiencies of vitamin included in formula (some contain multiple vitamins whose content varies among products; others contain only vitamins A, D and C).

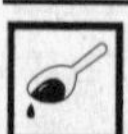

DOSAGE & USAGE INFORMATION

How to take:
- Chewable tablet—Chew or crush before swallowing.
- Oral liquid—Measure with specially marked dropper. May mix with food, fruit juice, cereal.

When to take:
- Bedtime or with or just after meals.
- If at bedtime, brush teeth first.

If you forget a dose:
Take as soon as you remember. If it is almost time for the next dose, wait for that dose (don't double this dose) and resume regular schedule.

Continued next column

OVERDOSE

SYMPTOMS:
Minor overdose—Black, brown or white spots on teeth.
Massive overdose—Shallow breathing, black or tarry stools, bloody vomit.
WHAT TO DO:
- **Dial 911 (emergency) for medical help or call poison control center 1-800-222-1222 for instructions.**
- **See emergency information on last 3 pages of this book.**

What drug does:
Provides supplemental fluoride to combat tooth decay.

Time lapse before drug works:
8 weeks to provide maximum benefit.

Don't take with:
- Other medicine at the same time.
- Any other medicine or any dietary supplement without consulting your doctor or pharmacist.

POSSIBLE ADVERSE REACTIONS OR SIDE EFFECTS

SYMPTOMS	WHAT TO DO
Life-threatening:	
Fainting, bloody vomit, bloody or black stool, breathing difficulty.	Discontinue. Seek emergency treatment.
Common:	
White, black or brown spots on teeth; nausea; vomiting.	Discontinue. Call doctor right away.
Infrequent:	
• Drowsiness; abdominal pain; increased salivation; watery eyes; weight loss; sore throat, fever, mouth sores; constipation; bone pain; rash; muscle stiffness; weakness; tremor; agitation.	Discontinue. Call doctor right away.
• Diarrhea.	Continue. Call doctor when convenient.
Rare:	
None expected.	

WARNINGS & PRECAUTIONS

Don't take if:

- Your water supply contains 0.7 parts fluoride per million. Too much fluoride stains teeth permanently.
- You are allergic to any fluoride-containing product.
- You have underactive thyroid.

Before you start, consult your doctor or dentist:
For proper dosage.

Over age 60:
No problems expected.

Pregnancy:
Risk factor determined by length of pregnancy and dosage amount. See category list on page xviii and consult doctor.

Breast-feeding:
No problems expected. Consult doctor.

Infants & children:
No problems expected in children over 3 years of age except in case of accidental overdose. Keep vitamin-mineral supplements out of children's reach.

Prolonged use:
Excess may cause discolored teeth and decreased calcium in blood.

Skin & sunlight:
No problems expected.

Driving, piloting or hazardous work:
No problems expected.

Discontinuing:
No problems expected.

Others:

- Store in original plastic container. Fluoride decomposes glass.
- Check with dentist once or twice a year to keep cavities at a minimum. Topical applications of fluoride may also be helpful.
- Fluoride probably not necessary if water contains about 1 part per million of fluoride or more. Check with health department.
- Don't freeze.
- Don't keep outdated medicine.

POSSIBLE INTERACTION WITH OTHER DRUGS

GENERIC NAME OR DRUG CLASS	COMBINED EFFECT
Anticoagulants*	Decreased effect of anticoagulant.
Iron supplements*	Decreased effect of any vitamin if iron is present in multivitamin product.
Vitamin A	May lead to vitamin A toxicity if vitamin A is in combination.
Vitamin D	May lead to vitamin D toxicity if vitamin D is in combination.

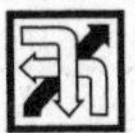

POSSIBLE INTERACTION WITH OTHER SUBSTANCES

INTERACTS WITH	COMBINED EFFECT
Alcohol:	None expected.
Beverages: Milk.	Prevents absorption of fluoride. Space dose 2 hours before or after milk.
Cocaine:	None expected.
Foods:	None expected.
Marijuana:	None expected.
Tobacco:	None expected.

XYLOMETAZOLINE

BRAND NAMES

Chlorohist-LA
Inspire
Neo-Synephrine II Long Acting Nasal Spray Adult Strength
Neo-Synephrine II Long Acting Nose Drops Adult Strength
Otrivin Decongestant Nose Drops
Otrivin Nasal Drops
Otrivin Nasal Spray
Otrivin Pediatric Decongestant Nose Drops
Otrivin Pediatric Nasal Drops
Otrivin Pediatric Nasal Spray
Otrivin with M-D Pump
Triaminic Decongestant Spray Nasal & Sinus Congestion

BASIC INFORMATION

Habit forming? No
Prescription needed? No
Available as generic? Yes
Drug class: Sympathomimetic

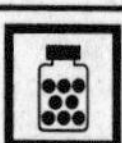

USES

Relieves congestion of nose, sinuses and throat from allergies and infections.

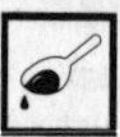

DOSAGE & USAGE INFORMATION

How to take:
Nasal solution, nasal spray—Use as directed on label. Avoid contamination. Don't use same container for more than 1 person.

When to take:
When needed, no more often than every 4 hours.

Continued next column

OVERDOSE

SYMPTOMS:
Headache, sweating, anxiety, agitation, rapid and irregular heartbeat (rare occurrence with systemic absorption).
WHAT TO DO:

- **Dial 911 (emergency) for medical help or call poison control center 1-800-222-1222 for instructions.**
- **If person is unconscious, check breathing and pulse. If not breathing, begin mouth-to-mouth rescue breathing. If heart is not beating, begin chest compressions.**
- **See emergency information on last 3 pages of this book.**

If you forget a dose:
Take as soon as you remember. Wait 4 hours for next dose.

What drug does:
Constricts walls of small arteries in nose, sinuses and eustachian tubes.

Time lapse before drug works:
5 to 30 minutes.

Don't take with:

- Nonprescription drugs for allergy, cough or cold without consulting doctor.
- Any other medicine or any dietary supplement without consulting your doctor or pharmacist.

POSSIBLE ADVERSE REACTIONS OR SIDE EFFECTS

SYMPTOMS	WHAT TO DO
Life-threatening:	
In case of overdose, see previous column.	
Common:	
None expected.	
Infrequent:	
Burning, dry or stinging nasal passages.	Continue. Call doctor when convenient.
Rare:	
Rebound congestion (increased runny or stuffy nose), headache, insomnia, nervousness (may occur with systemic absorption).	Discontinue. Call doctor when convenient.

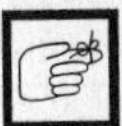

WARNINGS & PRECAUTIONS

Don't take if:
You are allergic to any sympathomimetic nasal spray.

Before you start, consult your doctor if:
- You have heart disease or high blood pressure.
- You have diabetes.
- You have overactive thyroid.
- You have taken a monoamine oxidase (MAO) inhibitor* in past 2 weeks.
- You have glaucoma.

Over age 60:
Adverse reactions and side effects may be more frequent and severe than in younger persons.

Pregnancy:
Decide with your doctor if drug benefits justify risk to unborn child. Risk category C (see page xviii).

Breast-feeding:
No proven problems. Consult doctor.

Infants & children:
Don't give to children younger than 2.

Prolonged use:
Drug may lose effectiveness, cause increased congestion (rebound effect*) and irritate nasal membranes.

Skin & sunlight:
No problems expected.

Driving, piloting or hazardous work:
No problems expected.

Discontinuing:
May be unnecessary to finish medicine. Follow doctor's instructions.

Others:
No problems expected.

POSSIBLE INTERACTION WITH OTHER DRUGS

GENERIC NAME OR DRUG CLASS	COMBINED EFFECT
Antidepressants, tricyclic*	Possible increased blood pressure.
Maprotiline	Possible increased blood pressure.
Monoamine oxidase (MAO) inhibitors*	Possible increased blood pressure.

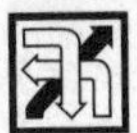

POSSIBLE INTERACTION WITH OTHER SUBSTANCES

INTERACTS WITH	COMBINED EFFECT
Alcohol:	None expected.
Beverages: Caffeine drinks.	Nervousness or insomnia.
Cocaine:	High risk of heartbeat irregularities and high blood pressure.
Foods:	None expected.
Marijuana:	Overstimulation. Avoid.
Tobacco:	None expected.

*See Glossary

ZALEPLON

BRAND NAMES

Sonata

BASIC INFORMATION

Habit forming? Yes
Prescription needed? Yes
Available as generic? Yes
Drug class: Anti-insomnia, hypnotic, sedative

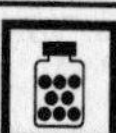

USES

Short-term treatment for insomnia (trouble sleeping).

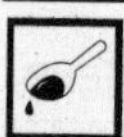

DOSAGE & USAGE INFORMATION

How to take:
Capsule—Swallow with liquid. If you can't swallow whole, open capsule and take with liquid or food.

When to take:
Take immediately before bedtime. Ensure that you can get at least 4 hours of rest after taking your medication. Zaleplon may be taken with or without food; however, if taken after a heavy or fatty meal, it may not work as fast as it should.

If you forget a dose:
Take as soon as you remember. If it is almost time for the next dose, wait for that dose (don't double this dose) and resume regular schedule.

What drug does:
Acts as a central nervous system depressant, decreasing sleep problems such as trouble falling asleep, waking up too often during the night and waking up too early in the morning.

Continued next column

OVERDOSE

SYMPTOMS:
Clumsiness, unsteadiness, stupor, severe dizziness or fainting, troubled breathing and sluggishness.
WHAT TO DO:

- **Dial 911 (emergency) for medical help or call poison control center 1-800-222-1222 for instructions.**
- **If person is unconscious, check breathing and pulse. If not breathing, begin mouth-to-mouth rescue breathing. If heart is not beating, begin chest compressions.**
- **See emergency information on last 3 pages of this book.**

Time lapse before drug works:
Within 2 hours.

Don't take with:
Any other medicine or any dietary supplement without consulting your doctor or pharmacist.

POSSIBLE ADVERSE REACTIONS OR SIDE EFFECTS

SYMPTOMS	WHAT TO DO
Life-threatening:	
Rare allergic reaction (hives, itching, rash, wheezing, tightness in chest, swelling of lips or tongue or throat).	Seek emergency treatment immediately.
Common:	
Dizziness, headache, muscle pain, nausea.	Continue. Call doctor when convenient.
Infrequent:	
• Anxiety, vision problems, not feeling like oneself.	Discontinue. Call doctor right away.
• Abdominal pain, burning or prickling or tingling, constipation, cough, dry mouth, eye pain, fever, indigestion, arthritis, amnesia, skin rash, menstrual pain, nervousness, sensitive hearing, tightness in chest, trembling or shaking, unusual weakness, depression or tiredness, wheezing.	Continue. Call doctor if symptoms persist.
Rare:	
• Nosebleed, hallucinations, sleep-induced behaviors.*	Discontinue. Call doctor right away.
• Loss of appetite, back pain, chest pain, ear pain, general feeling of discomfort, sense of smell difficulty, swelling, rapid weight gain, sensitivity of skin and eyes to sunlight, redness, burning, sunburn.	Continue. Call doctor if symptoms persist.

WARNINGS & PRECAUTIONS

Don't take if:
You have had an allergic reaction to zaleplon.

Before you start, consult your doctor if:
- You have a history of alcohol or drug abuse.
- You have impaired kidney or liver function.
- You are pregnant or nursing.
- You have been diagnosed with clinical depression.

Over age 60:
Adverse reactions and side effects may be more frequent and severe than in younger persons.

Pregnancy:
Decide with your doctor whether drug benefits justify risk to unborn child. Risk category C (see page xviii).

Breast-feeding:
Drug passes into milk. Avoid drug or discontinue nursing until you finish medicine. Consult doctor for advice on maintaining milk supply.

Infants & children:
Not recommended.

Prolonged use:
Not intended for long term use.

Skin & sunlight:
No problems expected.

Driving, piloting or hazardous work:
Don't drive or pilot aircraft, work around dangerous machinery, climb ladders or work in high places for at least 4 hours after taking this medication. Danger increases if you drink alcohol or take medicine affecting alertness and reflexes, such as antihistamines, tranquilizers, sedatives, pain medicine, narcotics and mind-altering drugs.

Discontinuing:
Dose may require gradual reduction. If drug has been taken for a long time, consult doctor before discontinuing. You may have trouble sleeping for the first few nights after you stop taking zaleplon.

Others:
Advise any doctor or dentist whom you consult that you take this medicine.

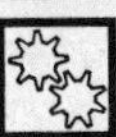

POSSIBLE INTERACTION WITH OTHER DRUGS

GENERIC NAME OR DRUG CLASS	COMBINED EFFECT
Antidepressants, tricyclic*	Increased effect of either drug. Avoid.
Central nervous system (CNS) depressants*	May increase effect of depressant.
Enzyme inducers*	Decreased zaleplon effect.
Enzyme inhibitors*	Increased zaleplon effect.

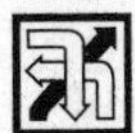

POSSIBLE INTERACTION WITH OTHER SUBSTANCES

INTERACTS WITH	COMBINED EFFECT
Alcohol:	Increased sedation. Avoid.
Beverages:	None expected.
Cocaine:	None expected.
Foods:	None expected.
Marijuana:	Increased sedation. Avoid.
Tobacco:	None expected.

***See Glossary**

ZINC SUPPLEMENTS

GENERIC AND BRAND NAMES

ZINC ACETATE	**ZINC SULFATE**
Galzin	**Egozinc**
ZINC GLUCONATE	**PMS Egozinc**
Orazinc	**Verazinc**
	Zinc-220
	Zincate

Many other multivitamins/mineral products.

BASIC INFORMATION

Habit forming? No
Prescription needed? No
Available as generic? Yes
Drug class: Nutritional supplement (mineral)

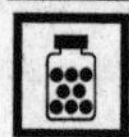

USES

- Treats zinc deficiency that may lead to growth retardation, appetite loss, changes in taste or smell, skin eruptions, slow wound healing, decreased immune function, diarrhea or impaired night vision.
- In absence of a deficiency, is used to treat burns, eating disorders, liver disorders, prematurity in infants, intestinal diseases, parasitism, kidney disorders, skin disorders and stress.
- May be useful as a supplement for those who are breast-feeding or pregnant (under a doctor's supervision).
- Zinc acetate is used for treatment of Wilson's disease.

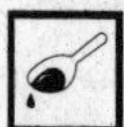

DOSAGE & USAGE INFORMATION

How to take:
Tablet or capsule—Swallow with liquid. If you can't swallow whole, crumble tablet or open capsule and take with liquid or food.

When to take:
At the same time each day, according to a doctor's instructions or the package label.

Continued next column

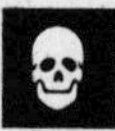

OVERDOSE

SYMPTOMS:
Dizziness, yellow eyes and skin, shortness of breath, chest pain, vomiting.
WHAT TO DO:
- **Have patient drink lots of water.**
- **Dial 911 (emergency) for medical help or call poison control center 1-800-222-1222 for instructions.**

If you forget a dose:
Take as soon as you remember. If it is almost time for the next dose, wait for that dose (don't double this dose) and resume regular schedule.

What drug does:
Required by the body for the utilization of many enzymes, nucleic acids and proteins and for cell growth.

Time lapse before drug works:
2 hours.

Don't take with:
Any other medicine or any dietary supplement without consulting your doctor or pharmacist.

POSSIBLE ADVERSE REACTIONS OR SIDE EFFECTS

SYMPTOMS	WHAT TO DO
Life-threatening: None expected.	
Common: None expected.	
Infrequent: None expected.	
Rare:	
• Indigestion, heartburn, nausea and vomiting (only with large doses).	Continue. Call doctor when convenient.
• Fever, chills, sore throat, ulcers in throat or mouth, unusual tiredness or weakness (only with large doses).	Discontinue. Call doctor right away.

WARNINGS & PRECAUTIONS

Don't take if:
You are allergic to zinc.

Before you start, consult your doctor if:
You are pregnant or breast-feeding.

Over age 60:
No special problems expected. Nutritional supplements may be helpful if the diet is restricted in any way.

Pregnancy:
Adequate zinc intake is important. Risk factor not designated. See category list on page xviii and consult doctor.

Breast-feeding:
Adequate zinc intake important. Consult a doctor.

Infants & children:
Normal daily requirements vary with age. Consult a doctor.

Prolonged use:
No special problems expected.

Skin & sunlight:
No special problems expected.

Driving, piloting or hazardous work:
No special problems expected.

Discontinuing:
No special problems expected.

Others:
The best natural sources of zinc are red meats, oysters, herring, peas and beans.

POSSIBLE INTERACTION WITH OTHER DRUGS

GENERIC NAME OR DRUG CLASS	COMBINED EFFECT
Copper supplements	Inhibited absorption of copper.
Diuretics, thiazide*	Increased need for zinc.
Folic acid	Increased need for zinc.
Iron supplements*	Increased need for zinc.
Tetracyclines*	Decreased absorption of tetracycline if taken within 2 hours of each other.

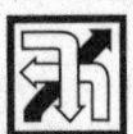

POSSIBLE INTERACTION WITH OTHER SUBSTANCES

INTERACTS WITH	COMBINED EFFECT
Alcohol:	May increase need for zinc.
Beverages:	None expected.
Cocaine:	None expected.
Foods:	
High-fiber.	May decrease zinc absorption.
Marijuana:	None expected.
Tobacco:	May increase need for zinc.

***See Glossary**

ZIPRASIDONE

BRAND NAMES

Geodon

BASIC INFORMATION

Habit forming? No
Prescription needed? Yes
Available as generic? Yes
Drug class: Antipsychotic

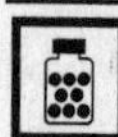

USES

- Treatment for schizophrenia.
- Treatment for bipolar disorder.

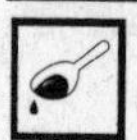

DOSAGE & USAGE INFORMATION

How to take:
Capsule—Swallow with liquid. Should be taken with food. Do not chew capsule.

When to take:
At the same times each day. The prescribed dosage may gradually be increased over the first few days or weeks of use.

If you forget a dose:
Take as soon as you remember. If it is almost time for the next dose, wait for the next scheduled dose (don't double this dose).

What drug does:
The exact mechanism is unknown. It appears to block certain nerve impulses between nerve cells.

Time lapse before drug works:
One to 7 days. A further increase in the dosage amount may be necessary to relieve symptoms for some patients.

Don't take with:
Any other medicine or any dietary supplement without consulting your doctor or pharmacist.

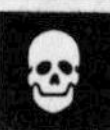

OVERDOSE

SYMPTOMS:
Extreme drowsiness, sleepiness, slurring of speech, high blood pressure.
WHAT TO DO:

- **If symptoms appear serious or severe, dial 911 (emergency) for medical help or call poison control center 1-800-222-1222 for instructions.**
- **See emergency information on last 3 pages of this book.**

POSSIBLE ADVERSE REACTIONS OR SIDE EFFECTS

SYMPTOMS	WHAT TO DO
Life-threatening:	
Rare allergic reaction (hives, itching, rash, wheezing, tightness in chest, swelling of lips or tongue or throat).	Seek emergency treatment immediately.
Common:	
Constipation or diarrhea, indigestion or heartburn, weight gain, rash, belching, stomach pain, nausea, drowsiness, dizziness, restlessness, feeling weak or a loss of strength, lack of muscle and balance control, coordination problems, trouble in speaking, drooling, twisting body movements (of face, neck and back), arms and legs or muscles feel stiff, muscles tremble, shuffling walk.	Continue. Call doctor when convenient.
Infrequent:	
Appetite loss and weight loss, runny or stuffy nose, dry mouth, sneezing, vision changes, red and itchy skin, dystonia (unable to move eyes, eyelid twitching, eyes blinking more, tongue wants to stick out, trouble in breathing or speaking or swallowing), muscles feel tight or ache, feel faint upon standing after sitting or lying.	Continue, but call doctor right away.
Rare:	
Faintness, persistent and painful erection, heartbeat irregular or fast or pounding, palpitations, convulsions, high blood sugar (thirstiness, frequent urination, increased hunger, weakness).	Discontinue. Call doctor right away.

WARNINGS & PRECAUTIONS

Don't take if:
You are allergic to ziprasidone.

Before you start, consult your doctor if:
- You have liver or kidney disease, heart disease, heart rhythm problems, QT prolongation, heart failure or recent heart attack.
- You have a history of seizures.
- The patient has Alzheimer's.
- You have a family history of, or have diabetes.
- You have tardive dyskinesia.
- You have hypokalemia (low potassium) or hypomagnesemia (low magnesium).
- You have neuroleptic malignant syndrome (serious or fatal problems may occur).

Over age 60:
- Adverse reactions and side effects may be more severe than in younger persons. A lower starting dosage is usually recommended until a response is determined.
- Use of antipsychotic drugs in elderly patients with dementia-related psychosis may increase risk of death. Consult doctor.

Pregnancy:
Decide with your doctor if drug benefits justify any possible risk to unborn child. Risk category C (see page xviii).

Breast-feeding:
It is unknown if drug passes into milk. Avoid nursing until you finish medicine. Consult doctor for advice on maintaining milk supply.

Infants & children:
Safety and efficacy has not been established. Use only under close medical supervision.

Prolonged use:
Consult with your doctor on a regular basis while taking this drug to check your progress or to discuss any increase or changes in side effects and the need for continued treatment. Also to check blood levels of potassium and magnesium and to monitor you for any heart problems.

Skin & sunlight:
Hot temperatures and exercise, hot baths can increase risk of heatstroke. Drug may affect body's ability to maintain normal temperature.

Driving, piloting or hazardous work:
Don't drive or pilot aircraft until you learn how medicine affects you. Don't work around dangerous machinery. Don't climb ladders or work in high places. Danger increases if you drink alcohol or take medicine affecting alertness and reflexes.

Discontinuing:
Don't discontinue this drug without consulting doctor. Dosage may require a gradual reduction before stopping.

Others:
- Get up slowly from a sitting or lying position to avoid dizziness, faintness or lightheadedness.
- Advise any doctor or dentist whom you consult that you take this medicine.
- Take medicine only as directed. Do not increase or reduce dosage without doctor's approval.

POSSIBLE INTERACTION WITH OTHER DRUGS

GENERIC NAME OR DRUG CLASS	COMBINED EFFECT
Antihypertensives*	Increased antihypertensive effect.
Carbamazepine	Decreased effect of ziprasidone.
Central nervous system (CNS) depressants*	Increased sedative effect. Increased effect of ziprasidone.
Central nervous system (CNS) stimulants*	Unknown effect. Avoid.
Dopamine agonists*	Decreased effect of dopamine agonist.
Enzyme inhibitors*	Increased effect of ziprasidone.
Levodopa	May decrease levodopa effect.
QT interval prolongation-causing drugs*	Heart rhythm problems. Avoid.

POSSIBLE INTERACTION WITH OTHER SUBSTANCES

INTERACTS WITH	COMBINED EFFECT
Alcohol:	Increased sedative affect. Avoid.
Beverages: Grapefruit juice.	May increase the effect of ziprasidone.
Cocaine:	Effect not known. Best to avoid.
Foods:	None expected.
Marijuana:	Effect not known. Best to avoid.
Tobacco:	None expected.

*See Glossary

ZOLPIDEM

BRAND NAMES

Ambien
Ambien CR
Edluar
Intermezzo
ZolpiMist

BASIC INFORMATION

Habit forming? Yes
Prescription needed? Yes
Available as generic? Yes
Drug class: Sedative-hypnotic agent

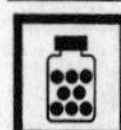

USES

- Short-term treatment for insomnia.
- May be used for other disorders as determined by your doctor.

DOSAGE & USAGE INFORMATION

How to take:
- Tablet—Swallow with liquid.
- Controlled-release tablet—Swallow tablet whole. Do not crumble, crush or chew tablet.
- Sublingual tablet—Place under tongue and let it dissolve. Do not take with a liquid and do not swallow tablet.
- Oral spray—Follow instructions provided with prescription.

When to take:
- Take immediately before bedtime. For best results, do not take with a meal or immediately after eating a meal.
- Take drug only when you are able to get 7 to 8 hours (4 hours for brand Intermezzo) of sleep before your daily activity begins.

Continued next column

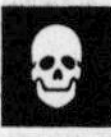

OVERDOSE

SYMPTOMS:
Drowsiness, weakness, stupor, coma.
WHAT TO DO:
- **Dial 911 (emergency) for medical help or call poison control center 1-800-222-1222 for instructions.**
- **If person is unconscious, check breathing and pulse. If not breathing, begin mouth-to-mouth rescue breathing. If heart is not beating, begin chest compressions.**
- **See emergency information on last 3 pages of this book.**

If you forget a dose:
Take as soon as you remember. Read How to Take for number of hours of sleep time needed. Do not exceed prescribed dosage.

What drug does:
Acts as a central nervous system depressant, decreasing sleep problems such as trouble falling asleep, waking up too often during the night and waking up too early in the morning.

Time lapse before drug works:
Within 1 to 2 hours.

Don't take with:
Any other medicine or any dietary supplement without consulting your doctor or pharmacist.

POSSIBLE ADVERSE REACTIONS OR SIDE EFFECTS

SYMPTOMS	WHAT TO DO
Life-threatening:	
Rare allergic reaction (hives, itching, rash, wheezing, tightness in chest, swelling of lips or tongue or throat).	Seek emergency treatment immediately.
Common:	
Daytime drowsiness, lightheadedness, dizziness, clumsiness, headache, diarrhea, nausea.	Continue. Call doctor when convenient.
Infrequent:	
Dry mouth, muscle aches or pain, tiredness, indigestion, joint pain, memory problems.	Continue. Call doctor when convenient.
Rare:	
Behavioral changes, agitation, confusion, hallucinations, worsening of depression, bloody or cloudy urine, painful or difficult urination, increased urge to urinate, skin rash or hives, itching, sleep-induced behaviors.*	Discontinue. Call doctor right away.

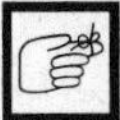

WARNINGS & PRECAUTIONS

Don't take if:
You are allergic to zolpidem.

Before you start, consult your doctor if:
- You have respiratory problems.
- You have kidney or liver disease.
- You suffer from depression.
- You are an active or recovering alcoholic or substance abuser.

Over age 60:
Adverse reactions and side effects may be more frequent and severe than in younger persons. You may need smaller doses for shorter periods of time.

Pregnancy:
Consult doctor. Risk category B (see page xviii).

Breast-feeding:
Drug passes into milk. Avoid drug or discontinue nursing until you finish medicine. Consult doctor for advice on maintaining milk supply.

Infants & children:
Not recommended for patients under age 18.

Prolonged use:
Not recommended for long-term usage. Don't take for longer than 1 to 2 weeks unless under doctor's supervision.

Skin & sunlight:
No special problems expected.

Driving, piloting or hazardous work:
Don't drive or pilot aircraft until you learn how medicine affects you. Don't work around dangerous machinery. Don't climb ladders or work in high places. Danger increases if you drink alcohol or take other medicines affecting alertness and reflexes.

Discontinuing:
- Don't discontinue without consulting doctor. Dose may require gradual reduction if you have taken drug for a long time.
- You may have sleeping problems for 1 or 2 nights after stopping drug.

Others:
- Advise any doctor or dentist whom you consult that you take this medicine.
- Don't take drug if you are traveling on an overnight airplane trip of less than 7 or 8 hours. A temporary memory loss may occur (traveler's amnesia).

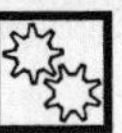

POSSIBLE INTERACTION WITH OTHER DRUGS

GENERIC NAME OR DRUG CLASS	COMBINED EFFECT
Central nervous system (CNS) depressants*	Increased sedative effect. Avoid.
Chlorpromazine	Increased sedative effect. Avoid.
Imipramine	Increased sedative effect. Avoid.

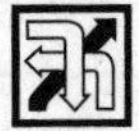

POSSIBLE INTERACTION WITH OTHER SUBSTANCES

INTERACTS WITH	COMBINED EFFECT
Alcohol:	Increased sedation. Avoid.
Beverages:	None expected.
Cocaine:	None expected.
Foods:	Decreased sedative effect if taken with a meal or right after a meal.
Marijuana:	None expected.
Tobacco:	None expected.

*See Glossary

ZONISAMIDE

BRAND NAMES

Zonegran

BASIC INFORMATION

Habit forming? No
Prescription needed? Yes
Available as generic? Yes
Drug class: Anticonvulsant, antiepileptic

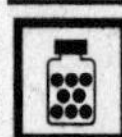

USES

Treatment for partial (focal) epileptic seizures. May be used alone or in combination with other antiepileptic drugs.

DOSAGE & USAGE INFORMATION

How to take:
Capsule—Swallow with liquid. Do not break or chew capsule. May be taken with or without food and on a full or empty stomach.

When to take:
Your doctor will determine the best schedule. Dosages will be increased rapidly over the first weeks of use. Further increases may be necessary to achieve maximum benefits.

If you forget a dose:
Take as soon as you remember. If it is almost time for the next dose, skip the missed dose and wait for your next scheduled dose (don't double this dose).

What drug does:
The exact mechanism is unknown. Studies have suggested different ways in which the drug provides anticonvulsant activity.

Time lapse before drug works:
May take several weeks for full effectiveness.

Don't take with:
Any other medicine or any dietary supplement without consulting your doctor or pharmacist.

OVERDOSE

SYMPTOMS:
Slow or irregular heartbeat, confusion, dizziness, faintness, unusual tiredness or weakness, blue skin or fingernails, breathing difficulty, coma.
WHAT TO DO:

- **Dial 911 (emergency) for medical help or call poison control center 1-800-222-1222 for instructions.**
- **See emergency information on last 3 pages of this book.**

POSSIBLE ADVERSE REACTIONS OR SIDE EFFECTS

SYMPTOMS	WHAT TO DO
Life-threatening:	
In case of overdose, see previous column.	
Common:	
• Unsteady walk, shakiness.	Continue, but call doctor right away.
• Sleepiness, dizziness, anxiety, restlessness, loss of appetite.	Continue. Call doctor when convenient.
Infrequent:	
• Agitation, delusions, hallucinations, bruising of the skin, depression, unusual mood or mental changes, double vision.	Continue, but call doctor right away.
• Constipation or diarrhea, heartburn, dry mouth, flu-like symptoms (chills, fever, headache, aching muscles and joints), problems with speech, difficulty in concentrating, sour stomach, belching, back and forth eye movement, nausea, runny or stuffy nose, tingling or burning sensations.	Continue. Call doctor when convenient.
Rare:	
Other symptoms.	Continue. Call doctor when convenient.

WARNINGS & PRECAUTIONS

Don't take if:
You are allergic to zonisamide or any other sulfonamides.*

Before you start, consult your doctor if:
- You have a history of liver disease.
- You have renal failure (inability of the kidneys to function properly).
- You are allergic to any medication, food or other substance.
- You have any other medical problems.

Over age 60:
No special problems expected.

Pregnancy:
Decide with your doctor if drug benefits justify risks to unborn child. Risk category C (see page xviii).

Breast-feeding:
Drug passes into milk. Avoid drug or discontinue nursing until you finish medicine. Consult doctor for advice on maintaining milk supply.

Infants & children:
Zonisamide has not been studied in children under age 16. Use only under medical supervision.

Prolonged use:
No special problems expected. Follow-up laboratory blood studies may be recommended by your doctor.

Skin & sunlight:
No problems expected.

Driving, piloting or hazardous work:
Don't drive or pilot aircraft until you learn how medicine affects you. Don't work around dangerous machinery. Don't climb ladders or work in high places. Danger increases if you drink alcohol or take other medicines affecting alertness and reflexes such as antihistamines, tranquilizers, sedatives, pain medicine, narcotics and mind-altering drugs.

Discontinuing:
Don't discontinue without doctor's approval due to risk of increased seizure activity. The dosage may need to be gradually decreased before stopping the drug completely.

Others:
- Advise any doctor or dentist whom you consult that you take this medicine.
- Zonisamide may be used with other anticonvulsant drugs and additional side effects may also occur. If they do, discuss them with your doctor.
- May alter some laboratory tests.
- Rarely, antiepileptic drugs may lead to suicidal thoughts and behaviors. Call doctor right away if suicidal symptoms or unusual behaviors occur.
- Wear or carry medical identification to show your seizure disorder and the drugs you take.

POSSIBLE INTERACTION WITH OTHER DRUGS

GENERIC NAME OR DRUG CLASS	COMBINED EFFECT
Anticonvulsants,* other	Decreased effect of zonisamide.
Central nervous system (CNS) depressants*	Increased sedative effect.

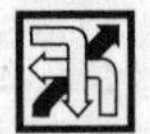

POSSIBLE INTERACTION WITH OTHER SUBSTANCES

INTERACTS WITH	COMBINED EFFECT
Alcohol:	Increased sedative effect. Decreased effect of zonisamide. Avoid.
Beverages:	None expected.
Cocaine:	Unknown effect. Avoid.
Foods:	None expected.
Marijuana:	Unknown effect. Avoid.
Tobacco:	None expected.

*See Glossary

Generic and Brand Name Directory

How to Read the Lists Below

On some of the drug charts in this book you are referred to this directory to see a listing of the generic and brand names of the drugs. There are just too many names to fit on the chart page itself, so they are listed here for your reference. It is almost impossible to list all brand names available. Those not listed should be considered as effective as those that are listed.

First, look up the drug chart name (printed in large capital letters). ACETAMINOPHEN is the first name listed in this directory. Under that name, you will find the brand names of drugs (in alphabetical order) that contain the generic drug acetaminophen.

The titles on some drug charts are *drug class* names, such as ADRENOCORTICOIDS (Systemic). In this directory, this *drug class* name is followed first by a numbered list of *generic drug names* in that class. Following that list is the *brand name* list. Each *brand name* has a small number at the end that can be used to match up to the number on the *generic name* list.

For example, under ADRENOCORTICOIDS (Systemic), you will find the brand-name drug **Aristocort**[9]. The number [9] means it contains the generic drug 9. TRIAMCINOLONE.

ACETAMINOPHEN

Abenol
Acephen
Aceta
AcetaDrink
Acetaminophen Uniserts
Aclophen
Actamin
Actamin Extra
Actamin Super
Actimol
Advanced Formula Dristan Caplets
Alba-Temp 300
Alka-Seltzer Plus Cold & Cough Effervescent
Alka-Seltzer Plus Cold & Sinus Liquid-Gels
Alka-Seltzer Plus Night-Time Effervescent
Alka-Seltzer Plus Night-Time Liquid-Gels
Alka-Seltzer Plus Original Effervescent
Alka-Seltzer PM
Allerest No-Drowsiness
All-Nite Cold Formula
Amaphen
Aminofen
Aminofen Max
Anacin-3
Anacin-3 Extra Strength
Anolor 300
Anoquan
Anuphen
Apacet Capsules
Apacet Elixir
Apacet Extra Strength Caplets
Apacet Extra Strength Tablets
Apacet Oral Solution
Apacet Regular Strength Tablets
APAP
Apo-Acetaminophen
Arcet
Aspirin Free Anacin Maximum Strength Caplets
Aspirin Free Anacin Maximum Strength Tablets
Aspirin Free Bayer Select Maximum Strength Headache Plus Caplets
Aspirin-Free Excedrin Caplets
Atasol Caplets
Atasol Drops
Atasol Forte
Atasol Forte Caplets
Atasol Forte Tablets
Atasol Oral Solution
Atasol Tablets
Bancap
Banesin
Bayer Select Maximum Strength Pain Relief Formula
Benadryl Allergy/Sinus Headache Caplets
Benylin All-In-One Cold & Flu Caplets
Benylin All-In-One Cold & Flu Night Caplets
Benylin All-In-One Cold & Flu Nightime Syrup
Benylin All-In-One Cold & Flu Syrup
Benylin All-In-One Day & Night Caplets
Benylin Cold & Sinus
Benylin Cold & Sinus Plus
Benylin Cold & Flu With Codeine Narcotic
Benylin DM 12 Hour Nightime Cough Syrup
Bromo-Seltzer
Bucet
Buffets
Campain
Children's Panadol
Children's Rapimed
Coldrine
Colrex Compound
Comtrex Deep Chest Cold
Conacetol
Conar-A
Congespirin
Congespirin for Children Cold Tablets
Congespirin for Children Liquid Cold Medicine
Congestant D
Contac Allergy/Sinus Day Caplets
Contac Allergy/Sinus Night Caplets
Contac Maximum Strength Sinus Caplets
Contac Night Caplets
Contac Non-Drowsy Formula Sinus Caplets
Contac Severe Cold Formula
Contac Severe Cold Formula Night Strength
Coricidin HBP
Dapa
Datril Extra Strength
Diabetic Tussin Cold & Flu
Diabetic Tussin Night Time Formula
Dolanex
Dolmar
Dristan AF
Dristan AF Plus
Dristan Cold and Flu
Dristan Cold Caplets
Dristan Cold Maximum Strength Caplets
Dristan Cold Multi-Symptom Formula
Dristan Juice Mix-in Cold, Flu, and Cough
Drixoral Cold and Flu
Drixoral Plus

Drixoral Sinus
Duradyne
Endolor
Esgic
Esgic Plus
Excedrin Caplets
Excedrin Extra Strength Caplets
Excedrin Back & Body
Excedrin Extra Strength Tablets
Excedrin Migraine
Excedrin Tension Headache
Exdol
Exdol Strong
Ezol
Febridyne
Femcet
Feverall Children's
Feverall Infants'
Feverall Junior Strength
Feverall Sprinkle Caps
Fioricet
Gelpirin
Gemnisyn
Genapap
Genapap Children's Elixir
Genapap Children's Tablets
Genapap Extra Strength
Genapap Infants'
Genapap Regular Strength Tablets
Gendecon
Gen-D-phen
Genebs
Genebs Extra Strength
Genebs Regular Strength Tablets
Genex
Goody's Extra Strength Tablets
Goody's Headache Powders
Halenol
Halenol Extra Strength
Histagesic Modified
Histosal
Hycomine Compound
Infants' Anacin-3
Infants' Apacet
Infants' Genapap
Infants' Panadol
Infants' Tylenol
Infants' Tylenol Suspension Drops
Isopap
Kolephrin
Kolephrin/DM Caplets
Liquiprin Children's Elixir
Liquiprin Infants' Drops
Mapap Infant Drops
Maximum Strength Tylenol Allergy Sinus Caplets
Maximum Strength Tylenol Flu Gelcaps
Meda Cap
Meda Tab
Medigesic
Myapap Elixir
Mucinex Adult Caplets - Cold & Sinus
Mucinex Adult Caplets - Cold, Flu, & Sore Throat
Mucinex Adult Caplets - Severe Congestion & Cold
Mucinex Fast-Max Cold, Flu & Sore Throat Liquid
Mucinex Maximum Strength Fast Max Cold, Flu & Sore Throat
ND-Gesic
Neocitrin Colds and Flu Calorie Reduced
NeoCitrin Extra Strength Colds and Flu
NeoCitrin Extra Strength Sinus
Neopap
Nighttime Pamprin
NyQuil Liquicaps
Nytcold Medicine
Oraphen-PD
Ornex Maximum Strength Caplets
Ornex No Drowsiness Caplets
Pacaps
Panadol
Panadol Extra Strength
Panadol Junior Strength Caplets
Panadol Maximum Strength Caplets
Panadol Maximum Strength Tablets
Panex
Panex 500
Paracetamol
Parafon Forte
PediaCare Children's Fever Reducer Plus Cough & Runny Nose
PediaCare Children's Fever Reducer Plus Cough & Sore Throat
PediaCare Children's Fever Reducer Plus Flu
PediaCare Fever Reducer Plus Multi-Symptom Cold
PediaCare Infants' Fever Reducer / Pain Reliever
Pedric
Pertussin All Night PM
Phenapap Sinus Headache & Congestion
Phenaphen
Phrenilin
Phrenilin Forte
Presalin
Redutemp
Refenesen Chest Congestion & Pain Relief PE
Remcol-C
Repan
Rid-A-Pain Compound
Robigesic
Robitussin Honey Flu
Robitussin Night Relief
Robitussin Night Relief Colds Formula Liquid
Rounox
Sedapap
Semcet
Sinubid
Sinus Relief
Slo-Phyllin GG
Snaplets-FR
St. Joseph Aspirin Free Fever Reducer for Children
Sudafed Multi-Symptom Cold & Cough
Summit
Supac
Suppap
Tapanol
Tapanol Extra Strength
Tapar
Tavist Allergy/Sinus/Headache
Tempra
Tempra Caplets
Tempra Chewable Tablets
Tempra Double Strength
Tempra Drops
Tempra D.S.
Tempra Infants
Tempra Syrup
Tencet
Tenol
Tenol Plus
Theracof Plus Multi-Symptom Cough and Cold Reliever
Theraflu Cold & Sore Throat Hot Liquid
Theraflu Daytime Severe Cold Caplets
Theraflu Flu & Chest Congestion Hot Liquid
Theraflu Flu & Sore Throat Hot Liquid
Theraflu Nighttime Severe Cold Caplets
Theraflu Nighttime Severe Cold Hot Liquid
Theraflu Warming Relief Daytime
Theraflu Warming Relief Nighttime
Triad
Triaminic Cough & Sore Throat
Triaminic Flu, Cough & Fever
Triaminic Softchews Cough & Sore Throat
Triaprin

Trigesic
Two-Dyne
Tylenol
Tylenol 8 Hour
Tylenol Allergy Multi-Symptom
Tylenol Allergy Multi-Symptom Nighttime
Tylenol Arthritis Pain
Tylenol Chest Congestion
Tylenol Cold Head Congestion Daytime
Tylenol Cold Head Congestion Nighttime
Tylenol Cold Head Congestion Severe
Tylenol Concentrated Infants' Drops
Tylenol Cough & Severe Congestion Daytime
Tylenol Cough & Sore Throat Daytime
Tylenol Cough & Sore Throat Nighttime
Tylenol Extra Strength
Tylenol Extra Strength Rapid Release Gels
Tylenol Junior Strength
Tylenol PM
Tylenol Severe Allergy
Tylenol Sinus Congestion & Pain Daytime
Tylenol Sinus Congestion & Pain Nighttime
Tylenol Sinus Congestion & Pain Severe
Tylenol Sinus Severe Congestion Daytime
Tylenol Sore Throat Daytime
Tylenol Sore Throat Nighttime
Ty-Pap
Ultracet
Valadol
Valadol Liquid
Valorin
Valorin Extra
Vanquis
Vicks DayQuil Cold/Flu Relief
Vicks DayQuil Cold & Flu Symptom Relief Plus Vitamin C
Vicks DayQuil Sinus LiquiCaps
Vicks Formula 44 Custom Care Body Aches
Vicks Formula 44 Custom Care Cough & Cold PM
Vicks NyQuil Cold & Flu Relief
Vicks NyQuil Cold & Flu Symptom Relief Plus Vitamin C
Vicks NyQuil D
Vicks NyQuil Less Drowsy Cold & Flu Relief Liquid
Vicks NyQuil Sinus LiquiCaps
Women's Tylenol Menstrual Relief Caplets

ADRENOCORTICOIDS (Systemic)

GENERIC NAMES

1. BETAMETHASONE
2. BUDESONIDE
3. CORTISONE
4. DEXAMETHASONE
5. FLUDROCORTISONE
6. HYDROCORTISONE (Cortisol)
7. METHYLPREDNISOLONE
8. PREDNISOLONE
9. PREDNISONE
10. TRIAMCINOLONE

BRAND NAMES

Apo-Prednisone[9]
Aristocort[10]
Betnelan[1]
Betnesol[1]
Celestone[1]
Cortef[6]
Cortenema[6]
Cortifoam[6]
Cortone[3]
Cortone Acetate[3]
Decadron[4]
Delta-Cortef8[7]
Deltasone[9]
Deronil[4]
Dexasone[4]
Dexone 0.5[4]
Dexone 0.75[4]
Dexone 1.5[4]
Dexone 4[4]
Entocort EC[2]
Flo-Pred[8]
Florinef[5]
Hexadrol[4]
Hydeltrasol8[7]
Hydrocortone[6]
Kenacort[10]
Kenacort Diacetate[10]
Medrol[7]
Meticorten[9]
Mymethasone[4]
Nor-Pred-TBA[8]
Oradexon[4]
Orapred[8]
Orapred ODT[8]
Orasone 1[9]
Orasone 5[9]
Orasone 10[9]
Orasone 20[9]
Orasone 50[9]
Pediapred[8]
Prednisone Intensol[9]
Prednicen-M[9]
Prelone[8]
Rayos[9]
Sterapred DS[9]
Solurex[4]
Solurex LA[4]
Uceris[2]
Winpred[9]

ADRENOCORTICOIDS (Topical)

GENERIC NAMES

1. ALCLOMETASONE (Topical)
2. AMCINONIDE (Topical)
3. BECLOMETHASONE (Topical)
4. BETAMETHASONE (Topical)
5. CLOBETASOL (Topical)
6. CLOBETASONE (Topical)
7. CLOCORTOLONE (Topical)
8. CORTISOL
9. DESONIDE (Topical)
10. DESOXIMETASONE (Topical)
11. DEXAMETHASONE (Topical)
12. DIFLORASONE (Topical)
13. DIFLUCORTOLONE (Topical)
14. FLUMETHASONE (Topical)
15. FLUOCINOLONE (Topical)
16. FLUOCINONIDE (Topical)
17. FLURANDRENOLIDE (Topical)
18. FLUTICASONE (Topical)
19. HALCINONIDE (Topical)
20. HALOBETASOL
21. HYDROCORTISONE (Dental)
22. HYDROCORTISONE (Topical)
23. MOMETASONE (Topical)
24. PREDNICARBATE
25. TRIAMCINOLONE (Topical)

BRAND NAMES

9-1-1[22]
Aclovate[1]
Acticort-100[22]
Adcortyl[25]
Aeroseb-Dex[11]
Aeroseb-HC[22]
Ala-Cort[22]
Ala-Scalp HP[22]
Allercort[22]
Alphaderm[22]
Alphatrex[4]
Anucort-HC[22]
Anusol-HC[22]
Anusol-HC 2.5%[22]
Aristocort[25]
Aristocort A[25]
Aristocort C[25]
Aristocort D[25]
Aristocort R[25]
Bactine[22]
Barriere-HC[22]
Beben[4]

Beta HC[22]
Betacort Scalp Lotion[4]
Betaderm[4]
Betaderm Scalp Lotion[4]
Betamethacot[4]
Betatrex[4]
Beta-Val[4]
Betnovate[4]
Betnovate 1/2[4]
Bio-Syn[15]
CaldeCORT Anti-Itch[22]
CaldeCORT-Light[22]
Carmol-HC[22]
Celestoderm-V[4]
Celestoderm-V/2[4]
Cetacort[22]
Cipro HC[22]
Clobex[5]
Cloderm[7]
Cloderm Pump[7]
Coraz Lotion[22]
Cordran[17]
Cordran SP[17]
Cormax[5]
Cortacet[22]
Cortaid[22]
Cortaid FastStick[22]
Cortate[22]
Cort-Dome[22]
Cort-Dome High Potency[22]
Cortef[22]
Cortef Feminine Itch[22]
Corticaine[22]
Corticreme[22]
Cortifair[22]
Cortiment-10[22]
Cortiment-40[22]
Cortoderm[22]
Cortril[22]
Cultivate[18]
Cyclocort[2]
Decaderm[11]
Decadron[11]
Decaspray[11]
Delacort[22]
Delta-Tritex[25]
Demarest DriCort[22]
Dermabet[4]
Dermacomb[25]
Dermacort[22]
Dermalleve[22]
DermAtop[24]
DermiCort[22]
Dermovate[5]
Dermovate Scalp Application[5]
Dermtex HC[22]
Desonate[9]
DesOwen[9]
Diprolene[4]
Diprolene AF[4]
Diprosone[4]
Drenison[17]
Drenison-1/4[17]
Ectosone[4]
Ectosone Regular[4]
Ectosone Scalp Lotion[4]
Efcortelan[22]
Elocon[23]
Emo-Cort[22]
Emo-Cort Scalp Solution[22]
Epifoam[8]
Eumovate[6]
Fludroxycortide[17]
Fluocet[15]
Fluocin[16]
Fluoderm[15]
Fluolar[15]
Fluonid[15]
Fluonide[15]
Flurosyn[15]
Flutex[25]
Foille Cort[22]
Gly-Cort[22]
Gynecort[22]
Gynecort 10[22]
Halciderm[19]
Halog[19]
Halog E[19]
Hi-Cor 1.0[22]
Hi-Cor 2.5[22]
Hyderm[22]
Hydro-Tex[22]
Hytone[22]
Kenac[25]
Kenalog[25]
Kenalog in Orabase[25]
Kenalog-H[25]
Kenonel[25]
Lacticare-HC[22]
Lanacort[22]
Lanacort 10[22]
Lemoderm[22]
Licon[16]
LidaMantle HC[22]
Lidemol[16]
Lidex[16]
Lidex-E[16]
Lipsovir[22]
Locacorten[14]
Locoid[22]
Lotrisone[4]
Lyderm[16]
Maxiflor[12]
Maximum Strength Cortaid[22]
Maxivate[4]
Metaderm Mild[4]
Metaderm Regular[4]
Metosyn[16]
Metosyn FAPG[16]
Myco II[25]
Mycogen II[25]
Mycolog II[25]
My Cort[22]
Myco-Triacet II[25]
Mytrex[25]
Nerisone[13]
Nerisone Oily[13]
Novobetamet[4]
Novohydrocort[22]
Nutracort[22]
Olux[5]
Olux-E[5]
Orabase HCA[22]
Oracort[25]
Oralone[25]
Pandel[22]
Penecort[22]
Pentacort[22]
Pharma-Cort[22]
Pramosone E Cream[22]
Prevex B[4]
Prevex HC[4]
Propaderm[3]
Psorcon[12]
Rederm[22]
Rhulicort[22]
Sarna HC[22]
Sential[22]
S-T Cort[22]
Synacort[22]
Synalar[15]
Synalar HP[15]
Synamol[15]
Synemol[15]
Taclonex[4]
Teladar[4]
Temovate[5]
Temovate E[5]
Temovate Emollient[5]
Temovate Gel[5]
Temovate Scalp Application[5]
Texacort[22]
Topicort[10]
Topicort LP[10]
Topicort Mild[10]
Topilene[4]
Topisone[4]
Topsyn[16]
Triacet[25]
Triaderm[25]
Trianex[25]
Trianide Mild[25]
Trianide Regular[25]
Tristatin II[25]
Triderm[25]
Tridesilon[9]
Tri-Luma[15]
Trymex[25]
Ultravate[20]
Unicort[22]
Uticort[4]
Valisone[4]
Valisone Reduced Strength[4]
Valisone Scalp Lotion[4]
Valnac[4]
Vanos[16]
Verdeso Foam[9]
Vioform-Hydrocortisone Lotion[22]
Westcort[22]
Xerese Cream[22]
Xyralid Cream[22]

Xyralid LP Lotion[22]
Zytopic Cream[25]

ANDROGENS

GENERIC NAMES

1. ETHYLESTRENOL
2. FLUOXYMESTERONE
3. METHYLTESTOSTERONE
4. NANDROLONE
5. OXANDROLONE
6. OXYMETHOLONE
7. STANOZOLOL
8. TESTOSTERONE

BRAND NAMES

Anabolin[4]
Anabolin LA 100[4]
Anadrol-50[6]
Anapolon 50[6]
Andro 100[8]
Andro-Cyp 100[8]
Andro-Cyp 200[8]
Androderm[8]
Androgel[8]
Android-10[3]
Android-25[3]
Android-T[8]
Andro-LA 200[8]
Androlone[4]
Andronaq-50[8]
Andronaq-LA[8]
Andronate 100[8]
Andronate 200[8]
Andropository 100[8]
Andryl 200[8]
Axiron[8]
Bio-T-Gel[8]
Deca-Durabolin[4]
Delatest[8]
Delatestryl[8]
Dep Andro 100[8]
Dep Andro 200[8]
Depotest[8]
Depo-Testosterone[8]
Durabolin[4]
Durabolin-50[4]
Duratest 100[8]
Duratest-200[8]
Durathate 200[8]
Everone[8]
Halotestin[2]
Histerone-50[8]
Histerone-100[8]
Hybolin Decanoate[4]
Dep-Androgyn[5]
Depo-Testadiol[5]
Depotestogen[5]
Duo-Cyp[5]
Duo-Gen L.A.[5]
Duogex L.A.[5]
Dura-Dumone 90/4[5]
Duratestin[5]
Estratest[3]
Estratest H.S.[3]
Fortesta[8]
Halodrin[4]
Menoject L.A.[5]
Neo-Pause[5]
OB[5]
Premarin with Methyltestosterone[1]
Striant[8]
Teev[5]
Tes Est Cyp[5]
Test-Estro Cypionate[5]
Testim[8]
Tylosterone[2]
Valertest No. 1[5]
Valertest No. 2[5]

ANESTHETICS (Topical)

GENERIC NAMES

1. BENZOCAINE
2. BENZOCAINE & MENTHOL
3. BUTAMBEN
4. DIBUCAINE
5. LIDOCAINE
6. LIDOCAINE & PRILOCAINE
7. PRAMOXINE
8. TETRACAINE
9. TETRACAINE & MENTHOL
10. TETRACAINE & LIDOCAINE

BRAND NAMES

Americaine[1]
Amercaine Topical Anesthetic First Aid Ointment[1]
Amercaine Topical Anesthetic Spray[1]
Anestafoam[5]
Benzocol[2]
Butesin Picrate[3]
Butyl Aminobenzoate[2]
Cinchocaine[4]
Dermoplast[2]
Emla[6]
Endocaine[1]
Ethyl Aminobenzoate[1]
Lagol[1]
LidaMantle[5]
Lidoderm[5]
Lidopatch[5]
Lignocaine[5]
Nupercainal Cream[4]
Nupercainal Ointment[4]
Pontocaine Cream[8]
Pontocaine Ointment[9]
Pramegel[7]
Pramosone E Cream[7]
Prax[7]
Synera[10]
Tronothane[7]
Unguentine[1]
Unguentine Plus[1]
Unguentine Spray[1]
Xylocaine[5]
Xyralid Cream[5]
Xyralid LP Lotion[5]
Zostrix Neuropathy Cream[5]

ANGIOTENSIN-CONVERTING ENZYME (ACE) INHIBITORS

GENERIC NAMES

1. BENAZEPRIL
2. CAPTOPRIL
3. ENALAPRIL
4. FOSINOPRIL
5. LISINOPRIL
6. MOEXIPRIL
7. PERINDOPRIL
8. QUINAPRIL
9. RAMIPRIL
10. TRANDOLAPRIL

BRAND NAMES

Accupril[8]
Aceon[7]
Altace[9]
Apo-Capto[2]
Capoten[2]
Lotensin[1]
Lotrel[1]
Mavik[10]
Monopril[4]
Novo-Captoril[2]
Prinivil[5]
Syn-Captopril[2]
Tarka[10]
Teczem[3]
Uniretic[6]
Univasc[6]
Vasotec[3]
Zestril[5]

ANGIOTENSIN-CONVERTING ENZYME (ACE) INHIBITORS & HYDROCHLOROTHIAZIDE

GENERIC NAMES

1. CAPTOPRIL & HYDROCHLOROTHIAZIDE
2. ENALAPRIL & HYDROCHLOROTHIAZIDE
3. LISINOPRIL & HYDROCHLOROTHIAZIDE
4. QUINAPRIL & HYDROCHLOROTHIAZIDE

BRAND NAMES

Accuretic[4]
Capozide[1]
Prinzide[3]
Vaseretic[2]
Zestoretic[3]

ANTACIDS

GENERIC NAMES

1. ALUMINA & MAGNESIA

2. ALUMINA & MAGNESIUM CARBONATE
3. ALUMINA & MAGNESIUM TRISILICATE
4. ALUMINA, MAGNESIA, & CALCIUM CARBONATE
5. ALUMINA, MAGNESIA, & SIMETHICONE
6. ALUMINA, MAGNESIUM, CALCIUM CARBONATE & SIMETHICONE
7. ALUMINA, MAGNESIUM TRISILICATE, & SODIUM BICARBONATE
8. ALUMINUM CARBONATE, BASIC
9. ALUMINUM HYDROXIDE
10. CALCIUM & MAGNESIUM CARBONATES
11. CALCIUM CARBONATE
12. CALCIUM CARBONATE & MAGNESIA
13. CALCIUM CARBONATE & MAGNESIUM HYDROXIDE
14. CALCIUM CARBONATE & SIMETHICONE
15. CALCIUM CARBONATE, MAGNESIA, & SIMETHICONE
16. MAGALDRATE
17. MAGALDRATE & SIMETHICONE
18. MAGNESIUM HYDROXIDE
19. MAGNESIUM OXIDE

BRAND NAMES

Acid + All[14]
Advanced Formula Di-Gel[15]
Alamag[1]
Algenic Alka[2]
Algenic Alka Improved[2]
Algicon[9]
Alka-Mints[11]
Alkets[11]
Alkets Extra Strength[11]
Almacone[5]
Almacone II[5]
Alma-Mag #4 Improved[5]
Alma-Mag Improved[5]
AlternaGEL[9]
Alu-Cap[9]
Aludrox[5]
Alu-Tab[9]
Amitone[12]
Amphojel[9]
Amphojel 500[1]
Amphojel Plus[4]
AntaGel[5]
AntaGel-II[5]
Basaljel[9]
Calglycine[11]
Camalox[4]
Chooz[11]
Dialume[9]
Di-Gel[5]
Diovol Ex[1]
Diovol Plus[5]
Duracid[9]
Equilet[11]
Foamicon[3]
Gas-X with Maalox[14]
Gaviscon[2]
Gaviscon Extra Strength Relief Formula[9]
Gaviscon-2[7]
Gelusil[5]
Gelusil Extra-Strength[1]
Genalac[11]
Genaton[2]
Genaton Extra Strength[2]
Glycate[11]
Kudrox Double Strength[5]
Losopan[16]
Losopan Plus[17]
Lowsium[16]
Lowsium Plus[17]
Maalox[1]
Maalox HRF[2]
Maalox Plus[5]
Maalox Plus, Extra Strength[5]
Maalox Quick Dissolving Chews[11]
Maalox TC[1]
Magnalox[5]
Magnalox Plus[5]
Mag-Ox 400[19]
Mallamint[11]
Maox[19]
Marblen[10]
Mi-Acid[5]
Mi-Acid Double Strength[5]
Mintox[1]
Mintox Extra Strength[5]
Mygel[5]
Mygel II[5]
Mylagen[5]
Mylagen II[5]
Mylanta[5]
Mylanta Calci Tabs[12]
Mylanta Double Strength[5]
Mylanta Double Strength Plain[5]
Mylanta Gelcaps[10]
Mylanta Maximum Strength[13]
Mylanta Night Time Strength[9]
Mylanta Regular Strength[5]
Mylanta Plain[5]
Mylanta-II[5]
Nephrox[9]
Neutralca-S[1]
Pepcid Complete[13]
Phillips' Milk of Magnesia[18]
Riopan[16]
Riopan Extra Strength[16]
Riopan Plus[17]
Riopan Plus Double Strength[17]
Riopan Plus Extra Strength[17]
Rolaids[12]
Rolaids Antacid Cool[12]
Rolaids Calcium Rich[11]
Rolaids Chewable[11]
Rolaids Extra Strength[12]
Rolaids Sodium Free[11]
Rulox[1]
Rulox No. 1[1]
Rulox No. 2[1]
Rulox Plus[5]
Simaal 2 Gel[5]
Simaal Gel[5]
Tempo[6]
Titralac[11]
Titralac Plus[11]
Triconsil[7]
Tums[11]
Tums Dual Action[13]
Tums E-X[11]
Tums Extra Strength[11]
Tums Kids[11]
Tums Lasting Effects[11]
Tums Liquid Extra Strength[11]
Tums Liquid Extra Strength with Simethicone[14]
Tums QuikPak[11]
Tums Freshers[11]
Tums Smooth Dissolve[11]
Univol[1]
Uro-Mag[19]
Zygerid Chewable Tablets[18]

ANTIBACTERIALS (Ophthalmic)

GENERIC NAMES

1. AZITHROMYCIN (Ophthalmic)
2. BACITRACIN & POLYMYXIN B
3. BESIFLOXACIN
4. CHLORAMPHENICOL (Ophthalmic)
5. CIPROFLOXACIN (Ophthalmic)
6. ERYTHROMYCIN (Ophthalmic)
7. GATIFLOXACIN (Ophthalmic)
8. GENTAMICIN (Ophthalmic)
9. LEVOFLOXACIN (Ophthalmic)
10. MOXIFLOXACIN (Ophthalmic)
11. NEOMYCIN, POLYMYXIN B
12. NEOMYCIN, POLYMYXIN B & BACITRACIN
13. NEOMYCIN, POLYMYXIN B & GRAMICIDIN
14. NORFLOXACIN (Ophthalmic)
15. OFLOXACIN (Ophthalmic)
16. SULFACETAMIDE (Ophthalmic)
17. SULFISOXAZOLE (Ophthalmic)

18. TOBRAMYCIN (Ophthalmic)

BRAND NAMES

Ak-Chlor Ophthalmic Ointment[4]
Ak-Chlor Ophthalmic Solution[4]
Ak-Spore[11]
Ak-Spore H.C.[11]
Ak-Sulf[16]
Aktob[18]
Alcomicin[7]
AzaSite[1]
Besivance[3]
Bleph-10[16]
Cetamide[16]
Chibroxin[14]
Chloracol Ophthalmic Solution (Ophthalmic)[4]
Chloromycetin Ophthalmic Ointment[4]
Chloromycetin Ophthalmic Solution[4]
Chloroptic Ophthalmic Solution[4]
Chloroptic S.O.P.[4]
Ciloxan[5]
Econochlor Ophthalmic Ointment[4]
Econochlor Ophthalmic Solution[4]
Fenicol Ophthalmic Ointment[4]
Gantrisin[17]
Garamycin[8]
Genoptic[8]
Gentacidin[8]
Gentafair[8]
Gentak[8]
Gentasol[8]
Gentrasul[8]
I-Chlor Ophthalmic Solution[4]
Ilotycin[6]
Iquix[9]
I-Sulfacet[16]
Moxeza[10]
Mycitracin[12]
Neocidin Ophthalmic Ointment[13]
Neo-Polycin[12]
Neo-Polycin HC[12]
Neosporin Ophthalmic Ointment[12]
Neosporin Ophthalmic Solution[12]
Neotal[12]
Neotricin HC[12]
Ocu-Chlor Ophthalmic Ointment[4]
Ocu-Chlor Ophthalmic Solution[4]
Ocuflox[15]
Ocu-Mycin[8]
Ocu-Spor-B[12]
Ocu-Spor-G[13]
Ocusporin[12]
Ocu-Sul-10[16]
Ocu-Sul-15[16]
Ocu-Sul-30[16]
Ocusulf-10[16]
Ocutricin Ophthalmic Ointment[12]
Ocutricin Ophthalmic Solution[12]
Ophthacet[16]
Ophthochlor Ophthalmic Solution[4]
Ophtho-Chloram Ophthalmic Solution[4]
Pentamycetin[4]
Pentamycetin Ophthalmic Ointment[4]
Pentamycetin Ophthalmic Solution[4]
P.N. Ophthalmic[13]
Polycin[2]
Quixin[9]
Sodium Sulamyd[16]
Sopamycetin Ophthalmic Ointment[4]
Sopamycetin Ophthalmic Solution[4]
Spectro-Chlor Ophthalmic Ointment[4]
Spectro-Chlor Ophthalmic Solution[4]
Spectro-Genta[8]
Spectro-Sporin[12]
Spectro-Sulf[16]
Steri-Units Sulfacetamide[16]
Sulamyd[16]
Sulf-10[16]
Sulfair[16]
Sulfair 10[16]
Sulfair 15[16]
Sulfair Forte[16]
Sulfamide[16]
Sulfex[16]
Sulten-10[16]
Tobradex[17]
Tobradex ST[17]
Tobrex[17]
Tribiotic[12]
Tri-Ophthalmic[13]
Vigamox[10]
Zylet[17]
Zymaxid[7]

ANTICHOLINERGICS

GENERIC NAMES

1. ANISOTROPINE
2. ATROPINE
3. HOMATROPINE
4. ISOPROPAMIDE
5. MEPENZOLATE
6. METHANTHELINE
7. METHSCOPOLAMINE
8. OXYPHENCYCLIMINE
9. PIRENZEPINE
10. TRIDIHEXETHYL

BRAND NAMES

AH-Chew[7]
AlleRx D[7]
AlleRx Dose Pack DF[7]
AlleRx Dose Pack PE[7]
Amdry-D[7]
Banthine[6]
Cantil[5]
Codan[3]
D.A. Chewable[7]
Dallergy[3]
Dallergy Caplets[3]
Darbid[4]
Daricon[8]
Durahist[7]
Dura-Vent/DA[7]
Extendryl[7]
Extendryl JR[7]
Extendryl SR[7]
Gastrozepin[9]
Hista-Vent PSE[7]
Homapin[3]
Hycodan[3]
Hydromet[3]
Hydropane[6]
OMNIhist L.A.[7]
Pamine[7]
Pamine Forte[7]
Pathilon[10]
Prehist D[7]
Tussigon[3]
Valpin 50[1]

ANTIDEPRESSANTS, TRICYCLIC

GENERIC NAMES

1. AMITRIPTYLINE
2. AMOXAPINE
3. CLOMIPRAMINE
4. DESIPRAMINE
5. DOXEPIN
6. IMIPRAMINE
7. NORTRIPTYLINE
8. PROTRIPTYLINE
9. TRIMIPRAMINE

BRAND NAMES

Adapin[5]
Anafranil[3]
Apo-Amitriptyline[1]
Apo-Imipramine[6]
Apo-Trimip[9]
Asendin[2]
Aventyl[7]
Endep[1]
Etrafon[1]
Etrafon-A[1]
Etrafon-D[1]
Etrafon-F[1]
Etrafon-Forte[1]
Impril[6]
Levate[1]
Norfranil[6]
Norpramin[4]

Novo-Doxepin[5]
Novopramine[6]
Novo-Tripramine[9]
Novotriptyn[1]
Pamelor[7]
PMS Amitriptyline[1]
PMS Impramine[6]
PMS Levazine[8]
Rhotrimine[9]
Silenor[5]
Sinequan[5]
Surmontil[9]
Tipramine[6]
Tofranil[6]
Tofranil-PM[6]
Triadapin[5]
Triavil[8]
Triptil[8]
Vivactil[8]

ANTIDYSKINETICS

GENERIC NAMES

1. BENZTROPINE
2. BIPERIDEN
3. ETHOPROPAZINE
4. PIMOZIDE
5. PROCYCLIDINE
6. TRIHEXYPHENIDYL

BRAND NAMES

Akineton[2]
Apo-Benztropine[1]
Apo-Trihex[6]
Artane[6]
Artane Sequels[6]
Cogentin[1]
Orap[4]
Parsidol[3]
Parsitan[3]
PMS Benztropine[1]
PMS Procyclidine[5]
PMS Trihexyphenidyl[6]
Procyclid[6]
Trihexane[6]
Trihexy[6]

ANTIFUNGALS (Topical)

GENERIC NAMES

1. AMPHOTERICIN B
2. BUTENAFINE
3. CICLOPIROX
4. CLOTRIMAZOLE
5. ECONAZOLE
6. FLUCONAZOLE
7. HALOPROGIN
8. KETOCONAZOLE (Topical)
9. MICONAZOLE
10. NAFTIFINE
11. NYSTATIN
12. OXICONAZOLE (Topical)
13. SERTACONAZOLE
14. SULCONAZOLE
15. TERBINAFINE
16. TOLNAFTATE
17. UNDECYLENIC ACID

BRAND NAMES

Aftate for Athlete's Foot Aerosol Spray Liquid[16]
Aftate for Athlete's Foot Aerosol Spray Powder[16]
Aftate for Athlete's Foot Gel[16]
Aftate for Athlete's Foot Sprinkle Powder[16]
Aftate for Jock Itch Aerosol Spray Powder[16]
Aftate for Jock Itch Gel[16]
Aftate for Jock Itch Sprinkle Powder[16]
Caldesene Medicated Powder[17]
Canesten Cream[4]
Canesten Solution[4]
Conazol[9]
Cruex Aerosol Powder[17]
Cruex Antifungal Cream[17]
Cruex Antifungal Powder[17]
Cruex Antifungal Spray Powder[17]
Cruex Cream[17]
Cruex Powder[17]
Decylenes[17]
Decylenes Powder[17]
Desenex Aerosol Powder[17]
Desenex Antifungal Cream[17]
Desenex Antifungal Liquid[17]
Desenex Antifungal Ointment[17]
Desenex Antifungal Penetrating Foam[17]
Desenex Antifungal Powder[17]
Desenex Antifungal Spray Powder[17]
Desenex Max Cream[17]
Desenex Ointment[17]
Desenex Powder[17]
Desenex Solution[17]
Ecostatin[5]
Ertazo[13]
Exelderm[14]
Extina[8]
Extina Foam[8]
Fungizone[1]
Genaspore Cream[16]
Gordochom Solution[17]
Halotex[7]
Lamisil[15]
Lamisil Solution 1%[15]
Loprox[3]
Lotriderm[4]
Lotrimin AF[4]
Lotrimin Cream[4]
Lotrimin Lotion[4]
Lotrimin Ointment[4]
Lotrimin Ultra[2]
Lotrisone[4]
Mentax[2]
Mentax TC[2]
Micatin[9]
Monistat-Derm[9]
Mycelex Cream[4]
Mycelex Solution[4]
Myclo Cream[4]
Myclo Solution[4]
Myclo Spray[4]
Mycostatin[11]
Nadostine[11]
Naftin[10]
Nilstat[11]
Nizoral A-D[8]
Nizoral Shampoo[8]
NP-27 Cream[16]
NP-27 Powder[16]
NP-27 Solution[16]
NP-27 Spray Powder[16]
Nyaderm[11]
Nystex[11]
Nystop[11]
Oravig[9]
Oxistat[12]
Penlac[3]
Pitrex Cream[16]
Spectazole[5]
Tinactin Aerosol Liquid[16]
Tinactin Aerosol Powder[16]
Tinactin Antifungal Deodorant Powder Aerosol[16]
Tinactin Cream[16]
Tinactin Jock Itch Aerosol Powder[16]
Tinactin Jock Itch Cream[16]
Tinactin Jock Itch Spray Powder[16]
Tinactin Plus Powder[16]
Tinactin Powder[16]
Tinactin Solution[16]
Ting Antifungal Cream[16]
Ting Antifungal Powder[16]
Ting Antifungal Spray Liquid[16]
Ting Antifungal Spray Powder[16]
Vusion[9]
Xolegel Gel[8]
Zeasorb-AF Powder[9]

ANTIFUNGALS (Vaginal)

GENERIC NAMES

1. BUTOCONAZOLE
2. CLOTRIMAZOLE
3. ECONAZOLE
4. GENTIAN VIOLET
5. MICONAZOLE
6. NYSTATIN
7. TERCONAZOLE
8. TIOCONAZOLE

BRAND NAMES

Canesten[2]
Canesten 1[2]
Canesten 3[2]
Canesten 10%[2]

Ecostatin[3]
FemCare[2]
Femizole Prefil[2]
Femizole-7[2]
Genapax[4]
Gynazole-1[1]
Gyne-Lotrimin[2]
Gyne-Lotrimin 3[2]
Gyno-Trosyd[8]
Monistat[5]
Monistat 1[8]
Monistat 3[5]
Monistat 5[5]
Monistat 7[5]
Mycelex-7[2]
Mycelex-G[2]
Myclo[2]
Mycostatin[6]
Nadostine[6]
Nilstat[6]
Nyaderm[6]
Terazol 3[7]
Terazol 7[7]
Three Day Cream[2]
Vagistat[8]
Vagistat-1[8]

ANTIHISTAMINES

GENERIC NAMES

1. ACRIVASTINE
2. AZATADINE
3. BROMODIPHENHYDRAMINE
4. BROMPHENIRAMINE
5. CARBINOXAMINE
6. CHLORPHENIRAMINE
7. CLEMASTINE FUMARATE
8. CYPROHEPTADINE
9. DEXBROMPHENIRAMINE
10. DEXCHLORPHENIRAMINE
11. DIMENHYDRINATE
12. DIPHENHYDRAMINE
13. DIPHENYLPYRALINE
14. DOXYLAMINE
15. PHENINDAMINE
16. PHENIRAMINE
17. PHENYLTOLOXAMINE
18. PYRILAMINE
19. TRIPELENNAMINE
20. TRIPROLIDINE

BRAND NAMES

Aclophen[6]
Actacin[20]
Actagen[20]
Actagen-C Cough[20]
Actidil[18]
Advil Multi-Symptom Cold[6]
AH-Chew[6]
Alersule[6]
Alka-Seltzer Plus Cold & Cough Liquid Gels[6]
Alka-Seltzer PM[12]
Allent[5]
Alleract[18]
Aller-Chlor[6]
Allercon[20]
Allerdryl[12]
Allerest Maximum Strength[6]
Allerfrim[20]
AllerMax Caplets[12]
Aller-med[12]
Allerphed[20]
Allert[6]
AlleRx Dose Pack DF[6]
AlleRx Dose Pack PE[6]
AlleRx Suspension[6]
All-Nite Cold Formula[14]
Ambay Cough[3]
Ambenyl Cough[3]
Ambophen Expectorant[3]
Anamine[6]
Anamine HD[6]
Anamine T. D.[6]
Apo-Dimenhydrinate[11]
Atrohist Pediatric[6]
Atrohist Pediatric Suspension Dye Free[6, 18]
Atrohist Sprinkle[6]
Banophen[12]
Banophen Caplets[12]
Beldin[12]
Belix[12]
Bena-D 10[12]
Bena-D 50[12]
Benadryl Allergy and Sinus Fastmelt[12]
Benadryl Allergy/Sinus Headache Caplets[12]
Benahist 10[12]
Benahist 50[12]
Ben-Allergin 50[12]
Benaphen[12]
Benoject-10[12]
Benoject-50[12]
Benylin All-In-One Cold & Flu Night Caplets[12]
Benylin All-In-One Cold & Flu Nightime Syrup[6]
Benylin Cold & Sinus Plus[6]
Brexin-L.A[6]
Brofed[5]
Bromanyl[3]
Bromatane DX Cough[5]
Bromfed[5]
Bromfed-DM[5]
Bromfed-PD[5]
Bydramine Cough[12]
Calm X[11]
Calmylin with Codeine[10]
Carbodec[5]
Carbodec DM Drops[5]
Carbodec TR[5]
Cenafed Plus[20]
Cerose-DM[6]
Children's Benadryl Allergy & Cold Fastmelt[12]
Children's Benadryl Perfect Measure[12]
Children's Dramamine[11]
Children's Triaminic Thin Strips Night Time Cold & Cough[12]
Chlo-Amine[6]
Chlor-100[6]
Chlorate[6]
Chlorgest-HD[6]
Chlor-Niramine[6]
Chlorphed[3]
Chlorphedrine SR[3]
Chlor-Pro[6]
Chlor-Pro 10[6]
Chlorspan-12[6]
Chlortab-4[6]
Chlortab-8[6]
Chlor-Trimeton 4 Hour Relief[6]
Chlor-Trimeton 12 Hour Relief[6]
Chlor-Tripolon[6]
CoActifed Expectorant[20]
Codehist DH[6]
Codeprex[6]
Codimal DH[18]
Codimal DM[6]
Codimal PH[18]
Codimal-A[5]
Codimal-L.A.[6]
Codimal-L.A. Half[6]
Colfed-A[6]
Colrex Compound[6]
Colrex Cough[6]
Coltab Children's[6]
Comhist[6]
Comhist LA[6]
Compoz[12]
Congestant D[6]
Conjec-B[5]
Contac 12-Hour[6]
Contac 12-Hour Allergy[7]
Contac Allergy/Sinus Night Caplets[7]
Contac Night Caplets[12]
Contac Severe Cold Formula[6]
Contac Severe Cold Formula Night Strength[6]
Coricidin HBP[6]
Cotridin[20]
D.A. Chewable[6]
Dallergy[6]
Dallergy Jr[5]
Decohistine DH[6]
Deconamine[6]
Deconamine SR[6]
Dexaphen SA[9]
Dexchlor[10]
Dexophed[9]
Diabetic Tussin Allergy Relief[6]
Diabetic Tussin Cold & Flu[6]
Diabetic Tussin Night Time Formula[12]
Diamine T.D.[5]
Dihistine[6]
Dihistine DH[6]
Dimetabs[11]

Dimetane[5]
Dimetapp Plus Caplets[5]
Dimetapp with Codeine[5]
Dimetapp-A[5]
Dimetapp-A Pediatric[5]
Dimetapp-DM[5]
Dimetapp-DM Cough and Cold[5]
Dimetapp-DM Elixir[5]
Dinate[11]
Diphen Cough[12]
Diphenacen-10[12]
Diphenacen-50[12]
Diphenadryl[12]
Disobrom[9]
Disophrol[9]
Disophrol Chronotabs[9]
Dommanate[11]
Donatussin[6]
Donatussin Drops[6]
Dondril[6]
Dormarex 2[12]
Dormin[12]
Dramamine[11]
Dramamine Chewable[11]
Dramamine Liquid[11]
Dramanate[11]
Dramocen[11]
Dramoject[11]
Dristan AF[6]
Dristan Cold and Flu[6]
Dristan Cold Maximum Strength Caplets[5]
Dristan Cold Multi-Symptom Formula[6]
Dristan Formula P[18]
Drixoral[9]
Drixoral Cold and Allergy[9]
Drixoral Cold and Flu[9]
Drixoral Plus[9]
Drixoral Sinus[9]
Drixtab[9]
Durahist[6]
Dura-Vent/DA[6]
Dymenate[11]
Ed A-Hist[6]
Endagen-HD[6]
Endal HD[6]
Endal-HD Plus[6]
Extendryl[6]
Extendryl JR[6]
Extendryl SR[6]
Father John's Medicine Plus[6]
Fedahist[6]
Fedahist Decongestant[6]
Fedahist Gyrocaps[6]
Fedahist Timecaps[6]
Fenylhist[12]
Fynex[12]
Genahist[12]
GenAllerate[6]
Gendecon[6]
Gen-D-phen[12]
Gravol[11]
Gravol L/A[11]
Hayfebrol[6]
Histafed C[18]
Histagesic Modified[6]
Histaject Modified[5]
Histalet[6]
Histalet-DM[6]
Histatab Plus[6]
Histatan[6]
Hista-Vent PSE[6]
Histex I/E[5]
Histor-D[6]
Histor-D Timecelles[6]
Hycomine Compound[6]
Hycomine-S Pediatric[6]
Hydramine[12]
Hydramine Cough[12]
Hydramyn[12]
Hydrate[11]
Hydril[12]
Hyrexin-50[12]
Insomnal[12]
Klerist-D[6]
Kolephrin[6]
Kolephrin/DM Caplets[6]
Kronofed-A[6]
Kronofed-A Jr.[6]
Lodrane D[4]
Lodrane LD[4]
Lodrane 12Hour ER[4]
Lodrane 24D[4]
Marmine[11]
Maximum Strength Tylenol Allergy Sinus Caplets[6]
Meda Syrup Forte[6]
Motion-Aid[12]
Myidil[20]
Nasahist B[5]
Nauseatol[11]
ND Clear T.D.[6]
ND Stat Revised[5]
ND-Gesic[6]
Neocitran A[16]
Neocitran Colds and Flu Calorie Reduced[16]
NeoCitran DM Coughs & Cold[16]
NeoCitran Extra Strength Colds and Flu[16]
Nervine Night-time Sleep-Aid[12]
Nico-Vert[11]
Nidryl[12]
Nisaval[17]
Nolahist[18]
Noradryl[12]
Norafed[18]
Nordryl[10]
Nordryl Cough[10]
Novodimenate[11]
Novopheniram[6]
NyQuil Cough[14]
Nytol Maximum Strength[12]
Nytol with DPH[12]
OMNIhist L.A.[6]
Optimine[2]
Oraminic II[5]
Palgic[5]
PBZ[19]
PBZ-SR[19]
PediaCare Children's Allergy[12]
PediaCare Children's Allergy & Cold[12]
PediaCare Children's Fever Reducer Plus Cough & Runny Nose[6]
PediaCare Children's Fever Reducer Plus Flu[6]
PediaCare Fever Reducer Plus Multi-Symptom Cold[6]
Pediacof Cough[6]
Pelamine[19]
Periactin[8]
Pertussin All Night PM[14]
Pfeiffer's Allergy[6]
Phenapap Sinus Headache & Congestion[6]
Phendry[12]
Phendry Children's Allergy Medicine[12]
Phenetron[6]
Phenetron Lanacaps[6]
PMS-Dimenhydrinate[11]
Poladex T.D.[10]
Prehist[6]
Prehist Cough Mixture 4[6]
Prehist D[6]
Pseudo-Chlor[6]
P-V-Tussin[6]
Pyribenzamine[19]
Pyrilamine Maleate Tablets[18]
Remcol-C[6]
Rescon-JR[6]
Rhinatate[6]
Rhinosyn[6]
Rhinosyn-DM[6]
Rhinosyn-PD[6]
Robitussin Children's Cough & Cold Long-Acting[6]
Robitussin Cough & Cold Long-Acting[6]
Robitussin Cough & Cold Nighttime[12]
Robitussin with Codeine[16]
Rolatuss Expectorant[6]
Rolatuss Plain[6]
R-Tannamine[6]
R-Tannamine Pediatric[6]
R-Tannate[6]
R-Tannate Pediatric[6]
Ryna[6]
Ryna-C Liquid[6]
Rynatan[6]
Rynatan Pediatric[6]
Rynatan-S Pediatric[6]
Rynatuss[6]
Rynatuss Pediatric[6]
Scot-Tussin DM[6]
Scot-Tussin Original 5-Action Cold Medicine[14]
Semprex-D[1]

Siladryl[12]
Silphen[12]
Simply Sleep[12]
Sleep-Eze 3[12]
Sominex Formula 2[12]
Sudafed PE Cold & Cough Caplets[12]
Tanoral[6]
Tavist[7]
Tavist-1[7]
Tavist Allergy/Sinus/Headache[7]
Tega-Vert[11]
Telachlor[6]
Teldrin[6]
Theraflu Cold & Cough Hot Liquid[16]
Theraflu Flu & Sore Throat Hot Liquid[16]
Theraflu Nighttime Severe Cold & Cough[12]
Theraflu Nighttime Severe Cold Hot Liquid[12]
Theraflu Thin Strips Multi Symptom[12]
Theraflu Thin Strips Nighttime Severe Cold & Cough[12]
Theraflu Warming Relief Nighttime Severe Cold & Cough[12]
Touro A&H[5]
Travamine[11]
Triafed[20]
Triafed with Codeine[20]
Triaminic-D Multi-Symptom Cold[6]
Triaminic Flu, Cough & Fever[6]
Triaminic Night Time Cough & Cold[6]
Triaminic Softchews Cough & Runny Nose[6]
Triaminic Thin Strips Cough & Runny Nose[12]
Triaminic Thin Strips Night Time Cold & Cough[12]
Tricodene Sugar Free[6]
Trimedine Liquid[6]
Tri-Nefrin Extra Strength[6]
Triotann[6]
Triotann Pediatric[6]
Trip-Tone[11]
Tritann Pediatric[6]
Tri-Tannate[6]
Tri-Tannate Plus Pediatric[6]
Trymegen[6]
Tussar DM[6]
TussiCaps[6]
Tussi-12[18]
Tussionex[6]
Tussirex with Codeine Liquid[16]
Tusstat[12]
Twilite[12]
Tylenol Allergy Multi-Symptom[6]
Tylenol Allergy Multi-Symptom Nighttime[12]
Tylenol Cold Head Congestion Nighttime[6]
Tylenol Cold Multi-Symptom Nighttime[14]
Tylenol Cough & Sore Throat Nighttime[14]
Tylenol Severe Allergy[12]
Tylenol Sinus Congestion & Pain Nighttime[6]
Uni-Bent Cough[12]
Unisom Nighttime Sleep Aid[14]
Unisom SleepGels Maximum Strength[12]
Vanex Forte R[6]
Vanex-HD[6]
Veltane[5]
Vertab[11]
Vicks Children's NyQuil[6]
Vicks Formula 44 Custom Care Cough & Cold PM[6]
Vicks NyQuil Cold & Flu Relief[14]
Vicks NyQuil Cold & Flu Symptom Relief Plus Vitamin C[14]
Vicks NyQuil Cough[14]
Vicks NyQuil D[14]
Vicks NyQuil Less Drowsy Cold & Flu Relief Liquid[6]
Vicks Pediatric Formula 44m Cough & Cold Relief[6]
Viravan DM[18]
Vituz[6]
Wehamine[11]
Wehdryl[12]
Wehdryl-10[12]
Wehdryl-50[12]
Zutripro[6]

ANTIHISTAMINES, NONSEDATING

GENERIC NAMES

1. CETIRIZINE
2. DESLORATADINE
3. FEXOFENADINE
4. LEVOCETIRIZINE
5. LORATADINE

BRAND NAMES

Alavert[5]
Alavert D-12[5]
Allegra[3]
Allegra ODT[3]
Allegra Oral Suspension[3]
Allegra-D[3]
Allegra-D 24 Hour[3]
Children's Allegra[3]
Children's Claritin Grape Chewable[5]
Children's Claritin Syrup, Grape[5]
Children's Zyrtec Allergy Bubble Gum Syrup[1]
Children's Zyrtec Perfect Measure[1]
Clarinex D 12 Hour[2]
Clarinex D 24 Hour[2]
Clarinex RediTabs[2]
Clarinex Syrup[2]
Clarinex[2]
Claritin RediTabs for Kids 24 Hour[5]
Claritin 12 Hour[5]
Claritin Extra[5]
Claritin Hives Relief[5]
Claritin Liqui-Gels[5]
Claritin RediTabs 24 Hour[5]
Claritin Syrup[5]
Claritin[5]
Claritin-D[5]
Claritin-D 12 Hour RediTabs for Kids[5]
Claritin-D 12 Hour[5]
Claritin-D 24 Hour[5]
Reactine[1]
Xyzal[4]
Zyrtec[1]
Zyrtec Allergy[1]
Zyrtec Children's Allergy Syrup[1]
Zyrtec Children's Chewable[1]
Zyrtec Children's Hives Relief Syrup[1]
Zyrtec-D[1]

ANTIHISTAMINES, PHENOTHIAZINE-DERIVATIVE

GENERIC NAMES

1. PROMETHAZINE
2. TRIMEPRAZINE

BRAND NAMES

Anergan 25[1]
Anergan 50[1]
Antinaus 50[1]
Histantil[1]
Mallergan-VC with Codeine[1]
Panectyl[2]
Penazine VC with Cough[1]
Pentazine[1]
Phenameth DM[1]
Phenameth VC with Codeine[1]
Phenazine 25[1]
Phenazine 50[1]
Phencen-50[1]
Phenergan[1]
Phenergan Fortis[1]
Phenergan Plain[1]
Phenergan VC[1]
Phenergan VC with Codeine[1]
Phenergan with Codeine[1]

Phenergan with
Dextromethorphan[1]
Phenoject-50[1]
Pherazine DM[1]
Pherazine VC[1]
Pherazine VC with Codeine[1]
Pherazine with Codeine[1]
PMS Promethazine[1]
Pro-Med 50[1]
Promehist with Codeine[1]
Promerhegan[1]
Promet[1]
Prometh VC with Codeine[1]
Prometh VC Plain[1]
Prometh with
Dextromethorphan[1]
Prometh-25[1]
Prometh-50[1]
Promethazine DM[1]
Promethazine VC[1]
Prorex-25[1]
Prorex-50[1]
Prothazine[1]
Prothazine Plain[1]
Shogan[1]
TV-Gan-25[1]
V-Gan-50[1]

ANTI-INFLAMMATORY DRUGS, NON-STEROIDAL (NSAIDs)

GENERIC NAMES

1. DICLOFENAC
2. DIFLUNISAL
3. ETODOLAC
4. FENOPROFEN
5. FLOCTAFENINE
6. FLURBIPROFEN
7. IBUPROFEN
8. INDOMETHACIN
9. KETOPROFEN
10. KETOROLAC
11. MECLOFENAMATE
12. MEFENAMIC ACID
13. NABUMETONE
14. NAPROXEN
15. OXAPROZIN
16. PHENYLBUTAZONE
17. PIROXICAM
18. SULINDAC
19. TENOXICAM
20. TIAPROFENIC ACID
21. TOLMETIN

BRAND NAMES

Aches-N-Pain[7]
Advil[7]
Advil Caplets[7]
Advil Chewable Tablets[7]
Advil Cold and Sinus Caplets[7]
Advil Cold and Sinus LiquiGels[7]
Advil Congestion Relief[7]
Advil First[7]
Advil Flu & Body Ache[7]
Advil Liqui-Gel[9]
Advil Migraine[7]
Albert Tiafen[20]
Aleve[14]
Aleve Liquid Gels[14]
Aleve-D Sinus & Cold[14]
Alka-Butazolidin[16]
Alkabutazone[16]
Alka-Phenylbutazone[16]
Alrheumat[9]
Amersol[7]
Anaprox[14]
Anaprox DS[14]
Ansaid[6]
Apo-Diclo[1]
Apo-Diflunisal[2]
Apo-Flurbiprofen[6]
Apo-Ibuprofen[7]
Apo-Indomethacin[8]
Apo-Keto[9]
Apo-Keto-E[9]
Apo-Naproxen[14]
Apo-Phenylbutazone[16]
Apo-Piroxicam[17]
Apsifen[7]
Apsifen-F[7]
Arthrotec[1]
Bayer Select Ibuprofen Caplets[7]
Bayer Select Pain Relief
Formula Caplets[7]
Brufen[7]
Butacote[16]
Butazone[16]
Cambia[1]
Cataflam[1]
Children's Advil[7]
Children's Motrin[7]
Clinoril[18]
CoAdvil Caplets[7]
Combunox[7]
Cotybutazone[16]
Cramp End[7]
Daypro[15]
Dimetapp Sinus Caplets[7]
Dolgesic[7]
Dolobid[2]
Dristan Sinus Caplets[7]
Duexis[7]
EC-Naprosyn[14]
Excedrin-IB Caplets[7]
Excedrin-IB Tablets[7]
Feldene[17]
Feldene Melt[17]
Fenopron[4]
Froben[6]
Froben SR[6]
Genpril[7]
Genpril Caplets[7]
Haltran[7]
Ibifon-600 Caplets[7]
Ibren[7]
Ibu[7]
Ibu-4[7]
Ibu-6[7]
Ibu-8[7]
Ibu-200[7]
Ibudone[7]
Ibumed[7]
Ibuprin[7]
Ibupro-600[7]
Ibu-Tab[7]
Ibutex[7]
Idarac[5]
Ifen[7]
Imbrilon[3]
Indameth[8]
Indocid[8]
Indocin[8]
Indocin SR[8]
Lodine[2]
Lodine XL[2]
Meclofen[11]
Meclomen[11]
Medipren[7]
Medipren Caplets[7]
Midol 200[7]
Midol-IB[7]
Mobiflex[19]
Motrin[7]
Motrin, Children's[7]
Motrin Cold and Flu[7]
Motrin, Infants[7]
Motrin-IB[7]
Motrin-IB Caplets[7]
Motrin-IB Cold & Sinus[7]
Motrin Migraine[7]
Nalfon[4]
Nalfon 200[4]
Naprelan[14]
Naprosyn[14]
Naprosyn-E[14]
Naprosyn-SR[14]
Naxen[14]
Nexcede[9]
Novobutazone[16]
Novo-Keto-EC[9]
Novomethacin[8]
Novonaprox[14]
Novopirocam[17]
Novoprofen[7]
Novo-Sundac[18]
Nu-Indo[8]
Nu-Pirox[17]
Nuprin[7]
Nuprin Caplets[7]
Orudis[9]
Orudis-E[9]
Orudis-KT[9]
Orudis-SR[9]
Oruvail[9]
Pamprin-IB[7]
Paxofen[7]
Pedia[7]
Phenylone Plus[16]
Ponstan[12]
Ponstel[12]
Prevacid NapraPac[14]
Progesic[4]

Reprexain[7]
Rhodis[9]
Rhodis-EC[9]
Ro-Profen[7]
Rufen[7]
Saleto-200[7]
Saleto-400[7]
Saleto-600[7]
Saleto-800[7]
Sine-Aid IB[7]
Sprix[10]
Surgam[20]
Surgam SR[20]
Synflex[14]
Synflex DS[14]
Telectin DS[21]
Toradol[10]
Trendar[7]
Treximet[14]
Vicoprofen[6]
Vimovo[14]
Voltaren[1]
Voltaren Rapide[1]
Voltaren SR[1]
Voltaren XR[1]
Voltarol[1]
Voltarol Retard[1]
Zipsor[1]

ANTI-INFLAMMATORY DRUGS, STEROIDAL (Ophthalmic)

GENERIC NAMES

1. BETAMETHASONE (Ophthalmic)
2. DEXAMETHASONE (Ophthalmic)
3. FLUOROMETHOLONE
4. HYDROCORTISONE (Ophthalmic)
5. LOTEPREDNOL
6. MEDRYSONE
7. PREDNISOLONE (Ophthalmic)
8. RIMEXOLONE

BRAND NAMES

Ak-Pred[7]
AK-Spore H.C.[4]
AK-Tate[7]
Alrex[5]
Baldex[2]
Betnesol[1]
Cortamed[4]
Decadron[2]
Dexair[2]
Dexotic[2]
Dexsone[2]
Diodex[2]
Econopred[7]
Econopred Plus[7]
Eflone[3]
Flarex[3]
Fluor-Op[3]
FML Forte[3]
FML Liquifilm[3]
FML S.O.P.[3]
HMS Liquifilm[6]
Inflamase Forte[7]
Inflamase-Mild[7]
Lite-Pred[7]
Lotemax[5]
Maxidex[2]
Neo-Polycin HC[4]
Neotricin[4]
Ocu-Dex[2]
Ocu-Pred[7]
Ocu-Pred Forte[7]
Ocu-Pred-A[7]
PMS-Dexamethasone Sodium Phosphate[2]
Pred Forte[7]
Pred Mild[7]
Predair[7]
Predair Forte[7]
Predair-A[7]
Spersadex[2]
Storz-Dexa[2]
Tobradex[2]
Tobradex ST[2]
Ultra Pred[7]
Vexol[8]
Zylet[5]

ANTISEBORRHEICS (Topical)

GENERIC NAMES

1. CHLOROXINE
2. PYRITHIONE
3. SALICYLIC ACID, SULFUR & COAL TAR
4. SELENIUM SULFIDE

BRAND NAMES

Capitrol[1]
Dan-Gard[2]
DHS Zinc Dandruff Shampoo[2]
Exsel[4]
Glo-Sel[4]
Head & Shoulders[2]
Head & Shoulders Antidandruff Cream Shampoo Normal to Dry Formula[2]
Head & Shoulders Antidandruff Cream Shampoo Normal to Oily Formula[2]
Head & Shoulders Antidandruff Lotion Shampoo 2 in 1 Formula[2]
Head & Shoulders Antidandruff Lotion Shampoo Normal to Dry Formula[2]
Head & Shoulders Antidandruff Lotion Shampoo Normal to Oily Formula[2]
Head & Shoulders Dry Scalp 2 in 1 Formula Lotion Shampoo[2]
Head & Shoulders Dry Scalp Conditioning Formula Lotion Shampoo[2]
Head & Shoulders Dry Scalp Regular Formula Lotion Shampoo[2]
Head & Shoulders Intensive Treatment 2 in 1 Formula Dandruff Lotion Shampoo[4]
Head & Shoulders Intensive Treatment Conditioning Formula Dandruff Lotion Shampoo[4]
Head & Shoulders Intensive Treatment Regular Formula Dandruff Lotion Shampoo[4]
Meted Maximum Strength Anti-Dandruff Shampoo with Conditioners[3]
Sebex-T Tar Shampoo[2]
Sebulex Conditioning Suspension Shampoo[3]
Sebulex Lotion Shampoo[3]
Sebulon[2]
Sebutone[3]
Selsun[4]
Selsun Blue[4]
Selsun Blue Dry Formula[4]
Selsun Blue Extra Conditioning Formula[4]
Selsun Blue Extra Medicated Formula[4]
Selsun Blue Oily Formula[4]
Selsun Blue Regular Formula[4]
Tersi Foam[4]
Theraplex Z[2]
Vanseb Cream Dandruff Shampoo[3]
Vanseb Lotion Dandruff Shampoo[3]
Vanseb-T[3]
Zincon[2]
ZNP[2]

APPETITE SUPPRESSANTS

GENERIC NAMES

1. BENZPHETAMINE
2. DIETHYLPROPION
3. MAZINDOL
4. PHENDIMETRAZINE
5. PHENTERMINE

BRAND NAMES

Adipex-P[5]
Adipost[4]
Adphen[4]
Anorex SR[4]
Appecon[4]
Bontril PDM[4]
Bontril Slow Release[4]
Dapex-37.5[5]
Didrex[1]
Dyrexan-OD[4]

Fastin[5]
Ionamin[5]
Mazanor[3]
Melfiat-105 Unicelles[4]
Metra[4]
Obalan[4]
Obezine[4]
Panshape[5]
Phendiet[4]
Phendimet[4]
Phentercot[5]
Phentra[5]
Phentride[5]
Phentrol[5]
Phenzine[4]
Plegine[4]
Prelu-2[4]
PT 105[4]
Qsymia[5]
Sanorex[3]
Statobex[4]
Suprenza[5]
T-Diet[5]
Tenuate[2]
Tenuate Dospan[2]
Tepanil[2]
Tepanil Ten-Tab[2]
Zantryl[5]

ASPIRIN

8-Hour Bayer Timed Release
217
217 Strong
Acetylsalicylic Acid
Alka-Seltzer Original
Alka-Seltzer Morning Relief Medicine
Alka-Seltzer Plus Flu Effervescent
Alka-Seltzer PM
Alpha-Phed
Anacin
APAC Improved
APF Arthritic Pain Formula
Arthrinol
Arthrisin
Arthritis Pain Formula
Artria S.R.
A.S.A.
A.S.A. Enseals
Ascriptin
Ascriptin A/D
Aspergum
Astrin
Axotal
Bayer
Bayer Advanced
Bayer Extra Strength Aspirin
Bayer Quick Release Crystals
Bayer Timed-Release Arthritic Pain Formula
Bayer Women's Caplets Aspirin Plus Calcium
Buffaprin
Bufferin
Buffets II
Buffinol
Butalgen
Cama Arthritis Reliever
Coryphen
Dristan Formula P
Duradyne
Easprin
Ecotrin
Empirin
Entrophen
Epromate-M
Equagesic
Equazine-M
Excedrin Back & Body
Excedrin Extra Strength Caplets
Excedrin Extra Strength Tablets
Excedrin Migraine
Extra Strength Bayer, Back & Body Pain
Extra Strength Bayer PM
Fasprin
Fiorgen PF
Fiorinal
Fiormor
Fortabs
Gelpirin
Gemnisyn
Goody's Extra Strength Tablets
Goody's Headache Powders
Halfprin
Headstart
Heptogesic
Isobutal
Isolin
Isollyl Improved
Laniroif
Lanorinal
Magnaprin
Magnaprin Arthritis Strength
Maprin
Marnal
Measurin
Meprogesic
Meprogesic Q
Micrainin
Nervine
Night-Time Effervescent Cold
Norwich Aspirin
Novasen
P-A-C Revised Formula
Pravigard PAC
Presalin
Riphen
Robaxisal
Sal-Adult
Salatin
Sal-Infant
Salocol
Soma Compound
St. Joseph Adult Chewable Aspirin
St. Joseph Companion Aspirin
Supac
Supasa
Synalgos-DC
Tecnal
Tenol Plus
Therapy Bayer
Triaphen
Trigesic
Ursinus Inlay
Vanquis
Vibutal
Viro-Med
Zorprin

BARBITURATES

GENERIC NAMES

1. AMOBARBITAL
2. APROBARBITAL
3. BUTABARBITAL
4. BUTALBITAL
5. MEPHOBARBITAL
6. METHARBITAL
7. PENTOBARBITAL
8. PHENOBARBITAL
9. SECOBARBITAL
10. SECOBARBITAL & AMOBARBITAL
11. TALBUTAL

BRAND NAMES

Alurate[2]
Amaphen[4]
Amytal[1]
Ancalixir[8]
Anolor-300[4]
Anoquan[4]
Arcet[4]
Axotal[4]
Bancap[4]
Barbita[8]
Bucet[4]
Busodium[3]
Butace[4]
Butalan[3]
Butalgen[4]
Butisol[3]
Cafergot PB[7]
Dolmar[4]
Endolor[4]
Esgic[4]
Esgic-Plus4[1]
Ezol[4]
Femcet[4]
Fiorgen PF[4]
Fioricet[4]
Fiorinal[4]
Fiormor[4]
Fortabs[4]
G-1[4]
Gemonil[6]
Isobutal[4]
Isocet[4]
Isolin[4]

Isollyl Improved[4]
Isopap[4]
Laniroif[4]
Lanorinal[4]
Luminal[8]
Marnal[4]
Medigesic[4]
Nembutal[7]
Nova Rectal[7]
Novopentobarb[7]
Novosecobarb[9]
Pacaps[4]
Phrenilin[4]
Phrenilin Forte[4]
Repan[4]
Sarisol No. 2[3]
Seconal[9]
Sedapap[4]
Solfoton[8]
Tecnal[4]
Tencet[4]
Theodrine[8]
Theodrine Pediatric[8]
Theofed[8]
Triad[4]
Triaprin[4]
Tuinal[10]
Two-Dyne[4]
Vibutal[4]

BARBITURATES, ASPIRIN & CODEINE (Also contains caffeine)

GENERIC NAMES
1. BUTALBITAL, ASPIRIN & CODEINE
2. PHENOBARBITAL, ASPIRIN & CODEINE

BRAND NAMES
Ascomp with Codeine No. 3[1]
B-A-C with Codeine[1]
Butalbital Compound with Codeine[1]
Butinal with Codeine No. 3[1]
Fiorgen with Codeine[1]
Fiorinal with Codeine[1]
Fiorinal with Codeine No. 3[1]
Fiorinal-C$^{1}/_{4}$[1]
Fiorinal-C$^{1}/_{2}$[1]
Fiormor with Codeine[1]
Idenal with Codeine[1]
Isollyl with Codeine[1]
Phenaphen with Codeine No. 2[2]
Phenaphen with Codeine No. 3[2]
Phenaphen with Codeine No. 4[2]

BELLADONNA ALKALOIDS & BARBITURATES

GENERIC NAMES
1. ATROPINE & PHENOBARBITAL
2. ATROPINE, HYOSCYAMINE, SCOPOLAMINE & BUTABARBITAL
3. ATROPINE, HYOSCYAMINE, SCOPOLAMINE & PHENOBARBITAL
4. BELLADONNA & AMOBARBITAL
5. BELLADONNA & BUTABARBITAL
6. BELLADONNA & PHENOBARBITAL
7. HYOSCYAMINE & PHENOBARBITAL

BRAND NAMES
Antrocol[1]
Barbidonna[3]
Barbidonna 2[3]
Barophen[3]
Belladenal[7]
Belladenal Spacetabs[6]
Belladenal-S[7]
Bellalphen[3]
Butibel[5]
Chardonna-2[6]
Donnamor[3]
Donnapine[3]
Donna-Sed[6]
Donnatal[3]
Donnatal Elixir[3]
Donnatal Extentabs[3]
Donnatal No. 2[3]
Donphen[3]
Hyosophen[3]
Kinesed[3]
Levsin with Phenobarbital[6]
Levsinex with Phenobarbital Timecaps[7]
Levsin-PB[7]
Malatal[3]
Pheno-Bella[6]
Relaxadon[3]
Spaslin[3]
Spasmolin[3]
Spasmophen[3]
Spasquid[3]
Susano[3]

BENZODIAZEPINES

GENERIC NAMES
1. ALPRAZOLAM
2. BROMAZEPAM
3. CHLORDIAZEPOXIDE
4. CLOBAZAM
5. CLONAZEPAM
6. CLORAZEPATE
7. DIAZEPAM
8. ESTAZOLAM
9. FLURAZEPAM
10. HALAZEPAM
11. KETAZOLAM
12. LORAZEPAM
13. MIDAZOLAM
14. NITRAZEPAM
15. OXAZEPAM
16. PRAZEPAM
17. QUAZEPAM
18. TEMAZEPAM

BRAND NAMES
Alprazolam Intensol[1]
Apo-Alpraz[1]
Apo-Chlordiazepoxide[3]
Apo-Clorazepate[6]
Apo-Diazepam[7]
Apo-Flurazepam[9]
Apo-Lorazepam[12]
Apo-Oxazepam[15]
Ativan[18]
Centrax[16]
Clindex[3]
Clinoxide[3]
Dalmane[9]
Diastat[7]
Diazemuls[7]
Diazepam Intensol[7]
Doral[17]
Klonopin[5]
Lectopam[2]
Librax[3]
Libritabs[3]
Librium[3]
Lidoxide[3]
Limbitrol[3]
Limbitrol DS[3]
Lipoxide[3]
Loftran[17]
Lorazepam Intensol[12]
Medilium[3]
Meval[7]
Mogadon[16]
Niravam[1]
Niravam Orally Disintegrating Tablets[1]
Novo-Alprazol[1]
Novoclopate[6]
Novodipam[7]
Novoflupam[9]
Novolorazem[12]
Novopoxide[3]
Novoxapam[15]
Nu-Alpraz[1]
Nu-Loraz[12]
Onfi[4]
Paxipam[10]
PMS Diazepam[7]
Restoril[18]
Rivotril[5]
Serax[15]
Solium[3]
Somnol[9]
T-Quil[7]
Tranxene[7]
Tranxene T-Tab[6]
Tranxene-SD[7]
Valium[7]
Valrelease[7]

Vivol[7]
Xanax[1]
Xanax XR[1]
Zapex[15]
Zebrax[3]
Zetran[7]

BENZOYL PEROXIDE

Acanya
Acetoxyl 2.5 Gel
Acetoxyl 5 Gel
Acetoxyl 10 Gel
Acetoxyl 20 Gel
Acne-5 Lotion
Acne-10 Lotion
Acne-Aid 10 Cream
Acne-Mask
Acnomel B.P. 5 Lotion
Ben-Aqua 2½ Gel
Ben-Aqua 2½ Lotion
Ben-Aqua 5 Gel
Ben-Aqua 5 Lotion
Ben-Aqua 10 Gel
Ben-Aqua 10 Lotion
Ben-Aqua Masque 5
Benoxyl 5 Lotion
Benoxyl 5 Wash
Benoxyl 10 Lotion
Benoxyl 10 Wash
Benoxyl 20 Lotion
Benzac Ac 2½ Gel
Benzac Ac 5 Gel
Benzac Ac 10 Gel
Benzac W 2½ Gel
Benzac W 5 Gel
Benzac W 10 Gel
Benzaclin
Benzagel 5 Acne Lotion
Benzagel 5 Acne Wash
Benzagel 5 Gel
Benzagel 10 Gel
Benzamycin
BenzaShave 5 Cream
BenzaShave 10 Cream
BenzEFoam
Brevoxyl 4 Gel
Buf-Oxal 10
Cleanse and Treat
Clear By Design 2.5 Gel
Clearasil BP Plus 5 Cream
Clearasil BP Plus 5 Lotion
Clearasil Maximum Strength Medicated Anti-Acne 10 Tinted Cream
Clearasil Maximum Strength Medicated Anti-Acne 10 Vanishing Cream
Clearasil Medicated Anti-Acne 10 Vanishing Lotion
Clinac BPO
Cuticura Acne 5 Cream
Del-Aqua-5 Gel
Del-Aqua-10 Gel
Del-Ray
Dermoxyl 2.5 Gel
Dermoxyl 5 Gel
Dermoxyl 10 Gel
Dermoxyl 20 Gel
Dermoxyl Aqua
Desquam-E 2.5 Gel
Desquam-E 5 Gel
Desquam-E 10 Gel
Desquam-X 2.5 Gel
Desquam-X 5 Gel
Desquam-X 5 Wash
Desquam-X 10 Gel
Desquam-X 10 Wash
Dry and Clear 5 Lotion
Dry and Clear Double Strength 10 Cream
Dryox 5 Gel
Dryox 10 Gel
Dryox 20 Gel
Dryox Wash 5
Dryox Wash 10
Duac Topical Gel
Epiduo
Fostex 5 Gel
Fostex 10 Bar
Fostex 10 Cream
Fostex 10 Gel
Fostex 10 Wash
H_2Oxyl 2.5 Gel
H_2Oxyl 5 Gel
H_2Oxyl 10 Gel
H_2Oxyl 20 Gel
Inova 8/2 ACT
Loroxide 5 Lotion with Flesh Tinted Base
Loroxide 5.5 Lotion
NeoBenz Micro
Neutrogena Acne Mask 5
Noxzema Clear-Ups Maximum Strength 10
Noxzema Clear-Ups On-the-Spot 10 Lotion
Oxy 5 Tinted Lotion
Oxy 5 Vanishing Formula Lotion
Oxy 5 Vanishing Lotion
Oxy 10
Oxy 10 Daily Face Wash
Oxy 10 Tinted Lotion
Oxy 10 Vanishing Lotion
Oxyderm 5 Lotion
Oxyderm 10 Lotion
Oxyderm 20 Lotion
PanOxyl 5 Bar
PanOxyl 5 Gel
PanOxyl 10 Bar
PanOxyl 10 Gel
PanOxyl 15 Gel
PanOxyl 20 Gel
PanOxyl Acne Creamy Wash
PanOxyl AQ 2½ Gel
PanOxyl AQ 5 Gel
Persa-Gel 5
Persa-Gel 10
Persa-Gel W 5
Persa-Gel W 10
pHisoAc BP 10
Propa P.H. 10 Acne Cover Stick
Propa P.H. 10 Liquid Acne Soap
Stri-Dex Maximum Strength Treatment 10 Cream
Theroxide 5 Lotion
Theroxide 10 Lotion
Theroxide 10 Wash
Topex 5 Lotion
Topex 10 Lotion
Vanoxide 5 Lotion
Xerac BP 5 Gel
Xerac BP 10 Gel
Zeroxin-5 Gel
Zeroxin-10 Gel
Zoderm
Zoderm Ready Pads

BETA-ADRENERGIC BLOCKING AGENTS

GENERIC NAMES

1. ACEBUTOLOL
2. ATENOLOL
3. BETAXOLOL
4. BISOPROLOL
5. CARTEOLOL
6. CARVEDILOL
7. LABETALOL
8. LEVOBETAXOLOL
9. METOPROLOL
10. NADOLOL
11. NEBIVOLOL
12. OXPRENOLOL
13. PENBUTOLOL
14. PINDOLOL
15. PROPRANOLOL
16. SOTALOL
17. TIMOLOL

BRAND NAMES

Apo-Atenolol[2]
Apo-Metoprolol[9]
Apo-Propranolol[15]
Apo-Timol[17]
Betaloc[9]
Betaxon[8]
Betapace[16]
Bystolic[11]
Blocadren[17]
Cartrol[5]
Coreg[6]
Coreg CR[6]
Corgard[10]
Detensol[15]
Inderal[15]
Inderal LA[15]
Kerlone[3]
Levatol[13]
Lopressor[9]
Lopressor SR[9]
Monitan[1]
Normodyne[7]

Novo-Atenol[2]
Novometoprol[9]
Novo-Pindol[14]
Novopranol[15]
Novo-Timol[17]
NuMetop[9]
Sectral[1]
Slow-Trasicor[12]
Sotacor[16]
Syn-Nadolol[10]
Syn-Pindolol[14]
Tenormin[2]
Toprol[9]
Toprol XL[9]
Toprol XL-XR[9]
Trandate[7]
Trasicor[12]
Visken[14]
Zebeta[4]

BETA-ADRENERGIC BLOCKING AGENTS & THIAZIDE DIURETICS

GENERIC NAMES

1. ATENOLOL & CHLORTHALIDONE
2. BETAXOLOL & CHLORTHALIDONE
3. BISOPROLOL & HYDROCHLOROTHIAZIDE
4. LABETALOL & HYDROCHLOROTHIAZIDE
5. METOPROLOL & HYDROCHLOROTHIAZIDE
6. NADOLOL & BENDROFLUMETHIAZIDE
7. PINDOLOL & HYDROCHLOROTHIAZIDE
8. PROPRANOLOL & HYDROCHLOROTHIAZIDE
9. TIMOLOL & HYDROCHLOROTHIAZIDE

BRAND NAMES

Co-Betaloc[5]
Corzide[6]
Dutoprol[5]
Inderide[8]
Inderide LA[8]
Kerledex[2]
Lopressor HCT[5]
Normozide[4]
Tenoretic[1]
Timolide[9]
Trandate HCT[4]
Viskazide[7]
Ziac[3]

BISPHOSPHONATES

GENERIC NAMES

1. ALENDRONATE
2. ETIDRONATE
3. IBANDRONATE
4. PAMIDRONATE
5. RISEDRONATE
6. TILUDRONATE
7. ZOLEDRONIC ACID

BRAND NAMES

Actonel[5]
Actonel with Calcium[5]
Aredia[4]
Atelvia[5]
Binosto[1]
Boniva[3]
Didronel[2]
Fosamax[1]
Fosamax Plus D[1]
Fosavance[1]
Reclast[7]
Skelid[6]
Zometa[7]

BRONCHODILATORS, ADRENERGIC

GENERIC NAMES

1. ALBUTEROL
2. ARFORMOTEROL
3. BITOLTEROL
4. EPHEDRINE SULFATE
5. EPINEPHRINE
6. ETHYLNOREPINEPHRINE
7. FENOTEROL
8. FORMOTEROL
9. INDACATEROL
10. ISOPROTERENOL
11. LEVALBUTEROL
12. METAPROTERENOL
13. PIRBUTEROL
14. PROCATEROL
15. RACEPINEPHRINE
16. SALMETEROL
17. TERBUTALINE

BRAND NAMES

Accuneb[1]
Adrenalin[5]
Advair Diskus[16]
Advair HFA[16]
Alupent[12]
Ana-Guard[5]
Arcapta[9]
Arm-a-Med Metaproterenol[12]
AsthmaHaler[5]
Asthmanefrin[15]
Berotec[7]
Brethaire[17]
Brethine[17]
Bricanyl[17]
Bronkaid Mist[5]
Bronkaid Mist Suspension[5]
Bronkaid Mistometer[5]
Brovana[3]
Combivent[1]
Combivent Respimat[1]
Dey-Dose Isoproterenol[10]
Dey-Dose Metaproterenol[12]
Dey-Dose Racepinephrine[15]
Dey-Lute Metaproterenol[12]
Dispos-a-Med Isoproterenol[10]
Dulera[8]
Duoneb[1]
Ephed II[4]
EpiPen Auto-Injector[5]
EpiPen Jr. Auto-Injector[5]
Foradil Aerolizer[8]
Foradil Certihaler[8]
Isuprel[10]
Isuprel Glossets[10]
Isuprel Mistometer[10]
Maxair[13]
Medihaler-Epi[5]
Medihaler-Iso[10]
microNEFRIN[15]
Nephron[5]
Novosalmol[1]
Perforomist Inhalation Solution[8]
Primatene HFC[5]
Primatene Mist Suspension[5]
Pro-Air[14]
Proventil[1]
Proventil HFA[1]
Proventil Repetabs[1]
Serevent[16]
Serevent Diskus[16]
Symbicort[8]
Tornalate[3]
Vapo-Iso[10]
Ventolin HFA[1]
Ventolin Rotocaps[1]
Volmax[1]
Xopenex[11]
Xopenex HFA[11]

BRONCHODILATORS, XANTHINE

GENERIC NAMES

1. AMINOPHYLLINE
2. DYPHYLLINE
3. OXTRIPHYLLINE
4. THEOPHYLLINE

BRAND NAMES

Accurbron[4]
Aerolate III[4]
Aerolate Jr.[4]
Aerolate Sr.[4]
Aerophyllin[1]
Aminophyllin[1]
Ami Rax[4]
Apo-Oxtriphylline[3]
Aquaphyllin[4]
Asbron G[4]
Asbron G Inlay Tablets[4]
Asmalix[4]
Bronchial[4]
Broncomar GG[4]
Bronkodyl[4]
Choledyl[3]

Choledyl Delayed-Release[3]
Choledyl SA[3]
Constant-T[4]
Corophyllin[1]
Dilor[2]
Dilor-400[2]
Duraphyl[4]
Dyflex 200[2]
Dyflex 400[2]
Ed-Bron G[4]
Elixicon[4]
Elixomin[1]
Elixophyllin[4]
Elixophyllin GG[4]
Elixophyllin SR[4]
Equibron G[4]
Glyceryl T[4]
Lanophyllin[4]
Lixolin[4]
Lufyllin[4]
Lufyllin-400[2]
Marax[4]
Marax D.F.[4]
Mudrane GG2[4]
Neothylline[2]
Novotriphyl[3]
Palaron[1]
Phyllocontin[1]
Phyllocontin-350[1]
PMS Theophylline[4]
Protophylline[2]
Pulmophylline[4]
Quibron[4]
Quibron 300[4]
Quibron-T[4]
Quibron-T Dividose[4]
Quibron-T/SR[4]
Quibron-T/SR Dividose[4]
Respbid[4]
Slo-Bid[4]
Slo-bid Gyrocaps[4]
Slo-phyllin[4]
Slo-Phyllin GG[4]
Slo-Phyllin Gyrocaps[4]
Solu-Phyllin[4]
Somophyllin[1]
Somophyllin-12[1]
Somophyllin-CRT[1]
Somophyllin-DF[1]
Somophyllin-T[1]
Sustaire[4]
Synophylate[4]
Theo-24[4]
Theobid Duracaps[4]
Theobid Jr. Duracaps[4]
Theochron[4]
Theoclear L.A. 130 Cenules[4]
Theoclear L.A. 260 Cenules[4]
Theoclear-80[4]
Theocot[4]
Theo-Dur[4]
Theo-Dur Sprinkle[4]
Theolair[4]
Theolair-SR[4]
Theolate[4]
Theomar[4]
Theon[4]
Theophylline SR[4]
Theo-Sav[4]
Theospan SR[4]
Theo-SR[4]
Theostat[4]
Theostat 80[4]
Theo-Time[4]
Theovent Long-acting[4]
Theox[4]
Thylline[2]
T-Phyl[4]
Truphylline[1]
Truxophyllin[4]
Unidur[4]
Uniphyl[4]

CAFFEINE

222
282
292
692
Actamin Super
Alka-Seltzer Morning Relief
Amaphen
Anacin
Anacin with Codeine
Anolor-300
Anoquan
A.P.C.
Aspirin Free Bayer Select
 Maximum Strength Headache
 Pain Relief Caplets
Aspirin-Free Excedrin Caplets
Bayer Quick Release Crystals
Cafergot
Cafergot PB
Cafertine
Cafetrate
Caffedrine
Caffefrine Caplets
Citrated Caffeine
Cotanal 65
Dexitac
Dristan AF
Dristan AF Plus
Dristan Formula P
Enerjets
Ercaf
Ergo-Caff
Esgic
Esgic-Plus
Excedrin Caplets
Excedrin Extra Strength
 Caplets
Excedrin Extra Strength
 Tablets
Excedrin Migraine
Excedrin Tension Headache
Extra Strength Bayer Back &
 Body Pain
Fiorinal
Gotamine
Keep Alert
Lucidex
Migergot
Novo-AC and C
P-A-C Revised Formula
Pacaps
PC-Cap
Pep-Back
Propoxyphene Compound-65
Quick Pep
Repan
Salatin
Salocol
Scot-tussin Original 5-Action
 Cold Medicine
Sinapils
Snap Back
Supac
Synalgos-DC
Tirend
Trigesic
Two-Dyne
Vanquish
Vivarin
Wake-Up
Wigraine

CALCIUM CHANNEL BLOCKERS

GENERIC NAMES
1. AMLODIPINE
2. BEPRIDIL
3. DILTIAZEM
4. FELODIPINE
5. FLUNARIZINE
6. ISRADIPINE
7. NICARDIPINE
8. NIFEDIPINE
9. NISOLDIPINE
10. VERAPAMIL

BRAND NAMES
Adalat[8]
Adalat CC[8]
Adalat FT[8]
Adalat P.A.[8]
Apo-Diltiaz[3]
Apo-Nifed[8]
Apo-Verap[10]
Amturnide[1]
Azor[1]
Bepadin[2]
Caduet[1]
Calan[10]
Calan SR[10]
Cardene[7]
Cardene SR[7]
Cardizem[3]
Cardizem CD[3]
Cardizem LA[3]
Cardizem SR[3]
Cartia XT[3]

Chronovera[10]
Dilacor-XR[3]
Dyna Circ[6]
Exforge[1]
Exforge HCT[1]
Isoptin[10]
Isoptin SR[10]
Ketorolac[3]
Lotrel[1]
Nifedical[3]
Norvasc[1]
Novo-Diltazem[3]
Novo-Nifedin[8]
Novo-Veramil[10]
Nu-Diltiaz[3]
Nu-Nifed[8]
Nu-Verap[10]
Plendil[4]
Procardia[8]
Procardia XL[8]
Renedil[4]
Sibelium[5]
Sular[9]
Syn-Diltiazem[3]
Tarka[10]
Teczem[3]
Tekamlo[1]
Tiazac[3]
Tribenzor[1]
Twynsta[1]
Vascor[2]
Verelan[10]
Verelan PM[10]

CALCIUM SUPPLEMENTS

GENERIC NAMES

1. CALCIUM CARBONATE
2. CALCIUM CITRATE
3. CALCIUM GLUBIONATE
4. CALCIUM GLUCONATE
5. CALCIUM GLYCEROPHOSPHATE & CALCIUM LACTATE
6. CALCIUM LACTATE
7. DIBASIC CALCIUM PHOSPHATE
8. TRIBASIC CALCIUM PHOSPHATE

BRAND NAMES

Actonel with Calcium[1]
Apo-Cal[1]
Bayer Women's Caplets Plus Calcium[1]
BioCal[1]
Calcarb 600[1]
Calci-Chew[1]
Calciday 667[1]
Calcilac[1]
Calcite 500[1]
Calcium Carbonate/600[1]
Calcium Stanley[4]
Calcium-600[1]
Calcium-Sandoz[3]
Calcium-Sandoz Forte[1,6]
Calglycine[1]
Calphosan[5]
Calsan[1]
Cal-sap[3]
Caltrate[1]
Caltrate-300[1]
Caltrate-600[1]
Caltrate Chewable[1]
Children's Pepto[1]
Chooz[1]
Citracal[2]
Citracal Liquitabs[2]
Gencalc 600[1]
Gramcal[1,6]
Mallamint[1]
Neo-Calglucon[3]
Nephro-Calci[1]
NutraCal[3]
Os-Cal[1]
Os-Cal 500[1]
Os-Cal Chewable[1]
Oysco[1]
Oysco 500 Chewable[1]
Oyst-Cal[1]
Oyst-Cal 500 Chewable[1]
Oystercal 500[1]
Posture[8]
Rolaids-Calcium Rich[1]
Titralac[1]
Tums[1]
Tums E-X[1]

COAL TAR (Topical)

Alphosyl
Aquatar
Balnetar
Balnetar Therapeutic Tar Bath
Cutar Water Dispersible Emollient Tar
Denorex
Denorex Extra Strength Medicated Shampoo
Denorex Extra Strength Medicated Shampoo with Conditioners
Denorex Medicated Shampoo
Denorex Medicated Shampoo and Conditioner
Denorex Mountain Fresh Herbal Scent Medicated Shampoo
DHS Tar Gel Shampoo
DHS Tar Shampoo
Doak Oil
Doak Oil Forte
Doak Oil Forte Therapeutic Bath Treatment
Doak Oil Therapeutic Bath Treatment For All-Over Body Care
Doak Tar Lotion
Doak Tar Shampoo
Doctar
Doctar Hair & Scalp Shampoo & Conditioner
Estar
Fototar
Ionil-T Plus
Lavatar
Liquor Carbonis Detergens
Medotar
Pentrax Extra-Strength Therapeutic Tar Shampoo
Pentrax Tar Shampoo
Psorent
psoriGel
PsoriNail
Scytera Foam
Tar Doak
Taraphilic
Tarbonis
Tarpaste
Tarpaste Doak
T/Derm Tar Emollient
Tegrin Lotion for Psoriasis
Tegrin Medicated Cream Shampoo
Tegrin Medicated Shampoo Concentrated Gel
Tegrin Medicated Shampoo Extra Conditioning Formula
Tegrin Medicated Shampoo Herbal Formula
Tegrin Medicated Shampoo Original Formula
Tegrin Medicated Soap for Psoriasis
Tegrin Skin Cream for Psoriasis
Tersa-Tar Mild Therapeutic Shampoo with Protein and Conditioner
Tersa-Tar Soapless Tar Shampoo
Tersa-Tar Therapeutic Shampoo
T-Gel
T/Gel Therapeutic Conditioner
T/Gel Therapeutic Shampoo
Theraplex T Shampoo
Zetar
Zetar Emulsion
Zetar Medicated Antiseborrheic Shampoo

CONTRACEPTIVES, ORAL & SKIN

GENERIC NAMES

1. DESOGESTREL & ETHINYL ESTRADIOL
2. DROSPIRENONE & ETHINYL ESTRADIOL
3. ESTRADIOL VALERATE & DIENOGEST
4. ETHYNODIOL DIACETATE & ETHINYL ESTRADIOL

5. LEVONORGESTREL & ETHINYL ESTRADIOL
6. NORELGESTROMIN & ETHINYL ESTRADIOL
7. NORETHINDRONE & ETHINYL ESTRADIOL
8. NORETHINDRONE & MESTRANOL
9. NORETHINDRONE ACETATE & ETHINYL ESTRADIOL
10. NORGESTIMATE & ETHINYL ESTRADIOL
11. NORGESTREL & ETHINYL ESTRADIOL

BRAND NAMES

Alesse[5]
Apri[1]
Aviane[5]
Beyaz[2]
Brevicon[7]
Brevicon 0.5/35[7]
Brevicon 1/35[7]
Camrese[5]
Cyclen[10]
Cyclessa[1]
Demulen 1/35[4]
Demulen 1/50[4]
Demulen 30[4]
Demulen 50[4]
Desogen 28[1]
Desogen Ortho-Cept[1]
Emoquette[1]
Estrostep[9]
Estrostep Fe[9]
Femcon Fe[7]
GenCept 0.5/35[7]
GenCept 1/35[7]
GenCept 10/11[7]
Generess Fe[7]
Genora 0.5/35[7]
Genora 1/35[7]
Genora 1/50[8]
Introvale[5]
Jenest-28[7]
Levlen[5]
Levlite[5]
Levora[5]
Loestrin 1/20[9]
Loestrin 1.5/30[9]
Loestrin 24 Fe[9]
Lo Loestrin Fe[9]
Lo/Ovral[11]
LoSeasonique[5]
Lybrel[5]
Marvelon[1]
Microgestin Fe[7]
Minestrin 1/20[9]
Min-Ovral[5]
Mircette[1]
ModiCon[7]
Myzilra[5]
Natazia[3]
Necon 0.5/35-21[7]
Necon 0.5/35-28[7]
Necon 1/35-21[7]
Necon 1/35-28[7]
Necon 1/50-21[8]
Necon 1/50-28[8]
Necon 10/11-21[7]
Necon 10/11-28[7]
N.E.E. 1/35[7]
N.E.E. 1/50[7]
Nelova 0.5/35E[7]
Nelova 1/35E[7]
Nelova 1/50M[8]
Nelova 10/11[7]
Nelulen 1/35E[4]
Nelulen 1/50E[4]
Norcept-E 1/35[9]
Nordette[5]
Norethin 1/35E[7]
Norethin 1/50M[8]
Norinyl 1+35[7]
Norinyl 1+50[8]
Norinyl 1/50[8]
Norlestrin 1/50[99]
Norlestrin 2.5/50[9]
Ocella[2]
Orsythia[5]
Ortho 0.5/35[7]
Ortho 1/35[7]
Ortho 7/7/7[7]
Ortho 10/11[7]
Ortho-Cept[1]
Ortho-Cyclen[10]
Orthro Evra[6]
Ortho-Novum 0.5[7]
Ortho-Novum 1/35[7]
Ortho-Novum 1/50[8]
Ortho-Novum 1/80[8]
Ortho-Novum 2[7]
Ortho-Novum 7/7/7[7]
Ortho-Novum 10/11[7]
Ortho-Tri-Cyclen 21[8]
Ortho-Tri-Cyclen 28[8]
Orthr-Tri-Cyclen Lo[10]
Ovcon-35[7]
Ovcon-50[7]
Ovral[11]
Previfem[10]
Quasense[5]
Safyral[2]
Seasonale[5]
Seasonique[5]
Symphasic[7]
Tri-Cyclen[10]
Tri-Levlen[5]
Tri-Norinyl[7]
Tri-Previfem[10]
Tri-Sprintec[10]
Triphasil[5]
Triquilar[5]
Trivora[5]
Yasmin[2]
Yaz[2]
Zovia 1/35E[4]
Zovia 1/50E[4]

CONTRACEPTIVES, VAGINAL

GENERIC NAMES

1. BENZALKONIUM CHLORIDE
2. ETONOGESTREL & ETHINYL ESTRADIOL
3. NONOXYNOL 9
4. OCTOXYNOL 9

BRAND NAMES

Advantage 24[3]
Because[3]
Conceptrol Gel[3]
Conceptrol-Contraceptive Inserts[3]
Delfen[3]
Emko[3]
Encare[3]
Gynol II Extra Strength[3]
Gynol II Original Formula[3]
Koromex Cream[3]
Koromex Crystal Gel[3]
Koromex Foam[3]
Koromex Jelly[3]
K-Y Plus[3]
NuvaRing[2]
Ortho-Creme[3]
Ortho-Gynol[4]
Pharmatex[1]
Pre-Fil[3]
Ramses Contraceptive Foam[3]
Ramses Contraceptive Vaginal Jelly[3]
Ramses Crystal Clear Gel[3]
Semicid[3]
Shur-Seal[3]
VCF[3]

DEXTROMETHORPHAN

2/G-DM Cough
Alka-Seltzer Plus Cold & Cough Effervescent
Alka-Seltzer Plus Cold & Cough Liquid
Alka-Seltzer Plus Cold & Cough Liquid-Gels
Alka-Seltzer Plus Day & Night Effervescent
Alka-Seltzer Plus Day & Night Liquid Gels
Alka-Seltzer Plus Day Cold Liquid
Alka-Seltzer Plus Flu Effervescent
Alka-Seltzer Plus Nighttime Cold Liquid
Alka-Seltzer Plus Night-Time Effervescent
Alka-Seltzer Plus Night-Time Liquid-Gels
All-Nite Cold Formula
Ambenyl-D Decongestant Cough Formula
Anatuss DM

Anti-Tuss DM Expectorant
Balminil DM
Baytussin DM
Benylin All-In-One Cold & Flu Caplets
Benylin All-In-One Cold & Flu Nightime Syrup
Benylin All-In-One Cold & Flu Syrup
Benylin All-In-One Day & Night Caplets
Benylin DM 12 Hour Nightime Cough Syrup
Benylin DM-D
Benylin DM-D for Children Cough & Cold Syrup
Benylin DM-D-E
Benylin DM-E Chest Cough Syrup
Benylin DM-D-E Extra Strength
Benylin DM-E
Benylin DM-E Chest Cough Syrup
Bromfed-DM
Broncho-Grippol-DM
Carbodec DM Drops
Cerose-DM
Cheracol D Cough
Children's Benylin DM-D
Children's Formula Cough
Children's Hold
Children's Tylenol Plus Cold & Cough
Children's Tylenol Plus Cough & Runny Nose
Children's Tylenol Plus Cough & Sore Throat
Children's Tylenol Plus Flu
Children's Tylenol Plus Multi-Symptom Plus Cold
Codimal DM
Codistan No. 1
Colrex Cough
Conar
Conar Expectorant
Conar-A
Concentrin
Congespirin
Contac Night Caplets
Contac Severe Cold Formula
Contac Severe Cold Formula Night Strength
Coricidin HBP
Coricidin HBP Chest Congestion & Cough
Cough X
Creo-Terpin
Delsym
Delsym Grape for Adults
Delsym Grape for Children
Diabetic Tussin Cold & Flu
Diabetic Tussin DM
Diabetic Tussin Night Time Formula
Dimetapp Children's Elixir Cold & Allergy PE
Dimetapp Children's Long Acting Cough Plus Cold
DM Cough
DM Syrup
Donatussin
Dondril
Dristan Cold and Flu
Dristan Juice Mix-in Cold, Flu, & Cough
Drixoral Cough
Efficol Cough Whip (Cough Suppressant/Decongestant)
Efficol Cough Whip (Cough Suppressant/Expectorant)
Extra Action Cough
Fast-Max DM Adult Liquid
Father John's Medicine Plus
Genatuss DM
Glycotuss-dM
Guiamid D.M. Liquid
Guiatuss-DM
Halotussin-DM Expectorant
Histalet-DM
Hold
Humibid DM Sprinkle
Koffex
Kolephrin GG/DM
Kolephrin/DM Caplets
Kophane Cough and Cold Formula
Maximum Strength Mucinex DM
Meda Syrup Forte
Medatussin
Mediquell
Mucinex Adult Caplets - Cold, Flu, & Sore Throat
Mucinex Adult Caplets - Severe Congestion & Cold
Mucinex Children's Cough, Expectorant & Suppressant
Mucinex Cough Mini-Melts
Mucinex Fast-Max Cold, Flu & Sore Throat Liquid
Mucinex Maximum Strength Fast Max Cold, Flu & Sore Throat
Mucinex Maximum Strength Fast Max Severe Congestion & Cough
Mytussin DM
Naldecon Senior DX
Naldecon-DX
NeoCitran DM Coughs & Colds
Neo-DM
Nytcold Medicine
Ornex DM 15
Ornex DM 30
Ornex Severe Cold No Drowsiness Caplets
Par Glycerol-DM
PediaCare Children's Cough & Congestion
PediaCare Children's Fever Reducer Plus Cough & Runny Nose
PediaCare Children's Fever Reducer Plus Cough & Sore Throat
PediaCare Children's Fever Reducer Plus Flu
PediaCare Children's Multi-Symptom Cold
PediaCare Fever Reducer Plus Multi-Symptom Cold
Pertussin All Night CS
Pertussin All Night PM
Pertussin Cough Suppressant
Pertussin CS
Pertussin ES
Phanatuss
Phenameth DM
Phenergan with Dextromethorphan
Pherazine DM
Prometh with Dextromethorphan
Promethazine DM
Queltuss
Remcol-C
Rhinosyn-DM
Rhinosyn-DMX Expectorant
Rhinosyn-X
Robafen DM
Robidex
Robitussin Children's Cough Long-Acting
Robitussin Children's Cough & Cold Long-Acting
Robitussin Cough & Chest Congestion
Robitussin Cough & Chest Congestion DM
Robitussin Cough & Chest Congestion DM Max
Robitussin Cough & Chest Congestion Sugar Free DM
Robitussin Cough & Cold CF
Robitussin Cough & Cold D
Robitussin Cough & Cold Long-Acting
Robitussin Cough Cold & Flu Nighttime
Robitussin Cough Gels Long Acting
Robitussin Cough Long Acting
Ru-Tuss Expectorant
SafeTussin 30
Scot-Tussin DM
Sedatuss
Silexin Cough
Simply Cough
Snaplets-DM

Snaplets-Multi
St. Joseph Cough Suppressant for Children
Sucrets Cough Control
Sudafed Multi-Symptom Cold & Cough
Sudafed PE Cold & Cough Caplets
Suppress Cough with Dextromethorphan
Terphan
Theracof Plus Multi-Symptom Cough and Cold Reliever
Theraflu Cold & Cough Hot Liquid
Theraflu Daytime Severe Cold Caplets
Theraflu Daytime Severe Cold Caplets
Theraflu Nighttime Severe Cold Caplets
Theraflu Thin Strips Daytime Cold & Cough
Theraflu Warming Relief Daytime
Tolu-Sed DM Cough
Touro DM
Triaminic Cough & Sore Throat
Triaminic-D Multi-Symptom Cold
Triaminic Day Time Cold & Cough
Triaminic Flu, Cough & Fever
Triaminic Long Acting Cough
Triaminic Softchews Cough & Runny Nose
Triaminic Softchews Cough & Sore Throat
Triaminic Thin Strips Daytime Cold & Cough
Triaminic Thin Strips Long Acting Cough
Tricodene Sugar Free
Trimedine Liquid
Trocal
Tussar DM
Tuss-DM
Tussi-Bid
Tylenol Cold Head Congestion Nighttime
Tylenol Cold Head Congestion Severe
Tylenol Cold Multi Symptom Daytime
Tylenol Cold Multi Symptom Nighttime
Tylenol Cold Multi Symptom Severe
Tylenol Cough & Severe Congestion Daytime
Tylenol Cough & Sore Throat Daytime
Tylenol Cough & Sore Throat Nighttime
Tylenol Sinus Severe Congestion Daytime
Uni-Tussin DM
Unproco
Vicks Children's NyQuil
Vicks DayQuil Cold/Flu Relief
Vicks DayQuil Cold & Flu Symptom Relief Plus Vitamin C
Vicks DayQuil Cough
Vicks DayQuil Mucus Control DM
Vicks Formula 44 Custom Care Chesty Cough
Vicks Formula 44 Custom Care Congestion
Vicks Formula 44 Custom Care Cough & Cold PM
Vicks Formula 44 Custom Care Dry Cough Suppressant
Vicks NyQuil Cold & Flu Relief
Vicks NyQuil Cold & Flu Symptom Relief Plus Vitamin C
Vicks NyQuil Cough
Vicks NyQuil D
Vicks NyQuil Less Drowsy Cold & Flu Relief Liquid
Vicks Pediatric Formula 44e Cough & Chest Congestion Relief
Vicks Pediatric Formula 44m Cough & Cold Relief
Viravan DM

DICYCLOMINE

Antispas
A-Spas
Bentyl
Bentylol
Byclomine
Dibent
Di-Cyclonex
Dilomine
Di-Spaz
Forulex
Lomine
Neoquess
Or-Tyl
Protylol
Spasmoban
Spasmoject
Viscerol

DIURETICS, THIAZIDE

GENERIC NAMES

1. BENDROFLUMETHIAZIDE
2. BENZTHIAZIDE
3. CHLOROTHIAZIDE
4. CHLORTHALIDONE
5. CYCLOTHIAZIDE
6. HYDROCHLOROTHIAZIDE
7. HYDROFLUMETHIAZIDE
8. METHYCLOTHIAZIDE
9. METOLAZONE
10. POLYTHIAZIDE
11. QUINETHAZONE
12. TRICHLORMETHIAZIDE

BRAND NAMES

Aldoclor[3]
Aldoril[6]
Anhydron[5]
Apo-Chlorthalidone[4]
Apo-Hydro[6]
Aquatensen[8]
Amturnide[6]
Atacand Plus[6]
Avalide[6]
Benicar HCT[6]
Demi-Regroton[4]
Diovan HCT[6]
Diucardin[7]
Diuchlor H[6]
Diulo[9]
Diupres[5]
Diurese R[12]
Diurigen with Reserpine[3]
Diuril[3]
Diutensen-R[8]
Duretic[8]
Dureticyl[8]
Edarbyclor[4]
Enduron[8]
Enduronyl[8]
Enduronyl Forte[8]
Exforge HCT[6]
Esidrix[6]
Exna[2]
Hydrex[2]
Hydro-D[6]
Hydrochlor[6]
HydroDIURIL[6]
Hydromox[11]
Hydropine[7]
Hydropine H.P.[7]
Hydropres[6]
Hygroton[4]
Hyzaar[6]
Metahydrin[12]
Micardis HCT[6]
Micardis Plus[6]
Microzide[6]
Minizide[10]
Mykrox[9]
Naqua[12]
Naturetin[1]
Neo-Codema[6]
Novodoparil[6]
Novo-Hydrazide[6]
Novo-Thalidone[4]
Oretic[6]
Oreticyl[6]
Oreticyl Forte[6]
PMS Dopazide[6]

Rauzide[1]
Regroton[4]
Renese[10]
Renese-R[10]
Saluron[7]
Salutensin[7]
Salutensin-Demi[7]
Supres[3]
Tekturna HCT[6]
Teveten HCT[6]
Thalitone[4]
Tribenzor[6]
Trichlorex[12]
Uniretic[6]
Uridon[4]
Urozide[6]
Zaroxolyn[9]

ERYTHROMYCINS

GENERIC NAMES

1. ERYTHROMYCIN ESTOLATE
2. ERYTHROMYCIN ETHYLSUCCINATE
3. ERYTHROMYCIN GLUCEPTATE
4. ERYTHROMYCIN LACTOBIONATE
5. ERYTHROMYCIN STEARATE
6. ERYTHROMYCIN-BASE

BRAND NAMES

Apo-Erythro[6]
Apo-Erythro E-C[6]
Apo-Erythro ES[2]
Apo-Erythro-S[5]
E-Base[6]
E.E.S.[2]
E/Gel[6]
Emgel[6]
E-Mycin[6]
Erybid[6]
ERYC[6]
EryPed[2]
Ery-Tab[6]
Erythraderm[6]
Erythro[2]
Erythrocin[5]
Erythrocot[5]
Erythromid[6]
Ilosone[1]
Ilotycin[3]
My-E[5]
Novorythro[5]
PCE Dispersatabs[5]
Pediazole[6]
Sulfimycin[6]
Wintrocin[5]

ESTROGENS

GENERIC NAMES

1. CONJUGATED ESTROGENS
2. DIETHYLSTILBESTROL
3. ESTERIFIED ESTROGENS
4. ESTRADIOL
5. ESTROGEN
6. ESTRONE
7. ESTROPIPATE
8. ETHINYL ESTRADIOL
9. QUINESTROL

BRAND NAMES

Activella[4]
Alora[4]
Angeliq[4]
Cenestin[1]
C.E.S.[1]
Climara[4]
Climara Pro[4]
Clinagen LA 40[4]
CombiPatch[4]
Congest[1]
Deladiol-40[4]
Delestrogen[4]
depGynogen[4]
Depo Estradiol[4]
Depogen[4]
DES[2]
Divigel[4]
Dura-Estrin[4]
Duragen[4]
Duragen-20[4]
Duragen-40[4]
E-Cypionate[4]
Elestrin[4]
Enjuvia[1]
Esclim[4]
Estinyl[8]
Estrace[4]
Estraderm[4]
Estragyn 5[6]
Estragyn LA 5[6]
Estra-L[4]
Estrasorb[4]
Estratab[3]
Estring[4]
Estro-A[6]
Estro-Cyp[4]
Estrofem[4]
Estrogel[4]
Estroject-L.A.[4]
Estro-L.A.[4]
Estro-Span[4]
EvaMist[4]
Femhrt[4]
Femogex[4]
Femring[4]
Femtrace[4]
Gynogen L.A. 20[4]
Gynogen L.A. 40[4]
Honvol [2]
Kestrone-5[6]
Mannest[2]
Menaval-20[4]
Menest[3]
Menostar[4]
Minivelle[4]
Neo-Estrone[3]
Ogen[7]
Ogen 1.25[7]
Ogen 2.5[7]
Ogen 6.25[7]
Ortho-Est[7]
Orthro-Prefest[4]
Premarin[1]
Premarin Vaginal Cream[1]
Premphase[1]
Prempro[1]
SCE-A Vaginal Cream[1]
Stilbestrol[2]
Stilphostrol[2]
Vagifem[4]
Valergen-10[4]
Valergen-20[4]
Valergen-40[4]
Vivelle[4]
Vivelle Dot[4]
Wehgen[6]

GUAIFENESIN

2/G-DM Cough
Adatuss D.C. Expectorant
Ambenyl-D Decongestant Cough Formula
Amonidrin
Anatuss DM
Anatuss LA
Anti-Tuss
Anti-Tuss DM Expectorant
Asbron G
Asbron G Inlay Tablets
Balminil Expectorant
Baytussin AC
Baytussin DM
Benylin All-In-One Cold & Flu Caplets
Benylin All-In-One Cold & Flu Nightime Syrup
Benylin All-In-One Cold & Flu Syrup
Benylin All-In-One Day & Night Caplets
Benylin Cold And Flu With Codeine Narcotic
Benylin DM-D-E
Benylin DM-D-E Extra Strength
Benylin DM-E Chest Cough Syrup
Breonesin
Bronchial
Broncholate
Broncomar GG
Brontex
Calmylin with Codeine
Cheracol D Cough
Children's Mucinex Cough
CoActifed Expectorant
Codiclear DH
Codimal Expectorant
Codistan No. 1
Colrex Expectorant

Comtrex Deep Chest Cold
Conar Expectorant
Conar-A
Concentrin
Congess JR
Congess SR
Congestac Caplets
Coricidin HBP Chest Congestion and Cough
Deconsal II
Detussin Expectorant
Diabetic Tussin DM
Diabetic Tussin EX
Diabetic Tussin Mucus Relief
Dihistine Expectorant
Dilaudid Cough
Donatussin
Donatussin DC
Donatussin Drops
Duratuss
Duratuss HD
Ed-Bron G
Efficol Cough Whip (Cough Suppressant/Decongestant)
Elixophyllin-GG
Entex PSE
Entuss Expectorant
Entuss Pediatric Expectorant
Entuss-D
Equibron G
Extra Action Cough
Fast-Max DM Adult Liquid
Father John's Medicine Plus
Fedahist Expectorant
Fedahist Expectorant Pediatric Drops
Fenesin
Gee-Gee
Genatuss
Genatuss DM
GG-CEN
Glyate
Glyceryl T
Glycotuss
Glycotuss-dM
Glydeine Cough
Glytuss
Guaifed
Guaifed-PD
GuaiMAX-D
Guiamid D.M. Liquid
Guiatuss A.C.
Guiatuss PE
Guiatuss-DM
Halotussin
Halotussin-DM Expectorant
Histalet X
Humibid L.A.
Humibid Sprinkle
Humibid-DM Sprinkle
Hycotuss Expectorant
Hytuss
Hytuss-2X
Kids-EEZE Chest Relief
Kolephrin GG/DM
Kwelcof Liquid
LiquiBid D
LiquiBid D-R
LiquiBid PD
Malotuss
Maximum Strength Mucinex
Maximum Strength Mucinex D
Maximum Strength Mucinex DM
Meda Syrup Forte
Medatussin
Medatussin Plus
Mucinex
Mucinex Adult Caplets - Cold & Sinus
Mucinex Adult Caplets - Cold, Flu, & Sore Throat
Mucinex Adult Caplets - Severe Congestion & Cold
Mucinex Children's Cough, Expectorant & Suppressant
Mucinex Children's Expectorant
Mucinex Cold Liquid
Mucinex Cough Mini-Melts
Mucinex D
Mucinex DM
Mucinex Fast-Max Cold, Flu & Sore Throat Liquid
Mucinex Junior Strength Expectorant
Mucinex Maximum Strength Fast Max Cold, Flu & Sore Throat
Mucinex Maximum Strength Fast Max Severe Congestion & Cough
Mucinex Mini-Melts
Mudrane GG2
Mytussin AC
Mytussin DAC
Mytussin DM
Naldecon Senior DX
Naldecon Senior EX
Nasatab LA
NeoCitrin DM Coughs & Colds
Nortussin
Nortussin with Codeine
Novahistine Expectorant
Organidin
PediaCare Children's Fever Reducer Plus Flu
Pertussin All Night CS
Phanatuss
Pneumomist
Poly-Histine Expectorant Plain
P-V-Tussin Tablets
Queltuss
Quibron
Quibron 300
Refenesen
Refenesen Chest Congestion & Pain Relief PE
Refenesen PE
Respaire-30
Resyl
Rhinosyn-DMX Expectorant
Rhinosyn-X
Robafen AC Cough
Robafen DAC
Robafen DM
Robafen Syrup
Robitussin Chest Congestion
Robitussin Cough & Chest Congestion
Robitussin Cough & Chest Congestion DM
Robitussin Cough & Chest Congestion DM Max
Robitussin Cough & Chest Congestion Sugar Free DM
Robitussin Cough & Cold CF
Robitussin Cough & Cold D
Robitussin with Codeine
Ru-Tuss DE
Ru-Tuss Expectorant
Ryna-CX Liquid
SafeTussin 30
Scot-Tussin
Silexin Cough
Sinumist-SR
Sinupan
Sinutab Non-Drying Liquid Caps
SINUvent PE
Slo-Phyllin GG
Stamoist E
Sudafed Multi-Symptom Cold & Cough
Sudafed Non-Drying Sinus Liquid Caps
Sudafed PE Cold & Cough Caplets
Theolate
Theracof Plus Multi-Symptom Cough and Cold Reliever
Theraflu Flu & Chest Congestion Hot Liquid
Tolu-Sed Cough
Tolu-Sed DM Cough
Touro DM
Touro Ex
Touro LA Caplets
Triaminic Chest & Nasal Congestion
Tussafed HCG Syrup
Tussafin Expectorant
Tussar SF
Tussar-2
Tuss-DM
Tussi-Bid
Tussi-organidin
Tylenol Chest Congestion
Tylenol Cold Head Congestion Severe
Tylenol Cold Multi Symptom Severe

Tylenol Cough & Severe Congestion Daytime
Tylenol Sinus Congestion & Pain Severe
Uni-Tussin
Uni-Tussin DM
Unproco
Versacaps
Vicks DayQuil Mucus Control DM
Vicks DayQuil Mucus Control Liquid
Vicks Formula 44 Custom Care Chesty Cough
Vicks Pediatric Formula 44e Cough & Chest Congestion Relief
Vicks VapoSyrup Severe Congestion Head & Chest Congestion Relief
Vicodin-Tuss

INSULIN

Humulin 70/30
Humulin N
Humulin R
Novolin 70/30
Novolin N
Novolin R

IRON SUPPLEMENTS

GENERIC NAMES

1. CARBONYL IRON
2. FERROUS FUMARATE
3. FERROUS GLUCONATE
4. FERROUS SULFATE
5. IRON DEXTRAN
6. IRON POLYSACCHARIDE
7. IRON SORBITOL

BRAND NAMES

Apo-Ferrous Gluconate[3]
Apo-Ferrous Sulfate[4]
Estrostep Fe[2]
Femiron[2]
Feosol[4]
Feosol Caplet[1]
Feostat[2]
Feostat Drops[2]
Fergon[3]
Fer-In-Sol[4]
Fer-In-Sol Drops[4]
Fer-In-Sol Syrup[4]
Fer-Iron[4]
Fero-folic 500[4]
Fero-Grad[4]
Fero-Gradumet[4]
FerraCap[1]
Ferralet[3]
Ferralet 90[1]
Ferralyn[4]
Ferra-TD[4]
Fertinic[4]
Generess Fe[2]
Hemocyte[2]
Hytinic[6]
Icar[1]
Ircon[2]
Jectofer[7]
Loestrin 24 Fe[2]
Lo Loestrin Fe[2]
Neo-Fer[2]
Novoferrogluc[6]
Novoferrosulfa[3]
Novofumar[4]
Nu-Iron[6]
Nu-Iron 150[6]
Palafer[2]
Palmiron[2]
PMS Ferrous Sulfate[4]
Simiron[3]
Slow Fe[4]
Span-FF[2]

KERATOLYTICS

GENERIC NAMES

1. RESORCINOL
2. RESORCINOL & SULFUR
3. SALICYLIC ACID
4. SALICYLIC ACID & SULFUR
5. SULFUR (Topical)

BRAND NAMES

Acne-Aid Gel[2]
AcnoAcnomel Cake[2]
Acnomel Cream[2]
Acnomel Vanishing Cream[2]
Acnomel-Acne Cream[2]
Acnotex[4]
Adult Acne Clearing Gel[3]
Antinea[3]
Aveeno Acne Bar[4]
Aveeno Cleansing Bar[4]
Bensulfoid Cream[2]
Buf-Puf Acne Cleansing Bar with Vitamin E[3]
Buf-Puf Medicated Maximum Strength Pads[3]
Buf-Puf Medicated Regular Strength Pads[3]
Calicylic[3]
Cleanse and Treat[4]
Clear Away[3]
Clear by Design Medicated Cleansing Pads[3]
Clearasil Adult Care Medicated Blemish Cream[2]
Clearasil Adult Care Medicated Blemish Stick[2]
Clearasil Clearstick Maximum Strength Topical Solution[3]
Clearasil Clearstick Regular Strength Topical Solution[3]
Clearasil Double Textured Pads Maximum Strength[3]
Clearasil Double Textured Pads Regular Strength[3]
Clearasil Medicated Deep Cleanser Topical Solution[3]
Compound W Gel[3]
Compound W Liquid[3]
Creamy SS Shampoo[4]
Cuplex Gel[3]
Cuticura Ointment[5]
Diasporal Cream[4]
Duofilm[3]
Duoplant[3]
Duoplant Topical Solution[3]
Finac[5]
Fostex CM[4]
Fostex Medicated Cleansing Bar[4]
Fostex Medicated Cleansing Cream[4]
Fostex Medicated Cleansing Liquid[4]
Fostex Regular Strength Medicated Cleansing Bar[4]
Fostex Regular Strength Medicated Cleansing Cream[4]
Fostex Regular Strength Medicated Cover-Up[4]
Fostril Cream[5]
Fostril Lotion[5]
Freezone[3]
Gordofilm[3]
Hydrisalic[3]
Inova 8/2 ACT[3]
Ionax Astringent Skin Cleanser Topical Solution[3]
Ionil Plus Shampoo[3]
Ionil Shampoo[3]
Keralyt[3]
Keratex Gel[3]
Lactisol[3]
Listerex Golden Scrub Lotion[3]
Listerex Herbal Scrub Lotion[3]
Lotio Asulfa[3]
Mediplast[3]
Meted Maximum Strength Anti-Dandruff Shampoo with Conditioners[4]
Night Cast R[4]
Night Cast Regular Formula Mask-Lotion[4]
Night Cast Special Formula Mask-Lotion[2]
Noxzema Anti-Acne Gel[3]
Noxzema Anti-Acne Pads Maximum Strength[3]
Noxzema Anti-Acne Pads Regular Strength[3]
Occlusal Topical Solution[3]
Occlusal-HP Topical Solution[3]
Off-Ezy Topical Solution Corn & Callus Removal Kit[3]
Off-Ezy Topical Solution Wart Removal Kit[3]
Oxy Clean Medicated Cleanser[3]

Oxy Clean Medicated Pads Maximum Strength[3]
Oxy Clean Medicated Pads Sensitive Skin[3]
Oxy Clean Regular Strength[3]
Oxy Clean Regular Strength Medicated Cleanser Topical Solution[3]
Oxy Clean Regular Strength Medicated Pads[3]
Oxy Clean Sensitive Skin Cleanser Topical Solution[3]
Oxy Clean Sensitive Skin Pads[3]
Oxy Night Watch Maximum Strength Lotion[3]
Oxy Night Watch Night Time Acne Medication Extra Strength Lotion[3]
Oxy Night Watch Night Time Acne Medication Regular Strength Lotion[3]
Oxy Night Watch Sensitive Skin Lotion[3]
Oxy Sensitive Skin Vanishing Formula Lotion[3]
P&S[3]
Paplex[3]
Paplex Ultra[3]
Pernox Lemon Medicated Scrub Cleanser[4]
Pernox Lotion Lathering Abradant Scrub Cleanser[4]
Pernox Lotion Lathering Scrub Cleanser[4]
Pernox Regular Medicated Scrub Cleanser[4]
Propa pH Medicated Acne Cream Maximum Strength[3]
Propa pH Medicated Cleansing Pads Maximum Strength[3]
Propa pH Medicated Cleansing Pads Sensitive Skin[3]
Propa pH Perfectly Clear Skin Cleanser Topical Solution Oily Skin[3]
Propa pH Perfectly Clear Skin Cleanser Topical Solution Sensitive Skin Formula[3]
R.A.[1]
Rezamid Lotion[2]
Salac[3]
Salacid[3]
Sal-Acid Plaster[3]
Salactic Film Topical Solution[3]
Sal-Clens Plus Shampoo[3]
Sal-Clens Shampoo[3]
Salex Shampoo[3]
Saligel[3]
Salonil[3]
Sal-Plant Gel Topical Solution[3]
Sastid (AL) Scrub[4]
Sastid Plain[4]
Sastid Plain Shampoo and Acne Wash[4]
Sastid Soap[4]
Sebasorb Liquid[4]
Sebex[4]
Sebucare[3]
Sebulex Antiseborrheic Treatment and Conditioning Shampoo[4]
Sebulex Antiseborrheic Treatment Shampoo[4]
Sebulex Conditioning Shampoo[4]
Sebulex Cream Medicated Shampoo[4]
Sebulex Medicated Dandruff Shampoo with Conditioners[4]
Sebulex Medicated Shampoo[4]
Sebulex Regular Medicated Dandruff Shampoo[4]
Sebulex Shampoo[4]
Stri-Dex[3]
Stri-Dex Dual Textured Pads Maximum Strength[3]
Stri-Dex Dual Textured Pads Regular Strength[3]
Stri-Dex Dual Textured Pads Sensitive Skin[3]
Stri-Dex Maximum Strength Pads[3]
Stri-Dex Regular Strength Pads[3]
Stri-Dex Super Scrub Pads[3]
Sulforcin[2]
Sulsal Soap[4]
Tersac Cleansing Gel[3]
Therac Lotion[4]
Trans-Plantar[3]
Trans-Ver-Sal[3]
Vanseb Cream Dandruff Shampoo[4]
Vanseb Lotion Dandruff Shampoo[4]
Verukan Topical Solution[3]
Verukan-HP Topical Solution[3]
Viranol[3]
Viranol Ultra[3]
Wart-Off Topical Solution[3]
X-Seb[3]

LAXATIVES, BULK-FORMING

GENERIC NAMES

1. CALCIUM POLYCARBOPHIL
2. CARBOXYMETHYLCELLUOSE SODIUM
3. MALT SOUP EXTRACT
4. METHYLCELLULOSE
5. POLYCARBOPHIL
6. PSYLLIUM

BRAND NAMES

Cillium[6]
Citrucel Orange Flavor[4]
Citrucel Sugar-Free Orange Flavor[4]
Cologel[4]
Disolan Forte[2]
Disoplex[2]
Effer-syllium[6]
Equalactin[5]
Fiberall[5]
Fibercon[5]
FiberNorm[5]
Fiberpur[6]
Hydrocil Instant[6]
Karacil[6]
Konsyl[5]
Konsyl Easy Mix Formula[6]
Konsyl-D[6]
Konsyl-Orange[6]
Maalox Daily Fiber Therapy[6]
Maalox Daily Fiber Therapy Citrus Flavor[6]
Maalox Daily Fiber Therapy Orange Flavor[6]
Maalox Sugar Free Citrus Flavor[6]
Maalox Sugar Free Orange Flavor[6]
Maltsupex[3]
Metamucil[6]
Metamucil Apple Crisp Fiber Wafers[6]
Metamucil Cinnamon Spice Fiber Wafers[6]
Metamucil Instant Mix, Orange Flavor[6]
Metamucil Smooth Citrus Flavor[6]
Metamucil Smooth Orange Flavor[6]
Metamucil Smooth, Sugar-Free Citrus Flavor[6]
Metamucil Smooth, Sugar-Free Orange Flavor[6]
Metamucil Smooth, Sugar-Free Regular Flavor[6]
Metamucil Sugar Free[6]
Metamucil Sugar Free Citrus Flavor[6]
Metamucil Sugar Free Lemon-Lime Flavor[6]
Metamucil Sugar Free Orange Flavor[6]
Mitrolan[5]
Modane Bulk[6]
Mylanta Natural Fiber Supplement[6]
Mylanta Sugar Free Natural Fiber Supplement[6]
Naturacil[6]
Natural Source Fibre Laxative[6]
Perdiem[6]
Perdiem Fiber[6]
Perdiem Plain[6]
Prodiem[6]
Prodiem Plain[6]
Prodiem Plus[6]
Pro-Lax[6]
Prompt[6]
Reguloid Natural[6]

Reguloid Orange[6]
Reguloid Orange Sugar Free[6]
SennaPrompt[6]
Serutan[6]
Serutan Toasted Granules[6]
Siblin[6]
Syllact[6]
Syllamalt[3]
Versabran[6]
Vitalax Super Smooth Sugar Free Orange Flavor[6]
Vitalax Unflavored[6]
V-Lax[6]

LAXATIVES, OSMOTIC

GENERIC NAMES

1. GLYCERIN
2. LACTULOSE
3. MAGNESIUM CITRATE
4. MAGNESIUM HYDROXIDE
5. MAGNESIUM OXIDE
6. MAGNESIUM SULFATE
7. MILK OF MAGNESIA
8. MINERAL OIL
9. POLYETHYLENE GLYCOL 3350
10. SODIUM PHOSPHATE

BRAND NAMES

Agarol Plain[7]
Agarol Strawberry[8]
Agarol Vanilla[8]
Bilagog[6]
Cholac[2]
Chronula[2]
Citroma[3]
Citro-Mag[3]
Citro-Nesia[3]
Constilac[2]
Constulose[2]
Duphalac[2]
Evalose[2]
Fleet Pedia Lax Liquid Gels[1]
Fleet Phospho-Soda[10]
Generlac[2]
Hayley's M-O[7]
HealthyLax[9]
Heptalac[2]
Kristalose[2]
Lactulax[2]
Magnolax[7]
Mag-Ox 400[5]
Maox[5]
Miralax[9]
Phillips' Chewable[4]
Phillips' Concentrated[4]
Phillips' Magnesia Tablets[4]
Phillips' Milk of Magnesia[4]
Portalac[2]

LAXATIVES, SOFTENER/LUBRICANT

GENERIC NAMES

1. CASANTHRANOL & DOCUSATE
2. DOCUSATE
3. DOCUSATE CALCIUM
4. DOCUSATE POTASSIUM
5. DOCUSATE SODIUM
6. MINERAL OIL
7. POLOXAMER 188

BRAND NAMES

Afko-Lube[2]
Afko-Lube Lax[2]
Agarol Plain[6]
Agarol Marshmallow[6]
Agarol Raspberry[6]
Agarol Strawberry[6]
Agarol Vanilla[6]
Alaxin[7]
Bilax[2]
Colace[5]
Colace Microenema[5]
Correctol Extra Gentle[2]
Dialose[2]
Diocto[2]
Diocto-C[1]
Diocto-K[2]
Diocto-K Plus[1]
Dioeze[2]
Diosuccin[2]
Dio-Sul[2]
Diothron[1]
Disanthrol[1]
Disolan[2]
Disolan Forte[1]
Disonate[2]
Disoplex[2]
Di-Sosul[2]
Di-Sosul Forte[1]
Docu-K Plus[1]
DOK[2]
DOK Softgels[2]
Doss[2]
Doss Tablets[2]
Doxinate[2]
DSMC Plus[1]
Dulcodos[2]
Duosol[2]
Fleet Enema Mineral Oil[7]
Fleet Pedia-Lax Childrens Liquid Stool Softener[5]
Gentlax-S[2]
Kasof[2]
Kondremul[7]
Kondremul with Cascara[7]
Kondremul Plain[7]
Lansoyl[7]
Laxinate 100[2]
Liqui-Doss[7]
Milkinol[7]
Modane Plus[2]
Modane Soft[2]
Molatoc[2]
Molatoc-CST[2]
Neo-Cultol[7]
Neolax[2]
Nujol[7]
Peri-Colase[1]
Pertrogalar Plain[7]
PMS-Docusate Calcium[2]
PMS-Docusate Sodium[2]
Pro-Cal-Sof[2]
Pro-Sof[1]
Pro-Sof Liquid Concentrate[1]
Pro-Sof Plus[1]
Regulace[2]
Regulax SS[2]
Regulex[2]
Regulex-D[2]
Regutol[2]
Senokot-S[2]
Stulex[2]
Sulfolax[2]
Surfak[2]
Therevac Plus[2]
Therevac-SB[2]
Trilax[2]
Zymenol[7]

LAXATIVES, STIMULANT

GENERIC NAMES

1. ALOE
2. BISACODYL
3. CASANTHRANOL
4. CASCARA
5. CASTOR OIL
6. DEHYDROCHOLIC ACID
7. SENNA
8. SENNOSIDES

BRAND NAMES

Afko-Lube Lax[3]
Alphamul[5]
Aromatic Cascara Fluidextract[4]
Bilax[6]
Bisac-Evac[2]
Bisacolax[2]
Bisco-Lax[2]
Black Draught[3]
Black-Draught Lax-Senna[7]
Caroid Laxative[2]
Carter's Little Pills[4]
Cascara Aromatic Fluidextract[4]
Cascara Sagrada[4]
Cholan-HMB[6]
Dacodyl[2]
Decholin[6]
Deficol[2]
Diocto-C[3]
Diocto-K Plus[1]
Diothron[3]
Disanthrol[3]
Disolan Forte[3]
Di-Sosul Forte[3]

Docu-K Plus[3]
Dosaflex[7]
Dr. Caldwell Senna Laxative[7]
DSMC Plus[3]
Dulcodos[2]
Dulcolax[2]
Dulcolax for Women[2]
Emulsoil[5]
Ex-Lax Gentle Nature[8]
Fleet Bisacodyl[2]
Fleet Bisacodyl Prep[2]
Fleet Flavored Castor Oil[5]
Fleet Laxative[2]
Fleet Pedia Lax Liquid Gels[8]
Fletcher's Castoria[7]
Gentlax S[7]
Gentle Nature[8]
Glysennid[8]
Hepahydrin[6]
Herbal Laxative[8]
Kellogg's Castor Oil[5]
Kondremul with Cascara[4]
Laxit[2]
Molatoc-CST[3]
Mucinum Herbal[8]
Nature's Remedy[4]
Neolax[6]
Neoloid[5]
Nytilax[8]
Perdiem[7]
Peri-Colace[3]
PMS-Bisacodyl[2]
PMS-Sennosides[8]
Prodiem Plus[7]
Prompt[8]
Pro-Sof Plus[3]
Purge[5]
Regulace[3]
Senexon[7]
SennaPrompt[8]
Senokot[7]
Senokot-S[7]
SenokotXTRA[7]
Senolax[7]
Theralax[2]
Trilax[6]
X-Prep Liquid[7]

MEPROBAMATE

Acabamate
Apo-Meprobamate
Epromate-M
Equagesic
Equanil
Equanil Wyseals
Equazine-M
Heptogesic
Medi-Tran
Meprogesic
Meprogesic Q
Meprospan 200
Meprospan 400
Micrainin
Miltown
Neuramate
Novo-Mepro
Pax 400
Probate
Sedabamate
Trancot
Tranmep

METFORMIN

ACTOplus Met
ACTOplus Met XR
Avandamet
Fortamet
Glucophage
Glucophage XR
Glucovance
Glumetza
Janumet
Kazano
Kombiglyze XR
Metaglip
Pazamet
PrandiMet
Riomet

NARCOTIC ANALGESICS

GENERIC NAMES

1. BUPRENORPHINE
2. CODEINE
3. CODEINE & TERPIN HYDRATE
4. DIHYDROCODEINE
5. FENTANYL
6. HYDROCODONE
7. HYDROCODONE & HOMATROPINE
8. HYDROMORPHONE
9. LEVORPHANOL
10. MEPERIDINE
11. METHADONE
12. MORPHINE
13. NALBUPHINE
14. OPIUM
15. OXYCODONE
16. OXYMORPHONE
17. PENTAZOCINE
18. PROPOXYPHENE

BRAND NAMES

642[18]
Abstral[5]
Actagen-C Cough[2]
Actifed with Codeine Cough[2]
Actiq[5]
Adatuss D.C. Expectorant[6]
Allerfrin with Codeine[2]
Ambay Cough[2]
Ambenyl Cough[2]
Ambophen Expectorant[2]
Anamine HD[6]
Anaplex HD[6]
Aprodrine with Codeine[2]
Astramorph[12]
Astramorph-PF[12]
Avinza[12]
Bayhistine DH[2]
Bayhistine Expectorant[2]
Baytussin AC[2]
Benylin Cold & Flu With Codeine Narcotic[2]
Bromanyl[2]
Brontex[2]
Buprenex[1]
Butrans[1]
Calcidrine[2]
Calmylin with Codeine[2]
Cheracol[2]
Chlorgest-HD[6]
CoActifed[2]
CoActifed Expectorant[2]
Codan[7]
Codehist DH[2]
Codeine Sulfate[2]
Codeprex[2]
Codiclear DH[6]
Codimal DH[6]
Codimal PH[2]
Colrex Compound[2]
Combunox[15]
Coristex-DH[6]
Coristine-DH[6]
Cotanal-65[18]
Cotridin[2]
C-Tussin Expectorant[2]
Decohistine DH[2]
Demerol[10]
Deproist Expectorant with Codeine[2]
De-Tuss[6]
Detussin Expectorant[6]
Detussin Liquid[6]
Dihistine DH[2]
Dihistine Expectorant[2]
Dihydromorphinone[8]
Dilaudid[8]
Dilaudid Cough[8]
Dilaudid-HP[8]
Dolophine[11]
Donatussin DC[6]
Doxaphene[18]
Duragesic[5]
Duragesic mc/hr[5]
Duramorph[12]
Duratuss HD[6]
Embeda[12]
Endagen-HD[6]
Endal-HD[6]
Endal-HD Plus[6]
Entuss Expectorant[6]
Entuss-D[6]
Epimorph[12]
Exalgo[8]
Fentora[5]
Fortral[17]
Glydeine Cough[2]
Guiatuss A.C.[2]

Guiatussin DAC[2]
Guiatussin with Codeine Liquid[2]
Histafed C[2]
Histussin HC[6]
Hycodan[6]
Hycomine Compound[6]
Hycomine-S Pediatric[6]
Hycotuss Expectorant[6]
Hydromet[7]
Hydropane[7]
Hydrostat IR[8]
Ibudone[6]
Isoclor Expectorant[2]
Kadian[12]
Kwelcof Liquid[6]
Laudanum[14]
Lazanda[5]
Levo-Dromoran[9]
Levorphan[9]
Mallergan-VC with Codeine[2]
Methadose[11]
Midahist DH[2]
Morphitec[12]
M.O.S.[12]
M.O.S.-SR[12]
MS Contin[12]
MSIR[12]
MST Continus[12]
Mytussin AC[2]
Mytussin DAC[2]
Nortussin with Codeine[2]
Novagest Expectorant with Codeine[2]
Novahistex C[2]
Novahistex DH[6]
Novahistex DH Expectorant[6]
Novahistine DH Expectorant[6]
Novahistine DH Liquid[2]
Novahistine Expectorant[2]
Nubain[13]
Nucochem[2]
Nucochem Expectorant[2]
Nucochem Pediatric Expectorant[2]
Nucofed[2]
Nucofed Expectorant[2]
Nucofed Pediatric Expectorant[2]
Numorphan[16]
Opana[16]
Opana ER[16]
Oramorph[12]
Oramorph-SR[12]
Oxecta[15]
Oxycontin SR[15]
Pantapon[14]
Paveral[2]
Pediacof Cough[2]
Penazine VC with Cough[2]
Phenameth VC with Codeine[2]
Phenergan VC with Codeine[2]
Phenergan with Codeine[2]
Phenhist DH with Codeine[2]
Phenhist Expectorant[2]
Pherazine VC with Codeine[2]
Pherazine with Codeine[2]
Physeptone[11]
Promehist with Codeine[2]
Prometh VC with Codeine[2]
Propoxycon[18]
Prunicodeine[2]
Pseudodine C Cough[2]
P-V-Tussin[6]
Reprexain[6]
Rezira[6]
RMS Uniserts[12]
Robafen AC Cough[2]
Robafen DAC[2]
Robidone[6]
Robitussin A-C[2]
Robitussin-DAC[2]
Rolatuss Expectorant[2]
Rolatuss with Hydrocodone[6]
Roxanol[12]
Roxanol SR[12]
Roxicodone[15]
Ryna-C Liquid[2]
Ryna-CX Liquid[2]
Soma Compound[2]
SRC Expectorant[6]
Statex[12]
Statuss Expectorant[2]
Subsys[5]
Supeudol[15]
Talwin[17]
Talwin-NX[17]
Temgesic[1]
Tolu-Sed Cough[2]
Triacin C Cough[2]
Triafed with Codeine[2]
Tricodene #1[2]
Trifed-C Cough[2]
Tussafed HCG Syrup[6]
Tussafin Expectorant[6]
Tussar SF[2]
Tussar-2[2]
TussiCaps[6]
Tussigon[7]
Tussionex[6]
Tussirex with Codeine Liquid[2]
Tyrodone[6]
Vanex Expectorant[6]
Vanex-HD[6]
Vicodin-Tuss[6]
Vicoprofen[8]
Vituz[6]
Zutripro[6]

NARCOTIC ANALGESICS & ACETAMINOPHEN

GENERIC NAMES

1. ACETAMINOPHEN & CODEINE
2. DIHYDROCODEINE & ACETAMINOPHEN
3. HYDROCODONE & ACETAMINOPHEN
4. MEPERIDINE & ACETAMINOPHEN
5. OXYCODONE & ACETAMINOPHEN
6. PENTAZOCINE & ACETAMINOPHEN
7. PROPOXYPHENE & ACETAMINOPHEN

BRAND NAMES

Allay[3]
Anexsia[3]
Anolor-DH5[3]
APAP with Codeine[1]
Atasol-8[1]
Atasol-15[1]
Atasol-30[1]
Balacet 325[7]
Bancap-HC[3]
Capital with Codeine[1]
Co-Gesic[3]
Compal[3]
Demerol-APAP[4]
DHCplus[2]
Dolacet[3]
Dolagesic[3]
Dolene-AP 65[7]
Duocet[3]
E-Lor[7]
Empracet 30[1]
Empracet 60[1]
Emtec[1]
Endocet[5]
Exdol-8[1]
Exdol-15[1]
Exdol-30[1]
EZ III[1]
Hycomed[3]
Hyco-Pap[3]
Hydrocet[2]
Hydrocodone with APAP[3]
Hydrogesic[3]
HY-PHEN[3]
Lenoltec with Codeine No. 1[1]
Lenoltec with Codeine No. 2[1]
Lenoltec with Codeine No. 3[1]
Lenoltec with Codeine No. 4[1]
Lorcet[3]
Lorcet 10/650[3]
Lorcet Plus[3]
Lorcet-HD[3]
Lortab[3]
Lortab 5[3]
Lortab 7[3]
Magnacet[5]
Margesic #3[1]
Margesic-H[3]
Maxidone[3]
Norco[3]
Novogesic[1]
Onset[3]
Oxycocet[5]

Panacet 5/500[3]
Panlor[3]
Percocet[5]
Percocet-Demi[5]
Phenaphen with Codeine[1]
Polygesic[3]
Pro Pox with APAP[7]
Propacet 100[7]
Pyregesic-C[1]
Roxicet[5]
Roxilox[5]
Stagesic[3]
Talacen[6]
T-gesic[3]
Tylaprin with Codeine[1]
Tylenol No.1[1]
Tylenol No.1 Forte[1]
Tylenol with Codeine[1]
Tylenol with Codeine No. 1[1]
Tylenol with Codeine No. 2[1]
Tylenol with Codeine No. 3[1]
Tylenol with Codeine No. 4[1]
Tylox[5]
Ugesic[3]
Ultragesic[3]
Vanacet[3]
Vapocet[3]
Veganin[1]
Vendone[3]
Vicodin[3]
Vicodin ES[3]
Wygesic[7]
Xodol[3]
Zydone[3]

NARCOTIC ANALGESICS & ASPIRIN

GENERIC NAMES

1. ASPIRIN & CODEINE
2. BUFFERED ASPIRIN & CODEINE
3. DIHYDROCODEINE & ASPIRIN
4. HYDROCODONE & ASPIRIN
5. OXYCODONE & ASPIRIN
6. PENTAZOCINE & ASPIRIN
7. PROPOXYPHENE & ASPIRIN

BRAND NAMES

222[1]
282[1]
292[1]
293[1]
692[7]
A.C.&C.[1]
Anacin with Codeine[1]
Azdone[1]
Cotanal 65[7]
Damason-P[4]
Drocade and Aspirin[3]
Emcodeine No. 2[1]
Emcodeine No. 3[1]
Emcodeine No. 4[1]
Empirin with Codeine[1]
Empirin with Codeine No. 3[1]
Empirin with Codeine No. 4[1]
Endodan[5]
Lortab ASA[4]
Novo-AC and C[1]
Oxycodan[5]
Panasal 5/500[4]
PC-Cap[7]
Percodan[5]
Percodan-Demi[5]
Propoxyphene Compound-65[7]
Roxiprin[5]
Synalgos-DC[3]
Talwin Compound[6]
Talwin Compound-50[6]

NITRATES

GENERIC NAMES

1. ERYTHRITYL TETRANITRATE
2. ISOSORBIDE DINITRATE
3. ISOSORBIDE MONONITRATE
4. NITROGLYCERIN (GLYCERYL TRINITRATE)
5. PENTAERYTHRITOL TETRANITRATE

BRAND NAMES

Apo-ISDN[2]
BiDil[2]
Cardilate[1]
Cedocard-SR[2]
Coradur[2]
Coronex[2]
Deponit[4]
Dilatrate-SR[2]
Duotrate[5]
Glyceryl Trinitrate[4]
IMDUR[3]
ISMO[3]
Iso-Bid[2]
Isonate[2]
Isorbid[2]
Isordil[2]
Isotrate[2]
Klavikordal[4]
Minitran[4]
Monoket[3]
Niong[4]
Nitro-Bid[4]
Nitrocap[4]
Nitrocap T.D.[4]
Nitrocine[4]
Nitrodisc[4]
Nitro-Dur[4]
Nitro-Dur II[4]
Nitrogard-SR[4]
Nitroglyn[4]
Nitrol[4]
Nitrolin[4]
Nitrolingual[4]
NitroMist[4]
Nitronet[4]
Nitrong[4]
Nitrong SR[4]
Nitrospan[4]
Nitrostat[4]
Novosorbide[2]
NTS[4]
Pentritol[5]
Pentylan[5]
Peritrate[5]
Peritrate Forte[5]
Peritrate SA[5]
P.E.T.N.[5]
Rectiv[4]
Sorbitrate[2]
Sorbitrate SA[2]
Transderm-Nitro[4]
Tridil[4]

OXYMETAZOLINE (Nasal)

4-Way Long Acting Nasal Spray
12-Hour Nostrilla Nasal Decongestant
Afrin 12 Hour Nasal Spray
Afrin 12 Hour Nose Drops
Afrin Cherry Scented Nasal Spray
Afrin Children's Strength 12 Hour Nose Drops
Afrin Children's Strength Nose Drops
Afrin Extra Moisturizing Nasal Decongestant Spray
Afrin Menthol Nasal Spray
Afrin Nasal Spray
Afrin No-Drip Extra Moisturizing
Afrin No-Drip Nasal Decongestant, Severe Congestion with Menthol
Afrin No-Drip Nasal Decongestant Sinus with Vapornase
Afrin No-Drip Sinus
Afrin Nose Drops
Afrin Sinus
Afrin Spray Pump
Allerest 12 Hour Nasal Spray
Cheracol Nasal Spray
Cheracol Nasal Spray Pump Cherry Scented
Coricidin Nasal Mist
Dristan 12-Hour Nasal Spray
Dristan Long Lasting Menthol Nasal Spray
Dristan Long Lasting Nasal Pump Spray
Dristan Long Lasting Nasal Spray
Dristan Long Lasting Nasal Spray 12 Hour Metered Dose Pump
Dristan Mentholated
Drixoral
Duramist Plus Up To 12 Hours Decongestant Nasal Spray
Duration 12 Hour Nasal Spray Pump

Mucinex Full Force Nasal Spray
Mucinex Moisture Smart Nasal Spray
Nasal Decongestant Spray
Nasal Relief
Nasal Spray 12-Hour
Nasal Spray Long Acting
Nasal-12 Hour
Neo-Synephrine 12 Hour Nasal Spray
Neo-Synephrine 12 Hour Nasal Spray Pump
Neo-Synephrine 12 Hour Nose Drops
Neo-Synephrine 12 Hour Vapor Nasal Spray
Nostril Nasal Decongestant Mild
Nostril Nasal Decongestant Regular
NTZ Long Acting Decongestant Nasal Spray
NTZ Long Acting Decongestant Nose Drops
Sinarest 12 Hour Nasal Spray
Vicks Sinex 12-Hour Nasal Spray
Vicks Sinex 12-Hour Ultra Fine Mist
Vicks Sinex Long-Acting 12 Hour Nasal Spray

PENICILLINS

GENERIC NAMES

1. AMOXICILLIN
2. AMPICILLIN
3. BACAMPICILLIN
4. CARBENICILLIN
5. CLOXACILLIN
6. DICLOXACILLIN
7. FLUCLOXACILLIN
8. NAFCILLIN
9. OXACILLIN
10. PENICILLIN G
11. PENICILLIN V
12. PIVAMPICILLIN
13. PIVMECILLINAM

BRAND NAMES

Amoxil[1]
Apo-Amoxi[1]
Apo-Ampi[2]
Apo-Cloxi[5]
Apo-Pen VK[11]
Bactocill[9]
Beepen-VK[11]
Betapen-VK[11]
Cloxapen[5]
DisperMax[1]
Dycill[6]
Dynapen[6]
Fluclox[7]
Geopen Oral[4]
Ledercillin-VK[11]
Megacillin[10]
Moxatag[1]
Nadopen-V[11]
Nadopen-V 200[11]
Nadopen-V 400[11]
Novamoxin[1]
Novo-Ampicillin[2]
Novo-Cloxin[5]
Novo-Pen VK[11]
Nu-Amoxi[11]
Nu-Ampi[2]
Nu-Cloxi[5]
Nu-Pen-VK[11]
Omnipen[2]
Omeclamox-Pak[1]
Orbenin[5]
Pathocil[6]
Pen Vee[11]
Pen Vee K[11]
Penbritin[2]
Penglobe[3]
Pentids[10]
Polycillin[2]
Pondocillin[12]
Principen[2]
Prostaphlin[9]
PVF[11]
PVF K[11]
Selexid[13]
Spectrobid[3]
Tegopen[5]
Totacillin[2]
Trimox[1]
Unipen[8]
V-Cillin K[11]
Veetids[11]
Wymox[1]

PHENOTHIAZINES

GENERIC NAMES

1. ACETOPHENAZINE
2. CHLORPROMAZINE
3. FLUPHENAZINE
4. MESORIDAZINE
5. METHOTRIMEPRAZINE
6. PERICYAZINE
7. PERPHENAZINE
8. PIPOTIAZINE
9. PROCHLORPERAZINE
10. PROMAZINE
11. THIOPROPAZATE
12. THIOPROPERAZINE
13. THIORIDAZINE
14. TRIFLUOPERAZINE
15. TRIFLUPROMAZINE

BRAND NAMES

Apo-Fluphenazine[3]
Apo-Perphenazine[7]
Apo-Thioridazine[13]
Apo-Trifluoperazine[14]
Chlorpromanyl-5[2]
Chlorpromanyl-20[2]
Chlorpromanyl-40[2]
Compazine[9]
Compazine Spansule[9]
Dartal[11]
Duo-Medihaler
Etrafon[7]
Etrafon-A[7]
Etrafon-D[7]
Etrafon-F[7]
Etrafon-Forte[7]
Largactil[2]
Largactil Liquid[2]
Largactil Oral Drops[2]
Levoprome[5]
Majeptil[12]
Mellaril[13]
Mellaril Concentrate[13]
Mellaril-S[13]
Modecate[3]
Modecate Concentrate[3]
Moditen Enanthate[3]
Moditen HCl[3]
Moditen HCl-H.P.[3]
Neuleptil[6]
Novo-Chlorpromazine[2]
Novo-Flurazine[14]
Novo-Ridazine[13]
Nozinan[5]
Nozinan Liquid[5]
Nozinan Oral Drops[5]
Permitil[3]
Permitil Concentrate[3]
Piportil L_4[8]
PMS Levazine[7]
PMS Thioridazine[13]
Prolixin[3]
Prolixin Concentrate[3]
Prolixin Decanoate[3]
Prolixin Enanthate[3]
Prorazin[9]
Prozine [10]
Serentil[4]
Serentil Concentrate[4]
Stemetil Liquid[9]
Suprazine[14]
Terfluzine[14]
Terfluzine Concentrate[14]
Thorazine[2]
Thorazine Concentrate[2]
Thorazine Spansule[2]
Thor-Prom[2]
Tindal[2]
Triavil[7]
Trilafon[7]
Trilafon Concentrate[7]
Ultrazine-10[9]
Vesprin[5]

PHENYLEPHRINE

Aclophen
Advil Congestion Relief
Advanced Formula Dristan Caplets
AH-Chew

Alersule
Alka-Seltzer Plus Cold & Sinus Effervescent
Alka-Seltzer Plus Night-Time Effervescent
Alka-Seltzer Plus Original Effervescent
AlleRx Dose Pack PE
AlleRx Suspension
Anamine HD
Atrohist Pediatric
Atrohist Pediatric Suspension Dye Free
Atrohist Sprinkle
Benylin All-In-One Cold & Flu Night Caplets
Benylin Cold & Sinus
Benylin Cold & Sinus Plus
Cerose-DM
Chlorgest-HD
Codimal DH
Codimal DM
Codimal PH
Colrex Compound
Colrex Cough
Coltab Children's
Comhist
Comhist LA
Conar
Conar Expectorant
Conar-A
Congespirin for Children Cold Tablets
Coristex-DH
Coristine-DH
D.A. Chewable
Dallergy
Dihistine
Doktors
Donatussin
Donatussin DC
Donatussin Drops
Dondril
Dristan Cold Multi-Symptom Formula
Dristan Formula P
Dristan-AF
Dristan-AF Plus
Dura-Vent/DA
Ed A-Hist
Endagen-HD
Endal-HD
Endal-HD Plus
Extendryl
Extendryl JR
Extendryl SR
Father John's Medicine Plus
Gendecon
Histagesic Modified
Histatab Plus
Histatan
Histor-D
Histor-D Timecelles
Hycomine Compound
LiquiBid D
LiquiBid D-R
LiquiBid PD
Mallergan-VC with Codeine
Meda Syrup Forte
Mucinex Adult Caplets - Cold & Sinus
Mucinex Adult Caplets - Cold, Flu, & Sore Throat
Mucinex Adult Caplets - Severe Congestion & Cold
Mucinex Cold Liquid
Mucinex Fast-Max Cold, Flu & Sore Throat Liquid
Mucinex Maximum Strength Fast Max Cold, Flu & Sore Throat
Mucinex Maximum Strength Fast Max Severe Congestion & Cough
ND-Gesic
Neocitran A
Neocitran Colds & Flu Calorie Reduced
NeoCitran DM Coughs & Colds
NeoCitran Extra Strength Colds & Flu
NeoCitran Extra Strength Sinus
Neo-Synephrine Nasal Drops
Neo-Synephrine Pediatric Nasal Drops
Nostril Spray Pump
OMNIhist L.A.
PediaCare Children's Allergy
PediaCare Children's Decongestant
PediaCare Children's Fever Reducer Plus Flu
PediaCare Children's Multi-Symptom Cold
PediaCare Fever Reducer Plus Multi-Symptom Cold
Pediacof Cough
Phenameth VC
Phenameth VC with Codeine
Pherazine VC
Pherazine VC with Codeine
Prehist
Prehist D
Prometh VC Plain
Prometh VC with Codeine
Promethazine VC
Refenesen Chest Congestion & Pain Relief PE
Refenesen PE
Rhinall
Rhinall Children's Flavored Nose Drops
Rhinatate
Robitussin Cough & Cold CF
Robitussin Cough & Cold Nighttime
Robitussin Cough Cold & Flu Nighttime
Rolatuss Expectorant
Rolatuss Plain
R-Tannamine
R-Tannamine Pediatric
R-Tannate
R-Tannate Pediatric
Rynatan
Rynatan Pediatric
Rynatan-S Pediatric
Rynatuss
Rynatuss Pediatric
Scot-Tussin
Scot-Tussin Original 5-Action Cold Medicine
Sinupan
SINUvent PE
Statuss Expectorant
Sudafed PE Cold & Cough Caplets
Tanoral
Theracof Plus Multi-Symptom Cough and Cold Reliever
TheraFlu Cold & Cough Hot Liquid
Theraflu Daytime Severe Cold Caplets
Theraflu Daytime Severe Cold Hot Liquid
Theraflu Flu & Sore Throat Hot Liquid
Theraflu Nighttime Severe Cold Caplets
Theraflu Nighttime Severe Cold Hot Liquid
Theraflu Thin Strips Daytime Cold & Cough
Theraflu Thin Strips Nighttime Severe Cold & Cough
Theraflu Warming Relief Daytime
Theraflu Warming Relief Nighttime
Triaminic Chest & Nasal Congestion
Triaminic Cold & Allergy
Triaminic Day Time Cold & Cough
Triaminic Night Time Cough & Cold
Triaminic Thin Strips Cold
Triaminic Thin Strips Daytime Cold & Cough
Triaminic Thin Strips Night Time Cold & Cough
Trimedine Liquid
Triotann
Triotann Pediatric
Tritann Pediatric
Tri-Tannate
Tri-Tannate Plus Pediatric
Tussafed HCG Syrup

Tussi-12
Tussirex with Codeine Liquid
Tylenol Allergy Multi-Symptom
Tylenol Allergy Multi-Symptom Nighttime
Tylenol Cold Head Congestion Daytime
Tylenol Cold Head Congestion Nighttime
Tylenol Cold Head Congestion Severe
Tylenol Cold Multi Symptom Daytime
Tylenol Cold Multi Symptom Nighttime
Tylenol Cold Multi Symptom Severe
Tylenol Cough & Severe Congestion Daytime
Tylenol Sinus Congestion & Pain Daytime
Tylenol Sinus Congestion & Pain Nighttime
Tylenol Sinus Congestion & Pain Severe
Vanex-HD
Vicks DayQuil Cold & Flu Symptom Relief Plus Vitamin C
Vicks DayQuil Sinus LiquiCaps
Vicks Formula 44 Custom Care Congestion
Vicks NyQuil Sinus LiquiCaps
Vicks Sinex Nasal Spray
Vicks VapoSyrup Severe Congestion Head & Chest Congestion Relief
Viravan DM

POTASSIUM SUPPLEMENTS

GENERIC NAMES

1. POTASSIUM ACETATE
2. POTASSIUM BICARBONATE
3. POTASSIUM BICARBONATE & POTASSIUM CHLORIDE
4. POTASSIUM BICARBONATE & POTASSIUM CITRATE
5. POTASSIUM CHLORIDE
6. POTASSIUM GLUCONATE
7. POTASSIUM GLUCONATE & POTASSIUM CHLORIDE
8. POTASSIUM GLUCONATE & POTASSIUM CITRATE
9. POTASSIUM TRIPLEX

BRAND NAMES

Apo-K[5]
Cambia[2]
Cena-K[5]
Effer-K[4]
Gen-K[5]
Glu-K[6]
K+10[5]
K-10[5]
K-8[5]
K+Care[5]
K+Care ET[2]
Kalium Durules[5]
Kaochlor[5]
Kaochlor S-F[5]
Kaochlor-10[5]
Kaochlor-20[5]
Kaochlor-Eff[5]
Kaon[6]
Kaon-Cl[5]
Kaon-Cl 10[5]
Kaon-Cl 20[5]
Kato[5]
Kay Ciel[5]
Kay Ciel Elixir[5]
Kaylixir[6]
KCL[5]
K-Dur[5]
K-Electrolyte[2]
K-G Elixir[6]
K-Lease[5]
K-Long[5]
K-Lor[5]
Klor-Con 8[5]
Klor-Con 10[5]
Klor-Con Powder[5]
Klor-Con/25[5]
Klor-Con/EF[2]
Klorvess[3]
Klorvess 10% Liquid[5]
Klorvess Effervescent Granules[5]
Klotrix[5]
K-Lyte[2]
K-Lyte DS[4]
K-Lyte/Cl[3]
K-Lyte/Cl 50[3]
K-Lyte/CL Powder[5]
K-Med 900[5]
K-Norm[5]
Kolyum[7]
K-Sol[5]
K-Tab[5]
K-Vescent[2]
Micro-K[5]
Micro-K 10[5]
Micro-K LS[5]
Neo-K[3]
Potasalan[5]
Potassium-Rougier[6]
Potassium-Sandoz[3]
Roychlor 10%[5]
Roychlor 20%[5]
Royonate[6]
Rum-K[5]
Slow-K[5]
Ten K[5]
Tri-K[9]
Twin-K[8]

PROGESTINS

GENERIC NAMES

1. DROSPIRENONE
2. ETONOGESTREL
3. HYDROXYPROGESTERONE
4. LEVONORGESTREL
5. MEDROXYPROGESTERONE
6. MEGESTROL
7. NORETHINDRONE
8. NORGESTIMATE
9. NORGESTREL
10. PROGESTERONE

BRAND NAMES

Activella[8]
Amen[5]
Angeliq[1]
Aygestin[7]
Climara Pro[4]
CombiPatch[7]
Crinone[10]
Curretab[5]
Cycrin[5]
Depo-Provera[5]
Duralutin[3]
Endometrin[10]
Femhrt[7]
Gesterol 50[10]
Gesterol L.A.[3]
Hy/Gestrone[3]
Hylutin[3]
Hyprogest[3]
Implanon[3]
Megace[6]
Megace ES[6]
Megace Oral Suspension[6]
Micronor[7]
Next Choice[4]
Norlutate[7]
Nor-Q.D.[7]
Ortho-Prefest[8]
Ovrette[9]
Plan B One Step[4]
Plan B OTC/Rx[4]
Premphase[5]
Prempro[5]
Prodrox[3]
Prometrium[10]
Provera[5]
ProveraPak[5]

PSEUDOEPHEDRINE

Actacin
Actagen
Actagen-C Cough
Advil Cold and Sinus Caplets
Advil Cold and Sinus LiquiGels
Advil Flu & Body Ache
Advil Multi-Symptom Cold
Alavert D-12
Aleve-D Sinus & Cold
Allegra-D
Allegra-D 24 Hour

Allent
Allercon
Allerest Maximum Strength
Allerest No-Drowsiness
Allerphed
AlleRx D
All-Nite Cold Formula
Ambenyl-D Decongestant Cough Formula
Amdry-D
Anamine
Anamine T.D.
Anatuss DM
Anatuss LA
Balminil Decongestant
Benylin All-In-One Cold & Flu Caplets
Benylin All-In-One Cold & Flu Nightime Syrup
Benylin All-In-One Cold & Flu Syrup
Benylin All-In-One Day & Night Caplets
Benylin Cold And Flu With Codeine Narcotic
Benylin DM-D
Benylin DM-D-E
Benylin DM-D-E Extra Strength
Brexin-L.A.
Brofed
Bromatane DX Cough
Bromfed
Bromfed-DM
Bromfed-PD
Carbodec
Carbodec DM Drops
Carbodec TR
Cenafed
Cenafed Plus
Children's Benadryl Allergy & Cold Fastmelt
Children's Motrin Cold
Chlorphedrine SR
Chlor-Trimeton 4 Hour Relief
Chlor-Trimeton 12 Hour Relief
Clarinex D 24 Hour
Claritin-D
Claritin-D 12 Hour
Claritin-D 24 Hour
CoActifed Expectorant
Codehist DH
Codimal-L.A.
Codimal-L.A. Half
Coldrine
Colfed-A
Concentrin
Congess JR
Congess SR
Congestac Caplets
Contac Allergy/Sinus Day Caplets
Contac Allergy/Sinus Night Caplets
Contac Maximum Strength Sinus Caplets
Contac Night Caplets
Contac Non-Drowsy Formula Sinus Caplets
Contac Severe Cold Formula
Contac Severe Cold Formula Night Strength
Cophene-XP
Cotridin
CoTylenol Cold Medication
Dallergy Jr.
Decohistine DH
Deconamine
Deconamine SR
Deconsal II
Detussin Expectorant
Detussin Liquid
Dexaphen SA
Dexophed
Dihistine DH
Dihistine Expectorant
Disophrol
Disophrol Chronotabs
Dristan Cold and Flu
Dristan Cold Caplets
Dristan Cold Maximum Strength Caplets
Dristan Juice Mix-in Cold, Flu, & Cough
Dristan Sinus Caplets
Drixoral
Drixoral Cold & Allergy
Drixoral Cold & Flu
Drixoral Nasal Decongestant
Drixoral Non-Drowsy Formula
Drixoral Plus
Drixoral Sinus
Drixtab
Durahist
Duratuss
Duratuss HD
Eltor-120
Entex PSE
Entuss Pediatric Expectorant
Entuss-D
Fedahist
Fedahist Decongestant
Fedahist Expectorant
Fedahist Expectorant Pediatric Drops
Fedahist Gyrocaps
Fedahist Timecaps
Genaphed
Guaifed
Guaifed-PD
GuaiMAX-D
Guiatuss PE
Hayfebrol
Histalet
Histalet X
Histalet-DM
Hista-Vent PSE
Isoclor Timesules
Klerist-D
Kolephrin
Kolephrin/DM Caplets
Kronofed-A
Kronofed-A Jr.
Lodrane D
Lodrane LD
Maxenal
Maximum Strength Mucinex D
Maximum Strength Tylenol Allergy Sinus Caplets
Motrin-IB Cold & Sinus
Mucinex D
Mucinex DM
Myfedrine
Mytussin DAC
Nasatab LA
ND Clear T.D.
Nexafed
Novahistine DH Liquid
Novahistine DMX Liquid
Novahistine Expectorant
Nucofed
Nytcold Medicine
Ornex Maximum Strength Caplets
Ornex No Drowsiness Caplets
Ornex Severe Cold No Drowsiness Caplets
Pertussin All Night PM
Phenapap Sinus Headache & Congestion
Phenergan-D
P-V-Tussin
Rescon-JR
Respaire-30
Rezira
Rhinosyn
Rhinosyn-DM
Rhinosyn-PD
Rhinosyn-X
Robafen DAC
Robafen DM
Robitussin Cough & Cold D
Ru-Tuss DE
Ru-Tuss Expectorant
Ryna
Ryna-C Liquid
Ryna-CX Liquid
Semprex-D
Simply Stuffy
Sinus Relief
Sinutab Non-Drying Liquid Caps
Stamoist E
Sudafed 12 Hour
Sudafed Multi-Symptom Cold & Cough
Sudafed Non-Drying Sinus Liquid Caps
Sufedrin
Tavist Allergy/Sinus/Headache

Touro A&H
Touro LA Caplets
Triafed
Triafed with Codeine
Triaminic-D Multi-Symptom Cold
Tussafin Expectorant
Tussar DM
Tussar-2
Tussend
Tussend Expectorant
Tussend Liquid
Tyrodone
Versacaps
Vicks NyQuil D
Zephrex-D
Zutripro
Zyrtec-D

RAUWOLFIA ALKALOIDS

GENERIC NAMES

1. DESERPIDINE
2. RAUWOLFIA SERPENTINA
3. RESERPINE

BRAND NAMES

Demi-Regroton[3]
Diupres[3]
Diurigen with Reserpine[3]
Diutensen-R[3]
Dureticyl[3]
Enduronyl[2]
Enduronyl Forte[2]
Harmonyl[1]
Hydropres[3]
Novoreserpine[3]
Oreticyl[1]
Oreticyl Forte[1]
Raudixin[2]
Rauval[2]
Rauverid[2]
Rauzide[2]
Regroton[3]
Reserfia[3]
Serpalan[3]
Serpasil[3]
Wolfina[2]

SALICYLATES

GENERIC NAMES

1. BALSALAZIDE
2. CHOLINE MAGNESIUM SALICYLATES
3. CHOLINE SALICYLATE
4. MAGNESIUM SALICYLATE
5. SALICYLAMIDE
6. SALSALATE
7. SODIUM SALICYLATE

BRAND NAMES

Amigesic[6]
Arthropan[3]
Choline Magnesium Trisalicylate[2]
Colazal[1]
Diagen[6]
Disalcid[6]
Doan's Pills[4]
Dodd's Pills[7]
Giazo[1]
Kolephrin[5]
Magan[4]
Mobidin[4]
Mono-Gesic[6]
Presalin[5]
Rid-A-Pain Compound[5]
Salflex[6]
Salgesic[5]
Salsitab[6]
Scot-tussin Original 5-Action Cold Medicine[7]
Tricosal[2]
Trilisate[2]
Tussirex with Codeine Liquid[7]
Uracel[7]

SCOPOLAMINE (Hyoscine)

Barbidonna
Barbidonna 2
Buscopan
Kinesed
Transderm-Scop
Transderm-V

SULFONAMIDES

GENERIC NAMES

1. SULFACYTINE
2. SULFADIAZINE
3. SULFAMETHIZOLE
4. SULFAMETHOXAZOLE
5. SULFISOXAZOLE

BRAND NAMES

Apo-Sulfamethoxazole[4]
Apo-Sulfatrim[4]
Apo-Sulfatrim DS[4]
Apo-Sulfisoxazole[5]
Bactrim[4]
Bactrim DS[4]
Cotrim[4]
Cotrim DS[4]
Co-trimoxazole[4]
Gantanol[4]
Gantrisin[5]
Novo-Soxazole[5]
Novotrimel[4]
Novotrimel DS[4]
Nu-Cotrimox[4]
Nu-Cotrimox DS[4]
Pediazole[5]
Protrin[4]
Renoquid[1]
Roubac[4]
Septra[4]
Septra DS[4]
SMZ-TMP[4]
Sulfamethoprim[4]
Sulfamethoprim DS[4]
Sulfaprim[4]
Sulfaprim DS[4]
Sulfatrim[4]
Sulfatrim DS[4]
Sulfimycin[5]
Sulfizole[5]
Sulfoxaprim[4]
Sulfoxaprim DS[4]
Sulmeprim[4]
Thiosulfil Forte[3]
Triazole[4]
Triazole DS[4]
Trimeth-Sulfa[4]
Trisulfam[4]
Urobak[4]
Uroplus DS[4]
Uroplus SS[4]

SULFONYLUREAS

GENERIC NAMES

1. ACETOHEXAMIDE
2. CHLORPROPAMIDE
3. GLIMEPIRIDE
4. GLIPIZIDE
5. GLYBURIDE
6. TOLAZAMIDE
7. TOLBUTAMIDE

BRAND NAMES

Albert Glyburide[5]
Amaryl[3]
Apo-Chlorpropamide[2]
Apo-Glyburide[5]
Apo-Tolbutamide[7]
Avandaryl[3]
DiaBeta[5]
Diabinese[2]
Duetact[3]
Euglucon[5]
Gen-Glybe[5]
Glucamide[2]
Glucotrol[4]
Glucotrol XL[4]
Glucovance[5]
Glynase PresTab[6]
Metaglip[4]
Micronase[5]
Novo-Butamide[7]
Novo-Glyburide[4]
Novo-Propamide[2]
Orinase[7]
Tolamide[6]
Tolinase[6]

TETRACYCLINES

GENERIC NAMES

1. DEMECLOCYCLINE
2. DOXYCYCLINE
3. MINOCYCLINE
4. OXYTETRACYCLINE
5. TETRACYCLINE

BRAND NAMES

Achromycin[5]
Achromycin V[5]
Apo-Doxy[2]
Apo-Tetra[5]
Arestin[3]
Declomycin[1]
Doryx[2]
Doxy-Caps[2]
Doxycin[2]
Doxy-Tabs[2]
E.P. Mycin[4]
Helidac[5]
Minocin[3]
Monodox[2]
Novodoxlin[2]
Novotetra[5]
Nu-Tetra[5]
Oracea[2]
Panmycin[5]
Periostat[5]
Pylera[5]
Robitet[5]
Solodyn[3]
Sumycin[5]
Terramycin[4]
Tetracyn[5]
Tija[4]
Vibramycin[2]
Ximino[3]

Additional Drug Interactions

The following lists of drugs and their interactions with other drugs are continuations of the POSSIBLE INTERACTIONS WITH OTHER DRUGS section found in the drug charts beginning on page 2. These lists are alphabetized by the drug chart name (shown in large capital letters). Only those lists too long for a particular drug chart are included in this section. For complete information about any generic drug, see the alphabetized charts.

GENERIC NAME OR DRUG CLASS	COMBINED EFFECT

ADRENOCORTICOIDS (Systemic)

GENERIC NAME OR DRUG CLASS	COMBINED EFFECT
Antivirals HIV/AIDS*	Increased adreno-corticoid effect or decreased antiviral effect.
Bupropion	Increased risk of seizures.
Carbamazepine	Decreased adreno-corticoid effect.
Carbonic anhydrase inhibitors	Increased risk of side effects.
Contraceptives, oral*	Increased adreno-corticoid effect or decreased contraceptive effect.
Cyclosporine	May increase effect of adrenocorticoid or cyclosporine.
Digitalis preparations*	Risk of heart rhythm problems. Possible digitalis toxicity.
Diuretics	Decreased levels of potassium.
Ephedrine	Decreased adreno-corticoid effect.
Estrogens*	Increased adreno-corticoid effect.
Insulin	Decreased insulin effect.
Insulin analogs	Decreased insulin analog effect.
Isoniazid	Decreased isoniazid effect.
Mifepristone	Variable. Consult doctor or pharmacist.
Mitotane	Decreased adreno-corticoid effect.
Phenobarbital	Decreased adreno-corticoid effect.
Phenytoin	Decreased adreno-corticoid effect.
Potassium supplements*	Decreased levels of potassium.
Primidone	Decreased adreno-corticoid effect.
Rifamycins	Decreased adreno-corticoid effect.
Salicylates*	Decreased salicylate effect.
Somatropin	Decreased effect of somatropin or adrenocorticoid
Thyroid hormones*	Effect can vary. Consult doctor or pharmacist.
Thyroid hormones*	Risk of viral infection or decreased vaccine effect.

AMPHETAMINES

GENERIC NAME OR DRUG CLASS	COMBINED EFFECT
Sympathomimetics*	Seizure risk.
Thyroid hormones*	Irregular heartbeat.

***See Glossary**

GENERIC NAME OR DRUG CLASS	COMBINED EFFECT	GENERIC NAME OR DRUG CLASS	COMBINED EFFECT

ANGIOTENSIN-CONVERTING ENZYME (ACE) INHIBITORS

GENERIC NAME OR DRUG CLASS	COMBINED EFFECT
Potassium supplements*	Possible increased potassium in blood.
Sotalol	Increased anti-hypertensive effects of both drugs. Dosages may require adjustment.
Spironolactone	Possible excessive potassium in blood.
Terazosin	Decreased effectiveness of terazosin.
Tiopronin	Increased risk of toxicity to kidneys.
Triamterene	Possible excessive potassium in blood.

ANGIOTENSIN-CONVERTING ENZYME (ACE) INHIBITORS & HYDROCHLOROTHIAZIDE

GENERIC NAME OR DRUG CLASS	COMBINED EFFECT
Diuretics*	Decreased blood pressure.
Lisinopril	Increased anti-hypertensive effect. Dosage of each may require adjustment.
Lithium	Increased lithium effect.
Monoamine oxidase (MAO) inhibitors*	Increased hydro-chlorothiazide effect.
Nicardipine	Blood pressure drop. Dosages may require adjustment.
Nimodipine	Possible irregular heartbeat. May worsen congestive heart failure.
Nitrates*	Excessive blood pressure drop.
Potassium supplements*	Excessive potassium in blood.
Probenecid	Decreased probenecid effect.
Sotalol	Increased antihypertensive effects of both drugs. Dosages may require adjustment.
Spironolactone	Possible excessive potassium in blood.
Triamterene	Possible excessive potassium in blood.

ANTIARRHYTHMICS, BENZOFURAN-TYPE

GENERIC NAME OR DRUG CLASS	COMBINED EFFECT
Cyclosporine	May increase effect of cyclosporine.
Digoxin	May increase digoxin effect.
Disopyramide	May increase risk of irregular heartbeat.
Enzyme inducers*	May decrease effect of benzofuran-type antiarrhythmic and enzyme inducer.
Enzyme inhibitors*	May increase effect and toxicity risk of benzofuran-type antiarrhythmic. May increase effect of enzyme inhibitor.
Fentanyl	May increase risk of low blood pressure.
Flecainide	May increase effect of flecainide.
HMG-CoA reductase inhibitors	Risk of muscle injury and kidney failure.
QT prolongation-causing drugs*	Increased risk of irregular heartbeat. Avoid.
Quinidine	May increase effect of quinidine.

ADDITIONAL DRUG INTERACTIONS

*See Glossary

GENERIC NAME OR DRUG CLASS	COMBINED EFFECT

ANTICONVULSANTS, HYDANTOIN

GENERIC NAME OR DRUG CLASS	COMBINED EFFECT
Central nervous system (CNS) depressants*	Oversedation.
Chloramphenicol	Increased anticonvulsant effect.
Cimetidine	Increased anti-convulsant toxicity.
Contraceptives, oral*	Increased seizures.
Cyclosporine	May decrease cyclosporine effect.
Digitalis preparations*	Decreased digitalis effect.
Disopyramide	Decreased disopyramide effect.
Disulfiram	Increased anticonvulsant effect.
Estrogens*	Increased estrogen effect.
Felbamate	Increased side effects and adverse reactions.
Furosemide	Decreased furosemide effect.
Gold compounds*	Increased anticon-vulsant blood levels. Hydantoin dose may require adjustment.
Griseofulvin	Increased griseofulvin effect.
Hypoglycemics, oral*	Possible decreased hypoglycemic effect.
Hypoglycemics,* other	Possible decreased hypoglycemic effect.
Isoniazid	Increased anticonvulsant effect.
Lamotrigine	Decreased lamotrigine effect with phenytoin.
Leucovorin	May counteract the effect of phenytoin or any hydantoin anticonvulsant.
Leukotriene modifiers	Increased phenytoin effect.
Loxapine	Decreased anticonvulsant effect.
Methadone	Decreased methadone effect.
Methotrexate	Increased methotrexate effect.
Methyldopa	Possible decreased methyldopa effect.
Methylphenidate	Increased anticonvulsant effect.
Mifepristone	Decreased effect of mifepristone.
Modafinil	Anticonvulsant dose may need adjustment.
Molindone	Increased phenytoin effect.
Monoamine oxidase (MAO) inhibitors*	Increased polythiazide effect.
Nicardipine	Increased anticonvulsant effect.
Nimodipine	Increased anticonvulsant effect.
Nitrates*	Excessive blood pressure drop.
Nitroimidazoles	Decreased effect of phenytoin.
Nizatidine	Increased effect and toxicity of phenytoin.
Omeprazole	Delayed excretion of phenytoin causing increased amount of phenytoin in blood.
Oxyphenbutazone	Increased anticonvulsant effect.
Para-aminosalicylic acid (PAS)	Increased anticonvulsant effect.
Paroxetine	Decreased anticonvulsant effect.
Phenacemide	Increased risk of paranoid symptoms.
Phenothiazines*	Increased anticonvulsant effect.
Phenylbutazone	Increased anticonvulsant effect.
Potassium supplements*	Decreased potassium effect.
Probenecid	Decreased probenecid effect.

*See Glossary

GENERIC NAME OR DRUG CLASS	COMBINED EFFECT	GENERIC NAME OR DRUG CLASS	COMBINED EFFECT

ANTICONVULSANTS, HYDANTOIN continued

GENERIC NAME OR DRUG CLASS	COMBINED EFFECT
Propafenone	Increased effect of both drugs and increased risk of toxicity.
Propranolol	Increased propranolol effect.
Quetiapine	Decreased quetiapine effect with phenytoin.
Quinidine	Increased quinidine effect.
Rifamycins	Decreased anticonvulsant effect.
Sedatives*	Increased sedative effect.
Sotalol	Decreased sotalol effect.
Sucralfate	Decreased anticonvulsant effect.
Sulfa drugs*	Increased anticonvulsant effect.
Theophylline	Reduced anticonvulsant effect.
Trimethoprim	Increased phenytoin effect.
Valproic acid*	Each drug may need dosage adjusted.
Xanthines*	Decreased effects of both drugs.
Zafirlukast	May increase effect of phenytoin.
Zaleplon	Decreased zaleplon effect.

ANTIDEPRESSANTS, TRICYCLIC

GENERIC NAME OR DRUG CLASS	COMBINED EFFECT
Benzodiazepines*	Increased sedation.
Bupropion	Increased risk of seizures.
Central nervous system (CNS) depressants*	Excessive sedation.
Cimetidine	Possible increased tricyclic anti-depressant effect and toxicity.
Citalopram	Increased tricyclic antidepressant effect and toxicity.
Clonidine	Blood pressure increase. Avoid combination.
Clozapine	Toxic effect on the central nervous system.
Contraceptives, oral*	Increased depression.
Desmopressin	Increased risk of thirstiness which may lead to drinking excess fluids.
Dextrothyroxine	Increased anti-depressant effect. Irregular heartbeat.
Disulfiram	Delirium.
Dofetilide	Increased risk of heart problems.
Ethchlorvynol	Delirium.
Fluoxetine	Increased effect of tricyclic antidepressant. Possible toxicity.
Fluvoxamine	Increased anti-depressant effect.
Furazolidone	Sudden, severe increase in blood pressure.
Guanabenz	Decreased guanabenz effect.
Guanadrel	Decreased guanadrel effect.
Guanethidine	Decreased guanethidine effect.
Leucovorin	High alcohol content of leucovorin may cause adverse effects.
Levodopa	May increase blood pressure. May decrease levodopa effect.
Lithium	Possible decreased seizure threshold.

*See Glossary

GENERIC NAME OR DRUG CLASS	COMBINED EFFECT	GENERIC NAME OR DRUG CLASS	COMBINED EFFECT

ANTIDEPRESSANTS, TRICYCLIC continued

GENERIC NAME OR DRUG CLASS	COMBINED EFFECT
Methyldopa	Possible decreased methyldopa effect.
Methylphenidate	Possible increased tricyclic anti-depressant effect and toxicity.
Modafinil	Increased anti-depressant effect.
Molindone	Increased molindone effect.
Monoamine oxidase (MAO) inhibitors*	Fever, delirium, convulsions.
Narcotics*	Oversedation.
Nicotine	Increased effect of antidepressant (with imipramine).
Phenothiazines*	Possible increased tricyclic anti-depressant effect and toxicity.
Phenytoin	Decreased phenytoin effect.
Procainamide	Possible irregular heartbeat.
Quinidine	Possible irregular heartbeat.
Serotonergics*	Increased risk of serotonin syndrome.*
Sertraline	Increased depressive effects of both drugs.
Sympathomimetics*	Increased sympatho-mimetic effect.
Thyroid hormones*	Irregular heartbeat.
Tolcapone	May increase incidence of adverse effects of tolcapone.
Zaleplon	Increased effect of either drug. Avoid.
Zolpidem	Increased sedative effect. Avoid.

ANTIDYSKINETICS

GENERIC NAME OR DRUG CLASS	COMBINED EFFECT
Imatinib	Increased effect of pimozide.
Levodopa	Possible increased levodopa effect.
Monoamine oxidase (MAO) inhibitors*	Increased antidyskinetic effect.
Telithromycin	Heart problem risk with pimozide. Avoid.

ANTIFUNGALS, AZOLES

GENERIC NAME OR DRUG CLASS	COMBINED EFFECT
Losartan	Decreased losartan effect.
Methscopolamine	Decreased azole effect.
Methylprednisolone	Increased effect of methylprednisolone.
Mifepristone	Decreased effect of mifepristone.
Nizatidine	Decreased azole effect.
Omeprazole	Decreased azole effect.
Phenytoin	May alter effect of both drugs.
Propantheline	Decreased azole effect.
Proton pump inhibitors	Decreased antifungal effect.
Quetiapine	Increased risk of quetiapine toxicity.
Ranitidine	Decreased azole effect.
Rifamycins	Decreased azole effect.
Ritonavir	Increased ritonavir effect.
Scopolamine	Decreased azole effect.
Sibutramine	Increased effect of sibutramine.
Sildenafil	Effects unknown. Consult doctor.
Sodium bicarbonate	Decreased azole effect.
Warfarin	Increased warfarin effect.

***See Glossary**

GENERIC NAME OR DRUG CLASS	COMBINED EFFECT	GENERIC NAME OR DRUG CLASS	COMBINED EFFECT

ANTIHISTAMINES, PHENOTHIAZINE-DERIVATIVE

GENERIC NAME OR DRUG CLASS	COMBINED EFFECT
Clozapine	Toxic effect on the central nervous system.
Dronabinol	Increased effects of both drugs. Avoid.
Epinephrine	Decreased epinephrine effect.
Ethinamate	Dangerous increased effects of ethinamate. Avoid combining.
Extrapyramidal reaction*-causing medicines	Increased frequency and severity of extra-pyramidal reactions.
Fluoxetine	Increased depressant effects of both drugs.
Guanethidine	Decreased guanethidine effect.
Guanfacine	May increase depressant effects of either medicine.
Leucovorin	High alcohol content of leucovorin may cause adverse effects.
Levodopa	Decreased levodopa effect.
Methyprylon	May increase sedative effect to dangerous level. Avoid.
Metyrosine	Increased likelihood of toxic symptoms of each.
Mind-altering drugs*	Increased effect of mind-altering drugs.
Molindone	Increased sedative and antihistamine effect.
Monoamine oxidase (MAO) inhibitors*	Increased anti-histamine effect.
Nabilone	Greater depression of central nervous system.
Narcotics*	Increased narcotic effect.
Sedatives*	Increased sedative effect.
Sertraline	Increased depressive effects of both drugs.
Sotalol	Increased antihistamine effect.
Tranquilizers*	Increased tranquilizer effect. Avoid.

ANTI-INFLAMMATORY DRUGS, NONSTEROIDAL (NSAIDs)

GENERIC NAME OR DRUG CLASS	COMBINED EFFECT
Diuretics*	May decrease diuretic effect.
Gold compounds*	Increased risk of kidney toxicity.
Lithium	Increased lithium effect.
Losartan	Decreased anti-hypertensive effect.
Meglitinides	Unknown effect. Avoid.
Meloxicam	Increased risk of side effects of meloxicam.
Methotrexate	Increased risk of side effects of methotrexate.
Minoxidil	Decreased minoxidil effect.
Potassium supplements	Increased risk of stomach problems.
Probenecid	Increased pain relief.
Terazosin	Decreased effectiveness of terazosin. Causes sodium and fluid retention.
Thyroid hormones*	Rapid heartbeat, blood pressure rise.
Tiopronin	Increased risk of toxicity to kidneys.
Triamterene	Reduced triamterene effect.

ADDITIONAL DRUG INTERACTIONS

*See Glossary

GENERIC NAME OR DRUG CLASS	COMBINED EFFECT	GENERIC NAME OR DRUG CLASS	COMBINED EFFECT

ASPIRIN

GENERIC NAME OR DRUG CLASS	COMBINED EFFECT
Dextrothyroxine (large doses, continuous use)	Increased dextrothyroxine effect.
Diclofenac	Increased risk of stomach ulcer.
Ethacrynic acid	Possible aspirin toxicity.
Furosemide	Possible aspirin toxicity. May decrease furosemide effect.
Gold compounds*	Increased likelihood of kidney damage.
Indomethacin	Risk of stomach bleeding and ulcers.
Ketoprofen	Increased risk of stomach ulcer.
Levamisole	Increased risk of bleeding.
Meloxicam	Increased risk of stomach ulcer.
Methotrexate	Increased methotrexate effect.
Minoxidil	Decreased minoxidil effect.
Oxprenolol	Decreased anti-hypertensive effect of oxprenolol.
Para-aminosalicylic acid	Possible aspirin toxicity.
Penicillins*	Increased effect of both drugs.
Phenobarbital	Decreased aspirin effect.
Phenytoin	Increased phenytoin effect.
Probenecid	Decreased probenecid effect.
Propranolol	Decreased aspirin effect.
Rauwolfia alkaloids*	Decreased aspirin effect.
Salicylates*	Likely aspirin toxicity.
Selective serotonin reuptake inhibitors (SSRIs)	Risk of bleeding problems.
Sotalol	Decreased anti-hypertensive effect of sotalol.
Spironolactone	Decreased spironolactone effect.
Sulfinpyrazone	Decreased sulfinpyrazone effect.
Terazosin	Decreased effectiveness of terazosin. Causes sodium and fluid retention.
Ticlopidine	Increased effect of both drugs.
Valproic acid*	May increase valproic acid effect.
Vitamin C (large doses)	Possible aspirin toxicity.

ATROPINE, HYOSCYAMINE, METHENAMINE, METHYLENE BLUE, PHENYLSALICYLATE & BENZOIC ACID

GENERIC NAME OR DRUG CLASS	COMBINED EFFECT
Cortisone drugs*	Increased internal eye pressure, increased cortisone effect. Risk of ulcers and stomach bleeding.
Diuretics, thiazide*	Decreased urine acidity.
Furosemide	Possible salicylate toxicity.
Gold compounds*	Increased likelihood of kidney damage.
Haloperidol	Increased internal eye pressure.
Indomethacin	Risk of stomach bleeding and ulcers.
Ketoconazole	Reduced ketoconazole effect.
Meperidine	Increased atropine and hyoscyamine effect.

*See Glossary

GENERIC NAME OR DRUG CLASS	COMBINED EFFECT	GENERIC NAME OR DRUG CLASS	COMBINED EFFECT

ATROPINE, HYOSCYAMINE, METHENAMINE, METHYLENE BLUE, PHENYLSALICYLATE & BENZOIC ACID continued

GENERIC NAME OR DRUG CLASS	COMBINED EFFECT
Methylphenidate	Increased atropine and hyoscyamine effect.
Minoxidil	Decreased minoxidil effect.
Monoamine oxidase (MAO) inhibitors*	Increased belladonna and atropine effect.
Orphenadrine	Increased atropine and hyoscyamine effect.
Oxprenolol	Decreased anti-hypertensive effect of oxprenolol.
Para-aminosalicylic acid (PAS)	Possible salicylate toxicity.
Penicillins*	Increased effect of both drugs.
Phenobarbital	Decreased salicylate effect.
Phenothiazines*	Increased atropine and hyoscyamine effect.
Phenytoin	Increased phenytoin effect.
Pilocarpine	Loss of pilocarpine effect in glaucoma treatment.
Potassium supplements*	Possible intestinal ulcers with oral potassium tablets.
Probenecid	Decreased probenecid effect.
Propranolol	Decreased salicylate effect.
Rauwolfia alkaloids*	Decreased salicylate effect.
Salicylates*	Likely salicylate toxicity.
Sedatives* or central nervous system (CNS) depressants*	Increased sedative effect of both drugs.
Serotonergics*	Serotonin syndrome.*
Sodium bicarbonate	Decreased methenamine effect.
Spironolactone	Decreased spironolactone effect.
Sulfa drugs*	Possible kidney damage.
Sulfinpyrazone	Decreased sulfinpyrazone effect.
Vitamin C (1 to 4 grams per day)	Increased effect of methenamine, contributing to urine acidity; decreased atropine effect; possible salicylate toxicity.

BARBITURATES

GENERIC NAME OR DRUG CLASS	COMBINED EFFECT
Meglitinides	Increased blood level of meglitinides.
Mifepristone	Decreased effect of mifepristone.
Mind-altering drugs*	Dangerous sedation. Avoid.
Modafinil	Increased modafinil effect.
Monoamine oxidase (MAO) inhibitors*	Increased barbiturate effect.
Narcotics*	Dangerous sedation. Avoid.
Nitroimidazoles	Decreased nitroimidazoles effect.
Sertraline	Increased depressive effects of both drugs.
Sotalol	Increased barbiturate effect. Dangerous sedation.
Valproic acid*	Increased barbiturate effect.
Zaleplon	Decreased zaleplon effect.

ADDITIONAL DRUG INTERACTIONS

*See Glossary

GENERIC NAME OR DRUG CLASS	COMBINED EFFECT	GENERIC NAME OR DRUG CLASS	COMBINED EFFECT

BARBITURATES, ASPIRIN & CODEINE (Also contains caffeine)

GENERIC NAME OR DRUG CLASS	COMBINED EFFECT
Anticoagulants, oral*	Increased anticoagulant effect. Abnormal bleeding.
Anticonvulsants*	Changed seizure patterns.
Antidepressants*	Decreased anti-depressant effect. Possible dangerous oversedation.
Antidiabetics, oral*	Increased butalbital effect. Low blood sugar.
Antihistamines*	Dangerous sedation. Avoid.
Anti-inflammatory drugs, nonsteroidal (NSAIDs)*	Risk of stomach bleeding and ulcers.
Aspirin, other	Likely aspirin toxicity.
Beta-adrenergic blocking agents*	Decreased effect of beta-adrenergic blocker.
Carteolol	Increased narcotic effect. Dangerous sedation.
Contraceptives, oral*	Decreased contraceptive effect.
Digitoxin	Decreased digitoxin effect.
Doxycycline	Decreased doxycycline effect.
Dronabinol	Increased effect of drugs.
Furosemide	Possible aspirin toxicity.
Gold compounds*	Increased likelihood of kidney damage.
Griseofulvin	Decreased griseofulvin effect.
Indapamide	Increased indapamide effect.
Indomethacin	Risk of stomach bleeding and ulcers.
Lamotrigine	Decreased lamotrigine effect.
Methotrexate	Increased methotrexate effect.
Mind-altering drugs*	Dangerous sedation. Avoid.
Minoxidil	Decreased minoxidil effect.
Monoamine oxidase (MAO) inhibitors*	Increased butalbital effect.
Naltrexone	Decreased analgesic effect.
Narcotics*	Dangerous sedation. Avoid.
Nitrates*	Excessive blood pressure drop.
Nitroimidazoles	Decreased nitroimidazole effect.
Pain relievers*	Dangerous sedation. Avoid.
Para-aminosalicylic acid	Possible aspirin toxicity.
Penicillins*	Increased effect of drugs.
Phenobarbital	Decreased aspirin effect.
Phenothiazines*	Increased phenothiazine effect.
Phenytoin	Increased phenytoin effect.
Probenecid	Decreased probenecid effect.
Propranolol	Decreased aspirin effect.
Rauwolfia alkaloids*	Decreased aspirin effect.
Salicylates*	Likely aspirin toxicity.
Sedatives*	Dangerous sedation. Avoid.
Sleep inducers*	Dangerous sedation. Avoid.
Sotalol	Increased narcotic effect. Dangerous sedation.
Spironolactone	Decreased spironolactone effect.
Sulfinpyrazone	Decreased sulfinpyrazone effect.

***See Glossary**

BARBITURATES, ASPIRIN & CODEINE (Also contains caffeine) continued

GENERIC NAME OR DRUG CLASS	COMBINED EFFECT
Tranquilizers*	Dangerous sedation. Avoid.
Valproic acid	Increased phenobarbital effect.
Vitamin C (large doses)	Possible aspirin toxicity.
Zidovudine	Increased toxicity of both.

BELLADONNA ALKALOIDS & BARBITURATES

GENERIC NAME OR DRUG CLASS	COMBINED EFFECT
Attapulgite	Decreased belladonna effect.
Beta-adrenergic blocking agents*	Decreased effects of beta-adrenergic blocker.
Carteolol	Increased barbiturate effect. Dangerous sedation.
Central nervous system (CNS) depressants*	Dangerous sedation. Avoid.
Contraceptives, oral*	Decreased contraceptive effect.
Digitoxin	Decreased digitoxin effect.
Doxycycline	Decreased doxycycline effect.
Dronabinol	Increased effects of both drugs. Avoid.
Furosemide	Possible orthostatic hypotension.*
Griseofulvin	Decreased griseofulvin effect.
Haloperidol	Increased internal eye pressure.
Indapamide	Increased indapamide effect.
Ketoconazole	Decreased ketoconazole effect.
Meperidine	Increased belladonna effect.
Methylphenidate	Increased belladonna effect.
Metronidazole	Decreased metronidazole effect.
Mind-altering drugs*	Dangerous sedation. Avoid.
Monoamine oxidase (MAO) inhibitors*	Increased belladonna and barbiturate effect.
Narcotics*	Dangerous sedation. Avoid.
Nitrates*	Increased internal eye pressure.
Nizatidine	Increased nizatidine effect.
Orphenadrine	Increased belladonna effect.
Pain relievers*	Dangerous sedation. Avoid.
Phenothiazines*	Increased belladonna effect. Danger of oversedation.
Pilocarpine	Loss of pilocarpine effect in glaucoma treatment.
Potassium supplements*	Possible intestinal ulcers with oral potassium tablets.
Quinidine	Increased belladonna effect.
Sedatives*	Dangerous sedation. Avoid.
Sleep inducers*	Dangerous sedation. Avoid.
Sotalol	Increased barbiturate effect. Dangerous sedation.
Tranquilizers*	Dangerous sedation. Avoid.
Valproic acid*	Increased barbiturate effect.
Vitamin C	Decreased belladonna effect. Avoid large doses of vitamin C.

ADDITIONAL DRUG INTERACTIONS

*See Glossary

GENERIC NAME OR DRUG CLASS	COMBINED EFFECT	GENERIC NAME OR DRUG CLASS	COMBINED EFFECT

BENZODIAZEPINES

GENERIC NAME OR DRUG CLASS	COMBINED EFFECT
Levodopa	Decreased levodopa effect.
Narcotics*	Increased sedative effect of both drugs.
Nefazodone	Increased effect of benzodiazepine.
Nicotine	Increased effect of benzodiazepine.
Omeprazole	Increased effect of benzodiazepine.
Probenecid	Increased effect of probenecid and risk of sedation.
Proton pump inhibitors	Increased effect of diazepam.
Rifamycins	Decreased effect of benzodiazepine.
Telithromycin	Increased effect of benzodiazepine.
Valproic acid*	Increased effect of benzodiazepines.
Zidovudine	Increased effect of zidovudine.

BETA-ADRENERGIC BLOCKING AGENTS

GENERIC NAME OR DRUG CLASS	COMBINED EFFECT
Diazoxide	Additional blood pressure drop.
Estrogens*	May cause blood pressure problems.
Flecainide	Increased effect of toxicity on heart muscle.
Fluvoxamine	Increased beta blocker effect.
Guanabenz	May cause blood pressure problems.
Insulin	Hypoglycemic effects may be prolonged.
Leukotriene modifiers	Increased beta blocker effect.
Meglitinides	Increased risk of low blood sugar.
Miglitol	Decreased effect of propranolol.
Molindone	Increased tranquilizer effect.
Monoamine oxidase (MAO) inhibitors*	High blood pressure following MAO discontinuation.
Nefazodone	Dosages of both drugs may require adjustment.
Nicotine	Increased effect of propranolol.
Nitrates*	Possible excessive blood pressure drop.
Phenothiazines	Increased effect of both drugs.
Phenytoin	Decreased beta blocker effect.
Propafenone	Increased beta blocker effect.
Quinidine	May cause heart problems.
Reserpine	Increased reserpine effect. Excessive sedation and depression. Additional blood pressure drop.
Sympathomimetics*	Decreased effects of both drugs.
Telithromycin	Various effects. Use with caution.
Warfarin	Increased warfarin effect.
Xanthines (aminophylline, theophylline)	Decreased effects of both drugs.

*See Glossary

GENERIC NAME OR DRUG CLASS	COMBINED EFFECT	GENERIC NAME OR DRUG CLASS	COMBINED EFFECT

BETA-ADRENERGIC BLOCKING AGENTS & THIAZIDE DIURETICS

GENERIC NAME OR DRUG CLASS	COMBINED EFFECT
Antidiabetics*	Increased antidiabetic effect.
Antihistamines*	Decreased antihistamine effect.
Antihypertensives*	Increased anti-hypertensive effect.
Anti-inflammatory drugs, nonsteroidal (NSAIDs)*	Decreased antiinflammatory effect.
Barbiturates*	Increased barbiturate effect. Dangerous sedation.
Bumetanide	Increased diuretic effect.
Calcium channel blockers*	Increased anti-hypertensive effect. Dosages of both drugs may require adjustments.
Cholestyramine	Decreased hydro-chlorothiazide effect.
Diclofenac	Decreased anti-hypertensive effect.
Digitalis preparations*	Excessive potassium loss that causes dangerous heart rhythms. Can either increase or decrease heart rate. Improves irregular heartbeat.
Diuretics, thiazide*	Increased effect of other thiazide diuretics.
Ethacrynic acid	Increased diuretic effect.
Furosemide	Increased diuretic effect.
Guanfacine	Increased effect of both drugs.
Hypoglycemics, oral*	Decreased ability to lower blood glucose.
Indapamide	Increased diuretic effect.
Insulin	Decreased ability to lower blood glucose.
Lisinopril	Increased anti-hypertensive effect. Dosage of each may require adjustment.
Metolazone	Increased diuretic effect.
Miglitol	Decreased effect of propranolol.
Monoamine oxidase (MAO) inhibitors*	Increased hydro-chlorothiazide effect.
Narcotics*	Increased narcotic effect. Dangerous sedation.
Nicardipine	Possible irregular heartbeat and congestive heart failure.
Nicotine	Increased beta blocker effect.
Nitrates*	Excessive blood pressure drop.
Phenytoin	Increased beta adrenergic effect.
Potassium supplements*	Decreased potassium effect.
Probenecid	Decreased probenecid effect.
Propafenone	Increased beta blocker effect.
Quinidine	Slows heart excessively.
Reserpine	Increased reserpine effect. Excessive sedation and depression.
Sympathomimetics*	Decreased effectiveness of both.
Theophylline	Decreased effectiveness of both.
Tocainide	May worsen congestive heart failure.
Zinc supplements	Increased need for zinc.

*See Glossary

GENERIC NAME OR DRUG CLASS	COMBINED EFFECT	GENERIC NAME OR DRUG CLASS	COMBINED EFFECT

BRONCHODILATORS, ADRENERGIC

Rauwolfia alkaloids	Decreased rauwolfia effect.	**Theophylline**	Increased gastro-intestinal intolerance.
Sympathomimetics,* other	Increased bronchodilator effect.	**Thyroid hormones***	Increased bronchodilator effect.
Terazosin	Decreased effectiveness of terazosin.	**Tolcapone**	May require adjustment in dosage.

BRONCHODILATORS, XANTHINE

Telithromycin	Increased effect of telithromycin.	**Zafirlukast**	May increase effect of zafirlukast.
Ticlopidine	Increased theophylline effect.	**Zileuton**	Increased theophylline effect.
Troleandomycin	Increased bronchodilator effect.		

CALCIUM CHANNEL BLOCKERS

Lithium	Possible decreased lithium effect.	**Nimodipine**	Dangerous blood pressure drop.
Metformin	Increased metformin effect.	**Nitrates***	Reduced angina attacks.
Nicardipine	Possible increased effect and toxicity of each drug.		

CALCIUM SUPPLEMENTS

Quinidine	Increased quinidine effect.	**Theophylline**	May increase effect and toxicity of theophylline.
Rifamycins	Decreased effect of calcium channel blocker.	**Vitamin A**	Decreased vitamin effect.
Salicylates*	Increased salicylate effect.	**Vitamin D**	Increased vitamin absorption, sometimes excessively; decreased effect of calcium channel blocker.
Sulfa drugs*	Decreased sulfa effect.	**Zafirlukast**	May increase calcium channel blocker effect.
Tetracyclines*	Decreased tetracycline effect.		

CARBAMAZEPINE

Antidepressants, tricyclic*	Confusion. Possible psychosis.	**Antifungals, azole**	Increased effect of carbamazepine. Decreased effect of antifungal.

*See Glossary

GENERIC NAME OR DRUG CLASS	COMBINED EFFECT	GENERIC NAME OR DRUG CLASS	COMBINED EFFECT
CARBAMAZEPINE continued			
Barbiturates*	Possible increased barbiturate metabolism.	**Guanfacine**	May increase depressant effects of either drug.
Benzodiazepines	Decreased effect of benzodiazepine.	**Haloperidol**	Decreased effect of haloperidol.
Bupropion	Decreased effect of bupropion.	**Isoniazid**	Increased effect of carbamazepine.
Carbonic anhydrase inhibitors (oral)	Increased risk of bone loss.	**Lamotrigine**	Decreased lamotrigine effect. Increased risk of side effects.
Central nervous system (CNS) depressants*	Increased sedative effect.	**Leucovorin**	High alcohol content of leucovorin may cause adverse effects.
Cimetidine	Increased carbamazepine effect.	**Leukotriene modifiers**	Increased effect of carbamazepine.
Citalopram	May lessen effect of citalopram.	**Lithium**	Increased risk of side effects.
Clozapine	Toxic effect on bone marrow and central nervous system.	**Meglitinides**	Blood sugar problems.
Contraceptives, oral*	Reduced contraceptive protection. Breakthrough bleeding.	**Methylphenidate**	Decreased effect of methylphenidate.
Cyclosporine	Decreased effect of cyclosporine.	**Mifepristone**	Decreased effect of mifepristone.
Danazol	Increased effect of carbamazepine.	**Monoamine oxidase (MAO) Inhibitors***	Dangerous overstimulation. Avoid.
Desmopressin	May increase desmopressin effect.	**Phenobarbital**	Decreased carbamazepine effect.
Digitalis preparations*	Decreased digitalis effect.	**Phenytoin**	Decreased effect of both drugs.
Diltiazem	Increased effect of carbamazepine.	**Primidone**	Decreased carbamazepine effect.
Doxycycline	Decreased doxycycline effect.	**Propoxyphene**	Increased toxicity of both. Avoid.
Estrogens*	Decreased estrogen effect.	**Rifampin**	Decreased carbamazepine effect.
Erythromycins*	Increased carbamazepine effect.	**Risperidone**	Decreased risperidone effect.
Felbamate	Increased side effects and adverse reactions.	**Theophylline**	Decreases effect of theophylline.
Felodipine	Decreased effect of felodipine.	**Ticlopidine**	Decreased effect of carbamazepine.
Fluoxetine	Increased carbamazepine effect.	**Tiopronin**	Increased risk of toxicity to bone marrow.
Fluvoxamine	Possible toxicity of carbamazepine.	**Valproic acid***	Decreased effect of valproic acid.

*See Glossary

GENERIC NAME OR DRUG CLASS	COMBINED EFFECT	GENERIC NAME OR DRUG CLASS	COMBINED EFFECT

CARBAMAZEPINE continued

GENERIC NAME OR DRUG CLASS	COMBINED EFFECT
Vasopressin	Increased effect of vasopressin.
Verapamil	Increased effect of carbamazepine.
Zafirlukast	Increased effect of carbamazepine.
Zaleplon	Decreased zaleplon effect.

CENTRAL ALPHA AGONISTS

GENERIC NAME OR DRUG CLASS	COMBINED EFFECT
Central nervous system (CNS) depressants*	Increased depressive effects of both drugs.
Monoamine oxidase (MAO) inhibitors*	Dangerous changes in blood pressure. Take at least 14 days apart.

CLONIDINE & CHLORTHALIDONE

GENERIC NAME OR DRUG CLASS	COMBINED EFFECT
Diuretics*	Excessive blood pressure drop.
Fenfluramine	Possible increased clonidine effect.
Guanfacine	Impaired blood pressure control.
Indapamide	Increased diuretic effect.
Lithium	Increased lithium effect.
Monoamine oxidase (MAO) inhibitors*	Increased chlorthalidone effect.
Nabilone	Greater depression of central nervous system.
Nicardipine	Blood pressure drop. Dosage may require adjustment.
Nitrates*	Possible excessive blood pressure drop.
Potassium supplements*	Decreased potassium effect.
Probenecid	Decreased probenecid effect.
Sedatives* or central nervous system (CNS) depressants*	Increased sedative effect of both drugs.
Sotalol	Decreased anti-hypertensive effect.
Terazosin	Decreased terazosin effect.

CONTRACEPTIVES, ORAL & SKIN

GENERIC NAME OR DRUG CLASS	COMBINED EFFECT
Dextrothyroxine	Decreased dextrothyroxine effect.
Guanethidine	Decreased guanethidine effect.
Hypoglycemics, oral*	Decreased effect of hypoglycemics.
Insulin	Possibly decreased insulin effect.
Insulin lispro	May need increased dosage of insulin.
Meperidine	Increased meperidine effect.
Meprobamate	Decreased contraceptive effect.
Mineral oil	Decreased contraceptive effect.
Non-nucleoside reverse transcriptase inhibitors	Decreased contraceptive effect. Use alternative birth control method.
Phenothiazines*	Increased phenothiazine effect.
Rifamycins	Decreased contraceptive effect.
Sulfadoxine and pyrimethamine	Reduced reliability of the pill.
Terazosin	Decreases terazosin effect.
Tetracyclines*	Decreased contraceptive effect.

*See Glossary

GENERIC NAME OR DRUG CLASS	COMBINED EFFECT

CONTRACEPTIVES, ORAL & SKIN continued

GENERIC NAME OR DRUG CLASS	COMBINED EFFECT
Thiazolidinediones	Decreased contraceptive effect.
Ursodiol	Decreased ursodiol effect.
Vitamin A	Vitamin A excess.
Vitamin C	Possible increased contraceptive effect.

CYCLOSPORINE

GENERIC NAME OR DRUG CLASS	COMBINED EFFECT
Nimodipine	Increased cyclosporine toxicity.
Nitroimidazoles	Increased cyclosporine effect
Orlistat	Unknown effect. Monitor closely.
Rifamycins	Decreased effect of cyclosporine.
Terbinafine (oral)	Decreased effect of cyclosporine.
Thiazolidinediones	Decreased effect of cyclosporine.
Tiopronin	Increased risk of toxicity to kidneys.
Vancomycin	Increased chance of hearing loss or kidney damage.
Virus vaccines	Increased adverse reactions to vaccine.
Zafirlukast	May increase effect of cyclosporine.

DIFENOXIN & ATROPINE

GENERIC NAME OR DRUG CLASS	COMBINED EFFECT
Nitrates*	Increased internal eye pressure.
Orphenadrine	Increased atropine effect.
Phenothiazines*	Increased atropine effect.
Pilocarpine	Loss of pilocarpine effect in glaucoma treatment.
Potassium supplements*	Possible intestinal ulcers with oral potassium tablets.
Procainamide	Increased atropine effect.
Sertraline	Increased depressive effects of both drugs.
Vitamin C	Decreased atropine effect. Avoid large doses of vitamin C.

DIGITALIS PREPARATIONS (Digitalis Glycosides)

GENERIC NAME OR DRUG CLASS	COMBINED EFFECT
Metoclopramide	Decreased digitalis absorption.
Mineral oil	Decreased digitalis effect.
Nefazodone	Increased effect of digoxin.
Nicardipine	Increased digitalis effect. May need to reduce dose.
Nizatidine	Increased digitalis effect.
Oxyphenbutazone	Decreased digitalis effect.
Paroxetine	Increased levels of paroxetine in blood.
Phenobarbital	Decreased digitalis effect.
Phenylbutazone	Decreased digitalis effect.
Potassium supplements*	Overdose of either drug may cause severe heartbeat irregularity.
Propafenone	Increased digitalis absorption.
Proton pump inhibitors	Increased effect of digoxin.

*See Glossary

GENERIC NAME OR DRUG CLASS	COMBINED EFFECT	GENERIC NAME OR DRUG CLASS	COMBINED EFFECT

DIGITALIS PREPARATIONS (Digitalis Glycosides) continued

GENERIC NAME OR DRUG CLASS	COMBINED EFFECT
Quinidine	Increased digitalis effect.
Ranolazine	Increased effect of digoxin.
Rauwolfia alkaloids*	Increased digitalis effect.
Rifamycins	Possible decreased digitalis effect.
Sotalol	Can either increase or decrease heart rate. Improves irregular heartbeat.
Spironolactone	Increased digitalis effect. May require digitalis dosage reduction.
Sulfasalazine	Decreased digitalis absorption.
Sympathomimetics*	Increased risk of heartbeat irregularities.
Telithromycin	May increase digoxin effect.
Tetracycline	May increase digitalis absorption.
Thyroid hormones*	Digitalis toxicity.
Ticlopidine	Slightly decreased digitalis effect (digoxin only).
Trazodone	Possible increased digitalis toxicity.
Triamterene	Possible decreased digitalis effect.
Verapamil	Increased digitalis effect.

DIURETICS, LOOP

GENERIC NAME OR DRUG CLASS	COMBINED EFFECT
Narcotics*	Dangerous low blood pressure. Avoid.
Nephrotoxics*	Increased risk of toxicity.
Nimodipine	Dangerous blood pressure drop.
Nitrates*	Excessive blood pressure drop.
Phenytoin	Decreased diuretic effect.
Potassium supplements*	Decreased potassium effect.
Probenecid	Decreased probenecid effect.
Salicylates* (including aspirin)	Dangerous salicylate retention.
Sedatives*	Increased diuretic effect.

DIURETICS, POTASSIUM-SPARING & HYDROCHLOROTHIAZIDE

GENERIC NAME OR DRUG CLASS	COMBINED EFFECT
Cholestyramine	Decreased diuretic effect. Take 1 hour before diuretic.
Colestipol	Decreased diuretic effect. Take 1 hour before diuretic.
Cyclosporine	Increased potassium levels.
Digitalis preparations*	Increased digitalis effect.
Diuretics,* other	Increased effect of both drugs.
Folic acid	Decreased effect of folic acid.
Lithium	Possible lithium toxicity.
Metformin	Increased metformin effect.
Potassium-containing medications	Increased potassium levels.

*See Glossary

GENERIC NAME OR DRUG CLASS	COMBINED EFFECT	GENERIC NAME OR DRUG CLASS	COMBINED EFFECT

DIURETICS, THIAZIDE

GENERIC NAME OR DRUG CLASS	COMBINED EFFECT
Indapamide	Increased diuretic effect.
Indomethacin	Decreased anti-hypertensive effect.
Lithium	Increased effect of lithium.
Meglitinides	Increased blood sugar levels.
Memantine	Increased effect of memantine and hydrochlorothiazide.
Monoamine oxidase (MAO) inhibitors*	Increased anti-hypertensive effect.
Nicardipine	Blood pressure drop. Dosages may require adjustment.
Nimodipine	Dangerous blood pressure drop.
Nitrates*	Excessive blood pressure drop.
Opiates*	Dizziness or weakness when standing up after sitting or lying down.
Pentoxifylline	Increased antihypertensive effect.
Potassium supplements*	Decreased potassium effect.
Probenecid	Decreased probenecid effect.
Sotalol	Increased antihypertensive effect.
Terazosin	Decreased terazosin effect.
Toremifene	Possible increased calcium.
Zinc supplements	Increased need for zinc.

FLUOROQUINOLONES

GENERIC NAME OR DRUG CLASS	COMBINED EFFECT
Cyclosporine	Increased cyclosporine effect.
Didanosine	Decreased fluoro-quinolone effect.
Digoxin	Increased digoxin effect.
Iron supplements	Decreased fluoro-quinolone effect.
Oxtriphylline	Increased risk of oxtriphylline toxicity.
Phenytoin	Decreased effect of phenytoin with ciprofloxacin.
Probenecid	Increased effect of fluoroquinolone.
QT interval prolongation causing drugs*	Heart rhythm problems.
Sucralfate	Decreased fluoro-quinolone effect.
Theophylline	Increased risk of theophylline toxicity.
Tizanidine	Dangerous increased tizanidine effect with ciprofloxacin
Warfarin	Increased warfarin effect.
Zinc supplements	Decreased fluoro-quinolone effect.

GLP-1 RECEPTOR AGONISTS

GENERIC NAME OR DRUG CLASS	COMBINED EFFECT
Warfarin	Increased risk of bleeding (with exenatide).

HALOPERIDOL

GENERIC NAME OR DRUG CLASS	COMBINED EFFECT
Fluoxetine	Increased depressant effects of both drugs.
Guanethidine	Decreased guanethidine effect.

*See Glossary

GENERIC NAME OR DRUG CLASS	COMBINED EFFECT	GENERIC NAME OR DRUG CLASS	COMBINED EFFECT

HALOPERIDOL continued

GENERIC NAME OR DRUG CLASS	COMBINED EFFECT
Guanfacine	May increase depressant effects of either drug.
Leucovorin	High alcohol content of leucovorin may cause adverse effects.
Levodopa	Decreased levodopa effect.
Lithium	Increased toxicity.
Loxapine	May increase toxic effects of both drugs.
Methyldopa	Possible psychosis.
Narcotics*	Excessive sedation.
Nefazodone	Unknown effect. May require dosage adjustment.
Pergolide	Decreased pergolide effect.
Procarbazine	Increased sedation.
QT interval prolongation-causing drugs*	Serious heart rhythm problems.
Sertraline	Increased depressive effects of both drugs.

HISTAMINE H_2 RECEPTOR ANTAGONISTS

GENERIC NAME OR DRUG CLASS	COMBINED EFFECT
Diazepam	Increased effect and toxicity of diazepam.
Digitalis preparations*	Increased digitalis effect.
Dofetilide	Increased risk of heart problems.
Encainide	Increased effect of histamine H_2 receptor antagonist.
Flurazepam	Increased effect and toxicity of flurazepam.
Glipizide	Increased effect and toxicity of glipizide.
Itraconazole	Decreased absorption of itraconazole.
Ketoconazole	Decreased ketoconazole absorption.
Labetalol	Increased anti-hypertensive effects.
Memantine	Increased effect of either drug.
Metformin	Increased metformin effect.
Methadone	Increased effect and toxicity of methadone.
Metoclopramide	Decreased absorption of histamine H_2 receptor antagonist.
Metoprolol	Increased effect and toxicity of metoprolol.
Miglitol	Decreased effect of ranitidine.
Moricizine	Increased concentration of H_2 receptor antagonist in the blood.
Morphine	Increased effect and toxicity of morphine.
Nicardipine	Possible increased effect and toxicity of nicardipine.
Nimodipine	Possible increased effect and toxicity of nimodipine.
Nitroimidazoles	Increased nitroimidazole effect
Paroxetine	Increased levels of paroxetine in blood.
Phenytoin	Increased effect and toxicity of phenytoin.
Propafenone	Increased effect of both drugs and increased risk of toxicity.
Propranolol	Possible increased propranolol effect.
Quinidine	Increased quinidine effect.
Tamoxifen	Decreased tamoxifen effect.
Terbinafine (oral)	Increased effect of terbinafine with cimetidine.

***See Glossary**

GENERIC NAME OR DRUG CLASS	COMBINED EFFECT	GENERIC NAME OR DRUG CLASS	COMBINED EFFECT

HISTAMINE H_2 RECEPTOR ANTAGONISTS continued

GENERIC NAME OR DRUG CLASS	COMBINED EFFECT
Theophylline	Increases theophylline effect.
Triazolam	Increased effect and toxicity of triazolam.
Varenicline	May increase effect of varenicline (with cimetidine).
Venlafaxine	With cimetidine—Increased risk of adverse reactions.
Verapamil	Increased effect and toxicity of verapamil.
Zaleplon	Increases zaleplon effect.

HYDRALAZINE

GENERIC NAME OR DRUG CLASS	COMBINED EFFECT
Lisinopril	Increased anti-hypertensive effect. Dosage of each may require adjustment.
Monoamine oxidase (MAO) inhibitors*	Increased hydralazine effect.
Nicardipine	Blood pressure drop. Dosages may require adjustment.
Nimodipine	Dangerous blood pressure drop.
Sotalol	Increased antihypertensive effect.
Terazosin	Decreased effectiveness of terazosin.

HYDRALAZINE & HYDROCHLOROTHIAZIDE

GENERIC NAME OR DRUG CLASS	COMBINED EFFECT
Antivirals, HIV/AIDS*	Increased risk of peripheral neuropathy.
Barbiturates*	Increased hydro-chlorothiazide effect.
Carteolol	Decreased anti-hypertensive effect.
Cholestyramine	Decreased hydro-chlorothiazide effect.
Cortisone drugs*	Excessive potassium loss that causes dangerous heart rhythms.
Diazoxide	Increased antihyper-tensive effect.
Digitalis preparations*	Excessive potassium loss that causes dangerous heart rhythms.
Diuretics,* oral	Increased effect of both drugs. When monitored carefully, combination may be beneficial in control-ling hypertension.
Indapamide	Increased diuretic effect.
Lisinopril	Increased anti-hypertensive effect. Dosage of each may require adjustment.
Lithium	Increased lithium effect.
Monoamine oxidase (MAO) inhibitors*	Increased effect of drugs.
Nimodipine	Dangerous blood pressure drop.
Nitrates*	Excessive blood pressure drop.
Potassium supplements*	Decreased potassium effect.
Probenecid	Decreased probenecid effect.

ADDITIONAL DRUG INTERACTIONS

*See Glossary

GENERIC NAME OR DRUG CLASS	COMBINED EFFECT	GENERIC NAME OR DRUG CLASS	COMBINED EFFECT

IMMUNOSUPPRESSIVE AGENTS

Probenecid	Increased effect of mycophenolate.	**Telithromycin**	Increased effect of tacrolimus.
Proton pump inhibitors	Increased effect of tacrolimus.	**Vaccinations**	Avoid unless doctor approves.

INDAPAMIDE

Probenecid	Decreased probenecid effect.	**Terazosin**	Decreased effectiveness of terazosin.
Sotalol	Increased antihypertensive effect.		

LITHIUM

Diuretics*	Increased lithium effect or toxicity.	**Oxyphenbutazone**	Increased lithium effect.
Fluvoxamine	Increased risk of seizure.	**Phenothiazines***	Decreased lithium effect.
Haloperidol	Increased toxicity of both drugs.	**Phenylbutazone**	Increased lithium effect.
Indomethacin	Increased lithium effect.	**Phenytoin**	Increased lithium effect.
Iodide salts	Increased lithium effects on thyroid function.	**Potassium iodide**	Increased potassium iodide effect.
Ketoprofen	May increase lithium in blood.	**Sodium bicarbonate**	Decreased lithium effect.
Meloxicam	Increased lithium effect.	**Sumatriptan**	Adverse effects unknown. Avoid.
Methyldopa	Increased lithium effect.	**Theophylline**	Decreased lithium effect.
Molindone	Brain changes.	**Tiopronin**	Increased risk of toxicity to kidneys.
Nitroimidazoles	Increased lithium effect		

LOXAPINE

Rauwolfia alkaloids*	May increase toxic effects of both drugs.	**Thioxanthenes***	May increase toxic effects of both drugs.
Sertraline	Increased depressive effects of both drugs.		

MAPROTILINE

Clonidine	Decreased clonidine effect.	**Clozapine**	Toxic effect on the central nervous system.

***See Glossary**

GENERIC NAME OR DRUG CLASS	COMBINED EFFECT	GENERIC NAME OR DRUG CLASS	COMBINED EFFECT

MAPROTILINE continued

GENERIC NAME OR DRUG CLASS	COMBINED EFFECT
Disulfiram	Delirium.
Diuretics, thiazide*	Increased maprotiline effect.
Ethchlorvynol	Delirium.
Fluoxetine	Increased depressant effects of both drugs.
Guanethidine	Decreased guanethidine effect.
Guanfacine	May increase depressant effects of either drug.
Leucovorin	High alcohol content of leucovorin may cause adverse effects.
Levodopa	Decreased levodopa effect.
Lithium	Possible decreased seizure threshold.
Methyldopa	Decreased methyldopa effect.
Methylphenidate	Possible increased antidepressant effect and toxicity.
Molindone	Increased tranquilizer effect.
Monoamine oxidase (MAO) inhibitors*	Fever, delirium, convulsions.
Narcotics*	Dangerous oversedation.
Phenothiazines*	Possible increased antidepressant effect and toxicity.
Phenytoin	Decreased phenytoin effect.
Quinidine	Irregular heartbeat.
Selegiline	Fever, delirium, convulsions.
Sertraline	Increased depressive effects of both drugs.
Sympathomimetics*	Increased sympathomimetic effect.
Thyroid hormones*	Irregular heartbeat.

METFORMIN

GENERIC NAME OR DRUG CLASS	COMBINED EFFECT
Quinine	Increased metformin effect.
Ranitidine	Increased metformin effect.
Trimethoprim	Increased metformin effect.
Vancomycin	Increased metformin effect.

METHOTREXATE

GENERIC NAME OR DRUG CLASS	COMBINED EFFECT
Sulfa drugs*	Possible methotrexate toxicity.
Sulfadoxine and pyrimethamine	Increased risk of toxicity.
Tetracyclines*	Possible methotrexate toxicity.
Tiopronin	Increased risk of toxicity to bone marrow and kidneys.
Vaccines, live or killed	Increased risk of toxicity or reduced effectiveness of vaccine.

METOCLOPRAMIDE

GENERIC NAME OR DRUG CLASS	COMBINED EFFECT
Phenothiazines*	Increased chance of muscle spasm and trembling.
Sertraline	Increased depressive effects of both drugs.
Tetracyclines*	Slow stomach emptying.
Thioxanthenes*	Increased chance of muscle spasm and trembling.

*See Glossary

MONOAMINE OXIDASE (MAO) INHIBITORS

GENERIC NAME OR DRUG CLASS	COMBINED EFFECT
Central nervous system (CNS) depressants*	Excessive depressant action.
Citalopram	Can cause a life-threatening reaction. Avoid.
Clozapine	Toxic effect on the central nervous system.
Doxepin (topical)	Potentially life-threatening. Allow 14 days between use of the 2 drugs.
Dexfenfluramine	Potentially life-threatening. Allow 14 days between use of 2 drugs.
Dextromethorphan	Very high blood pressure.
Diuretics*	Excessively low blood pressure.
Ephedrine	Increased blood pressure.
Fluoxetine	Potentially life-threatening. Avoid.
Fluvoxamine	Potentially life-threatening. Avoid.
Furazolidone	Sudden, severe increase in blood pressure.
Guanadrel	High blood pressure.
Guanethidine	Blood pressure rise.
Guanfacine	May increase depressant effects of either drug.
Indapamide	Increased indapamide effect.
Insulin	Increased hypoglycemic effect.
Leucovorin	High alcohol content of leucovorin may cause adverse effects.
Levodopa	Sudden, severe blood pressure rise.
Maprotiline	Dangerous blood pressure rise.
Meglitinides	Increased risk of low blood sugar.
Methyldopa	Sudden, severe blood pressure rise.
Methylphenidate	Increased blood pressure.
Mirtazapine	Potentially life-threatening. Allow 14 days between use of 2 drugs.
Monoamine oxidase (MAO) inhibitors (others, when taken together)	High fever, convulsions, death.
Narcotics*	Severe high blood pressure.
Nefazodone	Potentially life-threatening. Allow 14 days between use of the 2 drugs.
Paroxetine	Potentially life-threatening. Avoid.
Phenothiazines*	Possible increased phenothiazine toxicity.
Pseudoephedrine	Increased blood pressure.
Serotonergics*	Increased risk of serotonin syndrome.*
Sertraline	Potentially life-threatening. Avoid.
Sympathomimetics*	Blood pressure rise to life-threatening level.
Tolcapone	May reduce effectiveness of MAO inhibitor.
Tramadol	Increased risk of seizures.
Trazodone	Increased risk of mental status changes.
Venlafaxine	Increased risk and severity of side effects. Allow 4 weeks between use of the 2 drugs.

***See Glossary**

NARCOTIC ANALGESICS

GENERIC NAME OR DRUG CLASS	COMBINED EFFECT
Cimetidine	Possible increased narcotic effect and toxicity.
Clozapine	Toxic effect on the central nervous system.
Ethinamate	Dangerous increased effects of ethinamate. Avoid combining.
Fluoxetine	Increased depressant effects of both drugs.
Guanfacine	May increase depressant effects of either drug.
Leucovorin	High alcohol content of leucovorin may cause adverse effects.
Methyprylon	Increased sedative effect, perhaps to dangerous level. Avoid.
Metformin	Increased effect of metformin with morphine.
Mind-altering drugs*	Increased sedative effect.
Molindone	Increased narcotic effect.
Monoamine oxidase (MAO) inhibitors*	Serious toxicity (including death).
Nabilone	Greater depression of central nervous system.
Nalbuphine	Possibly precipitates withdrawal with chronic narcotic use.
Naltrexone	Precipitates withdrawal symptoms. May lead to respiratory arrest, coma and death.
Narcotics,* other	Increased narcotic effect.
Nicotine	Increased effect of pentazocine and propoxyphene.
Nitrates*	Excessive blood pressure drop.
Pentazocine	Possibly precipitates withdrawal with chronic narcotic use.
Phenothiazines*	Increased sedative effect.
Phenytoin	Possible decreased narcotic effect.
Rifamycins	Possible decreased narcotic effect.
Sedatives*	Increased sedative effect.
Selegiline	Severe toxicity characterized by breathing difficulties, seizures, coma.
Sertraline	Increased depressive effects of both drugs.
Sleep inducers*	Increased sedative effect.
Sotalol	Increased narcotic effect. Dangerous sedation.
Tramadol	Increased sedation.
Tranquilizers*	Increased sedative effect.

NARCOTIC ANALGESICS & ACETAMINOPHEN

GENERIC NAME OR DRUG CLASS	COMBINED EFFECT
Phenobarbital and other barbiturates*	Quicker elimination and decreased effect of acetaminophen.
Phenothiazines*	Increased phenothiazine effect.
Sedatives*	Increased sedative effect.
Selegiline	Severe toxicity characterized by breathing difficulty, seizures, coma.
Sertraline	Increased depressive effects of both drugs.

*See Glossary

GENERIC NAME OR DRUG CLASS	COMBINED EFFECT	GENERIC NAME OR DRUG CLASS	COMBINED EFFECT

NARCOTIC ANALGESICS & ACETAMINOPHEN continued

GENERIC NAME OR DRUG CLASS	COMBINED EFFECT
Sleep inducers*	Increased sedative effect.
Sotalol	Increased narcotic effect. Dangerous sedation.
Tetracyclines*	May slow tetracycline absorption. Space doses 2 hours apart.
Tramadol	Increased sedation.
Tranquilizers*	Increased sedative effect.
Zidovudine	Increased toxicity of zidovudine.

NARCOTIC ANALGESICS & ASPIRIN

GENERIC NAME OR DRUG CLASS	COMBINED EFFECT
Antidiabetics,* oral	Low blood sugar.
Anti-inflammatory drugs, nonsteroidal (NSAIDs)*	Risk of stomach bleeding and ulcers.
Aspirin, other	Likely aspirin toxicity.
Bumetanide	Possible aspirin toxicity.
Carteolol	Increased narcotic effect. Dangerous sedation.
Ethacrynic acid	Possible aspirin toxicity.
Furosemide	Possible aspirin toxicity. May decrease furosemide effect.
Gold compounds*	Increased likelihood of kidney damage.
Indomethacin	Risk of stomach bleeding and ulcers.
Methotrexate	Increased methotrexate effect.
Minoxidil	Decreased minoxidil effect.
Narcotics,* other	Increased narcotic effect.
Nitrates*	Excessive blood pressure drop.
Propranolol	Decreased aspirin effect.
Rauwolfia alkaloids*	Decreased aspirin effect.
Salicylates, other*	Likely aspirin toxicity.
Sedatives*	Increased sedative effect.
Selegiline	Severe toxicity characterized by breathing difficulties, seizures, coma.
Sleep inducers*	Increased sedative effect.
Sotalol	Increased narcotic effect. Dangerous sedation.
Spironolactone	Decreased spironolactone effect.
Sulfinpyrazone	Decreased sulfinpyrazone effect.
Ticlopidine	Decreased effects of both drugs.
Tramadol	Increased sedation.
Tranquilizers*	Increased sedative effect.
Valproic acid*	May increase valproic acid effect.
Vitamin C (large doses)	Possible aspirin toxicity.

NEFAZODONE

GENERIC NAME OR DRUG CLASS	COMBINED EFFECT
Haloperidol	Unknown. May need haloperidol dosage adjusted.
Monoamine oxidase (MAO) inhibitors*	Potentially life-threatening. Allow 14 days between use of 2 drugs.

***See Glossary**

NEFAZODONE continued

GENERIC NAME OR DRUG CLASS	COMBINED EFFECT
Pentazocine	Increased effect of pentazocine.
Pimozide	Increased effect of pimozide. Avoid.
Propranolol	Unknown effect. May need dosage adjustment of both drugs.
Terfenadine	Increased effect of terfenadine. Avoid.
Triazolam	Increased effect of triazolam.

NICOTINE

GENERIC NAME OR DRUG CLASS	COMBINED EFFECT
Phenylephrine	Decreased effect of phenylephrine.
Propoxyphene	Increased effect of propoxyphene.
Theophylline	Increased effect of theophylline.

NUCLEOSIDE REVERSE TRANSCRIPTASE INHIBITORS

GENERIC NAME OR DRUG CLASS	COMBINED EFFECT
Probenecid	Increased effect of zidovudine.
Rifamycins	Decreased zidovudine effect.
Tenofovir	Increased effect of didanosine. Take tenofovir 2 hours before or 1 hour after didanosine.
Tetracyclines	Decreased antibiotic effect.
Valproic acid*	Increased effect of zidovudine.

OLANZAPINE

GENERIC NAME OR DRUG CLASS	COMBINED EFFECT
Eszopiclone	Decreased alertness.
Hepatotoxics*	Risk of liver problems.
Levodopa	May decrease levodopa effect.

ORPHENADRINE, ASPIRIN & CAFFEINE

GENERIC NAME OR DRUG CLASS	COMBINED EFFECT
Adrenocorticoids, systemic	Increased risk of ulcers. Increased adrenocorticoid effect.
Allopurinol	Decreased allopurinol effect.
Antacids*	Decreased aspirin effect.
Anticholinergics*	Increased anticholinergic effect.
Anticoagulants*	Increased anticoagulant effect. Abnormal bleeding.
Antidepressants, tricyclic*	Increased sedation.
Antidiabetics, oral*	Low blood sugar.
Anti-inflammatory drugs, nonsteroidal (NSAIDs)*	Risk of stomach bleeding and ulcers.
Aspirin, other	Likely aspirin toxicity.

***See Glossary**

GENERIC NAME OR DRUG CLASS	COMBINED EFFECT	GENERIC NAME OR DRUG CLASS	COMBINED EFFECT

ORPHENADRINE, ASPIRIN & CAFFEINE continued

GENERIC NAME OR DRUG CLASS	COMBINED EFFECT
Chlorpromazine	Hypoglycemia (low blood sugar).
Contraceptives, oral*	Increased caffeine effect.
Furosemide	Possible aspirin toxicity.
Gold compounds*	Increased likelihood of kidney damage.
Griseofulvin	Decreased griseofulvin effect.
Indomethacin	Risk of stomach bleeding and ulcers.
Isoniazid	Increased caffeine effect.
Levodopa	Increased levodopa effect. (Improves effectiveness in treating Parkinson's disease.)
Methotrexate	Increased methotrexate effect.
Minoxidil	Decreased minoxidil effect.
Monoamine oxidase (MAO) inhibitors*	Dangerous blood pressure rise.
Nitrates*	Increased internal eye pressure.
Para-aminosalicylic acid (PAS)	Possible aspirin toxicity.
Penicillins*	Increased effect of drugs.
Phenobarbital	Decreased aspirin effect.
Potassium supplements*	Increased possibility of intestinal ulcers with oral potassium tablets.
Probenecid	Decreased probenecid effect.
Propoxyphene	Possible confusion, nervousness, tremors.
Propranolol	Decreased aspirin effect.
Rauwolfia alkaloids*	Decreased aspirin effect.
Salicylates, other*	Likely aspirin toxicity.
Sedatives*	Decreased sedative effect.
Sleep inducers*	Decreased sedative effect.
Spironolactone	Decreased spirono-lactone effect.
Sulfinpyrazone	Decreased sulfin-pyrazone effect.
Sympathomimetics*	Overstimulation.
Thyroid hormones*	Increased thyroid effect.
Tranquilizers*	Decreased tranquilizer effect.
Valproic acid*	May increase valproic acid effect.
Vitamin C (large doses)	Possible aspirin toxicity.

PHENOTHIAZINES

GENERIC NAME OR DRUG CLASS	COMBINED EFFECT
Doxepin (topical)	Increased risk of toxicity of both drugs.
Duloxetine	Increased effect of duloxetine.
Guanethidine	Increased guanethidine effect.
Isoniazid	Increased risk of liver damage.
Levodopa	Decreased levodopa effect.
Lithium	Decreased lithium effect
Mind-altering drugs*	Increased effect of mind-altering drug.
Molindone	Increased tranquilizer effect.
Narcotics*	Increased narcotic effect.
Procarbazine	Increased sedation.
Quetiapine	Decreased quetiapine effect.
Tramadol	Increased sedation.
Zolpidem	Increased sedation. Avoid.

***See Glossary**

GENERIC NAME OR DRUG CLASS	COMBINED EFFECT	GENERIC NAME OR DRUG CLASS	COMBINED EFFECT

POTASSIUM SUPPLEMENTS

GENERIC NAME OR DRUG CLASS	COMBINED EFFECT
Potassium-containing drugs*	Increased potassium levels.
Spironolactone	Dangerous rise in blood potassium.
Triamterene	Dangerous rise in blood potassium.
Vitamin B-12	Extended-release tablets may decrease vitamin B-12 absorption and increase vitamin B-12 requirements.

PRIMIDONE

GENERIC NAME OR DRUG CLASS	COMBINED EFFECT
Narcotics*	Increased narcotic effect.
Oxyphenbutazone	Decreased oxyphenbutazone effect.
Phenylbutazone	Decreased phenylbutazone effect.
Phenytoin	Possible increased primidone toxicity.
Rifamycins	Possible decreased primidone effect.
Sedatives*	Increased sedative effect.
Sertraline	Increased depressive effects of both drugs.
Sleep inducers*	Increased effect of sleep inducer.
Tranquilizers*	Increased tranquilizer effect.
Valproic acid*	Increased effect of primidone.

PROCARBAZINE

GENERIC NAME OR DRUG CLASS	COMBINED EFFECT
Diuretics*	Excessively low blood pressure.
Doxapram	Increased blood pressure.
Ethinamate	Dangerous increased effects of ethinamate. Avoid combining.
Fluoxetine	Increased depressant effects of both drugs.
Guanethidine	Blood pressure rise to life-threatening level.
Guanfacine	May increase depressant effects of either medicine.
Leucovorin	High alcohol content of leucovorin may cause adverse effects.
Levamisole	Increased risk of bone marrow depression.
Levodopa	Sudden, severe blood pressure rise.
Methyldopa	Severe high blood pressure.
Methylphenidate	Excessive high blood pressure.
Methyprylon	May increase sedative effect to dangerous level. Avoid.
Monoamine oxidase (MAO) inhibitors,* other	High fever, convulsions, death.
Nabilone	Greater depression of central nervous system.
Narcotics*	Increased sedation.
Phenothiazines*	Increased sedation.
Rauwolfia alkaloids*	Very high blood pressure.
Reserpine	Increased blood pressure, excitation.
Sertraline	Increased depressive effects of both drugs.

*See Glossary

PROCARBAZINE continued

GENERIC NAME OR DRUG CLASS	COMBINED EFFECT
Sumatriptan	Adverse effects unknown. Avoid.
Sympathomimetics*	Heartbeat abnormalities, severe high blood pressure.
Tiopronin	Increased risk of toxicity to bone marrow.

PROTEASE INHIBITORS

GENERIC NAME OR DRUG CLASS	COMBINED EFFECT
Protease inhibitor, other	Increased risk of severe heart problem if both saquinavir and ritonavir taken.
Proton pump inhibitors	May need dosage adjustment of protease inhibitor.
Rifabutin	Decreased effect of protease inhibitor.
Rifampin	Decreased protease inhibitor effect. Don't use with saquinavir.
Trazodone	Increased trazodone effect.
Warfarin	Increased or decreased warfarin effect.

QUETIAPINE

GENERIC NAME OR DRUG CLASS	COMBINED EFFECT
Levodopa or dopamine agonists*	Decreased effect of levodopa or dopamine agonist.
Phenytoin	Decreased quetiapine effect.
Thioridazine	Decreased quetiapine effect.

RAUWOLFIA ALKALOIDS

GENERIC NAME OR DRUG CLASS	COMBINED EFFECT
Lisinopril	Increased anti-hypertensive effect. Dosage of each may require adjustment.
Loxapine	May increase toxic effects of both drugs.
Methyprylon	May increase sedative effect to dangerous level. Avoid.
Mind-altering drugs*	Excessive sedation.
Monoamine oxidase (MAO) inhibitors*	Severe depression.
Nabilone	Greater depression of central nervous system.
Nicardipine	Blood pressure drop. Dosages may require adjustment.
Nimodipine	Dangerous blood pressure drop.
Pergolide	Decreased pergolide effect.
Pseudoephedrine	Increased effect of either drug.
Sertraline	Increased depressive effects of both drugs.
Sotalol	Decreased antihypertensive effect.
Terazosin	Decreased effectiveness of terazosin.

*See Glossary

RESERPINE, HYDRALAZINE & HYDROCHLOROTHIAZIDE

GENERIC NAME OR DRUG CLASS	COMBINED EFFECT
Amphetamines*	Decreased hydralazine effect.
Anticoagulants,* oral	Unpredictable increased or decreased effect of anticoagulant.
Anticonvulsants*	Serious change in seizure pattern.
Antidepressants, tricyclic*	Dangerous drop in blood pressure. Avoid combination unless under medical supervision.
Antihistamines*	Increased anti-histamine effect.
Antihypertensives, other*	Increased anti-hypertensive effect.
Anti-inflammatory drugs, nonsteroidal (NSAIDs)*	Decreased hydralazine effect.
Aspirin	Decreased aspirin effect.
Barbiturates*	Increased hydro-chlorothiazide effect.
Beta-adrenergic blocking agents*	Increased effect of reserpine. Excessive sedation.
Carteolol	Increased anti-hypertensive effect.
Cholestyramine	Decreased hydro-chlorothiazide effect.
Cortisone drugs*	Excessive potassium loss that causes dangerous heart rhythms.
Diazoxide	Increased anti-hypertensive effect.
Digitalis preparations*	Excessive potassium loss that causes dangerous heart rhythms.
Diuretics, oral*	Increased effects of drugs. When monitored carefully, combination may be beneficial in controlling hypertension.
Dronabinol	Increased effects of drugs.
Indapamide	Increased diuretic effect.
Levodopa	Decreased levodopa effect.
Lisinopril	Increased anti-hypertensive effect. Dosage of each may require adjustment.
Lithium	Increased lithium effect.
Mind-altering drugs*	Excessive sedation.
Monoamine oxidase (MAO) inhibitors*	Increased effects of both drugs. Severe depression.
Nicardipine	Blood pressure drop. Dosages may require adjustment.
Nimodipine	Dangerous blood pressure drop.
Nitrates*	Excessive blood pressure drop.
Oxprenolol	Increased anti-hypertensive effect. Dosages of drugs may require adjustments.
Pergolide	Decreased pergolide effect.
Potassium supplements*	Decreased potassium effect.
Probenecid	Decreased probenecid effect.
Sotalol	Decreased anti-hypertensive effect.
Terazosin	Decreased effectiveness of terazosin.

*See Glossary

GENERIC NAME OR DRUG CLASS	COMBINED EFFECT

RIFAMYCINS

GENERIC NAME OR DRUG CLASS	COMBINED EFFECT
Phenytoin	Decreased phenytoin effect.
Probenecid	Possible toxicity to liver.
Protease inhibitors	Decreased protease inhibitor effect.
Quinidine	Decreased effect of both drugs.
Quinine	Decreased quinine effect.
Sildenafil	Decreased sildenafil effect.
Tacrolimus	Decreased tacrolimus effect.
Telithromycin	Decreased effect of rifampin.
Theophylline	Decreased theophylline effect.
Tocainide	Possible decreased blood cell production in bone marrow.
Trimethoprim	Decreased trimethoprim effect.
Valproic acid*	Decreased effect of valproic acid with rifampin.
Zaleplon	Decreased zaleplon effect.
Zidovudine	Decreased zidovudine effect.

SALICYLATES

GENERIC NAME OR DRUG CLASS	COMBINED EFFECT
Insulin lispro	May need decreased dosage of insulin.
Ketoconazole	Decreased keto-conazole effect with buffered salicylates.
Methotrexate	Increased metho-trexate effect and toxicity.
Para-aminosalicylic acid	Possible salicylate toxicity.
Penicillins*	Increased effect of both drugs.
Phenobarbital	Decreased salicylate effect.
Phenytoin	Increased phenytoin effect.
Probenecid	Decreased probenecid effect.
Rauwolfia alkaloids*	Decreased salicylate effect.
Salicylates,* other	Likely salicylate toxicity.
Sotalol	Decreased antihypertensive effect of sotalol.
Spironolactone	Decreased spirono-lactone effect.
Sulfinpyrazone	Decreased sulfin-pyrazone effect.
Terazosin	Decreased effective-ness of terazosin. Causes sodium and fluid retention.
Urinary acidifiers*	Decreased excretion. Increased salicylate effect.
Urinary alkalizers*	Increased excretion. Decreased salicylate effect.
Vitamin C (large doses)	Possible salicylate toxicity.
Zidovudine	increased zidovudine effect.

SCOPOLAMINE (Hyoscine)

GENERIC NAME OR DRUG CLASS	COMBINED EFFECT
Nabilone	Greater depression of central nervous system.
Nitrates*	Increased internal eye pressure.
Nizatidine	Increased nizatidine effect.

*See Glossary

GENERIC NAME OR DRUG CLASS	COMBINED EFFECT	GENERIC NAME OR DRUG CLASS	COMBINED EFFECT

SCOPOLAMINE (Hyoscine) continued

GENERIC NAME OR DRUG CLASS	COMBINED EFFECT
Orphenadrine	Increased scopolamine effect.
Phenothiazines*	Increased scopolamine effect.
Pilocarpine	Loss of pilocarpine effect in glaucoma treatment.
Potassium supplements*	Possible intestinal ulcers with oral potassium tablets.
Quinidine	Increased scopolamine effect.
Sedatives* or central nervous system (CNS) depressants*	Increased sedative effect of both drugs.
Sertraline	Increased depressive effects of both drugs.
Vitamin C	Decreased scopolamine effect. Avoid large doses of vitamin C.

SELECTIVE SEROTONIN REUPTAKE INHIBITORS (SSRIs)

GENERIC NAME OR DRUG CLASS	COMBINED EFFECT
Benzodiazepines*	Increased benzo-diazepine effect.
Bromocriptine	Increased risk of serotonin syndrome.*
Buspirone	Increased risk of serotonin syndrome.*
Desmopressin	Increased risk of thirstiness which may lead to drinking excess fluids.
Dextromethorphan	Increased risk of serotonin syndrome.*
Digoxin	Increased risk of side effects of both drugs.
Levodopa	Increased risk of serotonin syndrome.*
Lithium	Increased risk of serotonin syndrome.*
Meperidine	Increased risk of serotonin syndrome.*
Moclobemide	Increased risk of side effects and serotonin syndrome.*
Monoamine oxidase (MAO) inhibitors*	Increased risk of adverse effects. May lead to convulsions and hypertensive crisis. Let 14 days elapse between taking the 2 drugs.
Nefazodone	Increased risk of serotonin syndrome.*
Pentazocine	Increased risk of serotonin syndrome.*
Phenytoin	Increased effect of phenytoin.
Propranolol	Increased effect of propranolol.
Ramelteon	Increased effect of ramelteon. Avoid.
Serotonergics*	Increased risk of serotonin syndrome.*
Sumatriptan	Increased risk of serotonin syndrome.*
Theophylline	Increased effect of theophylline.
Tizanidine	Dangerous increased tizanidine effect with fluvoxamine.

SEROTONIN & NOREPINEPHRINE REUPTAKE INHIBITORS (SNRIs)

GENERIC NAME OR DRUG CLASS	COMBINED EFFECT
Serotonergics*	Increased risk of serotonin syndrome.*
Tramadol	Increased risk of serotonin syndrome.*
Trazodone	Increased risk of serotonin syndrome.*
Tryptophan	Increased risk of serotonin syndrome.*

***See Glossary**

GENERIC NAME OR DRUG CLASS	COMBINED EFFECT	GENERIC NAME OR DRUG CLASS	COMBINED EFFECT

SEROTONIN & NOREPINEPHRINE REUPTAKE INHIBITORS (SNRIs) continued

GENERIC NAME OR DRUG CLASS	COMBINED EFFECT
Venlafaxine	Increased risk of serotonin syndrome.*

SULFONYLUREAS

GENERIC NAME OR DRUG CLASS	COMBINED EFFECT
Insulin	Increased blood sugar lowering.
Insulin lispro	Increased anti-diabetic effect.
Isoniazid	Decreased blood sugar lowering.
Labetalol	Increased blood sugar lowering, may mask hypoglycemia.
Leukotriene modifiers	Increased effect of tolbutamide.
MAO inhibitors*	Increased blood sugar lowering.
Nicotinic acid	Decreased blood sugar lowering.
Oxyphenbutazone	Increased blood sugar lowering.
Phenothiazines*	Decreased blood sugar lowering.
Phenylbutazone	Increased blood sugar lowering.
Phenyramidol	Increased blood sugar lowering.
Phenytoin	Decreased blood sugar lowering.
Probenecid	Increased blood sugar lowering.
Pyrazinamide	Decreased blood sugar lowering.
Ranitidine	Increased blood sugar lowering.
Rifamycins	Decreased blood sugar lowering.
Sulfa drugs*	Increased blood sugar lowering.
Sulfadoxine and pyrimethamine	Increased risk of toxicity.
Sulfaphenazole	Increased blood sugar lowering.
Thiazolidinediones*	May decrease plasma glucose concentrations.
Thyroid hormones*	Decreased blood sugar lowering.
Zafirlukast	May increase effect of tolbutamide.

TETRACYCLINES

GENERIC NAME OR DRUG CLASS	COMBINED EFFECT
Tiopronin	Increased risk of toxicity to kidneys (except with doxycycline and minocycline).
Vitamin A	Increased risk of intracranial hypertension.
Zinc supplements	Decreased tetracycline absorption if taken within 2 hours of each other.

THIOTHIXENE

GENERIC NAME OR DRUG CLASS	COMBINED EFFECT
Sertraline	Increased depressive effects of both drugs.
Tranquilizers*	Increased thiothixene effect. Excessive sedation.

VALPROIC ACID

GENERIC NAME OR DRUG CLASS	COMBINED EFFECT
Salicylates*	Increased effect of valproic acid.
Zidovudine	Increased effect of zidovudine.

***See Glossary**

Glossary

Many of the following medical terms are found in the drug charts. Where drug names are listed, they indicate the generic or drug class and not the brand names.

A

ACE Inhibitors—See Angiotensin-Converting Enzyme (ACE) Inhibitors.

Acne Preparations—Creams, lotions and liquids applied to the skin to treat acne. These include adapalene; alcohol and acetone; alcohol and sulfur; azelaic acid; benzoyl peroxide; clindamycin; erythromycin; erythromycin and benzoyl peroxide; isotretinoin; meclocycline; resorcinol; resorcinol and sulfur; salicylic acid gel USP; salicylic acid lotion; salicylic acid ointment; salicylic acid pads; salicylic acid soap; salicylic acid and sulfur bar soap; salicylic acid and sulfur cleansing lotion; salicylic acid and sulfur cleansing suspension; salicylic acid and sulfur lotion; sulfurated lime; sulfur bar soap; sulfur cream; sulfur lotion; tetracycline, oral; tetracycline hydrochloride for topical solution; tretinoin.

Acridine Derivatives—Dyes or stains (usually yellow or orange) used for some medical tests and as antiseptic agents.

Acute—Having a short and relatively severe course.

Addiction—Psychological or physiological dependence upon a drug.

Addictive Drugs—Any drug that can lead to physiological dependence on the drug. These include alcohol, cocaine, marijuana, nicotine, opium, morphine, codeine, heroin (and other narcotics) and others.

Addison's Disease—Changes in the body caused by a deficiency of hormones manufactured by the adrenal gland. Usually fatal if untreated.

Adrenal Cortex—Center of the adrenal gland.

Adrenal Gland—Gland next to the kidney that produces cortisone and epinephrine (adrenalin).

Agranulocytosis—A symptom complex characterized by (1) a sharply decreased number of granulocytes (one of the types of white blood cells), (2) lesions of the throat and other mucous membranes, (3) lesions of the gastrointestinal tract and (4) lesions of the skin. Sometimes also called granulocytopenia.

Alkalizers—These drugs neutralize acidic properties of the blood and urine by making them more alkaline (or basic). Systemic alkalizers include potassium citrate and citric acid, sodium bicarbonate, sodium citrate and citric acid, and tricitrates. Urinary alkalizers include potassium citrate, potassium citrate and citric acid, potassium citrate and sodium citrate, sodium citrate and citric acid.

Alkylating Agent—Chemical used to treat malignant diseases.

Allergy—Excessive sensitivity to a substance that is ordinarily harmless. Reactions include sneezing, stuffy nose, hives, itching.

Alpha-Adrenergic Blocking Agents—A group of drugs used to treat hypertension. These drugs include alfuzosin, prazosin, terazosin, doxazosin and labetalol (an alpha-adrenergic and beta-adrenergic combination drug). Also included are other drugs that produce an alpha-adrenergic blocking action such as haloperidol, loxapine, phenothiazines, thioxanthenes.

Amebiasis—Infection with amoebas, one-celled organisms. Causes diarrhea, fever and abdominal cramps.

Amenorrhea—Abnormal absence of menstrual periods.

Aminoglycosides—A family of antibiotics used for serious infections. Their usefulness is limited because of their relative toxicity compared to some other antibiotics. These drugs include amikacin, gentamicin, kanamycin, neomycin, netilmicin, streptomycin, tobramycin.

Amphetamines—A family of drugs that stimulates the central nervous system, prescribed to treat attention-deficit disorders in children and also for narcolepsy. They are habit-forming, are controlled under U.S. law and are no longer prescribed as appetite suppressants. These drugs include amphetamine, dextroamphetamine, lisdexamfetamine, methamphetamine. They may be ingredients of several combination drugs.

ANA Titers—A test to evaluate the immune system and to detect antinuclear antibodies (ANAs), substances that appear in the blood of some patients with autoimmune disease.

Analgesics—Agents that reduce pain without reducing consciousness.

Anaphylaxis—Severe allergic response to a substance. Symptoms are wheezing, itching, hives, nasal congestion, intense burning of hands and feet, collapse, loss of consciousness and cardiac arrest. Symptoms appear within a few seconds or minutes after exposure. Anaphylaxis is a severe medical emergency. Without appropriate treatment, it can cause death. Instructions for home treatment for anaphylaxis are at the end of the book.

Androgens—Male hormones, including fluoxymesterone, methyltestosterone, testosterone, DHEA.

Anemia—Not enough healthy red blood cells in the bloodstream or too little hemoglobin in the red blood cells. Anemia is caused by an imbalance between blood loss and blood production.

Anemia, Aplastic—A form of anemia in which the bone marrow is unable to manufacture adequate numbers of blood cells of all types—red cells, white cells, and platelets.

Anemia, Hemolytic—Anemia caused by a shortened lifespan of red blood cells. The body can't manufacture new cells fast enough to replace old cells.

Anemia, Iron-Deficiency—Anemia caused when iron necessary to manufacture red blood cells is not available.

Anemia, Pernicious—Anemia caused by a vitamin B-12 deficiency. Symptoms include weakness, fatigue, numbness and tingling of the hands or feet and degeneration of the central nervous system.

Anemia, Sickle-Cell—Anemia caused by defective hemoglobin that deprives red blood cells of oxygen, making them sickle-shaped.

Anesthesias, General—Gases that are used in surgery to render patients unconscious and able to withstand the pain of surgical cutting and manipulation. They include alfentanil, amobarbital, butabarbital, butorphanol, chloral hydrate, enflurane, etomidate, fentanyl, halothane, hydroxyzine, isoflurane, ketamine, levorphanol, meperidine, methohexital, methoxyflurane, midazolam, morphine parenteral, nalbuphine, nitrous oxide, oxymorphone, pentazocine, pentobarbital, phenobarbital, promethazine, propiomazine, propofol, scopolamine, secobarbital, sufentanil, thiamylal, thiopental.

Anesthetics—Drugs that eliminate the sensation of pain.

Angina (Angina Pectoris)—Chest pain with a sensation of suffocation and impending death. Caused by a temporary reduction in the amount of oxygen to the heart muscle through diseased coronary arteries. The pain may also occur in the left shoulder, jaw or arm.

Angiotensin-Converting Enzyme (ACE) Inhibitors—A family of drugs used to treat hypertension and congestive heart failure. Inhibitors decrease the rate of conversion of angiotensin I into angiotensin II, which is the normal process for the angiotensin-converting enzyme. These drugs include benazepril, captopril, enalapril, fosinopril, lisinopril, moexipril, perindopril, quinapril, ramipril, trandolapril.

Antacids—A large family of drugs prescribed to treat hyperacidity, peptic ulcer, esophageal reflux and other conditions. These drugs include alumina and magnesia; alumina, magnesia and calcium carbonate; alumina, magnesia and simethicone; alumina and magnesium carbonate; alumina and magnesium trisilicate; alumina, magnesium trisilicate and sodium bicarbonate; aluminum carbonate; aluminum hydroxide; bismuth subsalicylate; calcium carbonate; calcium carbonate and magnesia; calcium carbonate, magnesia and simethicone; calcium and magnesium carbonates; calcium and magnesium carbonates and magnesium oxide; calcium carbonate and simethicone; dihydroxyaluminum aminoacetate; dihydroxyaluminum sodium carbonate; magaldrate; magaldrate and simethicone; magnesium carbonate and sodium bicarbonate; magnesium hydroxide; magnesium oxide; magnesium trisilicate, alumina and magnesia; simethicone, alumina, calcium carbonate and magnesia; simethicone, alumina, magnesium carbonate and magnesia; sodium bicarbonate.

Antacids, Calcium Carbonate—These antacids include calcium carbonate and magnesium, calcium carbonate and simethicone, calcium carbonate and magnesium carbonates.

Antacids, Magnesium-Containing—These antacids include magnesium carbonate, magnesium hydroxide, magnesium oxide and magnesium trisilicate. All these medicines are designed to treat excess stomach acidity. In addition to being an effective antacid, magnesium can sometimes cause unpleasant side effects and drug interactions. Look for the presence of magnesium in nonprescription drugs.

Anthelmintics—A family of drugs used to treat intestinal parasites. Names of these drugs include niclosamide, piperazine, pyrantel, pyrvinium, quinacrine, mebendazole, metronidazole, oxamniquine, praziquantel, thiabendazole.

Antiacne Topical Preparations—See Acne Preparations.

Antiadrenals—Medicines or drugs that prevent the effects of the hormones produced by the adrenal glands.

Antianginals—A group of drugs used to treat angina pectoris (chest pain that comes and goes, caused by coronary artery disease). These drugs include acebutolol, amlodipine, amyl nitrite, atenolol, bepridil, carteolol, diltiazem, felodipine, isosorbide dinitrate, labetalol, metoprolol, nadolol, nicardipine, nifedipine, nitroglycerin, oxprenolol, penbutolol, pindolol, propranolol, sotalol, timolol, verapamil.

Antianxiety Drugs—A group of drugs prescribed to treat anxiety. These drugs include alprazolam, bromazepam, buspirone, chlordiazepoxide, chlorpromazine, clomipramine, clorazepate, diazepam, halazepam, hydroxyzine, imipramine, ketazolam, lorazepam, meprobamate, oxazepam, prazepam, prochlorperazine, thioridazine, trifluoperazine, venlafaxine.

Antiarrhythmics—A group of drugs used to treat heartbeat irregularities (arrhythmias). These drugs include acebutolol, adenosine, amiodarone, atenolol, atropine, bretylium, deslanoside, digitalis, digitoxin, diltiazem, disopyramide, dofetilide, edrophonium, encainide, esmolol, flecainide, glycopyrrolate, hyoscyamine, lidocaine, methoxamine, metoprolol, mexiletine, nadolol, oxprenolol, phenytoin, propafenone, propranolol, quinidine, scopolamine, sotalol, timolol, verapamil.

Antiasthmatics—Medicines used to treat asthma, which may be tablets, liquids or aerosols (to be inhaled to get directly to the bronchial tubes rather than through the bloodstream). These medicines include adrenocorticoids, glucocorticoid; albuterol; aminophylline; astemizole; beclomethasone; bitolterol; budesonide; cetirizine; corticotropin; cromolyn; dexamethasone; dyphylline; ephedrine; epinephrine; ethylnorepinephrine; fenoterol; flunisolide; fluticasone; ipratropium, isoetharine; isoproterenol; isoproterenol and phenylephrine; loratadine; metaproterenol; oxtriphylline; oxtriphylline and guaifenesin; pirbuterol; racepinephrine; terbutaline; theophylline; theophylline and guaifenesin; triamcinolone.

Antibacterials (Antibiotics)—A group of drugs prescribed to treat infections. These drugs include, amikacin, amoxicillin, amoxicillin and clavulanate, ampicillin, azithromycin, azlocillin, aztreonam, bacampicillin, carbenicillin, cefaclor, cefadroxil, cefamandole, cefazolin, cefonicid, cefoperazone, ceforanide, cefotaxime, cefotetan, cefoxitin, ceftazidime, ceftibuten, ceftizoxime, ceftriaxone, cefuroxime, cephalexin, cephalothin, cephapirin, cephradine, chloramphenicol, cinoxacin, clarithromycin, clindamycin, cloxacillin, cyclacillin, cycloserine, demeclocycline, dicloxacillin, dirithromycin, doxycycline, erythromycin, erythromycin and sulfisoxazole, fidaxomicin, flucloxacillin, fusidic acid, gentamicin, imipenem and cilastatin, kanamycin, lincomycin, methacycline, methenamine, methicillin, metronidazole, mezlocillin, minocycline, moxalactam, nafcillin, nalidixic acid, netilmicin, nitrofurantoin, norfloxacin, oxacillin, oxytetracycline, penicillin G, penicillin V, piperacillin, pivampicillin, rifabutin, rifampin, rifaximin, spectinomycin, streptomycin, sulfacytine, sulfadiazine and trimethoprim, sulfamethoxazole, sulfamethoxazole and trimethoprim, sulfisoxazole, telithromycin, tetracycline, ticarcillin, ticarcillin and clavulanate, tinidazole, tobramycin, trimethoprim, vancomycin.

Antibiotics—Chemicals that inhibit the growth of or kill germs. See Antibacterials.

Anticholinergics—Drugs that work against acetylcholine, a chemical found in many locations in the body, including connections between nerve cells and connections between muscle and nerve cells. Anticholinergic drugs include aclidinium. amantadine, anisotropine, atropine, belladonna, benztropine, biperiden, clidinium, darifenacin, dicyclomine, glycopyrrolate, homatropine, hyoscyamine, ipratropium, isopropamide, mepenzolate, methantheline, methscopolamine, oxybutynin, pirenzepine, propantheline, scopolamine, solifenacin, tolterodine, trihexyphenidyl, trospium.

Anticoagulants—A family of drugs prescribed to slow the rate of blood clotting. These drugs include acenocoumarol, anisindione, dicumarol, dihydroergotamine and heparin, heparin, warfarin.

Anticonvulsants—A group of drugs prescribed to treat or prevent seizures (convulsions). These drugs include these families: barbiturates, carbonic anhydrase inhibitors, diones, hydantoins and succinimides. These are the names of the generic drugs in these families: acetazolamide, amobarbital, carbamazepine, carbonic anhydrase inhibitors, clobazam, clonazepam, clorazepate, diazepam, dichlorphenamide, divalproex, ethosuximide, ethotoin, felbamate, fosphenytoin, gabapentin, lacosamide, lamotrigine, levetiracetam lorazepam, mephenytoin, mephobarbital, metharbital, methsuximide, nitrazepam, oxcarbazepine, paraldehyde, phenacemide, paramethadione, pentobarbital, phenobarbital, phenytoin, primidone, secobarbital, tiagabine, topiramate, trimethadione, valproic acid, zonisamide.

Antidepressants—A group of medicines prescribed to treat mental depression. These drugs include amitriptyline, amoxapine, bupropion, citalopram, clomipramine, desipramine, doxepin, duloxetine, escitalopram, fluoxetine, fluvoxamine, imipramine, isocarboxazid, lithium, maprotiline, mirtazapine, moclobemide, nefazodone, nortriptyline, paroxetine, phenelzine, protriptyline, sertraline, tranylcypromine, trazodone, trimipramine, venlafaxine.

Antidepressants, MAO (Monoamine Oxidase) Inhibitors—A special group of drugs prescribed for mental depression. These are not as popular as in years past because of a relatively high incidence of adverse effects. These drugs include isocarboxazid (Marplan), phenelzine (Nardil), tranylcypromine (Parnate).

Antidepressants, Tricyclic (TCAs)—A group of medicines with similar chemical structure and pharmacologic activity used to treat mental depression. These drugs include amitriptyline, amoxapine, clomipramine, desipramine, doxepin, imipramine, nortriptyline, protriptyline, trimipramine.

Antidiabetic Agents—A group of drugs used in the treatment of diabetes. These medicines all reduce blood sugar. These drugs include acarbose, acetohexamide, chlorpropamide, gliclazide, glimepiride, glipizide, glyburide, insulin, linagliptin, metformin, nateglinide, pioglitazone, repaglinide, rosiglitazone, saxagliptin, sitagliptin, tolazamide, tolbutamide, troglitazone.

Antidiarrheal Preparations—Medicines that treat diarrhea symptoms. Most do not cure the cause. Oral medicines include aluminum hydroxide; charcoal, activated; kaolin and pectin; loperamide; polycarbophil; psyllium hydrophilic mucilloid. Systemic medicines include carbohydrates; codeine; difenoxin and atropine; diphenoxylate and atropine; glucose and electrolytes; glycopyrrolate; kaolin, pectin, belladonna alkaloids and opium; kaolin, pectin and paregoric; nitazoxanide, opium tincture; paregoric, rifaximin.

Antidyskinetics—A group of drugs used for treatment of Parkinsonism (paralysis agitans) and drug-induced extrapyramidal reactions (see elsewhere in Glossary). These drugs include amantadine, benztropine, biperiden, bromocriptine, carbidopa and levodopa, diphenhydramine, entacapone, ethopropazine, levodopa, levodopa and benserazide, procyclidine, rasagiline, selegiline, trihexyphenidyl.

Antiemetics—A group of drugs used to treat nausea and vomiting. These drugs include buclizine, cyclizine, chlorpromazine, dimenhydrinate, diphenhydramine, diphenidol, domperidone, dronabinol, haloperidol, hydroxyzine, meclizine, metoclopramide, nabilone, ondansetron, perphenazine, prochlorperazine, promethazine, scopolamine, thiethylperazine, triflupromazine, trimethobenzamide.

Antifibrinolytic Drugs—Drugs that are used to treat serious bleeding. These drugs include aminocaproic acid and tranexamic acid.

Antifungals—A group of drugs used to treat fungus infections. Those listed as systemic are taken orally or given by injection. Those listed as topical are applied directly to the skin and include liquids, powders, creams, ointments and liniments. Those listed as vaginal are used topically inside the vagina and sometimes on the vaginal lips. These drugs include: Systemic—amphotericin B, miconazole, fluconazole, flucytosine, griseofulvin, itraconazole, ketoconazole, potassium iodide, posaconazole, terbinafine. Topical— amphotericin B, carbol-fuchsin, ciclopirox; clioquinol, clotrimazole, econazole, haloprogin, ketoconazole, mafenide, miconazole, naftifine, nystatin, oxiconazole, salicylic acid, silver sulfadiazine, sulconazole, sulfur and coal, terbinafine, tioconazole, tolnaftate, undecylenic acid. Vaginal—butoconazole, clotrimazole, econazole, gentian violet, miconazole, nystatin, terconazole, tioconazole.

Antifungals, Azole—Drugs used to treat certain types of fungal infections. These drugs include fluconazole, itraconazole, ketoconazole, miconazole, posaconazole, sertaconazole, voriconazole.

Antiglaucoma Drugs—Medicines used to treat glaucoma. Those listed as systemic are taken orally or given by injection. Those listed as ophthalmic are for external use. These drugs include: Systemic—acetazolamide, dichlorphenamide, glycerin, mannitol, methazolamide, timolol, urea. Ophthalmic—apraclonidine, betaxolol, bimatoprost, brimonidine, brinzolamide, carbachol ophthalmic solution, carteolol, demecarium, dipivefrin, dorzolamide, echothiophate, epinephrine, epinephrine bitartrate, epinephryl borate, isoflurophate, isopropyl unoprostone, latanoprost, levobetaxolol, levobunolol, metipranolol, physostigmine, pilocarpine, tafluprost, timolol, travoprost, unoprostone.

Antigout Drugs—Drugs to treat the metabolic disease called gout. Gout causes recurrent attacks of joint pain caused by deposits of uric acid in the joints. Antigout drugs include allopurinol, carprofen, colchicine, febuxostat, fenoprofen, ibuprofen, indomethacin, ketoprofen, naproxen, phenylbutazone, piroxicam, probenecid, probenecid and colchicine, sulfinpyrazone, sulindac.

Antihistamines—A family of drugs used to treat allergic conditions, such as hay fever, allergic conjunctivitis, itching, sneezing, runny nose, motion sickness, dizziness, sedation, insomnia and others. These drugs include astemizole, azatadine, brompheniramine, carbinoxamine, cetirizine, chlorpheniramine, clemastine, cyproheptadine, desloratadine, dexchlorpheniramine, dimenhydrinate, diphenhydramine, diphenylpyraline, doxylamine, fexofenadine, hydroxyzine, loratadine, phenindamine, promethazine, pyrilamine, trimeprazine, tripelennamine, triprolidine.

Antihyperammonemias—Medications that decrease the amount of ammonia in the blood. The ones with this pharmacological property that are available in the United States are lactulose, sodium benzoate and sodium phenylacetate.

Antihyperlipidemics—A group of drugs used to treat hyperlipidemia (high levels of lipids in the blood). These include atorvastatin, cerivastatin, cholestyramine, clofibrate, colesevelam, colestipol, ezetimibe, fenofibrate, fluvastatin, gemfibrozil, lovastatin, niacin, pitavastatin, pravastatin, probucol, simvastatin, sodium dichloroacetate.

Antihypertensives—Drugs used to help lower high blood pressure. These medicines can be used singly or in combination with other drugs. They work best if accompanied by a low-salt, low-fat diet plus an active exercise program. These drugs include acebutolol, amiloride, amiloride and hydrochlorothiazide, amlodipine, atenolol, atenolol and chlorthalidone, benazepril, bendroflumethiazide, benzthiazide, betaxolol, bisoprolol, bumetanide, candesartan, captopril, captopril and hydrochlorothiazide, carteolol, carvedilol, chlorothiazide, chlorthalidone, cilazapril, clonidine, clonidine and chlorthalidone, cyclothiazide, debrisoquine, deserpidine, deserpidine and hydrochlorothiazide, deserpidine and methyclothiazide, diazoxide, diltiazem, doxazosin, enalapril, enalapril and hydrochlorothiazide, eplerenone, eprosartan ethacrynic acid, felodipine, fosinopril, furosemide, guanabenz, guanadrel, guanethidine, guanethidine and hydrochlorothiazide, guanfacine, hydralazine, hydralazine and hydrochlorothiazide, hydrochlorothiazide, hydroflumethiazide, indapamide, irbesartan isradipine, labetalol, labetalol and hydrochlorothiazide, lisinopril, lisinopril and hydrochlorothiazide, losartan, losartan and hydrochlorothiazide, mecamylamine, methyclothiazide, methyldopa, methyldopa and chlorothiazide, methyldopa and hydrochlorothiazide, metolazone, metoprolol, metoprolol and hydrochlorothiazide, minoxidil, moexipril, nadolol, nadolol and bendroflumethiazide, nicardipine, nifedipine, nisoldipine, nitroglycerin, nitroprusside, olmesartan, oxprenolol, penbutolol, perindopril, pindolol, pindolol and hydrochlorothiazide, polythiazide, prazosin, prazosin and polythiazide, propranolol, propranolol and hydrochlorothiazide, quinapril, quinethazone, ramipril, rauwolfia serpentina, rauwolfia serpentina and bendroflumethiazide, reserpine, reserpine and chlorothiazide, reserpine and chlorthalidone, reserpine and hydralazine, reserpine, hydralazine and hydrochlorothiazide, reserpine and hydrochlorothiazide, reserpine and hydroflumethiazide, reserpine and methyclothiazide, reserpine and polythiazide, reserpine and quinethazone, reserpine and trichlormethiazide, sotalol, spironolactone, spironolactone and hydrochlorothiazide, telmisartan, terazosin, timolol, timolol and hydrochlorothiazide, torsemide, trandolapril, triamterene, triamterene and hydrochlorothiazide, trichlormethiazide, trimethaphan, valsartan, verapamil.

Anti-Inflammatory Drugs, Nonsteroidal (NSAIDs)—A family of drugs not related to cortisone or other steroids that decrease inflammation wherever it occurs in the body. Used for treatment of pain, fever, arthritis, gout, menstrual cramps and vascular headaches. These drugs include aspirin; aspirin, alumina and magnesia tablets; buffered aspirin; bufexamac; celecoxib; choline salicylate; choline and magnesium salicylates; diclofenac, diflunisal; fenoprofen; flurbiprofen, ibuprofen; indomethacin; ketoprofen; magnesium salicylate; meclofenamate; meloxicam; naproxen; piroxicam; rofecoxib; salsalate; sodium salicylate; sulindac; tolmetin.

Anti-Inflammatory Drugs, Steroidal—A family of drugs with pharmacologic characteristics similar to those of cortisone and cortisone-like drugs. They are used for many purposes to help the body deal with inflammation no matter what the cause. Steroidal drugs may be taken orally or by injection (systemic) or applied locally (topical) for the skin, eyes, ears, bronchial tubes and others. These drugs include: Nasal—beclomethasone, budesonide, dexamethasone, flunisolide, fluticasone, triamcinolone. Ophthalmic (eyes)—betamethasone, dexamethasone, fluorometholone, hydrocortisone, medrysone, prednisolone, rimexolone. Otic (ears)—betamethasone, desonide and acetic acid, dexamethasone, hydrocortisone, hydrocortisone and acetic acid, prednisolone. Systemic—betamethasone, corticotropin, cortisone, dexamethasone, hydrocortisone, methylprednisolone, paramethasone, prednisolone, prednisone, triamcinolone. Topical—alclometasone; amcinonide; beclomethasone; betamethasone; clobetasol; clobetasone; clocortolone; desonide; desoximetasone; dexamethasone; diflorasone; diflucortolone; flumethasone; fluocinolone; fluocinonide; fluocinonide; flurandrenolide; fluticasone; halcinonide; halobetasol; mometasone; procinonide and ciprocinonide; flurandrenolide; halcinonide; hydrocortisone; methylprednisolone; mometasone; triamcinolone.

Antimalarials (also called Antiprotozoals)—A group of drugs used to treat malaria. The choice depends on the precise type of malaria organism and its developmental state. These drugs include amphotericin B, atovaquone and proguanil, clindamycin, chloroquine, dapsone, demeclocycline, doxycycline, halofantrine; hydroxychloroquine, iodoquinol, methacycline, mefloquine, metronidazole, minocycline, oxytetracycline, pentamidine, primaquine, proguanil, pyrimethamine, quinacrine, quinidine, quinine, sulfadoxine and pyrimethamine, sulfamethoxazole, sulfamethoxazole and trimethoprim, sulfisoxazole, tetracycline.

Antimuscarinics—Drugs that relax smooth muscle such as the detrusor muscle in the bladder. They can also decrease the secretion of saliva, sweat and digestive juice. Some dilate the eyes.

Antimyasthenics—Medicines to treat myasthenia gravis, a muscle disorder (especially of the face and head) with increasing fatigue and weakness as muscles tire from use. These medicines include ambenonium, neostigmine, pyridostigmine.

Antineoplastics—Potent drugs used for malignant disease. Some of these are not described in this book, but they are listed here for completeness. These drugs include: Systemic—amifostine, altretamine, aminoglutethimide, amsacrine, anastrazole, antithyroid agents, asparaginase, azathioprine, bicalutamide, bleomycin, busulfan, capecitabine, carboplatin, carmustine, chlorambucil, chloramphenicol, chlorotrianisene, chromic phosphate, cisplatin, colchicine, cyclophosphamide, cyclosporine, cyproterone, cytarabine, dacarbazine, dactinomycin, daunorubicin, deferoxamine, diethylstilbestrol, docetaxel, doxorubicin, dromostanolone, epirubicin, estradiol, estradiol valerate, estramustine, estrogens (conjugated and esterified), estrone, ethinyl estradiol, etoposide, exemestane, floxuridine, flucytosine, fluorouracil, flutamide, fluoxymesterone, gemcitabine, gold compounds, goserelin, hexamethylmelamine, hydroxyprogesterone, hydroxyurea, ifosfamide, interferon alfa-2a and alfa-2b (recombinant), ketoconazole, letrozole, leucovorin, leuprolide, levamisole, levothyroxine, liothyronine, liotrix, lithium, lomustine, masoprocol, mechlorethamine, medroxyprogesterone, megestrol, melphalan, methyltestosterone, mercaptopurine, methotrexate, mitomycin, mitotane, mitoxantrone, nandrolone, paclitaxel, phenpropionate, penicillamine, plicamycin, porfimer, procarbazine, raltitrexed, sodium iodide I 131, sodium phosphate P 32, streptozocin, tamoxifen, temoporfin, teniposide, testolactone, testosterone, thioguanine, thiotepa, thyroglobulin, thyroid, thyrotropin, topotecan, toremifene, trastuzumab, trimetrexate, triptorelin, uracil mustard, valrubicin, vinblastine, vincristine, vindesine, vinorelbine, zidovudine. Topical—fluorouracil, mechlorethamine.

Antiparkinsonism Drugs—Drugs used to treat Parkinson's disease. A disease of the central nervous system in older adults, it is characterized by gradual progressive muscle rigidity, tremors and clumsiness. These drugs include amantadine, benztropine, biperiden, bromocriptine, carbidopa and levodopa, diphenhydramine, entacapone, ethopropazine, levodopa, levodopa and benserazide, orphenadrine, pramipexole, procyclidine, rasagiline, ropinirole, rotigotine, selegiline, trihexyphenidyl.

Antiplatelet Drugs—Drugs used to stop the platelets in the blood from sticking to one another and forming blood clots. These drugs include aspirin, clopidogrel, dipyridamole, prasugrel, rivaroxaban, ticagrelor, ticlopidine.

Antipsychotic Drugs—A group of drugs used to treat the mental disease of psychosis, including such variants as schizophrenia, manic-depressive illness, anxiety states, severe behavior problems and others. These drugs include acetophenazine, aripiprazole, asenapine, carbamazepine, chlorpromazine, chlorprothixene, fluphenazine, flupenthixol, fluspirilene, haloperidol, iloperidone, loxapine, mesoridazine, methotrimeprazine, molindone, paliperidone, pericyazine, perphenazine, pimozide, pipotiazine, prochlorperazine, promazine, risperidone, thioproperazine, thioridazine, thiothixene, trifluoperazine, triflupromazine.

Antitussives—A group of drugs used to suppress coughs. These drugs include benzonatate, chlophedianol, codeine (oral), dextromethorphan, diphenhydramine syrup, hydrocodone, hydromorphone, methadone, morphine.

Antiulcer Drugs—A group of medicines used to treat peptic ulcer in the stomach, duodenum or the lower end of the esophagus. These drugs include amitriptyline, antacids, anticholinergics, antispasmodics, bismuth subsalicylate, cimetidine, doxepin, famotidine, lansoprazole, misoprostol, nizatidine, omeprazole, ranitidine, sucralfate, trimipramine.

Antiurolithics—Medicines that prevent the formation of kidney stones.

Antiviral Drugs—A group of drugs used to treat viral infections. These drugs include: Ophthalmic (eye)—idoxuridine, trifluridine, vidarabine. Systemic—acyclovir, amantadine, didanosine, famciclovir, foscarnet, ganciclovir, oseltamivir, ribavirin, rilpivirine, rimantadine, stavudine, zalcitabine, zanamivir, zidovudine. Topical drugs—acyclovir, docosanol.

Antivirals, HIV/AIDS—A group of drugs used to treat human immunodeficiency virus (HIV) and acquired immune deficiency syndrome (AIDS). They work by suppressing the replication of HIV. These drugs include abacavir, darunavir, delavirdine, didanosine, efavirenz, indinavir, lamivudine, maraviroc, nelfinavir, nevirapine, raltegravir, ritonavir, saquinavir, stavudine, tipranavir, zalcitabine, zidovudine.

Appendicitis—Inflammation or infection of the appendix. Symptoms include loss of appetite, nausea, low-grade fever and tenderness in the lower right of the abdomen.

Appetite Suppressants—A group of drugs used to decrease the appetite as part of an overall treatment for obesity. These drugs include amphetamine and dextroamphetamine, benzphetamine, diethylpropion, fenfluramine, mazindol, phendimetrazine, phentermine, phenylpropanolamine, sibutramine.

Artery—Blood vessel carrying blood away from the heart.

Asthma—Recurrent attacks of breathing difficulty due to spasms and contractions of the bronchial tubes.

Attenuated Virus Vaccines—Liquid products of killed germs used for injections to prevent certain diseases.

B

Bacteria—Microscopic organisms. Some bacteria contribute to health; others (germs) cause disease and infection.

Barbiturates—Powerful drugs used for sedation, to help induce sleep and sometimes to prevent seizures. Except for use in seizures (phenobarbital), barbiturates are being used less and less because there are better, less hazardous drugs that produce the same or better effects. These drugs include amobarbital, aprobarbital, butabarbital, mephobarbital, metharbital, pentobarbital, phenobarbital, secobarbital, secobarbital and amobarbital, talbutal.

Basal Area of Brain—Part of the brain that regulates muscle control and tone.

Benzethonium Chloride—A compound used as a preservative in some drug preparations. It is also used in various concentrations for cleaning cooking and eating utensils and as a disinfectant.

Benzodiazepines—A family of drugs prescribed to treat anxiety and alcohol withdrawal and sometimes prescribed for sedation. These drugs include alprazolam, bromazepam, chlordiazepoxide, clobazam, clonazepam, clorazepate, diazepam, estazolam, flurazepam, halazepam, ketazolam, lorazepam, nitrazepam, oxazepam, prazepam, quazepam, triazolam.

Beta Agonists—A group of drugs that act directly on cells in the body (beta-adrenergic receptors) to relieve spasms of the bronchial tubes and other organs consisting of smooth muscles. These drugs include albuterol, bitolterol, indacaterol, isoetharine, isoproterenol, metaproterenol, terbutaline.

Beta-Adrenergic Blocking Agents—A family of drugs with similar pharmacological actions with some variations. These drugs are prescribed for angina, heartbeat irregularities (arrhythmias), high blood pressure, hypertrophic subaortic stenosis, vascular headaches (as a preventative, not to treat once the pain begins) and others. Timolol is prescribed for treatment of open-angle glaucoma. These drugs include acebutolol, atenolol, betaxolol, bisoprolol, carteolol, labetalol, levobetaxolol, metoprolol, nadolol, oxprenolol, penbutolol, pindolol, propranolol, sotalol, timolol.

Bile Acids—Components of bile that are derived from cholesterol and formed in the liver. Bile acids aid the digestion of fat.

Biologic Response Modifiers—Substances that are produced naturally in the body or manufactured as drugs designed to strengthen, direct, or restore the body's immune response. The drugs are used in treating disease such as rheumatoid arthritis, certain cancers and some infections. These drugs include abatacept, adalimumab, anakinra, atumumab, canakinumab, certolizumab, etanercept, infliximab, golimumab, interferon, interleukin-2, natalizumab, rilonacept, rituximab, tocilizumab, tofacitinib, ustekinumab, various types of colony-stimulating factors.

Blood Count—Laboratory studies to count white blood cells, red blood cells, platelets and other elements of the blood.

Blood Dyscrasia-Causing Medicines—Drugs which cause unpredictable damaging effects to human bone marrow. These effects occur in a small minority of patients and are not dependent upon dosage. These medicines include the following (some of which are not described in this book): ACE inhibitors, acetazolamide, aminopyrine, amodiaquine, anticonvulsants (dione, hydantoin, succinimide), antidepressants (tricyclic), antidiabetic agents (sulfonylurea), anti-inflammatory analgesics, antithyroid agents, bexarotene, captopril, carbamazepine, cephalosporins, chloramphenicol, cisplatin, clopidogrel, clozapine, dapsone, divalproex, felbamate, flecainide acetate, foscarnet, gold compounds, levamisole, loxapine, maprotiline, methicillin, methimazole, methsuximide, metronidazole, mirtazapine, pantoprazole, penicillins (some), penicillamine, pentamidine, phenacemide, phenothiazines, phensuximide, phenytoin, pimozide, primaquine, primidone, propafenone, propylthiouracil, pyrimethamine (large doses), rabeprazole, rifampin, rifapentine, rituximab, sulfamethoxazole and trimethoprim, sulfasalazine, sulfonamides, thioxanthenes, ticlopidine, tiopronin, topiramate, trastuzumab, trimethobenzamide, trimethoprim, valproic acid.

Blood Pressure, Diastolic—Pressure (usually recorded in millimeters of mercury) in the large arteries of the body when the heart muscle is relaxed and filling for the next contraction.

Blood Pressure, Systolic—Pressure (usually recorded in millimeters of mercury) in the large arteries of the body at the instant the heart muscle contracts.

Blood Sugar (Blood Glucose)—Necessary element in the blood to sustain life.

Bone Marrow Depressants—Medicines that affect the bone marrow to depress its normal function of forming blood cells. These medicines include the following (some of which are not described in this book): abacavir, alcohol, aldesleukin, altretamine, amphotericin B (systemic), anticancer drugs, antithyroid drugs, azathioprine, bexarotene, busulfan, capecitabine, carboplatin, carmustine, chlorambucil, chloramphenicol, chromic phosphate, cisplatin, cladribine, clozapine, colchicine, cyclophosphamide, cyproterone, cytarabine, dacarbazine, dactinomycin, daunorubicin, didanosine, docetaxel, doxorubicin, eflornithine, epirubicin, etoposide, floxuridine, flucytosine, fludarabine, fluorouracil, ganciclovir, gemcitabine, hydroxyurea, idarubicin, ifosfamide, imatinib, interferon, irinotecan, lomustine, mechlorethamine, melphalan, mercaptopurine, methotrexate, mitomycin, mitoxantrone, paclitaxel, pentostatin, plicamycin, procarbazine, sirolimus, streptozocin, sulfa drugs, temozolomide, teniposide, thioguanine, thiotepa, topotecan, trimetrexate, uracil mustard, valrubicin, vidarabine (large doses), vinblastine, vincristine, vindesine, vinorelbine, zidovudine, zoledronic acid.

Bone Marrow Depression—Reduction of the blood-producing capacity of human bone marrow. Can be caused by many drugs taken for long periods of time in high doses.

Brain Depressants—Any drug that depresses brain function, such as tranquilizers, narcotics, alcohol and barbiturates.

Bronchodilators—A group of drugs used to dilate the bronchial tubes to treat such problems as asthma, emphysema, bronchitis, bronchiectasis, allergies and others. These drugs include albuterol, aminophylline, arformoterol, bitolterol, cromolyn, dyphylline, ephedrine, epinephrine, ethylnorepinephrine, fenoterol, formoterol, indacaterol, ipratropium, isoetharine, isoproterenol, levalbuterol metaproterenol, nedocromil, oxtriphylline, oxtriphylline and guaifenesin, pirbuterol, procaterol, salmeterol, terbutaline, theophylline and guaifenesin.

Bronchodilators, Xanthine-Derivative—Drugs of similar chemical structure and pharmacological activity that are prescribed to dilate bronchial tubes in disorders such as asthma, bronchitis, emphysema and other chronic lung diseases. These drugs include aminophylline, dyphylline, oxtriphylline, theophylline.

BUN—Abbreviation for blood urea nitrogen. A test often used as a measurement of kidney function.

C

Calcium Channel Blockers—A group of drugs used to treat angina and heartbeat irregularities. These drugs include bepridil, diltiazem, felodipine, flunarizine, isradipine, nicardipine, nifedipine, nimodipine, verapamil.

Calcium Supplements—Supplements used to increase the calcium concentration in the blood in an attempt to make bones denser (as in osteoporosis). These supplements include calcium citrate, calcium glubionate, calcium gluconate, calcium glycerophosphate and calcium lactate, calcium lactate, dibasic calcium phosphate, tribasic calcium phosphate.

Carbamates—A group of drugs derived from carbamic acid and used for anxiety or as sedatives. They include meprobamate and ethinamate.

Carbetapentane—An antitussive (cough suppressing) drug similar to dextromethorphan in action. It is an ingredient in some cough and cold remedies.

Carbonic Anhydrase Inhibitors—Drugs used to treat glaucoma and seizures and to prevent high altitude sickness. They include acetazolamide, brinzolamide, dichlorphenamide, dorzolamide, methazolamide.

Cataract—Loss of transparency in the lens of the eye.

Catecholamines—A group of drugs, also found naturally in the body, used to treat low blood pressure or shock. These drugs include dopamine, norepinephrine and epinephrine.

Cationic Drugs—Drugs removed from the body by the kidneys (called renal tubular secretion). If two of these drugs are taken together, one of them may stay in the body longer and increase its effect. These drugs include digoxin, metformin, morphine, pancuronium, tenofovir, trospium, vancomycin.

Cell—Unit of protoplasm, the essential living matter of all plants and animals.

Central Nervous System (CNS) Depressants—These drugs cause sedation or otherwise diminish brain activity and other parts of the nervous system. These drugs include alcohol, aminoglutethimide, anesthetics (general and injection-local), anticonvulsants, antidepressants (MAO inhibitors, tricyclic), antidyskinetics (except amantadine), antihistamines, apomorphine, azelastine, baclofen, barbiturates, benzodiazepines, beta-adrenergic blocking agents, brimonidine, buclizine, carbamazepine, cetirizine, chlophedianol, chloral hydrate, chlorzoxazone, clonidine, clozapine, cyclizine, cytarabine, difenoxin and atropine, diphenoxylate and atropine, disulfiram, donepezil, dronabinol, droperidol, ethchlorvynol, ethinamate, etomidate, fenfluramine, fluoxetine, glutethimide, guanabenz, guanfacine, haloperidol, hydroxyzine, ifosfamide, interferon, loxapine, magnesium sulfate (injection), maprotiline, meclizine, meprobamate, methyldopa, methyprylon, metoclopramide, metyrosine, mirtazapine, mitotane, molindone, nabilone, nefazodone, olanzapine, opioid (narcotic) analgesics, oxcarbazepine, oxybutynin, paliperidone, paraldehyde, paregoric, pargyline, paroxetine, phenothiazines, pimozide, procarbazine, promethazine, propiomazine, propofol, quetiapine, rauwolfia alkaloids, risperidone, scopolamine, sertraline, skeletal muscle relaxants (centrally acting), tapentadol, thalidomide, thioxanthenes, tramadol, trazodone, trimeprazine, trimethobenzamide, zaleplon, zolpidem, zonisamide, zopiclone.

Central Nervous System (CNS) Stimulants— Drugs that cause excitation, anxiety and nervousness or otherwise stimulate the brain and other parts of the central nervous system. These drugs include amantadine, amphetamines, anesthetics (local), appetite suppressants (except fenfluramine), bronchodilators (xanthine-derivative), bupropion, caffeine, chlophedianol, cocaine, dextroamphetamine, diclofenac, doxapram, dronabinol, dyphylline, entacapone, ephedrine (oral), fluoroquinolones, fluoxetine, meropenem, methamphetamine, methylphenidate, moclobemide, modafinil, nabilone, pemoline, rasagiline, selegiline, sertraline, sympathomimetics, topiramate, tranylcypromine, zonisamide.

Cephalosporins—Antibiotics that kill many bacterial germs that penicillin and sulfa drugs can't destroy.

Cholinergics (Parasympathomimetics)— Chemicals that facilitate passage of nerve impulses through the parasympathetic nervous system.

Cholinesterase Inhibitors—Drugs that prevent the action of cholinesterase (an enzyme that breaks down acetylcholine in the body).

Chronic—Long-term, continuing. Chronic illnesses may not be curable, but they can often be prevented from becoming worse. Symptoms usually can be alleviated or controlled.

Cirrhosis—Disease that scars and destroys liver tissue resulting in abnormal function.

Citrates—Medicines taken orally to make urine more acid. Citrates include potassium citrate, potassium citrate and citric acid, potassium citrate and sodium citrate, sodium citrate and acid, tricitrates.

Coal Tar Preparations—Creams, ointments and lotions used on the skin for various skin ailments.

Cold Urticaria—Hives that appear in areas of the body exposed to the cold.

Colitis, Ulcerative—Chronic, recurring ulcers of the colon for unknown reasons.

Collagen—Support tissue of skin, tendon, bone, cartilage and connective tissue.

Colostomy—Surgical opening from the colon, the large intestine, to the outside of the body.

Coma—A sleeplike state from which a person cannot be aroused.

Compliance—The extent to which a person follows medical advice.

Congestive—Characterized by excess accumulation of fluid. In congestive heart failure, congestion occurs in the lungs, liver, kidneys and other parts of the body to cause shortness of breath, swelling of the ankles and feet, rapid heartbeat and other symptoms.

Constriction—Tightness or pressure.

Contraceptives, Hormonal—Any form of contraception (birth control) that contains hormones (such as ethinyl estradiol and others). These forms include oral, injectable, transdermal and implantable.

Contraceptives, Oral (Birth Control Pills)—A group of hormones used to prevent ovulation, therefore preventing pregnancy. These hormones include drospirenone and ethinyl estradiol, ethynodiol diacetate and ethinyl estradiol, ethynodiol diacetate and mestranol, etonogestrel, levonorgestrel and ethinyl estradiol, medroxyprogesterone, norethindrone tablets, norethindrone acetate and ethinyl estradiol, norethindrone and ethinyl estradiol, norethindrone and mestranol, norethynodrel and mestranol, norgestrel, norgestrel and ethinyl estradiol.

Contraceptives, Vaginal—Topical medications or devices applied inside the vagina to prevent pregnancy.

Convulsions—Violent, uncontrollable contractions of the voluntary muscles.

COPD (Chronic Obstructive Pulmonary Disease)—Lung conditions including emphysema and chronic bronchitis.

Corticosteroids (Adrenocorticosteroids)— Steroid hormones produced by the body's adrenal cortex or their synthetic equivalents.

Cortisone (Adrenocorticoids, Glucocorticoids) and Other Adrenal Steroids—Medicines that mimic the action of the steroid hormone cortisone, manufactured in the cortex of the adrenal gland. These drugs decrease the effects of inflammation within the body. They are available for injection, oral use, topical use for the skin, eyes and nose and inhalation for the bronchial tubes. These drugs include alclometasone; amcinonide; beclomethasone; benzyl benzoate; betamethasone; bismuth; ciclesonide; clobetasol; clobetasone 17-butyrate; clocortolone; cortisone; desonide; desoximetasone; desoxycorticosterone; dexamethasone; diflorasone; diflucortolone; fludrocortisone; flumethasone; flunisolide; fluocinonide; fluocinonide, procinonide and ciprocinonide; fluorometholone; fluprednisolone, flurandrenolide; halcinonide; hydrocortisone; medrysone; methylprednisolone; mometasone; paramethasone; Peruvian balsam; prednisolone; prednisone; triamcinolone; zinc oxide.

Cycloplegics—Eye drops that prevent the pupils from accommodating to varying degrees of light.

Cystitis—Inflammation of the urinary bladder.

D

Decongestants—Drugs used to relieve congestion by shrinking swollen membranes. These drugs include: Cough-suppressing—phenylephrine and dextromethorphan, phenylpropanolamine (phenylpropanolamine products are being discontinued) and caramiphen, phenylpropanolamine and dextromethorphan, phenylpropanolamine and hydrocodone, pseudoephedrine and codeine, pseudoephedrine and dextromethorphan, pseudoephedrine and hydrocodone.
Cough-suppressing and pain-relieving—phenylpropanolamine, dextromethorphan and acetaminophen.
Cough-suppressing and sputum-thinning—phenylephrine, dextromethorphan and guaifenesin; phenylephrine, hydrocodone and guaifenesin; phenylpropanolamine, codeine and guaifenesin; phenylpropanolamine, dextromethorphan and guaifenesin; pseudoephedrine, codeine and guaifenesin; pseudoephedrine, dextromethorphan and guaifenesin; pseudoephedrine, hydrocodone and guaifenesin; phenylephrine, dextromethorphan, guaifenesin and acetaminophen; pseudoephedrine, dextromethorphan, guaifenesin and acetaminophen.
Sputum-thinning—ephedrine and guaifenesin; ephedrine and potassium iodide; phenylephrine, phenylpropanolamine and guaifenesin; phenylpropanolamine and guaifenesin; pseudoephedrine and guaifenesin.
Nasal—ephedrine (oral), phenylpropanolamine, pseudoephedrine.
Ophthalmic (eye)—naphazoline, oxymetazoline, phenylephrine.
Topical—oxymetazoline, phenylephrine, xylometazoline.

Delirium—Temporary mental disturbance characterized by hallucinations, agitation and incoherence.

Diabetes—Metabolic disorder in which the body can't use carbohydrates efficiently. This leads to a dangerously high level of glucose (a carbohydrate) in the blood.

Dialysis—Procedure to filter waste products from the bloodstream of patients with kidney failure.

Digitalis Preparations (Digitalis Glycosides)—Important drugs to treat heart disease, such as congestive heart failure, heartbeat irregularities and cardiogenic shock. These drugs include digitoxin, digoxin.

Digoxin—One of the digitalis drugs used to treat heart disease. All digitalis products were originally derived from the foxglove plant.

Dilation—Enlargement.

Disulfiram Reaction—Disulfiram (Antabuse) is a drug to treat alcoholism. When alcohol in the bloodstream interacts with disulfiram, it causes a flushed face, severe headache, chest pains, shortness of breath, nausea, vomiting, sweating and weakness. Severe reactions may cause death. A disulfiram reaction is the interaction of any drug with alcohol or another drug to produce these symptoms.

Diuretics—Drugs that act on the kidneys to prevent reabsorption of electrolytes, especially chlorides. They are used to treat edema, high blood pressure, congestive heart failure, kidney and liver failure and others. These drugs include amiloride, amiloride and hydrochlorothiazide, bendroflumethiazide, benzthiazide, bumetanide, chlorothiazide, chlorthalidone, cyclothiazide, ethacrynic acid, furosemide, glycerin, hydrochlorothiazide, hydroflumethiazide, indapamide, mannitol, methyclothiazide, metolazone, polythiazide, quinethazone, spironolactone, spironolactone and hydrochlorothiazide, triamterene, triamterene and hydrochlorothiazide, trichlormethiazide, urea.

Diuretics, Loop—Drugs that act on the kidneys to prevent reabsorption of electrolytes, especially sodium. They are used to treat edema, high blood pressure, congestive heart failure, kidney and liver failure and others. These drugs include bumetanide, ethacrynic acid, furosemide.

Diuretics, Potassium-Sparing—Drugs that act on the kidneys to prevent reabsorption of electrolytes, especially sodium. They are used to treat edema, high blood pressure, congestive heart failure, kidney and liver failure and others. This particular group of diuretics does not allow the unwanted side effect of low potassium in the blood to occur. These drugs include amiloride, spironolactone, triamterene.

Diuretics, Thiazide—Drugs that act on the kidneys to prevent reabsorption of electrolytes, especially chlorides. They are used to treat edema, high blood pressure, congestive heart failure, kidney and liver failure and others. These drugs include bendroflumethiazide, benzthiazide, chlorothiazide, chlorthalidone, cyclothiazide, hydrochlorothiazide, hydroflumethiazide, methyclothiazide, metolazone, polythiazide, quinethazone, trichlormethiazide.

Dopamine Agonists—Drugs that stimulate activity of dopamine (a brain chemical that helps control movement). These include apomorphine, bromocriptine, cabergoline, pramipexole, quinagolide, ropinirole, rotigotine.

Dopamine Antagonists—Drugs that interfere with dopamine production (brain chemical that helps control movement). These drugs include haloperidol, metoclopramide, phenothiazines, procainamide, thioxanthenes and others.

Duodenum—The first 12 inches of the small intestine.

E

ECG (or EKG)—Abbreviation for electrocardiogram or electrocardiograph. An ECG is a graphic tracing representing the electrical current produced by impulses passing through the heart muscle. This is a useful test in the diagnosis of heart disease, but used alone it usually can't make a complete diagnosis. An ECG is most useful in two areas:
(1) demonstrating heart rhythm disturbances and
(2) demonstrating changes when there is a myocardial infarction (heart attack). It will detect enlargement of either heart chamber, but will not establish a diagnosis of heart failure or disease of the heart valves.

Eczema—Disorder of the skin with redness, itching, blisters, weeping and abnormal pigmentation.

EEG—Electroencephalogram or electro-encephalograph. An EEG is a graphic recording of electrical activity generated spontaneously from nerve cells in the brain. This test is useful in the diagnosis of brain dysfunction, particularly in studying seizure disorders.

Electrolytes—Substances that can transmit electrical impulses when dissolved in body fluids. These include sodium, potassium, chloride, bicarbonate, and carbon dioxide.

Embolism—Sudden blockage of an artery by a clot or foreign material in the blood.

Emphysema—An irreversible disease in which the lung's air sacs lose elasticity and air accumulates in the lungs.

Endometriosis—Condition in which uterus tissue is found outside the uterus. Can cause pain, abnormal menstruation and infertility.

Enzyme Inducers—Drugs that increase the metabolism of another drug in the liver, resulting in a decrease of that drug's effect. Ask your doctor or pharmacist about this possible interaction. Listed here are the more common used drugs in this category. These drugs include: alcohol (chronic use), barbiturates (especially phenobarbital), carbamazepine, darunavir, dexamethasone, efavirenz, glucocorticoids, glutethimide, griseofulvin, insulin, isoniazid, modafinil, nafcillin, nevirapine, norethindrone, omeprazole, oxcarbazepine, phenylbutazone, phenytoin, pioglitazone, prednisone, primidone, rifabutin, rifampin, rifapentine, saquinavir, secobarbital, St. John's wort, tipranavir, troglitazone. Also included are charbroiled meats, cruciferous vegetables (such as broccoli and cabbage) and smoking. There may be other drugs in this category. Consult doctor or pharmacist.

Enzyme Inducing Antiepileptic Drugs—Drugs used for seizure disorders that increase the metabolism of another drug in the liver, resulting in a decrease of that drug's effect. These drugs include carbamazepine, phenytoin, primidone and phenobarbital.

Enzyme Inhibitors—Drugs that decrease the metabolism of another drug in the liver, resulting in an increase of that drug's effect. Ask your doctor or pharmacist about this possible interaction. Listed here are the more common used drugs in this category. These drugs include: amiodarone, antipsychotics, aprepitant, asenapine, azole antifungals, bicalutamide, bupropion, celecoxib, chloramphenicol, chlorpheniramine, chlorpromazine, cimetidine, cinacalcet, ciprofloxacin, citalopram, clarithromycin, clemastine, clomipramine, cyclosporine, darunavir, delavirdine, diphenhydramine, diltiazem, disulfiram, doxepin, doxorubicin, duloxetine, enoxacin, erythromycins, escitalopram, fenofibrate, felbamate, fluoroquinolones, fluoxetine, fluvoxamine, gemfibrozil, glitazones, halofantrine, histamine H2 receptor antagonists, HIV antivirals (some), hydroxyzine, imatinib, indomethacin, isoniazid, itraconazole, ketoconazole, lansoprazole, levomepromazine, lorcaserin, lovastatin, methadone, methoxsalen, metoclopramide, metronidazole, mibefradil, midodrine, mifepristone, mirabegron, moclobemide, modafinil, montelukast, nefazodone, nelfinavir, norfloxacin, norfluoxetine, omeprazole, oxcarbazepine, pantoprazole, paroxetine, perphenazine, phenothiazines, phenylbutazone, probenecid, protease inhibitors, quercetin, quinidine, rabeprazole, ranitidine, ranolazine, ritonavir, saquinavir, selective serotonin reuptake inhibitors (SSRIs), sertraline, sulfamethoxazole, sulfaphenazole, telithromycin, teniposide, terbinafine, thiotepa, ticagrelor, ticlopidine, topiramate, trimethoprim, tripelennamine, valproic acid, venlafaxine, verapamil, voriconazole, zafirlukast; and grapefruit juice. There may be other drugs in this category. Consult doctor or pharmacist.

Enzymes—Protein chemicals that can accelerate chemical reactions in the body.

Epilepsy—Episodes of brain disturbance that cause convulsions and loss of consciousness.

Erectile Dysfunction Agents—Medicines used to treat male impotence (the inability to develop and sustain an erection). These drugs include: Alprostadil, papaverine, sildenafil citrate, tadalafil, vardenafil, yohimbine.

Ergot Preparations (Alkaloids)—Medicines used to treat migraine and other types of throbbing headaches. Also used after delivery of babies to make the uterus clamp down and reduce excessive bleeding. These drugs include dihydroergotamine, ergoloid mesylates, ergotamine.

Erythromycins—A group of drugs with similar structure used to treat infections. These drugs include erythromycin, erythromycin estolate, erythromycin ethylsuccinate, erythromycin gluceptate, erythromycin lactobionate, erythromycin stearate.

Esophagitis—Inflammation of the lower part of the esophagus, the tube connecting the throat and the stomach.

Estrogens—Female hormones used to replenish the body's stores after the ovaries have been removed or become nonfunctional after menopause. Also used with progesterone in some birth control pills and for other purposes. These drugs include:
Systemic— chlorotrianisene, diethylstilbestrol, estradiol, estrogens (conjugated and esterified), estrone, estropipate, ethinyl estradiol, quinestrol.
Vaginal—dienestrol, estradiol, estrogens (conjugated), estrone, estropipate.

Eustachian Tube—Small passage from the middle ear to the sinuses and nasal passages.

Extrapyramidal Reactions—Abnormal reactions in the power and coordination of posture and muscular movements. Movements are not under voluntary control. Some drugs associated with producing extrapyramidal reactions include amoxapine, antidepressants (tricyclic), droperidol, haloperidol, loxapine, metoclopramide, metyrosine, moclobemide, molindone, olanzapine, paliperidone, paroxetine, phenothiazines, pimozide, rauwolfia alkaloids, risperidone, tacrine, thioxanthenes.

Extremity—Arm, leg, hand or foot.

F

Fecal Impaction—Condition in which feces become firmly wedged in the rectum.

Fibrocystic Breast Disease—Overgrowth of fibrous tissue in the breast, producing non-malignant cysts.

Fibroid Tumors—Non-malignant tumors of the muscular layer of the uterus.

Flu (Influenza)—A virus infection of the respiratory tract that lasts three to ten days. Symptoms include headache, fever, runny nose, cough, tiredness and muscle aches.

Fluoroquinolones—A class of drugs used to treat bacterial infections, such as urinary tract infections and some types of bronchitis. These drugs include ciprofloxacin, enoxacin, gatifloxacin, gemifloxacin, levofloxacin, lomefloxacin, moxifloxacin, norfloxacin, ofloxacin, sparfloxacin.

Folate Antagonists—Drugs that impair the body's utilization of folic acid, which is necessary for cell growth. These drugs include dione anticonvulsants, hydantoin anticonvulsants, succinimide anticonvulsants, divalproex, methotrexate, oral contraceptives, phenobarbital (long-term use), pyrimethamine, sulfonamides, triamterene, trimethoprim, trimetrexate, valproic acid.

Folliculitis—Inflammation of a follicle.

Functional Dependence—The development of dependence on a drug for a normal body function. The primary example is the use of laxatives for a prolonged period so that there is a dependence on the laxative for normal bowel action.

G

G6PD—Deficiency of glucose 6-phosphate, which is necessary for glucose metabolism.

Ganglionic Blockers—Medicines that block the passage of nerve impulses through a part of the nerve cell called a ganglion. Ganglionic blockers are used to treat urinary retention and other medical problems. Bethanechol is one of the best ganglionic blockers.

Gastritis—Inflammation of the stomach.

Gastrointestinal—Of the stomach and intestinal tract.

Gland—Organ or group of cells that manufactures and excretes materials not required for its own metabolic needs.

Glaucoma—Eye disease in which increased pressure inside the eye damages the optic nerve, causes pain and changes vision.

Glucagon—Injectable drug that immediately elevates blood sugar by mobilizing glycogen from the liver.

Gold Compounds—Medicines which use gold as their base and are usually used to treat joint or arthritic disorders. These medicines include auranofin, aurothioglucose, gold sodium thiomalate.

H

H_2 Antagonists—Antihistamines that work against H_2 histamine. H_2 histamine may be liberated at any point in the body, but most often in the gastrointestinal tract.

Hangover Effect—The same feelings as a "hangover" after too much alcohol consumption. Symptoms include headache, irritability and nausea.

Hematocrit—A blood test that measure how much space in blood is occupied by red blood cells.

Hemochromatosis—Disorder of iron metabolism in which excessive iron is deposited in and damages body tissues, particularly of the liver and pancreas.

Hemoglobin—Pigment in blood that carries oxygen in red blood cells.

Hemolytics—Drugs that can destroy red blood cells and separate hemoglobin from the blood cells. These include acetohydroxamic acid, antidiabetic agents (sulfonylurea), doxapram, furazolidone, mefenamic acid, menadiol, methyldopa, nitrofurans, primaquine, quinidine, quinine, sulfonamides (systemic), sulfones, vitamin K.

Hemorrhage—Heavy bleeding.

Hemorheologic Agents—Medicines to help control bleeding.

Hemosiderosis—Increase of iron deposits in body tissues without tissue damage.

Hepatitis—Inflammation of liver cells, usually accompanied by jaundice.

Hepatotoxics—Medications that can possibly cause toxicity or decreased normal function of the liver. These drugs include the following (some of which are not described in this book): acetaminophen (with long-term use), abacavir, acitretin, alcohol, amiodarone, anabolic steroids, androgens, angiotensin-converting enzyme (ACE) inhibitors, acitretin, anti-inflammatory drugs, nonsteroidal (NSAIDs), antithyroid agents, asparaginase, azlocillin, bexarotene, carbamazepine, carmustine, clindamycin, clofibrate, colestipol, cox 2 inhibitors, cyproterone, cytarabine, danazol, dantrolene, dapsone, daunorubicin, disulfiram, divalproex, dofetilide, epirubicin, erythromycins, estrogens, ethionamide, etretinate, felbamate, fenofibrate, fluconazole, flutamide, gold compounds, halothane, HMG-CoA reductase inhibitors, imatinib, iron (overdose) isoniazid, itraconazole, ketoconazole (oral), labetalol, mercaptopurine, methimazole, methotrexate, methyldopa, metronidazole, naltrexone, nevirapine, niacin (high doses), nilutamide, nitrofurans, pemoline, phenothiazines, phenytoin, piperacillin, plicamycin, posaconazole, pravastatin, probucol, rifampin, rosiglitazone, sulfamethoxazole and trimethoprim, sulfonamides, tacrine, tenofovir, testosterone, tizanidine, tolcapone, toremifene, tretinoin, troglitazone, valproic acid, zidovudine, zidovudine and lamivudine.

Hiatal Hernia—Section of the stomach that protrudes into the chest cavity.

Histamine—Chemical in body tissues that dilates the smallest blood vessels, constricts the smooth muscle surrounding the bronchial tubes and stimulates stomach secretions.

History—Past medical events in a patient's life.

Hives—Elevated patches on the skin that are redder or paler than surrounding skin and often itch severely.

HMG-CoA Reductase Inhibitors—A group of prescription drugs used to lower cholesterol. These include Atorvastatin, fluvastatin, lovastatin, pravastatin, pravastatin & aspirin, and simvastatin.

Hoarseness—Husky, gruff, weak voice.

Hormone Replacement Therapy—A medication (estrogen) or combination of medications (estrogen and progestin or estrogen and androgen) used for treatment of premenopausal and menopausal symptoms and for prevention of diseases that affect women in their later years

Hormones—Chemical substances produced in the body to regulate other body functions.

Hypercalcemia—Too much calcium in the blood. This happens with some malignancies and in calcium overdose.

Hyperglycemia-Causing Medications—A group of drugs that may contribute to hyperglycemia (high blood sugar). These include oral estrogen-containing contraceptives, corticosteroids, estrogens, isoniazid, nicotinic acid, phenothiazines, phenytoin, sympathomimetics, thyroid hormones, thiazide diuretics.

Hyperkalemia-Causing Medications—Medicines that cause too much potassium in the bloodstream. These include ACE inhibitors; amiloride, anti-inflammatory drugs, nonsteroidal (NSAIDs); cyclosporine; digitalis glycosides; diuretics (potassium-sparing); pentamidine; spironolactone; succinylcholine chloride; tacrolimus; triamterene; trimethoprim; possibly any medicine that is combined with potassium.

Hypersensitivity—Serious reactions to many medications. The effects of hypersensitivity may be characterized by wheezing, shortness of breath, rapid heart rate, severe itching, faintness, unconsciousness and severe drop in blood pressure.

Hypertension—High blood pressure.

Hypervitaminosis—A condition due to an excess of one or more vitamins. Symptoms may include weakness, fatigue, loss of hair and changes in the skin.

Hypnotics—Drugs used to induce a sleeping state. See Barbiturates.

Hypocalcemia—Abnormally low level of calcium in the blood.

Hypoglycemia—Low blood sugar (blood glucose). A critically low blood sugar level will interfere with normal brain function and can damage the brain permanently.

Hypoglycemia-Causing Medications—A group of drugs that may contribute to hypoglycemia (low blood sugar). These include clofibrate, monoamine oxidase (MAO) inhibitors, probenecid, propranolol, rifabutin, rifampicin, salicylates, sulfonamides (long-acting), sulfonylureas.

Hypoglycemics—Drugs that reduce blood sugar. These include acetohexamide, chlorpropamide, gliclazide, glipizide, glyburide, insulin, metformin, tolazamide, tolbutamide.

Hypokalemia-Causing Medications—Medicines that cause a depletion of potassium in the bloodstream. These include adrenocorticoids (systemic), alcohol, amphotericin B (systemic), bronchodilators (adrenergic), capreomycin, carbonic anhydrase inhibitors, cisplatin, diuretics (loop and thiazide), edetate (long-term use), foscarnet, ifosfamide, indapamide, insulin, insulin lispro, laxatives (if dependent on), penicillins (some), salicylates, sirolimus, sodium bicarbonate, urea, vitamin D (overdose of).

Hypomagnesemia-Causing Drugs—Drugs that may increase the loss of magnesium in urine. The loss can lead to low blood levels of magnesium (hypomagnesemia). These drugs include busulfan, cyclosporine, digoxin, foscarnet, lenalidomide, loop diuretics, mycophenolate, nilotinib, proton-pump inhibitors, tacrolimus, thiazide diuretics, valganciclovir, voriconazole and others.

Hypotension—Blood pressure decrease below normal. Symptoms may include weakness, lightheadedness and dizziness.

Hypotension-Causing Drugs—Medications that might cause hypotension (low blood pressure). These include alcohol, alpha adrenergic blocking agents, alprostadil, amantadine, anesthetics (general), angiotensin-converting enzyme inhibitors (ACE inhibitors), angiotensin II receptor antagonists, antidepressants (MAO inhibitors, tricyclic), antihypertensives, benzodiazepines used as preanesthetics, beta-adrenergic blocking agents, brimonidine, bromocriptine, cabergoline, calcium channel-blocking agents, carbidopa and levodopa, clonidine, clozapine, dipyridamole and aspirin, diuretics, docetaxel, droperidol, edetate calcium disodium, edetate disodium, haloperidol, hydralazine, levodopa, lidocaine (systemic), loxapine, magnesium sulfate, maprotiline, mirtazapine, molindone, nabilone (high doses), nefazodone, nitrates, olanzapine, opioid analgesics (including fentanyl, fentanyl and sufentanil), oxcarbazepine, paclitaxel, paliperidone, pentamidine, pentoxifylline, phenothiazines, pimozide, pramipexole, propofol, quetiapine, quinidine, radiopaques (materials used in x-ray studies), ranitidine risperidone, rituximab, ropinirole, sildenafil, thioxanthenes, tizanidine, tolcapone, trazodone, vancomycin, venlafaxine. If you take any of these medications, be sure to tell a dentist, anesthesiologist or anyone else who intends to give you an anesthetic to put you to sleep.

Hypothermia-Causing Medications—Medicines that can cause a significant lowering of body temperature. These drugs include alcohol, alpha-adrenergic blocking agents (dihydroergotamine, ergotamine, labetalol, phenoxybenzamine, phentolamine, prazosin, tolazoline), barbiturates (large amounts), beta-adrenergic blocking agents, clonidine, insulin, minoxidil, narcotic analgesics (with overdose), phenothiazines, vasodilators.

I

Ichthyosis—Skin disorder with dryness, scaling and roughness.

Ileitis—Inflammation of the ileum, the last section of the small intestine.

Ileostomy—Surgical opening from the ileum, the end of the small intestine, to the outside of the body.

Immunosuppressants—Powerful drugs that suppress the immune system. Immunosuppressants are used in patients who have had organ transplants or severe disease associated with the immune system. These drugs include the following (some of which are not described in this book): azathioprine, basiliximab, betamethasone, chlorambucil, corticotropin, cortisone, cyclophosphamide, cyclosporine, dacliximab, dexamethasone, hydrocortisone, mercaptopurine, methylprednisolone, muromonab, muromonab-CD3, mycophenolate, prednisolone, prednisone, sirolimus, tacrolimus, thalidomide, triamcinolone, ursodiol.

Impotence—Male's inability to achieve or sustain erection of the penis for sexual intercourse.

Insomnia—Sleeplessness.

Interaction—Change in the body's response to one drug when another is taken. Interaction may decrease the effect of one or both drugs, increase the effect of one or both drugs or cause toxicity.

Iron Supplements—Products that contain iron in a form that can be absorbed from the intestinal tract. Supplements include ferrous fumarate, ferrous gluconate, ferrous sulfate, iron dextran, iron-polysaccharide.

J

Jaundice—Symptoms of liver damage, bile obstruction or destruction of red blood cells. Symptoms include yellowed whites of the eyes, yellow skin, dark urine and light stool.

K

Keratosis—Growth that is an accumulation of cells from the outer skin layers.

Kidney Stones—Small, solid stones made from calcium, cholesterol, cysteine and other body chemicals.

L

Laxatives—Medicines prescribed to treat constipation. These medicines include bisacodyl; bisacodyl and docusate; casanthranol; casanthranol and docusate; cascara sagrada; cascara sagrada and aloe; cascara sagrada and phenolphthalein; castor oil; danthron; danthron and docusate; danthron and poloxamer 188; dehydrocholic acid; dehydrocholic acid and docusate; docusate; docusate and phenolphthalein; docusate and mineral oil; docusate and phenolphthalein; docusate, carboxymethylcellulose and casanthranol; glycerin; lactulose; magnesium citrate; magnesium hydroxide; magnesium hydroxide and mineral oil; magnesium oxide; magnesium sulfate; malt soup extract; malt soup extract and psyllium; methylcellulose; mineral oil; mineral oil and cascara sagrada; mineral oil and phenolphthalein; mineral oil, glycerin and phenolphthalein; phenolphthalein; poloxamer; polycarbophil; potassium bitartrate and sodium bicarbonate; psyllium; psyllium and senna; psyllium hydrophilic mucilloid; psyllium hydrophilic mucilloid and carboxymethylcellulose; psyllium hydrophilic mucilloid and sennosides; psyllium hydrophilic mucilloid and senna; senna; senna and docusate; sennosides; sodium phosphate.

LDH—Abbreviation for lactate dehydrogenase. It is a measurement of cardiac enzymes used to confirm some heart conditions.

Lincomycins—A family of antibiotics used to treat certain infections.

Low-Purine Diet—A diet that avoids high-purine foods, such as liver, sweetbreads, kidneys, sardines, oysters and others. If you need a low-purine diet, request instructions from your doctor.

Lupus—Serious disorder of connective tissue that primarily affects women. Varies in severity with skin eruptions, joint inflammation, low white blood cell count and damage to internal organs, especially the kidneys.

Lymph Glands—Glands in the lymph vessels throughout the body that trap foreign and infectious matter and protect the bloodstream from infection.

M

Macrolides—A class of antibiotic (antibacterial) drugs. They include azithromycin, clarithromycin, dirithromycin, erythromycin, fidaxomicin, and telithromycin.

Male Hormones—Chemical substances secreted by the testicles, ovaries and adrenal glands in humans. Some male hormones used by humans are derived synthetically. Male hormones include testosterone cypionate and estradiol cypionate, testosterone enanthate and estradiol valerate.

Mania—A mood disturbance characterized by euphoria, agitation, elation, irritability, rapid and confused speech and excessive activity. Mania usually occurs as part of bipolar (manic-depressive) disorder.

Manic-Depressive Illness—Psychosis with alternating cycles of excessive enthusiasm and depression.

MAO Inhibitors—See Monoamine Oxidase (MAO) Inhibitors.

Mast Cell—Connective tissue cell.

Meglitinides—Drugs that stimulate the pancreas to produce insulin. Used to treat Type II (non-insulin dependent) diabetes. These drugs include repaglinide and nateglinide.

Menopause—The end of menstruation in the female, often accompanied by irritability, hot flashes, changes in the skin and bones and vaginal dryness.

Metabolism—Process of using nutrients and energy to build and break down wastes.

Migraine Headaches—Periodic headaches caused by constriction of arteries to the skull. Symptoms include severe pain, vision disturbances, nausea, vomiting and sensitivity to light.

Mind-Altering Drugs—Any drugs that decrease alertness, perception, concentration, contact with reality or muscular coordination.

Mineral Supplements—Mineral substances added to the diet to treat or prevent mineral deficiencies. They include iron, copper, magnesium, calcium, etc.

Monoamine Oxidase (MAO) Inhibitors—Drugs that prevent the activity of the enzyme monoamine oxidase (MAO) in brain tissue. MAO inhibitors include drugs that treat depression, Parkinson's and other conditions. MAOs can cause dangerous interactions with certain foods, beverages and other drugs. Drugs in this class include furazolidone, isocarboxazid, linezolid, methylene blue, phenelzine, procarbazine, rasagiline, selegiline, St. John's wort (acts similar to MAO inhibitors), tranylcypromine.

Muscle Blockers—Same as muscle relaxants or skeletal muscle relaxants.

Muscle Relaxants—Medicines used to lessen painful contractions and spasms of muscles. These include atracurium, carisoprodol, chlorphenesin, chlorzoxazone, cyclobenzaprine, metaxalone, methocarbamol, metocurine, orphenadrine citrate, orphenadrine hydrochloride, pancuronium, phenytoin, succinylcholine, tubocurarine, vecuronium.

Myasthenia Gravis—Disease of the muscles characterized by fatigue and progressive paralysis. It is usually confined to muscles of the face, lips, tongue and neck.

Mydriatics—Eye drops that cause the pupils to dilate (become larger) to a marked degree.

N

Narcotics—A group of habit-forming, addicting drugs used for treatment of pain, diarrhea, cough, acute pulmonary edema and others. They are all derived from opium, a milky exudate in capsules of papaver somniferum. Law requires licensed physicians to dispense by prescription. These drugs include alfentanil, buprenorphine, butorphanol, codeine, fentanyl, hydrocodone, hydromorphone, levorphanol, meperidine, methadone, morphine, nalbuphine, opium, oxycodone, oxymorphone, paregoric, pentazocine, propoxyphene, sufentanil.

Nephrotoxics—Under some circumstances, these medicines can be toxic to the kidneys. These medicines include acetaminophen (in high doses); acyclovir (injection of); aminoglycosides; amphotericin B (given internally); analgesic combinations containing acetaminophen and aspirin or other salicylates (with chronic high-dose use); anti-inflammatory analgesics (nonsteroidal); bacitracin (injection of); capreomycin; carmustine; chlorpropamide; cidofovir; ciprofloxacin; cisplatin; cox 2 inhibitors; cyclosporine; deferoxamine (long-term use); edetate calcium disodium (with high doses); edetate disodium (with high dose); foscarnet; gold compounds; ifosfamide; imipenem; lithium; methicillin, methotrexate (with high dose therapy); methoxyflurane; nafcillin; neomycin (oral); pamidronate; penicillamine; pentamidine; pentostatin, phenacetin; plicamycin; polymyxins (injection of); radiopaques (materials used for special x-ray examinations); rifampin; streptozocin; sulfonamides; tacrolimus; tetracyclines (except doxycycline and minocycline); tiopronin; tretinoin; vancomycin (injection of).

Neuroleptic Malignant Syndrome—Ceaseless involuntary, jerky movements of the tongue, facial muscles and hands.

Neuromuscular Blocking Agents—A group of drugs prescribed to relax skeletal muscles. They are all given by injection, and descriptions are not included in this book. These drugs include atracurium, edrophonium, gallamine, neostigmine, metocurine, pancuronium, pyridostigmine, succinylcholine, tubocurarine, vecuronium.

Neurotoxic Medications—Medicines that cause toxicity to the nerve tissues in the body. These drugs include alcohol (chronic use), allopurinol; altretamine, amantadine; amiodarone; anticonvulsants (hydantoin), capreomycin, carbamazepine, carboplatin, chloramphenicol (oral), chloroquine, cilastatin, ciprofloxacin, cisplatin, cycloserine, cyclosporine, cytarabine, didanosine, disulfiram, docetaxel, ethambutol, ethionamide, fludarabine, hydroxychloroquine, imipenem, interferon, isoniazid, lincomycins, lindane (topical), lithium, meperidine, methotrexate, metronidazole, mexiletine, nitrofurantoin, oxcarbazepine, paclitaxel, pemoline, pentostatin, pyridoxine (large amounts), quinacrine, quinidine, quinine, stavudine, tacrolimus, tetracyclines, thalidomide, vinblastine, vincristine, vindesine, zalcitabine.

Nitrates—Medicines made from a chemical with a nitrogen base. Nitrates include erythrityl tetranitrate, isosorbide dinitrate, nitroglycerin, pentaerythritol tetranitrate.

Nonsteroidal Anti-Inflammatory Drugs (NSAIDs)—See Anti-Inflammatory Drugs, Nonsteroidal.

Nutritional Supplements—Substances used to treat and prevent deficiencies when the body is unable to absorb them by eating a well-balanced, nutritional diet. These supplements include: Vitamins—ascorbic acid, ascorbic acid and sodium ascorbate, calcifediol, calcitriol, calcium pantothenate, cyanocobalamin, dihydrotachysterol, ergocalciferol, folate sodium, folic acid, hydroxocobalamin, niacin, niacinamide, pantothenic, pyridoxine, riboflavin, sodium ascorbate, thiamine, vitamin A, vitamin E. Minerals—calcium carbonate, calcium citrate, calcium glubionate, calcium gluconate, calcium lactate, calcium phosphate (dibasic and tribasic), sodium fluoride. Other—levocarnitine, omega-3 polyunsaturated fatty acids.

O

Opiates—See Narcotics.

Orthostatic Hypotension—Excess drop in blood pressure when arising from a sitting or lying position.

Osteoporosis—Softening of bones caused by a loss of calcium usually found in bone. Bones become brittle and fracture easily.

Ototoxic Medications—These medicines may possibly cause hearing damage. They include aminoglycosides, 4-aminoquinolines, anti-inflammatory analgesics (nonsteroidal), bumetanide (injected), capreomycin, carboplatin, chloroquine, cisplatin, deferoxamine, erythromycins, ethacrynic acid, furosemide, hydroxychloroquine, quinidine, quinine, salicylates, vancomycin (injected).

Ovary—Female sexual gland where eggs mature and ripen for fertilization.

P

Pain Relievers—Non-narcotic medicines used to treat pain.

Palpitations—Rapid, forceful or throbbing heartbeat noticeable to the patient.

Pancreatitis—Serious inflammation or infection of the pancreas that causes upper abdominal pain.

Pancreatitis-associated Drugs—Medications associated with the development of pancreatitis. These include alcohol, asparaginase, azathioprine, didanosine, estrogens, furosemide, methyldopa, nitrofurantoin, sulfonamides, tetracyclines, thiazide diuretics, valproic acid.

Parkinson's Disease or Parkinson's Syndrome—Disease of the central nervous system. Characteristics are a fixed, emotionless expression of the face, tremor, slower muscle movements, weakness, changed gait and a peculiar posture.

Pellagra—Disease caused by a deficiency of the water-soluble vitamin thiamine (vitamin B-1). Symptoms include brain disturbance, diarrhea and skin inflammation.

Penicillin—Chemical substance (antibiotic) originally discovered as a product of mold, that can kill some bacterial germs.

Peripheral Neuropathy (Peripheral Neuritis)—Inflammation and degeneration of the nerve endings or of the terminal nerves. It most often occurs in the nerve tissue of the muscles of the extremities (arms and legs). Symptoms include pain of varying intensity and sensations of numbness, tingling and burning in the hands and feet. It can be caused by certain medications or chemicals, infections, chronic inflammation or nutritive disease.

Peripheral-neuropathy Associated Drugs—Medications that are associated with the development of peripheral neuropathy. These include chloramphenicol, cisplatin, dapsone, didanosine, ethambutol, ethionamide, hydralazine, isoniazid, lithium, metronidazole, nitrofurantoin, nitrous oxide, phenytoin, stavudine, vincristine, zalcitabine.

P-glycoprotein Inducers—Drugs or supplements that can decrease the amount of another drug in the body's cells. These drugs and supplements include dexamethasone, morphine, phenobarbital, rifampin, St. John's wort, trazodone and others. Consult doctor or pharmacist about interaction.

P-glycoprotein Inhibitors—Drugs that can increase the amount of another drug in the body's cells. The interaction may be helpful by increasing a drug's effectiveness. The interaction may be harmful by increasing the risk of a drug's side effects or toxicity. These drugs include amiodarone, amprenavir, clarithromycin, colchicine, cyclosporine A, daunorubicin, digoxin, diltiazem, dronedarone, erythromycin, indinavir, itraconazole, ketoconazole, loperamide, nelfinavir, nicardipine, omeprazole, paroxetine, propafenone, propranolol, quinidine, saquinavir, sertraline, tacrolimus, tamoxifen, ticagrelor, valspodar, verapamil, vinblastine and others. Consult doctor or pharmacist about interaction.

Phenothiazines—Drugs used to treat mental, nervous and emotional conditions. These drugs include acetophenazine, chlorpromazine, fluphenazine, mesoridazine, methotrimeprazine, pericyazine, perphenazine, prochlorperazine, promazine, thiopropazate, thioproperazine, thioridazine, trifluoperazine, triflupromazine.

Pheochromocytoma—A tumor of the adrenal gland that produces chemicals that cause high blood pressure, headache, nervousness and other symptoms.

Phlegm—Thick mucus secreted by glands in the respiratory tract.

Photophobia—Increased sensitivity to light as perceived by the human eye. Drugs that can cause photophobia include antidiabetic drugs, atropine, belladonna, bromides, chloroquine, ciprofloxacin, chlordiazepoxide, clidinium, clomiphene, dicyclomine, digitalis drugs, doxepin, ethambutol, ethionamide, ethosuximide, etretinate, glycopyrrolate, hydroxychloroquine, hydroxyzine, hyoscyamine, isopropamide, mephenytoin, methenamine, methsuximide, monoamine oxidase (MAO) inhibitors, nalidixic acid, norfloxacin, oral contraceptives, orphenadrine, paramethadione, phenothiazines, propantheline, quinidine, quinine, scopolamine, tetracyclines, tridihexethyl, trimethadione.

Photosensitizing Medications—Medicines that can cause abnormally heightened skin reactions to the effects of sunlight and ultraviolet light. These medicines include acetazolamide, acetohexamide, alprazolam, amantadine, amiloride, amiodarone, amitriptyline, amoxapine, antidiabetic agents (oral), barbiturates, bendroflumethiazide, benzocaine, benzoyl peroxide, benzthiazide, captopril, carbamazepine, chlordiazepoxide, chloroquine, chlorothiazide, chlorpromazine, chlorpropamide, chlortetracycline, chlorthalidone, ciprofloxacin, clindamycin, clofazimine, clofibrate, clomipramine, coal tar, contraceptives (estrogen-containing), cyproheptadine, dacarbazine, dapsone, demeclocycline, desipramine, desoximetasone, diethylstilbestrol, diflunisal, diltiazem, diphenhydramine, disopyramide, doxepin, doxycycline, enoxacin, estrogens, etretinate, flucytosine, fluorescein, fluorouracil, fluphenazine, flutamide, furosemide, glipizide, glyburide, gold preparations, griseofulvin, haloperidol, hexachlorophene, hydrochlorothiazide, hydroflumethiazide, ibuprofen, imipramine, indomethacin, isotretinoin, ketoprofen, lincomycin, lomefloxacin, maprotiline, mesoridazine, methacycline, methotrexate, methoxsalen, methyclothiazide, methyldopa, metolazone, minocycline, minoxidil, nabumetone, nalidixic acid, naproxen, nifedipine, norfloxacin, nortriptyline, ofloxacin, oral contraceptives, oxyphenbutazone, oxytetracycline, perphenazine, phenelzine, phenobarbital, phenylbutazone, phenytoin, piroxicam, polythiazide, prochlorperazine, promazine, promethazine, protriptyline, pyrazinamide, quinidine, quinine, sulfonamides, sulindac, tetracycline, thiabendazole, thioridazine, thiothixene, tolazamide, tolbutamide, tranylcypromine, trazodone, tretinoin, triamterene, trichlormethiazide, trifluoperazine, triflupromazine, trimeprazine, trimethoprim, trimipramine, triprolidine, vinblastine.

Pinworms—Common intestinal parasites that cause rectal itching and irritation.

Pituitary Gland—Gland at the base of the brain that secretes hormones to stimulate growth and other glands to produce hormones.

Platelet—Disc-shaped element of the blood, smaller than a red or white blood cell, necessary for blood clotting.

Polymyxins—A family of antibiotics that kill bacteria.

Polyp—Growth on a mucous membrane.

Porphyria—Inherited metabolic disorder characterized by changes in the nervous system and kidneys.

Post-Partum—Following delivery of a baby.

Potassium—Important chemical found in body cells.

Potassium Foods—Foods high in potassium content, including dried apricots and peaches, lentils, raisins, citrus and whole-grain cereals.

Potassium Supplements—Medicines needed by people who don't have enough potassium in their diets or by those who develop a deficiency due to illness or taking diuretics and other medicines. These supplements include chloride; potassium acetate; potassium bicarbonate; potassium bicarbonate and potassium chloride; potassium bicarbonate and potassium citrate; potassium chloride; potassium chloride, potassium bicarbonate and potassium citrate; potassium gluconate; potassium gluconate and potassium chloride; potassium gluconate and potassium citrate; potassium gluconate, potassium citrate and ammonium; trikates.

Premenstrual Dysphoric Disorder (PMDD)—A severe form of premenstrual syndrome which is characterized by severe monthly mood swings as well as physical symptoms that interfere with everyday life, especially a woman's relationships with her family and friends.

Progesterone—A female steroid sex hormone that is responsible for preparing the uterus for pregnancy.

Progestin—A synthetic hormone that is designed to mimic the actions of progesterone. These include etonogestrel, hydroxy-progesterone, medroxyprogesterone, megestrol, norethindrone, norgestrel and progesterone.

Prostaglandins—A group of drugs used for a variety of therapeutic purposes. These drugs include alprostadil (treats newborns with congenital heart disease), carboprost and dinoprost (both used to induce labor) and dinoprostone (used to induce labor or to induce a late abortion).

Prostate—Gland in the male that surrounds the neck of the bladder and the urethra.

Protease Inhibitors—A class of anti-HIV drugs which inhibit the protease enzyme and stop virus replication. These drugs include: abacavir, atazanavir, darunavir, fosamprenavir, indinavir, lopinavir and ritonavir; nelfinavir, ritonavir, saquinavir and tipranavir.

Protein Bound Drugs—This protein is not to be confused with the protein in your food. If two highly protein bound drugs are given together, they will compete for protein carriers in the body and may possibly cause one or both of the drugs to be less effective and dosages may need to be adjusted. Some of these drugs are clofibrate, diazepam, diazoxide, fluoxetine, ibuprofen, indomethacin, naproxen, raloxifene, tiagabine, vilazodone.

Prothrombin—Blood substance essential in clotting.

Prothrombin Time (Pro Time)—Laboratory study used to follow prothrombin activity and keep coagulation safe.

Psoriasis—Chronic inherited skin disease. Symptoms are lesions with silvery scales on the edges.

Psychosis—Mental disorder characterized by deranged personality, loss of contact with reality and possible delusions, hallucinations or illusions.

Purine Foods—Foods that are metabolized into uric acid. Foods high in purines include anchovies, liver, brains, sweetbreads, sardines, kidneys, oysters, gravy and meat extracts.

Q

QT Interval Prolongation-Causing Drugs—A group of drugs that can cause serious heart rhythm problems. These drugs include amiodarone, asenapine, azithromycin, azole antifungals, calcium channel blockers (especially bepridil), chloroquine, chlorpromazine, clarithromycin, dirithromycin, disopyramide, dofetilide, domperidone, dronedarone, droperidol, erythromycins, flecainide, fluoroquinolones, halofantrine, haloperidol, ibutilide, macrolide antibiotics, maprotiline, mesoridazine, methadone, pentamidine, phenothiazines, pimozide, quinidine, ranolazine, sotalol, sparfloxacin, thioridazine, toremifene, tricyclic antidepressants and others.

R

Rauwolfia Alkaloids—Drugs that belong to the family of antihypertensives (drugs that lower blood pressure). Rauwolfia alkaloids are not used as extensively as in years past. They include alseroxylon, deserpidine, rauwolfia serpentina, reserpine.

RDA—Recommended daily allowance of a vitamin or mineral.

Rebound Effect—The worsening or return of symptoms when a drug (such as a decongestant) is discontinued or a patient no longer responds to it.

Renal—Pertaining to the kidney.

Retina—Innermost covering of the eyeball on which the image is formed.

Retinoids—A group of drugs that are synthetic vitamin A-like compounds used to treat skin conditions. These drugs include etretinate, isotretinoin and retinoic acid.

Retroperitoneal Imaging—Special x-rays or CT scans of the organs attached to the abdominal wall behind the peritoneum (the covering of the intestinal tract and lining of the walls of the abdominal and pelvic cavities).

Reye's Syndrome—Rare, sometimes fatal, disease of children that causes brain and liver damage.

Rickets—Bone disease caused by vitamin D deficiency. Bones become bent and distorted during infancy or childhood.

S

Salicylates—Medicines to relieve pain and reduce fever. These include aspirin, aspirin and caffeine, balsalazide, buffered aspirin, choline salicylate, choline and magnesium salicylates, magnesium salicylate, salicylamide, salsalate, sodium salicylate.

Sedatives—Drugs that reduce excitement or anxiety. They are used to produce sedation (calmness). These include alprazolam, amobarbital, aprobarbital, bromazepam, butalbital, chloral hydrate, clonazepam, clorazepate, chlordiazepoxide, diazepam, diphenhydramine, doxylamine, estazolam, ethchlorvynol, ethinamate, eszopiclone, flurazepam, glutethimide, halazepam, hydroxyzine, ketazolam, lorazepam, methotrimeprazine, midazolam, nitrazepam, oxazepam, pentobarbital, phenobarbital, prazepam, promethazine, propiomazine, propofol, quazepam, secobarbital, temazepam, triazolam, trimeprazine, zaleplon, zolpidem, zopiclone.

Seizure—A sudden attack of epilepsy or some other disease can cause changes of consciousness or convulsions.

Seizure threshold lowering drugs—Seizure threshold refers to the minimal conditions required to trigger a seizure. A number of drugs can lower the seizure threshold in susceptible patients and increase the risk for a seizure. These drugs include certain antibiotics, antiasthmatics, antidepressants, antipsychotics, phenothiazines, psychostimulants, hormones, local anesthetics, immunosuppressants, narcotics and others. Herbal remedies may also lower seizure threshold. Consult your doctor about your risks.

Selective Serotonin Reuptake Inhibitors (SSRIs)—Medications used for treatment of depression that work by increasing the serotonin levels in the brain. Serotonin is a neurotransmitter (brain chemical) having to do with mood and behavior. These drugs include fluoxetine, fluvoxamine, paroxetine, sertraline. More information can be found on the individual drug chart for each drug.

Serotonergics—Drugs that increase the levels of serotonin (a brain chemical). Excess serotonin can lead to serotonin syndrome (a possibly life-threatening condition). These drugs include almotriptan, amitriptyline, amphetamines, bromocriptine, buspirone, citalopram, clomipramine, desvenlafaxine, dextromethorphan, duloxetine, eletriptan, escitalopram, fenfluramine, fluoxetine, fluvoxamine, frovatriptan, imipramine, levodopa, linezolid, lithium, meperidine, moclobemide, monoamine oxidase (MAO) inhibitors, naratriptan, nefazodone, paroxetine, pentazocine, rizatriptan, sertraline, sibutramine, St. John's Wort, sumatriptan, tapentadol, tramadol, trazodone, tricyclic antidepressants, tryptophan, valproic acid, venlafaxine, vilazodone, zolmitriptan and some drugs of abuse (e.g., cocaine, LSD, ecstasy, marijuana and others). Other drugs or herbal supplements may be risk factors also. Ask your doctor or pharmacist about the safety of any drugs you are prescribed and advised them of any herbal supplements you take.

Serotonin Syndrome—A potentially very serious and life-threatening condition caused by drugs that increase serotonin levels in the brain. The syndrome can be caused by an overdose, interaction with other drugs, or rarely, with doses used in treatment. It is more likely to occur when starting a drug or increasing the dosage of a drug. Symptoms often come on quickly and progress rapidly. Symptoms may include confusion, agitation, headache, diarrhea, irritability, muscle rigidity, high body temperature, fast heart beat, rapid change in blood pressure, nausea or vomiting, poor coordination, dilated pupils, restlessness, hallucinations, overactive reflexes, sweating, shivering, tremor, and muscle twitching. More severe symptoms can include seizures, delirium, shock loss of consciousness and other major medical problems.

SGOT—Abbreviation for serum glutamic-oxaloacetic transaminase. Measuring the level in the blood helps demonstrate liver disorders and diagnose recent heart damage.

SGPT—Abbreviation for a laboratory study measuring the blood level of serum glutamic-pyruvic transaminase. Deviations from a normal level may indicate liver disease.

Sick Sinus Syndrome—A complicated, serious heartbeat rhythm disturbance characterized by a slow heart rate alternating with a fast or slow heart rate with heart block.

Sinusitis—Inflammation or infection of the sinus cavities in the skull.

Skeletal Muscle Relaxants (same as Skeletal Muscle Blockers)—A group of drugs prescribed to treat spasms of the skeletal muscles. These drugs include carisoprodol, chlorphenesin, chlorzoxazone, cyclobenzaprine, diazepam, lorazepam, metaxalone, methocarbamol, orphenadrine, phenytoin.

Sleep Inducers—Night-time sedatives to aid in falling asleep.

Sleep-Related Behaviors—Certain behaviors that can occur with the use of sedative-hypnotic drugs. The behaviors include: cooking and eating, using the telephone, having sex and sleep-driving (driving while not fully awake). Typically, the person has no memory of these actions.

Statins—See HMG-CoA Reductase Inhibitors.

Streptococci—A bacteria that can cause infections in the throat, respiratory system and skin. Improperly treated, can lead to disease in the heart, joints and kidneys.

Stroke—Sudden, severe attack, usually sudden paralysis, from injury to the brain or spinal cord caused by a blood clot or hemorrhage in the brain.

Stupor—Near unconsciousness.

Sublingual—Under the tongue. Some drugs are absorbed almost as quickly this way as by injection.

Sulfa Drugs—Shorthand for sulfonamide drugs, which are used to treat infections.

Sulfonamides—Sulfa drugs prescribed to treat infections. They include sulfacytine, sulfamethoxazole, sulfamethoxazole and trimethoprim, sulfasalazine, sulfisoxazole.

Sulfonylureas—A family of drugs that lower blood sugar (hypoglycemic agents). Used in the treatment of some forms of diabetes.

Sympatholytics—A group of drugs that block the action of the sympathetic nervous system. These drugs include beta-blockers, guanethidine, hydralazine and prazosin.

Sympathomimetics—A large group of drugs that mimic the effects of stimulation of the sympathetic part of the autonomic nervous system. These drugs include albuterol, amphetamine, benzphetamine, bitolterol, cocaine, dextroamphetamine, diethylpropion, dobutamine, ephedrine, epinephrine, ethylnorepinephrine, fenfluramine, indacaterol, ipratropium, isoproterenol, isoetharine, mazindol, mephentermine, metaproterenol, metaraminol, methoxamine, norepinephrine, phendimetrazine, phentermine, phenylephrine, pirbuterol, pseudoephedrine, ritodrine, terbutaline.

T

Tardive Dyskinesia—Slow, involuntary movements of the jaw, lips and tongue caused by an unpredictable drug reaction. Drugs that can cause this include haloperidol, phenothiazines, thiothixene.

Tartrazine Dye—A dye used in foods and medicine preparations that may cause an allergic reaction in some people.

Tetracyclines—A group of medicines with similar chemical structure used to treat infections. These drugs include demeclocycline, doxycycline, methacycline, minocycline, oxytetracycline, tetracycline.

Thiazides—A group of chemicals that cause diuresis (loss of water through the kidneys). Frequently used to treat high blood pressure and congestive heart failure. Thiazides include bendroflumethiazide, benzthiazide, chlorothiazide, chlorthalidone, cyclothiazide, hydrochlorothiazide, hydroflumethiazide, methyclothiazide, metolazone, polythiazide, quinethazone, trichlormethiazide.

Thiothixines—See Thioxanthenes.

Thioxanthenes—Drugs used to treat emotional, mental and nervous conditions. These drugs include chlorprothixene, flupenthixol, thiothixene.

Thrombocytopenias—Diseases characterized by inadequate numbers of blood platelets circulating in the bloodstream.

Thrombolytic Agents—Drugs that help to dissolve blood clots. They include alteplase, anistreplase, streptokinase, urokinase.

Thrombophlebitis—Inflammation of a vein caused by a blood clot in the vein.

Thyroid—Gland in the neck that manufactures and secretes several hormones.

Thyroid Hormones—Medications that mimic the action of the thyroid hormone made in the thyroid gland. They include dextrothyroxine, levothyroxine, liothyronine, liotrix, thyroglobulin, thyroid.

Tic Douloureux—Painful condition caused by inflammation of a nerve in the face.

Tolerance—A decreasing response to repeated constant doses of a drug or a need to increase doses to produce the same physical or mental response.

Toxicity—Poisonous reaction to a drug that impairs body functions or damages cells.

Tranquilizers—Drugs that calm a person without clouding consciousness.

Transdermal Patches—Medicated patches that stick to the skin. There are more and more medications in this form. This method produces a prolonged systemic effect. If you are using this form, follow these instructions: Choose an area of skin without cuts, scars or hair, such as the upper arm, chest or behind the ear. Thoroughly clean area where patch is to be applied. If patch gets wet and loose, cover with an additional piece of plastic. Apply a fresh patch if the first one falls off. Apply each dose to a different area of skin if possible.

Tremor—Involuntary trembling.

Trichomoniasis—Infestation of the vagina by trichomonas, an infectious organism. The infection causes itching, vaginal discharge and irritation.

Triglyceride—Fatty chemical manufactured from carbohydrates for storage in fat cells.

Tyramine—Normal chemical component of the body that helps sustain blood pressure. Can rise to fatal levels in combination with some drugs. Tyramine is found in many foods:

Beverages—Alcohol beverages, especially Chianti or robust red wines, vermouth, ale, beer.

Breads—Homemade bread with a lot of yeast and breads or crackers containing cheese.

Fats—Sour cream.

Fruits—Bananas, red plums, avocados, figs, raisins, raspberries.

Meats and meat substitutes—Aged game, liver (if not fresh), canned meats, salami, sausage, aged cheese, salted dried fish, pickled herring, meat tenderizers.

Vegetables—Italian broad beans, green bean pods, eggplant.

Miscellaneous—Yeast concentrates or extracts, marmite, soup cubes, commercial gravy, soy sauce, any protein food that has been stored improperly or is spoiled.

U

Ulcer, Peptic—Open sore on the mucous membrane of the esophagus, stomach or duodenum caused by stomach acid.

Urethra—Hollow tube through which urine (and semen in men) is discharged.

Urethritis—Inflammation or infection of the urethra.

Uricosurics—A group of drugs that promotes excretion of uric acid in the urine. These drugs include probenecid and sulfinpyrazone.

Urinary Acidifiers—Medications that cause urine to become acid. These include ascorbic acid, potassium phosphate, potassium and sodium phosphates, racemethionine.

Urinary Alkalizers—Medications that cause urine to become alkaline. These include potassium citrate, potassium citrate and citric acid, potassium citrate and sodium citrate, sodium bicarbonate, sodium citrate and citric acid, tricitrate.

Uterus—Also called the womb. A hollow muscular organ in the female in which the embryo develops into a fetus.

V

Valproic Acid Drugs—Anticonvulsant drugs that are used to prevent seizures in epilepsy, and as treatment for migraine and bipolar disorder. They include oral drugs divalproex and valproic acid and the injectable drug valproate.

Vascular—Pertaining to blood vessels.

Vascular Headache Preventatives—Medicines prescribed to prevent the occurrence of or reduce the frequency and severity of vascular headaches such as migraines. These drugs include atenolol; clonidine; ergotamine, belladonna alkaloids and phenobarbital; fenoprofen; flunarizine; ibuprofen; indomethacin; isocarboxazid, lithium; mefenamic acid; methysergide; metoprolol; nadolol; naproxen; phenelzine; pizotyline; propranolol; timolol, tranylcypromine, verapamil.

Vascular Headache Treatment—Medicine prescribed to treat vascular headaches such as migraines. These drugs include butalbital (combined with acetaminophen, aspirin, caffeine or codeine); cyproheptadine; diclofenac; diflunisal; dihydroergotamine; ergotamine; ergotamine and caffeine; ergotamine, caffeine, belladonna alkaloids and pentobarbital; etodolac; fenoprofen; ibuprofen; indomethacin (capsules, oral suspension, rectal); isometheptene, dichloralphenazone and acetaminophen; ketoprofen; meclofenamate; mefenamic acid; metoclopramide; naproxen; phenobarbital; triptans.

Vasoconstrictor—Any agent that causes a narrowing of the blood vessels.

Vasodilator—Any agent that causes a widening of the blood vessels.

Vertigo—A sensation of motion, usually dizziness or whirling either of oneself or one's surroundings.

Virus—Infectious organism that reproduces in the cells of the infected host. Viruses cause many diseases in humans including the common cold.

Xanthines—Substances that stimulate muscle tissue, especially that of the heart. Types of xanthines include aminophylline, caffeine, dyphylline, oxtriphylline, theophylline.

Yeast—A single-cell organism that can cause infections of the mouth, vagina, skin and parts of the gastrointestinal system.

INDEX

How to Find a Drug Name in the Index

Look it up by its brand name, such as Tylenol, or its generic name, such as acetaminophen (which is the generic name for Tylenol).

The drug names in the index appear in two different formats:

1. Drug brand (or trade) names. These names appear in ***bold italic***, and are followed by the drug chart name and a page number. (The drug chart name may be a single generic drug name or a drug family name.)

Example: ***Bayer*** - See ASPIRIN 152

Many brand name drugs contain two or more generic ingredients. These brand names will be followed by two or more drug chart names. Refer to all the drug charts listed for complete information on that particular brand name.

Example: ***Allent*** - See
ANTIHISTAMINES 106
PSEUDOEPHEDRINE 694

2. Drug generic names or drug family names (a group of similar generic drugs such as antihistamines). These names appear in all capital letters and are followed by their chart page number. An underlined name in the index indicates that it is a title of a drug chart in the book.

Example: HMG-CoA REDUCTASE INHIBITORS 424
Example: ATORVASTATIN - See HMG-CoA REDUCTASE INHIBITORS 424

Drug class names are also listed. The drug class is usually a treatment (therapeutic) name (e.g., antihypertensive). These names appear in regular type with capital and lowercase letters. The drug class name is followed by drug chart names that are in that class:

Example: Antifungal - See
ANTIFUNGALS, AZOLES 86
CLOTRIMAZOLE (Oral-Local) 262
GRISEOFULVIN 414
NYSTATIN 614

2/G-DM Cough - See
DEXTROMETHORPHAN 312
GUAIFENESIN 416
4-Way Long Acting Nasal Spray - See
OXYMETAZOLINE (Nasal) 630
5-ALPHA REDUCTASE INHIBITORS 2
5-ASA - See MESALAMINE 542
5-FU - See FLUOROURACIL (Topical) 394
6-MP - See MERCAPTOPURINE 540
8-Hour Bayer Timed Release - See ASPIRIN 152
12 Hour Nostrilla Nasal Decongestant - See
OXYMETAZOLINE (Nasal) 630
222 - See
CAFFEINE 216
NARCOTIC ANALGESICS & ASPIRIN 588
282 - See
CAFFEINE 216
NARCOTIC ANALGESICS & ASPIRIN 588
292 - See
CAFFEINE 216
NARCOTIC ANALGESICS & ASPIRIN 588
293 - See NARCOTIC ANALGESICS & ASPIRIN 588
642 - See NARCOTIC ANALGESICS 584
692 - See
CAFFEINE 216
NARCOTIC ANALGESICS & ASPIRIN 588

A

A-200 Gel - See PEDICULICIDES (Topical) 642
A-200 Shampoo - See PEDICULICIDES (Topical) 642
A/B Otic - See ANTIPYRINE & BENZOCAINE (Otic) 130
ABACAVIR - See NUCLEOSIDE REVERSE TRANSCRIPTASE INHIBITORS 610
Abenol - See ACETAMINOPHEN 8
Abilify - See ARIPIPRAZOLE 148
Abilify DiscMelt - See ARIPIPRAZOLE 148
Abilify Oral Solution - See ARIPIPRAZOLE 148
Abitrate - See FIBRATES 386
Abortifacient - See MIFEPRISTONE 556
Abraxane - See PACLITAXEL 632
Abreva - See ANTIVIRALS (Topical) 144

Absorica - See ISOTRETINOIN 462
Abstral - See NARCOTIC ANALGESICS 584
A.C.&C. - See NARCOTIC ANALGESICS & ASPIRIN 588
Acabamate - See MEPROBAMATE 538
ACAMPROSATE 4
Acanya - See
ANTIBACTERIALS FOR ACNE (Topical) 64
BENZOYL PEROXIDE 178
ACARBOSE 6
Accolate - See LEUKOTRIENE MODIFIERS 488
Accuneb - See BRONCHODILATORS, ADRENERGIC 200
Accupril - See ANGIOTENSIN-CONVERTING ENZYME (ACE) INHIBITORS 44
Accurbron - See BRONCHODILATORS, XANTHINE 204
Accuretic - See ANGIOTENSIN-CONVERTING ENZYME (ACE) INHIBITORS & HYDROCHLOROTHIAZIDE 46
ACEBUTOLOL - See BETA-ADRENERGIC BLOCKING AGENTS 182
Aceon - See ANGIOTENSIN-CONVERTING ENZYME (ACE) INHIBITORS 44
Acephen - See ACETAMINOPHEN 8
Aceta - See ACETAMINOPHEN 8
ACETAMINOPHEN 8
ACETAMINOPHEN & CODEINE - See NARCOTIC ANALGESICS & ACETAMINOPHEN 586
Acetaminophen Uniserts - See ACETAMINOPHEN 8
Acetasol HC - See ANTIBACTERIALS (Otic) 68
Acetazolam - See CARBONIC ANHYDRASE INHIBITORS 232
ACETAZOLAMIDE - See CARBONIC ANHYDRASE INHIBITORS 232
ACETIC ACID - See ANTIBACTERIALS (Otic) 68
ACETIC ACID & ALUMINUM ACETATE - See ANTIBACTERIALS (Otic) 68
ACETIC ACID & HYDROCORTISONE - See ANTIBACTERIALS (Otic) 68
ACETOHEXAMIDE - See SULFONYLUREAS 770
ACETOHYDROXAMIC ACID (AHA) 10
ACETOPHENAZINE - See PHENOTHIAZINES 656
Acetoxyl 2.5 Gel - See BENZOYL PEROXIDE 178
Acetoxyl 5 Gel - See BENZOYL PEROXIDE 178
Acetoxyl 10 Gel - See BENZOYL PEROXIDE 178
Acetoxyl 20 Gel - See BENZOYL PEROXIDE 178
Acetylsalicylic Acid - See ASPIRIN 152
Aches-N-Pain - See ANTI-INFLAMMATORY DRUGS, NONSTEROIDAL (NSAIDs) 116
Achromycin - See
ANTIBACTERIALS FOR ACNE (Topical) 64
TETRACYCLINES 782
Achromycin V - See TETRACYCLINES 782
Acid + All - See ANTACIDS 48
AcipHex - See PROTON PUMP INHIBITORS 692
ACITRETIN - See RETINOIDS (Oral) 720
ACLIDINIUM - See BRONCHODILATORS, ANTICHOLINERGIC 202
Aclophen - See
ACETAMINOPHEN 8
ANTIHISTAMINES 106
PHENYLEPHRINE 658
Aclovate - See ADRENOCORTICOIDS (Topical) 18
Acne-5 Lotion - See BENZOYL PEROXIDE 178
Acne-10 Lotion - See BENZOYL PEROXIDE 178
Acne-Aid 10 Cream - See BENZOYL PEROXIDE 178
Acne-Aid Gel - See KERATOLYTICS 470
Acne-Mask - See BENZOYL PEROXIDE 178
AcnoAcnomel Cake - See KERATOLYTICS 470
Acnomel B.P. 5 Lotion - See BENZOYL PEROXIDE 178
Acnomel Cream - See KERATOLYTICS 470
Acnomel Vanishing Cream - See KERATOLYTICS 470
Acnomel-Acne Cream - See KERATOLYTICS 470
Acnotex - See KERATOLYTICS 470
Acon - See VITAMIN A 834
ACRIVASTINE - See ANTIHISTAMINES 106
Acta-Char - See CHARCOAL, ACTIVATED 238
Acta-Char Liquid - See CHARCOAL, ACTIVATED 238
Actacin - See
ANTIHISTAMINES 106
PSEUDOEPHEDRINE 694
Actagen - See
ANTIHISTAMINES 106
PSEUDOEPHEDRINE 694
Actagen-C Cough - See
ANTIHISTAMINES 106
NARCOTIC ANALGESICS 584
PSEUDOEPHEDRINE 694
Actamin - See ACETAMINOPHEN 8
Actamin Extra - See ACETAMINOPHEN 8
Actamin Super - See
ACETAMINOPHEN 8
CAFFEINE 216
Acti-B-12 - See VITAMIN B-12 (Cyanocobalamin) 836
Acticin - See PEDICULICIDES (Topical) 642
Acticort-100 - See ADRENOCORTICOIDS (Topical) 18
Actidil - See ANTIHISTAMINES 106
Actidose with Sorbitol - See CHARCOAL, ACTIVATED 238

Actidose-Aqua - See CHARCOAL, ACTIVATED 238
Actifed Cold & Allergy Tablet - See
ANTIHISTAMINES 106
PHENYLEPHRINE 658
Actifed Cold & Sinus Caplet - See
ACETAMINOPHEN 8
ANTIHISTAMINES 106
Actigall - See URSODIOL 824
Actimol - See ACETAMINOPHEN 8
Actinex - See MASOPROCOL 524
Actiq - See NARCOTIC ANALGESICS 584
Activella - See
ESTROGENS 372
PROGESTINS 680
Actonel - See BISPHOSPHONATES 192
Actonel with Calcium - See
BISPHOSPHONATES 192
CALCIUM SUPPLEMENTS 222
ACTOplus met - See
METFORMIN 544
THIAZOLIDINEDIONES 786
ACTOplus Met XR - See
METFORMIN 544
THIAZOLIDINEDIONES 786
Actos - See THIAZOLIDINEDIONES 786
Acular - See ANTI-INFLAMMATORY DRUGS, NONSTEROIDAL (NSAIDs) (Ophthalmic) 120
Acular LS - See ANTI-INFLAMMATORY DRUGS NONSTEROIDAL (NSAIDs) (Ophthalmic) 120
ACYCLOVIR - See ANTIVIRALS FOR HERPES VIRUS 136
ACYCLOVIR (Topical) - See ANTIVIRALS (Topical) 144
Aczone - See DAPSONE 304
Adalat - See CALCIUM CHANNEL BLOCKERS 220
Adalat CC - See CALCIUM CHANNEL BLOCKERS 220
Adalat FT - See CALCIUM CHANNEL BLOCKERS 220
Adalat P.A. - See CALCIUM CHANNEL BLOCKERS 220
ADALIMUMAB - See TUMOR NECROSIS FACTOR BLOCKERS 822
ADAPALENE - See RETINOIDS (Topical) 722
Adapin - See ANTIDEPRESSANTS, TRICYCLIC 80
Adatuss D.C. Expectorant - See
GUAIFENESIN 416
NARCOTIC ANALGESICS 584
Adcortyl - See ADRENOCORTICOIDS (Topical) 18
Adderall - See AMPHETAMINES 28
Adderall XR - See AMPHETAMINES 28
Adeflor - See VITAMINS & FLUORIDE 848
Adipex-P - See APPETITE SUPPRESSANTS 146
Adipost - See APPETITE SUPPRESSANTS 146
Adoxa - See ANTIBACTERIALS FOR ACNE (Topical) 64
Adoxa Pak - See ANTIBACTERIALS FOR ACNE (Topical) 64
Adphen - See APPETITE SUPPRESSANTS 146
Adrenal steroid - See DEHYDROEPIANDROSTERONE (DHEA) 308
Adrenalin - See BRONCHODILATORS, ADRENERGIC 200
Adrenocorticoid (Nasal) - See ADRENOCORTICOIDS (Nasal Inhalation) 12
Adrenocorticoid (Ophthalmic) - See ANTI-INFLAMMATORY DRUGS, STEROIDAL (Ophthalmic) 122
Adrenocorticoid (Otic) - See ANTI-INFLAMMATORY DRUGS, STEROIDAL (Otic) 124
Adrenocorticoid (Topical) - See ADRENOCORTICOIDS (Topical) 18
<u>ADRENOCORTICOIDS (Nasal Inhalation)</u> 12
<u>ADRENOCORTICOIDS (Oral Inhalation)</u> 14
<u>ADRENOCORTICOIDS (Systemic)</u> 16
<u>ADRENOCORTICOIDS (Topical)</u> 18
Adsorbocarpine - See ANTIGLAUCOMA, CHOLINERGIC AGONISTS 100
Adult Acne Clearing Gel - See KERATOLYTICS 470
Advair Diskus - See
ADRENOCORTICOIDS (Oral Inhalation) 14
BRONCHODILATORS, ADRENERGIC 200
Advair HFA - See
ADRENOCORTICOIDS (Oral Inhalation) 14
BRONCHODILATORS, ADRENERGIC 200
Advanced Formula Di-Gel - See ANTACIDS 48
Advanced Formula Dristan Caplets - See
ACETAMINOPHEN 8
PHENYLEPHRINE 658
Advantage 24 - See CONTRACEPTIVES, VAGINAL 280
Advicor - See
HMG-CoA REDUCTASE INHIBITORS 424
NIACIN 596
Advil - See ANTI-INFLAMMATORY DRUGS, NONSTEROIDAL (NSAIDs) 116
Advil Allergy Sinus - See
ANTIHISTAMINES 106
ANTI-INFLAMMATORY DRUGS, NON-STEROIDAL (NSAIDs) 116
PSEUDOEPHEDRINE 694

Advil Cold and Sinus LiquiGels - See
ANTI-INFLAMMATORY DRUGS, NONSTEROIDAL (NSAIDs) 116
PSEUDOEPHEDRINE 694
Advil Congestion Relief - See
ANTI-INFLAMMATORY DRUGS, NON-STEROIDAL (NSAIDs) 120
PHENYLEPHRINE 658
Advil Congestion Relief - See
ANTI-INFLAMMATORY DRUGS, NON-STEROIDAL (NSAIDs) 116
PHENYLEPHRINE 658
Advil Flu and Body Ache - See
ANTI-INFLAMMATORY DRUGS, NONSTEROIDAL (NSAIDs) 116
PSEUDOEPHEDRINE 694
Advil Migraine - See
ANTI-INFLAMMATORY DRUGS, NONSTEROIDAL (NSAIDs) 116
Advil Multi-Symptom Cold - See
ANTIHISTAMINES 106
ANTI-INFLAMMATORY DRUGS, NONSTEROIDAL (NSAIDs) 116
PSEUDOEPHEDRINE 694
Advil PM - See
ANTIHISTAMINES 106
ANTI-INFLAMMATORY DRUGS, NON-STEROIDAL (NSAIDs) 116
Aerolate III - See BRONCHODILATORS, XANTHINE 204
Aerolate Jr. - See BRONCHODILATORS, XANTHINE 204
Aerolate Sr. - See BRONCHODILATORS, XANTHINE 204
Aerophyllin - See BRONCHODILATORS, XANTHINE 204
Aeroseb-Dex - See ADRENOCORTICOIDS (Topical) 18
Aeroseb-HC - See ADRENOCORTICOIDS (Topical) 18
Afaxin - See VITAMIN A 834
Afko-Lube - See LAXATIVES, SOFTENER/LUBRICANT 480
Afko-Lube Lax - See
LAXATIVES, SOFTENER/LUBRICANT 480
LAXATIVES, STIMULANT 482
Afrin 12 Hour Nasal Spray - See OXYMETAZOLINE (Nasal) 630
Afrin 12 Hour Nose Drops - See OXYMETAZOLINE (Nasal) 630
Afrin Cherry Scented Nasal Spray - See OXYMETAZOLINE (Nasal) 630
Afrin Children's Strength 12 Hour Nose Drops - See OXYMETAZOLINE (Nasal) 630
Afrin Children's Strength Nose Drops - See OXYMETAZOLINE (Nasal) 630
Afrin Extra Moisturizing Nasal Decongestant Spray - See OXYMETAZOLINE (Nasal) 630
Afrin Menthol Nasal Spray - See OXYMETAZOLINE (Nasal) 630
Afrin Nasal Spray - See OXYMETAZOLINE (Nasal) 630
Afrin No Drip Extra Moisturizing - See OXYMETAZOLINE (Nasal) 630
Afrin No Drip Nasal Decongestant, Severe Congestion with Menthol - See OXYMETAZOLINE (Nasal) 630
Afrin No Drip Nasal Decongestant, Sinus with Vapornase - See OXYMETAZOLINE (Nasal) 630
Afrin No Drip Sinus - See OXYMETAZOLINE (Nasal) 630
Afrin Nose Drops - See OXYMETAZOLINE (Nasal) 630
Afrin Sinus - See OXYMETAZOLINE (Nasal) 630
Afrin Spray Pump - See OXYMETAZOLINE (Nasal) 630
Aftate for Athlete's Foot Aerosol Spray Liquid - See ANTIFUNGALS (Topical) 88
Aftate for Athlete's Foot Aerosol Spray Powder - See ANTIFUNGALS (Topical) 88
Aftate for Athlete's Foot Gel - See ANTIFUNGALS (Topical) 88
Aftate for Athlete's Foot Sprinkle Powder - See ANTIFUNGALS (Topical) 88
Aftate for Jock Itch Aerosol Spray Powder - See ANTIFUNGALS (Topical) 88
Aftate for Jock Itch Gel - See ANTIFUNGALS (Topical) 88
Aftate for Jock Itch Sprinkle Powder - See ANTIFUNGALS (Topical) 88
Agarol - See
LAXATIVES, SOFTENER/LUBRICANT 480
LAXATIVES, STIMULANT 482
Agarol Marshmallow - See
LAXATIVES, SOFTENER/LUBRICANT 480
LAXATIVES, STIMULANT 482
Agarol Plain - See
LAXATIVES, OSMOTIC 478
LAXATIVES, SOFTENER/LUBRICANT 480
Agarol Raspberry - See
LAXATIVES, SOFTENER/LUBRICANT 480
LAXATIVES, STIMULANT 482
Agarol Strawberry - See
LAXATIVES, OSMOTIC 478
LAXATIVES, STIMULANT 482
Agarol Vanilla - See
LAXATIVES, OSMOTIC 478
LAXATIVES, STIMULANT 482

Aggrenox - See DIPYRIDAMOLE 326
Agrylin - See ANAGRELIDE 30
AH-Chew - See
ANTICHOLINERGICS 72
ANTIHISTAMINES 106
PHENYLEPHRINE 658
AK Homatropine - See CYCLOPLEGIC, MYDRIATIC (Ophthalmic) 292
Akarpine - See ANTIGLAUCOMA, CHOLINERGIC AGONISTS 100
AKBeta - See ANTIGLAUCOMA, BETA BLOCKERS 96
Ak-Chlor Ophthalmic Ointment - See ANTIBACTERIALS (Ophthalmic) 66
Ak-Chlor Ophthalmic Solution - See ANTIBACTERIALS (Ophthalmic) 66
Ak-Con - See DECONGESTANTS (Ophthalmic) 306
Ak-Dilate - See PHENYLEPHRINE (Ophthalmic) 660
Akineton - See ANTIDYSKINETICS 82
Ak-Nefrin - See PHENYLEPHRINE (Ophthalmic) 660
Akne-Mycin - See ANTIBACTERIALS FOR ACNE (Topical) 64
Ak-Pentolate - See CYCLOPENTOLATE (Ophthalmic) 288
Ak-Pred - See ANTI-INFLAMMATORY DRUGS, STEROIDAL (Ophthalmic) 122
AKPro - See ANTIGLAUCOMA, ADRENERGIC AGONISTS 92
Ak-Spore - See
ANTIBACTERIALS (Ophthalmic) 66
ANTI-INFLAMMATORY DRUGS, STEROIDAL (Ophthalmic) 122
Ak-Spore HC - See ANTIBACTERIALS (Ophthalmic) 66
Ak-Sulf - See ANTIBACTERIALS (Ophthalmic) 66
AK-Tate - See ANTI-INFLAMMATORY DRUGS, STEROIDAL (Ophthalmic) 122
Aktob - See ANTIBACTERIALS (Ophthalmic) 66
Ak-Zol - See CARBONIC ANHYDRASE INHIBITORS 232
Ala-Cort - See ADRENOCORTICOIDS (Topical) 18
Alamag - See ANTACIDS 48
Alamast - See ANTIALLERGIC AGENTS (Ophthalmic) 56
Ala-Scalp HP - See ADRENOCORTICOIDS (Topical) 18
Alavert - See ANTIHISTAMINES, NONSEDATING 110
Alavert D-12 - See
ANTIHISTAMINES, NONSEDATING 110
PSEUDOEPHEDRINE 694
Alaway - See ANTIALLERGIC AGENTS (Ophthalmic) 56
Alaxin - See LAXATIVES, SOFTENER/ LUBRICANT 480
Albalon - See DECONGESTANTS (Ophthalmic) 306
Albalon Liquifilm - See DECONGESTANTS (Ophthalmic) 306
Alba-Temp 300 - See ACETAMINOPHEN 8
ALBENDAZOLE - See ANTHELMINTICS 50
Albenza - See ANTHELMINTICS 50
Albert Glyburide - See SULFONYLUREAS 770
Albert Tiafen - See ANTI-INFLAMMATORY DRUGS, NONSTEROIDAL (NSAIDs) 116
Albright's Solution - See CITRATES 254
ALBUTEROL - See BRONCHODILATORS, ADRENERGIC 200
ALCAFTADINE - See ANTIALLERGIC AGENTS (Ophthalmic) 56
ALCLOMETASONE (Topical) - See ADRENOCORTICOIDS (Topical) 18
ALCOHOL & ACETONE - See ANTIACNE, CLEANSING (Topical) 54
ALCOHOL & SULFUR - See ANTIACNE, CLEANSING (Topical) 54
Alcohol-abuse deterrent - See ACAMPROSATE 4
Alcomicin - See ANTIBACTERIALS (Ophthalmic) 66
Aldactazide - See DIURETICS, POTASSIUM-SPARING & HYDROCHLOROTHIAZIDE 336
Aldactone - See DIURETICS, POTASSIUM-SPARING 334
Aldara - See CONDYLOMA ACUMINATUM AGENTS 276
Aldoclor - See
CENTRAL ALPHA AGONISTS 234
DIURETICS, THIAZIDE 338
Aldomet - See CENTRAL ALPHA AGONISTS 234
Aldoril - See
CENTRAL ALPHA AGONISTS 234
DIURETICS, THIAZIDE 338
ALENDRONATE - See BISPHOSPHONATES 192
Alersule - See
ANTIHISTAMINES 106
PHENYLEPHRINE 658
Alertec - See STIMULANTS, AMPHETAMINE RELATED 756
Alesse - See CONTRACEPTIVES, ORAL & SKIN 278
Aleve - See ANTI-INFLAMMATORY DRUGS, NONSTEROIDAL (NSAIDs) 116

Aleve-D Sinus & Cold - See
ANTI-INFLAMMATORY DRUGS, NONSTEROIDAL (NSAIDs) 116
PSEUDOEPHEDRINE 694
Aleve Liquid Gels - See ANTI-INFLAMMATORY DRUGS, NONSTEROIDAL (NSAIDs) 116
ALFACALCIDOL - See VITAMIN D 840
ALFUZOSIN - See ALPHA ADRENERGIC RECEPTOR BLOCKERS 20
Algenic Alka - See ANTACIDS 48
Algenic Alka Improved - See ANTACIDS 48
Algicon - See ANTACIDS 48
Alinia - See NITAZOXANIDE 600
ALISKIREN - See RENIN INHIBITORS 716
Alka-Butazolidin - See ANTI-INFLAMMATORY DRUGS, NONSTEROIDAL (NSAIDs) 116
Alkabutazone - See ANTI-INFLAMMATORY DRUGS, NONSTEROIDAL (NSAIDs) 116
Alkalizer - See SODIUM BICARBONATE 750
Alka-Mints - See ANTACIDS 48
Alka-Phenylbutazone - See ANTI-INFLAMMATORY DRUGS, NONSTEROIDAL (NSAIDs) 116
Alka-Seltzer Gas Relief - See SIMETHICONE 748
Alka-Seltzer Morning Relief - See
ASPIRIN 152
CAFFEINE 216
Alka-Seltzer Original - See
ASPIRIN 152
SODIUM BICARBONATE 750
Alka-Seltzer Plus Cold & Cough Effervescent - See
ACETAMINOPHEN 8
ANTIHISTAMINES 106
DEXTROMETHORPHAN 312
PHENYLEPHRINE 658
Alka-Seltzer Plus Cold & Cough Liquid - See
ACETAMINOPHEN 8
ANTIHISTAMINES 106
DEXTROMETHORPHAN 312
PHENYLEPHRINE 658
Alka-Seltzer Plus Cold & Cough Liquid-Gels - See
ACETAMINOPHEN 8
ANTIHISTAMINES 106
DEXTROMETHORPHAN 312
PHENYLEPHRINE 658
Alka-Seltzer Plus Day & Night Effervescent - See
ACETAMINOPHEN 8
DEXTROMETHORPHAN 312
PHENYLEPHRINE 658
Alka-Seltzer Plus Day & Night Liquid Gels - See
ACETAMINOPHEN 8
DEXTROMETHORPHAN 312
PHENYLEPHRINE 658
Alka-Seltzer Plus Day Cold Liquid - See
ACETAMINOPHEN 8
DEXTROMETHORPHAN 312
PHENYLEPHRINE 658
Alka-Seltzer Plus Flu Effervescent - See
ANTIHISTAMINES 106
ASPIRIN 152
DEXTROMETHORPHAN 312
Alka-Seltzer Plus Night Cold Liquid - See
ACETAMINOPHEN 8
ANTIHISTAMINES 106
DEXTROMETHORPHAN 312
PHENYLEPHRINE 658
Alka-Seltzer Plus Night-Time Effervescent - See
ACETAMINOPHEN 8
ANTIHISTAMINES 106
DEXTROMETHORPHAN 312
PHENYLEPHRINE 658
Alka-Seltzer Plus Night-Time Liquid-Gels - See
ACETAMINOPHEN 8
ANTIHISTAMINES 106
DEXTROMETHORPHAN 312
Alka-Seltzer Plus Original Effervescent - See
ACETAMINOPHEN 8
ANTIHISTAMINES 106
PHENYLEPHRINE 658
Alka-Seltzer PM - See
ANTIHISTAMINES 106
ASPIRIN 152
Alkeran - See MELPHALAN 534
Alkets - See ANTACIDS 48
Alkets Extra Strength - See ANTACIDS 48
Allay - See NARCOTIC ANALGESICS & ACETAMINOPHEN 586
Allegra - See ANTIHISTAMINES, NONSEDATING 110
Allegra-D - See
ANTIHISTAMINES, NONSEDATING 110
PSEUDOEPHEDRINE 694
Allegra-D 24 Hour - See
ANTIHISTAMINES, NONSEDATING 110
PSEUDOEPHEDRINE 694
Allegra ODT - See ANTIHISTAMINES, NONSEDATING 110
Allegra Oral Suspension - See ANTIHISTAMINES, NONSEDATING 110
Allent - See
ANTIHISTAMINES 106
PSEUDOEPHEDRINE 694

Alleract - See ANTIHISTAMINES 106
Aller-Chlor - See ANTIHISTAMINES 106
Allercon - See
ANTIHISTAMINES 106
PSEUDOEPHEDRINE 694
Allercort - See ADRENOCORTICOIDS (Topical) 18
Allerdryl - See ANTIHISTAMINES 106
Allerest - See DECONGESTANTS (Ophthalmic) 306
Allerest 12 Hour Nasal Spray - See OXYMETAZOLINE (Nasal) 630
Allerest Maximum Strength - See
ANTIHISTAMINES 106
PSEUDOEPHEDRINE 694
Allerest No-Drowsiness - See
ACETAMINOPHEN 8
PSEUDOEPHEDRINE 694
Allerfrim - See ANTIHISTAMINES 106
Allergen - See ANTIPYRINE & BENZOCAINE (Otic) 130
AllerMax Caplets - See ANTIHISTAMINES 106
Aller-med - See ANTIHISTAMINES 106
AllerNaze - See ADRENOCORTICOIDS (Nasal Inhalation) 12
Allerphed - See
ANTIHISTAMINES 106
PSEUDOEPHEDRINE 694
Allert - See ANTIHISTAMINES 106
AlleRx D - See
ANTICHOLINERGICS 72
PSEUDOEPHEDRINE 694
AlleRx Dose Pack DF - See
ANTICHOLINERGICS 72
ANTIHISTAMINES 106
AlleRx Dose Pack PE - See
ANTICHOLINERGICS 72
ANTIHISTAMINES 106
PHENYLEPHRINE 658
AlleRx Suspension - See
ANTIHISTAMINES 106
PHENYLEPHRINE 658
Alli- See ORLISTAT 622
All-Nite Cold Formula - See
ACETAMINOPHEN 8
ANTIHISTAMINES 106
DEXTROMETHORPHAN 312
PSEUDOEPHEDRINE 694
Alloprin - See ANTIGOUT DRUGS 104
ALLOPURINOL - See ANTIGOUT DRUGS 104
Almacone - See ANTACIDS 48
Almacone II - See ANTACIDS 48
Alma-Mag #4 Improved - See ANTACIDS 48
Alma-Mag Improved - See ANTACIDS 48
Almocarpine - See ANTIGLAUCOMA, CHOLINERGIC AGONISTS 100
ALMOTRIPTAN MALATE - See TRIPTANS 820
Alocril - See ANTIALLERGIC AGENTS (Ophthalmic) 56
ALOGLIPTIN - See DPP-4 INHIBITORS 348
ALOE - See LAXATIVES, STIMULANT 482
Alomide - See ANTIALLERGIC AGENTS (Ophthalmic) 56
Alora - See ESTROGENS 372
ALPHA ADRENERGIC RECEPTOR BLOCKERS 20
Alpha Redisol - See VITAMIN B-12 (Cyanocobalamin) 836
Alphaderm - See ADRENOCORTICOIDS (Topical) 18
Alphagan - See ANTIGLAUCOMA, ADRENERGIC AGONISTS 92
Alphagan P - See ANTIGLAUCOMA, ADRENERGIC AGONISTS 92
Alphalin - See VITAMIN A 834
Alphamin - See VITAMIN B-12 (Cyanocobalamin) 836
Alphamul - See LAXATIVES, STIMULANT 482
Alpha-Tamoxifen - See TAMOXIFEN 772
Alphatrex - See ADRENOCORTICOIDS (Topical) 18
Alphosyl - See COAL TAR (Topical) 266
Alprazolam Intensol - See BENZODIAZEPINES 176
ALPRAZOLAM - See BENZODIAZEPINES 176
ALPROSTADIL 22
Alrex - See ANTI-INFLAMMATORY DRUGS, STEROIDAL (Ophthalmic) 122
Alrheumat - See ANTI-INFLAMMATORY DRUGS, NONSTEROIDAL (NSAIDs) 116
Alsuma - See TRIPTANS 820
Altabax - See ANTIBACTERIALS (Topical) 70
Altace - See ANGIOTENSIN-CONVERTING ENZYME (ACE) INHIBITORS 44
AlternaGEL - See ANTACIDS 48
Alti-Acyclovir - See ANTIVIRALS FOR HERPES VIRUS 136
Alti-Bromocriptine - See BROMOCRIPTINE 198
Altocor - See HMG-CoA REDUCTASE INHIBITORS 424
Alu-Cap - See ANTACIDS 48
Aludrox - See ANTACIDS 48
ALUMINA & MAGNESIA - See ANTACIDS 48
ALUMINA & MAGNESIUM CARBONATE - See ANTACIDS 48
ALUMINA & MAGNESIUM TRISILICATE - See ANTACIDS 48
ALUMINA, MAGNESIA, & CALCIUM CARBONATE - See ANTACIDS 48
ALUMINA, MAGNESIA, & SIMETHICONE - See ANTACIDS 48

ALUMINA, MAGNESIUM, CALCIUM CARBONATE & SIMETHICONE - See ANTACIDS 48
ALUMINA, MAGNESIUM TRISILICATE, & SODIUM BICARBONATE - See ANTACIDS 48
ALUMINUM CARBONATE, BASIC - See ANTACIDS 48
ALUMINUM HYDROXIDE - See ANTACIDS 48
Alupent - See BRONCHODILATORS, ADRENERGIC 200
Alurate - See BARBITURATES 168
Alu-Tab - See ANTACIDS 48
Alvesco Inhalation - See ADRENOCORTICOIDS (Oral Inhalation) 14
AMANTADINE - See ANTIVIRALS FOR INFLUENZA 138
Amandron - See ANTIANDROGENS, NONSTEROIDAL 58
Amaphen - See
ACETAMINOPHEN 8
BARBITURATES 168
CAFFEINE 216
Amaryl - See SULFONYLUREAS 770
Ambay Cough - See
ANTIHISTAMINES 106
NARCOTIC ANALGESICS 584
Ambenyl Cough - See
ANTIHISTAMINES 106
NARCOTIC ANALGESICS 584
Ambenyl-D Decongestant Cough Formula - See
DEXTROMETHORPHAN 312
GUAIFENESIN 416
PSEUDOEPHEDRINE 694
Ambien - See ZOLPIDEM 858
Ambien CR - See ZOLPIDEM 858
Ambophen Expectorant - See
ANTIHISTAMINES 106
NARCOTIC ANALGESICS 584
AMBRISENTAN - See ENDOTHELIN RECEPTOR ANTAGONISTS 354
AMCINONIDE (Topical) - See ADRENOCORTICOIDS (Topical) 18
Amdry-D - See
ANTICHOLINERGICS 72
PSEUDOEPHEDRINE 694
Amen - See PROGESTINS 680
Amerge - See TRIPTANS 820
Americaine - See ANESTHETICS (Topical) 40
Americaine Hemorrhoidal - See ANESTHETICS (Rectal) 38
Americaine Topical Anesthetic First Aid Ointment - See ANESTHETICS (Topical) 40
Americaine Topical Anesthetic Spray - See ANESTHETICS (Topical) 40
Amersol - See ANTI-INFLAMMATORY DRUGS, NONSTEROIDAL (NSAIDs) 116
Amethopterin - See METHOTREXATE 548
Amicar - See ANTIFIBRINOLYTIC AGENTS 84
Amigesic - See SALICYLATES 736
AMILORIDE - See DIURETICS, POTASSIUM-SPARING 334
AMILORIDE & HYDROCHLOROTHIAZIDE - See DIURETICS, POTASSIUM-SPARING & HYDROCHLOROTHIAZIDE 336
AMINOCAPROIC ACID - See ANTIFIBRINOLYTIC AGENTS 84
Aminofen - See ACETAMINOPHEN 8
Aminofen Max - See ACETAMINOPHEN 8
AMINOGLUTETHIMIDE 24
Aminophyllin - See BRONCHODILATORS, XANTHINE 204
AMINOPHYLLINE - See BRONCHODILATORS, XANTHINE 204
AMIODARONE - See ANTIARRHYTHMICS, BENZOFURAN-TYPE 60
Ami Rax - See
BRONCHODILATORS, XANTHINE 204
EPHEDRINE 356
HYDROXYZINE 436
Amitiza - See LUBIPROSTONE 514
Amitone - See ANTACIDS 48
AMITRIPTYLINE - See ANTIDEPRESSANTS, TRICYCLIC 80
AMLEXANOX 26
AMLODIPINE - See CALCIUM CHANNEL BLOCKERS 220
Amnesteem - See ISOTRETINOIN 462
AMOBARBITAL - See BARBITURATES 168
Amonidrin - See GUAIFENESIN 416
AMOXAPINE - See ANTIDEPRESSANTS, TRICYCLIC 80
AMOXICILLIN - See PENICILLINS 646
AMOXICILLIN & CLAVULANATE - See PENICILLINS & BETA-LACTAMASE INHIBITORS 648
Amoxil - See PENICILLINS 646
AMPHETAMINE & DEXTROAMPHETAMINE - See AMPHETAMINES 28
AMPHETAMINES 28
Amphojel - See ANTACIDS 48
Amphojel 500 - See ANTACIDS 48
Amphojel Plus - See ANTACIDS 48
AMPHOTERICIN B - See ANTIFUNGALS (Topical) 88
AMPICILLIN - See PENICILLINS 646
Amrix - See CYCLOBENZAPRINE 286
Amturnide - See
CALCIUM CHANNEL BLOCKERS 220
DIURETICS, THIAZIDE 338
RENIN INHIBITORS 716

Amyotrophic lateral sclerosis therapy agent - See
RILUZOLE 732
Amylinomimetic - See PRAMLINTIDE 668
Amytal - See BARBITURATES 168
Anabolin - See ANDROGENS 34
Anabolin LA 100 - See ANDROGENS 34
Anacin - See
ASPIRIN 152
CAFFEINE 216
Anacin with Codeine - See
CAFFEINE 216
NARCOTIC ANALGESICS & ASPIRIN 588
Anacin-3 - See ACETAMINOPHEN 8
Anacin-3 Extra Strength - See
ACETAMINOPHEN 8
Anadrol-50 - See ANDROGENS 34
Anafranil - See ANTIDEPRESSANTS,
TRICYCLIC 80
ANAGRELIDE 30
Ana-Guard - See BRONCHODILATORS,
ADRENERGIC 200
ANAKINRA 32
Analgesic - See
ACETAMINOPHEN 8
ANTI-INFLAMMATORY DRUGS,
NONSTEROIDAL (NSAIDs) 116
ANTI-INFLAMMATORY DRUGS,
NONSTEROIDAL (NSAIDs) COX-2
INHIBITORS 118
ASPIRIN 152
BARBITURATES, ASPIRIN & CODEINE (Also
contains caffeine) 170
CARBAMAZEPINE 228
NARCOTIC ANALGESICS &
ACETAMINOPHEN 586
NARCOTIC ANALGESICS & ASPIRIN 588
ORPHENADRINE, ASPIRIN & CAFFEINE 626
SALICYLATES 736
TAPENTADOL 774
TRAMADOL 808
Analgesic (Otic) - See ANTIPYRINE &
BENZOCAINE (Otic) 130
Analgesic (Topical) - See CAPSAICIN 226
Analgesic (Urinary) - See
ATROPINE, HYOSCYAMINE,
METHENAMINE, METHYLENE BLUE,
PHENYLSALICYLATE & BENZOIC ACID 158
PHENAZOPYRIDINE 654
SULFONAMIDES & PHENAZOPYRIDINE 768
Analgesic Ear Drops - See ANTIPYRINE &
BENZOCAINE (Otic) 130
Anamantle HC Cream Kit - See
ANESTHETICS (Rectal) 38
HYDROCORTISONE (Rectal) 430
Anamine - See
ANTIHISTAMINES 106
PSEUDOEPHEDRINE 694
Anamine HD - See
ANTIHISTAMINES 106
NARCOTIC ANALGESICS 584
PHENYLEPHRINE 658
Anamine T.D. - See
ANTIHISTAMINES 106
PSEUDOEPHEDRINE 694
Anapolon 50 - See ANDROGENS 34
Anaprox - See ANTI-INFLAMMATORY DRUGS,
NONSTEROIDAL (NSAIDs) 116
Anaprox DS - See ANTI-INFLAMMATORY
DRUGS, NONSTEROIDAL (NSAIDs) 116
Anaspaz - See HYOSCYAMINE 438
Anaspaz PB - See HYOSCYAMINE 438
Anatuss DM - See
DEXTROMETHORPHAN 312
GUAIFENESIN 416
PSEUDOEPHEDRINE 694
Anatuss LA - See
GUAIFENESIN 416
PSEUDOEPHEDRINE 694
Anbesol Baby Gel - See ANESTHETICS
(Mucosal-Local) 36
Anbesol Gel - See ANESTHETICS (Mucosal-
Local) 36
Anbesol Liquid - See ANESTHETICS (Mucosal-
Local) 36
Anbesol Maximum Strength Gel - See
ANESTHETICS (Mucosal-Local) 36
Anbesol Maximum Strength Liquid - See
ANESTHETICS (Mucosal-Local) 36
Anbesol Regular Strength Gel - See
ANESTHETICS (Mucosal-Local) 36
Anbesol Regular Strength Liquid - See
ANESTHETICS (Mucosal-Local) 36
Ancalixir - See BARBITURATES 168
Andro 100 - See ANDROGENS 34
Andro-Cyp 100 - See ANDROGENS 34
Andro-Cyp 200 - See ANDROGENS 34
Androderm - See ANDROGENS 34
Androgel - See ANDROGENS 34
Androgen - See ANDROGENS 34
ANDROGENS 34
Android-10 - See ANDROGENS 34
Android-25 - See ANDROGENS 34
Android-T - See ANDROGENS 34
Andro-LA 200 - See ANDROGENS 34
Androlone - See ANDROGENS 34
Andronaq-50 - See ANDROGENS 34
Andronaq-LA - See ANDROGENS 34
Andronate 100 - See ANDROGENS 34
Andronate 200 - See ANDROGENS 34

Andropository 100 - See ANDROGENS 34
Andryl 200 - See ANDROGENS 34
Anergan 25 - See ANTIHISTAMINES, PHENOTHIAZINE-DERIVATIVE 112
Anergan 50 - See ANTIHISTAMINES, PHENOTHIAZINE-DERIVATIVE 112
Anestafoam - See ANESTHETICS (Topical) 40
Anesthetic - See ANTIPYRINE & BENZOCAINE (Otic) 130
Anesthetic (Mucosal-Local) - See ANESTHETICS (Mucosal-Local) 36
Anesthetic (Rectal) - See
ANESTHETICS (Rectal) 38
HYDROCORTISONE (Rectal) 430
Anesthetic (Topical) - See ANESTHETICS (Topical) 40
ANESTHETICS (Mucosal-Local) 36
ANESTHETICS (Rectal) 38
ANESTHETICS (Topical) 40
Anexsia - See NARCOTIC ANALGESICS & ACETAMINOPHEN 586
Angeliq - See
ESTROGENS 372
PROGESTINS 680
ANGIOTENSIN II RECEPTOR ANTAGONISTS 42
ANGIOTENSIN-CONVERTING ENZYME (ACE) INHIBITORS 44
ANGIOTENSIN-CONVERTING ENZYME (ACE) INHIBITORS & HYDROCHLOROTHIAZIDE 46
Anhydron - See DIURETICS, THIAZIDE 338
ANISOTROPINE - See ANTICHOLINERGICS 72
Anocobin - See VITAMIN B-12 (Cyanocobalamin) 836
Anolor 300 - See
ACETAMINOPHEN 8
BARBITURATES 168
CAFFEINE 216
Anolor-DH5 - See NARCOTIC ANALGESICS & ACETAMINOPHEN 586
Anoquan - See
ACETAMINOPHEN 8
BARBITURATES 168
CAFFEINE 216
Anorex SR - See APPETITE SUPPRESSANTS 146
Anorexiant - See LORCASERIN 510
Ansaid - See ANTI-INFLAMMATORY DRUGS, NONSTEROIDAL (NSAIDs) 116
Anspor - See CEPHALOSPORINS 236
Antabuse - See DISULFIRAM 330
Antacid - See
ANTACIDS 48
BISMUTH SALTS 190
SODIUM BICARBONATE 750
ANTACIDS 48
AntaGel - See ANTACIDS 48
AntaGel-II - See ANTACIDS 48
Antara - See FIBRATES 386
ANTAZOLINE - See DECONGESTANTS (Ophthalmic) 306
Anthelmintics - See ANTHELMINTICS 50
ANTHELMINTICS 50
Anthra-Derm - See ANTHRALIN (Topical) 52
Anthraforte - See ANTHRALIN (Topical) 52
ANTHRALIN (Topical) 52
Anthranol - See ANTHRALIN (Topical) 52
Anthrascalp - See ANTHRALIN (Topical) 52
Antiacne - See TETRACYCLINES 782
Antiacne agent - See
AZELAIC ACID 164
ERYTHROMYCINS 368
Antiacne agent, cleansing agent - See ANTIACNE, CLEANSING (Topical) 54
ANTIACNE, CLEANSING (Topical) 54
Antiacne (Systemic) - See ISOTRETINOIN 462
Antiacne (Topical) - See
BENZOYL PEROXIDE 178
KERATOLYTICS 470
RETINOIDS (Topical) 722
Antiadrenal - See
AMINOGLUTETHIMIDE 24
METYRAPONE 552
TRILOSTANE 814
Antiadrenergic - See BETA-ADRENERGIC BLOCKING AGENTS 182
ANTIALLERGIC AGENTS (Ophthalmic) 56
ANTIANDROGENS, NONSTEROIDAL 58
Antianemic - See LEUCOVORIN 486
Antianginal - See
BETA-ADRENERGIC BLOCKING AGENTS 182
CALCIUM CHANNEL BLOCKERS 220
RANOLAZINE 712
Antianginal (Nitrate) - See NITRATES 602
Antianxiety agent - See
BUSPIRONE 210
MEPROBAMATE 538
SELECTIVE SEROTONIN REUPTAKE INHIBITORS (SSRIs) 742
Antiaphthous ulcer agent - See AMLEXANOX 26
Antiarrhythmic - See
ANTIARRHYTHMICS, BENZOFURAN-TYPE 60
BETA-ADRENERGIC BLOCKING AGENTS 182
CALCIUM CHANNEL BLOCKERS 220
DISOPYRAMIDE 328
DOFETILIDE 342
FLECAINIDE ACETATE 390
MEXILETINE 554
PROPAFENONE 684
QUINIDINE 704

ANTIARRHYTHMICS, BENZOFURAN-TYPE 60
Antiasthmatic - See
ADRENOCORTICOIDS (Oral Inhalation) 14
LEUKOTRIENE MODIFIERS 488
Antibacterial - See
CEPHALOSPORINS 236
CHLORAMPHENICOL 242
CLINDAMYCIN 258
CYCLOSERINE 294
ERYTHROMYCINS 368
FLUOROQUINOLONES 392
LINCOMYCIN 500
LINEZOLID 502
NEOMYCIN (Oral) 592
NITROIMIDAZOLES 606
PENICILLINS 646
PENICILLINS & BETA-LACTAMASE INHIBITORS 648
RIFAMYCINS 728
RIFAXIMIN 730
TELITHROMYCIN 778
TETRACYCLINES 782
VANCOMYCIN 828
Antibacterial (Antibiotic) - See
ACETOHYDROXAMIC ACID (AHA) 10
FURAZOLIDONE 398
NITROFURANTOIN 604
SULFONAMIDES 766
Antibacterial (Antileprosy) - See DAPSONE 304
Antibacterial (Dental) - See CHLORHEXIDINE 244
Antibacterial (Ophthalmic) - See
ANTIBACTERIALS (Ophthalmic) 66
Antibacterial (Otic) - See ANTIBACTERIALS (Otic) 68
Antibacterial (Topical) - See
ANTIBACTERIALS, ANTIFUNGALS (Topical) 62
ANTIBACTERIALS FOR ACNE (Topical) 64
ANTIBACTERIALS (Topical) 70
NEOMYCIN (Topical) 594
ANTIBACTERIALS, ANTIFUNGALS (Topical) 62
ANTIBACTERIALS FOR ACNE (Topical) 64
ANTIBACTERIALS (Ophthalmic) 66
ANTIBACTERIALS (Otic) 68
ANTIBACTERIALS (Topical) 70
Antiben - See ANTIPYRINE & BENZOCAINE (Otic) 130
Antibiotic Ear - See ANTIBACTERIALS (Otic) 68
Antibiotic (Erythromycin) - See MACROLIDE ANTIBIOTICS 518
Antibiotic (Ketolide) - See TELITHROMYCIN 778
Antibiotic (Macrolide) - See MACROLIDE ANTIBIOTICS 518
Antibiotic (Oxazolidinone) - See LINEZOLID 502
Anticancer treatment adjunct - See
LEVAMISOLE 490
Anticholelithic - See URSODIOL 824
Anticholinergic - See
ANTICHOLINERGICS 72
BELLADONNA ALKALOIDS & BARBITURATES 174
BRONCHODILATORS, ANTICHOLINERGIC 202
CLIDINIUM 256
DICYCLOMINE 316
GLYCOPYRROLATE 410
HYOSCYAMINE 438
IPRATROPIUM 456
MUSCARINIC RECEPTOR ANTAGONISTS 574
ORPHENADRINE 624
PROPANTHELINE 686
SCOPOLAMINE (Hyoscine) 738
ANTICHOLINERGICS 72
Anticoagulant - See
ANTICOAGULANTS (Oral)74
DABIGATRAN 298
FACTOR Xa INHIBITORS 382
ANTICOAGULANTS (Oral) 74
Anticonvulsant - See
BARBITURATES 168
BENZODIAZEPINES 176
CARBAMAZEPINE 228
DIVALPROEX 340
FELBAMATE 384
GABAPENTIN 402
LACOSAMIDE 472
LAMOTRIGINE 474
LEVETIRACETAM 492
OXCARBAZEPINE 628
PRIMIDONE 674
TIAGABINE 794
TOPIRAMATE 804
VALPROIC ACID 826
ZONISAMIDE 860
Anticonvulsant (Hydantoin) - See
ANTICONVULSANTS, HYDANTOIN 76
Anticonvulsant (Succinimide) - See
ANTICONVULSANTS, SUCCINIMIDE 78
ANTICONVULSANTS, HYDANTOIN 76
ANTICONVULSANTS, SUCCINIMIDE 78
Antidepressant - See
BUPROPION 208
LOXAPINE 512
MAPROTILINE 520
MIRTAZAPINE 566
MONOAMINE OXIDASE (MAO) INHIBITORS 570
SEROTONIN & NOREPINEPHRINE REUPTAKE INHIBITORS (SNRIs) 746
VILAZODONE 832

Antidepressant (Nontricyclic) - See
TRAZODONE 810
Antidepressant (Phenylpiperazine) - See
NEFAZODONE 590
Antidepressant (Selective Serotonin Reuptake Inhibitor) - See SELECTIVE SEROTONIN REUPTAKE INHIBITORS (SSRIs) 742
Antidepressant (Tricyclic) - See
ANTIDEPRESSANTS, TRICYCLIC 80
ANTIDEPRESSANTS, TRICYCLIC 80
Antidiabetic - See
ACARBOSE 6
BROMOCRIPTINE 198
DPP-4 INHIBITORS 348
GLP-1 RECEPTOR AGONISTS 406
INSULIN 446
INSULIN ANALOGS 448
MEGLITINIDES 528
METFORMIN 544
MIGLITOL 558
PRAMLINTIDE 668
THIAZOLIDINEDIONES 786
Antidiabetic (Oral), sulfonylurea - See
SULFONYLUREAS 770
Antidiarrheal - See
ATTAPULGITE 160
BISMUTH SALTS 190
DIFENOXIN & ATROPINE 318
DIPHENOXYLATE & ATROPINE 324
KAOLIN & PECTIN 468
LOPERAMIDE 508
NITAZOXANIDE 600
PAREGORIC 640
RIFAXIMIN 730
Antidiuretic - See DESMOPRESSIN 310
Antidote (Adsorbent) - See CHARCOAL, ACTIVATED 238
Antidote (Heavy Metal) - See PENICILLAMINE 644
Antidyskinetic - See
ANTIDYSKINETICS 82
MONOAMINE OXIDASE TYPE B (MAO-B) INHIBITORS 572
ANTIDYSKINETICS 82
Antiemetic - See
ANTIHISTAMINES, PIPERAZINE (Antinausea) 114
DIPHENIDOL 322
DRONABINOL (THC, Marijuana) 350
METOCLOPRAMIDE 550
NABILONE 578
TRIMETHOBENZAMIDE 816
Antiemetic (Phenothiazine) - See
PHENOTHIAZINES 656
Antiepileptic - See
GABAPENTIN 402
LACOSAMIDE 472
LAMOTRIGINE 474
LEVETIRACETAM 492
OXCARBAZEPINE 628
PREGABALIN 670
TIAGABINE 794
TOPIRAMATE 804
ZONISAMIDE 860
Antifibrinolytic - See ANTIFIBRINOLYTIC AGENTS 84
ANTIFIBRINOLYTIC AGENTS 84
Antiflatulent - See SIMETHICONE 748
Antifungal - See
ANTIFUNGALS, AZOLES 86
CLOTRIMAZOLE (Oral-Local) 262
GRISEOFULVIN 414
NYSTATIN 614
TERBINAFINE (Oral) 780
ANTIFUNGALS, AZOLES 86
Antifungal (Topical) - See
ANTIBACTERIALS, ANTIFUNGALS (Topical) 62
ANTIFUNGALS (Topical) 88
ANTIFUNGALS (Topical) 88
Antifungal (Vaginal) - See ANTIFUNGALS (Vaginal) 90
ANTIFUNGALS (Vaginal) 90
Antiglaucoma - See
ANTIGLAUCOMA, ADRENERGIC AGONISTS 92
ANTIGLAUCOMA, ANTICHOLINESTERASES 94
ANTIGLAUCOMA, BETA BLOCKERS 96
ANTIGLAUCOMA, CARBONIC ANHYDRASE INHIBITORS 98
ANTIGLAUCOMA, CHOLINERGIC AGONISTS 100
ANTIGLAUCOMA, PROSTAGLANDINS 102
ANTIGLAUCOMA, ADRENERGIC AGONISTS 92
ANTIGLAUCOMA, ANTICHOLINESTERASES 94
ANTIGLAUCOMA, BETA BLOCKERS 96
ANTIGLAUCOMA, CARBONIC ANHYDRASE INHIBITORS 98
ANTIGLAUCOMA, CHOLINERGIC AGONISTS 100
ANTIGLAUCOMA, PROSTAGLANDINS 102
Antigout - See
ANTIGOUT DRUGS 104
ANTI-INFLAMMATORY DRUGS, NONSTEROIDAL (NSAIDs) 116
COLCHICINE 268
PROBENECID 676
SULFINPYRAZONE 764

ANTIGOUT DRUGS 104
Antihemorrhagic - See
ANTIFIBRINOLYTIC AGENTS 84
DESMOPRESSIN 310
Antihistamine - See
ANTIHISTAMINES 106
ANTIHISTAMINES (Nasal) 108
ANTIHISTAMINES, NONSEDATING 110
ANTIHISTAMINES, PIPERAZINE (Antinausea) 114
HYDROXYZINE 436
ORPHENADRINE 624
ANTIHISTAMINES 106
ANTIHISTAMINES (Nasal) 108
ANTIHISTAMINES, NONSEDATING 110
ANTIHISTAMINES, PHENOTHIAZINE-DERIVATIVE 112
ANTIHISTAMINES, PIPERAZINE (Antinausea) 114
Antihistaminic - See ANTIALLERGIC AGENTS (Ophthalmic) 56
Antihyperglycemic - See
ACARBOSE 6
METFORMIN 544
Antihyperlipidemic - See
CHOLESTYRAMINE 248
COLESEVELAM 270
COLESTIPOL 272
EZETIMIBE 380
FIBRATES 386
GEMFIBROZIL 404
HMG-CoA REDUCTASE INHIBITORS 424
NIACIN (Vitamin B-3, Nicotinic Acid, Nicotinamide) 596
OMEGA-3 ACID ETHYL ESTERS 620
Antihypertensive - See
ALPHA ADRENERGIC RECEPTOR BLOCKERS 20
ANGIOTENSIN II RECEPTOR ANTAGONISTS 42
BETA-ADRENERGIC BLOCKING AGENTS 182
CENTRAL ALPHA AGONISTS 234
DIURETICS, LOOP 332
DIURETICS, POTASSIUM-SPARING 334
DIURETICS, POTASSIUM-SPARING & HYDROCHLOROTHIAZIDE 336
DIURETICS, THIAZIDE 338
EPLERENONE 358
GUANADREL 418
HYDRALAZINE 426
HYDRALAZINE & HYDROCHLOROTHIAZIDE 428
INDAPAMIDE 444
MINOXIDIL 560
RAUWOLFIA ALKALOIDS 714
RENIN INHIBITORS 716
RESERPINE, HYDRALAZINE & HYDROCHLOROTHIAZIDE 718
Antihypertensive, ACE inhibitor - See
ANGIOTENSIN-CONVERTING ENZYME (ACE) INHIBITORS 44
Antihypertensive, angiotensin II receptor antagonist - See ANGIOTENSIN II RECEPTOR ANTAGONISTS 42
Antihypertensive, diuretic (Thiazide), ACE inhibitor - See ANGIOTENSIN-CONVERTING ENZYME (ACE) INHIBITORS & HYDROCHLOROTHIAZIDE 46
Antihypertensive (pulmonary) - See
ENDOTHELIN RECEPTOR ANTAGONISTS 354
Antihyperthyroid - See ANTITHYROID DRUGS 134
Antihypocalcemic - See CALCIUM SUPPLEMENTS 222
Antihypoglycemic - See GLUCAGON 408
Antihypokalemic - See
DIURETICS, POTASSIUM-SPARING 334
DIURETICS, POTASSIUM-SPARING & HYDROCHLOROTHIAZIDE 336
Anti-infective (Urinary) - See
ATROPINE, HYOSCYAMINE, METHENAMINE, METHYLENE BLUE, PHENYLSALICYLATE & BENZOIC ACID 158
CINOXACIN 252
METHENAMINE 546
ANTI-INFLAMMATORY DRUGS, NONSTEROIDAL (NSAIDs) 116
ANTI-INFLAMMATORY DRUGS, NONSTEROIDAL (NSAIDs) COX-2 INHIBITORS 118
ANTI-INFLAMMATORY DRUGS, NONSTEROIDAL (NSAIDs) (Ophthalmic) 120
ANTI-INFLAMMATORY DRUGS, STEROIDAL (Ophthalmic) 122
ANTI-INFLAMMATORY DRUGS, STEROIDAL (Otic) 124
Anti-inflammatory (Inhalation) - See
ADRENOCORTICOIDS (Oral Inhalation) 14

Anti-inflammatory (Nonsteroidal) - See
ANTI-INFLAMMATORY DRUGS, NONSTEROIDAL (NSAIDs) 116
ANTI-INFLAMMATORY DRUGS, NONSTEROIDAL (NSAIDs) COX-2 INHIBITORS 118
ASPIRIN 152
CROMOLYN 282
MELOXICAM 532
MESALAMINE 542
NARCOTIC ANALGESICS & ASPIRIN 588
ORPHENADRINE, ASPIRIN & CAFFEINE 626
SALICYLATES 736
Anti-inflammatory (Steroidal) - See ADRENOCORTICOIDS (Systemic) 16
Anti-inflammatory (Steroidal), nasal - See ADRENOCORTICOIDS (Nasal Inhalation) 12
Anti-inflammatory, steroidal (Ophthalmic) - See ANTI-INFLAMMATORY DRUGS, STEROIDAL (Ophthalmic) 122
Anti-inflammatory, steroidal (Otic) - See ANTI-INFLAMMATORY DRUGS, STEROIDAL (Otic) 124
Anti-inflammatory, steroidal (Rectal) - See HYDROCORTISONE (Rectal) 430
Anti-influenza - See ANTIVIRALS FOR INFLUENZA, NEURAMINIDASE INHIBITORS 140
Anti-insomnia - See ZALEPLON 852
Antimalarial - See
ANTIMALARIAL 126
ATOVAQUONE 156
PROGUANIL 682
<u>ANTIMALARIAL</u> 126
Antimanic agent - See CARBAMAZEPINE 228
Antimetabolite - See METHOTREXATE 548
Antimicrobial - See NITROFURANTOIN 604
Antimicrobial (Antibacterial) - See TRIMETHOPRIM 818
Antimigraine - See
ERGOT DERIVATIVES 366
TRIPTANS 820
Antiminth - See ANTHELMINTICS 50
Antimotion sickness - See ANTIHISTAMINES, PIPERAZINE (Antinausea) 114
Antimyasthenic - See ANTIMYASTHENICS 128
<u>ANTIMYASTHENICS</u> 128
Antimycobacterial (Antituberculosis) - See ETHIONAMIDE 376
Antinarcoleptic - See STIMULANTS, AMPHETAMINE-RELATED 756
Antinaus 50 - See ANTIHISTAMINES, PHENOTHIAZINE-DERIVATIVE 112
Antinea - See KERATOLYTICS 470
Antineoplastic - See
AMINOGLUTETHIMIDE 24
ANTIANDROGENS, NONSTEROIDAL 58
BUSULFAN 212
CAPECITABINE 224
CHLORAMBUCIL 240
CYCLOPHOSPHAMIDE 290
ESTRAMUSTINE 370
ETOPOSIDE 378
HYDROXYUREA 434
IMATINIB 440
LOMUSTINE 506
MELPHALAN 534
MERCAPTOPURINE 540
PACLITAXEL 632
PROCARBAZINE 678
TAMOXIFEN 772
THIOGUANINE 788
TOREMIFENE 806
Antineoplastic (Topical) - See
FLUOROURACIL (Topical) 394
MASOPROCOL 524
MECHLORETHAMINE (Topical) 526
Antiobesity - See ORLISTAT 622
Antiobsessional agent - See SELECTIVE SEROTONIN REUPTAKE INHIBITORS (SSRIs) 742
Antiparasitic - See
ANTHELMINTICS 50
ANTIMALARIAL 126
IODOQUINOL 454
Antiparkinsonism - See
ANTIDYSKINETICS 82
ANTIVIRALS FOR INFLUENZA 138
BROMOCRIPTINE 198
CARBIDOPA & LEVODOPA 230
COMT Inhibitors 274
LEVODOPA 496
MONOAMINE OXIDASE TYPE B (MAO-B) INHIBITORS 572
ORPHENADRINE 624
Antiprotozoal - See
ANTIMALARIAL 126
ATOVAQUONE 156
CHLOROQUINE 246
FURAZOLIDONE 398
HYDROXYCHLOROQUINE 432
IODOQUINOL 454
NITAZOXANIDE 600
NITROIMIDAZOLES 606
PENTAMIDINE 650
QUINACRINE 702
QUININE 706
SULFADOXINE & PYRIMETHAMINE 760
SULFONAMIDES 766

Antiprotozoal (Antimalarial) - See PRIMAQUINE 672
Antipruritic - See CHOLESTYRAMINE 248
Antipruritic (Topical) - See DOXEPIN (Topical) 346
Antipsoriatic - See
ANTHRALIN (Topical) 52
BIOLOGICS FOR PSORIASIS 188
COAL TAR (Topical) 266
METHOTREXATE 548
RETINOIDS (Oral) 720
RETINOIDS (Topical) 722
VITAMIN D (Topical) 842
Antipsychotic - See
ARIPIPRAZOLE 148
ASENAPINE 150
CLOZAPINE 264
HALOPERIDOL 420
LURASIDONE 516
OLANZAPINE 616
PHENOTHIAZINES 656
QUETIAPINE 700
SEROTONIN-DOPAMINE ANTAGONISTS 744
ZIPRASIDONE 856
Antipsychotic (Thioxanthine) - See
THIOTHIXENE 790
ANTIPYRINE & BENZOCAINE (Otic) 130
Antirheumatic - See
ANAKINRA 32
AZATHIOPRINE 162
CHLOROQUINE 246
HYDROXYCHLOROQUINE 432
LEFLUNOMIDE 484
MELOXICAM 532
PENICILLAMINE 644
TUMOR NECROSIS FACTOR BLOCKERS 822
Antiseborrheic - See
ANTISEBORRHEICS (Topical) 132
COAL TAR (Topical) 266
KERATOLYTICS 470
ANTISEBORRHEICS (Topical) 132
Antismoking agent - See
NICOTINE 598
VARENICLINE 830
Antispas - See DICYCLOMINE 316
Antispasmodic - See
ANTICHOLINERGICS 72
ATROPINE, HYOSCYAMINE, METHENAMINE, METHYLENE BLUE, PHENYLSALICYLATE & BENZOIC ACID 158
BELLADONNA ALKALOIDS & BARBITURATES 174
CLIDINIUM 256
DICYCLOMINE 316
GLYCOPYRROLATE 410
HYOSCYAMINE 438
MUSCARINIC RECEPTOR ANTAGONISTS 574
PROPANTHELINE 686
SCOPOLAMINE (Hyoscine) 738
Antispasmodic (Urinary Tract) - See
FLAVOXATE 388
MIRABEGRON 564
Antispastic - See
DANTROLENE 302
TIZANIDINE 800
Antithrombocythemia - See ANAGRELIDE 30
Antithrombotic - See PLATELET INHIBITORS 664
ANTITHYROID DRUGS 134
Antitubercular - See
ISONIAZID 460
RIFAMYCINS 728
Anti-Tuss - See GUAIFENESIN 416
Anti-Tuss DM Expectorant - See
DEXTROMETHORPHAN 312
GUAIFENESIN 416
Antiulcer agent - See
MISOPROSTOL 568
PROTON PUMP INHIBITORS 692
SUCRALFATE 758
Antiurolithic - See
ACETOHYDROXAMIC ACID (AHA) 10
CITRATES 254
TIOPRONIN 798
Antitussive - See DEXTROMETHORPHAN 312
Antivert - See ANTIHISTAMINES, PIPERAZINE (Antinausea) 114
Antivert/25 - See ANTIHISTAMINES, PIPERAZINE (Antinausea) 114
Antivert/50 - See ANTIHISTAMINES, PIPERAZINE (Antinausea) 114
Antivertigo - See DIPHENIDOL 322
Antiviral - See
ANTIVIRALS FOR HERPES VIRUS 136
ANTIVIRALS FOR INFLUENZA 138
ANTIVIRALS (Topical) 144
INTEGRASE INHIBITORS 450
MARAVIROC 522
NUCLEOSIDE REVERSE TRANSCRIPTASE INHIBITORS 610
NUCLEOTIDE REVERSE TRANSCRIPTASE INHIBITORS 612
RIBAVIRIN 724
Antiviral, HIV and AIDS - See
NON-NUCLEOSIDE REVERSE TRANSCRIPTASE INHIBITORS 608
Antiviral (Ophthalmic) - See ANTIVIRALS (Ophthalmic) 142
ANTIVIRALS FOR HERPES VIRUS 136
ANTIVIRALS FOR INFLUENZA 138
ANTIVIRALS FOR INFLUENZA, NEURAMINIDASE INHIBITORS 140

ANTIVIRALS (Ophthalmic) 142
ANTIVIRALS (Topical) 144
Antrocol - See BELLADONNA ALKALOIDS & BARBITURATES 174
Anturan - See SULFINPYRAZONE 764
Anturane - See SULFINPYRAZONE 764
Anturol - See MUSCARINIC RECEPTOR ANTAGONISTS 574
Anucort - See HYDROCORTISONE (Rectal) 430
Anucort-HC - See ADRENOCORTICOIDS (Topical) 18
Anuphen - See ACETAMINOPHEN 8
Anusol-HC - See
ADRENOCORTICOIDS (Topical) 18
HYDROCORTISONE (Rectal) 430
Anusol-HC 2.5% - See ADRENOCORTICOIDS (Topical) 18
Anxanil - See HYDROXYZINE 436
APAC Improved - See ASPIRIN 152
Apacet Capsules - See ACETAMINOPHEN 8
Apacet Elixir - See ACETAMINOPHEN 8
Apacet Extra Strength Caplets - See ACETAMINOPHEN 8
Apacet Extra Strength Tablets - See ACETAMINOPHEN 8
Apacet Oral Solution - See ACETAMINOPHEN 8
Apacet Regular Strength Tablets - See ACETAMINOPHEN 8
APAP - See ACETAMINOPHEN 8
APAP with Codeine - See NARCOTIC ANALGESICS & ACETAMINOPHEN 586
A.P.C. - See CAFFEINE 216
APF Arthritic Pain Formula - See ASPIRIN 152
Aphthasol - See AMLEXANOX 26
Apidra - See INSULIN ANALOGS 448
Apidra SoloStar - See INSULIN ANALOGS 448
APIXABAN - See FACTOR Xa INHIBITORS 382
Aplenzin - See BUPROPION 208
Apo Acetazolamide - See CARBONIC ANHYDRASE INHIBITORS 232
Apo-Acetaminophen - See ACETAMINOPHEN 8
Apo-Allopurinol - See ANTIGOUT DRUGS 104
Apo-Alpraz - See BENZODIAZEPINES 176
Apo-Amitriptyline - See ANTIDEPRESSANTS, TRICYCLIC 80
Apo-Amoxi - See PENICILLINS 646
Apo-Ampi - See PENICILLINS 646
Apo-Atenolol - See BETA-ADRENERGIC BLOCKING AGENTS 182
Apo-Benztropine - See ANTIDYSKINETICS 82
Apo-Bromocriptine - See BROMOCRIPTINE 198
Apo-Cal - See CALCIUM SUPPLEMENTS 222
Apo-Capto - See ANGIOTENSIN-CONVERTING ENZYME (ACE) INHIBITORS 44
Apo-Carbamazepine - See CARBAMAZEPINE 228
Apo-Cephalex - See CEPHALOSPORINS 236
Apo-Chlorax - See CLIDINIUM 256
Apo-Chlordiazepoxide - See BENZODIAZEPINES 176
Apo-Chlorpropamide - See SULFONYLUREAS 770
Apo-Chlorthalidone - See DIURETICS, THIAZIDE 338
Apo-Cimetidine - See HISTAMINE H_2 RECEPTOR ANTAGONISTS 422
Apo-Clorazepate - See BENZODIAZEPINES 176
Apo-Cloxi - See PENICILLINS 646
Apo-Diazepam - See BENZODIAZEPINES 176
Apo-Diclo - See ANTI-INFLAMMATORY DRUGS, NONSTEROIDAL (NSAIDs) 116
Apo-Diflunisal - See ANTI-INFLAMMATORY DRUGS, NONSTEROIDAL (NSAIDs) 116
Apo-Diltiaz - See CALCIUM CHANNEL BLOCKERS 220
Apo-Dimenhydrinate - See ANTIHISTAMINES 106
Apo-Dipyridamole - See DIPYRIDAMOLE 326
Apo-Doxy - See TETRACYCLINES 782
Apo-Erythro - See ERYTHROMYCINS 368
Apo-Erythro E-C - See ERYTHROMYCINS 368
Apo-Erythro ES - See ERYTHROMYCINS 368
Apo-Erythro-S - See ERYTHROMYCINS 368
Apo-Ferrous Gluconate - See IRON SUPPLEMENTS 458
Apo-Ferrous Sulfate - See IRON SUPPLEMENTS 458
Apo-Fluphenazine - See PHENOTHIAZINES 656
Apo-Flurazepam - See BENZODIAZEPINES 176
Apo-Flurbiprofen - See ANTI-INFLAMMATORY DRUGS, NONSTEROIDAL (NSAIDs) 116
Apo-Folic - See FOLIC ACID (Vitamin B-9) 396
Apo-Furosemide - See DIURETICS, LOOP 332
Apo-Glyburide - See SULFONYLUREAS 770
Apo-Haloperidol - See HALOPERIDOL 420
Apo-Hydro - See DIURETICS, THIAZIDE 338
Apo-Hydroxyzine - See HYDROXYZINE 436
Apo-Ibuprofen - See ANTI-INFLAMMATORY DRUGS, NONSTEROIDAL (NSAIDs) 116
Apo-Imipramine - See ANTIDEPRESSANTS, TRICYCLIC 80
Apo-Indomethacin - See ANTI-INFLAMMATORY DRUGS, NONSTEROIDAL (NSAIDs) 116
Apo-Ipravent - See IPRATROPIUM 456
Apo-ISDN - See NITRATES 602
Apo-K - See POTASSIUM SUPPLEMENTS 666
Apo-Keto - See ANTI-INFLAMMATORY DRUGS, NONSTEROIDAL (NSAIDs) 116
Apo-Keto-E - See ANTI-INFLAMMATORY DRUGS, NONSTEROIDAL (NSAIDs) 116

Apo-Loperamide Caplets - See LOPERAMIDE 508
Apo-Lorazepam - See BENZODIAZEPINES 176
Apo-Meprobamate - See MEPROBAMATE 538
Apo-Methyldopa - See CENTRAL ALPHA AGONISTS 234
Apo-Metoclop - See METOCLOPRAMIDE 550
Apo-Metoprolol - See BETA-ADRENERGIC BLOCKING AGENTS 182
Apo-Metronidazole - See NITROIMIDAZOLES 606
Apo-Naproxen - See ANTI-INFLAMMATORY DRUGS, NONSTEROIDAL (NSAIDs) 116
Apo-Nifed - See CALCIUM CHANNEL BLOCKERS 220
Apo-Nitrofurantoin - See NITROFURANTOIN 604
Apo-Oxazepam - See BENZODIAZEPINES 176
Apo-Oxtriphylline - See BRONCHODILATORS, XANTHINE 204
Apo-Pen VK - See PENICILLINS 646
Apo-Perphenazine - See PHENOTHIAZINES 656
Apo-Phenylbutazone - See ANTI-INFLAMMATORY DRUGS, NONSTEROIDAL (NSAIDs) 116
Apo-Piroxicam - See ANTI-INFLAMMATORY DRUGS, NONSTEROIDAL (NSAIDs) 116
Apo-Prednisone - See ADRENOCORTICOIDS (Systemic) 16
Apo-Primidone - See PRIMIDONE 674
Apo-Propranolol - See BETA-ADRENERGIC BLOCKING AGENTS 182
Apo-Quinidine - See QUINIDINE 704
Apo-Ranitidine - See HISTAMINE H_2 RECEPTOR ANTAGONISTS 422
Apo-Selegiline - See MONOAMINE OXIDASE TYPE B (MAO-B) INHIBITORS 572
Apo-Sulfamethoxazole - See SULFONAMIDES 766
Apo-Sulfatrim - See
SULFONAMIDES 766
TRIMETHOPRIM 818
Apo-Sulfatrim DS - See
SULFONAMIDES 766
TRIMETHOPRIM 818
Apo-Sulfinpyrazone - See SULFINPYRAZONE 764
Apo-Sulfisoxazole - See SULFONAMIDES 766
Apo-Tetra - See TETRACYCLINES 782
Apo-Thioridazine - See PHENOTHIAZINES 656
Apo-Timol - See BETA-ADRENERGIC BLOCKING AGENTS 182
Apo-Timop - See ANTIGLAUCOMA, BETA BLOCKERS 96
Apo-Tolbutamide - See SULFONYLUREAS 770
Apo-Triazide - See DIURETICS, POTASSIUM-SPARING & HYDROCHLOROTHIAZIDE 336
Apo-Triazo - See TRIAZOLAM 812
Apo-Trifluoperazine - See PHENOTHIAZINES 656
Apo-Trihex - See ANTIDYSKINETICS 82
Apo-Trimip - See ANTIDEPRESSANTS, TRICYCLIC 80
Apo-Verap - See CALCIUM CHANNEL BLOCKERS 220
Apo-Zidovudine - See NUCLEOSIDE REVERSE TRANSCRIPTASE INHIBITORS 610
Appecon - See APPETITE SUPPRESSANTS 146
Appetite suppressant - See APPETITE SUPPRESSANTS 146
<u>APPETITE SUPPRESSANTS</u> 146
APRACLONIDINE - See ANTIGLAUCOMA, ADRENERGIC AGONISTS 92
Apresazide - See HYDRALAZINE & HYDROCHLOROTHIAZIDE 428
Apresoline - See HYDRALAZINE 426
Apresoline-Esidrix - See HYDRALAZINE & HYDROCHLOROTHIAZIDE 428
Apri - See CONTRACEPTIVES, ORAL & SKIN 278
Apriso - See MESALAMINE 542
APROBARBITAL - See BARBITURATES 168
Aprozide - See HYDRALAZINE & HYDROCHLOROTHIAZIDE 428
Apsifen - See ANTI-INFLAMMATORY DRUGS, NONSTEROIDAL (NSAIDs) 116
Apsifen-F - See ANTI-INFLAMMATORY DRUGS, NONSTEROIDAL (NSAIDs) 116
Aptivus - See PROTEASE INHIBITORS 688
Aquaphyllin - See BRONCHODILATORS, XANTHINE 204
Aquasol A - See VITAMIN A 834
Aquasol E - See VITAMIN E 844
Aquatar - See COAL TAR (Topical) 266
Aquatensen - See DIURETICS, THIAZIDE 338
Aqueous Charcodote - See CHARCOAL, ACTIVATED 238
Aralen - See CHLOROQUINE 246
Arava - See LEFLUNOMIDE 484
Arcapta - See BRONCHODILATORS, ADRENERGIC 200
Arcet - See
ACETAMINOPHEN 8
BARBITURATES 168
Aredia - See BISPHOSPHONATES 192
ARFORMOTEROL - See BRONCHODILATORS, ADRENERGIC 200

Aricept - See CHOLINESTERASE INHIBITORS 250
Aricept ODT - See CHOLINESTERASE INHIBITORS 250
ARIPIPRAZOLE 148
Aristocort - See ADRENOCORTICOIDS (Systemic) 16
Aristocort A - See ADRENOCORTICOIDS (Topical) 18
Aristocort C - See ADRENOCORTICOIDS (Topical) 18
Aristocort D - See ADRENOCORTICOIDS (Topical) 18
Aristocort R - See ADRENOCORTICOIDS (Topical) 18
Arm & Hammer Pure Baking Soda - See SODIUM BICARBONATE 750
Arm-a-Med Metaproterenol - See BRONCHODILATORS, ADRENERGIC 200
ARMODAFINIL - See STIMULANTS, AMPHETAMINE-RELATED 756
Armour Thyroid - See THYROID HORMONES 792
Aromatic Cascara Fluidextract - See LAXATIVES, STIMULANT 482
Artane - See ANTIDYSKINETICS 82
Artane Sequels - See ANTIDYSKINETICS 82
ArthriCare - See CAPSAICIN 226
Arthrinol - See ASPIRIN 152
Arthrisin - See ASPIRIN 152
Arthritis Pain Formula - See ASPIRIN 152
Arthropan - See SALICYLATES 736
Arthrotec - See
ANTI-INFLAMMATORY DRUGS, NONSTEROIDAL (NSAIDs) 116
MISOPROSTOL 568
ARTH-RX - See CAPSAICIN 226
Artificial tears - See PROTECTANT (Ophthalmic) 690
Artificial Tears - See PROTECTANT (Ophthalmic) 690
Artria S.R. - See ASPIRIN 152
A.S.A. - See ASPIRIN 152
A.S.A. Enseals - See ASPIRIN 152
Asacol - See MESALAMINE 542
Asacol HD - See MESALAMINE 542
Asbron G - See
BRONCHODILATORS, XANTHINE 204
GUAIFENESIN 416
Asbron G Inlay Tablets - See
BRONCHODILATORS, XANTHINE 204
GUAIFENESIN 416
Ascomp with Codeine No. 3 - See BARBITURATES, ASPIRIN & CODEINE (Also contains caffeine) 170
Ascorbicap - See VITAMIN C (Ascorbic Acid) 838
Ascriptin - See ASPIRIN 152
Ascriptin A/D - See ASPIRIN 152
ASENAPINE 150
Asendin - See ANTIDEPRESSANTS, TRICYCLIC 80
Asmalix - See BRONCHODILATORS, XANTHINE 204
Asmanex - See ADRENOCORTICOIDS (Nasal Inhalation) 12
A-Spas - See DICYCLOMINE 316
Aspergum - See ASPIRIN 152
ASPIRIN 152
ASPIRIN & CODEINE - See NARCOTIC ANALGESICS & ASPIRIN 588
Aspirin Free Anacin Maximum Strength Caplets - See ACETAMINOPHEN 8
Aspirin Free Anacin Maximum Strength Tablets - See ACETAMINOPHEN 8
Aspirin Free Bayer Select Maximum Strength Headache Pain Relief Caplets - See CAFFEINE 216
Aspirin Free Bayer Select Maximum Strength Headache Plus Caplets - See ACETAMINOPHEN 8
Aspirin-Free Excedrin Caplets - See
ACETAMINOPHEN 8
CAFFEINE 216
Astelin - See ANTIHISTAMINES (Nasal) 108
Astepro - See ANTIHISTAMINES (Nasal) 108
AsthmaHaler - See BRONCHODILATORS, ADRENERGIC 200
AsthmaNefrin - See BRONCHODILATORS, ADRENERGIC 200
Astramorph - See NARCOTIC ANALGESICS 584
Astramorph-PF - See NARCOTIC ANALGESICS 584
Astrin - See ASPIRIN 152
Atabrine - See QUINACRINE 702
Atacand - See ANGIOTENSIN II RECEPTOR ANTAGONISTS 42
Atapryl - See MONOAMINE OXIDASE TYPE B (MAO-B) INHIBITORS 572
Atarax - See HYDROXYZINE 436
Atasol Caplets - See ACETAMINOPHEN 8
Atasol Drops - See ACETAMINOPHEN 8
Atasol Forte - See ACETAMINOPHEN 8
Atasol Forte Caplets - See ACETAMINOPHEN 8
Atasol Forte Tablets - See ACETAMINOPHEN 8
Atasol Oral Solution - See ACETAMINOPHEN 8
Atasol Tablets - See ACETAMINOPHEN 8
Atasol-8 - See NARCOTIC ANALGESICS & ACETAMINOPHEN 586

Atasol-15 - See NARCOTIC ANALGESICS & ACETAMINOPHEN 586
Atasol-30 - See NARCOTIC ANALGESICS & ACETAMINOPHEN 586
ATAZANAVIR - See PROTEASE INHIBITORS 688
Atelvia - See BISPHOSPHONATES 192
ATENOLOL - See BETA-ADRENERGIC BLOCKING AGENTS 182
ATENOLOL & CHLORTHALIDONE - See BETA-ADRENERGIC BLOCKING AGENTS & THIAZIDE DIURETICS 184
Ativan - See BENZODIAZEPINES 176
<u>ATOMOXETINE</u> 154
ATORVASTATIN - See HMG-CoA REDUCTASE INHIBITORS 424
<u>ATOVAQUONE</u> 156
Atralin Gel - See RETINOIDS (Topical) 722
Atripla - See
NON-NUCLEOSIDE REVERSE TRANSCRIPTASE INHIBITORS 608
NUCLEOSIDE REVERSE TRANSCRIPTASE INHIBITORS 610
NUCLEOTIDE REVERSE TRANSCRIPTASE INHIBITORS 612
Atrohist Pediatric - See
ANTIHISTAMINES 106
PHENYLEPHRINE 658
Atrohist Pediatric Suspension Dye Free - See
ANTIHISTAMINES 106
PHENYLEPHRINE 658
Atrohist Sprinkle - See
ANTIHISTAMINES 106
PHENYLEPHRINE 658
Atromid-S - See FIBRATES 386
Atropair - See CYCLOPLEGIC, MYDRIATIC (Ophthalmic) 292
ATROPINE - See ANTICHOLINERGICS 72
ATROPINE & PHENOBARBITAL - See BELLADONNA ALKALOIDS & BARBITURATES 174
ATROPINE (Ophthalmic) - See CYCLOPLEGIC, MYDRIATIC (Ophthalmic) 292
Atropine Care Eye Drops and Ointment - See CYCLOPLEGIC, MYDRIATIC (Ophthalmic) 292
<u>ATROPINE, HYOSCYAMINE, METHENAMINE, METHYLENE BLUE, PHENYLSALICYLATE & BENZOIC ACID</u> 158
ATROPINE, HYOSCYAMINE, SCOPOLAMINE & BUTABARBITAL - See BELLADONNA ALKALOIDS & BARBITURATES 174
ATROPINE, HYOSCYAMINE, SCOPOLAMINE & PHENOBARBITAL - See BELLADONNA ALKALOIDS & BARBITURATES 174
Atropine Sulfate S.O.P. - See CYCLOPLEGIC, MYDRIATIC (Ophthalmic) 292
Atropisol - See CYCLOPLEGIC, MYDRIATIC (Ophthalmic) 292
Atrosept - See ATROPINE, HYOSCYAMINE, METHENAMINE, METHYLENE BLUE, PHENYLSALICYLATE & BENZOIC ACID 158
Atrosulf - See CYCLOPLEGIC, MYDRIATIC (Ophthalmic) 292
Atrovent - See IPRATROPIUM 456
Atrovent Inhalation Aerosol - See IPRATROPIUM 456
A/T/S - See ANTIBACTERIALS FOR ACNE (Topical) 64
<u>ATTAPULGITE</u> 160
Augmentin - See PENICILLINS & BETA-LACTAMASE INHIBITORS 648
Augmentin ES-600 - See PENICILLINS & BETA-LACTAMASE INHIBITORS 648
Augmentin XR - See PENICILLINS & BETA-LACTAMASE INHIBITORS 648
Auralgan - See ANTIPYRINE & BENZOCAINE (Otic) 130
AURANOFIN - See GOLD COMPOUNDS 412
Aureomycin - See ANTIBACTERIALS FOR ACNE (Topical) 64
Aurodex - See ANTIPYRINE & BENZOCAINE (Otic) 130
Aut - See ANTHELMINTICS 50
Avage - See RETINOIDS (Topical) 722
Avalide - See
ANGIOTENSIN II RECEPTOR ANTAGONISTS 42
DIURETICS, THIAZIDE 338
AVANAFIL- See ERECTILE DYSFUNCTION AGENTS 360
Avandamet - See
METFORMIN 544
THIAZOLIDINEDIONES 786
Avandaryl - See
SULFONYLUREAS 770
THIAZOLIDINEDIONES 786
Avandia - See THIAZOLIDINEDIONES 786
Avapro - See ANGIOTENSIN II RECEPTOR ANTAGONISTS 42
Aveeno Acne Bar - See KERATOLYTICS 470
Aveeno Cleansing Bar - See KERATOLYTICS 470
Avelox - See FLUOROQUINOLONES 392
Aventyl - See ANTIDEPRESSANTS, TRICYCLIC 80
Aviane - See CONTRACEPTIVES, ORAL & SKIN 278
Avinza - See NARCOTIC ANALGESICS 584
Avirax - See ANTIVIRALS FOR HERPES VIRUS 136

Avita - See RETINOIDS (Topical) 722
Avlosulfon - See DAPSONE 304
Avodart - See 5-ALPHA REDUCTASE INHIBITORS 2
Axert - See TRIPTANS 820
Axid - See HISTAMINE H_2 RECEPTOR ANTAGONISTS 422
Axiron - See ANDROGENS 34
Axotal - See
ASPIRIN 152
BARBITURATES 168
Axsain - See CAPSAICIN 226
Aygestin - See PROGESTINS 680
Azaline - See SULFASALAZINE 762
Azasan - See AZATHIOPRINE 162
AzaSite - See ANTIBACTERIALS (Ophthalmic) 66
AZATADINE - See ANTIHISTAMINES 106
AZATHIOPRINE 162
Azdone - See NARCOTIC ANALGESICS & ASPIRIN 588
AZELAIC ACID 164
AZELASTINE - See ANTIHISTAMINES (Nasal) 108
AZELASTINE (Ophthalmic) - See ANTI-ALLERGIC AGENTS (Ophthalmic) 56
Azelex - See AZELAIC ACID 164
Azilect - See MONOAMINE OXIDASE TYPE B (MAO-B) INHIBITORS 572
AZILSARTAN - See ANGIOTENSIN II RECEPTOR ANTAGONISTS 42
AZITHROMYCIN - See MACROLIDE ANTIBIOTICS 518
AZITHROMYCIN (Ophthalmic) - See ANTIBACTERIALS (Ophthalmic) 66
Azmacort - See ADRENOCORTICOIDS (Oral Inhalation) 14
Azo Gantanol - See SULFONAMIDES & PHENAZOPYRIDINE 768
Azo-Cheragan - See PHENAZOPYRIDINE 654
Azo-Gantrisin - See
PHENAZOPYRIDINE 654
SULFONAMIDES & PHENAZOPYRIDINE 768
Azopt - See ANTIGLAUCOMA, CARBONIC ANHYDRASE INHIBITORS 98
Azor - See
ANGIOTENSIN II RECEPTOR ANTAGONISTS 42
CALCIUM CHANNEL BLOCKERS 220
Azo-Standard - See PHENAZOPYRIDINE 654
Azo-Sulfamethoxazole - See SULFONAMIDES & PHENAZOPYRIDINE 768
Azo-Sulfisoxazol - See SULFONAMIDES & PHENAZOPYRIDINE 768
Azo-Truxazole - See SULFONAMIDES & PHENAZOPYRIDINE 768
AZT - See NUCLEOSIDE REVERSE TRANSCRIPTASE INHIBITORS 610
Azulfidine - See SULFASALAZINE 762
Azulfidine En-Tabs - See SULFASALAZINE 762

B

Baby Anbesol - See ANESTHETICS (Mucosal-Local) 36
Baby Orabase - See ANESTHETICS (Mucosal-Local) 36
Baby Oragel - See ANESTHETICS (Mucosal-Local) 36
Baby Oragel Nighttime Formula - See ANESTHETICS (Mucosal-Local) 36
B-A-C with Codeine - See BARBITURATES, ASPIRIN & CODEINE (Also contains caffeine) 170
BACAMPICILLIN - See PENICILLINS 646
BACLOFEN 166
Bactine - See ADRENOCORTICOIDS (Topical) 18
Bactine First Aid - See ANTIBACTERIALS (Topical) 70
Bactocill - See PENICILLINS 646
Bactrim - See
SULFONAMIDES 766
TRIMETHOPRIM 818
Bactrim DS - See
SULFONAMIDES 766
TRIMETHOPRIM 818
Bactroban - See ANTIBACTERIALS (Topical) 70
Bactroban Nasal - See ANTIBACTERIALS (Topical) 70
Balacet 325 - See NARCOTIC ANALGESICS & ACETAMINOPHEN 586
Baldex - See ANTI-INFLAMMATORY DRUGS, STEROIDAL (Ophthalmic) 122
Balminil Decongestant - See PSEUDOEPHEDRINE 694
Balminil DM - See DEXTROMETHORPHAN 312
Balminil Expectorant - See GUAIFENESIN 416
Balnetar - See COAL TAR (Topical) 266
Balnetar Therapeutic Tar Bath - See COAL TAR (Topical) 266
BALSALAZIDE - See SALICYLATES 736
Bancap - See
ACETAMINOPHEN 8
BARBITURATES 168
Bancap-HC - See NARCOTIC ANALGESICS & ACETAMINOPHEN 586
Banesin - See ACETAMINOPHEN 8
Banflex - See ORPHENADRINE 624
Banophen - See ANTIHISTAMINES 106
Banophen Caplets - See ANTIHISTAMINES 106
Banthine - See ANTICHOLINERGICS 72

Barbidonna - See
BELLADONNA ALKALOIDS & BARBITURATES 174
HYOSCYAMINE 438
SCOPOLAMINE (Hyoscine) 738
Barbidonna 2 - See
BELLADONNA ALKALOIDS & BARBITURATES 174
HYOSCYAMINE 438
SCOPOLAMINE (Hyoscine) 738
Barbita - See BARBITURATES 168
Barbiturate - See
BARBITURATES 168
BARBITURATES, ASPIRIN & CODEINE (Also contains caffeine) 170
BARBITURATES 168
BARBITURATES, ASPIRIN & CODEINE (Also contains caffeine) 170
Barc - See PEDICULICIDES (Topical) 642
Baridium - See PHENAZOPYRIDINE 654
Barophen - See BELLADONNA ALKALOIDS & BARBITURATES 174
Barr - See NALTREXONE 582
Barriere-HC - See ADRENOCORTICOIDS (Topical) 18
Basaljel - See ANTACIDS 48
Bayer - See ASPIRIN 152
Bayer Advanced - See ASPIRIN 152
Bayer Extra Strength Aspirin - See ASPIRIN 152
Bayer Quick Release Crystals - See
ASPIRIN 152
CAFFEINE 216
Bayer Select Maximum Strength Pain Relief Formula - See ACETAMINOPHEN 8
Bayer Timed-Release Arthritic Pain Formula - See ASPIRIN 152
Bayer Women's Caplets, Aspirin Plus Calcium - See
ASPIRIN 152
CALCIUM SUPPLEMENTS 222
Baytussin AC - See
GUAIFENESIN 416
NARCOTIC ANALGESICS 584
Baytussin DM - See
DEXTROMETHORPHAN 312
GUAIFENESIN 416
Beben - See ADRENOCORTICOIDS (Topical) 18
BECAPLERMIN 172
Because - See CONTRACEPTIVES, VAGINAL 280
Beclodisk - See ADRENOCORTICOIDS (Oral Inhalation) 14
Becloforte - See ADRENOCORTICOIDS (Oral Inhalation) 14
BECLOMETHASONE (Nasal) - See ADRENOCORTICOIDS (Nasal Inhalation) 12
BECLOMETHASONE (Oral Inhalation) - See ADRENOCORTICOIDS (Oral Inhalation) 14
BECLOMETHASONE (Topical) - See ADRENOCORTICOIDS (Topical) 18
Beconase - See ADRENOCORTICOIDS (Nasal Inhalation) 12
Beconase AQ - See ADRENOCORTICOIDS (Nasal Inhalation) 12
Bedoz - See VITAMIN B-12 (Cyanocobalamin) 836
Beepen-VK - See PENICILLINS 646
Beesix - See PYRIDOXINE (Vitamin B-6) 698
Beldin - See ANTIHISTAMINES 106
Belix - See ANTIHISTAMINES 106
Belladenal - See
BELLADONNA ALKALOIDS & BARBITURATES 174
HYOSCYAMINE 438
Belladenal Spacetabs - See BELLADONNA ALKALOIDS & BARBITURATES 174
Belladenal-S - See BELLADONNA ALKALOIDS & BARBITURATES 174
BELLADONNA & AMOBARBITAL - See BELLADONNA ALKALOIDS & BARBITURATES 174
BELLADONNA & BUTABARBITAL - See BELLADONNA ALKALOIDS & BARBITURATES 174
BELLADONNA & PHENOBARBITAL - See BELLADONNA ALKALOIDS & BARBITURATES 174
BELLADONNA ALKALOIDS & BARBITURATES 174
Bellalphen - See BELLADONNA ALKALOIDS & BARBITURATES 174
Bell/ans - See SODIUM BICARBONATE 750
Belviq - See LORCASERIN 510
Bena-D 10 - See ANTIHISTAMINES 106
Bena-D 50 - See ANTIHISTAMINES 106
Benadryl Allergy & Cold Caplet - See
ACETAMINOPHEN 8
ANTIHISTAMINES 106
PHENYLEPHRINE 658
Benadryl Allergy & Sinus Headache Gelcap - See
ACETAMINOPHEN 8
ANTIHISTAMINES 106
PSEUDOEPHEDRINE 694
Benadryl Allergy Dye-Free Liqui-gel - See ANTIHISTAMINES 106
Benadryl Allergy Kapseals - See ANTIHISTAMINES 106

Benadryl Allergy Quick Dissolve Strips - See ANTIHISTAMINES 106
Benadryl Allergy Ultratab Tablets - See ANTIHISTAMINES 106
Benadryl Severe Allergy & Sinus Headache Caplet - See
ACETAMINOPHEN 8
ANTIHISTAMINES 106
PSEUDOEPHEDRINE 694
Benadryl Severe Allergy & Sinus Headache w/ PE Caplet - See
ACETAMINOPHEN 8
ANTIHISTAMINES 106
PHENYLEPHRINE 658
Benadryl Allergy/Sinus Headache Caplets - See
ACETAMINOPHEN 8
ANTIHISTAMINES 106
PSEUDOEPHEDRINE 694
Benadryl-D Allergy & Sinus Fastmelt Tablet - See
ANTIHISTAMINES 106
PSEUDOEPHEDRINE 694
Benadryl-D Allergy & Sinus Tablet - See
ANTIHISTAMINES 106
PSEUDOEPHEDRINE 694
Benahist 10 - See ANTIHISTAMINES 106
Benahist 50 - See ANTIHISTAMINES 106
Ben-Allergin 50 - See ANTIHISTAMINES 106
Benaphen - See ANTIHISTAMINES 106
Ben-Aqua 5 Gel - See BENZOYL PEROXIDE 178
Ben-Aqua 5 Lotion - See BENZOYL PEROXIDE 178
Ben-Aqua 10 Gel - See BENZOYL PEROXIDE 178
Ben-Aqua 10 Lotion - See BENZOYL PEROXIDE 178
Ben-Aqua 21/2 Gel - See BENZOYL PEROXIDE 178
Ben-Aqua 21/2 Lotion - See BENZOYL PEROXIDE 178
Ben-Aqua Masque 5 - See BENZOYL PEROXIDE 178
BENAZEPRIL - See ANGIOTENSIN-CONVERTING ENZYME (ACE) INHIBITORS 44
BENDROFLUMETHIAZIDE - See DIURETICS, THIAZIDE 338
Benemid - See PROBENECID 676
Benicar - See ANGIOTENSIN II RECEPTOR ANTAGONISTS 42
Benicar HCT - See
ANGIOTENSIN II RECEPTOR ANTAGONISTS 42
DIURETICS, THIAZIDE 338
Benoject-10 - See ANTIHISTAMINES 106
Benoject-50 - See ANTIHISTAMINES 106
Benoxyl 5 Lotion - See BENZOYL PEROXIDE 178
Benoxyl 5 Wash - See BENZOYL PEROXIDE 178
Benoxyl 10 Lotion - See BENZOYL PEROXIDE 178
Benoxyl 10 Wash - See BENZOYL PEROXIDE 178
Benoxyl 20 Lotion - See BENZOYL PEROXIDE 178
Bensulfoid Cream - See KERATOLYTICS 470
Bentyl - See DICYCLOMINE 316
Bentylol - See DICYCLOMINE 316
Benuryl - See PROBENECID 676
Benylin All-In-One Cold & Flu Caplets - See
ACETAMINOPHEN 8
DEXTROMETHORPHAN 312
GUAIFENESIN 416
PSEUDOEPHEDRINE 694
Benylin All-In-One Cold & Flu Night Caplets - See
ACETAMINOPHEN 8
ANTIHISTAMINES 106
PHENYLEPHRINE 658
Benylin All-In-One Cold & Flu Nightime Syrup - See
ACETAMINOPHEN 8
ANTIHISTAMINES 106
DEXTROMETHORPHAN 312
GUAIFENESIN 416
PSEUDOEPHEDRINE 694
Benylin All-In-One Cold & Flu Syrup - See
ACETAMINOPHEN 8
DEXTROMETHORPHAN 312
GUAIFENESIN 416
PSEUDOEPHEDRINE 694
Benylin All-In-One Day & Night Caplets - See
ACETAMINOPHEN 8
DEXTROMETHORPHAN 312
GUAIFENESIN 416
PSEUDOEPHEDRINE 694
Benylin Cold & Sinus - See
ACETAMINOPHEN 8
PHENYLEPHRINE 658
Benylin Cold & Sinus Plus - See
ACETAMINOPHEN 8
ANTIHISTAMINES 106
PHENYLEPHRINE 658
Benylin Cold & Flu With Codeine Narcotic - See
GUAIFENESIN 416
NARCOTIC ANALGESICS 584
PSEUDOEPHEDRINE 694

Benylin DM 12 Hour Nightime Cough Syrup - See DEXTROMETHORPHAN 312
Benylin DM-D - See
DEXTROMETHORPHAN 312
PSEUDOEPHEDRINE 694
Benylin DM-D for Children Cough & Cold Syrup - See
DEXTROMETHORPHAN 312
PSEUDOEPHEDRINE 694
Benylin DM-D-E - See
DEXTROMETHORPHAN 312
GUAIFENESIN 416
PSEUDOEPHEDRINE 694
Benylin DM-D-E Extra Strength - See
DEXTROMETHORPHAN 312
GUAIFENESIN 416
PSEUDOEPHEDRINE 694
Benylin DM Dry Cough Syrup - See
DEXTROMETHORPHAN 312
Benylin DM-E Chest Cough Syrup - See
DEXTROMETHORPHAN 312
GUAIFENESIN 416
Benylin DM for Children Dry Cough Syrup - See DEXTROMETHORPHAN 312
Benzac Ac 5 Gel - See BENZOYL PEROXIDE 178
Benzac Ac 10 Gel - See BENZOYL PEROXIDE 178
Benzac Ac 21/2 Gel - See BENZOYL PEROXIDE 178
Benzac W 5 Gel - See BENZOYL PEROXIDE 178
Benzac W 10 Gel - See BENZOYL PEROXIDE 178
Benzac W 21/2 Gel - See BENZOYL PEROXIDE 178
Benzaclin - See
ANTIBACTERIALS FOR ACNE (Topical) 64
BENZOYL PEROXIDE 178
Benzagel 5 Acne Lotion - See BENZOYL PEROXIDE 178
Benzagel 5 Acne Wash - See BENZOYL PEROXIDE 178
Benzagel 5 Gel - See BENZOYL PEROXIDE 178
Benzagel 10 Gel - See BENZOYL PEROXIDE 178
BENZALKONIUM CHLORIDE - See CONTRACEPTIVES, VAGINAL 280
Benzamycin - See
ANTIBACTERIALS FOR ACNE (Topical) 64
BENZOYL PEROXIDE 178
BenzaShave 5 Cream - See BENZOYL PEROXIDE 178
BenzaShave 10 Cream - See BENZOYL PEROXIDE 178
BenzEFoam - See BENZOYL PEROXIDE 178
BENZOCAINE - See
ANESTHETICS (Mucosal-Local) 36
ANESTHETICS (Rectal) 38
ANESTHETICS (Topical) 40
BENZOCAINE & MENTHOL - See
ANESTHETICS (Mucosal-Local) 36
ANESTHETICS (Topical) 40
BENZOCAINE & PHENOL - See ANESTHETICS (Mucosal-Local) 36
Benzocol - See ANESTHETICS (Topical) 40
Benzodent - See ANESTHETICS (Mucosal Local) 36
BENZODIAZEPINES 176
BENZOYL PEROXIDE 178
BENZPHETAMINE - See APPETITE SUPPRESSANTS 146
BENZTHIAZIDE - See DIURETICS, THIAZIDE 338
BENZTROPINE - See ANTIDYSKINETICS 82
BENZYL ALCOHOL - See PEDICULICIDES (Topical) 642
Bepadin - See CALCIUM CHANNEL BLOCKERS 220
BEPOTASTINE - See ANTIALLERGIC AGENTS (Ophthalmic) 56
Bepreve - See ANTIALLERGIC AGENTS (Ophthalmic) 56
BEPRIDIL - See CALCIUM CHANNEL BLOCKERS 220
Berotec - See BRONCHODILATORS, ADRENERGIC 200
Berubigen - See VITAMIN B-12 (Cyanocobalamin) 836
BESIFLOXACIN - See ANTIBACTERIALS (Ophthalmic) 66
Besivance - See ANTIBACTERIALS (Ophthalmic) 66
BETA CAROTENE 180
Beta HC - See ADRENOCORTICOIDS (Topical) 18
Beta-adrenergic blocker - See BETA-ADRENERGIC BLOCKING AGENTS & THIAZIDE DIURETICS 184
BETA-ADRENERGIC BLOCKING AGENTS 182
BETA-ADRENERGIC BLOCKING AGENTS & THIAZIDE DIURETICS 184
Betacort Scalp Lotion - See
ADRENOCORTICOIDS (Topical) 18
Betaderm - See ADRENOCORTICOIDS (Topical) 18
Betaderm Scalp Lotion - See
ADRENOCORTICOIDS (Topical) 18
Betagen C Cap B.I.D. - See ANTIGLAUCOMA, BETA BLOCKERS 96
Betagen C Cap Q.D. - See ANTIGLAUCOMA, BETA BLOCKERS 96
Betagen Standard Cap - See
ANTIGLAUCOMA, BETA BLOCKERS 96

Betalin 12 - See VITAMIN B-12 (Cyanocobalamin) 836
Betalin S - See THIAMINE (Vitamin B-1) 784
Betaloc - See BETA-ADRENERGIC BLOCKING AGENTS 182
Betamethacot - See ADRENOCORTICOIDS (Topical) 18
BETAMETHASONE - See ADRENOCORTICOIDS (Systemic) 16
BETAMETHASONE (Ophthalmic) - See ANTI-INFLAMMATORY DRUGS, STEROIDAL (Ophthalmic) 122
BETAMETHASONE (Otic) - See ANTI-INFLAMMATORY DRUGS, STEROIDAL (Otic) 124
BETAMETHASONE (Topical) - See ADRENOCORTICOIDS (Topical) 18
Betapace - See BETA-ADRENERGIC BLOCKING AGENTS 182
Betapen-VK - See PENICILLINS 646
Beta-Tim - See ANTIGLAUCOMA, BETA BLOCKERS 96
Betatrex - See ADRENOCORTICOIDS (Topical) 18
Beta-Val - See ADRENOCORTICOIDS (Topical) 18
Betaxin - See THIAMINE (Vitamin B-1) 784
BETAXOLOL - See BETA-ADRENERGIC BLOCKING AGENTS 182
BETAXOLOL & CHLORTHALIDONE - See BETA-ADRENERGIC BLOCKING AGENTS & THIAZIDE DIURETICS 184
BETAXOLOL (Ophthalmic) - See ANTIGLAUCOMA, BETA BLOCKERS 96
Betaxon - See BETA-ADRENERGIC BLOCKING AGENTS 182
BETHANECHOL 186
Bethaprim - See TRIMETHOPRIM 818
Betimol - See ANTIGLAUCOMA, BETA BLOCKERS 96
Betnelan - See ADRENOCORTICOIDS (Systemic) 16
Betnesol - See
  ADRENOCORTICOIDS (Systemic) 16
  ANTI-INFLAMMATORY DRUGS, STEROIDAL (Ophthalmic) 122
  ANTI-INFLAMMATORY DRUGS, STEROIDAL (Otic) 124
Betnovate - See ADRENOCORTICOIDS (Topical) 18
Betnovate 1/2 - See ADRENOCORTICOIDS (Topical) 18
Betoptic - See ANTIGLAUCOMA, BETA BLOCKERS 96
Betoptic S - See ANTIGLAUCOMA, BETA BLOCKERS 96
Bewon - See THIAMINE (Vitamin B-1) 784
BEXAROTENE - See RETINOIDS (Topical) 722
Beyaz - See
  CONTRACEPTIVES, ORAL & SKIN 278
  FOLIC ACID (Vitamin B-9) 396
Biamine - See THIAMINE (Vitamin B-1) 784
Biaxin - See MACROLIDE ANTIBIOTICS 518
BICALUTAMIDE - See ANTIANDROGENS, NONSTEROIDAL 58
Bicitra - See CITRATES 254
BiDil - See
  HYDRALAZINE 426
  NITRATES 602
Bifera - See IRON SUPPLEMENTS 458
Bilagog - See LAXATIVES, OSMOTIC 478
Bilax - See
  LAXATIVES, SOFTENER/LUBRICANT 480
  LAXATIVES, STIMULANT 482
BIMATOPROST - See ANTIGLAUCOMA, PROSTAGLANDINS 102
Binosto - See BISPHOSPHONATES 192
BioCal - See CALCIUM SUPPLEMENTS 222
Biologic response modifier - See
  ANAKINRA 32
  TUMOR NECROSIS FACTOR BLOCKERS 822
BIOLOGICS FOR PSORIASIS 188
Bion Tears - See PROTECTANT (Ophthalmic) 690
Bio-Syn - See ADRENOCORTICOIDS (Topical) 18
Bio-T-Gel - See ANDROGENS 34
BIPERIDEN - See ANTIDYSKINETICS 82
Bisac-Evac - See LAXATIVES, STIMULANT 482
BISACODYL - See LAXATIVES, STIMULANT 482
Bisacolax - See LAXATIVES, STIMULANT 482
Bisco-Lax - See LAXATIVES, STIMULANT 482
BISKALCITRATE - See BISMUTH SALTS 190
Bismatrol - See BISMUTH SALTS 190
BISMUTH SALTS 190
BISMUTH SUBSALICYLATE - See BISMUTH SALTS 190
BISOPROLOL - See BETA-ADRENERGIC BLOCKING AGENTS 182
BISOPROLOL & HYDROCHLOROTHIAZIDE - See BETA-ADRENERGIC BLOCKING AGENTS & THIAZIDE DIURETICS 184
BISPHOSPHONATES 192
BITOLTEROL - See BRONCHODILATORS, ADRENERGIC 200
Black Draught - See LAXATIVES, STIMULANT 482
Black-Draught Lax-Senna - See LAXATIVES, STIMULANT 482

Blanex - See ORPHENADRINE 624
Bleph-10 - See ANTIBACTERIALS (Ophthalmic) 66
Blocadren - See BETA-ADRENERGIC BLOCKING AGENTS 182
Blue - See PEDICULICIDES (Topical) 642
Bonamine - See ANTIHISTAMINES, PIPERAZINE (Antinausea) 114
BONE FORMATION AGENTS 194
Bonine - See ANTIHISTAMINES, PIPERAZINE (Antinausea) 114
Boniva - See BISPHOSPHONATES 192
Bontril PDM - See APPETITE SUPPRESSANTS 146
Bontril Slow Release - See APPETITE SUPPRESSANTS 146
BOSENTAN - See ENDOTHELIN RECEPTOR ANTAGONISTS 354
Botox - See BOTULINUM TOXIN TYPE A 196
Botox Cosmetic - See BOTULINUM TOXIN TYPE A 196
BOTULINUM TOXIN TYPE A 196
Bowel preparation - See KANAMYCIN 466
Breonesin - See GUAIFENESIN 416
Brethaire - See BRONCHODILATORS, ADRENERGIC 200
Brethine - See BRONCHODILATORS, ADRENERGIC 200
Brevicon - See CONTRACEPTIVES, ORAL & SKIN 278
Brevicon 0.5/35 - See CONTRACEPTIVES, ORAL & SKIN 278
Brevicon 1/35 - See CONTRACEPTIVES, ORAL & SKIN 278
Brevoxyl 4 Gel - See BENZOYL PEROXIDE 178
Bricanyl - See BRONCHODILATORS, ADRENERGIC 200
Brilinta - See TICAGRELOR 796
BRIMONIDINE - See ANTIGLAUCOMA, ADRENERGIC AGONISTS 92
BRINZOLAMIDE - See ANTIGLAUCOMA, CARBONIC ANHYDRASE INHIBITORS 98
Brofed - See
ANTIHISTAMINES 106
PSEUDOEPHEDRINE 694
Bromanyl - See
ANTIHISTAMINES 106
NARCOTIC ANALGESICS 584
Bromatane DX Cough - See
ANTIHISTAMINES 106
PSEUDOEPHEDRINE 694
BROMAZEPAM - See BENZODIAZEPINES 176
Bromfed - See
ANTIHISTAMINES 106
PSEUDOEPHEDRINE 694
Bromfed-DM - See
ANTIHISTAMINES 106
DEXTROMETHORPHAN 312
PSEUDOEPHEDRINE 694
Bromfed-PD - See
ANTIHISTAMINES 106
PSEUDOEPHEDRINE 694
BROMFENAC - See ANTI-INFLAMMATORY DRUGS, NONSTEROIDAL (NSAIDs) (Ophthalmic) 120
BROMOCRIPTINE 198
BROMODIPHENHYDRAMINE - See ANTIHISTAMINES 106
Bromo-Seltzer - See
ACETAMINOPHEN 8
SODIUM BICARBONATE 750
BROMPHENIRAMINE - See ANTIHISTAMINES 106
Bronchial - See
BRONCHODILATORS, XANTHINE 204
GUAIFENESIN 416
Bronchodilator - See
BARBITURATES 168
BRONCHODILATORS, ADRENERGIC 200
BRONCHODILATORS, ANTICHOLINERGIC 202
BRONCHODILATORS, XANTHINE 204
GUAIFENESIN 416
IPRATROPIUM 456
BRONCHODILATORS, ADRENERGIC 200
BRONCHODILATORS, ANTICHOLINERGIC 202
BRONCHODILATORS, XANTHINE 204
Broncho-Grippol-DM - See DEXTROMETHORPHAN 312
Broncholate - See
EPHEDRINE 356
GUAIFENESIN 416
Broncomar GG - See
BRONCHODILATORS, XANTHINE 204
GUAIFENESIN 416
Bronitin Mist - See BRONCHODILATORS, ADRENERGIC 200
Bronkaid Mist Suspension - See BRONCHODILATORS, ADRENERGIC 200
Bronkaid Mistometer - See BRONCHODILATORS, ADRENERGIC 200
Bronkodyl - See BRONCHODILATORS, XANTHINE 204
Brontex - See
GUAIFENESIN 416
NARCOTIC ANALGESICS 584
Brovana - See BRONCHODILATORS, ADRENERGIC 200

Brown Mixture - See PAREGORIC 640
Brufen - See ANTI-INFLAMMATORY DRUGS, NONSTEROIDAL (NSAIDs) 116
Bucet - See
ACETAMINOPHEN 8
BARBITURATES 168
BUDESONIDE - See ADRENOCORTICOIDS (Systemic) 16
BUDESONIDE (Nasal) - See ADRENOCORTICOIDS (Nasal Inhalation) 12
BUDESONIDE (Oral Inhalation) - See ADRENOCORTICOIDS (Oral Inhalation) 14
Buffaprin - See ASPIRIN 152
BUFFERED ASPIRIN & CODEINE - See NARCOTIC ANALGESICS & ASPIRIN 588
Bufferin - See ASPIRIN 152
Buffets II - See
ACETAMINOPHEN 8
ASPIRIN 152
Buffinol - See ASPIRIN 152
Buf-Oxal 10 - See BENZOYL PEROXIDE 178
Buf-Puf Acne Cleansing Bar with Vitamin E - See KERATOLYTICS 470
Buf-Puf Medicated Maximum Strength Pads - See KERATOLYTICS 470
Buf-Puf Medicated Regular Strength Pads - See KERATOLYTICS 470
BUMETANIDE - See DIURETICS, LOOP 332
Bumex - See DIURETICS, LOOP 332
Buprenex - See NARCOTIC ANALGESICS 584
BUPRENORPHINE - See NARCOTIC ANALGESICS 584
BUPRENORPHINE & NALOXONE 206
BUPROPION 208
Buscopan - See SCOPOLAMINE (Hyoscine) 738
Busodium - See BARBITURATES 168
BuSpar - See BUSPIRONE 210
BUSPIRONE 210
BUSULFAN 212
BUTABARBITAL - See BARBITURATES 168
Butace - See BARBITURATES 168
Butacote - See ANTI-INFLAMMATORY DRUGS, NONSTEROIDAL (NSAIDs) 116
Butalan - See BARBITURATES 168
BUTALBITAL - See BARBITURATES 168
BUTALBITAL, ASPIRIN & CODEINE - See BARBITURATES, ASPIRIN & CODEINE (Also contains caffeine) 170
Butalbital Compound with Codeine - See BARBITURATES, ASPIRIN & CODEINE (Also contains caffeine) 170
Butalgen - See
ASPIRIN 152
BARBITURATES 168
BUTAMBEN - See ANESTHETICS (Topical) 40
Butazone - See ANTI-INFLAMMATORY DRUGS, NONSTEROIDAL (NSAIDs) 116
BUTENAFINE - See ANTIFUNGALS (Topical) 88
Butesin Picrate - See ANESTHETICS (Topical) 40
Butibel - See BELLADONNA ALKALOIDS & BARBITURATES 174
Butinal with Codeine No. 3 - See BARBITURATES, ASPIRIN & CODEINE (Also contains caffeine) 170
Butisol - See BARBITURATES 168
BUTOCONAZOLE - See ANTIFUNGALS (Vaginal) 90
BUTORPHANOL 214
Butorphanol Tartrate Nasal Spray - See BUTORPHANOL 214
Butrans - See NARCOTIC ANALGESICS 584
Butyl Aminobenzoate - See ANESTHETICS (Topical) 40
Byclomine - See DICYCLOMINE 316
Bydramine Cough - See ANTIHISTAMINES 106
Bydureon - See GLP-1 RECEPTOR AGONISTS 406
Byetta - See GLP-1 RECEPTOR AGONISTS 406
Bystolic - See BETA-ADRENERGIC BLOCKING AGENTS 182

C

Caduet - See
CALCIUM CHANNEL BLOCKERS 220
HMG-CoA REDUCTASE INHIBITORS 424
Caffedrine - See
CAFFEINE 216
ERGOT DERIVATIVES 366
Cane - See CAFFEINE 216
Caffefrine Caplets - See CAFFEINE 216
CAFFEINE 216
Calan - See CALCIUM CHANNEL BLOCKERS 220
Calan SR - See CALCIUM CHANNEL BLOCKERS 220
Calcarb 600 - See CALCIUM SUPPLEMENTS 222
Calci-Chew - See CALCIUM SUPPLEMENTS 222
Calciday 667 - See CALCIUM SUPPLEMENTS 222
Calcidrine - See NARCOTIC ANALGESICS 584
CALCIFEDIOL - See VITAMIN D 840
Calciferol - See VITAMIN D 840
Calcilac - See CALCIUM SUPPLEMENTS 222
CALCIPOTRIENE - See VITAMIN D (Topical) 842

Calcite 500 - See CALCIUM SUPPLEMENTS 222
<u>CALCITONIN</u> 218
CALCITRIOL - See VITAMIN D 840
CALCITRIOL (Topical) - See VITAMIN D (Topical) 842
CALCIUM & MAGNESIUM CARBONATES - See ANTACIDS 48
CALCIUM CARBONATE - See
ANTACIDS 48
CALCIUM SUPPLEMENTS 222
CALCIUM CARBONATE & MAGNESIA - See ANTACIDS 48
CALCIUM CARBONATE & SIMETHICONE - See ANTACIDS 48
CALCIUM CARBONATE, MAGNESIA, & SIMETHICONE - See ANTACIDS 48
Calcium Carbonate/600 - See CALCIUM SUPPLEMENTS 222
Calcium channel blocker - See CALCIUM CHANNEL BLOCKERS 220
<u>CALCIUM CHANNEL BLOCKERS</u> 220
CALCIUM CITRATE - See CALCIUM SUPPLEMENTS 222
CALCIUM GLUBIONATE - See CALCIUM SUPPLEMENTS 222
CALCIUM GLUCONATE - See CALCIUM SUPPLEMENTS 222
CALCIUM GLYCEROPHOSPHATE & CALCIUM LACTATE - See CALCIUM SUPPLEMENTS 222
CALCIUM LACTATE - See CALCIUM SUPPLEMENTS 222
CALCIUM, MAGNESIUM CARBONATES & MAGNESIUM OXIDE - See ANTACIDS 48
CALCIUM PANTOTHENATE - See PANTOTHENIC ACID (Vitamin B-5) 636
CALCIUM POLYCARBOPHIL - See LAXATIVES, BULK-FORMING 476
Calcium Stanley - See CALCIUM SUPPLEMENTS 222
<u>CALCIUM SUPPLEMENTS</u> 222
Calcium-600 - See CALCIUM SUPPLEMENTS 222
Calcium-Sandoz - See CALCIUM SUPPLEMENTS 222
Calcium-Sandoz Forte - See CALCIUM SUPPLEMENTS 222
CaldeCORT Anti-Itch - See ADRENOCORTICOIDS (Topical) 18
CaldeCORT-Light - See ADRENOCORTICOIDS (Topical) 18
Calderol - See VITAMIN D 840
Caldesene Medicated Powder - See ANTIFUNGALS (Topical) 88
Calglycine - See
ANTACIDS 48
CALCIUM SUPPLEMENTS 222
Calicylic - See KERATOLYTICS 470
Calm X - See ANTIHISTAMINES 106
Calmylin with Codeine - See
ANTIHISTAMINES 106
GUAIFENESIN 416
NARCOTIC ANALGESICS 584
PSEUDOEPHEDRINE 694
CaloMist - See VITAMIN B-12 (Cyanocobalamin) 836
Calphosan - See CALCIUM SUPPLEMENTS 222
Calsan - See CALCIUM SUPPLEMENTS 222
Cal-Sap - See CALCIUM SUPPLEMENTS 222
Caltrate - See CALCIUM SUPPLEMENTS 222
Caltrate Chewable - See CALCIUM SUPPLEMENTS 222
Caltrate-300 - See CALCIUM SUPPLEMENTS 222
Caltrate-600 - See CALCIUM SUPPLEMENTS 222
Cama Arthritis Reliever - See ASPIRIN 152
Camalox - See ANTACIDS 48
Cam-Ap-Es - See RESERPINE, HYDRALAZINE & HYDROCHLOROTHIAZIDE 718
Cambia - See
ANTI-INFLAMMATORY DRUGS, NONSTEROIDAL (NSAIDs) 116
POTASSIUM SUPPLEMENTS 666
Campain - See ACETAMINOPHEN 8
Camphorated Opium Tincture - See PAREGORIC 640
Campral - See ACAMPROSATE 4
Camrese - See CONTRACEPTIVES, ORAL & SKIN 278
Canasa - See MESALAMINE 542
CANDESARTAN - See ANGIOTENSIN II RECEPTOR ANTAGONISTS 42
Canesten - See ANTIFUNGALS (Vaginal) 90
Canesten 1 - See ANTIFUNGALS (Vaginal) 90
Canesten 3 - See ANTIFUNGALS (Vaginal) 90
Canesten 10% - See ANTIFUNGALS (Vaginal) 90
Canesten Cream - See ANTIFUNGALS (Topical) 88
Canesten Solution - See ANTIFUNGALS (Topical) 88
Cantil - See ANTICHOLINERGICS 72
<u>CAPECITABINE</u> 224
Capen - See TIOPRONIN 798
Capital with Codeine - See NARCOTIC ANALGESICS & ACETAMINOPHEN 586
Capitrol - See ANTISEBORRHEICS (Topical) 132

Capoten - See ANGIOTENSIN-CONVERTING ENZYME (ACE) INHIBITORS 44
Capozide - See ANGIOTENSIN-CONVERTING ENZYME (ACE) INHIBITORS & HYDROCHLOROTHIAZIDE 46
Capsagel - See CAPSAICIN 226
CAPSAICIN 226
Captimer - See TIOPRONIN 798
CAPTOPRIL - See ANGIOTENSIN-CONVERTING ENZYME (ACE) INHIBITORS 44
CAPTOPRIL & HYDROCHLOROTHIAZIDE - See ANGIOTENSIN-CONVERTING ENZYME (ACE) INHIBITORS & HYDROCHLOROTHIAZIDE 46
Carafate - See SUCRALFATE 758
CARBACHOL - See ANTIGLAUCOMA, CHOLINERGIC AGONISTS 100
Carbacot - See MUSCLE RELAXANTS, SKELETAL 576
CARBAMAZEPINE 228
Carbastat - See ANTIGLAUCOMA, CHOLINERGIC AGONISTS 100
Carbatrol - See CARBAMAZEPINE 228
CARBENICILLIN - See PENICILLINS 646
Carbex - See MONOAMINE OXIDASE TYPE B (MAO-B) INHIBITORS 572
CARBIDOPA & LEVODOPA 230
CARBINOXAMINE - See ANTIHISTAMINES 106
Carbodec - See
ANTIHISTAMINES 106
PSEUDOEPHEDRINE 694
Carbodec DM Drops - See
ANTIHISTAMINES 106
DEXTROMETHORPHAN 312
PSEUDOEPHEDRINE 694
Carbodec TR - See
ANTIHISTAMINES 106
PSEUDOEPHEDRINE 694
Carbolith - See LITHIUM 504
Carbonic anhydrase inhibitor - See CARBONIC ANHYDRASE INHIBITORS 232
CARBONIC ANHYDRASE INHIBITORS 232
CARBONYL IRON - See IRON SUPPLEMENTS 458
Carboptic - See ANTIGLAUCOMA, CHOLINERGIC AGONISTS 100
CARBOXYMETHYLCELLULOSE SODIUM - See LAXATIVES, BULK-FORMING 476
Cardene - See CALCIUM CHANNEL BLOCKERS 220
Cardene SR - See CALCIUM CHANNEL BLOCKERS 220
Cardilate1 - See NITRATES 602
Cardioquin - See QUINIDINE 704
Cardizem - See CALCIUM CHANNEL BLOCKERS 220
Cardizem CD - See CALCIUM CHANNEL BLOCKERS 220
Cardizem LA - See CALCIUM CHANNEL BLOCKERS 220
Cardizem SR - See CALCIUM CHANNEL BLOCKERS 220
Cardura - See ALPHA ADRENERGIC RECEPTOR BLOCKERS 20
Cardura XL- See ALPHA ADRENERGIC RECEPTOR BLOCKERS 20
CARISOPRODOL - See MUSCLE RELAXANTS, SKELETAL 576
Cari-Tab - See VITAMINS & FLUORIDE 848
Carmol-HC - See ADRENOCORTICOIDS (Topical) 18
Carnitor - See LEVOCARNITINE 494
Carnitor Sugar-free Oral Solution - See LEVOCARNITINE 494
Caroid Laxative - See LAXATIVES, STIMULANT 482
Carpine - See ANTIGLAUCOMA, CHOLINERGIC AGONISTS 100
CARTEOLOL - See BETA-ADRENERGIC BLOCKING AGENTS 182
CARTEOLOL (Ophthalmic) - See ANTIGLAUCOMA, BETA BLOCKERS 96
Carter's Little Pills - See LAXATIVES, STIMULANT 482
Cartia XT - See CALCIUM CHANNEL BLOCKERS 220
Cartrol - See BETA-ADRENERGIC BLOCKING AGENTS 182
CARVEDILOL - See BETA-ADRENERGIC BLOCKING AGENTS 182
CASANTHRANOL - See LAXATIVES, STIMULANT 482
CASANTHRANOL & DOCUSATE - See LAXATIVES, SOFTENER/LUBRICANT 480
CASCARA - See LAXATIVES, STIMULANT 482
Cascara Aromatic Fluidextract - See LAXATIVES, STIMULANT 482
Cascara Sagrada - See LAXATIVES, STIMULANT 482
Casodex - See ANTIANDROGENS, NONSTEROIDAL 58
CASTOR OIL - See LAXATIVES, STIMULANT 482
Cataflam - See ANTI-INFLAMMATORY DRUGS, NONSTEROIDAL (NSAIDs) 116
Catapres - See CENTRAL ALPHA AGONISTS 234
Catapres-TTS - See CENTRAL ALPHA AGONISTS 234

Caverject - See ALPROSTADIL 22
CCNU - See LOMUSTINE 506
Ceclor - See CEPHALOSPORINS 236
Ceclor CD - See CEPHALOSPORINS 236
Cecon - See VITAMIN C (Ascorbic Acid) 838
Cedax - See CEPHALOSPORINS 236
Cedocard-SR - See NITRATES 602
CeeNU - See LOMUSTINE 506
CEFACLOR - See CEPHALOSPORINS 236
CEFADROXIL - See CEPHALOSPORINS 236
Cefanex - See CEPHALOSPORINS 236
CEFDINIR - See CEPHALOSPORINS 236
CEFDITOREN - See CEPHALOSPORINS 236
CEFIXIME - See CEPHALOSPORINS 236
Cefotan - See CEPHALOSPORINS 236
CEFOTETAN - See CEPHALOSPORINS 236
CEFPODOXIME - See CEPHALOSPORINS 236
CEFPROZIL - See CEPHALOSPORINS 236
CEFTIBUTEN - See CEPHALOSPORINS 236
Ceftin - See CEPHALOSPORINS 236
CEFUROXIME - See CEPHALOSPORINS 236
Cefzil - See CEPHALOSPORINS 236
Celebrex - See ANTI-INFLAMMATORY DRUGS, NONSTEROIDAL (NSAIDs) COX-2 INHIBITORS 118
CELECOXIB - See ANTI-INFLAMMATORY DRUGS, NONSTEROIDAL (NSAIDs) COX-2 INHIBITORS 118
Celestoderm-V - See ADRENOCORTICOIDS (Topical) 18
Celestoderm-V/2 - See ADRENOCORTICOIDS (Topical) 18
Celestone - See ADRENOCORTICOIDS (Systemic) 16
Celexa - See SELECTIVE SEROTONIN REUPTAKE INHIBITORS (SSRIs) 742
Celontin - See ANTICONVULSANTS, SUCCINIMIDE 78
Cemill - See VITAMIN C (Ascorbic Acid) 838
Cenafed - See PSEUDOEPHEDRINE 694
Cenafed Plus - See
ANTIHISTAMINES 106
PSEUDOEPHEDRINE 694
Cena-K - See POTASSIUM SUPPLEMENTS 666
Cenestin - See ESTROGENS 372
Cenolate - See VITAMIN C (Ascorbic Acid) 838
<u>CENTRAL ALPHA AGONISTS</u> 234
Central nervous system stimulant - See
AMPHETAMINES 28
LORCASERIN 510
STIMULANT MEDICATIONS 754
STIMULANTS, AMPHETAMINE-RELATED 756
Centrax - See BENZODIAZEPINES 176
CEPHALEXIN - See CEPHALOSPORINS 236
<u>CEPHALOSPORINS</u> 236
CEPHRADINE - See CEPHALOSPORINS 236
Ceporex - See CEPHALOSPORINS 236
Cerespan - See PAPAVERINE 638
Cerose-DM - See
ANTIHISTAMINES106
DEXTROMETHORPHAN 312
PHENYLEPHRINE 658
CERTOLIZUMAB - See TUMOR NECROSIS FACTOR BLOCKERS 822
C.E.S. - See ESTROGENS 372
Cesamet - See NABILONE 578
Cetacort - See ADRENOCORTICOIDS (Topical) 18
Cetamide - See ANTIBACTERIALS (Ophthalmic) 66
Cetane - See VITAMIN C (Ascorbic Acid) 838
CETIRIZINE - See ANTIHISTAMINES, NONSEDATING 110
Cetraxal - See ANTIBACTERIALS (Otic) 58
Cevalin - See VITAMIN C (Ascorbic Acid) 838
Cevi-Bid - See VITAMIN C (Ascorbic Acid) 838
Ce-Vi-Sol - See VITAMIN C (Ascorbic Acid) 838
Cevita - See VITAMIN C (Ascorbic Acid) 838
Chantix - See VARENICLINE 830
Charac-50 - See CHARCOAL, ACTIVATED 238
Charac-tol 50 - See CHARCOAL, ACTIVATED 238
Charcoaid - See CHARCOAL, ACTIVATED 238
<u>CHARCOAL, ACTIVATED</u> 238
Charcocaps - See CHARCOAL, ACTIVATED 238
Charcodote - See CHARCOAL, ACTIVATED 238
Charcodote TFS - See CHARCOAL, ACTIVATED 238
Chardonna-2 - See BELLADONNA ALKALOIDS & BARBITURATES 174
Chelating agent - See PENICILLAMINE 644
Cheracol D Cough - See
DEXTROMETHORPHAN 312
GUAIFENESIN 416
Cherapas - See RESERPINE, HYDRALAZINE & HYDROCHLOROTHIAZIDE 718
Chew-E - See VITAMIN E 844
Chibroxin - See ANTIBACTERIALS (Ophthalmic) 66
Children's Advil - See ANTI-INFLAMMATORY DRUGS, NONSTEROIDAL (NSAIDs) 116
Children's Allegra - See ANTIHISTAMINES, NONSEDATING 110
Children's Benadryl Allergy & Cold Fastmelt - See
ANTIHISTAMINES 106
PSEUDOEPHEDRINE 694
Children's Benadryl Allergy Fastmelt - See ANTIHISTAMINES 106

Children's Benadryl Allergy Liquid - See ANTIHISTAMINES 106
Children's Benadryl Allergy Quick Dissolve Strips - See ANTIHISTAMINES 106
Children's Benadryl-D Allergy & Sinus Liquid - See
ANTIHISTAMINES 106
PSEUDOEPHEDRINE 694
Children's Benadryl Perfect Measure - See ANTIHISTAMINES 106
Children's Claritin Grape Chewable - See ANTIHISTAMINES, NONSEDATING 110
Children's Claritin Syrup Grape - See ANTIHISTAMINES, NONSEDATING 110
Children's Cloraseptic Lozenges - See ANESTHETICS (Mucosal-Local) 36
Children's Dramamine - See ANTIHISTAMINES 106
Children's Hold - See DEXTROMETHORPHAN 312
Children's Motrin - See ANTI-INFLAMMATORY DRUGS, NONSTEROIDAL (NSAIDs) 116
Children's Motrin Cold - See
ANTI-INFLAMMATORY DRUGS, NONSTEROIDAL (NSAIDs) 116
PSEUDOEPHEDRINE 694
Children's Mucinex Cough - See GUAIFENESIN 416
Children's Panadol - See ACETAMINOPHEN 8
Children's Pepto - See CALCIUM SUPPLEMENTS 222
Children's Rapimed - See ACETAMINOPHEN 8
Children's Sucrets - See ANESTHETICS (Mucosal-Local) 36
Children's Sudafed Nasal Decongestant Chewables - See PSEUDOEPHEDRINE 694
Children's Sudafed Nasal Decongestant Liquid - See PSEUDOEPHEDRINE 694
Children's Triaminic Thin Strips Night Time Cold & Cough - See
ANTIHISTAMINES 106
PHENYLEPHRINE 658
Children's Tylenol - See ACETAMINOPHEN 8
Children's Tylenol Plus Cold - See
ACETAMINOPHEN 8
ANTIHISTAMINES 106
PHENYLEPHRINE 658
Children's Tylenol Plus Cold & Allergy - See
ACETAMINOPHEN 8
ANTIHISTAMINES 106
PHENYLEPHRINE 658
Children's Tylenol Plus Cold & Cough - See
ACETAMINOPHEN 8
ANTIHISTAMINES 106
DEXTROMETHORPHAN 312
PSEUDOEPHEDRINE 694
Children's Tylenol Plus Cold Fruit Flavor - See
ACETAMINOPHEN 8
PSEUDOEPHEDRINE 694
Children's Tylenol Plus Cold Grape - See
ACETAMINOPHEN 8
ANTIHISTAMINES 106
PHENYLEPHRINE 658
Children's Tylenol Plus Cold Nighttime - See
ACETAMINOPHEN 8
ANTIHISTAMINES 106
PSEUDOEPHEDRINE 694
Children's Tylenol Plus Cough & Runny Nose - See
ACETAMINOPHEN 8
ANTIHISTAMINES 106
DEXTROMETHORPHAN 312
Children's Tylenol Plus Cough & Sore Throat - See
ACETAMINOPHEN 8
DEXTROMETHORPHAN 312
Children's Tylenol Plus Flu - See
ACETAMINOPHEN 8
ANTIHISTAMINES 106
DEXTROMETHORPHAN 312
PHENYLEPHRINE 658
Children's Tylenol Plus Multi-Symptom Cold - See
ACETAMINOPHEN 8
ANTIHISTAMINES 106
DEXTROMETHORPHAN 312
PHENYLEPHRINE 658
Children's Zyrtec Allergy Bubble Gum Syrup - See ANTIHISTAMINES, NONSEDATING 110
Children's Zyrtec Perfext Measure - See ANTIHISTAMINES, NONSEDATING 110
Chlo-Amine - See ANTIHISTAMINES 106
Chlor-100 - See ANTIHISTAMINES 106
Chloracol Ophthalmic Solution (Ophthalmic) - See ANTIBACTERIALS (Ophthalmic) 66
CHLORAMBUCIL 240
CHLORAMPHENICOL 242
CHLORAMPHENICOL (Ophthalmic) - See ANTIBACTERIALS (Ophthalmic) 66
CHLORAMPHENICOL (Topical) - See ANTIBACTERIALS (Topical) 70
Chloraseptic Lozenges Cherry Flavor - See ANESTHETICS (Mucosal-Local) 36
Chlorate - See ANTIHISTAMINES 106
CHLORDIAZEPOXIDE - See BENZODIAZEPINES 176

Chlorgest-HD - See
ANTIHISTAMINES 106
NARCOTIC ANALGESICS 584
PHENYLEPHRINE 658
CHLORHEXIDINE 244
Chlor-Niramine - See ANTIHISTAMINES 106
Chlorohist-LA - See XYLOMETAZOLINE 850
Chloromycetin - See
ANTIBACTERIALS (Topical) 70
CHLORAMPHENICOL 242
Chloromycetin Ophthalmic Ointment - See ANTIBACTERIALS (Ophthalmic) 66
Chloromycetin Ophthalmic Solution - See ANTIBACTERIALS (Ophthalmic) 66
Chloroptic Ophthalmic Solution - See ANTIBACTERIALS (Ophthalmic) 66
Chloroptic S.O.P. - See ANTIBACTERIALS (Ophthalmic) 66
CHLOROQUINE 246
CHLOROTHIAZIDE - See DIURETICS, THIAZIDE 338
CHLOROXINE - See ANTISEBORRHEICS (Topical) 132
Chlorphed - See ANTIHISTAMINES 106
Chlorphedrine SR - See
ANTIHISTAMINES 106
PSEUDOEPHEDRINE 694
CHLORPHENESIN - See MUSCLE RELAXANTS, SKELETAL 576
CHLORPHENIRAMINE - See ANTIHISTAMINES 106
Chlor-Pro - See ANTIHISTAMINES 106
Chlor-Pro 10 - See ANTIHISTAMINES 106
Chlorpromanyl-5 - See PHENOTHIAZINES 656
Chlorpromanyl-20 - See PHENOTHIAZINES 656
Chlorpromanyl-40 - See PHENOTHIAZINES 656
CHLORPROMAZINE - See PHENOTHIAZINES 656
CHLORPROPAMIDE - See SULFONYLUREAS 770
Chlorspan-12 - See ANTIHISTAMINES 106
Chlortab-4 - See ANTIHISTAMINES 106
Chlortab-8 - See ANTIHISTAMINES 106
CHLORTETRACYCLINE (Topical) - See ANTIBACTERIALS FOR ACNE (Topical) 64
CHLORTHALIDONE - See DIURETICS, THIAZIDE 338
Chlor-Trimeton 4 Hour Relief - See
ANTIHISTAMINES 106
PSEUDOEPHEDRINE 694
Chlor-Trimeton 12 Hour Relief - See
ANTIHISTAMINES 106
PSEUDOEPHEDRINE 694
Chlor-Tripolon - See ANTIHISTAMINES 106
CHLORZOXAZONE - See MUSCLE RELAXANTS, SKELETAL 576
Cholac - See LAXATIVES, OSMOTIC 478
Cholan-HMB - See LAXATIVES, STIMULANT 482
CHOLECALCIFEROL - See VITAMIN D 840
Choledyl - See BRONCHODILATORS, XANTHINE 204
Choledyl Delayed-Release - See BRONCHODILATORS, XANTHINE 204
Choledyl SA - See BRONCHODILATORS, XANTHINE 204
CHOLESTYRAMINE 248
CHOLINE MAGNESIUM SALICYLATES - See SALICYLATES 736
Choline Magnesium Trisalicylate - See SALICYLATES 736
Cholinergic - See
ANTIMYASTHENICS 128
BETHANECHOL 186
PILOCARPINE (Oral) 662
CHOLINE SALICYLATE - See SALICYLATES 736
Cholinesterase inhibitor - See CHOLINESTERASE INHIBITORS 250
CHOLINESTERASE INHIBITORS 250
Cholybar - See CHOLESTYRAMINE 248
Chooz - See
ANTACIDS 48
CALCIUM SUPPLEMENTS 222
Chronovera - See CALCIUM CHANNEL BLOCKERS 220
Chronula - See LAXATIVES, OSMOTIC 478
Cialis - See ERECTILE DYSFUNCTION AGENTS 360
Cibalith-S - See LITHIUM 504
CICLESONIDE (Nasal) - See ADRENOCORTICOIDS (Nasal Inhalation) 12
CICLESONIDE (Oral Inhalation) - See ADRENOCORTICOIDS (Oral Inhalation) 14
CICLOPIROX - See ANTIFUNGALS (Topical) 88
Cillium - See LAXATIVES, BULK-FORMING 476
CILOSTAZOL - See INTERMITTENT CLAUDICATION AGENTS 452
Ciloxan - See ANTIBACTERIALS (Ophthalmic) 66
CIMETIDINE - See HISTAMINE H_2 RECEPTOR ANTAGONISTS 422
Cimzia - See TUMOR NECROSIS FACTOR BLOCKERS 822
Cinchocaine - See ANESTHETICS (Topical) 40
Cinobac - See CINOXACIN 252
CINOXACIN 252
Cin-Quin - See QUINIDINE 704
Cipro - See FLUOROQUINOLONES 392
Cipro HC - See ANTIBACTERIALS (Otic) 68
Cipro XR - See FLUOROQUINOLONES 392

INDEX

Ciprodex - See ANTIBACTERIALS (Otic) 68
CIPROFLOXACIN - See
FLUOROQUINOLONES 392
CIPROFLOXACIN (Ophthalmic) - See
ANTIBACTERIALS (Ophthalmic) 66
CIPROFLOXACIN (Otic) - See
ANTIBACTERIALS (Otic) 68
CIPROFLOXACIN & DEXAMETHASONE - See
ANTIBACTERIALS (Otic) 68
CIPROFLOXACIN & HYDROCORTISONE
(Otic) - See ANTIBACTERIALS (Otic) 68
CIP-Tramadol ER - See TRAMADOL 808
CITALOPRAM - See SELECTIVE SEROTONIN
REUPTAKE INHIBITORS (SSRIs) 742
Citracal - See CALCIUM SUPPLEMENTS 222
Citracal Liquitabs - See CALCIUM
SUPPLEMENTS 222
Citrated Caffeine - See CAFFEINE 216
Citra-Forte - See CITRATES 254
CITRATES 254
Citrocarbonate - See SODIUM BICARBONATE
750
Citrocovorin Calcium - See LEUCOVORIN 486
Citrolith - See CITRATES 254
Citroma - See LAXATIVES, OSMOTIC 478
Citro-Mag - See LAXATIVES, OSMOTIC 478
Citro-Nesia - See LAXATIVES, OSMOTIC 478
Citrovorum Factor - See LEUCOVORIN 486
Citrucel Orange Flavor - See LAXATIVES,
BULK-FORMING 476
Citrucel Sugar-Free Orange Flavor - See
LAXATIVES, BULK-FORMING 476
Claravis - See ISOTRETINOIN 462
Clarinex - See ANTIHISTAMINES,
NONSEDATING 110
Clarinex-D 12 Hour - See
ANTIHISTAMINES, NONSEDATING 110
PSEUDOEPHEDRINE 694
Clarinex-D 24 Hour - See
ANTIHISTAMINES, NONSEDATING 110
PSEUDOEPHEDRINE 694
Clarinex RediTabs - See ANTIHISTAMINES,
NONSEDATING 110
Clarinex Syrup - See ANTIHISTAMINES,
NONSEDATING 110
Claripex - See FIBRATES 386
CLARITHROMYCIN - See MACROLIDE
ANTIBIOTICS 518
Claritin - See ANTIHISTAMINES,
NONSEDATING 110
Claritin 12 Hour RediTabs - See
ANTIHISTAMINES, NONSEDATING 110
Claritin-D - See
ANTIHISTAMINES, NONSEDATING 110
PSEUDOEPHEDRINE 694
Claritin-D 12 Hour - See
ANTIHISTAMINES, NONSEDATING 110
PSEUDOEPHEDRINE 694
Claritin-D 12 Hour RediTabs for Kids - See
ANTIHISTAMINES, NONSEDATING 110
Claritin-D 24 Hour - See
ANTIHISTAMINES, NONSEDATING 110
PSEUDOEPHEDRINE 694
Claritin Extra - See ANTIHISTAMINES,
NONSEDATING 110
Claritin Eye - See ANTIALLERGIC AGENTS
(Ophthalmic) 56
Claritin Hives Relief - See ANTIHISTAMINES,
NONSEDATING 110
Claritin Liqui-Gels - See ANTIHISTAMINES,
NONSEDATING 110
Claritin RediTabs - See ANTIHISTAMINES,
NONSEDATING 110
Claritin RediTabs for Kids 24 Hour - See
ANTIHISTAMINES, NONSEDATING 110
Claritin Syrup - See ANTIHISTAMINES,
NONSEDATING 110
Clavulin - See PENICILLINS &
BETALACTAMASE INHIBITORS 648
Cleanse and Treat - See
BENZOYL PEROXIDE 178
KERATOLYTICS 470
Clear Away - See KERATOLYTICS 470
Clear by Design 2.5 Gel - See BENZOYL
PEROXIDE 178
Clear by Design Medicated Cleansing Pads
- See KERATOLYTICS 470
Clear Eyes - See DECONGESTANTS
(Ophthalmic) 306
*Clearasil Adult Care Medicated Blemish
Cream* - See KERATOLYTICS 470
Clearasil Adult Care Medicated Blemish Stick
- See KERATOLYTICS 470
Clearasil BP Plus 5 Cream - See BENZOYL
PEROXIDE 178
Clearasil BP Plus 5 Lotion - See BENZOYL
PEROXIDE 178
*Clearasil Clearstick Maximum Strength
Topical Solution* - See KERATOLYTICS 470
*Clearasil Clearstick Regular Strength Topical
Solution* - See KERATOLYTICS 470
*Clearasil Double Textured Pads Maximum
Strength* - See KERATOLYTICS 470
*Clearasil Double Textured Pads Regular
Strength* - See KERATOLYTICS 470
*Clearasil Maximum Strength Medicated Anti-
Acne 10 Tinted Cream* - See BENZOYL
PEROXIDE 178

Clearasil Maximum Strength Medicated Anti-Acne 10 Vanishing Cream - See BENZOYL PEROXIDE 178
Clearasil Medicated Anti-Acne 10 Vanishing Lotion - See BENZOYL PEROXIDE 178
Clearasil Medicated Deep Cleanser Topical Solution - See KERATOLYTICS 470
CLEMASTINE FUMARATE - See ANTIHISTAMINES 106
Cleocin - See CLINDAMYCIN 258
Cleocin Pediatric - See CLINDAMYCIN 258
Cleocin T Gel - See ANTIBACTERIALS FOR ACNE (Topical) 64
Cleocin T Lotion - See ANTIBACTERIALS FOR ACNE (Topical) 64
Cleocin T Topical Solution - See ANTIBACTERIALS FOR ACNE (Topical) 64
Cleocin (Vaginal) - See CLINDAMYCIN 258
C-Lexin - See CEPHALOSPORINS 236
CLIDINIUM 256
Climara - See ESTROGENS 372
Climara Pro - See
ESTROGENS 372
PROGESTINS 680
Clinac BPO - See BENZOYL PEROXIDE 178
Clinagen LA 40 - See ESTROGENS 372
Clinda-Derm - See ANTIBACTERIALS FOR ACNE (Topical) 64
CLINDAMYCIN 258
CLINDAMYCIN (Topical) - See ANTIBACTERIALS FOR ACNE (Topical) 64
ClindaReach - See ANTIBACTERIALS FOR ACNE (Topical) 64
Clindesse Vaginal Cream - See CLINDAMYCIN 258
Clindex - See
BENZODIAZEPINES 176
CLIDINIUM 256
Clinoril - See ANTI-INFLAMMATORY DRUGS, NONSTEROIDAL (NSAIDs) 116
Clinoxide - See
BENZODIAZEPINES 176
CLIDINIUM 256
CLIOQUINOL & HYDROCORTISONE - See ANTIBACTERIALS, ANTIFUNGALS (Topical) 62
CLOBAZAM - See BENZODIAZEPINES 176
CLOBETASOL (Topical) - See ADRENOCORTICOIDS (Topical) 18
CLOBETASONE (Topical) - See ADRENOCORTICOIDS (Topical) 18
Clobex - See ADRENOCORTICOIDS (Topical) 18
CLOCORTOLONE (Topical) - See ADRENOCORTICOIDS (Topical) 18
Cloderm - See ADRENOCORTICOIDS (Topical) 18
Cloderm Pump - See ADRENOCORTICOIDS (Topical) 18
CLOFIBRATE - See FIBRATES 386
Clomid - See CLOMIPHENE 260
CLOMIPHENE 260
CLOMIPRAMINE - See ANTIDEPRESSANTS, TRICYCLIC 80
CLONAZEPAM - See BENZODIAZEPINES 176
CLONIDINE - See CENTRAL ALPHA AGONISTS 234
CLOPIDOGREL- See PLATELET INHIBITORS 664
Clopra - See METOCLOPRAMIDE 550
CLORAZEPATE - See BENZODIAZEPINES 176
CLOTRIMAZOLE - See ANTIFUNGALS (Topical) 88
CLOTRIMAZOLE (Vaginal) - See ANTIFUNGALS (Vaginal) 90
CLOTRIMAZOLE (Oral-Local) 262
CLOXACILLIN - See PENICILLINS 646
Cloxapen - See PENICILLINS 646
CLOZAPINE 264
Clozaril - See CLOZAPINE 264
Clysodrast - See LAXATIVES, STIMULANT 482
CoActifed Expectorant - See
ANTIHISTAMINES 106
GUAIFENESIN 416
NARCOTIC ANALGESICS 584
PSEUDOEPHEDRINE 694
COAL TAR (Topical) 266
Cobantril - See ANTHELMINTICS 50
Co-Betaloc - See BETA-ADRENERGIC BLOCKING AGENTS & THIAZIDE DIURETICS 184
Codan - See
ANTICHOLINERGICS 72
NARCOTIC ANALGESICS 584
Codehist DH - See
ANTIHISTAMINES 106
NARCOTIC ANALGESICS 584
PSEUDOEPHEDRINE 694
CODEINE - See NARCOTIC ANALGESICS 584
CODEINE & TERPIN HYDRATE - See NARCOTIC ANALGESICS 584
Codeine Sulfate - See NARCOTIC ANALGESICS 584
Codeprex - See
ANTIHISTAMINES 106
NARCOTIC ANALGESIC 584
Codiclear DH - See
GUAIFENESIN 416
NARCOTIC ANALGESICS 584

Codimal DH - See
ANTIHISTAMINES 106
NARCOTIC ANALGESICS 584
PHENYLEPHRINE 658
Codimal DM - See
ANTIHISTAMINES 106
DEXTROMETHORPHAN 312
PHENYLEPHRINE 658
Codimal PH - See
ANTIHISTAMINES 106
NARCOTIC ANALGESICS 584
PHENYLEPHRINE 658
Codimal-A - See ANTIHISTAMINES 106
Codimal-L.A. - See
ANTIHISTAMINES 106
PSEUDOEPHEDRINE 694
Codimal-L.A. Half - See
ANTIHISTAMINES 106
PSEUDOEPHEDRINE 694
Codistan No. 1 - See
DEXTROMETHORPHAN 312
GUAIFENESIN 416
Codroxomin - See VITAMIN B-12 (Cyanocobalamin) 836
Cogentin - See ANTIDYSKINETICS 82
Co-Gesic - See NARCOTIC ANALGESICS & ACETAMINOPHEN 586
Colace - See LAXATIVES, SOFTENER/ LUBRICANT 480
Colace Microenema - See LAXATIVES, SOFTENER/LUBRICANT 480
Colax - See
LAXATIVES, SOFTENER/LUBRICANT 480
LAXATIVES, STIMULANT 482
Colazal - See SALICYLATES 736
COLCHICINE 268
Colcrys - See COLCHICINE 268
Coldrine - See
ACETAMINOPHEN 8
PSEUDOEPHEDRINE 694
COLESEVELAM 270
Colestid - See COLESTIPOL 272
COLESTIPOL 272
Colfed-A - See
ANTIHISTAMINES 106
PSEUDOEPHEDRINE 694
Cologel - See LAXATIVES, BULK-FORMING 476
Col-Probenecid - See
COLCHICINE 268
PROBENECID 676
Colrex Compound - See
ACETAMINOPHEN 8
ANTIHISTAMINES 106
NARCOTIC ANALGESICS 584
PHENYLEPHRINE 658
Colrex Cough - See
ANTIHISTAMINES 106
DEXTROMETHORPHAN 312
PHENYLEPHRINE 658
Colrex Expectorant - See GUAIFENESIN 416
Coltab Children's - See
ANTIHISTAMINES 106
PHENYLEPHRINE 658
Coly-Mycin S - See ANTIBACTERIALS (Otic) 68
Combigan - See
ANTIGLAUCOMA, ADRENERGIC AGONISTS 92
ANTIGLAUCOMA, BETA BLOCKERS 96
Combipatch - See
ESTROGENS 372
PROGESTINS 680
Combivent Respimat - See
BRONCHODILATORS, ADRENERGIC 200
IPRATROPIUM 456
Combivir - See NUCLEOSIDE REVERSE TRANSCRIPTASE INHIBITORS 610
Combunox - See
ANTI-INFLAMMATORY DRUGS, NONSTEROIDAL (NSAIDs) 116
NARCOTIC ANALGESICS 584
Comfort Eye Drops - See DECONGESTANTS (Ophthalmic) 306
Comhist - See
ANTIHISTAMINES 106
PHENYLEPHRINE 658
Comhist LA - See
ANTIHISTAMINES 106
PHENYLEPHRINE 658
Commit - See NICOTINE 598
Compal - See NARCOTIC ANALGESICS & ACETAMINOPHEN 586
Compazine - See PHENOTHIAZINES 656
Compazine Spansule - See PHENOTHIAZINES 656
Complera - See
NON-NUCLEOSIDE REVERSE TRANSCRIPTASE INHIBITORS 608
NUCLEOSIDE REVERSE TRANSCRIPTASE INHIBITORS 610
NUCLEOTIDE REVERSE TRANSCRIPTASE INHIBITORS 612
Compound W Gel - See KERATOLYTICS 470
Compound W Liquid - See KERATOLYTICS 470
Compoz - See ANTIHISTAMINES 106
COMT INHIBITORS 274
Comtan - See COMT INHIBITORS 274
Comtrex Acute Head Cold Nighttime - See
ACETAMINOPHEN 8
ANTIHISTAMINES 106
PSEUDOEPHEDRINE 694

Comtrex Cold & Cough Day/Night - See
ACETAMINOPHEN 8
ANTIHISTAMINES 106
DEXTROMETHORPHAN 312
PSEUDOEPHEDRINE 694
Comtrex Deep Chest Cold - See
ACETAMINOPHEN 8
GUAIFENESIN 416
Comtrex Flu Therapy - See
ACETAMINOPHEN 8
ANTIHISTAMINES 106
PSEUDOEPHEDRINE 694
Conacetol - See ACETAMINOPHEN 8
Conar - See
DEXTROMETHORPHAN 312
PHENYLEPHRINE 658
Conar Expectorant - See
DEXTROMETHORPHAN 312
GUAIFENESIN 416
PHENYLEPHRINE 658
Conar-A - See
ACETAMINOPHEN 8
DEXTROMETHORPHAN 312
GUAIFENESIN 416
PHENYLEPHRINE 658
Conazol - See ANTIFUNGALS (Topical) 88
Concentrin - See
DEXTROMETHORPHAN 312
GUAIFENESIN 416
PSEUDOEPHEDRINE 694
Conceptrol Gel - See CONTRACEPTIVES, VAGINAL 280
Conceptrol-Contraceptive Inserts - See CONTRACEPTIVES, VAGINAL 280
Concerta - See STIMULANT MEDICATIONS 754
CONDYLOMA ACUMINATUM AGENTS 276
Condylox - See CONDYLOMA ACUMINATUM AGENTS 276
Congespirin - See
ACETAMINOPHEN 8
DEXTROMETHORPHAN 312
Congespirin for Children Cold Tablets - See
ACETAMINOPHEN 8
PHENYLEPHRINE 658
Congespirin for Children Liquid Cold Medicine - See ACETAMINOPHEN 8
Congess JR - See
GUAIFENESIN 416
PSEUDOEPHEDRINE 694
Congess SR - See
GUAIFENESIN 416
PSEUDOEPHEDRINE 694
Congest - See ESTROGENS 372
Congestac Caplets - See
GUAIFENESIN 416
PSEUDOEPHEDRINE 694
Congestant D - See
ACETAMINOPHEN 8
ANTIHISTAMINES 106
CONJUGATED ESTROGENS - See ESTROGENS 372
Constant-T - See BRONCHODILATORS, XANTHINE 204
Constilac - See LAXATIVES, OSMOTIC 478
Constulose - See LAXATIVES, OSMOTIC 478
Contac 12-Hour Allergy - See ANTIHISTAMINES 106
Contac Allergy/Sinus Day Caplets - See
ACETAMINOPHEN 8
PSEUDOEPHEDRINE 694
Contac Allergy/Sinus Night Caplets - See
ACETAMINOPHEN 8
ANTIHISTAMINES 106
PSEUDOEPHEDRINE 694
Contac Maximum Strength Sinus Caplets - See
ACETAMINOPHEN 8
PSEUDOEPHEDRINE 694
Contac Night Caplets - See
ACETAMINOPHEN 8
ANTIHISTAMINES 106
DEXTROMETHORPHAN 312
PSEUDOEPHEDRINE 694
Contac Non-Drowsy Formula Sinus Caplets - See
ACETAMINOPHEN 8
PSEUDOEPHEDRINE 694
Contac Severe Cold Formula - See
ACETAMINOPHEN 8
ANTIHISTAMINES 106
DEXTROMETHORPHAN 312
PSEUDOEPHEDRINE 694
Contac Severe Cold Formula Night Strength - See
ACETAMINOPHEN 8
ANTIHISTAMINES 106
DEXTROMETHORPHAN 312
PSEUDOEPHEDRINE 694
Contraceptive - See
CONTRACEPTIVES, ORAL & SKIN 278
CONTRACEPTIVES, VAGINAL 280
SELECTIVE PROGESTERONE RECEPTOR MODULATORS 740
CONTRACEPTIVES, ORAL & SKIN 278
CONTRACEPTIVES, VAGINAL 280
Coradur - See NITRATES 602
Coraz Lotion - See ADRENOCORTICOIDS (Topical) 18

Cordarone - See ANTIARRHYTHMICS, BENZOFURAN-TYPE 60
Cordran - See ADRENOCORTICOIDS (Topical) 18
Cordran SP - See ADRENOCORTICOIDS (Topical) 18
Coreg - See BETA-ADRENERGIC BLOCKING AGENTS 182
Coreg CR - See BETA-ADRENERGIC BLOCKING AGENTS 182
Corgard - See BETA-ADRENERGIC BLOCKING AGENTS 182
Coricidin HBP - See
ANTIHISTAMINES 106
DEXTROMETHORPHAN 312
Coricidin HBP Chest Congestion & Cough - See
DEXTROMETHORPHAN 312
GUAIFENESIN 416
Coricidin Nasal Mist - See OXYMETAZOLINE (Nasal) 630
Coristex-DH - See
NARCOTIC ANALGESICS 584
PHENYLEPHRINE 658
Coristine-DH - See
NARCOTIC ANALGESICS 584
PHENYLEPHRINE 658
Corium - See CLIDINIUM 256
Cormax - See ADRENOCORTICOIDS (Topical) 18
Coronex - See NITRATES 602
Corophyllin - See BRONCHODILATORS, XANTHINE 204
Correctol - See
LAXATIVES, SOFTENER/LUBRICANT 480
LAXATIVES, STIMULANT 482
Correctol Caplets - See
LAXATIVES, SOFTENER/LUBRICANT 480
LAXATIVES, STIMULANT 482
Correctol Extra Gentle - See LAXATIVES, SOFTENER/LUBRICANT 480
Cortacet - See ADRENOCORTICOIDS (Topical) 18
Cortaid - See ADRENOCORTICOIDS (Topical) 18
Cortaid FastStick - See ADRENOCORTICOIDS (Topical) 18
Cortamed - See ANTI-INFLAMMATORY DRUGS, STEROIDAL (Ophthalmic) 122
Cortarigen Modified Ear Drops - See ANTIBACTERIALS (Otic) 68
Cortate - See ADRENOCORTICOIDS (Topical) 18
Cort-Biotic - See ANTIBACTERIALS (Otic) 68
Cort-Dome - See ADRENOCORTICOIDS (Topical) 18
Cort-Dome High Potency - See
ADRENOCORTICOIDS (Topical) 18
HYDROCORTISONE (Rectal) 430
Cortef - See
ADRENOCORTICOIDS (Systemic) 16
ADRENOCORTICOIDS (Topical) 18
Cortef Feminine Itch - See ADRENOCORTICOIDS (Topical) 18
Cortenema - See ADRENOCORTICOIDS (Systemic) 16
Corticaine - See
ADRENOCORTICOIDS (Topical) 18
HYDROCORTISONE (Rectal) 430
Corticosteroid - See ADRENOCORTICOIDS (Systemic) 16
Corticreme - See ADRENOCORTICOIDS (Topical) 18
Cortifair - See ADRENOCORTICOIDS (Topical) 18
Cortifoam - See ADRENOCORTICOIDS (Systemic) 16
Cortiment-10 - See
ADRENOCORTICOIDS (Topical) 18
HYDROCORTISONE (Rectal) 430
Cortiment-40 - See
ADRENOCORTICOIDS (Topical) 18
HYDROCORTISONE (Rectal) 430
CORTISOL - See ADRENOCORTICOIDS (Topical) 18
CORTISONE - See ADRENOCORTICOIDS (Systemic) 16
Cortoderm - See ADRENOCORTICOIDS (Topical) 18
Cortone - See ADRENOCORTICOIDS (Systemic) 16
Cortone Acetate - See ADRENOCORTICOIDS (Systemic) 16
Cortril - See ADRENOCORTICOIDS (Topical) 18
Coryphen - See ASPIRIN 152
Corzide - See BETA-ADRENERGIC BLOCKING AGENTS & THIAZIDE DIURETICS 184
Cosopt - See
ANTIGLAUCOMA, BETA BLOCKERS 96
ANTIGLAUCOMA, CARBONIC ANHYDRASE INHIBITORS 98
Cosopt PF - See
ANTIGLAUCOMA, BETA BLOCKERS 96
ANTIGLAUCOMA, CARBONIC ANHYDRASE INHIBITORS 98
Cotanal-65 - See
NARCOTIC ANALGESICS 584
Cotridin - See
ANTIHISTAMINES 106
NARCOTIC ANALGESICS 584
PSEUDOEPHEDRINE 694

Cotrim - See
SULFONAMIDES 766
TRIMETHOPRIM 818
Cotrim DS - See
SULFONAMIDES 766
TRIMETHOPRIM 818
Co-trimoxazole - See
SULFONAMIDES 766
TRIMETHOPRIM 818
Cotybutazone - See ANTI-INFLAMMATORY DRUGS, NONSTEROIDAL (NSAIDs) 116
Cough/cold preparation - See
BARBITURATES 168
GUAIFENESIN 416
Cough suppressant - See DEXTROMETHORPHAN 312
Cough X - See DEXTROMETHORPHAN 312
Coumadin - See ANTICOAGULANTS (Oral) 74
Cozaar - See ANGIOTENSIN II RECEPTOR ANTAGONISTS 42
Cramp End - See ANTI-INFLAMMATORY DRUGS, NONSTEROIDAL (NSAIDs) 116
Creamy SS Shampoo - See KERATOLYTICS 470
Creon - See PANCRELIPASE 634
Creo-Terpin - See DEXTROMETHORPHAN 312
Crestor - See HMG-CoA REDUCTASE INHIBITORS 424
Crinone - See PROGESTINS 680
Crixivan - See PROTEASE INHIBITORS 688
Crolom - See CROMOLYN 282
CROMOLYN 282
Cruex Aerosol Powder - See ANTIFUNGALS (Topical) 88
Cruex Antifungal Cream - See ANTIFUNGALS (Topical) 88
Cruex Antifungal Powder - See ANTIFUNGALS (Topical) 88
Cruex Antifungal Spray Powder - See ANTIFUNGALS (Topical) 88
Cruex Cream - See ANTIFUNGALS (Topical) 88
Cruex Powder - See ANTIFUNGALS (Topical) 88
Crystodigin - See DIGITALIS PREPARATIONS (Digitalis Glycosides) 320
C-Span - See VITAMIN C (Ascorbic Acid) 838
Cultivate - See ADRENOCORTICOIDS (Topical) 18
Cuplex Gel - See KERATOLYTICS 470
Cuprimine - See PENICILLAMINE 644
Curretab - See PROGESTINS 680
Cutar Water Dispersible Emollient Tar - See COAL TAR (Topical) 266
Cuticura Acne 5 Cream - See BENZOYL PEROXIDE 178
Cuticura Ointment - See KERATOLYTICS 470
Cyanabin - See VITAMIN B-12 (Cyanocobalamin) 836
CYANOCOBALAMIN - See VITAMIN B-12 (Cyanocobalamin) 836
Cyantin - See NITROFURANTOIN 604
CYCLANDELATE 284
Cyclen - See CONTRACEPTIVES, ORAL & SKIN 278
Cyclessa - See CONTRACEPTIVES, ORAL & SKIN 278
CYCLIZINE - See ANTIHISTAMINES, PIPERAZINE (Antinausea) 114
CYCLOBENZAPRINE 286
Cyclocort - See ADRENOCORTICOIDS (Topical) 18
Cyclogyl - See CYCLOPENTOLATE (Ophthalmic) 288
Cyclomen - See DANAZOL 300
CYCLOPENTOLATE (Ophthalmic) 288
CYCLOPHOSPHAMIDE 290
CYCLOPLEGIC, MYDRIATIC (Ophthalmic) 292
CYCLOSERINE 294
Cycloset- See BROMOCRIPTINE 198
Cyclospasmol - See CYCLANDELATE 284
Cycloplegic - See
CYCLOPENTOLATE (Ophthalmic) 288
CYCLOPLEGIC, MYDRIATIC (Ophthalmic) 292
CYCLOSPORINE 296
CYCLOTHIAZIDE - See DIURETICS, THIAZIDE 338
Cycoflex - See CYCLOBENZAPRINE 286
Cycrin - See PROGESTINS 680
Cyklokapron - See ANTIFIBRINOLYTIC AGENTS 84
Cymbalta - See SEROTONIN & NOREPINEPHRINE REUPTAKE INHIBITORS (SNRIs) 746
CYPROHEPTADINE - See ANTIHISTAMINES 106
Cyraso-400 - See CYCLANDELATE 284
Cystospaz - See HYOSCYAMINE 438
Cystospaz-M - See HYOSCYAMINE 438
Cytadren - See AMINOGLUTETHIMIDE 24
Cytomel - See THYROID HORMONES 792
Cytotec - See MISOPROSTOL 568
Cytotoxic (Topical) - See CONDYLOMA ACUMINATUM AGENTS 276
Cytovene - See ANTIVIRALS FOR HERPES VIRUS 136

D

d4T - See NUCLEOSIDE REVERSE TRANSCRIPTASE INHIBITORS 610
D.A. Chewable - See
ANTICHOLINERGICS 72
ANTIHISTAMINES 106
PHENYLEPHRINE 658
DABIGATRAN 298
Dacodyl - See LAXATIVES, STIMULANT 482
Dalacin C - See CLINDAMYCIN 258
Dalacin C Palmitate - See CLINDAMYCIN 258
Dalacin C Phosphate - See CLINDAMYCIN 258
Dalacin T Topical Solution - See ANTIBACTERIALS FOR ACNE (Topical) 64
Daliresp - See ROFLUMILAST 734
Dallergy - See
ANTICHOLINERGICS 72
ANTIHISTAMINES 106
PHENYLEPHRINE 658
Dallergy Jr. - See
ANTIHISTAMINES 106
PSEUDOEPHEDRINE 694
Dalmane - See BENZODIAZEPINES 176
Damason-P - See NARCOTIC ANALGESICS & ASPIRIN 588
DANAZOL 300
Dan-Gard - See ANTISEBORRHEICS (Topical) 132
Danocrine - See DANAZOL 300
Dantrium - See DANTROLENE 302
DANTROLENE 302
Dapa - See ACETAMINOPHEN 8
Dapex-37.5 - See APPETITE SUPPRESSANTS 146
DAPSONE 304
Daranide - See CARBONIC ANHYDRASE INHIBITORS 232
Darbid - See ANTICHOLINERGICS 72
Daricon - See ANTICHOLINERGICS 72
DARIFENACIN - See - See MUSCARINIC RECEPTOR ANTAGONISTS 574
Dartal - See PHENOTHIAZINES 656
DARUNAVIR - See PROTEASE INHIBITORS 688
Datril Extra Strength - See ACETAMINOPHEN 8
Dayhist Allergy - See
ANTIHISTAMINES 106
Daypro - See ANTI-INFLAMMATORY DRUGS, NONSTEROIDAL (NSAIDs) 116
DayTime Liquid - See
ACETAMINOPHEN 8
DEXTROMETHORPHAN 312
PSEUDOEPHEDRINE 694
Daytrana - See STIMULANT MEDICATIONS 754
Dazamide - See CARBONIC ANHYDRASE INHIBITORS 232
DDAVP - See DESMOPRESSIN 310
DDS - See DAPSONE 304
Decadron - See ADRENOCORTICOIDS (Systemic) 16
Decaderm - See ADRENOCORTICOIDS (Topical) 18
Decadron - See ANTI-INFLAMMATORY DRUGS, STEROIDAL (Ophthalmic) 122
Decadron - See ANTI-INFLAMMATORY DRUGS, STEROIDAL (Otic) 124
Decadron Respihaler - See ADRENOCORTICOIDS (Oral Inhalation) 14
Deca-Durabolin - See ANDROGENS 34
Decaspray - See ADRENOCORTICOIDS (Topical) 18
Decholin - See LAXATIVES, STIMULANT 482
Declomycin - See TETRACYCLINES 782
Decohistine DH - See
ANTIHISTAMINES 106
NARCOTIC ANALGESICS 584
PSEUDOEPHEDRINE 694
Deconamine - See
ANTIHISTAMINES 106
PSEUDOEPHEDRINE 694
Deconamine SR - See
ANTIHISTAMINES 106
PSEUDOEPHEDRINE 694
Decongestant - See
PHENYLEPHRINE 658
PSEUDOEPHEDRINE 694
Decongestant (Ophthalmic) - See
DECONGESTANTS (Ophthalmic) 306
PHENYLEPHRINE (Ophthalmic) 660
DECONGESTANTS (Ophthalmic) 306
Deconsal CT Tannate Chewable Tablets - See
ANTIHISTAMINES 106
PHENYLEPHRINE 658
Deconsal DM Tannate Chewable Tablets - See
ANTIHISTAMINES 106
DEXTROMETHORPHAN 312
PHENYLEPHRINE 658
Deconsal II - See
GUAIFENESIN 416
PSEUDOEPHEDRINE 694
Decylenes - See ANTIFUNGALS (Topical) 88
Decylenes Powder - See ANTIFUNGALS (Topical) 88
Deficol - See LAXATIVES, STIMULANT 482
Degas - See SIMETHICONE 748
Degest 2 - See DECONGESTANTS (Ophthalmic) 306

DEHYDROCHOLIC ACID - See LAXATIVES, STIMULANT 482
DEHYDROEPIANDROSTERONE (DHEA) 308
Delacort - See ADRENOCORTICOIDS (Topical) 18
Deladiol-40 - See ESTROGENS 372
Del-Aqua-5 Gel - See BENZOYL PEROXIDE 178
Del-Aqua-10 Gel - See BENZOYL PEROXIDE 178
Delatest - See ANDROGENS 34
Delatestryl - See ANDROGENS 34
DELAVIRDINE - See NON-NUCLEOSIDE REVERSE TRANSCRIPTASE INHIBITORS 608
Delaxin - See MUSCLE RELAXANTS, SKELETAL 576
Delestrogen - See ESTROGENS 372
Delfen - See CONTRACEPTIVES, VAGINAL 280
Del-Ray - See BENZOYL PEROXIDE 178
Delsym - See DEXTROMETHORPHAN 312
Delsym Grape for Adults - See DEXTROMETHORPHAN 312
Delsym Grape for Children - See DEXTROMETHORPHAN 312
Delta-Cortef - See ADRENOCORTICOIDS (Systemic) 16
Deltasone - See ADRENOCORTICOIDS (Systemic) 16
Delta-Tritex - See ADRENOCORTICOIDS (Topical) 18
Delzicol - See MESALAMINE 542
DEMECARIUM - See ANTIGLAUCOMA, ANTICHOLINESTERASES 94
Demadex - See DIURETICS, LOOP 332
Demarest DriCort - See ADRENOCORTICOIDS (Topical) 18
DEMECLOCYCLINE - See TETRACYCLINES 782
Demerol - See NARCOTIC ANALGESICS 584
Demerol-APAP - See NARCOTIC ANALGESICS & ACETAMINOPHEN 586
Demi-Regroton - See
DIURETICS, THIAZIDE 338
RAUWOLFIA ALKALOIDS 714
Demulen 1/35 - See CONTRACEPTIVES, ORAL & SKIN 278
Demulen 1/50 - See CONTRACEPTIVES, ORAL & SKIN 278
Demulen 30 - See CONTRACEPTIVES, ORAL & SKIN 278
Demulen 50 - See CONTRACEPTIVES, ORAL & SKIN 278
Denavir - See ANTIVIRALS (Topical) 144
Denorex - See COAL TAR (Topical) 266
Denorex Extra Strength Medicated Shampoo - See COAL TAR (Topical) 266
Denorex Extra Strength Medicated Shampoo with Conditioners - See COAL TAR (Topical) 266
Denorex Medicated Shampoo - See COAL TAR (Topical) 266
Denorex Medicated Shampoo and Conditioner - See COAL TAR (Topical) 266
Denorex Mountain Fresh Herbal Scent Medicated Shampoo - See COAL TAR (Topical) 266
Dentapaine - See ANESTHETICS (Mucosal-Local) 36
Dentocaine - See ANESTHETICS (Mucosal-Local) 36
Dent-Zel-Ite - See ANESTHETICS (Mucosal-Local) 36
Dep Andro 100 - See ANDROGENS 34
Dep Andro 200 - See ANDROGENS 34
Depakene - See VALPROIC ACID 826
Depakote - See DIVALPROEX 340
Depakote ER - See DIVALPROEX 340
Depakote Sprinkle - See DIVALPROEX 340
Depen - See PENICILLAMINE 644
depGynogen - See ESTROGENS 372
Depo Estradiol - See ESTROGENS 372
Depogen - See ESTROGENS 372
Deponit - See NITRATES 602
Depo-Provera - See PROGESTINS 680
Depotest - See ANDROGENS 34
Depo-Testosterone - See ANDROGENS 34
Derbac - See PEDICULICIDES (Topical) 642
Dermabet - See ADRENOCORTICOIDS (Topical) 18
Dermacomb - See
ADRENOCORTICOIDS (Topical) 18
NYSTATIN 614
Dermacort - See ADRENOCORTICOIDS (Topical) 18
Dermal - See MINOXIDIL (Topical) 562
Dermalleve - See ADRENOCORTICOIDS (Topical) 18
DermAtop - See ADRENOCORTICOIDS (Topical) 18
DermiCort - See ADRENOCORTICOIDS (Topical) 18
Dermolate - See HYDROCORTISONE (Rectal) 430
Dermoplast - See ANESTHETICS (Topical) 40
Dermovate - See ADRENOCORTICOIDS (Topical) 18
Dermovate Scalp Application - See ADRENOCORTICOIDS (Topical) 18

Dermoxyl 2.5 Gel - See BENZOYL PEROXIDE 178
Dermoxyl 5 Gel - See BENZOYL PEROXIDE 178
Dermoxyl 10 Gel - See BENZOYL PEROXIDE 178
Dermoxyl 20 Gel - See BENZOYL PEROXIDE 178
Dermoxyl Aqua - See BENZOYL PEROXIDE 178
Dermtex HC - See ADRENOCORTICOIDS (Topical) 18
Deronil - See ADRENOCORTICOIDS (Systemic) 16
DES - See ESTROGENS 372
Desenex Aerosol Powder - See ANTIFUNGALS (Topical) 88
Desenex Antifungal Cream - See ANTIFUNGALS (Topical) 88
Desenex Antifungal Liquid - See ANTIFUNGALS (Topical) 88
Desenex Antifungal Ointment - See ANTIFUNGALS (Topical) 88
Desenex Antifungal Penetrating Foam - See ANTIFUNGALS (Topical) 88
Desenex Antifungal Powder - See ANTIFUNGALS (Topical) 88
Desenex Antifungal Spray Powder - See ANTIFUNGALS (Topical) 88
Desenex Ointment - See ANTIFUNGALS (Topical) 88
Desenex Powder - See ANTIFUNGALS (Topical) 88
Desenex Solution - See ANTIFUNGALS (Topical) 88
DESERPIDINE - See RAUWOLFIA ALKALOIDS 714
DESIPRAMINE - See ANTIDEPRESSANTS, TRICYCLIC 80
DESLORATADINE - See ANTIHISTAMINES, NONSEDATING 110
DESMOPRESSIN 310
Desogen 28 - See CONTRACEPTIVES, ORAL & SKIN 278
Desogen Ortho-Cept - See CONTRACEPTIVES, ORAL & SKIN 278
DESOGESTREL & ETHINYL ESTRADIOL - See CONTRACEPTIVES, ORAL & SKIN 278
Desonate - See ADRENOCORTICOIDS (Topical) 18
DESONIDE (Topical) - See ADRENOCORTICOIDS (Topical) 18
DesOwen - See ADRENOCORTICOIDS (Topical) 18
DESOXIMETASONE (Topical) - See ADRENOCORTICOIDS (Topical) 18
Desoxyn - See AMPHETAMINES 28
Desoxyn Gradumet - See AMPHETAMINES 28
Desquam-E 2.5 Gel - See BENZOYL PEROXIDE 178
Desquam-E 5 Gel - See BENZOYL PEROXIDE 178
Desquam-E 10 Gel - See BENZOYL PEROXIDE 178
Desquam-X 2.5 Gel - See BENZOYL PEROXIDE 178
Desquam-X 5 Gel - See BENZOYL PEROXIDE 178
Desquam-X 5 Wash - See BENZOYL PEROXIDE 178
Desquam-X 10 Gel - See BENZOYL PEROXIDE 178
Desquam-X 10 Wash - See BENZOYL PEROXIDE 178
DESVENLAFAXINE- See SEROTONIN & NOREPINEPHRINE REUPTAKE INHIBITORS (SNRIs) 746
Detensol - See BETA-ADRENERGIC BLOCKING AGENTS 182
Detrol - See - See MUSCARINIC RECEPTOR ANTAGONISTS 574
Detrol LA - See MUSCARINIC RECEPTOR ANTAGONISTS 574
Detussin Expectorant - See
GUAIFENESIN 416
NARCOTIC ANALGESICS 584
PSEUDOEPHEDRINE 694
Detussin Liquid - See
NARCOTIC ANALGESICS 584
PSEUDOEPHEDRINE 694
Dexacort Turbinaire - See ADRENOCORTICOIDS (Nasal Inhalation) 12
Dexair - See ANTI-INFLAMMATORY DRUGS, STEROIDAL (Ophthalmic) 122
DEXAMETHASONE - See ADRENOCORTICOIDS (Systemic) 16
DEXAMETHASONE (Nasal) - See ADRENOCORTICOIDS (Nasal Inhalation) 12
DEXAMETHASONE (Ophthalmic) - See ANTI-INFLAMMATORY DRUGS, STEROIDAL (Ophthalmic) 122
DEXAMETHASONE (Oral Inhalation) - See ADRENOCORTICOIDS (Oral Inhalation) 14
DEXAMETHASONE (Otic) - See ANTI-INFLAMMATORY DRUGS, STEROIDAL (Otic) 124
DEXAMETHASONE (Topical) - See ADRENOCORTICOIDS (Topical) 18
Dexaphen SA - See
ANTIHISTAMINES 106
PSEUDOEPHEDRINE 694

Dexasone - See ADRENOCORTICOIDS (Systemic) 16
DEXBROMPHENIRAMINE - See ANTIHISTAMINES 106
Dexchlor - See ANTIHISTAMINES 106
DEXCHLORPHENIRAMINE - See ANTIHISTAMINES 106
Dexedrine - See AMPHETAMINES 28
Dexedrine Spansule - See AMPHETAMINES 28
Dexilant - See PROTON PUMP INHIBITORS 692
Dexitac - See CAFFEINE 216
DEXLANSOPRAZOLE - See PROTON PUMP INHIBITORS 692
DEXMETHYLPHENIDATE - See STIMULANT MEDICATIONS 754
Dexol T.D. - See PANTOTHENIC ACID (Vitamin B-5) 636
Dexone 0.5 - See ADRENOCORTICOIDS (Systemic) 16
Dexone 0.75 - See ADRENOCORTICOIDS (Systemic) 16
Dexone 1.5 - See ADRENOCORTICOIDS (Systemic) 16
Dexone 4 - See ADRENOCORTICOIDS (Systemic) 16
Dexophed - See
ANTIHISTAMINES 106
PSEUDOEPHEDRINE 694
Dexotic - See ANTI-INFLAMMATORY DRUGS, STEROIDAL (Ophthalmic) 122
Dexsone - See ANTI-INFLAMMATORY DRUGS, STEROIDAL (Ophthalmic) 122
DEXTROAMPHETAMINE - See AMPHETAMINES 28
<u>DEXTROMETHORPHAN</u> 312
Dey-Dose Isoetharine - See BRONCHODILATORS, ADRENERGIC 200
Dey-Dose Isoetharine S/F - See BRONCHODILATORS, ADRENERGIC 200
Dey-Dose Isoproterenol - See BRONCHODILATORS, ADRENERGIC 200
Dey-Dose Metaproterenol - See BRONCHODILATORS, ADRENERGIC 200
Dey-Dose Racepinephrine - See BRONCHODILATORS, ADRENERGIC 200
Dey-Lute Metaproterenol - See BRONCHODILATORS, ADRENERGIC 200
DHCplus - See NARCOTIC ANALGESICS & ACETAMINOPHEN 586
DHEA - See DEHYDROEPIANDROSTERONE (DHEA) 308
DHS Tar Gel Shampoo - See COAL TAR (Topical) 266
DHS Tar Shampoo - See COAL TAR (Topical) 266
DHS Zinc Dandruff Shampoo - See ANTISEBORRHEICS (Topical) 132
DHT - See VITAMIN D 840
DHT Intensol - See VITAMIN D 840
DiaBeta - See SULFONYLUREAS 770
Diabetic Tussin Allergy Relief - See ANTIHISTAMINES 106
Diabetic Tussin Cold & Flu - See
ACETAMINOPHEN 8
ANTIHISTAMINES 106
DEXTROMETHORPHAN 312
Diabetic Tussin DM - See
DEXTROMETHORPHAN 312
GUAIFENESIN 416
Diabetic Tussin EX - See GUAIFENESIN 416
Diabetic Tussin Mucus Relief - See GUAIFENESIN 416
Diabetic Tussin Night Time Formula - See
ACETAMINOPHEN 8
ANTIHISTAMINES 106
DEXTROMETHORPHAN 312
Diabinese - See SULFONYLUREAS 770
Diagen - See SALICYLATES 736
Diagnostic aid - See GLUCAGON 408
Dialose - See LAXATIVES, SOFTENER/ LUBRICANT 480
Dialose Plus - See
LAXATIVES, SOFTENER/LUBRICANT 480
LAXATIVES, STIMULANT 482
Dialume - See ANTACIDS 48
Diamine T.D. - See ANTIHISTAMINES 106
Diamox - See CARBONIC ANHYDRASE INHIBITORS 232
Diar-Aid - See ATTAPULGITE 160
Diasorb - See ATTAPULGITE 160
Diasporal Cream - See KERATOLYTICS 470
Diastat - See BENZODIAZEPINES 176
Diazemuls - See BENZODIAZEPINES 176
DIAZEPAM - See BENZODIAZEPINES 176
Diazepam Intensol - See BENZODIAZEPINES 176
Diazide - See DIURETICS, POTASSIUM-SPARING & HYDROCHLOROTHIAZIDE 336
DIBASIC CALCIUM PHOSPHATE - See CALCIUM SUPPLEMENTS 222
Dibent - See DICYCLOMINE 316
DIBUCAINE - See ANESTHETICS (Rectal) 38
DIBUCAINE - See ANESTHETICS (Topical) 40
Dicarbosil - See
ANTACIDS 48
CALCIUM SUPPLEMENTS 222
DICHLORPHENAMIDE - See CARBONIC ANHYDRASE INHIBITORS 232

DICLOFENAC - See
ANTI-INFLAMMATORY DRUGS, NONSTEROIDAL (NSAIDs) 116
ANTI-INFLAMMATORY DRUGS, NONSTEROIDAL (NSAIDs) (Ophthalmic) 120
DICLOFENAC (Topical) 314
DICLOXACILLIN - See PENICILLINS 646
DICYCLOMINE 316
Di-Cyclonex - See DICYCLOMINE 316
DIDANOSINE - See NUCLEOSIDE REVERSE TRANSCRIPTASE INHIBITORS 610
Didrex - See APPETITE SUPPRESSANTS 146
Didronel - See BISPHOSPHONATES 192
Dietary replacement - See CALCIUM SUPPLEMENTS 222
DIETHYLPROPION - See APPETITE SUPPRESSANTS 146
DIETHYLSTILBESTROL - See ESTROGENS 372
DIFENOXIN & ATROPINE 318
Differin - See RETINOIDS (Topical) 722
Dificid - See MACROLIDE ANTIBIOTICS 518
DIFLORASONE (Topical) - See ADRENOCORTICOIDS (Topical) 18
Diflucan - See ANTIFUNGALS, AZOLES 86
DIFLUCORTOLONE (Topical) - See ADRENOCORTICOIDS (Topical) 18
DIFLUNISAL - See ANTI-INFLAMMATORY DRUGS, NONSTEROIDAL (NSAIDs) 116
Di-Gel - See
ANTACIDS 48
SIMETHICONE 748
Digitalis Glycosides - See DIGITALIS PREPARATIONS (Digitalis Glycosides) 320
Digitalis preparation - See DIGITALIS PREPARATIONS (Digitalis Glycosides) 320
DIGITALIS PREPARATIONS (Digitalis Glycosides) 320
DIGITOXIN - See DIGITALIS PREPARATIONS (Digitalis Glycosides) 320
DIGOXIN - See DIGITALIS PREPARATIONS (Digitalis Glycosides) 320
Dihistine - See
ANTIHISTAMINES 106
PHENYLEPHRINE 658
Dihistine DH - See
ANTIHISTAMINES 106
NARCOTIC ANALGESICS 584
PSEUDOEPHEDRINE 694
Dihistine Expectorant - See
GUAIFENESIN 416
NARCOTIC ANALGESICS 584
PSEUDOEPHEDRINE 694
DIHYDROCODEINE - See NARCOTIC ANALGESICS 584
DIHYDROCODEINE & ACETAMINOPHEN - See NARCOTIC ANALGESICS & ACETAMINOPHEN 586
DIHYDROCODEINE & ASPIRIN - See NARCOTIC ANALGESICS & ASPIRIN 588
DIHYDROERGOTAMINE - See ERGOT DERIVATIVES 366
Dihydromorphinone - See NARCOTIC ANALGESICS 584
DIHYDROTACHYSTEROL - See VITAMIN D 840
Dihydrotestosterone inhibitor - See 5-ALPHA REDUCTASE INHIBITORS 2
Diiodohydroxyquin - See IODOQUINOL 454
Dilacor-XR - See CALCIUM CHANNEL BLOCKERS 220
Dilantin - See ANTICONVULSANTS, HYDANTOIN 76
Dilantin 30 - See ANTICONVULSANTS, HYDANTOIN 76
Dilantin 125 - See ANTICONVULSANTS, HYDANTOIN 76
Dilantin Infatabs - See ANTICONVULSANTS, HYDANTOIN 76
Dilantin Kapseals - See ANTICONVULSANTS, HYDANTOIN 76
Dilatair - See PHENYLEPHRINE (Ophthalmic) 660
Dilatrate-SR - See NITRATES 602
Dilaudid - See NARCOTIC ANALGESICS 584
Dilaudid Cough - See
GUAIFENESIN 416
NARCOTIC ANALGESICS 584
Dilaudid-HP - See NARCOTIC ANALGESICS 584
Dilomine - See DICYCLOMINE 316
Dilor - See BRONCHODILATORS, XANTHINE 204
Dilor-400 - See BRONCHODILATORS, XANTHINE 204
DILTIAZEM - See CALCIUM CHANNEL BLOCKERS 220
Dimaphen DM Elixir - See
ANTIHISTAMINES 106
DEXTROMETHORPHAN 312
PSEUDOEPHEDRINE 694
Dimaphen Elixir - See
ANTIHISTAMINES 106
PSEUDOEPHEDRINE 694
DIMENHYDRINATE - See ANTIHISTAMINES 106
Dimetabs - See ANTIHISTAMINES 106
Dimetane - See ANTIHISTAMINES 106
Dimetapp Children's DM Elixir Cough & Cold - See
ANTIHISTAMINES 106
PHENYLEPHRINE 658

Dimetapp Children's Elixir Cold & Allergy PE - See
ANTIHISTAMINES 106
PHENYLEPHRINE 658
Dimetapp Children's Long Acting Cough Plus Cold - See
ANTIHISTAMINES 106
DEXTROMETHORPHAN 312
Dimetapp Cold & Allergy - See
ANTIHISTAMINES 106
PHENYLEPHRINE 658
Dimetapp Cold & Cough DM Elixir - See
ANTIHISTAMINES 106
DEXTROMETHORPHAN 312
PHENYLEPHRINE 658
Dimetapp Long Acting Cough Plus Cold - See
ANTIHISTAMINES 106
DEXTROMETHORPHAN 312
Dimetapp Nighttime Flu Syrup - See
ACETAMINOPHEN 8
ANTIHISTAMINES 106
DEXTROMETHORPHAN 312
PHENYLEPHRINE 658
Dinate - See ANTIHISTAMINES 106
Diocto - See LAXATIVES, SOFTENER/LUBRICANT 480
Diocto-C - See
LAXATIVES, SOFTENER/LUBRICANT 480
LAXATIVES, STIMULANT 482
Diocto-K - See LAXATIVES, SOFTENER/LUBRICANT 480
Diocto-K Plus - See
LAXATIVES, SOFTENER/LUBRICANT 480
LAXATIVES, STIMULANT 482
Diodex - See ANTI-INFLAMMATORY DRUGS, STEROIDAL (Ophthalmic) 122
Diodoquin - See IODOQUINOL 454
Dioeze - See LAXATIVES, SOFTENER/LUBRICANT 480
Dionephrine - See PHENYLEPHRINE (Ophthalmic) 660
Diosuccin - See LAXATIVES, SOFTENER/LUBRICANT 480
Dio-Sul - See LAXATIVES, SOFTENER/LUBRICANT 480
Diothron - See
LAXATIVES, SOFTENER/LUBRICANT 480
LAXATIVES, STIMULANT 482
Diovan - See ANGIOTENSIN II RECEPTOR ANTAGONISTS 42
Diovan HCT - See
ANGIOTENSIN II RECEPTOR ANTAGONISTS 42
DIURETICS, THIAZIDE 338
Diovan Oral - See ANGIOTENSIN II RECEPTOR ANTAGONISTS 42
Diovol Ex - See ANTACIDS 48
Diovol Plus - See ANTACIDS 48
Dipentum - See OLSALAZINE 618
Diphen Cough - See ANTIHISTAMINES 106
Diphenacen-10 - See ANTIHISTAMINES 106
Diphenacen-50 - See ANTIHISTAMINES 106
Diphenadryl - See ANTIHISTAMINES 106
Diphenatol - See DIPHENOXYLATE & ATROPINE 324
DIPHENHYDRAMINE - See ANTIHISTAMINES 106
DIPHENIDOL 322
DIPHENOXYLATE & ATROPINE 324
Diphenylan - See ANTICONVULSANTS, HYDANTOIN 76
DIPHENYLPYRALINE - See ANTIHISTAMINES 106
Dipimol - See DIPYRIDAMOLE 326
DIPIVEFRIN - See ANTIGLAUCOMA, ADRENERGIC AGONISTS 92
Dipridacot - See DIPYRIDAMOLE 326
Diprolene - See ADRENOCORTICOIDS (Topical) 18
Diprolene AF - See ADRENOCORTICOIDS (Topical) 18
Diprosone - See ADRENOCORTICOIDS (Topical) 18
DIPYRIDAMOLE 326
Diquinol - See IODOQUINOL 454
DIRITHROMYCIN - See MACROLIDE ANTIBIOTICS 518
Disalcid - See SALICYLATES 736
Disanthrol - See
LAXATIVES, SOFTENER/LUBRICANT 480
LAXATIVES, STIMULANT 482
Disipal - See ORPHENADRINE 624
Disolan - See LAXATIVES, SOFTENER/LUBRICANT 480
Disolan Forte - See
LAXATIVES, BULK-FORMING 476
LAXATIVES, SOFTENER/LUBRICANT 480
LAXATIVES, STIMULANT 482
Disonate - See LAXATIVES, SOFTENER/LUBRICANT 480
Disophrol - See
ANTIHISTAMINES 106
PSEUDOEPHEDRINE 694
Disophrol Chronotabs - See
ANTIHISTAMINES 106
PSEUDOEPHEDRINE 694
Disoplex - See
LAXATIVES, BULK-FORMING 476
LAXATIVES, SOFTENER/LUBRICANT 480

INDEX

DISOPYRAMIDE 328
Di-Sosul - See LAXATIVES, SOFTENER/ LUBRICANT 480
Di-Sosul Forte - See
LAXATIVES, SOFTENER/LUBRICANT 480
LAXATIVES, STIMULANT 482
Dispatabs - See VITAMIN A 834
Di-Spaz - See DICYCLOMINE 316
DisperMox - See PENICILLINS 646
Dispos-a-Med Isoproterenol - See BRONCHODILATORS, ADRENERGIC 200
DISULFIRAM 330
Dithranol - See ANTHRALIN (Topical) 52
Ditropan - See - See MUSCARINIC RECEPTOR ANTAGONISTS 574
Ditropan XL - See - See MUSCARINIC RECEPTOR ANTAGONISTS 574
Diucardin - See DIURETICS, THIAZIDE 338
Diuchlor H - See DIURETICS, THIAZIDE 338
Diulo - See DIURETICS, THIAZIDE 338
Diupres - See
DIURETICS, THIAZIDE 338
RAUWOLFIA ALKALOIDS 714
Diuretic - See
DIURETICS, POTASSIUM-SPARING 334
DIURETICS, POTASSIUM-SPARING & HYDROCHLOROTHIAZIDE 336
HYDRALAZINE & HYDROCHLOROTHIAZIDE 428
INDAPAMIDE 444
Diuretic (Loop) - See DIURETICS, LOOP 332
Diuretic (Thiazide) - See
BETA-ADRENERGIC BLOCKING AGENTS & THIAZIDE DIURETICS 184
DIURETICS, THIAZIDE 338
DIURETICS, LOOP 332
DIURETICS, POTASSIUM-SPARING 334
DIURETICS, POTASSIUM-SPARING & HYDROCHLOROTHIAZIDE 336
DIURETICS, THIAZIDE 338
Diurigen with Reserpine - See
DIURETICS, THIAZIDE 338
RAUWOLFIA ALKALOIDS 714
Diuril - See DIURETICS, THIAZIDE 338
Diutensen-R - See
DIURETICS, THIAZIDE 338
RAUWOLFIA ALKALOIDS 714
DIVALPROEX 340
Divigel - See ESTROGENS 372
Dixarit - See CENTRAL ALPHA AGONISTS 234
DM Cough - See DEXTROMETHORPHAN 312
DM Syrup - See DEXTROMETHORPHAN 312
Doak Oil - See COAL TAR (Topical) 266
Doak Oil Forte - See COAL TAR (Topical) 266
Doak Oil Forte Therapeutic Bath Treatment - See COAL TAR (Topical) 266
Doak Oil Therapeutic Bath Treatment For All-Over Body Care - See COAL TAR (Topical) 266
Doak Tar Lotion - See COAL TAR (Topical) 266
Doak Tar Shampoo - See COAL TAR (Topical) 266
Doan's Pills - See SALICYLATES 736
DOCOSANOL (Topical) - See ANTIVIRALS (Topical) 144
Doctar - See COAL TAR (Topical) 266
Doctar Hair & Scalp Shampoo & Conditioner - See COAL TAR (Topical) 266
Docucal-P - See
LAXATIVES, SOFTENER/LUBRICANT 480
LAXATIVES, STIMULANT 482
Docu-K Plus - See
LAXATIVES, SOFTENER/LUBRICANT 480
LAXATIVES, STIMULANT 482
DOCUSATE - See LAXATIVES, SOFTENER/ LUBRICANT 480
DOCUSATE CALCIUM - See LAXATIVES, SOFTENER/LUBRICANT 480
DOCUSATE POTASSIUM - See LAXATIVES, SOFTENER/LUBRICANT 480
DOCUSATE SODIUM - See LAXATIVES, SOFTENER/LUBRICANT 480
Dodd's Pills - See SALICYLATES 736
DOFETILIDE 342
DOK - See LAXATIVES, SOFTENER/ LUBRICANT 480
DOK Softgels - See LAXATIVES, SOFTENER/ LUBRICANT 480
Doktors - See PHENYLEPHRINE 658
Dolacet - See NARCOTIC ANALGESICS & ACETAMINOPHEN 586
Dolagesic - See NARCOTIC ANALGESICS & ACETAMINOPHEN 586
Dolanex - See ACETAMINOPHEN 8
Dolene-AP 65 - See NARCOTIC ANALGESICS & ACETAMINOPHEN 586
Dolgesic - See ANTI-INFLAMMATORY DRUGS, NONSTEROIDAL (NSAIDs) 116
Dolmar - See
ACETAMINOPHEN 8
BARBITURATES 168
Dolobid - See ANTI-INFLAMMATORY DRUGS, NONSTEROIDAL (NSAIDs) 116
Dolophine - See NARCOTIC ANALGESICS 584
Dolotic - See ANTIPYRINE & BENZOCAINE (Otic) 130
Dolsed - See ATROPINE, HYOSCYAMINE, METHENAMINE, METHYLENE BLUE, PHENYLSALICYLATE & BENZOIC ACID 158

Domeboro - See ANTIBACTERIALS (Otic) 68
Dommanate - See ANTIHISTAMINES 106
Donatussin - See
ANTIHISTAMINES 106
DEXTROMETHORPHAN 312
GUAIFENESIN 416
PHENYLEPHRINE 658
Donatussin DC - See
GUAIFENESIN 416
NARCOTIC ANALGESICS 584
PHENYLEPHRINE 658
Donatussin Drops - See
ANTIHISTAMINES 106
GUAIFENESIN 416
PHENYLEPHRINE 658
Dondril - See
ANTIHISTAMINES 106
DEXTROMETHORPHAN 312
PHENYLEPHRINE 658
DONEPEZIL - See CHOLINESTERASE INHIBITORS 250
Donnagel-MB - See KAOLIN & PECTIN 468
Donnamor - See BELLADONNA ALKALOIDS & BARBITURATES 174
Donnapine - See BELLADONNA ALKALOIDS & BARBITURATES 174
Donna-Sed - See BELLADONNA ALKALOIDS & BARBITURATES 174
Donnatal - See BELLADONNA ALKALOIDS & BARBITURATES 174
Donnatal Elixir - See BELLADONNA ALKALOIDS & BARBITURATES 174
Donnatal Extentabs - See BELLADONNA ALKALOIDS & BARBITURATES 174
Donnatal No. 2 - See BELLADONNA ALKALOIDS & BARBITURATES 174
Donphen - See BELLADONNA ALKALOIDS & BARBITURATES 174
Dopamet - See CENTRAL ALPHA AGONISTS 234
Dopamine agonists - See DOPAMINE AGONISTS, NONERGOT 344
DOPAMINE AGONISTS, NONERGOT 344
Dopaminergic blocker - See METOCLOPRAMIDE 550
Dopar - See LEVODOPA 496
Dormarex 2 - See ANTIHISTAMINES 106
Dormin - See ANTIHISTAMINES 106
Doryx - See TETRACYCLINES 782
DORZOLAMIDE - See ANTIGLAUCOMA, CARBONIC ANHYDRASE INHIBITORS 98
Dosaflex - See LAXATIVES, STIMULANT 482
Doss - See LAXATIVES, SOFTENER/ LUBRICANT 480
Doss Tablets - See LAXATIVES, SOFTENER/ LUBRICANT 480
Dovonex - See VITAMIN D (Topical) 842
Doxaphene - See NARCOTIC ANALGESICS 584
DOXAZOSIN - See ALPHA ADRENERGIC RECEPTOR BLOCKERS 20
DOXEPIN - See ANTIDEPRESSANTS, TRICYCLIC 80
DOXEPIN (Topical) 346
DOXERCALCIFEROL - See VITAMIN D 840
Doxidan - See
LAXATIVES, SOFTENER/LUBRICANT 480
LAXATIVES, STIMULANT 482
Doxidan Liqui-Gels - See
LAXATIVES, SOFTENER/LUBRICANT 480
LAXATIVES, STIMULANT 482
Doxinate - See LAXATIVES, SOFTENER/ LUBRICANT 480
Doxy-Caps - See TETRACYCLINES 782
Doxycin - See TETRACYCLINES 782
DOXYCYCLINE - See ANTIBACTERIALS FOR ACNE (Topical) 64
DOXYCYCLINE - See TETRACYCLINES 782
DOXYLAMINE - See ANTIHISTAMINES 106
Doxy-Tabs - See TETRACYCLINES 782
DPE - See ANTIGLAUCOMA, ADRENERGIC AGONISTS 92
DPP-4 INHIBITORS 348
Dr. Caldwell Senna Laxative - See LAXATIVES, STIMULANT 482
Dramamine - See ANTIHISTAMINES 106
Dramamine Chewable - See ANTIHISTAMINES 106
Dramamine II - See ANTIHISTAMINES, PIPERAZINE (Antinausea) 114
Dramamine Liquid - See ANTIHISTAMINES 106
Dramanate - See ANTIHISTAMINES 106
Dramocen - See ANTIHISTAMINES 106
Dramoject - See ANTIHISTAMINES 106
Drenison - See ADRENOCORTICOIDS (Topical) 18
Drenison-1/4 - See ADRENOCORTICOIDS (Topical) 18
Drisdol - See VITAMIN D 840
Dristan 12-Hour Nasal Spray - See OXYMETAZOLINE (Nasal) 630
Dristan Cold and Flu - See
ACETAMINOPHEN 8
ANTIHISTAMINES 106
DEXTROMETHORPHAN 312
PSEUDOEPHEDRINE 694
Dristan Cold Caplets - See
ACETAMINOPHEN 8
PSEUDOEPHEDRINE 694

INDEX

Dristan Cold Maximum Strength Caplets - See
ACETAMINOPHEN 8
ANTIHISTAMINES 106
PSEUDOEPHEDRINE 694
Dristan Cold Multi-Symptom Formula - See
ACETAMINOPHEN 8
ANTIHISTAMINES 106
PHENYLEPHRINE 658
Dristan Formula P - See
ANTIHISTAMINES 106
ASPIRIN 152
CAFFEINE 216
PHENYLEPHRINE 658
Dristan Juice Mix-in Cold, Flu, & Cough - See
ACETAMINOPHEN 8
DEXTROMETHORPHAN 312
PSEUDOEPHEDRINE 694
Dristan Long Lasting Menthol Nasal Spray - See OXYMETAZOLINE (Nasal) 630
Dristan Long Lasting Nasal Pump Spray - See OXYMETAZOLINE (Nasal) 630
Dristan Long Lasting Nasal Spray - See OXYMETAZOLINE (Nasal) 630
Dristan Long Lasting Nasal Spray 12 Hour Metered Dose Pump - See OXYMETAZOLINE (Nasal) 630
Dristan Mentholated - See OXYMETAZOLINE (Nasal) 630
Dristan Sinus Caplets - See
ANTI-INFLAMMATORY DRUGS, NONSTEROIDAL (NSAIDs) 116
PSEUDOEPHEDRINE 694
Dristan-AF - See
ACETAMINOPHEN 8
ANTIHISTAMINES 106
CAFFEINE 216
PHENYLEPHRINE 658
Dristan-AF Plus - See
ACETAMINOPHEN 8
CAFFEINE 216
PHENYLEPHRINE 658
Drithocreme - See ANTHRALIN (Topical) 52
Drithocreme HP - See ANTHRALIN (Topical) 52
Dritho-Scalp - See ANTHRALIN (Topical) 52
Drixoral - See
ANTIHISTAMINES 106
OXYMETAZOLINE (Nasal) 630
PSEUDOEPHEDRINE 694
Drixoral Cold and Allergy - See
ANTIHISTAMINES 106
PSEUDOEPHEDRINE 694
Drixoral Cold and Flu - See
ACETAMINOPHEN 8
ANTIHISTAMINES 106
PSEUDOEPHEDRINE 694
Drixoral Cough - See DEXTROMETHORPHAN 312
Drixoral Nasal Decongestant - See PSEUDOEPHEDRINE 694
Drixoral Non-Drowsy Formula - See PSEUDOEPHEDRINE 694
Drixoral Plus - See
ACETAMINOPHEN 8
ANTIHISTAMINES 106
PSEUDOEPHEDRINE 694
Drixoral Sinus - See
ACETAMINOPHEN 8
ANTIHISTAMINES 106
PSEUDOEPHEDRINE 694
Drixtab - See
ANTIHISTAMINES 106
PSEUDOEPHEDRINE 694
Drocade and Aspirin - See NARCOTIC ANALGESICS & ASPIRIN 588
DRONABINOL (THC, Marijuana) 350
DRONEDARONE - See ANTIARRHYTHMICS, BENZOFURAN-TYPE 60
DROSPIRENONE - See PROGESTINS 680
DROSPIRENONE & ETHINYL ESTRADIOL - See CONTRACEPTIVES, ORAL & SKIN 278
Drotic - See ANTIBACTERIALS (Otic) 68
Droxia - See HYDROXYUREA 434
Droxomin - See VITAMIN B-12 (Cyanocobalamin) 836
Dry and Clear 5 Lotion - See BENZOYL PEROXIDE 178
Dry and Clear Double Strength 10 Cream - See BENZOYL PEROXIDE 178
Dryox 5 Gel - See BENZOYL PEROXIDE 178
Dryox 10 Gel - See BENZOYL PEROXIDE 178
Dryox 20 Gel - See BENZOYL PEROXIDE 178
Dryox Wash 5 - See BENZOYL PEROXIDE 178
Dryox Wash 10 - See BENZOYL PEROXIDE 178
Dryphen - See
ACETAMINOPHEN 8
ANTIHISTAMINES 106
PHENYLEPHRINE 658
DSMC Plus - See
LAXATIVES, SOFTENER/LUBRICANT 480
LAXATIVES, STIMULANT 482
DUAC Topical Gel - See
ANTIBACTERIALS FOR ACNE (Topical) 64
BENZOYL PEROXIDE 178
Duagen - See 5-ALPHA REDUCTASE INHIBITORS 2
Duetact - See
SULFONYLUREAS 770
THIAZOLIDINEDIONES 786

Duexis - See
ANTI-INFLAMMATORY DRUGS, NONSTEROIDAL (NSAIDs) 116
HISTAMINE H2 RECEPTOR ANTAGONISTS 422
Dulcodos - See
LAXATIVES, SOFTENER/LUBRICANT 480
LAXATIVES, STIMULANT 482
Dulcolax - See LAXATIVES, STIMULANT 482
Dulcolax for Women - See LAXATIVES, STIMULANT 482
Dulera - See
ADRENOCORTICOIDS (Oral Inhalation) 14
BRONCHODILATORS, ADRENERGIC 200
DULOXETINE - See SEROTONIN & NOREPINEPHRINE REUPTAKE INHIBITORS (SNRIs) 746
Duocet - See NARCOTIC ANALGESICS & ACETAMINOPHEN 586
Duofilm - See KERATOLYTICS 470
Duo-Medihaler - See PHENYLEPHRINE 658
Duoneb - See
BRONCHODILATORS, ADRENERGIC 200
IPRATROPIUM 456
Duoplant - See KERATOLYTICS 470
Duoplant Topical Solution - See KERATOLYTICS 470
Duosol - See LAXATIVES, SOFTENER/ LUBRICANT 480
Duotrate - See NITRATES 602
Duphalac - See LAXATIVES, OSMOTIC 478
Durabolin - See ANDROGENS 34
Durabolin-50 - See ANDROGENS 34
Duracid - See ANTACIDS 48
Duradyne - See
ACETAMINOPHEN 8
ASPIRIN 152
Dura-Estrin - See ESTROGENS 372
Duragen - See ESTROGENS 372
Duragen-20 - See ESTROGENS 372
Duragen-40 - See ESTROGENS 372
Duragesic - See NARCOTIC ANALGESICS 584
Duragesic 12 mc/hr - See NARCOTIC ANALGESICS 584
Durahist - See
ANTICHOLINERGICS 72
ANTIHISTAMINES 106
PSEUDOEPHEDRINE 694
Duralith - See LITHIUM 504
Duralutin - See PROGESTINS 680
Duramist Plus Up To 12 Hours Decongestant Nasal Spray - See OXYMETAZOLINE (Nasal) 630
Duramorph - See NARCOTIC ANALGESICS 584
Dura-Patch - See CAPSAICIN 226
Dura-Patch Joint - See CAPSAICIN 226
Duraphyl - See BRONCHODILATORS, XANTHINE 204
Duraquin - See QUINIDINE 704
Duratest 100 - See ANDROGENS 34
Duratest-200 - See ANDROGENS 34
Durathate 200 - See ANDROGENS 34
Duration 12 Hour Nasal Spray Pump - See OXYMETAZOLINE (Nasal) 630
Duratuss - See
GUAIFENESIN 416
PSEUDOEPHEDRINE 694
Duratuss HD - See
GUAIFENESIN 416
NARCOTIC ANALGESICS 584
PSEUDOEPHEDRINE 694
Dura-Vent/DA - See
ANTICHOLINERGICS 72
ANTIHISTAMINES 106
PHENYLEPHRINE 658
Duretic - See DIURETICS, THIAZIDE 338
Dureticyl - See
DIURETICS, THIAZIDE 338
RAUWOLFIA ALKALOIDS 714
Duricef - See CEPHALOSPORINS 236
DUTASTERIDE - See 5-ALPHA REDUCTASE INHIBITORS 2
Dutoprol - See BETA-ADRENERGIC BLOCKING AGENTS & THIAZIDE DIURETICS 184
Duvoid - See BETHANECHOL 186
D-Vert 15 - See ANTIHISTAMINES, PIPERAZINE (Antinausea) 114
D-Vert 30 - See ANTIHISTAMINES, PIPERAZINE (Antinausea) 114
Dycill - See PENICILLINS 646
DYCLONINE - See ANESTHETICS (Mucosal-Local) 36
Dyflex 200 - See BRONCHODILATORS, XANTHINE 204
Dyflex 400 - See BRONCHODILATORS, XANTHINE 204
Dymenate - See ANTIHISTAMINES 106
Dymista - See
ADRENOCORTICOIDS (Nasal Inhalation) 12
ANTIHISTAMINES (Nasal) 108
Dyna Circ - See CALCIUM CHANNEL BLOCKERS 220
Dynabac - See MACROLIDE ANTIBIOTICS 518
Dynapen - See PENICILLINS 646
DYPHYLLINE - See BRONCHODILATORS, XANTHINE 204
Dyrenium - See DIURETICS, POTASSIUM-SPARING 334
Dyrexan-OD - See APPETITE SUPPRESSANTS 146

Dysport - See BOTULINUM TOXIN TYPE A 196

E

Earache Drops - See ANTIPYRINE & BENZOCAINE (Otic) 130
Ear-Eze - See ANTIBACTERIALS (Otic) 68
Earocol - See ANTIPYRINE & BENZOCAINE (Otic) 130
Easprin - See ASPIRIN 152
E-Base - See ERYTHROMYCINS 368
ECHOTHIOPHATE - See ANTIGLAUCOMA, ANTICHOLINESTERASES 94
EC-Naprosyn - See ANTI-INFLAMMATORY DRUGS, NONSTEROIDAL (NSAIDs) 116
ECONAZOLE - See ANTIFUNGALS (Topical) 88
ECONAZOLE - See ANTIFUNGALS (Vaginal) 90
Econochlor Ophthalmic Ointment - See ANTIBACTERIALS (Ophthalmic) 66
Econochlor Ophthalmic Solution - See ANTIBACTERIALS (Ophthalmic) 66
Econopred - See ANTI-INFLAMMATORY DRUGS, STEROIDAL (Ophthalmic) 122
Econopred Plus - See ANTI-INFLAMMATORY DRUGS, STEROIDAL (Ophthalmic) 122
Ecostatin - See
ANTIFUNGALS (Topical) 88
ANTIFUNGALS (Vaginal) 90
Ecotrin - See ASPIRIN 152
Ectosone - See ADRENOCORTICOIDS (Topical) 18
Ectosone Regular - See ADRENOCORTICOIDS (Topical) 18
Ectosone Scalp Lotion - See ADRENOCORTICOIDS (Topical) 18
E-Cypionate - See ESTROGENS 372
Ed A-Hist - See
ANTIHISTAMINES 106
PHENYLEPHRINE 658
Edarbi - See ANGIOTENSIN II RECEPTOR ANTAGONISTS 42
Edarbyclor - See
ANGIOTENSIN II RECEPTOR 42 ANTAGONISTS
DIURETICS, THIAZIDE 338
Ed-Bron G - See
BRONCHODILATORS, XANTHINE 204
GUAIFENESIN 416
Edecrin - See DIURETICS, LOOP 332
Edex - See ALPROSTADIL 22
Edluar - See ZOLPIDEM 858
Edurant - See NON-NUCLEOSIDE REVERSE TRANSCRIPTASE INHIBITORS 608
E.E.S. - See ERYTHROMYCINS 368
EFAVIRENZ - See NON-NUCLEOSIDE REVERSE TRANSCRIPTASE INHIBITORS 608
Efcortelan - See ADRENOCORTICOIDS (Topical) 18
Effer-K - See POTASSIUM SUPPLEMENTS 666
Effer-K-10 - See POTASSIUM SUPPLEMENTS 666
Effer-syllium - See LAXATIVES, BULK-FORMING 476
Effexor - See SEROTONIN & NOR-EPINEPHRINE REUPTAKE INHIBITORS (SNRIs) 746
Effexor XR - See SEROTONIN & NOR-EPINEPHRINE REUPTAKE INHIBITORS (SNRIs) 746
Efficol Cough Whip (Cough Suppressant/ Expectorant) - See
DEXTROMETHORPHAN 312
GUAIFENESIN 416
Effient - See PLATELET INHIBITORS 664
Eflone - See ANTI-INFLAMMATORY DRUGS, STEROIDAL (Ophthalmic) 122
EFLORNITHINE (Topical) 352
Efudex - See FLUOROURACIL (Topical) 394
E/Gel - See ERYTHROMYCINS 368
Egozinc - See ZINC SUPPLEMENTS 854
Eldepryl - See MONOAMINE OXIDASE TYPE B (MAO-B) INHIBITORS 572
Elestat - See ANTIALLERGIC AGENTS (Ophthalmic) 56
Elestrin - See ESTROGENS 372
ELETRIPTAN - See TRIPTANS 820
Elimite Cream - See PEDICULICIDES (Topical) 642
Eliquis - See FACTOR Xa INHIBITORS 382
Elixicon - See BRONCHODILATORS, XANTHINE 204
Elixomin - See BRONCHODILATORS, XANTHINE 204
Elixophyllin - See BRONCHODILATORS, XANTHINE 204
Elixophyllin SR - See BRONCHODILATORS, XANTHINE 204
Elixophyllin-GG - See
BRONCHODILATORS, XANTHINE 204
GUAIFENESIN 416
Ella - See SELECTIVE PROGESTERONE RECEPTOR MODULATORS 740
Elocon - See ADRENOCORTICOIDS (Topical) 18
E-Lor - See NARCOTIC ANALGESICS & ACETAMINOPHEN 586
Eltor-122 - See PSEUDOEPHEDRINE 694
Eltroxin - See THYROID HORMONES 792

Emadine - See ANTIALLERGIC AGENTS (Ophthalmic) 56
Embeda - See
NALTREXONE 582
NARCOTIC ANALGESICS 584
EMEDASTINE - See ANTIALLERGIC AGENTS (Ophthalmic) 56
Emcodeine No. 2 - See NARCOTIC ANALGESICS & ASPIRIN 588
Emcodeine No. 3 - See NARCOTIC ANALGESICS & ASPIRIN 588
Emcodeine No. 4 - See NARCOTIC ANALGESICS & ASPIRIN 588
Emcyt - See ESTRAMUSTINE 370
Emex - See METOCLOPRAMIDE 550
Emgel - See ERYTHROMYCINS 368
Emko - See CONTRACEPTIVES, VAGINAL 280
Emla - See ANESTHETICS (Topical) 40
Emo-Cort - See ADRENOCORTICOIDS (Topical) 18
Emo-Cort Scalp Solution - See ADRENOCORTICOIDS (Topical) 18
Emoquette - See CONTRACEPTIVES, ORAL & SKIN 278
Empirin - See ASPIRIN 152
Empirin with Codeine - See NARCOTIC ANALGESICS & ASPIRIN 588
Empirin with Codeine No. 3 - See NARCOTIC ANALGESICS & ASPIRIN 588
Empirin with Codeine No. 4 - See NARCOTIC ANALGESICS & ASPIRIN 588
Empracet 30 - See NARCOTIC ANALGESICS & ACETAMINOPHEN 586
Empracet 60 - See NARCOTIC ANALGESICS & ACETAMINOPHEN 586
Emsam - See MONOAMINE OXIDASE TYPE B (MAO-B) INHIBITORS 572
Emtec - See NARCOTIC ANALGESICS & ACETAMINOPHEN 586
EMTRICITABINE - See NUCLEOSIDE REVERSE TRANSCRIPTASE INHIBITORS 610
Emtriva - See NUCLEOSIDE REVERSE TRANSCRIPTASE INHIBITORS 610
Emulsoil - See LAXATIVES, STIMULANT 482
E-Mycin - See ERYTHROMYCINS 368
Enablex - See MUSCARINIC RECEPTOR ANTAGONISTS 574
ENALAPRIL - See ANGIOTENSIN-CONVERTING ENZYME (ACE) INHIBITORS 44
ENALAPRIL & HYDROCHLOROTHIAZIDE - See ANGIOTENSIN-CONVERTING ENZYME (ACE) INHIBITORS & HYDROCHLOROTHIAZIDE 46
Enbrel - See TUMOR NECROSIS FACTOR BLOCKERS 822
Encare - See CONTRACEPTIVES, VAGINAL 280
Endagen-HD - See
ANTIHISTAMINES 106
NARCOTIC ANALGESICS 584
PHENYLEPHRINE 658
Endal-HD - See
ANTIHISTAMINES 106
NARCOTIC ANALGESICS 584
PHENYLEPHRINE 658
Endal-HD Plus - See
ANTIHISTAMINES 106
NARCOTIC ANALGESICS 584
PHENYLEPHRINE 658
Endep - See ANTIDEPRESSANTS, TRICYCLIC 80
Endocaine - See ANESTHETICS (Topical) 40
Endocet - See NARCOTIC ANALGESICS & ACETAMINOPHEN 586
Endodan - See NARCOTIC ANALGESICS & ASPIRIN 588
Endolor - See
ACETAMINOPHEN 8
BARBITURATES 168
Endometrin - See PROGESTINS 680
ENDOTHELIN RECEPTOR ANTAGONISTS 354
Endur-Acin - See NIACIN (Vitamin B-3, Nicotinic Acid, Nicotinamide) 596
Enduron - See DIURETICS, THIAZIDE 338
Enduronyl - See
DIURETICS, THIAZIDE 338
RAUWOLFIA ALKALOIDS 714
Enduronyl Forte - See
DIURETICS, THIAZIDE 338
RAUWOLFIA ALKALOIDS 714
Enerjets - See CAFFEINE 216
ENFUVIRTIDE - See FUSION INHIBITOR 400
Enjuvia - See ESTROGENS 372
ENOXACIN - See FLUOROQUINOLONES 392
ENTACAPONE - See COMT INHIBITORS 274
Entex PSE - See
GUAIFENESIN 416
PSEUDOEPHEDRINE 694
Entocort EC - See ADRENOCORTICOIDS (Systemic) 16
ETRAVIRINE - See NON-NUCLEOSIDE REVERSE TRANSCRIPTASE INHIBITORS 608
Entrophen - See ASPIRIN 152
Entuss Expectorant - See
GUAIFENESIN 416
NARCOTIC ANALGESICS 584
Entuss Pediatric Expectorant - See
GUAIFENESIN 416
PSEUDOEPHEDRINE 694

Entuss-D - See
GUAIFENESIN 416
NARCOTIC ANALGESICS 584
PSEUDOEPHEDRINE 694
Enzyme (Pancreatic) - See PANCRELIPASE 634
Enzyme Inhibitor (topical) - See EFLORNITHINE (Topical) 352
E.P. Mycin - See TETRACYCLINES 782
Epatiol - See TIOPRONIN 798
Ephed II - See BRONCHODILATORS, ADRENERGIC 200
EPHEDRINE 356
EPHEDRINE SULFATE - See BRONCHODILATORS, ADRENERGIC 200
Epiduo - See
BENZOYL PEROXIDE 178
RETINOIDS (Topical) 722
Epifoam - See ADRENOCORTICOIDS (Topical) 18
Epifren - See ANTIGLAUCOMA, ADRENERGIC AGONISTS 92
EPINASTINE - See ANTIALLERGIC AGENTS (Ophthalmic) 56
Epimorph - See NARCOTIC ANALGESICS 584
EPINEPHRINE - See ANTIGLAUCOMA, ADRENERGIC AGONISTS 92
Epinal - See ANTIGLAUCOMA, ADRENERGIC AGONISTS 92
Eppy/N - See ANTIGLAUCOMA, ADRENERGIC AGONISTS 92
EpiPen Auto-Injector - See BRONCHODILATORS, ADRENERGIC 200
EpiPen Jr. Auto-Injector - See BRONCHODILATORS, ADRENERGIC 200
Epistatin - See HMG-CoA REDUCTASE INHIBITORS 424
Epitol - See CARBAMAZEPINE 228
Epival - See DIVALPROEX 340
Epivir - See NUCLEOSIDE REVERSE TRANSCRIPTASE INHIBITORS 610
EPLERENONE 358
Eprolin - See VITAMIN E 844
Epromate-M - See
ASPIRIN 152
MEPROBAMATE 538
EPROSARTAN - See ANGIOTENSIN II RECEPTOR ANTAGONISTS 42
Epsilan-M - See VITAMIN E 844
Eptastatin - See HMG-CoA REDUCTASE INHIBITORS 424
Epzicom - See NUCLEOSIDE REVERSE TRANSCRIPTASE INHIBITORS 610
Equagesic - See
ASPIRIN 152
MEPROBAMATE 538
Equalactin - See LAXATIVES, BULK-FORMING 476
Equanil - See MEPROBAMATE 538
Equanil Wyseals - See MEPROBAMATE 538
Equazine-M - See
ASPIRIN 152
MEPROBAMATE 538
Equetro - See CARBAMAZEPINE 228
Equibron G - See
BRONCHODILATORS, XANTHINE 204
GUAIFENESIN 416
Equilet - See ANTACIDS 48
ERECTILE DYSFUNCTION AGENTS 360
Ergamisol - See LEVAMISOLE 490
ERGOCALCIFEROL - See VITAMIN D 840
ERGOLOID MESYLATES 362
Ergomar - See ERGOT DERIVATIVES 366
Ergometrine - See ERGOT ALKALOIDS 364
ERGOT ALKALOIDS 364
ERGOT DERIVATIVES 366
Ergot preparation - See
ERGOLOID MESYLATES 362
ERGOT DERIVATIVES 366
Ergot preparation (Uterine Stimulant) - See ERGOT ALKALOIDS 364
Ergotrate - See ERGOT ALKALOIDS 364
Ergotrate Maleate - See ERGOT ALKALOIDS 364
Eridium - See PHENAZOPYRIDINE 654
Ertaczo - See ANTIFUNGALS (Topical) 88
Erybid - See ERYTHROMYCINS 368
ERYC - See ERYTHROMYCINS 368
Erycette - See ANTIBACTERIALS FOR ACNE (Topical) 64
EryDerm - See ANTIBACTERIALS FOR ACNE (Topical) 64
EryGel - See ANTIBACTERIALS FOR ACNE (Topical) 64
EryMax - See ANTIBACTERIALS FOR ACNE (Topical) 64
EryPed - See ERYTHROMYCINS 368
ErySol - See ANTIBACTERIALS FOR ACNE (Topical) 64
Ery-Tab - See ERYTHROMYCINS 368
Erythraderm - See ERYTHROMYCINS 368
ERYTHRITYL TETRANITRATE - See NITRATES 602
Erythro - See ERYTHROMYCINS 368
Erythrocin - See ERYTHROMYCINS 368
Erythrocot - See ERYTHROMYCINS 368
Erythromid - See ERYTHROMYCINS 368
ERYTHROMYCIN ESTOLATE - See ERYTHROMYCINS 368
ERYTHROMYCIN ETHYLSUCCINATE - See ERYTHROMYCINS 368

ERYTHROMYCIN GLUCEPTATE - See ERYTHROMYCINS 368
ERYTHROMYCIN LACTOBIONATE - See ERYTHROMYCINS 368
ERYTHROMYCIN (Ophthalmic) - See ANTIBACTERIALS (Ophthalmic) 66
ERYTHROMYCIN STEARATE - See ERYTHROMYCINS 368
ERYTHROMYCIN (Topical) - See ANTIBACTERIALS FOR ACNE (Topical) 64
ERYTHROMYCIN-BASE - See ERYTHROMYCINS 368
ERYTHROMYCINS 368
Erythro-statin - See ANTIBACTERIALS FOR ACNE (Topical) 64
ESCITALOPRAM - See SELECTIVE SEROTONIN REUPTAKE INHIBITORS (SSRIs) 742
Esclim - See ESTROGENS 372
Esgic - See
ACETAMINOPHEN 8
BARBITURATES 168
CAFFEINE 216
Esgic Plus - See
ACETAMINOPHEN 8
BARBITURATES 168
CAFFEINE 216
Esidrix - See DIURETICS, THIAZIDE 338
Eskalith - See LITHIUM 504
Eskalith CR - See LITHIUM 504
ESOMEPRAZOLE - See PROTON PUMP INHIBITORS 692
Estar - See COAL TAR (Topical) 266
ESTAZOLAM - See BENZODIAZEPINES 176
ESTERIFIED ESTROGENS - See ESTROGENS 372
Estinyl - See ESTROGENS 372
Estivin II - See DECONGESTANTS (Ophthalmic) 306
Estrace - See ESTROGENS 372
Estraderm - See ESTROGENS 372
ESTRADIOL - See ESTROGENS 372
ESTRADIOL VALERATE & DIENOGEST - See CONTRACEPTIVES, ORAL & SKIN 278
Estragen 5 - See ESTROGENS 372
Estragen LA 5 - See ESTROGENS 372
Estra-L - See ESTROGENS 372
ESTRAMUSTINE 370
Estrasorb - See ESTROGENS 372
Estratab - See ESTROGENS 372
Estring - See ESTROGENS 372
Estro-A - See ESTROGENS 372
Estro-Cyp - See ESTROGENS 372
Estrofem - See ESTROGENS 372
Estrogel - See ESTROGENS 372
ESTROGENS 372
Estroject-L.A. - See ESTROGENS 372
Estro-L.A. - See ESTROGENS 372
ESTRONE - See ESTROGENS 372
ESTROPIPATE - See ESTROGENS 372
Estro-Span - See ESTROGENS 372
Estrostep - See CONTRACEPTIVES, ORAL & SKIN 278
Estrostep Fe - See
CONTRACEPTIVES, ORAL & SKIN 278
IRON SUPPLEMENTS 458
Estrovis - See ESTROGENS 372
ESZOPICLONE 374
ETANERCEPT - See TUMOR NECROSIS FACTOR BLOCKERS 822
ETHACRYNIC ACID - See DIURETICS, LOOP 332
ETHINYL ESTRADIOL - See ESTROGENS 372
ETHIONAMIDE 376
ETHOPROPAZINE - See ANTIDYSKINETICS 82
ETHOSUXIMIDE - See ANTICONVULSANTS, SUCCINIMIDE 78
ETHOTOIN - See ANTICONVULSANTS, HYDANTOIN 76
Ethyl Aminobenzoate - See
ANESTHETICS (Rectal) 38
ANESTHETICS (Topical) 40
ETHYLESTRENOL - See ANDROGENS 34
ETHYLNOREPINEPHRINE - See BRONCHODILATORS, ADRENERGIC 200
ETHYNODIOL DIACETATE & ETHINYL ESTRADIOL - See CONTRACEPTIVES, ORAL & SKIN 278
ETIDRONATE - See BISPHOSPHONATES 192
ETODOLAC - See ANTI-INFLAMMATORY DRUGS, NONSTEROIDAL (NSAIDs) 116
ETONOGESTREL - See PROGESTINS 680
ETONOGESTREL & ETHINYL ESTRADIOL - See CONTRACEPTIVES, VAGINAL 280
ETOPOSIDE 378
Etrafonl - See
ANTIDEPRESSANTS, TRICYCLIC 80
PHENOTHIAZINES 656
Etrafon-A - See
ANTIDEPRESSANTS, TRICYCLIC 80
PHENOTHIAZINES 656
Etrafon-D - See
ANTIDEPRESSANTS, TRICYCLIC 80
PHENOTHIAZINES 656
Etrafon-F - See
ANTIDEPRESSANTS, TRICYCLIC 80
PHENOTHIAZINES 656
Etrafon-Forte I - See
ANTIDEPRESSANTS, TRICYCLIC 80
PHENOTHIAZINES 656

ETS - See ANTIBACTERIALS FOR ACNE (Topical) 64
Euflex - See ANTIANDROGENS, NONSTEROIDAL 58
Euglucon - See SULFONYLUREAS 770
Eulexin - See ANTIANDROGENS, NON-STEROIDAL 58
Eumovate - See ADRENOCORTICOIDS (Topical) 18
Euthroid - See THYROID HORMONES 792
Evac-U-Lax - See LAXATIVES, STIMULANT 482
Evalose - See LAXATIVES, OSMOTIC 478
EvaMist - See ESTROGENS 372
Everone - See ANDROGENS 34
Evista - See RALOXIFENE 708
Evoclin Foam - See ANTIBACTERIALS FOR ACNE (Topical) 64
Exalgo - See NARCOTIC ANALGESICS 584
Excedrin Back & Body - See
ACETAMINOPHEN 8
ASPIRIN 152
Excedrin Caplets - See
ACETAMINOPHEN 8
CAFFEINE 216
Excedrin Extra Strength Caplets - See
ACETAMINOPHEN 8
ASPIRIN 152
CAFFEINE 216
Excedrin Extra Strength Tablets - See
ACETAMINOPHEN 8
ASPIRIN 152
CAFFEINE 216
Excedrin Migraine - See
ACETAMINOPHEN 8
ASPIRIN 152
CAFFEINE 216
Excedrin-IB Caplets - See ANTI-INFLAMMATORY DRUGS, NONSTEROIDAL (NSAIDs) 116
Excedrin-IB Tablets - See ANTI-INFLAMMATORY DRUGS, NONSTEROIDAL (NSAIDs) 116
Excedrin Sinus Headache - See
ACETAMINOPHEN 8
PHENYLEPHRINE 658
Excedrin Tension Headache - See
ACETAMINOPHEN 8
CAFFEINE 216
Exdol - See ACETAMINOPHEN 8
Exdol Strong - See ACETAMINOPHEN 8
Exdol-8 - See NARCOTIC ANALGESICS & ACETAMINOPHEN 586
Exdol-15 - See NARCOTIC ANALGESICS & ACETAMINOPHEN 586
Exdol-30 - See NARCOTIC ANALGESICS & ACETAMINOPHEN 586
Exelderm - See ANTIFUNGALS (Topical) 88
Exelon - See CHOLINESTERASE INHIBITORS 250
Exelon Patch - See CHOLINESTERASE INHIBITORS 250
EXENATIDE - See GLP-1 RECEPTOR AGONISTS 406
Exforge - See
ANGIOTENSIN II RECEPTOR ANTAGONISTS 42
CALCIUM CHANNEL BLOCKERS 220
Exforge HCT - See
ANGIOTENSIN II RECEPTOR ANTAGONISTS 42
CALCIUM CHANNEL BLOCKERS 220
DIURETICS, THIAZIDE 338
Ex-Lax - See LAXATIVES, STIMULANT 482
Ex-Lax Chocolate - See LAXATIVES, STIMULANT 482
Ex-Lax Gentle Nature - See LAXATIVES, STIMULANT 482
Ex-Lax Light Formula - See
LAXATIVES, SOFTENER/LUBRICANT 480
LAXATIVES, STIMULANT 482
Ex-Lax Maximum Relief Formula - See LAXATIVES, STIMULANT 482
Ex-Lax Pills - See LAXATIVES, STIMULANT 482
Exna - See DIURETICS, THIAZIDE 338
Expectorant - See GUAIFENESIN 416
Exsel - See ANTISEBORRHEICS (Topical) 132
Extendryl - See
ANTICHOLINERGICS 72
ANTIHISTAMINES 106
PHENYLEPHRINE 658
Extendryl JR - See
ANTICHOLINERGICS 72
ANTIHISTAMINES 106
PHENYLEPHRINE 658
Extendryl SR - See
ANTICHOLINERGICS 72
ANTIHISTAMINES 106
PHENYLEPHRINE 658
Extina - See ANTIFUNGALS (Topical) 88
Extina Foam - See ANTIFUNGALS (Topical) 88
Extra Action Cough - See
DEXTROMETHORPHAN 312
GUAIFENESIN 416
Extra Gentle Ex-Lax - See
LAXATIVES, SOFTENER/LUBRICANT 480
LAXATIVES, STIMULANT 482
Extra Strength Bayer Back & Body Pain - See
ASPIRIN 152
CAFFEINE 216

Extra Strength Bayer PM - See ASPIRIN 152
Extra Strength Gas-X - See SIMETHICONE 748
Extra Strength Maalox Anti-Gas - See SIMETHICONE 748
Extra Strength Maalox GRF Gas Relief Formula - See SIMETHICONE 748
Eye Lube - See PROTECTANT (Ophthalmic) 690
EZ III - See NARCOTIC ANALGESICS & ACETAMINOPHEN 586
EZETIMIBE 380
Ezol - See
ACETAMINOPHEN 8
BARBITURATES 168

F

Fabior - See RETINOIDS (Topical) 722
Factive - See FLUOROQUINOLONES 392
FACTOR Xa INHIBITORS 382
FAMCICLOVIR - See ANTIVIRALS FOR HERPES VIRUS 136
FAMOTIDINE - See HISTAMINE H_2 RECEPTOR ANTAGONISTS 422
Famvir - See ANTIVIRALS FOR HERPES VIRUS 136
Fanapt - See SEROTONIN-DOPAMINE ANTAGONISTS 744
Fansidar - See SULFADOXINE & PYRIMETHAMINE 760
Fareston - See TOREMIFENE 806
Fasprin - See ASPIRIN 152
Fast-Max DM Adult Liquid- See
DEXTROMETHORPHAN 312
GUAIFENESIN 416
Father John's Medicine Plus - See
ANTIHISTAMINES 106
DEXTROMETHORPHAN 312
GUAIFENESIN 416
PHENYLEPHRINE 658
FazaClo - See CLOZAPINE 264
FBM - See FELBAMATE 384
Febridyne - See ACETAMINOPHEN 8
FEBUXOSTAT - See ANTIGOUT DRUGS 104
Fedahist - See
ANTIHISTAMINES 106
PSEUDOEPHEDRINE 694
Fedahist Decongestant - See
ANTIHISTAMINES 106
PSEUDOEPHEDRINE 694
Fedahist Expectorant - See
GUAIFENESIN 416
PSEUDOEPHEDRINE 694
Fedahist Expectorant Pediatric Drops - See
GUAIFENESIN 416
PSEUDOEPHEDRINE 694
Fedahist Gyrocaps - See
ANTIHISTAMINES 106
PSEUDOEPHEDRINE 694
Fedahist Timecaps - See
ANTIHISTAMINES 106
PSEUDOEPHEDRINE 694
Feen-a-Mint - See
LAXATIVES, SOFTENER/LUBRICANT 480
LAXATIVES, STIMULANT 482
Feen-a-Mint Gum - See LAXATIVES, STIMULANT 482
Feen-a-Mint Pills - See
LAXATIVES, SOFTENER/LUBRICANT 480
LAXATIVES, STIMULANT 482
FELBAMATE 384
Felbatol - See FELBAMATE 384
Feldene - See ANTI-INFLAMMATORY DRUGS, NONSTEROIDAL (NSAIDs) 116
Feldene Melt - See ANTI-INFLAMMATORY DRUGS, NONSTEROIDAL (NSAIDs) 116
FELODIPINE - See CALCIUM CHANNEL BLOCKERS 220
Female sex hormone - See CONTRACEPTIVES, ORAL & SKIN 278
Female sex hormone (Estrogen) - See ESTROGENS 372
Female sex hormone (Progestin) - See PROGESTINS 680
FemCare - See ANTIFUNGALS (Vaginal) 90
Femcet - See
ACETAMINOPHEN 8
BARBITURATES 168
Femcon Fe - See CONTRACEPTIVES, ORAL & SKIN 278
Femhrt - See
ESTROGENS 372
PROGESTINS 680
Femilax - See
LAXATIVES, SOFTENER/LUBRICANT 480
LAXATIVES, STIMULANT 482
Femiron - See IRON SUPPLEMENTS 458
Femizole Prefil - See ANTIFUNGALS (Vaginal) 90
Femizole-7 - See ANTIFUNGALS (Vaginal) 90
Femogex - See ESTROGENS 372
Femring - See ESTROGENS 372
Femstat 3 - See ANTIFUNGALS (Vaginal) 90
Femtrace - See ESTROGENS 372
Fenesin - See GUAIFENESIN 416
Fenicol Ophthalmic Ointment - See ANTIBACTERIALS (Ophthalmic) 66
FENOFIBRATE - See FIBRATES 386
FENOFIBRIC ACID - See FIBRATES 386
Fenoglide - See FIBRATES 386
FENOPROFEN - See ANTI-INFLAMMATORY DRUGS, NONSTEROIDAL (NSAIDs) 116

Fenopron - See ANTI-INFLAMMATORY DRUGS, NONSTEROIDAL (NSAIDs) 116
FENOTEROL - See BRONCHODILATORS, ADRENERGIC 200
FENTANYL - See NARCOTIC ANALGESICS 584
Fentora - See NARCOTIC ANALGESICS 584
Fenylhist - See ANTIHISTAMINES 106
Feosol - See IRON SUPPLEMENTS 458
Feosol Caplets - See IRON SUPPLEMENTS 458
Feostat - See IRON SUPPLEMENTS 458
Feostat Drops - See IRON SUPPLEMENTS 458
Fergon - See IRON SUPPLEMENTS 458
Fer-In-Sol - See IRON SUPPLEMENTS 458
Fer-In-Sol Drops - See IRON SUPPLEMENTS 458
Fer-In-Sol Syrup - See IRON SUPPLEMENTS 458
Fer-Iron - See IRON SUPPLEMENTS 458
Fero-folic 500 - See IRON SUPPLEMENTS 458
Fero-Grad - See IRON SUPPLEMENTS 458
Fero-Gradumet - See IRON SUPPLEMENTS 458
FerraCap - See IRON SUPPLEMENTS 458
Ferralet - See IRON SUPPLEMENTS 458
Ferralet 90 - See IRON SUPPLEMENTS 458
Ferralyn - See IRON SUPPLEMENTS 458
Ferra-TD - See IRON SUPPLEMENTS 458
FERROUS FUMARATE - See IRON SUPPLEMENTS 458
FERROUS GLUCONATE - See IRON SUPPLEMENTS 458
FERROUS SULFATE - See IRON SUPPLEMENTS 458
Fertinic - See IRON SUPPLEMENTS 458
FESOTERODINE - See MUSCARINIC RECEPTOR ANTAGONISTS 574
Feverall Children's - See ACETAMINOPHEN 8
Feverall Infants' - See ACETAMINOPHEN 8
Feverall Junior Strength - See ACETAMINOPHEN 8
Feverall Sprinkle Caps - See ACETAMINOPHEN 8
Fever reducer - See
ACETAMINOPHEN 8
ANTI-INFLAMMATORY DRUGS, NONSTEROIDAL (NSAIDs) 116
ANTI-INFLAMMATORY DRUGS, NONSTEROIDAL (NSAIDs) COX-2 INHIBITORS 118
NARCOTIC ANALGESICS & ACETAMINOPHEN 586
FEXOFENADINE - See ANTIHISTAMINES, NONSEDATING 110
Fiberall - See LAXATIVES, BULK-FORMING 476
Fibercon - See LAXATIVES, BULK-FORMING 476
FiberNorm - See LAXATIVES, BULK-FORMING 476
Fiberpur - See LAXATIVES, BULK-FORMING 476
<u>FIBRATES</u> 386
Fibricor - See FIBRATES 386
FIDAXOMICIN - See MACROLIDE ANTIBIOTICS 518
Finac - See KERATOLYTICS 470
Finacea - See AZELAIC ACID 164
FINASTERIDE - See 5-ALPHA REDUCTASE INHIBITORS 2
Finevin - See AZELAIC ACID 164
Fiorgen PF - See
ASPIRIN 152
BARBITURATES 168
Fiorgen with Codeine - See BARBITURATES, ASPIRIN & CODEINE (Also contains caffeine) 170
Fioricet - See
ACETAMINOPHEN 8
BARBITURATES 168
Fiorinal - See
ASPIRIN 152
BARBITURATES 168
CAFFEINE 216
Fiorinal with Codeine - See BARBITURATES, ASPIRIN & CODEINE (Also contains caffeine) 170
Fiorinal with Codeine No. 3 - See BARBITURATES, ASPIRIN & CODEINE (Also contains caffeine) 170
Fiorinal-C1/4 - See BARBITURATES, ASPIRIN & CODEINE (Also contains caffeine) 170
Fiorinal-C1/2 - See BARBITURATES, ASPIRIN & CODEINE (Also contains caffeine) 170
Fiormor - See
ASPIRIN 152
BARBITURATES 168
Fiormor with Codeine - See BARBITURATES, ASPIRIN & CODEINE (Also contains caffeine) 170
Fivent - See CROMOLYN 282
Flagyl - See NITROIMIDAZOLES 606
Flamazine - See ANTIBACTERIALS, ANTIFUNGALS (Topical) 62
Flarex - See ANTI-INFLAMMATORY DRUGS, STEROIDAL (Ophthalmic) 122
Flatulex - See SIMETHICONE 748
Flavorcee - See VITAMIN C (Ascorbic Acid) 838
<u>FLAVOXATE</u> 388

FLECAINIDE ACETATE 390
Flector Patch - See DICLOFENAC (Topical) 314
Fleet Bisacodyl - See LAXATIVES, STIMULANT 482
Fleet Bisacodyl Prep - See LAXATIVES, STIMULANT 482
Fleet Enema Mineral Oil - See LAXATIVES, SOFTENER/LUBRICANT 480
Fleet Flavored Castor Oil - See LAXATIVES, STIMULANT 482
Fleet Laxative - See LAXATIVES, STIMULANT 482
Fleet Pedia-Lax Childrens Liquid Stool Softener - See LAXATIVES, SOFTENER/LUBRICANT 480
Fleet Pedia Lax Liquid Gels - See LAXATIVES, OSMOTIC 478
Fleet Phospho-Soda - See LAXATIVES, OSMOTIC 478
Fleet Relief - See ANESTHETICS (Rectal) 38
Fletcher's Castoria - See LAXATIVES, STIMULANT 482
Flexagin - See ORPHENADRINE 624
Flexain - See ORPHENADRINE 624
Flexeril - See CYCLOBENZAPRINE 286
Flexoject - See ORPHENADRINE 624
Flexon - See ORPHENADRINE 624
Flint SSD - See ANTIBACTERIALS, ANTIFUNGALS (Topical) 62
FLOCTAFENINE - See ANTI-INFLAMMATORY DRUGS, NONSTEROIDAL (NSAIDs) 116
Flomax - See ALPHA ADRENERGIC RECEPTOR BLOCKERS 20
Flonase - See ADRENOCORTICOIDS (Nasal Inhalation) 12
Flo-Pred - See ADRENOCORTICOIDS (Systemic) 16
Florinef - See ADRENOCORTICOIDS (Systemic) 16
Flovent - See ADRENOCORTICOIDS (Oral Inhalation) 14
Flovent HFA - See ADRENOCORTICOIDS (Oral Inhalation) 14
Floxin - See FLUOROQUINOLONES 392
Floxin Otic - See ANTIBACTERIALS (Otic) 68
Fluclox - See PENICILLINS 646
FLUCLOXACILLIN - See PENICILLINS 646
FLUCONAZOLE - See
ANTIFUNGALS, AZOLES 86
ANTIFUNGALS (Topical) 88
FLUDROCORTISONEt - See ADRENOCORTICOIDS (Systemic) 16
Fludroxycortide - See ADRENOCORTICOIDS (Topical) 18
Flumadine - See ANTIVIRALS FOR INFLUENZA 138
FLUMETHASONE (Topical) - See ADRENOCORTICOIDS (Topical) 18
FLUNARIZINE - See CALCIUM CHANNEL BLOCKERS 220
Fluocet - See ADRENOCORTICOIDS (Topical) 18
Fluocin - See ADRENOCORTICOIDS (Topical) 18
FLUOCINOLONE (Topical) - See ADRENOCORTICOIDS (Topical) 18
FLUOCINONIDE (Topical) - See ADRENOCORTICOIDS (Topical) 18
Fluoderm - See ADRENOCORTICOIDS (Topical) 18
Fluolar - See ADRENOCORTICOIDS (Topical) 18
Fluonid - See ADRENOCORTICOIDS (Topical) 18
Fluonide - See ADRENOCORTICOIDS (Topical) 18
FLUOROMETHOLONE - See ANTI-INFLAMMATORY DRUGS, STEROIDAL (Ophthalmic) 122
Fluor-Op - See ANTI-INFLAMMATORY DRUGS, STEROIDAL (Ophthalmic) 122
Fluoroplex - See FLUOROURACIL (Topical) 394
FLUOROQUINOLONES 392
FLUOROURACIL (Topical) 394
FLUOXETINE - See SELECTIVE SEROTONIN REUPTAKE INHIBITORS (SSRIs) 742
FLUOXYMESTERONE - See ANDROGENS 34
FLUPHENAZINE - See PHENOTHIAZINES 656
FLURANDRENOLIDE (Topical) - See ADRENOCORTICOIDS (Topical) 18
FLURAZEPAM - See BENZODIAZEPINES 176
FLURBIPROFEN - See
ANTI-INFLAMMATORY DRUGS, NONSTEROIDAL (NSAIDs) 116
ANTI-INFLAMMATORY DRUGS, NONSTEROIDAL (NSAIDs) (Ophthalmic) 120
Flurosyn - See ADRENOCORTICOIDS (Topical) 18
FLUTAMIDE - See ANTIANDROGENS, NONSTEROIDAL 58
Flutex - See ADRENOCORTICOIDS (Topical) 18
FLUTICASONE - See ADRENOCORTICOIDS (Topical) 18
FLUTICASONE (Nasal) - See ADRENOCORTICOIDS (Nasal Inhalation) 12
FLUTICASONE (Oral Inhalation) - See ADRENOCORTICOIDS (Oral Inhalation) 14
FLUVASTATIN - See HMG-CoA REDUCTASE INHIBITORS 424
FLUVOXAMINE - See SELECTIVE SEROTONIN REUPTAKE INHIBITORS (SSRIs) 742

Fluxid - See HISTAMINE H_2 RECEPTOR ANTAGONISTS 422
FML Forte - See ANTI-INFLAMMATORY DRUGS, STEROIDAL (Ophthalmic) 122
FML Liquifilm - See ANTI-INFLAMMATORY DRUGS, STEROIDAL (Ophthalmic) 122
FML S.O.P. - See ANTI-INFLAMMATORY DRUGS, STEROIDAL (Ophthalmic) 122
Foamicon - See ANTACIDS 48
Focalin - See STIMULANT MEDICATIONS 754
Focalin XR - See STIMULANT MEDICATIONS 754
Foille - See ANTIBACTERIALS (Topical) 70
Foille Cort - See ADRENOCORTICOIDS (Topical) 18
Foldan - See ANTHELMINTICS 50
Folex - See METHOTREXATE 548
Folex PFS - See METHOTREXATE 548
FOLIC ACID (Vitamin B-9) 396
Folinic Acid - See LEUCOVORIN 486
Folvite - See FOLIC ACID (Vitamin B-9) 396
Foradil Aerolizer - See BRONCHODILATORS, ADRENERGIC 200
Foradil Certihaler - See BRONCHODILATORS, ADRENERGIC 200
Forfivo XL - See BUPROPION 208
FORMOTEROL - See BRONCHODILATORS, ADRENERGIC 200
Fortabs - See
ASPIRIN 152
BARBITURATES 168
Fortamet - See METFORMIN 544
Forteo - See BONE FORMATION AGENTS 194
Fortesta - See ANDROGENS 34
Fortical - See CALCITONIN 218
Fortral - See NARCOTIC ANALGESICS 584
Forulex - See DICYCLOMINE 316
Fosamax - See BISPHOSPHONATES 192
Fosamax Plus D - See
BISPHOSPHONATES 192
VITAMIN D 840
FOSAMPRENAVIR - See PROTEASE INHIBITORS 688
Fosavance - See
BISPHOSPHONATES 192
VITAMIN D 840
FOSINOPRIL - See ANGIOTENSIN-CONVERTING ENZYME (ACE) INHIBITORS 44
Fostex 5 Gel - See BENZOYL PEROXIDE 178
Fostex 10 Bar - See BENZOYL PEROXIDE 178
Fostex 10 Cream - See BENZOYL PEROXIDE 178
Fostex 10 Gel - See BENZOYL PEROXIDE 178
Fostex 10 Wash - See BENZOYL PEROXIDE 178
Fostex CM - See KERATOLYTICS 470
Fostex Medicated Cleansing Bar - See KERATOLYTICS 470
Fostex Medicated Cleansing Cream - See KERATOLYTICS 470
Fostex Medicated Cleansing Liquid - See KERATOLYTICS 470
Fostex Regular Strength Medicated Cleansing Bar - See KERATOLYTICS 470
Fostex Regular Strength Medicated Cleansing Cream - See KERATOLYTICS 470
Fostex Regular Strength Medicated Cover-Up - See KERATOLYTICS 470
Fostril Cream - See KERATOLYTICS 470
Fostril Lotion - See KERATOLYTICS 470
Fototar - See COAL TAR (Topical) 266
Fowlers Diarrhea Tablets - See ATTAPULGITE 160
Freezone - See KERATOLYTICS 470
Froben - See ANTI-INFLAMMATORY DRUGS, NONSTEROIDAL (NSAIDs) 116
Froben SR - See ANTI-INFLAMMATORY DRUGS, NONSTEROIDAL (NSAIDs) 116
Frova - See TRIPTANS 820
FROVATRIPTAN - See TRIPTANS 820
Fulvicin P/G - See GRISEOFULVIN 414
Fulvicin U/F - See GRISEOFULVIN 414
Fungizone - See ANTIFUNGALS (Topical) 88
Furadantin - See NITROFURANTOIN 604
Furalan - See NITROFURANTOIN 604
Furaloid - See NITROFURANTOIN 604
Furan - See NITROFURANTOIN 604
Furanite - See NITROFURANTOIN 604
Furantoin - See NITROFURANTOIN 604
Furatine - See NITROFURANTOIN 604
Furaton - See NITROFURANTOIN 604
FURAZOLIDONE 398
FUROSEMIDE - See DIURETICS, LOOP 332
Furoside - See DIURETICS, LOOP 332
Furoxone - See FURAZOLIDONE 398
Furoxone Liquid - See FURAZOLIDONE 398
FUSION INHIBITOR 400
Fusion inhibitor - See FUSION INHIBITOR 400
Fuzeon - See FUSION INHIBITOR 400
Fynex - See ANTIHISTAMINES 106

G

G-1 - See BARBITURATES 168
GABAPENTIN 402
Gabitril - See TIAGABINE 794
GALANTAMINE - See CHOLINESTERASE INHIBITORS 250
Galzin - See ZINC SUPPLEMENTS 854
GANCICLOVIR - See ANTIVIRALS FOR HERPES VIRUS 136

GANCICLOVIR (Ophthalmic) - See ANTIVIRALS (Ophthalmic) 142
Gantanol - See SULFONAMIDES 766
Gantrisin - See
ANTIBACTERIALS (Ophthalmic) 66
SULFONAMIDES 766
Garamycin - See
ANTIBACTERIALS (Ophthalmic) 66
ANTIBACTERIALS (Topical) 70
Gas Aid - See SIMETHICONE 748
Gas Relief - See SIMETHICONE 748
Gastrocrom - See CROMOLYN 282
Gastrointestinal selective receptor agonist - See TEGASEROD 776
Gastrosed - See HYOSCYAMINE 438
Gastrozepin - See ANTICHOLINERGICS 72
Gas-X - See SIMETHICONE 748
Gas-X Extra Strength - See SIMETHICONE 748
Gas-X Thin Strips - See SIMETHICONE 748
Gas-X with Maalox - See
ANTACIDS 48
SIMETHICONE 748
GATIFLOXACIN (Ophthalmic) - See ANTIBACTERIALS (Ophthalmic) 66
Gaviscon - See ANTACIDS 48
Gaviscon Extra Strength Relief Formula - See ANTACIDS 48
Gaviscon-2 - See ANTACIDS 48
GBH - See PEDICULICIDES (Topical) 642
Gee-Gee - See GUAIFENESIN 416
Gelnique - See MUSCARINIC RECEPTOR ANTAGONISTS 574
Gelpirin - See
ACETAMINOPHEN 8
ASPIRIN 152
Gelusil - See
ANTACIDS 48
SIMETHICONE 748
Gelusil Extra-Strength - See ANTACIDS 48
GEMFIBROZIL 404
GEMIFLOXACIN - See FLUOROQUINOLONES 392
Gemnisyn - See
ACETAMINOPHEN 8
ASPIRIN 152
Gemonil - See BARBITURATES 168
Genabid - See PAPAVERINE 638
Genahist - See ANTIHISTAMINES 106
Genalac - See ANTACIDS 48
GenAllerate - See ANTIHISTAMINES 106
Genapap - See ACETAMINOPHEN 8
Genapap Children's Elixir - See ACETAMINOPHEN 8
Genapap Children's Tablets - See ACETAMINOPHEN 8
Genapap Extra Strength - See ACETAMINOPHEN 8
Genapap Infants' - See ACETAMINOPHEN 8
Genapap Regular Strength Tablets - See ACETAMINOPHEN 8
Genapax - See ANTIFUNGALS (Vaginal) 90
Genaphed - See PSEUDOEPHEDRINE 694
Genaspore Cream - See ANTIFUNGALS (Topical) 88
Genasyme - See SIMETHICONE 748
Genaton - See ANTACIDS 48
Genaton Extra Strength - See ANTACIDS 48
Genatuss - See GUAIFENESIN 416
Genatuss DM - See
DEXTROMETHORPHAN 312
GUAIFENESIN 416
Gencalc 600 - See CALCIUM SUPPLEMENTS 222
GenCept 0.5/35 - See CONTRACEPTIVES, ORAL & SKIN 278
GenCept 1/35 - See CONTRACEPTIVES, ORAL & SKIN 278
GenCept 10/11 - See CONTRACEPTIVES, ORAL & SKIN 278
Gendecon - See
ACETAMINOPHEN 8
ANTIHISTAMINES 106
PHENYLEPHRINE 658
Gen-D-phen - See
ACETAMINOPHEN 8
ANTIHISTAMINES 106
Genebs - See ACETAMINOPHEN 8
Genebs Extra Strength - See ACETAMINOPHEN 8
Genebs Regular Strength Tablets - See ACETAMINOPHEN 8
Generess Fe - See
CONTRACEPTIVES, ORAL & SKIN 278
IRON SUPPLEMENTS 458
Generlac - See LAXATIVES, OSMOTIC 478
Gen-Glybe - See SULFONYLUREAS 770
Gengraf- See CYCLOSPORINE 296
Gen-K - See POTASSIUM SUPPLEMENTS 666
Genoptic - See ANTIBACTERIALS (Ophthalmic) 66
Genora 0.5/35 - See CONTRACEPTIVES, ORAL & SKIN 278
Genora 1/35 - See CONTRACEPTIVES, ORAL & SKIN 278
Genora 1/50 - See CONTRACEPTIVES, ORAL & SKIN 278
Genpril - See ANTI-INFLAMMATORY DRUGS, NONSTEROIDAL (NSAIDs) 116
Genpril Caplets - See ANTI-INFLAMMATORY DRUGS, NONSTEROIDAL (NSAIDs) 116

Gen-Selegiline - See MONOAMINE OXIDASE TYPE B (MAO-B) INHIBITORS 572
Gentacidin - See ANTIBACTERIALS (Ophthalmic) 66
Gentafair - See ANTIBACTERIALS (Ophthalmic) 66
Gentak - See ANTIBACTERIALS (Ophthalmic) 66
Gentamar - See ANTIBACTERIALS (Topical) 70
GENTAMICIN - See ANTIBACTERIALS (Topical) 70
GENTAMICIN (Ophthalmic) - See ANTIBACTERIALS (Ophthalmic) 66
Gentasol - See ANTIBACTERIALS (Ophthalmic) 66
GENTIAN VIOLET - See ANTIFUNGALS (Vaginal) 90
Gen-Timolol - See ANTIGLAUCOMA, BETA BLOCKERS 96
Gentlax-S - See
LAXATIVES, SOFTENER/LUBRICANT 480
LAXATIVES, STIMULANT 482
Gentle Nature - See LAXATIVES, STIMULANT 482
Gentrasul - See ANTIBACTERIALS (Ophthalmic) 66
Geodon - See ZIPRASIDONE 856
Geopen Oral - See PENICILLINS 646
Geridium - See PHENAZOPYRIDINE 654
Gerimal - See ERGOLOID MESYLATES 362
Gesterol 50 - See PROGESTINS 680
Gesterol L.A. - See PROGESTINS 680
GG-CEN - See GUAIFENESIN 416
Giazo - See SALICYLATES 736
Glaucon - See ANTIGLAUCOMA, ADRENERGIC AGONISTS 92
Gleevec - See IMATINIB 440
GLIMEPIRIDE - See SULFONYLUREAS 770
GLIPIZIDE - See SULFONYLUREAS 770
Glo-Sel - See ANTISEBORRHEICS (Topical) 132
GLP-1 RECEPTOR AGONISTS 406
GLUCAGON 408
Glucagon for Injection - See GLUCAGON 408
Glucamide - See SULFONYLUREAS 770
Glucophage - See METFORMIN 544
Glucophage XR - See METFORMIN 544
Glucotrol - See SULFONYLUREAS 770
Glucotrol XL - See SULFONYLUREAS 770
Glucovance - See
METFORMIN 544
SULFONYLUREAS 770
Glu-K - See POTASSIUM SUPPLEMENTS 666
Glumetza - See METFORMIN 544
Glyate - See GUAIFENESIN 416
GLYBURIDE - See SULFONYLUREAS 770
Glycate - See ANTACIDS 48
GLYCERIN - See LAXATIVES, OSMOTIC 478
Glyceryl T - See
BRONCHODILATORS, XANTHINE 204
GUAIFENESIN 416
Glyceryl Trinitrate - See NITRATES 602
GLYCOPYRROLATE 410
Gly-Cort - See ADRENOCORTICOIDS (Topical) 18
Glycotuss - See GUAIFENESIN 416
Glycotuss-dM - See
DEXTROMETHORPHAN 312
GUAIFENESIN 416
Glydeine Cough - See
GUAIFENESIN 416
NARCOTIC ANALGESICS 584
Glynase PresTab - See SULFONYLUREAS 770
Glysennid - See LAXATIVES, STIMULANT 482
Glyset - See MIGLITOL 558
Glytuss - See GUAIFENESIN 416
G-Myticin Antibiotic - See ANTIBACTERIALS (Topical) 70
Gold compounds - See GOLD COMPOUNDS 412
GOLD COMPOUNDS 412
GOLD SODIUM THIOMALATE - See GOLD COMPOUNDS 412
GOLIMUMAB - See TUMOR NECROSIS FACTOR BLOCKERS 822
Gonad stimulant - See CLOMIPHENE 260
Gonadotropin inhibitor - See
DANAZOL 300
NAFARELIN 580
Gonak - See PROTECTANT (Ophthalmic) 690
Goniosoft - See PROTECTANT (Ophthalmic) 690
Goniosol - See PROTECTANT (Ophthalmic) 690
Goody's Extra Strength Tablet - See
ACETAMINOPHEN 8
ASPIRIN 152
Goody's Headache Powders - See
ACETAMINOPHEN 8
ASPIRIN 152
Gordochom Solution - See ANTIFUNGALS (Topical) 88
Gordofilm - See KERATOLYTICS 470
Gralise - See GABAPENTIN 402
Gramcal - See CALCIUM SUPPLEMENTS 222
Gravol - See ANTIHISTAMINES 106
Gravol L/A - See ANTIHISTAMINES 106
Grifulvin V - See GRISEOFULVIN 414
Grisactin - See GRISEOFULVIN 414
Grisactin Ultra - See GRISEOFULVIN 414
GRISEOFULVIN 414
Grisovin-FP - See GRISEOFULVIN 414
Gris-PEG - See GRISEOFULVIN 414

Guaifed - See
GUAIFENESIN 416
PSEUDOEPHEDRINE 694
Guaifed-PD - See
GUAIFENESIN 416
PSEUDOEPHEDRINE 694
GUAIFENESIN 416
GuaiMAX-D - See
GUAIFENESIN 416
PSEUDOEPHEDRINE 694
GUANABENZ - See CENTRAL ALPHA AGONISTS 234
GUANADREL 418
GUANFACINE - See CENTRAL ALPHA AGONISTS 234
Guanylate cyclase-C agonist - See LINACLOTIDE 498
Guanylate cyclase-C agonist - See LINACLOTIDE 498
Guiamid D.M. Liquid - See
DEXTROMETHORPHAN 312
GUAIFENESIN 416
Guiatuss A.C. - See
GUAIFENESIN 416
NARCOTIC ANALGESICS 584
Guiatuss PE - See
GUAIFENESIN 416
PSEUDOEPHEDRINE 694
Guiatuss-DM - See
DEXTROMETHORPHAN 312
GUAIFENESIN 416
G-Well - See PEDICULICIDES (Topical) 642
Gynazole-1 - See ANTIFUNGALS (Vaginal) 90
Gynecort - See ADRENOCORTICOIDS (Topical) 18
Gynecort 10 - See ADRENOCORTICOIDS (Topical) 18
Gyne-Lotrimin - See ANTIFUNGALS (Vaginal) 90
Gyne-Lotrimin 3 - See ANTIFUNGALS (Vaginal) 90
Gyno-Trosyd - See ANTIFUNGALS (Vaginal) 90
Gynogen L.A. 20 - See ESTROGENS 372
Gynogen L.A. 40 - See ESTROGENS 372
Gynol II Extra Strength - See CONTRACEPTIVES, VAGINAL 280
Gynol II Original Formula - See CONTRACEPTIVES, VAGINAL 280

H

H_2Oxyl 2.5 Gel - See BENZOYL PEROXIDE 178
H_2Oxyl 5 Gel - See BENZOYL PEROXIDE 178
H_2Oxyl 10 Gel - See BENZOYL PEROXIDE 178
Habitrol - See NICOTINE 598
Hair growth stimulant - See
ANTHRALIN (Topical) 52
MINOXIDIL (Topical) 562
HALAZEPAM - See BENZODIAZEPINES 176
Halciderm - See ADRENOCORTICOIDS (Topical) 18
HALCINONIDE (Topical) - See ADRENOCORTICOIDS (Topical) 18
Halcion - See TRIAZOLAM 812
Haldol - See HALOPERIDOL 420
Haldol Decanoate - See HALOPERIDOL 420
Haldol LA - See HALOPERIDOL 420
Halenol - See ACETAMINOPHEN 8
Halenol Extra Strength - See ACETAMINOPHEN 8
Halfan - See ANTIMALARIAL 126
Halfprin - See ASPIRIN 152
HALOBETASOL - See ADRENOCORTICOIDS (Topical) 18
HALOFANTRINE - See ANTIMALARIAL 126
Halog - See ADRENOCORTICOIDS (Topical) 18
Halog E - See ADRENOCORTICOIDS (Topical) 18
HALOPERIDOL 420
HALOPROGIN - See ANTIFUNGALS (Topical) 88
Halotestin - See ANDROGENS 34
Halotex - See ANTIFUNGALS (Topical) 88
Halotussin - See GUAIFENESIN 416
Halotussin-DM Expectorant - See
DEXTROMETHORPHAN 312
GUAIFENESIN 416
Halperon - See HALOPERIDOL 420
Haltran - See ANTI-INFLAMMATORY DRUGS, NONSTEROIDAL (NSAIDs) 116
Harmonyl - See RAUWOLFIA ALKALOIDS 714
Hayfebrol - See
ANTIHISTAMINES 106
PSEUDOEPHEDRINE 694
Hayley's M-O - See LAXATIVES, OSMOTIC 478
Head & Shoulders - See ANTISEBORRHEICS (Topical) 132
Head & Shoulders Antidandruff Cream Shampoo Normal to Dry Formula - See ANTISEBORRHEICS (Topical) 132
Head & Shoulders Antidandruff Cream Shampoo Normal to Oily Formula - See ANTISEBORRHEICS (Topical) 132
Head & Shoulders Antidandruff Lotion Shampoo 2 in 1 Formula - See ANTISEBORRHEICS (Topical) 132
Head & Shoulders Antidandruff Lotion Shampoo Normal to Dry Formula - See ANTISEBORRHEICS (Topical) 132

Head & Shoulders Antidandruff Lotion Shampoo Normal to Oily Formula - See ANTISEBORRHEICS (Topical) 132
Head & Shoulders Dry Scalp 2 in 1 Formula Lotion Shampoo - See ANTISEBORRHEICS (Topical) 132
Head & Shoulders Dry Scalp Conditioning Formula Lotion Shampoo - See ANTISEBORRHEICS (Topical) 132
Head & Shoulders Dry Scalp Regular Formula Lotion Shampoo - See ANTISEBORRHEICS (Topical) 132
Head & Shoulders Intensive Treatment 2 in 1 Formula Dandruff Lotion Shampoo - See ANTISEBORRHEICS (Topical) 132
Head & Shoulders Intensive Treatment Conditioning Formula Dandruff Lotion Shampoo - See ANTISEBORRHEICS (Topical) 132
Head & Shoulders Intensive Treatment Regular Formula Dandruff Lotion Shampoo - See ANTISEBORRHEICS (Topical) 132
Headstart - See ASPIRIN 152
HealthyLax - See LAXATIVES, OSMOTIC 478
Hectorol - See VITAMIN D 840
Helidac - See
BISMUTH SALTS 190
NITROIMIDAZOLES 606
TETRACYCLINES 782
Helmex - See ANTHELMINTICS 50
Hemocyte - See IRON SUPPLEMENTS 458
Hemorheologic agent - See PENTOXIFYLLINE 652
Hemril-HC - See HYDROCORTISONE (Rectal) 430
Hepahydrin - See LAXATIVES, STIMULANT 482
Heptalac - See LAXATIVES, OSMOTIC 478
Heptogesic - See
ASPIRIN 152
MEPROBAMATE 538
Herbal Laxative - See LAXATIVES, STIMULANT 482
Herplex Eye Drops - See ANTIVIRALS (Ophthalmic) 142
Hexa-Betalin - See PYRIDOXINE (Vitamin B-6) 698
Hexadrol - See ADRENOCORTICOIDS (Systemic) 16
Hexalol - See ATROPINE, HYOSCYAMINE, METHENAMINE, METHYLENE BLUE, PHENYLSALICYLATE & BENZOIC ACID 158
Histafed C - See ANTIHISTAMINES 106
Hi-Cor 1.0 - See ADRENOCORTICOIDS (Topical) 18
Hi-Cor 2.5 - See ADRENOCORTICOIDS (Topical) 18
Hiprex - See METHENAMINE 546
Histagesic Modified - See
ACETAMINOPHEN 8
ANTIHISTAMINES 106
PHENYLEPHRINE 658
Histaject Modified - See ANTIHISTAMINES 106
Histalet - See
ANTIHISTAMINES 106
PSEUDOEPHEDRINE 694
Histalet X - See
GUAIFENESIN 416
PSEUDOEPHEDRINE 694
Histalet-DM - See
ANTIHISTAMINES 106
DEXTROMETHORPHAN 312
PSEUDOEPHEDRINE 694
Histamine H_2 antagonist - See HISTAMINE H_2 RECEPTOR ANTAGONISTS 422
HISTAMINE H_2 RECEPTOR ANTAGONISTS 422
Histantil - See ANTIHISTAMINES, PHENOTHIAZINE-DERIVATIVE 112
Histatab Plus - See
ANTIHISTAMINES 106
PHENYLEPHRINE 658
Histatan - See
ANTIHISTAMINES 106
PHENYLEPHRINE 658
Hista-Vent PSE- See
ANTICHOLINERGICS 72
ANTIHISTAMINES 106
PSEUDOEPHEDRINE 694
Histerone-50 - See ANDROGENS 34
Histerone-100 - See ANDROGENS 34
Histex I/E - See ANTIHISTAMINES 106
Histor-D - See
ANTIHISTAMINES 106
PHENYLEPHRINE 658
Histor-D Timecelles - See
ANTIHISTAMINES 106
PHENYLEPHRINE 658
HMG-CoA REDUCTASE INHIBITORS 424
HMS Liquifilm - See ANTI-INFLAMMATORY DRUGS, STEROIDAL (Ophthalmic) 122
Hold - See DEXTROMETHORPHAN 312
Homapin - See ANTICHOLINERGICS 72
HOMATROPINE - See ANTICHOLINERGICS 72
HOMATROPINE (Ophthalmic) - See CYCLOPLEGIC, MYDRIATIC (Ophthalmic) 292
Honvol - See ESTROGENS 372
Horizant - See GABAPENTIN 402
Hormone - See MELATONIN 530
Humalog - See INSULIN ANALOGS 448

Humalog Mix 50/50- See INSULIN ANALOGS 448
Humalog Mix 75/25 - See INSULIN ANALOGS 448
Humibid L.A. - See GUAIFENESIN 416
Humibid Sprinkle - See GUAIFENESIN 416
Humibid-DM Sprinkle - See
DEXTROMETHORPHAN 312
GUAIFENESIN 416
Humira - See TUMOR NECROSIS FACTOR BLOCKERS 822
Humorsol - See ANTIGLAUCOMA, ANTICHOLINESTERASES 94
Humulin BR - See INSULIN 446
Humulin L - See INSULIN 446
Humulin N - See INSULIN 446
Humulin R - See INSULIN 446
Humulin U - See INSULIN 446
Hurricaine - See ANESTHETICS (Mucosal-Local) 36
Hybolin Decanoate - See ANDROGENS 34
Hybolin-Improved - See ANDROGENS 34
Hycodan - See
ANTICHOLINERGICS 72
NARCOTIC ANALGESICS 584
Hycomed - See NARCOTIC ANALGESICS & ACETAMINOPHEN 586
Hycomine Compound - See
ACETAMINOPHEN 8
ANTIHISTAMINES 106
NARCOTIC ANALGESICS 584
PHENYLEPHRINE 658
Hycomine-S Pediatric - See
ANTIHISTAMINES 106
NARCOTIC ANALGESICS 584
PHENYLEPHRINE 658
Hyco-Pap - See NARCOTIC ANALGESICS & ACETAMINOPHEN 586
Hycotuss Expectorant - See
GUAIFENESIN 416
NARCOTIC ANALGESICS 584
Hydeltrasol - See ADRENOCORTICOIDS (Systemic) 16
Hydergine - See ERGOLOID MESYLATES 362
Hydergine LC - See ERGOLOID MESYLATES 362
Hyderm - See ADRENOCORTICOIDS (Topical) 18
HYDRALAZINE 426
HYDRALAZINE & HYDROCHLOROTHIAZIDE 428
Hydramine - See ANTIHISTAMINES 106
Hydramine Cough - See ANTIHISTAMINES 106
Hydramyn - See ANTIHISTAMINES 106
Hydrate - See ANTIHISTAMINES 106
Hydra-Zide - See HYDRALAZINE & HYDROCHLOROTHIAZIDE 428
Hydrea - See HYDROXYUREA 434
Hydrex - See DIURETICS, THIAZIDE 338
Hydril - See ANTIHISTAMINES 106
Hydrisalic - See KERATOLYTICS 470
Hydrocet - See NARCOTIC ANALGESICS & ACETAMINOPHEN 586
HYDROCHLOROTHIAZIDE - See DIURETICS, THIAZIDE 338
Hydrocil Instant - See LAXATIVES, BULK-FORMING 476
HYDROCODONE - See NARCOTIC ANALGESICS 584
HYDROCODONE & ACETAMINOPHEN - See NARCOTIC ANALGESICS & ACETAMINOPHEN 586
HYDROCODONE & ASPIRIN - See NARCOTIC ANALGESICS & ASPIRIN 588
HYDROCODONE & HOMATROPINE - See NARCOTIC ANALGESICS 584
Hydrocodone with APAP - See NARCOTIC ANALGESICS & ACETAMINOPHEN 586
HYDROCORTISONE (Cortisol) - See ADRENOCORTICOIDS (Systemic) 16
HYDROCORTISONE (Dental) - See ADRENOCORTICOIDS (Topical) 18
HYDROCORTISONE (Ophthalmic) - See ANTI-INFLAMMATORY DRUGS, STEROIDAL (Ophthalmic) 122
HYDROCORTISONE (Rectal) 430
HYDROCORTISONE (Topical) - See ADRENOCORTICOIDS (Topical) 18
Hydrocortone - See ADRENOCORTICOIDS (Systemic) 16
Hydro-D - See DIURETICS, THIAZIDE 338
HydroDIURIL - See DIURETICS, THIAZIDE 338
HYDROFLUMETHIAZIDE - See DIURETICS, THIAZIDE 338
Hydrogesic - See NARCOTIC ANALGESICS & ACETAMINOPHEN 586
Hydromet - See
ANTICHOLINERGICS 72
NARCOTIC ANALGESICS 584
HYDROMORPHONE - See NARCOTIC ANALGESICS 584
Hydromox - See DIURETICS, THIAZIDE 338
Hydropane - See
ANTICHOLINERGICS 72
NARCOTIC ANALGESICS 584
Hydropres - See
DIURETICS, THIAZIDE 338
RAUWOLFIA ALKALOIDS 714
Hydrostal IR - See NARCOTIC ANALGESICS 584

INDEX

Hydro-Tex - See ADRENOCORTICOIDS (Topical) 18
HYDROXOCOBALAMIN - See VITAMIN B-12 (Cyanocobalamin) 836
HYDROXYCHLOROQUINE 432
HYDROXYPROGESTERONE - See PROGESTINS 680
HYDROXYPROPYL CELLULOSE - See PROTECTANT (Ophthalmic) 690
HYDROXYPROPYL METHYLCELLULOSE - See PROTECTANT (Ophthalmic) 690
HYDROXYUREA 434
HYDROXYZINE 436
Hy/Gestrone - See PROGESTINS 680
Hygroton - See DIURETICS, THIAZIDE 338
Hylorel - See GUANADREL 418
Hylutin - See PROGESTINS 680
HYOSCYAMINE 438
HYOSCYAMINE & PHENOBARBITAL - See BELLADONNA ALKALOIDS & BARBITURATES 174
Hyosophen - See BELLADONNA ALKALOIDS & BARBITURATES 174
Hyperosmotic - See LAXATIVES, OSMOTIC 478
HY-PHEN - See NARCOTIC ANALGESICS & ACETAMINOPHEN 586
Hypnotic - See ZALEPLON 852
Hypopigmentation agent - See AZELAIC ACID 164
Hyprogest - See PROGESTINS 680
Hyrexin-50 - See ANTIHISTAMINES 106
Hytakerol - See VITAMIN D 840
Hytinic - See IRON SUPPLEMENTS 458
Hytone - See ADRENOCORTICOIDS (Topical) 18
Hytrin - See ALPHA ADRENERGIC RECEPTOR BLOCKERS 20
Hytuss - See GUAIFENESIN 416
Hytuss-2X - See GUAIFENESIN 416
Hyzaar - See
ANGIOTENSIN II RECEPTOR ANTAGONISTS 42
DIURETICS, THIAZIDE 338

I

IBANDRONATE - See BISPHOSPHONATES 192
Ibifon-600 Caplets - See ANTI-INFLAMMATORY DRUGS, NONSTEROIDAL (NSAIDs) 116
Ibren - See ANTI-INFLAMMATORY DRUGS, NONSTEROIDAL (NSAIDs) 116
Ibu - See ANTI-INFLAMMATORY DRUGS, NONSTEROIDAL (NSAIDs) 116
Ibu-4 - See ANTI-INFLAMMATORY DRUGS, NONSTEROIDAL (NSAIDs) 116
Ibu-6 - See ANTI-INFLAMMATORY DRUGS, NONSTEROIDAL (NSAIDs) 116
Ibu-8 - See ANTI-INFLAMMATORY DRUGS, NONSTEROIDAL (NSAIDs) 116
Ibu-200 - See ANTI-INFLAMMATORY DRUGS, NONSTEROIDAL (NSAIDs) 116
Ibudone - See
ANTI-INFLAMMATORY DRUGS, NONSTEROIDAL (NSAIDs) 116
NARCOTIC ANALGESICS 584
Ibumed - See ANTI-INFLAMMATORY DRUGS, NONSTEROIDAL (NSAIDs) 116
Ibuprin - See ANTI-INFLAMMATORY DRUGS, NONSTEROIDAL (NSAIDs) 116
Ibupro-600 - See ANTI-INFLAMMATORY DRUGS, NONSTEROIDAL (NSAIDs) 116
IBUPROFEN - See ANTI-INFLAMMATORY DRUGS, NONSTEROIDAL (NSAIDs) 116
Ibu-profen Cold & Sinus Caplets - See
ANTI-INFLAMMATORY DRUGS, NONSTEROIDAL (NSAIDs) 116
PSEUDOEPHEDRINE 694
Ibu-Tab - See ANTI-INFLAMMATORY DRUGS, NONSTEROIDAL (NSAIDs) 116
Ibutex - See ANTI-INFLAMMATORY DRUGS, NONSTEROIDAL (NSAIDs) 116
Icar - See IRON SUPPLEMENTS 458
I-Chlor Ophthalmic Solution - See ANTIBACTERIALS (Ophthalmic) 66
Idarac - See ANTI-INFLAMMATORY DRUGS, NONSTEROIDAL (NSAIDs) 116
Idenal with Codeine - See BARBITURATES, ASPIRIN & CODEINE (Also contains caffeine) 170
IDOXURIDINE - See ANTIVIRALS (Ophthalmic) 142
Ifen - See ANTI-INFLAMMATORY DRUGS, NONSTEROIDAL (NSAIDs) 116
I-Homatrine - See CYCLOPLEGIC, MYDRIATIC (Ophthalmic) 292
I-Homatropine - See CYCLOPLEGIC, MYDRIATIC (Ophthalmic) 292
Ilevro - See ANTI-INFLAMMATORY DRUGS, NONSTEROIDAL (NSAIDs) (Ophthalmic) 120
ILOPERIDONE - See SEROTONIN-DOPAMINE ANTAGONISTS 744
Ilosone - See ERYTHROMYCINS 368
Ilotycin - See
ANTIBACTERIALS (Ophthalmic) 66
ERYTHROMYCINS 368
IMATINIB 440
Imbrilon - See ANTI-INFLAMMATORY DRUGS, NONSTEROIDAL (NSAIDs) 116
IMDUR - See NITRATES 602

IMIPRAMINE - See ANTIDEPRESSANTS, TRICYCLIC 80
IMIQUIMOD - See CONDYLOMA ACUMINATUM AGENTS 276
Imitrex - See TRIPTANS 820
Imitrex Nasal Spray- See TRIPTANS 820
Immunosuppressant - See
ADRENOCORTICOIDS (Systemic) 16
AZATHIOPRINE 162
BIOLOGICS FOR PSORIASIS 188
BUSULFAN 212
CHLORAMBUCIL 240
CYCLOPHOSPHAMIDE 290
CYCLOSPORINE 296
IMMUNOSUPPRESSIVE AGENTS 442
MERCAPTOPURINE 540
IMMUNOSUPPRESSIVE AGENTS 442
Imodium - See LOPERAMIDE 508
Imodium A-D - See LOPERAMIDE 508
Imodium Advanced - See
LOPERAMIDE 508
SIMETHICONE 748
Imodium Multi-Symptom Relief - See
LOPERAMIDE 508
SIMETHICONE 748
Implanon - See PROGESTINS 680
Impotence therapy - See
ALPROSTADIL 22
ERECTILE DYSFUNCTION AGENTS 360
Impril - See ANTIDEPRESSANTS, TRICYCLIC 80
Imuran - See AZATHIOPRINE 162
I-Naphline - See DECONGESTANTS (Ophthalmic) 306
Incretin mimetic - See
DPP-4 INHIBITORS 348
GLP-1 RECEPTOR AGONISTS 406
INDACATEROL - See BRONCHODILATORS, ADRENERGIC 200
Indameth - See ANTI-INFLAMMATORY DRUGS, NONSTEROIDAL (NSAIDs) 116
INDAPAMIDE 444
Inderal - See BETA-ADRENERGIC BLOCKING AGENTS 182
Inderal LA - See BETA-ADRENERGIC BLOCKING AGENTS 182
Inderide - See BETA-ADRENERGIC BLOCKING AGENTS & THIAZIDE DIURETICS 184
Inderide LA - See BETA-ADRENERGIC BLOCKING AGENTS & THIAZIDE DIURETICS 184
INDINAVIR - See PROTEASE INHIBITORS 688
Indocid - See ANTI-INFLAMMATORY DRUGS, NONSTEROIDAL (NSAIDs) 116
Indocid Ophthalmic - See ANTI-INFLAMMATORY DRUGS, NONSTEROIDAL (NSAIDs) (Ophthalmic) 120
Indocin - See ANTI-INFLAMMATORY DRUGS, NONSTEROIDAL (NSAIDs) 116
Indocin SR - See ANTI-INFLAMMATORY DRUGS, NONSTEROIDAL (NSAIDs) 116
INDOMETHACIN - See
ANTI-INFLAMMATORY DRUGS, NONSTEROIDAL (NSAIDs) 116
Infants' Advil - See ANTI-INFLAMMATORY DRUGS, NONSTEROIDAL (NSAIDs) 116
Infants' Anacin-3 - See ACETAMINOPHEN 8
Infants' Apacet - See ACETAMINOPHEN 8
Infants' Genapap - See ACETAMINOPHEN 8
Infants' Panadol - See ACETAMINOPHEN 8
Infants' Tylenol - See ACETAMINOPHEN 8
Infants' Tylenol Suspension Drops - See ACETAMINOPHEN 8
Inflamase Forte - See ANTI-INFLAMMATORY DRUGS, STEROIDAL (Ophthalmic) 122
Inflamase-Mild - See ANTI-INFLAMMATORY DRUGS, STEROIDAL (Ophthalmic) 122
Inflammatory bowel disease suppressant - See OLSALAZINE 618
INFLIXIMAB - See TUMOR NECROSIS FACTOR BLOCKERS 822
INH - See ISONIAZID 460
Inova 8/2 ACT - See
BENZOYL PEROXIDE 178
KERATOLYTICS 470
Insomnal - See ANTIHISTAMINES 106
Inspire - See XYLOMETAZOLINE 850
Inspra - See EPLERENONE 358
Insta-Char - See CHARCOAL, ACTIVATED 238
INSULIN 446
INSULIN ANALOGS 448
INSULIN ASPART - See INSULIN ANALOGS 448
INSULIN DETEMIR - See INSULIN ANALOGS 448
INSULIN GLARGINE - See INSULIN ANALOGS 448
INSULIN GLULISINE - See INSULIN ANALOGS 448
INSULIN LISPRO - See INSULIN ANALOGS 448
INTEGRASE INHIBITORS 450
Intelence - See NON-NUCLEOSIDE REVERSE TRANSCRIPTASE INHIBITORS 608
Intermezzo - See ZOLPIDEM 858
INTERMITTENT CLAUDICATION AGENTS 452
Introvale - See CONTRACEPTIVES, ORAL & SKIN 278
Intuniv - See CENTRAL ALPHA AGONISTS 234

Invega - See SEROTONIN-DOPAMINE ANTAGONISTS 744
Invega Sustenna - See SEROTONIN-DOPAMINE ANTAGONISTS 744
Invirase - See PROTEASE INHIBITORS 688
IODOQUINOL 454
Ionamin - See APPETITE SUPPRESSANTS 146
Ionax Astringent Skin Cleanser Topical Solution - See KERATOLYTICS 470
Ionil Plus Shampoo - See KERATOLYTICS 470
Ionil Shampoo - See KERATOLYTICS 470
Ionil-T Plus - See COAL TAR (Topical) 266
Iopidine - See ANTIGLAUCOMA, ADRENERGIC AGONISTS 92
I-Pentolate - See CYCLOPENTOLATE (Ophthalmic) 288
I-Phrine - See PHENYLEPHRINE (Ophthalmic) 660
IPRATROPIUM 456
Iquix - See ANTIBACTERIALS (Ophthalmic) 66
IRBESARTAN - See ANGIOTENSIN II RECEPTOR ANTAGONISTS 42
Ircon - See IRON SUPPLEMENTS 458
IRON DEXTRAN - See IRON SUPPLEMENTS 458
IRON POLYSACCHARIDE - See IRON SUPPLEMENTS 458
IRON SORBITOL - See IRON SUPPLEMENTS 458
IRON SUPPLEMENTS 458
Isentress - See INTEGRASE INHIBITORS 450
ISMO - See NITRATES 602
Iso-Bid - See NITRATES 602
Isobutal - See
ASPIRIN 152
BARBITURATES 168
ISOCARBOXAZID - See MONOAMINE OXIDASE (MAO) INHIBITORS 570
Isocet - See BARBITURATES 168
Isolin - See
ASPIRIN 152
BARBITURATES 168
Isollyl Improved - See
ASPIRIN 152
BARBITURATES 168
Isollyl with Codeine - See BARBITURATES, ASPIRIN & CODEINE (Also contains caffeine) 170
Isonate - See NITRATES 602
ISONIAZID 460
Isopap - See
ACETAMINOPHEN 8
BARBITURATES 168
ISOPROPAMIDE - See ANTICHOLINERGICS 72
ISOPROPYL UNOPROSTONE - See ANTIGLAUCOMA, PROSTAGLANDINS 102
ISOPROTERENOL - See BRONCHODILATORS, ADRENERGIC 200
Isoptin - See CALCIUM CHANNEL BLOCKERS 220
Isoptin SR - See CALCIUM CHANNEL BLOCKERS 220
Isopto Alkaline - See PROTECTANT (Ophthalmic) 690
Isopto Atropine - See CYCLOPLEGIC, MYDRIATIC (Ophthalmic) 292
Isopto Carpine - See ANTIGLAUCOMA, CHOLINERGIC AGONISTS 100
Isopto Frin - See PHENYLEPHRINE (Ophthalmic) 660
Isopto Plain - See PROTECTANT (Ophthalmic) 690
Isopto Tears - See PROTECTANT (Ophthalmic) 690
Isorbid - See NITRATES 602
Isordil - See NITRATES 602
ISOSORBIDE DINITRATE - See NITRATES 602
ISOSORBIDE MONONITRATE - See NITRATES 602
Isotamine - See ISONIAZID 460
Isotrate - See NITRATES 602
ISOTRETINOIN 462
ISOXSUPRINE 464
ISRADIPINE - See CALCIUM CHANNEL BLOCKERS 220
Istalol - See ANTIGLAUCOMA, BETA BLOCKERS 96
I-Sulfacet - See ANTIBACTERIALS (Ophthalmic) 66
Isuprel - See BRONCHODILATORS, ADRENERGIC 200
Isuprel Glossets - See BRONCHODILATORS, ADRENERGIC 200
Isuprel Mistometer - See BRONCHODILATORS, ADRENERGIC 200
ITRACONAZOLE - See ANTIFUNGALS, AZOLES 86
I-Tropine - See CYCLOPLEGIC, MYDRIATIC (Ophthalmic) 292
IVERMECTIN - See ANTHELMINTICS 50
IVERMECTIN (Topical) - See PEDICULICIDES (Topical) 642

J

JAK (Janus kinase) inhibitor - See TOFACITINIB 802

Jalyn - See
5-ALPHA REDUCTASE INHIBITORS 2
ALPHA ADRENERGIC RECEPTOR BLOCKERS 20
Janumet - See
DPP-4 INHIBITORS 348
METFORMIN 544
Janumet XR - See
DPP-4 INHIBITORS 348
METFORMIN 544
Januvia - See DPP-4 INHIBITORS 348
Jectofer - See IRON SUPPLEMENTS 458
Jenest-28 - See CONTRACEPTIVES, ORAL & SKIN 278
Jenloga - See CENTRAL ALPHA AGONISTS 234
Jentadueto - See
DPP-4 INHIBITORS 348
METFORMIN 544
Junior Strength Advil - See ANTI-INFLAMMATORY DRUGS, NONSTEROIDAL (NSAIDs) 116
Junior Tylenol - See ACETAMINOPHEN 8
Just Tears - See PROTECTANT (Ophthalmic) 690
Juvisync - See
DPP-4 INHIBITORS 348
HMG-CoA REDUCTASE INHIBITORS 424

K

K-10 - See POTASSIUM SUPPLEMENTS 666
K+10 - See POTASSIUM SUPPLEMENTS 666
K+Care - See POTASSIUM SUPPLEMENTS 666
K+Care ET - See POTASSIUM SUPPLEMENTS 666
Kabolin - See ANDROGENS 34
Kadian - See NARCOTIC ANALGESICS 584
Kaletra - See PROTEASE INHIBITORS 688
Kalium Durules - See POTASSIUM SUPPLEMENTS 666
KANAMYCIN 466
Kantrex - See KANAMYCIN 466
Kaochlor - See POTASSIUM SUPPLEMENTS 666
Kaochlor S-F - See POTASSIUM SUPPLEMENTS 666
Kaochlor-10 - See POTASSIUM SUPPLEMENTS 666
Kaochlor-20 - See POTASSIUM SUPPLEMENTS 666
Kaochlor-Eff - See POTASSIUM SUPPLEMENTS 666
Kao-Con - See KAOLIN & PECTIN 468
KAOLIN & PECTIN 468
Kaon - See POTASSIUM SUPPLEMENTS 666
Kaon-Cl - See POTASSIUM SUPPLEMENTS 666
Kaon-Cl 10 - See POTASSIUM SUPPLEMENTS 666
Kaon-Cl 20 - See POTASSIUM SUPPLEMENTS 666
Kaopectate - See ATTAPULGITE 160
Kaopectate Advanced Formula - See ATTAPULGITE 160
Kaopectate II Caplets - See LOPERAMIDE 508
Kaopectate Maximum Strength - See ATTAPULGITE 160
Kaotin - See KAOLIN & PECTIN 468
Kapectolin - See KAOLIN & PECTIN 468
Kapectolin with Paregoric - See
KAOLIN & PECTIN 468
PAREGORIC 640
Kapvay - See CENTRAL ALPHA AGONISTS 234
Karacil - See LAXATIVES, BULK-FORMING 476
Kasof - See LAXATIVES, SOFTENER/ LUBRICANT 480
Kato - See POTASSIUM SUPPLEMENTS 666
Kay Ciel - See POTASSIUM SUPPLEMENTS 666
Kay Ciel Elixir - See POTASSIUM SUPPLEMENTS 666
Kaybovite - See VITAMIN B-12 (Cyanocobalamin) 836
Kaybovite-1000 - See VITAMIN B-12 (Cyanocobalamin) 836
Kaylixir - See POTASSIUM SUPPLEMENTS 666
Kazano - See
DPP-4 INHIBITORS 348
METFORMIN 544
K-C - See KAOLIN & PECTIN 468
KCL - See POTASSIUM SUPPLEMENTS 666
K-Dur - See POTASSIUM SUPPLEMENTS 666
Keep Alert - See CAFFEINE 216
Keflex - See CEPHALOSPORINS 236
Keftab - See CEPHALOSPORINS 236
K-Electrolyte - See POTASSIUM SUPPLEMENTS 666
Kellogg's Castor Oil - See LAXATIVES, STIMULANT 482
Kemstro - See BACLOFEN 166
Kenac - See ADRENOCORTICOIDS (Topical) 18
Kenacort - See ADRENOCORTICOIDS (Systemic) 16
Kenacort Diacetate - See ADRENOCORTICOIDS (Systemic) 16
Kenalog - See ADRENOCORTICOIDS (Topical) 18
Kenalog in Orabase - See ADRENOCORTICOIDS (Topical) 18

Kenalog-H - See ADRENOCORTICOIDS (Topical) 18
Kendral-Ipratropium - See IPRATROPIUM 456
Kenonel - See ADRENOCORTICOIDS (Topical) 18
Keppra - See LEVETIRACETAM 492
Keppra XR - See LEVETIRACETAM 492
Keralyt - See KERATOLYTICS 470
Keratex Gel - See KERATOLYTICS 470
Keratolytic - See
COAL TAR (Topical) 266
KERATOLYTICS 470
KERATOLYTICS 470
Kerledex - See BETA-ADRENERGIC BLOCKING AGENTS & THIAZIDE DIURETICS 184
Kerlone - See BETA-ADRENERGIC BLOCKING AGENTS 182
Kestrone-5 - See ESTROGENS 372
KETAZOLAM - See BENZODIAZEPINES 176
Ketek- See TELITHROMYCIN 778
KETOCONAZOLE - See ANTIFUNGALS, AZOLES 86
KETOCONAZOLE (Topical) - See ANTIFUNGALS (Topical) 88
KETOPROFEN - See ANTI-INFLAMMATORY DRUGS, NONSTEROIDAL (NSAIDs) 116
KETOROLAC - See ANTI-INFLAMMATORY DRUGS, NONSTEROIDAL (NSAIDs) 116
KETOROLAC - See ANTI-INFLAMMATORY DRUGS, NONSTEROIDAL (NSAIDs) (Ophthalmic) 120
KETOTIFEN - See ANTIALLERGIC AGENTS (Ophthalmic) 56
K-Flex - See ORPHENADRINE 624
K-G Elixir - See POTASSIUM SUPPLEMENTS 666
KI - See POTASSIUM SUPPLEMENTS 666
Kids-EEZE Chest Relief - See GUAIFENESIN 416
Kineret - See ANAKINRA 32
Kinesed - See
BELLADONNA ALKALOIDS & BARBITURATES 174
HYOSCYAMINE 438
SCOPOLAMINE (Hyoscine) 738
Klavikordal - See NITRATES 602
K-Lease - See POTASSIUM SUPPLEMENTS 666
Klerist-D - See
ANTIHISTAMINES 106
PSEUDOEPHEDRINE 694
K-Long - See POTASSIUM SUPPLEMENTS 666
Klonopin - See BENZODIAZEPINES 176
K-Lor - See POTASSIUM SUPPLEMENTS 666
Klor-Con 8 - See POTASSIUM SUPPLEMENTS 666
Klor-Con 10 - See POTASSIUM SUPPLEMENTS 666
Klor-Con Powder - See POTASSIUM SUPPLEMENTS 666
Klor-Con/25 - See POTASSIUM SUPPLEMENTS 666
Klor-Con/EF - See POTASSIUM SUPPLEMENTS 666
Klorvess - See POTASSIUM SUPPLEMENTS 666
Klorvess 10% Liquid - See POTASSIUM SUPPLEMENTS 666
Klorvess Effervescent Granules - See POTASSIUM SUPPLEMENTS 666
Klotrix - See POTASSIUM SUPPLEMENTS 666
K-Lyte - See POTASSIUM SUPPLEMENTS 666
K-Lyte DS - See POTASSIUM SUPPLEMENTS 666
K-Lyte/Cl - See POTASSIUM SUPPLEMENTS 666
K-Lyte/Cl 50 - See POTASSIUM SUPPLEMENTS 666
K-Lyte/CL Powder - See POTASSIUM SUPPLEMENTS 666
K-Med 900 - See POTASSIUM SUPPLEMENTS 666
K-Norm - See POTASSIUM SUPPLEMENTS 666
Koffex - See DEXTROMETHORPHAN 312
Kolephrin - See
ACETAMINOPHEN 8
ANTIHISTAMINES 106
PSEUDOEPHEDRINE 694
Kolephrin GG/DM - See
DEXTROMETHORPHAN 312
GUAIFENESIN 416
Kolephrin/DM Caplets - See
ACETAMINOPHEN 8
ANTIHISTAMINES 106
DEXTROMETHORPHAN 312
PSEUDOEPHEDRINE 694
Kolyum - See POTASSIUM SUPPLEMENTS 666
Kombiglyze XR - See METFORMIN 544
Kondremul - See LAXATIVES, SOFTENER/ LUBRICANT 480
Kondremul Plain - See LAXATIVES, SOFTENER/LUBRICANT 480
Kondremul with Cascara - See
LAXATIVES, SOFTENER/LUBRICANT 480
LAXATIVES, STIMULANT 482

Kondremul with Phenolphthalein - See
LAXATIVES, SOFTENER/LUBRICANT 480
LAXATIVES, STIMULANT 482
Konsyl - See LAXATIVES, BULK-FORMING 476
Konsyl Easy Mix Formula - See LAXATIVES, BULK-FORMING 476
Konsyl-D - See LAXATIVES, BULK-FORMING 476
Konsyl-Orange - See LAXATIVES, BULK-FORMING 476
Koromex Cream - See CONTRACEPTIVES, VAGINAL 280
Koromex Crystal Gel - See CONTRACEPTIVES, VAGINAL 280
Koromex Foam - See CONTRACEPTIVES, VAGINAL 280
Koromex Jelly - See CONTRACEPTIVES, VAGINAL 280
K-P - See KAOLIN & PECTIN 468
K-Pek - See KAOLIN & PECTIN 468
K-Phos 2 - See POTASSIUM SUPPLEMENTS 666
K-Phos M.F. - See POTASSIUM SUPPLEMENTS 666
K-Phos Neutral - See POTASSIUM SUPPLEMENTS 666
K-Phos Original - See POTASSIUM
Kristalose - See LAXATIVES, OSMOTIC 478
Kronofed-A - See
ANTIHISTAMINES 106
PSEUDOEPHEDRINE 694
Kronofed-A Jr. - See
ANTIHISTAMINES 106
PSEUDOEPHEDRINE 694
K-Tab - See POTASSIUM SUPPLEMENTS 666
Kudrox Double Strength - See ANTACIDS 48
K-Vescent - See POTASSIUM SUPPLEMENTS 666
Kwelcof Liquid - See
GUAIFENESIN 416
NARCOTIC ANALGESICS 584
Kwellada - See PEDICULICIDES (Topical) 642
Kwildane - See PEDICULICIDES (Topical) 642
K-Y-Plus - See CONTRACEPTIVES, VAGINAL 280

L

LABETALOL - See BETA-ADRENERGIC BLOCKING AGENTS 182
LABETALOL & HYDROCHLOROTHIAZIDE - See BETA-ADRENERGIC BLOCKING AGENTS & THIAZIDE DIURETICS 184
LACOSAMIDE 472
Lacril - See PROTECTANT (Ophthalmic) 690
Lacrisert - See PROTECTANT (Ophthalmic) 690
Lacticare-HC - See ADRENOCORTICOIDS (Topical) 18
Lactisol - See KERATOLYTICS 470
Lactulax - See LAXATIVES, OSMOTIC 478
LACTULOSE - See LAXATIVES, OSMOTIC 478
Lagol - See ANESTHETICS (Topical) 40
Lamictal - See LAMOTRIGINE 474
Lamictal Chewable Dispersible Tablets - See LAMOTRIGINE 474
Lamictal ODT - See LAMOTRIGINE 474
Lamictal XR - See LAMOTRIGINE 474
Lamisil - See ANTIFUNGALS (Topical) 88
Lamisil Oral Granules - See TERBINAFINE (Oral) 780
Lamisil Solution 1% - See ANTIFUNGALS (Topical) 88
Lamisil Tablets - See TERBINAFINE (Oral) 780
LAMIVUDINE - See NUCLEOSIDE REVERSE TRANSCRIPTASE INHIBITORS 610
LAMOTRIGINE 474
Lanacort - See ADRENOCORTICOIDS (Topical) 18
Lanacort 10 - See ADRENOCORTICOIDS (Topical) 18
Laniazid - See ISONIAZID 460
Laniroif - See
ASPIRIN 152
BARBITURATES 168
Lanophyllin - See BRONCHODILATORS, XANTHINE 204
Lanorinal - See
ASPIRIN 152
BARBITURATES 168
Lanoxicaps - See DIGITALIS PREPARATIONS (Digitalis Glycosides) 320
Lanoxin - See DIGITALIS PREPARATIONS (Digitalis Glycosides) 320
Lansoyl - See LAXATIVES, SOFTENER/LUBRICANT 480
LANSOPRAZOLE - See PROTON PUMP INHIBITORS 692
Lantus - See INSULIN ANALOGS 448
Lantus OptiClik - See INSULIN ANALOGS 448
Lantus Solostar Pen - See INSULIN ANALOGS 448
Lanvis - See THIOGUANINE 788
Largactil - See PHENOTHIAZINES 656
Largactil Liquid - See PHENOTHIAZINES 656
Largactil Oral Drops - See PHENOTHIAZINES 656
Lariam - See ANTIMALARIAL 126
Larodopa - See LEVODOPA 496
Lasan - See ANTHRALIN (Topical) 52
Lasan HP - See ANTHRALIN (Topical) 52
Lasan Pomade - See ANTHRALIN (Topical) 52

Lasan Unguent - See ANTHRALIN (Topical) 52
Lasix - See DIURETICS, LOOP 332
Lasix Special - See DIURETICS, LOOP 332
Lastacaft - See ANTIALLERGIC AGENTS (Ophthalmic) 56
LATANOPROST - See ANTIGLAUCOMA, PROSTAGLANDINS 102
Latuda - See LURASIDONE 516
Laudanum - See NARCOTIC ANALGESICS 584
Lavatar - See COAL TAR (Topical) 266
Laxative - See
LAXATIVES, OSMOTIC 478
LUBIPROSTONE 514
Laxative, bulk-forming - See LAXATIVES, BULK-FORMING 476
Laxative (Stimulant) - See LAXATIVES, STIMULANT 482
Laxative (Stool Softener-emollient) - See LAXATIVES, SOFTENER/LUBRICANT 480
LAXATIVES, BULK-FORMING 476
LAXATIVES, OSMOTIC 478
LAXATIVES, SOFTENER/LUBRICANT 480
LAXATIVES, STIMULANT 482
Laxinate 100 - See LAXATIVES, SOFTENER/ LUBRICANT 480
Laxit - See LAXATIVES, STIMULANT 482
Lazanda - See NARCOTIC ANALGESICS 584
LazerSporin - See ANTIBACTERIALS (Otic) 68
L-Carnitine - See LEVOCARNITINE 494
Lectopam - See BENZODIAZEPINES 176
Ledercillin-VK - See PENICILLINS 646
LEFLUNOMIDE 484
Lemoderm - See ADRENOCORTICOIDS (Topical) 18
Lenoltec with Codeine No. 1 - See NARCOTIC ANALGESICS & ACETAMINOPHEN 586
Lenoltec with Codeine No. 2 - See NARCOTIC ANALGESICS & ACETAMINOPHEN 586
Lenoltec with Codeine No. 3 - See NARCOTIC ANALGESICS & ACETAMINOPHEN 586
Lenoltec with Codeine No. 4 - See NARCOTIC ANALGESICS & ACETAMINOPHEN 586
Leponex - See CLOZAPINE 264
Lescol - See HMG-CoA REDUCTASE INHIBITORS 424
Lescol XL - See HMG-CoA REDUCTASE INHIBITORS 424
Letairis - See ENDOTHELIN RECEPTOR ANTAGONISTS 354
LEUCOVORIN 486
Leukeran - See CHLORAMBUCIL 240
LEUKOTRIENE MODIFIERS 488
Levadex - See ERGOT DERIVATIVES 366
LEVALBUTEROL - See BRONCHODILATORS, ADRENERGIC 200
LEVAMISOLE 490
Levaquin - See FLUOROQUINOLONES 392
Levate - See ANTIDEPRESSANTS, TRICYCLIC 80
Levatol - See BETA-ADRENERGIC BLOCKING AGENTS 182
Levbid - See HYOSCYAMINE 438
Levemir - See INSULIN ANALOGS 448
LEVETIRACETAM 492
Levitra - See ERECTILE DYSFUNCTION AGENTS 360
Levlen - See CONTRACEPTIVES, ORAL & SKIN 278
Levlite - See CONTRACEPTIVES, ORAL & SKIN 278
LEVOBETAXOLOL - See BETA-ADRENERGIC BLOCKING AGENTS 182
LEVOBUNOLOL (Ophthalmic) - See ANTIGLAUCOMA, BETA BLOCKERS 96
LEVOCABASTINE - See ANTIALLERGIC AGENTS (Ophthalmic) 56
LEVOCARNITINE 494
LEVOCETIRIZINE - See ANTIHISTAMINES, NONSEDATING 110
LEVODOPA 496
Levo-Dromoran - See NARCOTIC ANALGESICS 584
LEVOFLOXACIN - See FLUOROQUINOLONES 392
LEVOFLOXACIN (Ophthalmic) - See ANTIBACTERIALS (Ophthalmic) 66
LEVONORGESTREL - See PROGESTINS 680
LEVONORGESTREL & ETHINYL ESTRADIOL - See CONTRACEPTIVES, ORAL & SKIN 278
Levoprome - See PHENOTHIAZINES 656
Levora - See CONTRACEPTIVES, ORAL & SKIN 278
Levorphan - See NARCOTIC ANALGESICS 584
LEVORPHANOL - See NARCOTIC ANALGESICS 584
Levo-T - See THYROID HORMONES 792
Levothroid - See THYROID HORMONES 792
LEVOTHYROXINE - See THYROID HORMONES 792
Levoxyl - See THYROID HORMONES 792
Levsin - See HYOSCYAMINE 438
Levsin S/L - See HYOSCYAMINE 438
Levsin with Phenobarbital - See BELLADONNA ALKALOIDS & BARBITURATES 174
Levsinex - See HYOSCYAMINE 438

Levsinex Timecaps - See HYOSCYAMINE 438
Levsinex with Phenobarbital Timecaps - See BELLADONNA ALKALOIDS & BARBITURATES 174
Levsin-PB - See BELLADONNA ALKALOIDS & BARBITURATES 174
Lexapro - See SELECTIVE SEROTONIN REUPTAKE INHIBITORS (SSRIs) 742
Lexiva - See PROTEASE INHIBITORS 688
Lialda - See MESALAMINE 542
Librax - See
BENZODIAZEPINES 176
CLIDINIUM 256
Libritabs - See BENZODIAZEPINES 176
Librium - See BENZODIAZEPINES 176
Lice-Enz Foam And Comb Lice Killing Shampoo Kit - See PEDICULICIDES (Topical) 642
Licon - See ADRENOCORTICOIDS (Topical) 18
LidaMantle - See ANESTHETICS (Topical) 40
LidaMantle HC - See ADRENOCORTICOIDS (Topical) 18
Lidemol - See ADRENOCORTICOIDS (Topical) 18
Lidex - See ADRENOCORTICOIDS (Topical) 18
Lidex-E - See ADRENOCORTICOIDS (Topical) 18
LIDOCAINE - See
ANESTHETICS (Mucosal-Local) 36
ANESTHETICS (Rectal) 38
ANESTHETICS (Topical) 40
LIDOCAINE & PRILOCAINE - See ANESTHETICS (Topical) 40
Lidoderm - See ANESTHETICS (Topical) 40
Lidopatch - See ANESTHETICS (Topical) 40
Lidox - See CLIDINIUM 256
Lidoxide - See BENZODIAZEPINES 176
Lignocaine - See ANESTHETICS (Topical) 40
Limbitrol - See BENZODIAZEPINES 176
Limbitrol DS - See BENZODIAZEPINES 176
LINACLOTIDE 498
LINAGLIPTIN - See DPP-4 INHIBITORS 348
Lincocin - See LINCOMYCIN 500
LINCOMYCIN 500
LINDANE - See PEDICULICIDES (Topical) 642
LINEZOLID 502
Linzess - See LINACLOTIDE 498
Lioresal - See BACLOFEN 166
LIOTHYRONINE - See THYROID HORMONES 792
LIOTRIX - See THYROID HORMONES 792
Lipase inhibitor - See ORLISTAT 622
Lipidil - See FIBRATES 386
Lipitor - See HMG-CoA REDUCTASE INHIBITORS 424
Lipofen - See FIBRATES 386
Lipoxide - See BENZODIAZEPINES 176
Lipsovir - See
ADRENOCORTICOIDS (Topical) 18
ANTIVIRALS (Topical) 144
Liquadd - See AMPHETAMINES 28
LiquiBid D - See
GUAIFENESIN 416
PHENYLEPHRINE 658
LiquiBid D-R - See
GUAIFENESIN/ 416
PHENYLEPHRINE 658
LiquiBid PD - See
GUAIFENESIN 416
PHENYLEPHRINE 658
Liqui-Char - See CHARCOAL, ACTIVATED 238
Liqui-Doss - See LAXATIVES, SOFTENER/ LUBRICANT 480
Liquid Tagamet - See HISTAMINE H_2 RECEPTOR ANTAGONISTS 422
Liquimat - See ANTIACNE, CLEANSING (Topical) 54
Liquiprin Children's Elixir - See ACETAMINOPHEN 8
Liquiprin Infants' Drops - See ACETAMINOPHEN 8
Liquor Carbonis Detergens - See COAL TAR (Topical) 266
LIRAGLUTIDE - See GLP-1 RECEPTOR AGONISTS 406
LISDEXAMFETAMINE - See AMPHETAMINES 28
LISINOPRIL - See ANGIOTENSIN-CONVERTING ENZYME (ACE) INHIBITORS 44
LISINOPRIL & HYDROCHLOROTHIAZIDE - See ANGIOTENSIN-CONVERTING ENZYME (ACE) INHIBITORS & HYDROCHLOROTHIAZIDE 46
Listerex Golden Scrub Lotion - See KERATOLYTICS 470
Listerex Herbal Scrub Lotion - See KERATOLYTICS 470
Lite-Pred - See ANTI-INFLAMMATORY DRUGS, STEROIDAL (Ophthalmic) 122
Lithane - See LITHIUM 504
LITHIUM 504
Lithizine - See LITHIUM 504
Lithobid - See LITHIUM 504
Lithonate - See LITHIUM 504
Lithostat - See ACETOHYDROXAMIC ACID (AHA) 10
Lithotabs - See LITHIUM 504
Livalo - See HMG-CoA REDUCTASE INHIBITORS 424

Livostin - See ANTIALLERGIC AGENTS (Ophthalmic) 56
Lixolin - See BRONCHODILATORS, XANTHINE 204
Locacorten - See ADRENOCORTICOIDS (Topical) 18
Locoid - See ADRENOCORTICOIDS (Topical) 18
Lodine - See ANTI-INFLAMMATORY DRUGS, NONSTEROIDAL (NSAIDs) 116
Lodine XL - See ANTI-INFLAMMATORY DRUGS, NONSTEROIDAL (NSAIDs) 116
LODOXAMIDE - See ANTIALLERGIC AGENTS (Ophthalmic) 56
Lodoxide - See CLIDINIUM 256
Lodrane D - See
ANTIHISTAMINES 106
PSEUDOEPHEDRINE 694
Lodrane LD - See
ANTIHISTAMINES 106
PSEUDOEPHEDRINE 694
Lodrane 12Hour ER - See ANTIHISTAMINES 106
Lodrane 24D - See ANTIHISTAMINES 106
Loestrin 1/20 - See CONTRACEPTIVES, ORAL & SKIN 278
Loestrin 1.5/30 - See CONTRACEPTIVES, ORAL & SKIN 278
Loestrin 24 Fe - See
CONTRACEPTIVES, ORAL & SKIN 278
IRON SUPPLEMENTS 458
Lofene - See DIPHENOXYLATE & ATROPINE 324
Lofibra - See FIBRATES 386
Loftran - See BENZODIAZEPINES 176
Logen - See DIPHENOXYLATE & ATROPINE 324
Lo Loestrin Fe - See
CONTRACEPTIVES, ORAL & SKIN 278
IRON SUPPLEMENTS 458
Lomanate - See DIPHENOXYLATE & ATROPINE 324
Lombriareu - See ANTHELMINTICS 50
LOMEFLOXACIN - See FLUOROQUINOLONES 392
Lomine - See DICYCLOMINE 316
Lomotil - See DIPHENOXYLATE & ATROPINE 324
LOMUSTINE 506
Loniten - See MINOXIDIL 560
Lonox - See DIPHENOXYLATE & ATROPINE 324
Lo/Ovral - See CONTRACEPTIVES, ORAL & SKIN 278
LOPERAMIDE 508
Lopid - See GEMFIBROZIL 404
LOPINAVIR - See PROTEASE INHIBITORS 688
Lopressor - See BETA-ADRENERGIC BLOCKING AGENTS 182
Lopressor HCT - See BETA-ADRENERGIC BLOCKING AGENTS & THIAZIDE DIURETICS 184
Lopressor SR - See BETA-ADRENERGIC BLOCKING AGENTS 182
Loprox - See ANTIFUNGALS (Topical) 88
Lopurin - See ANTIGOUT DRUGS 104
LORATADINE - See ANTIHISTAMINES, NONSEDATING 110
LORAZEPAM - See BENZODIAZEPINES 176
Lorazepam Intensol - See BENZODIAZEPINES 176
LORCASERIN 510
Lorcet - See NARCOTIC ANALGESICS & ACETAMINOPHEN 586
Lorcet 10/646 - See NARCOTIC ANALGESICS & ACETAMINOPHEN 586
Lorcet Plus - See NARCOTIC ANALGESICS & ACETAMINOPHEN 586
Lorcet-HD - See NARCOTIC ANALGESICS & ACETAMINOPHEN 586
Loroxide 5 Lotion with Flesh Tinted Base - See BENZOYL PEROXIDE 178
Loroxide 5.5 Lotion - See BENZOYL PEROXIDE 178
Lortab - See NARCOTIC ANALGESICS & ACETAMINOPHEN 586
Lortab 5 - See NARCOTIC ANALGESICS & ACETAMINOPHEN 586
Lortab 7 - See NARCOTIC ANALGESICS & ACETAMINOPHEN 586
Lortab ASA - See NARCOTIC ANALGESICS & ASPIRIN 588
LOSARTAN - See ANGIOTENSIN II RECEPTOR ANTAGONISTS 42
LoSeasonique - See CONTRACEPTIVES, ORAL & SKIN 278
Losec - See PROTON PUMP INHIBITORS 692
Losopan - See ANTACIDS 48
Losopan Plus - See ANTACIDS 48
Lotemax - See ANTI-INFLAMMATORY DRUGS, STEROIDAL (Ophthalmic) 122
Lotensin - See ANGIOTENSIN-CONVERTING ENZYME (ACE) INHIBITORS 44
LOTEPREDNOL - See ANTI-INFLAMMATORY DRUGS, STEROIDAL (Ophthalmic) 122
Lotio Asulfa - See KERATOLYTICS 470
Lotrel - See
ANGIOTENSIN-CONVERTING ENZYME (ACE) INHIBITORS 44
CALCIUM CHANNEL BLOCKERS 220
Lotriderm - See ANTIFUNGALS (Topical) 88

Lotrimin AF - See ANTIFUNGALS (Topical) 88
Lotrimin Cream - See ANTIFUNGALS (Topical) 88
Lotrimin Lotion - See ANTIFUNGALS (Topical) 88
Lotrimin Ointment - See ANTIFUNGALS (Topical) 88
Lotrimin Ultra - See ANTIFUNGALS (Topical) 88
Lotrisone - See
ADRENOCORTICOIDS (Topical) 18
ANTIFUNGALS (Topical) 88
Lo-Trol - See DIPHENOXYLATE & ATROPINE 324
LOVASTATIN - See HMG-CoA REDUCTASE INHIBITORS 424
Lovaza - See OMEGA-3 ACID ETHYL ESTERS 620
Lowsium - See ANTACIDS 48
Lowsium Plus - See ANTACIDS 48
Loxapac - See LOXAPINE 512
LOXAPINE 512
Loxitane - See LOXAPINE 512
Loxitane C - See LOXAPINE 512
Lozide - See INDAPAMIDE 444
Lozol - See INDAPAMIDE 444
L-PAM - See MELPHALAN 534
L-Thyroxine - See THYROID HORMONES 792
LUBIPROSTONE 514
Lucidex - See CAFFEINE 216
Ludiomil - See MAPROTILINE 520
Lufyllin - See BRONCHODILATORS, XANTHINE 204
Lufyllin-400 - See BRONCHODILATORS, XANTHINE 204
Lumigan - See ANTIGLAUCOMA, PROSTAGLANDINS 102
Luminal - See BARBITURATES 168
Lunesta - See ESZOPICLONE 374
LURASIDONE 516
Luvox - See SELECTIVE SEROTONIN REUPTAKE INHIBITORS (SSRIs) 742
Luvox CR - See SELECTIVE SEROTONIN REUPTAKE INHIBITORS (SSRIs) 742
Lybrel - See CONTRACEPTIVES, ORAL & SKIN 278
Lyderm - See ADRENOCORTICOIDS (Topical) 18
Lyrica - See PREGABALIN 670
Lysteda - See ANTIFIBRINOLYTIC AGENTS 84

M

Maalox - See ANTACIDS 48
Maalox Anti-Gas - See SIMETHICONE 748
Maalox Daily Fiber Therapy - See LAXATIVES, BULK-FORMING 476
Maalox Daily Fiber Therapy Citrus Flavor - See LAXATIVES, BULK-FORMING 476
Maalox Daily Fiber Therapy Orange Flavor - See LAXATIVES, BULK-FORMING 476
Maalox GRF Gas Relief Formula - See SIMETHICONE 748
Maalox HRF - See ANTACIDS 48
Maalox Max - See ANTACIDS 48
Maalox Plus - See ANTACIDS 48
Maalox Plus, Extra Strength - See ANTACIDS 48
Maalox Quick Dissolving Chews - See ANTACIDS 48
Maalox Sugar Free Citrus Flavor - See LAXATIVES, BULK-FORMING 476
Maalox Sugar Free Orange Flavor - See LAXATIVES, BULK-FORMING 476
Maalox TC - See ANTACIDS 48
Maalox Total Stomach Relief - See BISMUTH SALTS 190
Macrobid - See NITROFURANTOIN 604
Macrodantin - See NITROFURANTOIN 604
MACROLIDE ANTIBIOTICS 518
MAGALDRATE - See ANTACIDS 48
MAGALDRATE & SIMETHICONE - See ANTACIDS 48
Magan - See SALICYLATES 736
Magnacet - See NARCOTIC ANALGESICS & ACETAMINOPHEN 586
Magnalox - See ANTACIDS 48
Magnalox Plus - See ANTACIDS 48
Magnaprin - See ASPIRIN 152
Magnaprin Arthritis Strength - See ASPIRIN 152
MAGNESIUM CITRATE - See LAXATIVES, OSMOTIC 478
MAGNESIUM HYDROXIDE - See
ANTACIDS 48
LAXATIVES, OSMOTIC 478
MAGNESIUM OXIDE - See
ANTACIDS 48
LAXATIVES, OSMOTIC 478
MAGNESIUM SALICYLATE - See SALICYLATES 736
MAGNESIUM SULFATE - See LAXATIVES, OSMOTIC 478
Magnolax - See LAXATIVES, OSMOTIC 478
Mag-Ox 400 - See
ANTACIDS 48
LAXATIVES, OSMOTIC 478
Majeptil - See PHENOTHIAZINES 656
Malarone - See
ATOVAQUONE 156
PROGUANIL 682

Malatal - See BELLADONNA ALKALOIDS & BARBITURATES 174
MALATHION - See PEDICULICIDES (Topical) 642
Mallamint - See
ANTACIDS 48
CALCIUM SUPPLEMENTS 222
Mallergan-VC with Codeine - See
ANTIHISTAMINES, PHENOTHIAZINE-DERIVATIVE 112
NARCOTIC ANALGESICS 584
PHENYLEPHRINE 658
Malogen - See ANDROGENS 34
Malogex - See ANDROGENS 34
Malotuss - See GUAIFENESIN 416
MALT SOUP EXTRACT - See LAXATIVES, BULK-FORMING 476
Maltsupex - See LAXATIVES, BULK-FORMING 476
Mandelamine - See METHENAMINE 546
Mannest - See ESTROGENS 372
MAO (Monoamine Oxidase) inhibitor - See MONOAMINE OXIDASE (MAO) INHIBITORS 570
Maolate - See MUSCLE RELAXANTS, SKELETAL 576
Maox - See
ANTACIDS 48
LAXATIVES, OSMOTIC 478
Mapap Infant Drops - See ACETAMINOPHEN 8
Mapap Sinus - See
ACETAMINOPHEN 8
PSEUDOEPHEDRINE 694
Maprin - See ASPIRIN 152
MAPROTILINE 520
MARAVIROC 522
Marax - See
BRONCHODILATORS, XANTHINE 204
EPHEDRINE 356
HYDROXYZINE 436
Marax D.F. - See
BRONCHODILATORS, XANTHINE 204
EPHEDRINE 356
HYDROXYZINE 436
Marbaxin - See MUSCLE RELAXANTS, SKELETAL 576
Marblen - See ANTACIDS 48
Marezine - See ANTIHISTAMINES, PIPERAZINE (Antinausea) 114
Marflex - See ORPHENADRINE 624
Margesic #3 - See NARCOTIC ANALGESICS & ACETAMINOPHEN 586
Margesic-H - See NARCOTIC ANALGESICS & ACETAMINOPHEN 586
Marinol - See DRONABINOL (THC, Marijuana) 350
Marmine - See ANTIHISTAMINES 106
Marnal - See
ASPIRIN 152
BARBITURATES 168
Marplan - See MONOAMINE OXIDASE (MAO) INHIBITORS 570
Marvelon - See CONTRACEPTIVES, ORAL & SKIN 278
MASOPROCOL 524
Masporin Otic - See ANTIBACTERIALS (Otic) 68
Matulane - See PROCARBAZINE 678
Mavik - See ANGIOTENSIN-CONVERTING ENZYME (ACE) INHIBITORS 44
Maxair10 - See BRONCHODILATORS, ADRENERGIC 200
Maxalt - See TRIPTANS 820
Maxalt-MLT - See TRIPTANS 820
Maxaquin - See FLUOROQUINOLONES 392
Maxenal - See PSEUDOEPHEDRINE 694
Maxeran - See METOCLOPRAMIDE 550
Maxibolin - See ANDROGENS 34
Maxidex - See ANTI-INFLAMMATORY DRUGS, STEROIDAL (Ophthalmic) 122
Maxidone - See NARCOTIC ANALGESICS & ACETAMINOPHEN 586
Maxiflor - See ADRENOCORTICOIDS (Topical) 18
Maximum Strength Cortaid - See ADRENOCORTICOIDS (Topical) 18
Maximum Strength Mucinex D - See
GUAIFENESIN 416
PSEUDOEPHEDRINE 694
Maximum Strength Mucinex DM - See
DEXTROMETHORPHAN 312
GUAIFENESIN 416
Maximum Strength Mucinex SE - See GUAIFENESIN 416
Maximum Strength Mylanta Gas Relief - See SIMETHICONE 748
Maximum Strength Phazyme - See SIMETHICONE 748
Maximum Strength Tylenol Allergy Sinus Caplets - See
ACETAMINOPHEN 8
ANTIHISTAMINES 106
PSEUDOEPHEDRINE 694
Maxivate - See ADRENOCORTICOIDS (Topical) 18
Maxzide - See DIURETICS, POTASSIUM-SPARING & HYDROCHLOROTHIAZIDE 336
Mazanor - See APPETITE SUPPRESSANTS 146

Mazepine - See CARBAMAZEPINE 228
MAZINDOL - See APPETITE SUPPRESSANTS 146
Measurin - See ASPIRIN 152
MECHLORETHAMINE (Topical) 526
Meclan - See ANTIBACTERIALS FOR ACNE (Topical) 64
MECLIZINE - See ANTIHISTAMINES, PIPERAZINE (Antinausea) 114
MECLOCYCLINE (Topical)- See ANTI-BACTERIALS FOR ACNE (Topical) 64
Meclofen - See ANTI-INFLAMMATORY DRUGS, NONSTEROIDAL (NSAIDs) 116
MECLOFENAMATE - See ANTI-INFLAMMATORY DRUGS, NONSTEROIDAL (NSAIDs) 116
Meclomen - See ANTI-INFLAMMATORY DRUGS, NONSTEROIDAL (NSAIDs) 116
Med Tamoxifen - See TAMOXIFEN 772
Meda Cap - See ACETAMINOPHEN 8
Meda Syrup Forte - See
ANTIHISTAMINES 106
DEXTROMETHORPHAN 312
GUAIFENESIN 416
PHENYLEPHRINE 658
Meda Tab - See ACETAMINOPHEN 8
Medatussin - See
DEXTROMETHORPHAN 312
GUAIFENESIN 416
Medatussin Plus - See GUAIFENESIN 416
Meclicot - See ANTIHISTAMINES, PIPERAZINE (Antinausea) 114
Medigesic - See
ACETAMINOPHEN 8
BARBITURATES 168
Medihaler-Epi - See BRONCHODILATORS, ADRENERGIC 200
Medihaler-Iso - See BRONCHODILATORS, ADRENERGIC 200
Medilium - See BENZODIAZEPINES 176
Mediplast - See KERATOLYTICS 470
Medipren - See ANTI-INFLAMMATORY DRUGS, NONSTEROIDAL (NSAIDs) 116
Medipren Caplets - See ANTI-INFLAMMATORY DRUGS, NONSTEROIDAL (NSAIDs) 116
Mediquell - See DEXTROMETHORPHAN 312
Medi-Tran - See MEPROBAMATE 538
Medivert - See ANTIHISTAMINES, PIPERAZINE (Antinausea) 114
Medotar - See COAL TAR (Topical) 266
Medrol - See ADRENOCORTICOIDS (Systemic) 16
MEDROXYPROGESTERONE - See PROGESTINS 680
MEDRYSONE - See ANTI-INFLAMMATORY DRUGS, STEROIDAL (Ophthalmic) 122
Med-Timolol - See ANTIGLAUCOMA, BETA BLOCKERS 96
MEFENAMIC ACID - See ANTI-INFLAMMATORY DRUGS, NONSTEROIDAL (NSAIDs) 116
MEFLOQUINE - See ANTIMALARIAL 126
Megace - See PROGESTINS 680
Megace ES - See PROGESTINS 680
Megace Oral Suspension - See PROGESTINS 680
Megacillin - See PENICILLINS 646
MEGESTROL - See PROGESTINS 680
MEGLITINIDES 528
MELATONIN 530
Melatonin receptor agonist - See RAMELTEON 710
Melfiat-105 Unicelles - See APPETITE SUPPRESSANTS 146
Mellaril - See PHENOTHIAZINES 656
Mellaril Concentrate - See PHENOTHIAZINES 656
Mellaril-S - See PHENOTHIAZINES 656
MELOXICAM 532
MELPHALAN 534
MEMANTINE 536
MENADIOL - See VITAMIN K 846
Menaval-20 - See ESTROGENS 372
Menest - See ESTROGENS 372
Menostar - See ESTROGENS 372
Men's Rogaine Topical Foam - See MINOXIDIL (Topical) 562
Mentax - See ANTIFUNGALS (Topical) 88
Mentax TC - See ANTIFUNGALS (Topical) 88
MEPENZOLATE - See ANTICHOLINERGICS 72
MEPERIDINE - See NARCOTIC ANALGESICS 584
MEPERIDINE & ACETAMINOPHEN - See NARCOTIC ANALGESICS & ACETAMINOPHEN 586
MEPHOBARBITAL - See BARBITURATES 168
Mephyton - See VITAMIN K 846
MEPROBAMATE 538
Meprogesic - See
ASPIRIN 152
MEPROBAMATE 538
Meprogesic Q - See
ASPIRIN 152
MEPROBAMATE 538
Meprolonel - See ADRENOCORTICOIDS (Systemic) 16
Mepron - See ATOVAQUONE 156
Meprospan 200 - See MEPROBAMATE 538
Meprospan 400 - See MEPROBAMATE 538
MERCAPTOPURINE 540
MESALAMINE 542
Mesalazine - See MESALAMINE 542

MESORIDAZINE - See PHENOTHIAZINES 656
Mestinon - See ANTIMYASTHENICS 128
Mestinon Timespans - See ANTIMYASTHENICS 128
Metadate CD - See STIMULANT MEDICATIONS 754
Metadate ER - See STIMULANT MEDICATIONS 754
Metaderm Mild - See ADRENOCORTICOIDS (Topical) 18
Metaderm Regular (Topical) - See ADRENOCORTICOIDS (Topical) 18
Metaglip - See
METFORMIN 544
SULFONYLUREAS 770
Metahydrin - See DIURETICS, THIAZIDE 338
Metamucil - See LAXATIVES, BULK-FORMING 476
Metamucil Apple Crisp Fiber Wafers - See LAXATIVES, BULK-FORMING 476
Metamucil Cinnamon Spice Fiber Wafers - See LAXATIVES, BULK-FORMING 476
Metamucil Instant Mix, Orange Flavor - See LAXATIVES, BULK-FORMING 476
Metamucil Smooth Citrus Flavor - See LAXATIVES, BULK-FORMING 476
Metamucil Smooth Orange Flavor - See LAXATIVES, BULK-FORMING 476
Metamucil Smooth, Sugar-Free Citrus Flavor - See LAXATIVES, BULK-FORMING 476
Metamucil Smooth, Sugar-Free Orange Flavor - See LAXATIVES, BULK-FORMING 476
Metamucil Smooth, Sugar-Free Regular Flavor - See LAXATIVES, BULK-FORMING 476
Metamucil Sugar Free - See LAXATIVES, BULK-FORMING 476
Metamucil Sugar Free Citrus Flavor - See LAXATIVES, BULK-FORMING 476
Metamucil Sugar Free Lemon-Lime Flavor - See LAXATIVES, BULK-FORMING 476
Metamucil Sugar Free Orange Flavor - See LAXATIVES, BULK-FORMING 476
Metandren - See ANDROGENS 34
METAPROTERENOL - See BRONCHODILATORS, ADRENERGIC 200
METAXALONE - See MUSCLE RELAXANTS, SKELETAL 576
Meted Maximum Strength Anti-Dandruff Shampoo with Conditioners - See
ANTISEBORRHEICS (Topical) 132
KERATOLYTICS 470
METFORMIN 544
Methacin - See CAPSAICIN 226
METHADONE - See NARCOTIC ANALGESICS 584
Methadose - See NARCOTIC ANALGESICS 584
METHAMPHETAMINE - See AMPHETAMINES 28
METHANTHELINE - See ANTICHOLINERGICS 72
METHARBITAL - See BARBITURATES 168
METHAZOLAMIDE - See CARBONIC ANHYDRASE INHIBITORS 232
METHENAMINE 546
METHIMAZOLE - See ANTITHYROID DRUGS 134
METHOCARBAMOL - See MUSCLE RELAXANTS, SKELETAL 576
Methocel - See PROTECTANT (Ophthalmic) 690
METHOTREXATE 548
METHOTRIMEPRAZINE - See PHENOTHIAZINES 656
METHOXSALEN - See PSORALENS 696
METHSCOPOLAMINE - See ANTICHOLINERGICS 72
METHSUXIMIDE - See ANTICONVULSANTS, SUCCINIMIDE 78
METHYCLOTHIAZIDE - See DIURETICS, THIAZIDE 338
METHYLCELLULOSE - See LAXATIVES, BULK-FORMING 476
METHYLDOPA - See CENTRAL ALPHA AGONISTS 234
Methylergometrine - See ERGOT ALKALOIDS 364
METHYLERGONOVINE - See ERGOT ALKALOIDS 364
Methylin Chewable - See STIMULANT MEDICATIONS 754
Methylin ER - See STIMULANT MEDICATIONS 754
Methylin Oral Suspension - See STIMULANT MEDICATIONS 754
METHYLPHENIDATE - See STIMULANT MEDICATIONS 754
METHYLPREDNISOLONE - See
ADRENOCORTICOIDS (Systemic) 16
ADRENOCORTICOIDS (Topical) 18
METHYLTESTOSTERONE - See ANDROGENS 34
Meticorten - See ADRENOCORTICOIDS (Systemic) 16
METIPRANOLOL (Ophthalmic) - See ANTIGLAUCOMA, BETA BLOCKERS 96
Metizol - See NITROIMIDAZOLES 606
METOCLOPRAMIDE 550

METOLAZONE - See DIURETICS, THIAZIDE 338
Metopirone - See METYRAPONE 552
METOPROLOL - See BETA-ADRENERGIC BLOCKING AGENTS 182
METOPROLOL & HYDROCHLOROTHIAZIDE - See BETA-ADRENERGIC BLOCKING AGENTS & THIAZIDE DIURETICS 184
Metosyn - See ADRENOCORTICOIDS (Topical) 18
Metosyn FAPG - See ADRENOCORTICOIDS (Topical) 18
Metozolv ODT - See METOCLOPRAMIDE 550
Metra - See APPETITE SUPPRESSANTS 146
Metric 21 - See NITROIMIDAZOLES 606
Metro Cream - See NITROIMIDAZOLES 606
MetroGel - See NITROIMIDAZOLES 606
MetroGel-Vaginal - See NITROIMIDAZOLES 606
METRONIDAZOLE - See NITROIMIDAZOLES 606
METYRAPONE 552
Mevacor - See HMG-CoA REDUCTASE INHIBITORS 424
Meval - See BENZODIAZEPINES 176
Mevinolin - See HMG-CoA REDUCTASE INHIBITORS 424
Mexate - See METHOTREXATE 548
Mexate AQ - See METHOTREXATE 548
MEXILETINE 554
Mexitil - See MEXILETINE 554
Miacalcin - See CALCITONIN 218
Mi-Acid - See ANTACIDS 48
Mi-Acid Double Strength - See ANTACIDS 48
Micanol - See ANTHRALIN (Topical) 52
Micardis - See ANGIOTENSIN II RECEPTOR ANTAGONISTS 42
Micardis HCT - See
ANGIOTENSIN II RECEPTOR ANTAGONISTS 42
DIURETICS, THIAZIDE 338
Micardis Plus - See
ANGIOTENSIN II RECEPTOR ANTAGONISTS 42
DIURETICS, THIAZIDE 338
Micatin - See ANTIFUNGALS (Topical) 88
MICONAZOLE - See
ANTIFUNGALS (Topical) 88
ANTIFUNGALS (Vaginal) 90
Micrainin - See
ASPIRIN 152
MEPROBAMATE 538
Microgestin Fe - See CONTRACEPTIVES, ORAL & SKIN 278
Micro-K - See POTASSIUM SUPPLEMENTS 666
Micro-K 10 - See POTASSIUM SUPPLEMENTS 666
Micro-K LS - See POTASSIUM SUPPLEMENTS 666
Micronase - See SULFONYLUREAS 770
microNEFRIN - See BRONCHODILATORS, ADRENERGIC 200
Micronor - See PROGESTINS 680
Midamor - See DIURETICS, POTASSIUM-SPARING 334
MIDAZOLAM - See BENZODIAZEPINES 176
Midol 200 - See ANTI-INFLAMMATORY DRUGS, NONSTEROIDAL (NSAIDs) 116
Midol-IB - See ANTI-INFLAMMATORY DRUGS, NONSTEROIDAL (NSAIDs) 116
Mifeprex - See MIFEPRISTONE 556
MIFEPRISTONE 556
Migergot - See
CAFFEINE 216
ERGOT DERIVATIVES 366
MIGLITOL 558
Migranal - See ERGOT DERIVATIVES 366
MILK OF MAGNESIA - See LAXATIVES, OSMOTIC 478
Milkinol - See LAXATIVES, SOFTENER/LUBRICANT 480
MILNACIPRAN - See SEROTONIN & NOREPINEPHRINE REUPTAKE INHIBITORS (SNRIs) 746
Milophene - See CLOMIPHENE 260
Miltown - See MEPROBAMATE 538
MINERAL OIL - See
LAXATIVES, OSMOTIC 478
LAXATIVES, SOFTENER/LUBRICANT 480
Mineral supplement - See
IRON SUPPLEMENTS 458
SODIUM FLUORIDE 752
Mineral supplement (Potassium) - See POTASSIUM SUPPLEMENTS 666
Minestrin 1/20 - See CONTRACEPTIVES, ORAL & SKIN 278
Minims Atropine - See CYCLOPLEGIC, MYDRIATIC (Ophthalmic) 292
Minims Cyclopentolate - See CYCLOPENTOLATE (Ophthalmic) 288
Minims Homatropine - See CYCLOPLEGIC, MYDRIATIC (Ophthalmic) 292
Minims Phenylephrine - See PHENYLEPHRINE (Ophthalmic) 660
Minims - See ANTIGLAUCOMA, CHOLINERGIC AGONISTS 100
Minipress - See ALPHA ADRENERGIC RECEPTOR BLOCKERS 20

Minitran - See NITRATES 602
Minivelle - See ESTROGENS 372
Minizide - See
ALPHA ADRENERGIC RECEPTOR BLOCKERS 20
DIURETICS, THIAZIDE 338
Minocin - See TETRACYCLINES 782
MINOCYCLINE - See TETRACYCLINES 782
Min-Ovral - See CONTRACEPTIVES, ORAL & SKIN 278
MINOXIDIL 560
MINOXIDIL (Topical) 562
Mintezol - See ANTHELMINTICS 50
Mintezol Topical - See ANTHELMINTICS 50
Mintox - See ANTACIDS 48
Mintox Extra Strength - See ANTACIDS 48
Minzolum - See ANTHELMINTICS 50
Miocarpine - See ANTIGLAUCOMA, CHOLINERGIC AGONISTS 100
Miostat - See ANTIGLAUCOMA, CHOLINERGIC AGONISTS 100
MIRABEGRON 564
Miralax - See LAXATIVES, OSMOTIC 478
Mirapex - See DOPAMINE AGONISTS NONERGOT 344
Mirapex ER - See DOPAMINE AGONISTS NONERGOT 344
Mircette- See CONTRACEPTIVES, ORAL & SKIN 278
MIRTAZAPINE 566
MISOPROSTOL 568
Mitrolan - See LAXATIVES, BULK-FORMING 476
Mobic - See MELOXICAM 532
Mobidin - See SALICYLATES 736
Mobiflex - See ANTI-INFLAMMATORY DRUGS, NONSTEROIDAL (NSAIDs) 116
MODAFINIL- See STIMULANTS, AMPHETAMINE-RELATED 756
Modane Bulk - See LAXATIVES, BULK-FORMING 476
Modane Plus - See LAXATIVES, SOFTENER/ LUBRICANT 480
Modane Soft - See LAXATIVES, SOFTENER/ LUBRICANT 480
Modecate - See PHENOTHIAZINES 656
Modecate Concentrate - See PHENOTHIAZINES 656
ModiCon - See CONTRACEPTIVES, ORAL & SKIN 278
Modified Shohl's Solution - See CITRATES 254
Moditen Enanthate - See PHENOTHIAZINES 656
Moditen HCl - See PHENOTHIAZINES 656
Moditen HCl-H.P - See PHENOTHIAZINES 656
Modrastane - See TRILOSTANE 814
Moduret - See DIURETICS, POTASSIUM-SPARING & HYDROCHLOROTHIAZIDE 336
Moduretic - See DIURETICS, POTASSIUM-SPARING & HYDROCHLOROTHIAZIDE 336
MOEXIPRIL - See ANGIOTENSIN-CONVERTING ENZYME (ACE) INHIBITORS 44
Mogadon - See BENZODIAZEPINES 176
Moisture Drops - See PROTECTANT (Ophthalmic) 690
Molatoc - See LAXATIVES, SOFTENER/ LUBRICANT 480
Molatoc-CST - See
LAXATIVES, SOFTENER/LUBRICANT 480
LAXATIVES, STIMULANT 482
MOMETASONE (Nasal) - See ADRENOCORTICOIDS (Nasal Inhalation) 12
MOMETASONE (Oral Inhalation) - See ADRENOCORTICOIDS (Oral Inhalation) 14
MOMETASONE (Topical) - See ADRENOCORTICOIDS (Topical) 18
Monistat - See ANTIFUNGALS (Vaginal) 90
Monistat 1 - See ANTIFUNGALS (Vaginal) 90
Monistat 3 - See ANTIFUNGALS (Vaginal) 90
Monistat 5 - See ANTIFUNGALS (Vaginal) 90
Monistat 7 - See ANTIFUNGALS (Vaginal) 90
Monistat-Derm - See ANTIFUNGALS (Topical) 88
Monitan - See BETA-ADRENERGIC BLOCKING AGENTS 182
MONOAMINE OXIDASE (MAO) INHIBITORS 570
MONOAMINE OXIDASE TYPE B (MAO-B) INHIBITORS 572
Monodox - See TETRACYCLINES 782
Mono-Gesic - See SALICYLATES 736
Monoket - See NITRATES 602
Monopril - See ANGIOTENSIN-CONVERTING ENZYME (ACE) INHIBITORS 44
MONTELUKAST - See LEUKOTRIENE MODIFIERS 488
Mood stabilizer - See LITHIUM 504
MORPHINE - See NARCOTIC ANALGESICS 584
Morphitec - See NARCOTIC ANALGESICS 584
M.O.S. - See NARCOTIC ANALGESICS 584
M.O.S.-SR - See NARCOTIC ANALGESICS 584
Motion-Aid - See ANTIHISTAMINES 106
Motofen - See DIFENOXIN & ATROPINE 318
Motrin-IB - See ANTI-INFLAMMATORY DRUGS, NONSTEROIDAL (NSAIDs) 116

Motrin-IB Cold & Sinus - See
ANTI-INFLAMMATORY DRUGS, NONSTEROIDAL (NSAIDs) 116
PSEUDOEPHEDRINE 694
Movergan - See MONOAMINE OXIDASE TYPE B (MAO-B) INHIBITORS 572
Moxatag - See PENICILLINS 646
Moxeza - See ANTIBACTERIALS (Ophthalmic) 66
MOXIFLOXACIN - See FLUOROQUINOLONES 392
MOXIFLOXACIN (Ophthalmic) - See ANTIBACTERIALS (Ophthalmic) 66
MS Contin - See NARCOTIC ANALGESICS 584
MSIR - See NARCOTIC ANALGESICS 584
MST Continus - See NARCOTIC ANALGESICS 584
Mucinex - See GUAIFENESIN 416
Mucinex Adult Caplets - Cold & Sinus - See
ACETAMINOPHEN 8
GUAIFENESIN 416
PHENYLEPHRINE 658
Mucinex Adult Caplets - Cold, Flu, & Sore Throat - See
ACETAMINOPHEN 8
DEXTROMETHORPHAN 312
GUAIFENESIN 416
PHENYLEPHRINE 658
Mucinex Adult Caplets - Severe Congestion & Cold - See
ACETAMINOPHEN 8
DEXTROMETHORPHAN 312
GUAIFENESIN 416
PHENYLEPHRINE 658
Mucinex Children's Cough, Expectorant and Suppressant - See
DEXTROMETHORPHAN 312
GUAIFENESIN 416
Mucinex Children's Expectorant - See
GUAIFENESIN 416
Mucinex Cold Liquid - See
GUAIFENESIN 416
PHENYLEPHRINE 658
Mucinex Cough Mini-Melts - See
DEXTROMETHORPHAN 312
GUAIFENESIN 416
Mucinex D - See
GUAIFENESIN 416
PSEUDOEPHEDRINE 694
Mucinex DM - See
DEXTROMETHORPHAN 312
GUAIFENESIN 416
Mucinex Fast-Max Cold, Flu & Sore Throat Liquid - See
ACETAMINOPHEN 8
DEXTROMETHORPHAN 312
GUAIFENESIN 416
PHENYLEPHRINE 658
Mucinex Full Force Nasal Spray - See
OXYMETAZOLINE (Nasal) 630
Mucinex Junior Strength Expectorant - See
GUAIFENESIN 416
Mucinex Maximum Strength Fast Max Cold, Flu & Sore Throat - See
ACETAMINOPHEN 8
DEXTROMETHORPHAN 312
GUAIFENESIN 416
PHENYLEPHRINE 658
Mucinex Maximum Strength - Fast Max Severe Congestion & Cough - See
DEXTROMETHORPHAN 312
GUAIFENESIN 416
PHENYLEPHRINE 658
Mucinex Mini-Melts - See GUAIFENESIN 416
Mucinex Moisture Smart Nasal Spray - See
OXYMETAZOLINE (Nasal) 630
Mucinum - See LAXATIVES, STIMULANT 482
Mucinum Herbal - See LAXATIVES, STIMULANT 482
Mucolysin - See TIOPRONIN 798
Mudrane GG2 - See
BRONCHODILATORS, XANTHINE 204
GUAIFENESIN 416
Multaq - See ANTIARRHYTHMICS, BENZOFURAN-TYPE 60
Multipax - See HYDROXYZINE 436
Mulvidren-F - See VITAMINS & FLUORIDE 848
MUPIROCIN - See ANTIBACTERIALS (Topical) 70
Murine Plus - See DECONGESTANTS (Ophthalmic) 306
Muro's Opcon - See DECONGESTANTS (Ophthalmic) 306
<u>MUSCARINIC RECEPTOR ANTAGONISTS</u> 574
Muscle relaxant - See
BACLOFEN 166
CYCLOBENZAPRINE 286
DANTROLENE 302
MUSCLE RELAXANTS, SKELETAL 576
ORPHENADRINE 624
ORPHENADRINE, ASPIRIN & CAFFEINE 626
TIZANIDINE 800
<u>MUSCLE RELAXANTS, SKELETAL</u> 576
Muse - See ALPROSTADIL 22
Mustargen - See MECHLORETHAMINE (Topical) 526
My Cort - See ADRENOCORTICOIDS (Topical) 18
Myapap Elixir - See ACETAMINOPHEN 8

Mycelex Cream - See ANTIFUNGALS (Topical) 88
Mycelex Solution - See ANTIFUNGALS (Topical) 88
Mycelex Troches - See CLOTRIMAZOLE (Oral-Local) 262
Mycelex-7 - See ANTIFUNGALS (Vaginal) 90
Mycelex-G - See ANTIFUNGALS (Vaginal) 90
Mycifradin - See NEOMYCIN (Oral) 592
Myciguent - See NEOMYCIN (Topical) 594
Mycitracin - See ANTIBACTERIALS (Topical) 70
Myclo - See ANTIFUNGALS (Vaginal) 90
Myclo Cream - See ANTIFUNGALS (Topical) 88
Myclo Solution - See ANTIFUNGALS (Topical) 88
Myclo Spray - See ANTIFUNGALS (Topical) 88
Myco II - See
ADRENOCORTICOIDS (Topical) 18
NYSTATIN 614
Mycobiotic II - See NYSTATIN 614
Mycogen II - See
ADRENOCORTICOIDS (Topical) 18
NYSTATIN 614
Mycolog II - See
ADRENOCORTICOIDS (Topical) 18
NYSTATIN 614
MYCOPHENOLATE - See IMMUNOSUPPRESSIVE AGENTS 442
Mycostatin - See
ANTIFUNGALS (Topical) 88
ANTIFUNGALS (Vaginal) 90
NYSTATIN 614
Myco-Triacet II - See
ADRENOCORTICOIDS (Topical) 18
NYSTATIN 614
Mydfrin - See PHENYLEPHRINE (Ophthalmic) 660
Mydriatic - See
CYCLOPENTOLATE (Ophthalmic) 288
CYCLOPLEGIC, MYDRIATIC (Ophthalmic) 292
PHENYLEPHRINE (Ophthalmic) 660
My-E - See ERYTHROMYCINS 368
Myfedrine - See PSEUDOEPHEDRINE 694
Myfortic - See IMMUNOSUPPRESSIVE AGENTS 442
Myfortic Delayed-Release - See IMMUNOSUPPRESSIVE AGENTS 442
Mygel - See
ANTACIDS 48
SIMETHICONE 748
Mygel II - See ANTACIDS 48
Myidil - See ANTIHISTAMINES 106
Myidone - See PRIMIDONE 674
Mykacet - See NYSTATIN 614
Mykacet II - See NYSTATIN 614
Mykrox - See DIURETICS, THIAZIDE 338
Mylagen - See ANTACIDS 48
Mylagen II - See ANTACIDS 48
Mylanta - See ANTACIDS 48
Mylanta Calci Tabs - See ANTACIDS 48
Mylanta Double Strength - See ANTACIDS 48
Mylanta Double Strength Plain - See ANTACIDS 48
Mylanta Gas - See SIMETHICONE 748
Mylanta Gelcaps - See ANTACIDS 48
Mylanta Maximum Strength - See ANTACIDS 48
Mylanta Natural Fiber Supplement - See LAXATIVES, BULK-FORMING 476
Mylanta Nighttime Strength - See ANTACIDS 48
Mylanta Plain - See ANTACIDS 48
Mylanta Regular Strength - See ANTACIDS 48
Mylanta Sugar Free Natural Fiber Supplement - See LAXATIVES, BULK-FORMING 476
Mylanta-AR - See HISTAMINE H_2 RECEPTOR ANTAGONISTS 422
Mylanta-II - See ANTACIDS 48
Myleran - See BUSULFAN 212
Mylicon - See SIMETHICONE 748
Mylicon-80 - See SIMETHICONE 748
Mylicon-125 - See SIMETHICONE 748
Mymethasone - See ADRENOCORTICOIDS (Systemic) 16
Myobloc - See BOTULINUM TOXIN TYPE A 196
Myocrisin - See GOLD COMPOUNDS 412
Myolin - See ORPHENADRINE 624
Myotrol - See ORPHENADRINE 624
Myrbetriq - See MIRABEGRON 564
Myrosemide - See DIURETICS, LOOP 332
Mysoline - See PRIMIDONE 674
Mytrex - See
ADRENOCORTICOIDS (Topical) 18
NYSTATIN 614
Mytussin AC - See
GUAIFENESIN 416
NARCOTIC ANALGESICS 584
Mytussin DAC - See
GUAIFENESIN 416
NARCOTIC ANALGESICS 584
PSEUDOEPHEDRINE 694
Mytussin DM - See
DEXTROMETHORPHAN 312
GUAIFENESIN 416
Myzilra - See CONTRACEPTIVES, ORAL & SKIN 278
MZM - See CARBONIC ANHYDRASE INHIBITORS 232

N

N3 Gesic - See ORPHENADRINE, ASPIRIN & CAFFEINE 626
N3 Gesic Forte - See ORPHENADRINE, ASPIRIN & CAFFEINE 626
NABILONE 578
NABUMETONE - See ANTI-INFLAMMATORY DRUGS, NONSTEROIDAL (NSAIDs) 116
NADOLOL - See BETA-ADRENERGIC BLOCKING AGENTS 182
NADOLOL & BENDROFLUMETHIAZIDE - See BETA-ADRENERGIC BLOCKING AGENTS & THIAZIDE DIURETICS 184
Nadopen-V - See PENICILLINS 646
Nadopen-V 200 - See PENICILLINS 646
Nadopen-V 400 - See PENICILLINS 646
Nadostine - See
ANTIFUNGALS (Topical) 88
ANTIFUNGALS (Vaginal) 90
NYSTATIN 614
NAFARELIN 580
Nafazair - See DECONGESTANTS (Ophthalmic) 306
NAFCILLIN - See PENICILLINS 646
NAFTIFINE - See ANTIFUNGALS (Topical) 88
Naftin - See ANTIFUNGALS (Topical) 88
NALBUPHINE - See NARCOTIC ANALGESICS 584
Nalcrom - See CROMOLYN 282
Naldecon Senior DX - See
DEXTROMETHORPHAN 312
GUAIFENESIN 416
Naldecon Senior EX - See GUAIFENESIN 416
Naldecon-DX - See DEXTROMETHORPHAN 312
Nalfon - See ANTI-INFLAMMATORY DRUGS, NONSTEROIDAL (NSAIDs) 116
Nalfon 200 - See ANTI-INFLAMMATORY DRUGS, NONSTEROIDAL (NSAIDs) 116
NALTREXONE 582
Namenda - See MEMANTINE 536
Namenda Oral Solution - See MEMANTINE 536
Namenda XR - See MEMANTINE 536
Nandrobolic - See ANDROGENS 34
Nandrobolic L.A. - See ANDROGENS 34
NANDROLONE - See ANDROGENS 34
NAPHAZOLINE - See DECONGESTANTS (Ophthalmic) 306
Naphcon - See DECONGESTANTS (Ophthalmic) 306
Naphcon A - See DECONGESTANTS (Ophthalmic) 306
Naphcon Forte - See DECONGESTANTS (Ophthalmic) 306
Naprelan - See ANTI-INFLAMMATORY DRUGS, NONSTEROIDAL (NSAIDs) 116
Naprosyn - See ANTI-INFLAMMATORY DRUGS, NONSTEROIDAL (NSAIDs) 116
Naprosyn-E - See ANTI-INFLAMMATORY DRUGS, NONSTEROIDAL (NSAIDs) 116
Naprosyn-SR - See ANTI-INFLAMMATORY DRUGS, NONSTEROIDAL (NSAIDs) 116
NAPROXEN - See ANTI-INFLAMMATORY DRUGS, NONSTEROIDAL (NSAIDs) 116
Naqua - See DIURETICS, THIAZIDE 338
NARATRIPTAN - See TRIPTANS 820
Narcotic - See
BARBITURATES, ASPIRIN & CODEINE (Also contains caffeine) 170
NARCOTIC ANALGESICS 584
NARCOTIC ANALGESICS & ACETAMINOPHEN 586
NARCOTIC ANALGESICS & ASPIRIN 588
PAREGORIC 640
Narcotic analgesic - See
BUPRENORPHINE & NALOXONE 206
BUTORPHANOL 214
NARCOTIC ANALGESICS 584
NARCOTIC ANALGESICS & ACETAMINOPHEN 586
NARCOTIC ANALGESICS & ASPIRIN 588
Narcotic antagonist - See NALTREXONE 582
Nardil - See MONOAMINE OXIDASE (MAO) INHIBITORS 570
Nasacort AQ - See ADRENOCORTICOIDS (Nasal Inhalation) 12
Nasacort HFA - See ADRENOCORTICOIDS (Nasal Inhalation) 12
Nasahist B - See ANTIHISTAMINES 106
Nasal decongestant - See CROMOLYN 282
Nasal Decongestant Spray - See OXYMETAZOLINE (Nasal) 630
Nasal Relief - See OXYMETAZOLINE (Nasal) 630
Nasal Spray 12-Hour - See OXYMETAZOLINE (Nasal) 630
Nasal Spray Long Acting - See OXYMETAZOLINE (Nasal) 630
Nasal-12 Hour - See OXYMETAZOLINE (Nasal) 630
Nasalcrom Nasal Spray - See CROMOLYN 282
Nasatab LA - See
GUAIFENESIN 416
PSEUDOEPHEDRINE 694
Nascobal - See VITAMIN B-12 (Cyanocobalamin) 836
Nasonex - See ADRENOCORTICOIDS (Nasal Inhalation) 12

INDEX

Nasonex Aqueous Nasal Spray - See ADRENOCORTICOIDS (Nasal Inhalation) 12
Natazia - See CONTRACEPTIVES, ORAL & SKIN 278
NATEGLINIDE - See MEGLITINIDES 528
Natroba Topical Suspension - See PEDICULICIDES (Topical) 642
Natulan - See PROCARBAZINE 678
Naturacil - See LAXATIVES, BULK-FORMING 476
Natural Source Fibre Laxative - See LAXATIVES, BULK-FORMING 476
Nature's Remedy - See LAXATIVES, STIMULANT 482
Nature's Tears - See PROTECTANT (Ophthalmic) 690
Naturetin - See DIURETICS, THIAZIDE 338
Nauseatol - See ANTIHISTAMINES 106
Navane - See THIOTHIXENE 790
Naxen - See ANTI-INFLAMMATORY DRUGS, NONSTEROIDAL (NSAIDs) 116
ND Clear T.D. - See
ANTIHISTAMINES 106
PSEUDOEPHEDRINE 694
ND Stat Revised - See ANTIHISTAMINES 106
ND-Gesic - See
ACETAMINOPHEN 8
ANTIHISTAMINES 106
PHENYLEPHRINE 658
NEBIVOLOL - See BETA-ADRENERGIC BLOCKING AGENTS 182
NebuPent - See PENTAMIDINE 650
Necon 0.5/35-21 - See CONTRACEPTIVES, ORAL & SKIN 278
Necon 0.5/35-28 - See CONTRACEPTIVES, ORAL & SKIN 278
Necon 1/35-21 - See CONTRACEPTIVES, ORAL & SKIN 278
Necon 1/35-28 - See CONTRACEPTIVES, ORAL & SKIN 278
Necon 1/50-21 - See CONTRACEPTIVES, ORAL & SKIN 278
Necon 1/50-28 - See CONTRACEPTIVES, ORAL & SKIN 278
Necon 10/11-21 - See CONTRACEPTIVES, ORAL & SKIN 278
Necon 10/11-28 - See CONTRACEPTIVES, ORAL & SKIN 278
NEDOCROMIL (Ophthalmic) - See ANTIALLERGIC AGENTS (Ophthalmic) 56
N.E.E. 1/35 - See CONTRACEPTIVES, ORAL & SKIN 278
N.E.E. 1/50 - See CONTRACEPTIVES, ORAL & SKIN 278
<u>NEFAZODONE</u> 590
NELFINAVIR - See PROTEASE INHIBITORS 688
Nelova 0.5/35E - See CONTRACEPTIVES, ORAL & SKIN 278
Nelova 1/35E - See CONTRACEPTIVES, ORAL & SKIN 278
Nelova 1/50M - See CONTRACEPTIVES, ORAL & SKIN 278
Nelova 10/11 - See CONTRACEPTIVES, ORAL & SKIN 278
Nelulen 1/35E - See CONTRACEPTIVES, ORAL & SKIN 278
Nelulen 1/50E - See CONTRACEPTIVES, ORAL & SKIN 278
Nembutal - See BARBITURATES 168
NeoBenz Micro- See BENZOYL PEROXIDE 178
Neo-Calglucon - See CALCIUM SUPPLEMENTS 222
Neocidin Ophthalmic Ointment - See ANTIBACTERIALS (Ophthalmic) 66
NeoCitran A - See
ANTIHISTAMINES 106
PHENYLEPHRINE 658
NeoCitran Colds & Flu Calorie Reduced - See
ACETAMINOPHEN 8
ANTIHISTAMINES 106
PHENYLEPHRINE 658
NeoCitran DM Coughs & Colds - See
ANTIHISTAMINES 106
DEXTROMETHORPHAN 312
GUAIFENESIN 416
PHENYLEPHRINE 658
NeoCitran Extra Strength Colds and Flu - See
ACETAMINOPHEN 8
ANTIHISTAMINES 106
PHENYLEPHRINE 658
NeoCitran Extra Strength Sinus - See
ACETAMINOPHEN 8
PHENYLEPHRINE 658
Neo-Codema - See DIURETICS, THIAZIDE 338
Neo-Cultol - See LAXATIVES, SOFTENER/ LUBRICANT 480
Neocyten - See ORPHENADRINE 624
Neo-DM - See DEXTROMETHORPHAN 312
Neo-Durabolic - See ANDROGENS 34
Neo-Estrone - See ESTROGENS 372
Neo-Fer - See IRON SUPPLEMENTS 458
Neofrin - See PHENYLEPHRINE (Ophthalmic) 660
Neo-K - See POTASSIUM SUPPLEMENTS 666
Neolax - See
LAXATIVES, SOFTENER/LUBRICANT 480
LAXATIVES, STIMULANT 482
Neoloid - See LAXATIVES, STIMULANT 482

Neo-Metric - See NITROIMIDAZOLES 606
NEOMYCIN (Oral) 592
NEOMYCIN (Topical) 594
NEOMYCIN & POLYMYXIN B - See
ANTIBACTERIALS (Ophthalmic) 66
ANTIBACTERIALS (Topical) 70
NEOMYCIN, COLISTIN & HYDROCORTISONE - See ANTIBACTERIALS (Otic) 68
NEOMYCIN, POLYMIXIN B & BACITRACIN - See
ANTIBACTERIALS (Ophthalmic) 66
ANTIBACTERIALS (Topical) 70
NEOMYCIN, POLYMIXIN B & GRAMICIDIN - See ANTIBACTERIALS (Ophthalmic) 66
Neopap - See ACETAMINOPHEN 8
Neo-Polycin - See ANTIBACTERIALS (Topical) 70
Neo-Polycin - See ANTIBACTERIALS (Ophthalmic) 66
Neo-Polycin HC - See
ANTIBACTERIALS (Ophthalmic) 66
ANTI-INFLAMMATORY DRUGS, STEROIDAL (Ophthalmic) 122
Neoquess - See
DICYCLOMINE 316
HYOSCYAMINE 438
Neoral - See CYCLOSPORINE 296
Neosar - See CYCLOPHOSPHAMIDE 290
Neosporin Cream - See ANTIBACTERIALS (Topical) 70
Neosporin Ointment - See ANTIBACTERIALS (Topical) 70
Neosporin Ophthalmic Ointment - See ANTIBACTERIALS (Ophthalmic) 66
Neosporin Ophthalmic Solution - See ANTIBACTERIALS (Ophthalmic) 66
NEOSTIGMINE - See ANTIMYASTHENICS 128
Neo-Synephrine 12 Hour Nasal Spray - See OXYMETAZOLINE (Nasal) 630
Neo-Synephrine 12 Hour Nasal Spray Pump - See OXYMETAZOLINE (Nasal) 630
Neo-Synephrine 12 Hour Nose Drops - See OXYMETAZOLINE (Nasal) 630
Neo-Synephrine 12 Hour Vapor Nasal Spray - See OXYMETAZOLINE (Nasal) 630
Neo-Synephrine II Long Acting Nasal Spray Adult Strength - See XYLOMETAZOLINE 850
Neo-Synephrine II Long Acting Nose Drops Adult Strength - See XYLOMETAZOLINE 850
Neo-Synephrine Nasal Drops - See PHENYLEPHRINE 658
Neo-Synephrine Pediatric Nasal Drops - See PHENYLEPHRINE 658
Neotal - See ANTIBACTERIALS (Ophthalmic) 66
Neothylline - See BRONCHODILATORS, XANTHINE 204
Neotricin HC- See
ANTIBACTERIALS (Ophthalmic) 66
ANTI-INFLAMMATORY DRUGS, STEROIDAL (Ophthalmic) 122
NEPAFENAC - See ANTI-INFLAMMATORY DRUGS, NONSTEROIDAL (NSAIDs) (Ophthalmic) 120
Nephro-Calci - See CALCIUM SUPPLEMENTS 222
Nephron - See BRONCHODILATORS, ADRENERGIC 200
Nephronex - See NITROFURANTOIN 604
Nephrox - See ANTACIDS 48
Neptazane - See CARBONIC ANHYDRASE INHIBITORS 232
Nerisone - See ADRENOCORTICOIDS (Topical) 18
Nerisone Oily - See ADRENOCORTICOIDS (Topical) 18
Nervine - See ASPIRIN 152
Nervine Night-time Sleep-Aid - See ANTIHISTAMINES 106
Nesina - See DPP-4 INHIBITORS 348
Neuleptil - See PHENOTHIAZINES 656
Neupro - See DOPAMINE AGONISTS NONERGOT 344
Neuramate - See MEPROBAMATE 538
Neuromuscular blocking agent - See BOTULINUM TOXIN TYPE A 196
Neurontin - See GABAPENTIN 402
Neutralca-S - See ANTACIDS 48
Neutra-Phos K - See POTASSIUM SUPPLEMENTS 666
Neutrogena Acne Mask 5 - See BENZOYL PEROXIDE 178
Nevanac - See ANTI-INFLAMMATORY DRUGS, NONSTEROIDAL (NSAIDs) (Ophthalmic) 120
NEVIRAPINE - See NON-NUCLEOSIDE REVERSE TRANSCRIPTASE INHIBITORS 608
Nexafed - See PSEUDOEPHEDRINE 694
Nexcede - See ANTI-INFLAMMATORY DRUGS, NONSTEROIDAL (NSAIDs) 116
Nexiclon XR - See CENTRAL ALPHA AGONISTS 234
Nexium Delayed Release Capsules - See PROTON PUMP INHIBITORS 692
Nexium For Delayed-Release Oral Suspension - See PROTON PUMP INHIBITORS 692

Next Choice - See PROGESTINS 680

Nia-Bid - See NIACIN (Vitamin B-3, Nicotinic Acid, Nicotinamide) 596

Niac - See NIACIN (Vitamin B-3, Nicotinic Acid, Nicotinamide) 596

Niacels - See NIACIN (Vitamin B-3, Nicotinic Acid, Nicotinamide) 596

Niacin - See NIACIN (Vitamin B-3, Nicotinic Acid, Nicotinamide) 596

NIACIN (Vitamin B-3, Nicotinic Acid, Nicotinamide) 596

Niacor - See NIACIN (Vitamin B-3, Nicotinic Acid, Nicotinamide) 596

Niaspan - See NIACIN (Vitamin B-3, Nicotinic Acid, Nicotinamide) 596

NICARDIPINE - See CALCIUM CHANNEL BLOCKERS 220

Nico-400 - See NIACIN (Vitamin B-3, Nicotinic Acid, Nicotinamide) 596

Nicobid - See NIACIN (Vitamin B-3, Nicotinic Acid, Nicotinamide) 596

Nicoderm - See NICOTINE 598

Nicoderm CQ - See NICOTINE 598

NicoDerm CQ ThinFlex Patch - See NICOTINE 598

Nicolar - See NIACIN (Vitamin B-3, Nicotinic Acid, Nicotinamide) 596

Nicorette - See NICOTINE 598

Nicorette DS - See NICOTINE 598

Nicorette Fresh Mint - See NICOTINE 598

Nicorrette Lozenge - See NICOTINE 598

NICOTINAMIDE - See NIACIN (Vitamin B-3, Nicotinic Acid, Nicotinamide) 596

NICOTINE 598

Nicotinex - See NIACIN (Vitamin B-3, Nicotinic Acid, Nicotinamide) 596

NICOTINIC ACID - See NIACIN (Vitamin B-3, Nicotinic Acid, Nicotinamide) 596

Nicotinyl alcohol - See NIACIN (Vitamin B-3, Nicotinic Acid, Nicotinamide) 596

Nicotrol - See NICOTINE 598

Nicotrol NS - See NICOTINE 598

Nico-Vert - See ANTIHISTAMINES 106

Nidryl - See ANTIHISTAMINES 106

Nifedical XL - See CALCIUM CHANNEL BLOCKERS 220

NIFEDIPINE - See CALCIUM CHANNEL BLOCKERS 220

Nifuran - See NITROFURANTOIN 604

Night Cast R - See KERATOLYTICS 470

Night Cast Regular Formula Mask-Lotion - See KERATOLYTICS 470

Night Cast Special Formula Mask-Lotion - See KERATOLYTICS 470

Nighttime Pamprin - See ACETAMINOPHEN 8

Nilandron - See ANTIANDROGENS, NONSTEROIDAL 58

Niloric - See ERGOLOID MESYLATES 362

Nilstat - See
ANTIFUNGALS (Topical) 88
ANTIFUNGALS (Vaginal) 90
NYSTATIN 614

NILUTAMIDE - See ANTIANDROGENS, NONSTEROIDAL 58

Niong - See NITRATES 602

Niravam - See BENZODIAZEPINES 176

Niravam Orally Disintegrating Tablets - See BENZODIAZEPINES 176

Nisaval - See ANTIHISTAMINES 106

NISOLDIPINE - See CALCIUM CHANNEL BLOCKERS 220

NITAZOXANIDE 600

NITRATES 602

NITRAZEPAM - See BENZODIAZEPINES 176

Nitrex - See NITROFURANTOIN 604

Nitro-Bid - See NITRATES 602

Nitrocap - See NITRATES 602

Nitrocap T.D. - See NITRATES 602

Nitrocine - See NITRATES 602

Nitrodisc - See NITRATES 602

Nitro-Dur - See NITRATES 602

Nitro-Dur II - See NITRATES 602

Nitrofan - See NITROFURANTOIN 604

Nitrofor - See NITROFURANTOIN 604

Nitrofuracot - See NITROFURANTOIN 604

NITROFURANTOIN 604

Nitrogard-SR - See NITRATES 602

NITROGLYCERIN (GLYCERYL TRINITRATE) - See NITRATES 602

Nitroglyn - See NITRATES 602

NITROIMIDAZOLES 606

Nitrol - See NITRATES 602

Nitrolin - See NITRATES 602

Nitrolingual - See NITRATES 602

NitroMist - See NITRATES 602

Nitronet - See NITRATES 602

Nitrong - See NITRATES 602

Nitrong SR - See NITRATES 602

Nitrospan - See NITRATES 602

Nitrostat - See NITRATES 602

Nix Cream Rinse - See PEDICULICIDES (Topical) 642

NIZATIDINE - See HISTAMINE H_2 RECEPTOR ANTAGONISTS 422

Nizoral - See ANTIFUNGALS, AZOLES 86

Nizoral A-D - See ANTIFUNGALS (Topical) 88

Nizoral Shampoo - See ANTIFUNGALS (Topical) 88

N-methyl-D-aspartate (NMDA) receptor antagonist - See MEMANTINE 536

Nolahist - See ANTIHISTAMINES 106
Nonbenzodiazepine hypnotic - See RAMELTEON 710
NON-NUCLEOSIDE REVERSE TRANSCRIPTASE INHIBITORS 608
NONOXYNOL 9 - See CONTRACEPTIVES, VAGINAL 280
Nonsteroidal anti-inflammatory drug (NSAID), topical - See DICLOFENAC (Topical) 314
Noradex - See ORPHENADRINE 624
Noradryl - See ANTIHISTAMINES 106
Norafed - See ANTIHISTAMINES 106
Norcept-E 1/35 - See CONTRACEPTIVES, ORAL & SKIN 278
Norco - See NARCOTIC ANALGESICS & ACETAMINOPHEN 586
Nordette - See CONTRACEPTIVES, ORAL & SKIN 278
Nordryl - See ANTIHISTAMINES 106
Nordryl Cough - See ANTIHISTAMINES 106
NORELGESTROMIN & ETHINYL ESTRADIOL - See CONTRACEPTIVES, ORAL & SKIN 278
Norethin 1/35E - See CONTRACEPTIVES, ORAL & SKIN 278
Norethin 1/50M - See CONTRACEPTIVES, ORAL & SKIN 278
NORETHINDRONE - See PROGESTINS 680
NORETHINDRONE & ETHINYL ESTRADIOL - See CONTRACEPTIVES, ORAL & SKIN 278
NORETHINDRONE & MESTRANOL - See CONTRACEPTIVES, ORAL & SKIN 278
NORETHINDRONE ACETATE & ETHINYL ESTRADIOL - See CONTRACEPTIVES, ORAL & SKIN 278
Norflex - See ORPHENADRINE 624
NORFLOXACIN - See FLUOROQUINOLONES 392
NORFLOXACIN (Ophthalmic) - See ANTIBACTERIALS (Ophthalmic) 66
Norfranil - See ANTIDEPRESSANTS, TRICYCLIC 80
Norgesic - See ORPHENADRINE, ASPIRIN & CAFFEINE 626
Norgesic Forte - See ORPHENADRINE, ASPIRIN & CAFFEINE 626
NORGESTIMATE - See PROGESTINS 680
NORGESTIMATE & ETHINYL ESTRADIOL - See CONTRACEPTIVES, ORAL & SKIN 278
NORGESTREL - See PROGESTINS 680
NORGESTREL & ETHINYL ESTRADIOL - See CONTRACEPTIVES, ORAL & SKIN 278
Norinyl 1+35 - See CONTRACEPTIVES, ORAL & SKIN 278
Norinyl 1+50 - See CONTRACEPTIVES, ORAL & SKIN 278
Norinyl 1/50 - See CONTRACEPTIVES, ORAL & SKIN 278
Noritate - See NITROIMIDAZOLES 606
Norlestrin 1/50 - See CONTRACEPTIVES, ORAL & SKIN 278
Norlestrin 2.5/50 - See CONTRACEPTIVES, ORAL & SKIN 278
Norlutate - See PROGESTINS 680
Nor-Mil - See DIPHENOXYLATE & ATROPINE 324
Normodyne - See BETA-ADRENERGIC BLOCKING AGENTS 182
Normozide - See BETA-ADRENERGIC BLOCKING AGENTS & THIAZIDE DIURETICS 184
Noroxin - See FLUOROQUINOLONES 392
Norpace - See DISOPYRAMIDE 328
Norpace CR - See DISOPYRAMIDE 328
Norphadrine - See ORPHENADRINE, ASPIRIN & CAFFEINE 626
Norphadrine Forte - See ORPHENADRINE, ASPIRIN & CAFFEINE 626
Norpramin - See ANTIDEPRESSANTS, TRICYCLIC 80
Nor-Pred-TBA - See ADRENOCORTICOIDS (Systemic) 16
Nor-Q.D. - See PROGESTINS 680
NORTRIPTYLINE - See ANTIDEPRESSANTS, TRICYCLIC 80
Nortussin - See GUAIFENESIN 416
Nortussin with Codeine - See
GUAIFENESIN 416
NARCOTIC ANALGESICS 584
Norvasc - See CALCIUM CHANNEL BLOCKERS 220
Norvir - See PROTEASE INHIBITORS 688
Norwich Aspirin - See ASPIRIN 152
Nostril Nasal Decongestant Mild - See OXYMETAZOLINE (Nasal) 630
Nostril Nasal Decongestant Regular - See OXYMETAZOLINE (Nasal) 630
Nostril Spray Pump - See PHENYLEPHRINE 658
Nova Rectal - See BARBITURATES 168
Novamoxin - See PENICILLINS 646
Novasen - See ASPIRIN 152
Novo-AC and C - See
CAFFEINE 216
NARCOTIC ANALGESICS & ASPIRIN 588
Novo-Alprazol - See BENZODIAZEPINES 176
Novo-Ampicillin - See PENICILLINS 646
Novo-Atenol - See BETA-ADRENERGIC BLOCKING AGENTS 182

Novo-AZT - See NUCLEOSIDE REVERSE TRANSCRIPTASE INHIBITORS 610
Novobetamet - See ADRENOCORTICOIDS (Topical) 18
Novo-Butamide - See SULFONYLUREAS 770
Novobutazone - See ANTI-INFLAMMATORY DRUGS, NONSTEROIDAL (NSAIDs) 116
Novo-Captoril - See ANGIOTENSIN-CONVERTING ENZYME (ACE) INHIBITORS 44
Novocarbamaz - See CARBAMAZEPINE 228
Novochlorocap - See CHLORAMPHENICOL 242
Novo-Chlorpromazine - See PHENOTHIAZINES 656
Novocimetine - See HISTAMINE H_2 RECEPTOR ANTAGONISTS 422
Novoclopate - See BENZODIAZEPINES 176
Novo-Cloxin - See PENICILLINS 646
Novo-Cromolyn - See CROMOLYN 282
Novodigoxin - See DIGITALIS PREPARATIONS (Digitalis Glycosides) 320
Novo-Diltazem - See CALCIUM CHANNEL BLOCKERS 220
Novodimenate - See ANTIHISTAMINES 106
Novodipam - See BENZODIAZEPINES 176
Novodipiradol - See DIPYRIDAMOLE 326
Novodoparil - See
CENTRAL ALPHA AGONISTS 234
DIURETICS, THIAZIDE 338
Novo-Doxepin - See ANTIDEPRESSANTS, TRICYCLIC 80
Novodoxlin - See TETRACYCLINES 782
Novoferrogluc - See IRON SUPPLEMENTS 458
Novoferrosulfa - See IRON SUPPLEMENTS 458
Novofibrate - See FIBRATES 386
Novoflupam - See BENZODIAZEPINES 176
Novo-Flurazine - See PHENOTHIAZINES 656
Novo-Folacid - See FOLIC ACID (Vitamin B-9) 396
Novofumar - See IRON SUPPLEMENTS 458
Novofuran - See NITROFURANTOIN 604
Novogesic - See NARCOTIC ANALGESICS & ACETAMINOPHEN 586
Novo-Glyburide - See SULFONYLUREAS 770
Novo-Hydrazide - See DIURETICS, THIAZIDE 338
Novohydrocort - See ADRENOCORTICOIDS (Topical) 18
Novo-Hydroxyzin - See HYDROXYZINE 436
Novo-Hylazin - See HYDRALAZINE 426
Novo-Keto-EC - See ANTI-INFLAMMATORY DRUGS, NONSTEROIDAL (NSAIDs) 116
Novolexin - See CEPHALOSPORINS 236
Novolin 70/30 - See INSULIN 446
Novolin N - See INSULIN 446
Novolin R - See INSULIN 446
Novolog - See INSULIN ANALOGS 448
NovoLog FlexPen - See INSULIN ANALOGS 448
Novolog Mix 50/50 - See INSULIN ANALOGS 448
Novolorazem - See BENZODIAZEPINES 176
Novomedopa - See CENTRAL ALPHA AGONISTS 234
Novo-Mepro - See MEPROBAMATE 538
Novomethacin - See ANTI-INFLAMMATORY DRUGS, NONSTEROIDAL (NSAIDs) 116
Novometoprol - See BETA-ADRENERGIC BLOCKING AGENTS 182
Novonaprox - See ANTI-INFLAMMATORY DRUGS, NONSTEROIDAL (NSAIDs) 116
Novonidazol - See NITROIMIDAZOLES 606
Novo-Nifedin - See CALCIUM CHANNEL BLOCKERS 220
Novo-Pen VK - See PENICILLINS 646
Novopentobarb - See BARBITURATES 168
Novo-Peridol - See HALOPERIDOL 420
Novopheniram - See ANTIHISTAMINES 106
Novo-Pindol - See BETA-ADRENERGIC BLOCKING AGENTS 182
Novopirocam - See ANTI-INFLAMMATORY DRUGS, NONSTEROIDAL (NSAIDs) 116
Novopoxide - See BENZODIAZEPINES 176
Novopramine - See ANTIDEPRESSANTS, TRICYCLIC 80
Novopranol - See BETA-ADRENERGIC BLOCKING AGENTS 182
Novoprofen - See ANTI-INFLAMMATORY DRUGS, NONSTEROIDAL (NSAIDs) 116
Novo-Propamide - See SULFONYLUREAS 770
Novopural - See ANTIGOUT DRUGS 104
Novopyrazone - See SULFINPYRAZONE 764
Novoquinidin - See QUINIDINE 704
Novoreserpine - See
DIURETICS, THIAZIDE 338
RAUWOLFIA ALKALOIDS 714
Novo-Ridazine - See PHENOTHIAZINES 656
Novorythro - See ERYTHROMYCINS 368
Novosalmol - See BRONCHODILATORS, ADRENERGIC 200
Novosecobarb - See BARBITURATES 168
Novo-Selegiline - See MONOAMINE OXIDASE TYPE B (MAO-B) INHIBITORS 572
Novosemide - See DIURETICS, LOOP 332
Novosorbide - See NITRATES 602
Novo-Soxazole - See SULFONAMIDES 766
Novospiroton - See DIURETICS, POTASSIUM-SPARING 334

Novo-Sundac - See ANTI-INFLAMMATORY DRUGS, NONSTEROIDAL (NSAIDs) 116
Novo-Tamoxifen - See TAMOXIFEN 772
Novotetra - See TETRACYCLINES 782
Novo-Thalidone - See DIURETICS, THIAZIDE 338
Novothyrox - See THYROID HORMONES 792
Novo-Timol - See BETA-ADRENERGIC BLOCKING AGENTS 182
Novo-Timolol - See ANTIGLAUCOMA, BETA BLOCKERS 96
Novo-Triamzide - See DIURETICS, POTASSIUM-SPARING & HYDROCHLOROTHIAZIDE 336
Novotrimel - See
SULFONAMIDES 766
TRIMETHOPRIM 818
Novotrimel DS - See
SULFONAMIDES 766
TRIMETHOPRIM 818
Novo-Triolam - See TRIAZOLAM 812
Novotriphyl - See BRONCHODILATORS, XANTHINE 204
Novo-Tripramine - See ANTIDEPRESSANTS, TRICYCLIC 80
Novotriptyn - See ANTIDEPRESSANTS, TRICYCLIC 80
Novo-Veramil - See CALCIUM CHANNEL BLOCKERS 220
Novoxapam - See BENZODIAZEPINES 176
Noxafil - See ANTIFUNGALS, AZOLES 86
Noxzema Anti-Acne Gel - See KERATOLYTICS 470
Noxzema Anti-Acne Pads Maximum Strength - See KERATOLYTICS 470
Noxzema Anti-Acne Pads Regular Strength - See KERATOLYTICS 470
Noxzema Clear-Ups Maximum Strength 10 - See BENZOYL PEROXIDE 178
Noxzema Clear-Ups On-the-Spot 10 Lotion - See BENZOYL PEROXIDE 178
Nozinan - See PHENOTHIAZINES 656
Nozinan Liquid - See PHENOTHIAZINES 656
Nozinan Oral Drops - See PHENOTHIAZINES 656
NP-27 Cream - See ANTIFUNGALS (Topical) 88
NP-27 Powder - See ANTIFUNGALS (Topical) 88
NP-27 Solution - See ANTIFUNGALS (Topical) 88
NP-27 Spray Powder - See ANTIFUNGALS (Topical) 88
NPH - See INSULIN 446
NPH Iletin I - See INSULIN 446
NPH Iletin II - See INSULIN 446
NSAIDs - See
ANTI-INFLAMMATORY DRUGS, NONSTEROIDAL (NSAIDs) 116
ANTI-INFLAMMATORY DRUGS, NONSTEROIDAL (NSAIDs) COX-2 INHIBITORS 118
ANTI-INFLAMMATORY DRUGS, NONSTEROIDAL (NSAIDs) (Ophthalmic) 120
NTS - See NITRATES 602
NTZ Long Acting Decongestant Nasal Spray - See OXYMETAZOLINE (Nasal) 630
NTZ Long Acting Decongestant Nose Drops - See OXYMETAZOLINE (Nasal) 630
Nu-Alpraz - See BENZODIAZEPINES 176
Nu-Amoxi - See PENICILLINS 646
Nu-Ampi - See PENICILLINS 646
Nubain - See NARCOTIC ANALGESICS 584
NuCarbamazepine- See CARBAMAZEPINE 228
Nu-Cephalex - See CEPHALOSPORINS 236
NUCLEOSIDE REVERSE TRANSCRIPTASE INHIBITORS 610
NUCLEOTIDE REVERSE TRANSCRIPTASE INHIBITORS 612
Nu-Cloxi - See PENICILLINS 646
Nucofed - See
NARCOTIC ANALGESICS 584
PSEUDOEPHEDRINE 694
Nu-Cotrimox - See
SULFONAMIDES 766
TRIMETHOPRIM 818
Nu-Cotrimox DS - See
SULFONAMIDES 766
TRIMETHOPRIM 818
Nucynta - See TAPENTADOL 774
Nucynta ER- See TAPENTADOL 774
Nu-Diltiaz - See CALCIUM CHANNEL BLOCKERS 220
Nu-Indo - See ANTI-INFLAMMATORY DRUGS, NONSTEROIDAL (NSAIDs) 116
Nu-Iron - See IRON SUPPLEMENTS 458
Nu-Iron 150 - See IRON SUPPLEMENTS 458
Nujol - See LAXATIVES, SOFTENER/ LUBRICANT 480
Nulev - See HYOSCYAMINE 438
Nu-Loraz - See BENZODIAZEPINES 176
Nu-Medopa - See CENTRAL ALPHA AGONISTS 234
NuMetop - See BETA-ADRENERGIC BLOCKING AGENTS 182
Numorphan - See NARCOTIC ANALGESICS 584
Numzident - See ANESTHETICS (Mucosal-Local) 36

Num-Zit Gel - See ANESTHETICS (Mucosal-Local) 36
Num-Zit Lotion - See ANESTHETICS (Mucosal-Local) 36
Nu-Nifed - See CALCIUM CHANNEL BLOCKERS 220
Nu-Pen-VK - See PENICILLINS 646
Nupercainal - See ANESTHETICS (Rectal) 38
Nupercainal Cream - See ANESTHETICS (Topical) 40
Nupercainal Ointment - See ANESTHETICS (Topical) 40
Nu-Pirox - See ANTI-INFLAMMATORY DRUGS, NONSTEROIDAL (NSAIDs) 116
Nuprin - See ANTI-INFLAMMATORY DRUGS, NONSTEROIDAL (NSAIDs) 116
Nuprin Caplets - See ANTI-INFLAMMATORY DRUGS, NONSTEROIDAL (NSAIDs) 116
Nu-Selegiline - See MONOAMINE OXIDASE TYPE B (MAO-B) INHIBITORS 572
Nu-Tetra - See TETRACYCLINES 782
Nu-Timolol - See ANTIGLAUCOMA, BETA BLOCKERS 96
NutraCal - See CALCIUM SUPPLEMENTS 222
Nutracort - See ADRENOCORTICOIDS (Topical) 18
Nu-Triazo - See TRIAZOLAM 812
Nutritional supplement - See
BETA CAROTENE 180
LEVOCARNITINE 494
Nutritional supplement (Mineral) - See ZINC SUPPLEMENTS 854
NuvaRing - See CONTRACEPTIVES, VAGINAL 280
Nu-Verap - See CALCIUM CHANNEL BLOCKERS 220
Nuvigil - See STIMULANTS, AMPHETAMINE RELATED 756
Nyaderm - See
ANTIFUNGALS (Topical) 88
ANTIFUNGALS (Vaginal) 90
Nydrazid - See ISONIAZID 460
Nystaform - See NYSTATIN 614
NYSTATIN 614
NYSTATIN - See
ANTIFUNGALS (Topical) 88
ANTIFUNGALS (Vaginal) 90
Nystex - See
ANTIFUNGALS (Topical) 88
NYSTATIN 614
Nystop - See ANTIFUNGALS (Topical) 88
Nytcold Medicine - See
ACETAMINOPHEN 8
DEXTROMETHORPHAN 312
PSEUDOEPHEDRINE 694
Nytilax - See LAXATIVES, STIMULANT 482
Nytol Maximum Strength - See ANTIHISTAMINES 106
Nytol with DPH - See ANTIHISTAMINES 106

O

Obalan - See APPETITE SUPPRESSANTS 146
Occlusal Topical Solution - See KERATOLYTICS 470
Occlusal-HP Topical Solution - See KERATOLYTICS 470
Ocella - See CONTRACEPTIVES, ORAL & SKIN 278
Octamide - See METOCLOPRAMIDE 550
Octamide PFS - See METOCLOPRAMIDE 550
Octigen - See ANTIBACTERIALS (Otic) 68
OCTOXYNOL 9 - See CONTRACEPTIVES, VAGINAL 280
Ocu-Carpine - See ANTIGLAUCOMA, CHOLINERGIC AGONISTS 100
Ocu-Chlor Ophthalmic Ointment - See ANTIBACTERIALS (Ophthalmic) 66
Ocu-Chlor Ophthalmic Solution - See ANTIBACTERIALS (Ophthalmic) 66
OcuClear - See DECONGESTANTS (Ophthalmic) 306
Ocu-Dex - See ANTI-INFLAMMATORY DRUGS, STEROIDAL (Ophthalmic) 122
Ocufen - See ANTI-INFLAMMATORY DRUGS, NONSTEROIDAL (NSAIDs) (Ophthalmic) 120
Ocuflox - See ANTIBACTERIALS (Ophthalmic) 66
Ocugestrin - See PHENYLEPHRINE (Ophthalmic) 660
Ocu-Mycin - See ANTIBACTERIALS (Ophthalmic) 66
Ocu-Pentolate - See CYCLOPENTOLATE (Ophthalmic) 288
Ocu-Phrin - See PHENYLEPHRINE (Ophthalmic) 660
Ocu-Pred - See ANTI-INFLAMMATORY DRUGS, STEROIDAL (Ophthalmic) 122
Ocu-Pred Forte - See ANTI-INFLAMMATORY DRUGS, STEROIDAL (Ophthalmic) 122
Ocu-Pred-A - See ANTI-INFLAMMATORY DRUGS, STEROIDAL (Ophthalmic) 122
Ocupress - See ANTIGLAUCOMA, BETA BLOCKERS 96
Ocusert Pilo - See ANTIGLAUCOMA, CHOLINERGIC AGONISTS 100
Ocu-Spor-B - See ANTIBACTERIALS (Ophthalmic) 66
Ocu-Spor-G - See ANTIBACTERIALS (Ophthalmic) 66

Ocusporin - See ANTIBACTERIALS (Ophthalmic) 66
Ocu-Sul-10 - See ANTIBACTERIALS (Ophthalmic) 66
Ocu-Sul-15 - See ANTIBACTERIALS (Ophthalmic) 66
Ocu-Sul-30 - See ANTIBACTERIALS (Ophthalmic) 66
Ocusulf-10 - See ANTIBACTERIALS (Ophthalmic) 66
Ocutears - See PROTECTANT (Ophthalmic) 690
Ocutricin Ophthalmic Ointment - See ANTIBACTERIALS (Ophthalmic) 66
Ocutricin Ophthalmic Solution - See ANTIBACTERIALS (Ophthalmic) 66
Ocu-Tropine - See CYCLOPLEGIC, MYDRIATIC (Ophthalmic) 292
Ocu-Zoline - See DECONGESTANTS (Ophthalmic) 306
Off-Ezy Topical Solution Corn & Callus Removal Kit - See KERATOLYTICS 470
Off-Ezy Topical Solution Wart Removal Kit - See KERATOLYTICS 470
O-Flex - See ORPHENADRINE 624
OFLOXACIN - See FLUOROQUINOLONES 392
OFLOXACIN (Ophthalmic) - See ANTIBACTERIALS (Ophthalmic) 66
OFLOXACIN (Otic) - See ANTIBACTERIALS (Otic) 68
Ogen - See ESTROGENS 372
Ogen 1.25 - See ESTROGENS 372
Ogen 2.5 - See ESTROGENS 372
Ogen 6.25 - See ESTROGENS 372
<u>OLANZAPINE</u> 616
Oleptro - See TRAZODONE 810
OLMESARTAN - See ANGIOTENSIN II RECEPTOR ANTAGONISTS 42
OLOPATADINE - See ANTIALLERGIC AGENTS (Ophthalmic) 56
OLOPATADINE (Nasal) - See ANTIHISTAMINES (Nasal) 108
<u>OLSALAZINE</u> 618
Olux - See ADRENOCORTICOIDS (Topical) 18
Olux-E - See ADRENOCORTICOIDS (Topical) 18
Omeclamox-Pak - See
MACROLIDE ANTIBIOTICS 518
PENICILLINS 646
PROTON PUMP INHIBITORS 692
<u>OMEGA-3 ACID ETHYL ESTERS</u> 620
OMEPRAZOLE - See PROTON PUMP INHIBITORS 692
Omnaris - See ADRENOCORTICOIDS (Nasal Inhalation) 12
Omnicef - See CEPHALOSPORINS 236
OMNIhist L.A. - See
ANTICHOLINERGICS 72
ANTIHISTAMINES 106
PHENYLEPHRINE 658
Omnipen - See PENICILLINS 646
One-Alpha - See VITAMIN D 840
Onfi - See BENZODIAZEPINES 174
Onglyza - See DPP-4 INHIBITORS 348
Onset - See NARCOTIC ANALGESICS & ACETAMINOPHEN 586
Opana - See NARCOTIC ANALGESICS 584
Opana ER - See NARCOTIC ANALGESICS 584
Ophthacet - See ANTIBACTERIALS (Ophthalmic) 66
Ophthalmic - See ANTIBACTERIALS (Ophthalmic) 66
Ophthalmic antiallergic agents - See ANTIALLERGIC AGENTS (Ophthalmic) 56
Ophthalmic anti-inflammatory agents, nonsteroidal - See ANTI-INFLAMMATORY DRUGS, NONSTEROIDAL (NSAIDs) (Ophthalmic) 120
Ophthochlor Ophthalmic Solution - See ANTIBACTERIALS (Ophthalmic) 66
Ophtho-Chloram Ophthalmic Solution - See ANTIBACTERIALS (Ophthalmic) 66
Ophtho-Dipivefrin - See ANTIGLAUCOMA, ADRENERGIC AGONISTS 92
OPIUM - See NARCOTIC ANALGESICS 584
Opticrom - See CROMOLYN 282
Optimine - See ANTIHISTAMINES 106
OptiPranolol - See ANTIGLAUCOMA, BETA BLOCKERS 96
Optivar - See ANTIALLERGIC AGENTS (Ophthalmic) 56
Orabase HCA - See ADRENOCORTICOIDS (Topical) 18
Orabase-B with Benzocaine - See ANESTHETICS (Mucosal-Local) 36
Oracea - See TETRACYCLINES 782
Oracit - See CITRATES 254
Oracort - See ADRENOCORTICOIDS (Topical) 18
Oradexon - See ADRENOCORTICOIDS (Systemic) 16
OraDisc - See AMLEXANOX 26
Orajel Extra Strength - See ANESTHETICS (Mucosal-Local) 36
Orajel Liquid - See ANESTHETICS (Mucosal-Local) 36
Orajel Maximum Strength - See ANESTHETICS (Mucosal-Local) 36
Oralone - See ADRENOCORTICOIDS (Topical) 18

INDEX

Oraminic II - See ANTIHISTAMINES 106
Oramorph - See NARCOTIC ANALGESICS 584
Oramorph-SR - See NARCOTIC ANALGESICS 584
Oraphen-PD - See ACETAMINOPHEN 8
Orapred - See ADRENOCORTICOIDS (Systemic) 16
Orapred ODT - See ADRENOCORTICOIDS (Systemic) 16
Orasone 1 - See ADRENOCORTICOIDS (Systemic) 16
Orasone 5 - See ADRENOCORTICOIDS (Systemic) 16
Orasone 10 - See ADRENOCORTICOIDS (Systemic) 16
Orasone 20 - See ADRENOCORTICOIDS (Systemic) 16
Orasone 50 - See ADRENOCORTICOIDS (Systemic) 16
Oratect Gel - See ANESTHETICS (Mucosal-Local) 36
Ora-Testryl - See ANDROGENS 34
Orazinc - See ZINC SUPPLEMENTS 854
Orbenin - See PENICILLINS 646
Oretic - See DIURETICS, THIAZIDE 338
Oreticyl - See
DIURETICS, THIAZIDE 338
RAUWOLFIA ALKALOIDS 714
Oreticyl Forte - See
DIURETICS, THIAZIDE 338
RAUWOLFIA ALKALOIDS 714
Oreton - See ANDROGENS 34
Orflagen - See ORPHENADRINE 624
Orfro - See ORPHENADRINE 624
Organidin - See GUAIFENESIN 416
Orinase - See SULFONYLUREAS 770
ORLISTAT 622
Ornex DM 15 - See DEXTROMETHORPHAN 312
Ornex DM 30 - See DEXTROMETHORPHAN 312
Ornex Maximum Strength Caplets - See
ACETAMINOPHEN 8
PSEUDOEPHEDRINE 694
Ornex No Drowsiness Caplets - See
ACETAMINOPHEN 8
PSEUDOEPHEDRINE 694
Ornex Severe Cold No Drowsiness Caplets - See
DEXTROMETHORPHAN 312
PSEUDOEPHEDRINE 694
Oravig - See ANTIFUNGALS (Topical) 88
ORPHENADRINE 624
ORPHENADRINE, ASPIRIN & CAFFEINE 626
Orphenagesic - See ORPHENADRINE, ASPIRIN & CAFFEINE 626
Orphenagesic Forte - See ORPHENADRINE, ASPIRIN & CAFFEINE 626
Orphenate - See ORPHENADRINE 624
Orsythia - See CONTRACEPTIVES, ORAL & SKIN 278
Ortho 0.5/35 - See CONTRACEPTIVES, ORAL & SKIN 278
Ortho 1/35 - See CONTRACEPTIVES, ORAL & SKIN 278
Ortho 7/7/7 - See CONTRACEPTIVES, ORAL & SKIN 278
Ortho 10/11 - See CONTRACEPTIVES, ORAL & SKIN 278
Ortho-Cept - See CONTRACEPTIVES, ORAL & SKIN 278
Ortho-Creme - See CONTRACEPTIVES, VAGINAL 280
Ortho-Cyclen - See CONTRACEPTIVES, ORAL & SKIN 278
Ortho-Est - See ESTROGENS 372
Ortho Evra - See CONTRACEPTIVES, ORAL & SKIN 278
Ortho-Gynol - See CONTRACEPTIVES, VAGINAL 280
Ortho-Novum 0.5 - See CONTRACEPTIVES, ORAL & SKIN 278
Ortho-Novum 1/35 - See CONTRACEPTIVES, ORAL & SKIN 278
Ortho-Novum 1/50 - See CONTRACEPTIVES, ORAL & SKIN 278
Ortho-Novum 1/80 - See CONTRACEPTIVES, ORAL & SKIN 278
Ortho-Novum 2 - See CONTRACEPTIVES, ORAL & SKIN 278
Ortho-Novum 7/7/7 - See CONTRACEPTIVES, ORAL & SKIN 278
Ortho-Novum 10/11 - See CONTRACEPTIVES, ORAL & SKIN 278
Ortho-Prefest - See
ESTROGENS 372
PROGESTINS 680
Ortho-Tri-Cyclen 21 - See CONTRACEPTIVES, ORAL & SKIN 278
Ortho-Tri-Cyclen 28 - See CONTRACEPTIVES, ORAL & SKIN 278
Ortho Tri-Cyclen Lo - See CONTRACEPTIVES, ORAL & SKIN 278
Or-Tyl - See DICYCLOMINE 316
Orudis - See ANTI-INFLAMMATORY DRUGS, NONSTEROIDAL (NSAIDs) 116
Orudis-E - See ANTI-INFLAMMATORY DRUGS, NONSTEROIDAL (NSAIDs) 116

Orudis-KT - See ANTI-INFLAMMATORY DRUGS, NONSTEROIDAL (NSAIDs) 116
Orudis-SR - See ANTI-INFLAMMATORY DRUGS, NONSTEROIDAL (NSAIDs) 116
Oruvail - See ANTI-INFLAMMATORY DRUGS, NONSTEROIDAL (NSAIDs) 116
Os-Cal - See CALCIUM SUPPLEMENTS 222
Os-Cal 500 - See CALCIUM SUPPLEMENTS 222
Os-Cal Chewable - See CALCIUM SUPPLEMENTS 222
OSELTAMIVIR - See ANTIVIRALS FOR INFLUENZA, NEURAMINIDASE INHIBITORS 140
Oseni - See
DPP-4 INHIBITORS 348
THIAZOLIDINEDIONES 786
Osteopenia therapy - See BISPHOSPHONATES 192
Osteoporosis therapy - See
BONE FORMATION AGENTS 194
CALCITONIN 218
RALOXIFENE 708
Osteoporosis therapy, bisphosphonate - See BISPHOSPHONATES 192
Osto Forte - See VITAMIN D 840
Oticair - See ANTIBACTERIALS (Otic) 68
Otimar - See ANTIBACTERIALS (Otic) 68
Otiprin - See ANTIPYRINE & BENZOCAINE (Otic) 130
Otobione - See ANTIBACTERIALS (Otic) 68
Otocalm - See ANTIPYRINE & BENZOCAINE (Otic) 130
Otocidin - See ANTIBACTERIALS (Otic) 68
Otocort - See ANTIBACTERIALS (Otic) 68
Otrivin Decongestant Nose Drops - See XYLOMETAZOLINE 850
Otrivin Nasal Drops - See XYLOMETAZOLINE 850
Otrivin Nasal Spray - See XYLOMETAZOLINE 850
Otrivin Pediatric Decongestant Nose Drops - See XYLOMETAZOLINE 850
Otrivin Pediatric Nasal Drops - See XYLOMETAZOLINE 850
Otrivin Pediatric Nasal Spray - See XYLOMETAZOLINE 850
Otrivin with M-D Pump - See XYLOMETAZOLINE 850
Ovcon-35 - See CONTRACEPTIVES, ORAL & SKIN 278
Ovcon-50 - See CONTRACEPTIVES, ORAL & SKIN 278
Ovide - See PEDICULICIDES (Topical) 642
Ovol - See SIMETHICONE 748
Ovol-40 - See SIMETHICONE 748
Ovol-80 - See SIMETHICONE 748
Ovral - See CONTRACEPTIVES, ORAL & SKIN 278
Ovrette - See PROGESTINS 680
OXACILLIN - See PENICILLINS 646
OXANDROLONE - See ANDROGENS 34
OXAPROZIN - See ANTI-INFLAMMATORY DRUGS, NONSTEROIDAL (NSAIDs) 116
OXAZEPAM - See BENZODIAZEPINES 176
OXCARBAZEPINE 628
Oxecta - See NARCOTIC ANALGESICS 584
OXICONAZOLE (Topical) - See ANTIFUNGALS (Topical) 88
Oxistat - See ANTIFUNGALS (Topical) 88
OXPRENOLOL - See BETA-ADRENERGIC BLOCKING AGENTS 182
Oxsoralen - See PSORALENS 696
Oxsoralen Topical - See PSORALENS 696
Oxsoralen Ultra - See PSORALENS 696
Oxtellar XR - See OXCARBAZEPINE 628
OXTRIPHYLLINE - See BRONCHODILATORS, XANTHINE 204
Oxy 5 Tinted Lotion - See BENZOYL PEROXIDE 178
Oxy 5 Vanishing Formula Lotion - See BENZOYL PEROXIDE 178
Oxy 5 Vanishing Lotion - See BENZOYL PEROXIDE 178
Oxy 10 - See BENZOYL PEROXIDE 178
Oxy 10 Daily Face Wash - See BENZOYL PEROXIDE 178
Oxy 10 Tinted Lotion - See BENZOYL PEROXIDE 178
Oxy 10 Vanishing Lotion - See BENZOYL PEROXIDE 178
Oxy Clean Medicated Cleanser - See KERATOLYTICS 470
Oxy Clean Medicated Pads Maximum Strength - See KERATOLYTICS 470
Oxy Clean Medicated Pads Sensitive Skin - See KERATOLYTICS 470
Oxy Clean Regular Strength - See KERATOLYTICS 470
Oxy Clean Regular Strength Medicated Cleanser Topical Solution - See KERATOLYTICS 470
Oxy Clean Regular Strength Medicated Pads - See KERATOLYTICS 470
Oxy Clean Sensitive Skin Cleanser Topical Solution - See KERATOLYTICS 470
Oxy Clean Sensitive Skin Pads - See KERATOLYTICS 470
Oxy Night Watch Maximum Strength Lotion - See KERATOLYTICS 470

Oxy Night Watch Night Time Acne Medication Extra Strength Lotion - See KERATOLYTICS 470
Oxy Night Watch Night Time Acne Medication Regular Strength Lotion - See KERATOLYTICS 470
Oxy Night Watch Sensitive Skin Lotion - See KERATOLYTICS 470
Oxy Sensitive Skin Vanishing Formula Lotion - See KERATOLYTICS 470
OXYBUTYNIN - See MUSCARINIC RECEPTOR ANTAGONISTS 574
Oxycocet - See NARCOTIC ANALGESICS & ACETAMINOPHEN 586
Oxycodan - See NARCOTIC ANALGESICS & ASPIRIN 588
OXYCODONE - See NARCOTIC ANALGESICS 584
OXYCODONE & ACETAMINOPHEN - See NARCOTIC ANALGESICS & ACETAMINOPHEN 586
OXYCODONE & ASPIRIN - See NARCOTIC ANALGESICS & ASPIRIN 588
Oxycontin SR - See NARCOTIC ANALGESICS 584
Oxyderm 5 Lotion - See BENZOYL PEROXIDE 178
Oxyderm 10 Lotion - See BENZOYL PEROXIDE 178
Oxyderm 20 Lotion - See BENZOYL PEROXIDE 178
Oxydess - See AMPHETAMINES 28
OXYMETAZOLINE - See DECONGESTANTS (Ophthalmic) 306
<u>OXYMETAZOLINE (Nasal)</u> 630
OXYMETHOLONE - See ANDROGENS 34
OXYMORPHONE - See NARCOTIC ANALGESICS 584
OXYPHENCYCLIMINE - See ANTICHOLINERGICS 72
OXYTETRACYCLINE - See TETRACYCLINES 782
Oxytrol - See MUSCARINIC RECEPTOR ANTAGONISTS 574
Oxytrol for Women - See MUSCARINIC RECEPTOR ANTAGONISTS 573
Oysco - See CALCIUM SUPPLEMENTS 222
Oysco 500 Chewable - See CALCIUM SUPPLEMENTS 222
Oyst-Cal - See CALCIUM SUPPLEMENTS 222
Oyst-Cal 500 Chewable - See CALCIUM SUPPLEMENTS 222
Oystercal 500 - See CALCIUM SUPPLEMENTS 222

P

P&S - See KERATOLYTICS 470
P-A-C Revised Formula - See
ASPIRIN 152
CAFFEINE 216
Pacaps - See
ACETAMINOPHEN 8
BARBITURATES 168
CAFFEINE 216
<u>PACLITAXEL</u> 632
Palafer - See IRON SUPPLEMENTS 458
Palaron - See BRONCHODILATORS, XANTHINE 204
Palgic - See ANTIHISTAMINES 106
PALIPERIDONE - See SEROTONIN-DOPAMINE ANTAGONISTS 744
Palladone - See NARCOTIC ANALGESICS 584
Palmiron - See IRON SUPPLEMENTS 458
Paludrine - See PROGUANIL 682
Pamelor - See ANTIDEPRESSANTS, TRICYCLIC 80
PAMIDRONATE - See BISPHOSPHONATES 192
Pamine - See ANTICHOLINERGICS 72
Pamine Forte - See ANTICHOLINERGICS 72
Pamprin-IB - See ANTI-INFLAMMATORY DRUGS, NONSTEROIDAL (NSAIDs) 116
Panacet 5/500 - See NARCOTIC ANALGESICS & ACETAMINOPHEN 586
Panadol - See ACETAMINOPHEN 8
Panadol Extra Strength - See ACETAMINOPHEN 8
Panadol Junior Strength Caplets - See ACETAMINOPHEN 8
Panadol Maximum Strength Caplets - See ACETAMINOPHEN 8
Panadol Maximum Strength Tablets - See ACETAMINOPHEN 8
Panasal 5/500 - See NARCOTIC ANALGESICS & ASPIRIN 588
Pancreaze - See PANCRELIPASE 634
<u>PANCRELIPASE</u> 634
Pandel - See ADRENOCORTICOIDS (Topical) 18
Panectyl - See ANTIHISTAMINES, PHENOTHIAZINE-DERIVATIVE 112
Panex - See ACETAMINOPHEN 8
Panex 500 - See ACETAMINOPHEN 8
Panlor - See NARCOTIC ANALGESICS & ACETAMINOPHEN 586
Panmycin - See TETRACYCLINES 782
PanOxyl 5 Bar - See BENZOYL PEROXIDE 178
PanOxyl 10 Bar - See BENZOYL PEROXIDE 178

PanOxyl 5 Gel - See BENZOYL PEROXIDE 178
PanOxyl 10 Gel - See BENZOYL PEROXIDE 178
PanOxyl 15 Gel - See BENZOYL PEROXIDE 178
PanOxyl 20 Gel - See BENZOYL PEROXIDE 178
PanOxyl Acne Creamy Wash - See BENZOYL PEROXIDE 178
PanOxyl AQ 21/2 Gel - See BENZOYL PEROXIDE 178
PanOxyl AQ 5 Gel - See BENZOYL PEROXIDE 178
Panshape - See APPETITE SUPPRESSANTS 146
Pantapon - See NARCOTIC ANALGESICS 584
Pantoloc - See PROTON PUMP INHIBITORS 692
PANTOPRAZOLE - See PROTON PUMP INHIBITORS 692
<u>PANTOTHENIC ACID (Vitamin B-5)</u> 636
Panwarfarin - See ANTICOAGULANTS (Oral) 74
<u>PAPAVERINE</u> 638
Paplex - See KERATOLYTICS 470
Paplex Ultra - See KERATOLYTICS 470
Papulex - See NIACIN (Vitamin B-3, Nicotinic Acid, Nicotinamide) 596
Par Glycerol-DM - See DEXTROMETHORPHAN 312
Paracetamol - See ACETAMINOPHEN 8
Paraflex - See MUSCLE RELAXANTS, SKELETAL 576
Parafon Forte - See
ACETAMINOPHEN 8
MUSCLE RELAXANTS, SKELETAL 576
Parepectolin - See
KAOLIN & PECTIN 468
PAREGORIC 640
Parcopa - See CARBIDOPA & LEVODOPA 230
<u>PAREGORIC</u> 640
Parlodel - See BROMOCRIPTINE 198
Parlodel Snaptabs - See BROMOCRIPTINE 198
Parnate - See MONOAMINE OXIDASE (MAO) INHIBITORS 570
PAROXETINE - See SELECTIVE SEROTONIN REUPTAKE INHIBITORS (SSRIs) 742
Parsidol - See ANTIDYSKINETICS 82
Parsitan - See ANTIDYSKINETICS 82
Pataday - See ANTIALLERGIC AGENTS (Ophthalmic) 56
Patanase - See ANTIHISTAMINES (Nasal) 108
Patanol - See ANTIALLERGIC AGENTS (Ophthalmic) 56
Pathilon - See ANTICHOLINERGICS 72
Pathocil - See PENICILLINS 646
Pavabid - See PAPAVERINE 638
Pavabid Plateau Caps - See PAPAVERINE 638
Pavacot - See PAPAVERINE 638
Pavagen - See PAPAVERINE 638
Pavarine - See PAPAVERINE 638
Pavased - See PAPAVERINE 638
Pavatine - See PAPAVERINE 638
Pavatym - See PAPAVERINE 638
Paveral - See NARCOTIC ANALGESICS 584
Paverolan - See PAPAVERINE 638
Pax 400 - See MEPROBAMATE 538
Paxil - See SELECTIVE SEROTONIN REUPTAKE INHIBITORS (SSRIs) 742
Paxil CR - See SELECTIVE SEROTONIN REUPTAKE INHIBITORS (SSRIs) 742
Paxipam - See BENZODIAZEPINES 176
Paxofen - See ANTI-INFLAMMATORY DRUGS, NONSTEROIDAL (NSAIDs) 116
Pazamet - See METFORMIN 544
PBZ - See ANTIHISTAMINES 106
PBZ-SR - See ANTIHISTAMINES 106
PC-Cap - See
CAFFEINE 216
NARCOTIC ANALGESICS & ASPIRIN 588
PCE Dispersatabs - See ERYTHROMYCINS 368
Pedia - See ANTI-INFLAMMATORY DRUGS, NONSTEROIDAL (NSAIDs) 116
PediaCare Children's Allergy - See
ANTIHISTAMINES 106
PHENYLEPHRINE 658
PediaCare Children's Allergy & Cold - See ANTIHISTAMINES 106
PediaCare Children's Cough & Congestion - See
DEXTROMETHORPHAN 312
GUAIFENESIN 416
PediaCare Children's Decongestant - See PHENYLEPHRINE 658
PediaCare Children's Fever Reducer Plus Cough & Runny Nose - See
ACETAMINOPHEN 8
ANTIHISTAMINES 10
DEXTROMETHORPHAN 312
PediaCare Children's Fever Reducer Plus Cough & Sore Throat - See
ACETAMINOPHEN 8
DEXTROMETHORPHAN 312
PediaCare Children's Fever Reducer Plus Flu - See
ACETAMINOPHEN 8
ANTIHISTAMINES 106
DEXTROMETHORPHAN 312
PHENYLEPHRINE 658

PediaCare Children's Multi-Symptom Cold - See
DEXTROMETHORPHAN 312
PHENYLEPHRINE 658
PediaCare Fever Reducer Plus Multi-Symptom Cold - See
ACETAMINOPHEN 8
ANTIHISTAMINES 106
DEXTROMETHORPHAN 312
PHENYLEPHRINE 658
PediaCare Infants' Fever Reducer / Pain Reliever - See
ACETAMINOPHEN 8
PediaCare Infants' Gas Relief - See
SIMETHICONE 748
Pediacof Cough - See
ANTIHISTAMINES 106
NARCOTIC ANALGESICS 584
PHENYLEPHRINE 658
Pediapred - See ADRENOCORTICOIDS (Systemic) 16
Pediatric Aqueous Charcodote - See CHARCOAL, ACTIVATED 238
Pediatric Charcodote - See CHARCOAL, ACTIVATED 238
Pediazole - See
ERYTHROMYCINS 368
SULFONAMIDES 766
Pediculicide - See PEDICULICIDES (Topical) 642
PEDICULICIDES (Topical) 642
Pediotic - See ANTIBACTERIALS (Otic) 68
Pedric - See ACETAMINOPHEN 8
Peganone - See ANTICONVULSANTS, HYDANTOIN 76
Pelamine - See ANTIHISTAMINES 106
PEMIROLAST - See ANTIALLERGIC AGENTS (Ophthalmic) 56
Pen Vee - See PENICILLINS 646
Pen Vee K - See PENICILLINS 646
Penazine VC with Cough - See
ANTIHISTAMINES, PHENOTHIAZINE-DERIVATIVE 112
NARCOTIC ANALGESICS 584
Penbritin - See PENICILLINS 646
PENBUTOLOL - See BETA-ADRENERGIC BLOCKING AGENTS 182
PENCICLOVIR (Topical) - See ANTIVIRALS (Topical) 144
Penecort - See ADRENOCORTICOIDS (Topical) 18
Penetrex - See FLUOROQUINOLONES 392
Penglobe - See PENICILLINS 646
PENICILLAMINE 644
PENICILLIN G - See PENICILLINS 646
PENICILLIN V - See PENICILLINS 646
PENICILLINS 646
PENICILLINS & BETA-LACTAMASE INHIBITORS 648
Penlac - See ANTIFUNGALS (Topical) 88
Pennsaid - See DICLOFENAC (Topical) 314
Pentacarinat - See PENTAMIDINE 650
Pentacort - See ADRENOCORTICOIDS (Topical) 18
PENTAERYTHRITOL TETRANITRATE - See NITRATES 602
PENTAMIDINE 650
Pentamycetin - See ANTIBACTERIALS (Ophthalmic) 66
Pentamycetin Ophthalmic Ointment - See ANTIBACTERIALS (Ophthalmic) 66
Pentamycetin Ophthalmic Solution - See ANTIBACTERIALS (Ophthalmic) 66
Pentasa - See MESALAMINE 542
Pentazine - See ANTIHISTAMINES, PHENOTHIAZINE-DERIVATIVE 112
PENTAZOCINE - See NARCOTIC ANALGESICS 584
PENTAZOCINE & ACETAMINOPHEN - See NARCOTIC ANALGESICS & ACETAMINOPHEN 586
PENTAZOCINE & ASPIRIN - See NARCOTIC ANALGESICS & ASPIRIN 588
Pentids - See PENICILLINS 646
PENTOBARBITAL - See BARBITURATES 168
Pentolair - See CYCLOPENTOLATE (Ophthalmic) 288
PENTOXIFYLLINE 652
Pentrax Extra-Strength Therapeutic Tar Shampoo - See COAL TAR (Topical) 266
Pentrax Tar Shampoo - See COAL TAR (Topical) 266
Pentritol - See NITRATES 602
Pentylan - See NITRATES 602
Pep-Back - See CAFFEINE 216
Pepcid - See HISTAMINE H_2 RECEPTOR ANTAGONISTS 422
Pepcid AC - See HISTAMINE H_2 RECEPTOR ANTAGONISTS 422
Pepcid Complete - See
ANTACIDS 48
HISTAMINE H_2 RECEPTOR ANTAGONISTS 422
Pepcid RPD - See HISTAMINE H_2 RECEPTOR ANTAGONISTS 422
Pepto Diarrhea Control - See LOPERAMIDE 508
Pepto-Bismol - See BISMUTH SALTS 190
Peptol - See HISTAMINE H_2 RECEPTOR ANTAGONISTS 422

Peranex HC Cream - See
ANESTHETICS (Rectal) 38
HYDROCORTISONE (Rectal) 430
Percocet - See NARCOTIC ANALGESICS & ACETAMINOPHEN 586
Percocet-Demi - See NARCOTIC ANALGESICS & ACETAMINOPHEN 586
Percodan - See NARCOTIC ANALGESICS & ASPIRIN 588
Percodan-Demi - See NARCOTIC ANALGESICS & ASPIRIN 588
Perdiem - See
LAXATIVES, BULK-FORMING 476
LAXATIVES, STIMULANT 482
Perdiem Fiber - See LAXATIVES, BULK-FORMING 476
Perdiem Plain - See LAXATIVES, BULK-FORMING 476
Perforomist Inhalation Solution - See BRONCHODILATORS, ADRENERGIC 200
Periactin - See ANTIHISTAMINES 106
Peri-Colace - See LAXATIVES, STIMULANT 482
Peri-Colase - See LAXATIVES, SOFTENER/ LUBRICANT 480
PERICYAZINE - See PHENOTHIAZINES 656
Peridex - See CHLORHEXIDINE 244
Peridol - See HALOPERIDOL 420
PERINDOPRIL - See ANGIOTENSIN-CONVERTING ENZYME (ACE) INHIBITORS 44
Periochip - See CHLORHEXIDINE 244
Periogard - See CHLORHEXIDINE 244
Periostat - See TETRACYCLINES 782
Peritrate - See NITRATES 602
Peritrate Forte - See NITRATES 602
Peritrate SA - See NITRATES 602
PERMETHRIN - See PEDICULICIDES (Topical) 642
Permitil - See PHENOTHIAZINES 656
Permitil Concentrate - See PHENOTHIAZINES 656
Pernox Lemon Medicated Scrub Cleanser - See KERATOLYTICS 470
Pernox Lotion Lathering Abradant Scrub Cleanser - See KERATOLYTICS 470
Pernox Lotion Lathering Scrub Cleanser - See KERATOLYTICS 470
Pernox Regular Medicated Scrub Cleanser - See KERATOLYTICS 470
PERPHENAZINE - See PHENOTHIAZINES 656
Persa-Gel 5 - See BENZOYL PEROXIDE 178
Persa-Gel 10 - See BENZOYL PEROXIDE 178
Persa-Gel W 5 - See BENZOYL PEROXIDE 178
Persa-Gel W 10 - See BENZOYL PEROXIDE 178
Persantine - See DIPYRIDAMOLE 326
Pertofrane - See ANTIDEPRESSANTS, TRICYCLIC 80
Pertrogalar Plain - See LAXATIVES, SOFTENER/LUBRICANT 480
Pertussin All Night CS - See
DEXTROMETHORPHAN 312
GUAIFENESIN 416
Pertussin All Night PM - See
ACETAMINOPHEN 8
ANTIHISTAMINES 106
DEXTROMETHORPHAN 312
PSEUDOEPHEDRINE 694
Pertussin Cough Suppressant - See DEXTROMETHORPHAN 312
Pertussin CS - See DEXTROMETHORPHAN 312
Pertussin ES - See DEXTROMETHORPHAN 312
Pertyze - See PANCRELIPASE 634
P.E.T.N. - See NITRATES 602
Pfeiffer's Allergy - See ANTIHISTAMINES 106
Phanatuss - See
DEXTROMETHORPHAN 312
GUAIFENESIN 416
Pharma-Cort - See ADRENOCORTICOIDS (Topical) 18
Pharmatex - See CONTRACEPTIVES, VAGINAL 280
Phazyme - See SIMETHICONE 748
Phazyme 55 - See SIMETHICONE 748
Phazyme 95 - See SIMETHICONE 748
Phenameth DM - See
ANTIHISTAMINES, PHENOTHIAZINE-DERIVATIVE 112
DEXTROMETHORPHAN 312
Phenameth VC - See PHENYLEPHRINE 658
Phenameth VC with Codeine - See
ANTIHISTAMINES, PHENOTHIAZINE-DERIVATIVE 112
NARCOTIC ANALGESICS 584
PHENYLEPHRINE 658
Phenapap Sinus Headache & Congestion - See
ACETAMINOPHEN 8
ANTIHISTAMINES 106
PSEUDOEPHEDRINE 694
Phenaphen - See ACETAMINOPHEN 8
Phenaphen with Codeine - See NARCOTIC ANALGESICS & ACETAMINOPHEN 586
Phenaphen with Codeine No. 2 - See BARBITURATES, ASPIRIN & CODEINE (Also contains caffeine) 170

Phenaphen with Codeine No. 3 - See BARBITURATES, ASPIRIN & CODEINE (Also contains caffeine) 170
Phenaphen with Codeine No. 4 - See BARBITURATES, ASPIRIN & CODEINE (Also contains caffeine) 170
Phenazine 25 - See ANTIHISTAMINES, PHENOTHIAZINE-DERIVATIVE 112
Phenazine 50 - See ANTIHISTAMINES, PHENOTHIAZINE-DERIVATIVE 112
Phen-Azo - See PHENAZOPYRIDINE 654
Phenazodine - See PHENAZOPYRIDINE 654
PHENAZOPYRIDINE 654
Phencen-50 - See ANTIHISTAMINES, PHENOTHIAZINE-DERIVATIVE 112
Phendiet - See APPETITE SUPPRESSANTS 146
Phendimet - See APPETITE SUPPRESSANTS 146
PHENDIMETRAZINE - See APPETITE SUPPRESSANTS 146
Phendry - See ANTIHISTAMINES 106
Phendry Children's Allergy Medicine - See ANTIHISTAMINES 106
PHENELZINE - See MONOAMINE OXIDASE (MAO) INHIBITORS 570
Phenergan - See ANTIHISTAMINES, PHENOTHIAZINE-DERIVATIVE 112
Phenergan with Dextromethorphan - See
ANTIHISTAMINES, PHENOTHIAZINE-DERIVATIVE 112
DEXTROMETHORPHAN 312
Phenergan-D - See PSEUDOEPHEDRINE 694
Phenetron - See ANTIHISTAMINES 106
Phenetron Lanacaps - See ANTIHISTAMINES 106
PHENINDAMINE - See ANTIHISTAMINES 106
PHENIRAMINE - See ANTIHISTAMINES 106
PHENOBARBITAL - See BARBITURATES 168
PHENOBARBITAL, ASPIRIN & CODEINE - See BARBITURATES, ASPIRIN & CODEINE (Also contains caffeine) 170
Pheno-Bella - See BELLADONNA ALKALOIDS & BARBITURATES 174
Phenoject-50 - See ANTIHISTAMINES, PHENOTHIAZINE-DERIVATIVE 112
Phenolax - See LAXATIVES, STIMULANT 482
Phenolphthalein Petrogalar - See
LAXATIVES, SOFTENER/LUBRICANT 480
LAXATIVES, STIMULANT 482
Phenoptic - See PHENYLEPHRINE (Ophthalmic) 660
PHENOTHIAZINES 656
Phentercot - See APPETITE SUPPRESSANTS 146
PHENTERMINE - See APPETITE SUPPRESSANTS 146
Phentride - See APPETITE SUPPRESSANTS 146
Phenylalanine Mustard - See MELPHALAN 534
PHENYLBUTAZONE - See ANTI-INFLAMMATORY DRUGS, NONSTEROIDAL (NSAIDs) 116
PHENYLEPHRINE 658
PHENYLEPHRINE (Ophthalmic) 660
PHENYLTOLOXAMINE - See ANTIHISTAMINES 106
PHENYTOIN - See ANTICONVULSANTS, HYDANTOIN 76
Phenzine - See APPETITE SUPPRESSANTS 146
Pherazine DM - See
ANTIHISTAMINES, PHENOTHIAZINE-DERIVATIVE 112
DEXTROMETHORPHAN 312
Pherazine VC - See
ANTIHISTAMINES, PHENOTHIAZINE-DERIVATIVE 112
PHENYLEPHRINE 658
Pherazine VC with Codeine - See
ANTIHISTAMINES, PHENOTHIAZINE-DERIVATIVE 112
NARCOTIC ANALGESICS 584
PHENYLEPHRINE 658
Pherazine with Codeine - See
ANTIHISTAMINES, PHENOTHIAZINE-DERIVATIVE 112
NARCOTIC ANALGESICS 584
Pheryl-E - See VITAMIN E 844
Phillips' Chewable - See LAXATIVES, OSMOTIC 478
Phillips' Concentrated - See LAXATIVES, OSMOTIC 478
Phillips' Gelcaps - See LAXATIVES, STIMULANT 482
Phillips' LaxCaps - See
LAXATIVES, SOFTENER/LUBRICANT 480
LAXATIVES, STIMULANT 482
Phillips' Magnesia Tablets - See LAXATIVES, OSMOTIC 478
Phillips' Milk of Magnesia - See
ANTACIDS 48
LAXATIVES, OSMOTIC 478
pHisoAc BP 10 - See BENZOYL PEROXIDE 178
Phosphodiesterase-4 (PDE4) inhibitor - See ROFLUMILAST 734
Phospholine Iodide - See ANTIGLAUCOMA, ANTICHOLINESTERASES 94

Phrenilin - See
ACETAMINOPHEN 8
BARBITURATES 168
Phrenilin Forte - See
ACETAMINOPHEN 8
BARBITURATES 168
Phyllocontin - See BRONCHODILATORS, XANTHINE 204
Phyllocontin-350 - See BRONCHODILATORS, XANTHINE 204
Physeptone - See NARCOTIC ANALGESICS 584
PHYTONADIONE - See VITAMIN K 846
PILOCARPINE (Oral) 662
PILOCARPINE - See ANTIGLAUCOMA, CHOLINERGIC AGONISTS 100
Pilocarpine Pilocar - See ANTIGLAUCOMA, CHOLINERGIC AGONISTS 100
Pilopine HS - See ANTIGLAUCOMA, CHOLINERGIC AGONISTS 100
Piloptic - See ANTIGLAUCOMA, CHOLINERGIC AGONISTS 100
Pilostat - See ANTIGLAUCOMA, CHOLINERGIC AGONISTS 100
Pima - See POTASSIUM SUPPLEMENTS 666
PINDOLOL - See BETA-ADRENERGIC BLOCKING AGENTS 182
PINDOLOL & HYDROCHLOROTHIAZIDE - See BETA-ADRENERGIC BLOCKING AGENTS & THIAZIDE DIURETICS 184
PIOGLITAZONE - See THIAZOLIDINEDIONES 786
Piperazine - See ESTROGENS 372
Piportil L4 - See PHENOTHIAZINES 656
PIPOTIAZINE - See PHENOTHIAZINES 656
PIRBUTEROL - See BRONCHODILATORS, ADRENERGIC 200
PIRENZEPINE - See ANTICHOLINERGICS 72
PIROXICAM - See ANTI-INFLAMMATORY DRUGS, NONSTEROIDAL (NSAIDs) 116
PITAVASTATIN - See HMG-CoA REDUCTASE INHIBITORS 424
Pitrex Cream - See ANTIFUNGALS (Topical) 88
PIVAMPICILLIN - See PENICILLINS 646
PIVMECILLINAM - See PENICILLINS 646
Plan B One-Step - See PROGESTINS 680
Plan B OTC/Rx - See PROGESTINS 680
Plaquenil - See HYDROXYCHLOROQUINE 432
Platelet aggregation inhibitor - See
DIPYRIDAMOLE 326
PLATELET INHIBITORS 664
TICAGRELOR 796
Platelet count-reducing agent - See
ANAGRELIDE 30
Platelet-derived growth factor - See
BECAPLERMIN 172
PLATELET INHIBITORS 664
Plavix- See PLATELET INHIBITORS 664
Plegine - See APPETITE SUPPRESSANTS 146
Plendil - See CALCIUM CHANNEL BLOCKERS 220
Pletal - See INTERMITTENT CLAUDICATION AGENTS 452
PMS Amitriptyline - See ANTIDEPRESSANTS, TRICYCLIC 80
PMS Benztropine - See ANTIDYSKINETICS 82
PMS-Bisacodyl - See LAXATIVES, STIMULANT 482
PMS Carbamazepine - See CARBAMAZEPINE 228
PMS-Dexamethasone Sodium Phosphate - See ANTI-INFLAMMATORY DRUGS, STEROIDAL (Ophthalmic) 122
PMS-Dimenhydrinate - See ANTIHISTAMINES 106
PMS-Docusate Calcium - See LAXATIVES, SOFTENER/LUBRICANT 480
PMS-Docusate Sodium - See LAXATIVES, SOFTENER/LUBRICANT 480
PMS Diazepam - See BENZODIAZEPINES 176
PMS Dopazide - See
CENTRAL ALPHA AGONISTS 234
DIURETICS, THIAZIDE 338
PMS Egozinc - See ZINC SUPPLEMENTS 854
PMS Ferrous Sulfate - See IRON SUPPLEMENTS 458
PMS Haloperidol - See HALOPERIDOL 420
PMS Impramine - See ANTIDEPRESSANTS, TRICYCLIC 80
PMS Isoniazid - See ISONIAZID 460
PMS Levazine - See
ANTIDEPRESSANTS, TRICYCLIC 80
PHENOTHIAZINES 656
PMS Lindane - See PEDICULICIDES (Topical) 642
PMS Methylphenidate - See STIMULANT MEDICATIONS 754
PMS Metronidazole - See NITROIMIDAZOLES 606
PMS Primidone - See PRIMIDONE 674
PMS Procyclidine - See ANTIDYSKINETICS 82
PMS Promethazine - See ANTIHISTAMINES, PHENOTHIAZINE-DERIVATIVE 112
PMS-Sennosides - See LAXATIVES, STIMULANT 482
PMS-Sodium Cromoglycate - See CROMOLYN 282
PMS Sulfasalazine - See SULFASALAZINE 762

PMS Sulfasalazine EC - See SULFASALAZINE 762
PMS Theophylline - See BRONCHODILATORS, XANTHINE 204
PMS Thioridazine - See PHENOTHIAZINES 656
PMS Trihexyphenidyl - See ANTIDYSKINETICS 82
P.N. Ophthalmic - See ANTIBACTERIALS (Ophthalmic) 66
Pneumomist - See GUAIFENESIN 416
Pneumopent - See PENTAMIDINE 650
PODOFILOX - See CONDYLOMA ACUMINATUM AGENTS 276
Podofin - See CONDYLOMA ACUMINATUM AGENTS 276
PODOPHYLLUM - See CONDYLOMA ACUMINATUM AGENTS 276
Poladex T.D. - See ANTIHISTAMINES 106
POLOXAMER 188 - See LAXATIVES, SOFTENER/LUBRICANT 480
POLYCARBOPHIL - See LAXATIVES, BULK-FORMING 476
Polycillin - See PENICILLINS 646
Polycin - See ANTIBACTERIALS (Ophthalmic) 66
Polycitra - See CITRATES 254
Polycitra LC - See CITRATES 254
Polycitra-K - See CITRATES 254
POLYETHYLENE GLYCOL 3350 - See LAXATIVES, OSMOTIC 478
Polygesic - See NARCOTIC ANALGESICS & ACETAMINOPHEN 586
Poly-Histine Expectorant Plain - See GUAIFENESIN 416
Polymox - See PENICILLINS 646
POLYMYXIN B - See ANTIBACTERIALS (Ophthalmic) 66
POLYTHIAZIDE - See DIURETICS, THIAZIDE 338
Poly-Vi-Flor - See VITAMINS & FLUORIDE 848
Pondocillin - See PENICILLINS 646
Ponstan - See ANTI-INFLAMMATORY DRUGS, NONSTEROIDAL (NSAIDs) 116
Ponstel - See ANTI-INFLAMMATORY DRUGS, NONSTEROIDAL (NSAIDs) 116
Pontocaine Cream - See
ANESTHETICS (Rectal) 38
ANESTHETICS (Topical) 40
Pontocaine Ointment - See
ANESTHETICS (Rectal) 38
ANESTHETICS (Topical) 40
Portalac - See LAXATIVES, OSMOTIC 478
POSACONAZOLE - See ANTIFUNGALS, AZOLES 86
Postacne - See ANTIACNE, CLEANSING (Topical) 54
Posture - See CALCIUM SUPPLEMENTS 222
Potasalan - See POTASSIUM SUPPLEMENTS 666
POTASSIUM ACETATE - See POTASSIUM SUPPLEMENTS 666
POTASSIUM BICARBONATE - See POTASSIUM SUPPLEMENTS 666
POTASSIUM BICARBONATE & POTASSIUM CHLORIDE - See POTASSIUM SUPPLEMENTS 666
POTASSIUM BICARBONATE & POTASSIUM CITRATE - See POTASSIUM SUPPLEMENTS 666
POTASSIUM CHLORIDE - See POTASSIUM SUPPLEMENTS 666
POTASSIUM CITRATE - See CITRATES 254
POTASSIUM CITRATE & CITRIC ACID - See CITRATES 254
POTASSIUM CITRATE & SODIUM CITRATE - See CITRATES 254
POTASSIUM GLUCONATE - See POTASSIUM SUPPLEMENTS 666
POTASSIUM GLUCONATE & POTASSIUM CHLORIDE - See POTASSIUM SUPPLEMENTS 666
POTASSIUM GLUCONATE & POTASSIUM CITRATE - See POTASSIUM SUPPLEMENTS 666
POTASSIUM GLUCONATE, POTASSIUM CITRATE & AMMONIUM - See POTASSIUM SUPPLEMENTS 666
POTASSIUM SUPPLEMENTS 666
Potassium-Rougier - See POTASSIUM SUPPLEMENTS 666
Potassium-Sandoz - See POTASSIUM SUPPLEMENTS 666
Pradaxa - See DABIGATRAN 298
Pramegel - See ANESTHETICS (Topical) 40
PRAMIPEXOLE - See DOPAMINE AGONISTS NONERGOT 344
PRAMLINTIDE 668
Pramosone E Cream - See
ADRENOCORTICOIDS (Topical) 18
ANESTHETICS (Topical) 40
PRAMOXINE - See
ANESTHETICS (Rectal) 38
ANESTHETICS (Topical) 40
PrandiMet - See
MEGLITINIDES 528
METFORMIN 544
Prandin - See MEGLITINIDES 528
PRASUGREL - See PLATELET INHIBITORS 664

Pravachol - See HMG-CoA REDUCTASE INHIBITORS 424
PRAVASTATIN - See HMG-CoA REDUCTASE INHIBITORS 424
Pravigard PAC - See
ASPIRIN 152
HMG-CoA REDUCTASE INHIBITORS 424
Prax - See ANESTHETICS (Topical) 40
PRAZEPAM - See BENZODIAZEPINES 176
PRAZOSIN - See ALPHA ADRENERGIC RECEPTOR BLOCKERS 20
Precose - See ACARBOSE 6
Pred Forte - See ANTI-INFLAMMATORY DRUGS, STEROIDAL (Ophthalmic) 122
Pred Mild - See ANTI-INFLAMMATORY DRUGS, STEROIDAL (Ophthalmic) 122
Predair - See ANTI-INFLAMMATORY DRUGS, STEROIDAL (Ophthalmic) 122
Predair Forte - See ANTI-INFLAMMATORY DRUGS, STEROIDAL (Ophthalmic) 122
Predair-A - See ANTI-INFLAMMATORY DRUGS, STEROIDAL (Ophthalmic) 122
PREDNICARBATE - See ADRENOCORTICOIDS (Topical) 18
Prednicen-M - See ADRENOCORTICOIDS (Systemic) 16
PREDNISOLONE - See ADRENOCORTICOIDS (Systemic) 16
PREDNISOLONE (Ophthalmic) - See ANTI-INFLAMMATORY DRUGS, STEROIDAL (Ophthalmic) 122
PREDNISONE - See ADRENOCORTICOIDS (Systemic) 16
Prednisone Intensol - See ADRENOCORTICOIDS (Systemic) 16
Pre-Fil - See CONTRACEPTIVES, VAGINAL 280
Prefrin Liquifilm - See PHENYLEPHRINE (Ophthalmic) 660
<u>PREGABALIN</u> 670
Prehist - See
ANTIHISTAMINES 106
PHENYLEPHRINE 658
Prehist Cough Mixture 4 - See ANTIHISTAMINES 106
Prehist D - See
ANTICHOLINERGICS 72
ANTIHISTAMINES 106
PHENYLEPHRINE 658
Prelone - See ADRENOCORTICOIDS (Systemic) 16
Prelu-2 - See APPETITE SUPPRESSANTS 146
Premarin - See ESTROGENS 372
Premarin Vaginal Cream - See ESTROGENS 372
Premphase - See
ESTROGENS 372
PROGESTINS 680
Prempro - See
ESTROGENS 372
PROGESTINS 680
Presalin - See
ACETAMINOPHEN 8
ASPIRIN 152
SALICYLATES 736
Prevacid - See PROTON PUMP INHIBITORS 692
Prevacid 24 Hour - See PROTON PUMP INHIBITORS 692
Prevacid Napra PAC - See
ANTI-INFLAMMATORY DRUGS NONSTEROIDAL (NSAIDs) 116
PROTON PUMP INHIBITORS 692
Prevacid SoluTab - See PROTON PUMP INHIBITORS 692
Prevex B - See ADRENOCORTICOIDS (Topical) 18
Prevex HC - See ADRENOCORTICOIDS (Topical) 18
Previfem - See CONTRACEPTIVES, ORAL & SKIN 278
Prezista - See PROTEASE INHIBITORS 688
Priftin - See RIFAMYCINS 728
Prilosec - See PROTON PUMP INHIBITORS 692
Prilosec OTC - See PROTON PUMP INHIBITORS 692
<u>PRIMAQUINE</u> 672
Primatene Mist HFC - See BRONCHODILATORS, ADRENERGIC 200
<u>PRIMIDONE</u> 674
Principen - See PENICILLINS 646
Prinivil - See ANGIOTENSIN-CONVERTING ENZYME (ACE) INHIBITORS 44
Prinzide - See ANGIOTENSIN-CONVERTING ENZYME (ACE) INHIBITORS & HYDROCHLOROTHIAZIDE 46
Pristiq - See SEROTONIN & NOREPINEPHRINE REUPTAKE INHIBITORS (SNRIs) 746
Pro Pox with APAP - See NARCOTIC ANALGESICS & ACETAMINOPHEN 586
Pro-Air - See BRONCHODILATORS, ADRENERGIC 200
Probalan - See PROBENECID 676
Pro-Banthine - See PROPANTHELINE 686
Probate - See MEPROBAMATE 538
<u>PROBENECID</u> 676
Pro-Cal-Sof - See LAXATIVES, SOFTENER/ LUBRICANT 480

PROCARBAZINE 678
Procardia - See CALCIUM CHANNEL BLOCKERS 220
Procardia XL - See CALCIUM CHANNEL BLOCKERS 220
PROCATEROL - See BRONCHODILATORS, ADRENERGIC 200
PROCHLORPERAZINE - See PHENOTHIAZINES 656
ProCort - See
ANESTHETICS (Rectal) 38
HYDROCORTISONE (Rectal) 430
Proctocort - See HYDROCORTISONE (Rectal) 430
Proctofoam - See ANESTHETICS (Rectal) 38
Procyclid - See ANTIDYSKINETICS 82
PROCYCLIDINE - See ANTIDYSKINETICS 82
Procytox - See CYCLOPHOSPHAMIDE 290
Prodiem - See LAXATIVES, BULK-FORMING 476
Prodiem Plain - See LAXATIVES, BULK-FORMING 476
Prodiem Plus - See
LAXATIVES, BULK-FORMING 476
LAXATIVES, STIMULANT 482
Prodrox - See PROGESTINS 680
Profenal - See ANTI-INFLAMMATORY DRUGS, NONSTEROIDAL (NSAIDs) (Ophthalmic) 120
Progesic - See ANTI-INFLAMMATORY DRUGS, NONSTEROIDAL (NSAIDs) 116
Progestaject - See PROGESTINS 680
PROGESTERONE - See PROGESTINS 680
PROGESTINS 680
Prograf - See IMMUNOSUPPRESSIVE AGENTS 442
PROGUANIL 682
Pro-Lax - See LAXATIVES, BULK-FORMING 476
Prolixin - See PHENOTHIAZINES 656
Prolixin Concentrate - See PHENOTHIAZINES 656
Prolixin Decanoate - See PHENOTHIAZINES 656
Prolixin Enanthate - See PHENOTHIAZINES 656
Proloid - See THYROID HORMONES 792
Proloprim - See TRIMETHOPRIM 818
PROMAZINE - See PHENOTHIAZINES 656
Pro-Med 50 - See ANTIHISTAMINES, PHENOTHIAZINE-DERIVATIVE 112
Promehist with Codeine - See
ANTIHISTAMINES, PHENOTHIAZINE-DERIVATIVE 112
NARCOTIC ANALGESICS 584
Promerhegan - See ANTIHISTAMINES, PHENOTHIAZINE-DERIVATIVE 112
Promet - See ANTIHISTAMINES, PHENOTHIAZINE-DERIVATIVE 112
Prometh VC Plain - See
ANTIHISTAMINES, PHENOTHIAZINE-DERIVATIVE 112
PHENYLEPHRINE 658
Prometh VC with Codeine - See
ANTIHISTAMINES, PHENOTHIAZINE-DERIVATIVE 112
NARCOTIC ANALGESICS 584
PHENYLEPHRINE 658
Prometh with Dextromethorphan - See
ANTIHISTAMINES, PHENOTHIAZINE-DERIVATIVE 112
DEXTROMETHORPHAN 312
Prometh-25 - See ANTIHISTAMINES, PHENOTHIAZINE-DERIVATIVE 112
Prometh-50 - See ANTIHISTAMINES, PHENOTHIAZINE-DERIVATIVE 112
PROMETHAZINE - See ANTIHISTAMINES, PHENOTHIAZINE-DERIVATIVE 112
Promethazine DM - See
ANTIHISTAMINES, PHENOTHIAZINE-DERIVATIVE 112
DEXTROMETHORPHAN 312
Promethazine VC - See
ANTIHISTAMINES, PHENOTHIAZINE-DERIVATIVE 112
PHENYLEPHRINE 658
Prometrium - See PROGESTINS 680
Prompt - See
LAXATIVES, BULK-FORMING 476
LAXATIVES, STIMULANT 482
Propa P.H. 10 Acne Cover Stick - See BENZOYL PEROXIDE 178
Propa P.H. 10 Liquid Acne Soap - See BENZOYL PEROXIDE 178
Propa pH Medicated Acne Cream Maximum Strength - See KERATOLYTICS 470
Propa pH Medicated Cleansing Pads Maximum Strength - See KERATOLYTICS 470
Propa pH Medicated Cleansing Pads Sensitive Skin - See KERATOLYTICS 470
Propa pH Perfectly Clear Skin Cleanser Topical Solution Oily Skin - See KERATOLYTICS 470
Propa pH Perfectly Clear Skin Cleanser Topical Solution Sensitive Skin Formula - See KERATOLYTICS 470
Propacet 100 - See NARCOTIC ANALGESICS & ACETAMINOPHEN 586

Propaderm - See ADRENOCORTICOIDS (Topical) 18
PROPAFENONE 684
Propanthel - See PROPANTHELINE 686
PROPANTHELINE 686
Propecia - See 5-ALPHA REDUCTASE INHIBITORS 2
Propine - See ANTIGLAUCOMA, ADRENERGIC AGONISTS 92
Propine C Cap - See ANTIGLAUCOMA, ADRENERGIC AGONISTS 92
PROPOXYPHENE - See NARCOTIC ANALGESICS 584
PROPOXYPHENE & ACETAMINOPHEN - See NARCOTIC ANALGESICS & ACETAMINOPHEN 586
PROPOXYPHENE & ASPIRIN - See NARCOTIC ANALGESICS & ASPIRIN 588
Propoxyphene Compound-65 - See
CAFFEINE 216
NARCOTIC ANALGESICS & ASPIRIN 588
PROPRANOLOL - See BETA-ADRENERGIC BLOCKING AGENTS 182
PROPRANOLOL & HYDROCHLOROTHIAZIDE - See BETA-ADRENERGIC BLOCKING AGENTS & THIAZIDE DIURETICS 184
PROPYLTHIOURACIL - See ANTITHYROID DRUGS 134
Propyl-Thyracil - See ANTITHYROID DRUGS 134
Proquin XR - See FLUOROQUINOLONES 392
Prorazin - See PHENOTHIAZINES 656
Prorex-25 - See ANTIHISTAMINES, PHENOTHIAZINE-DERIVATIVE 112
Prorex-50 - See ANTIHISTAMINES, PHENOTHIAZINE-DERIVATIVE 112
Proscar - See 5-ALPHA REDUCTASE INHIBITORS 2
Prosed/DS - See ATROPINE, HYOSCYAMINE, METHENAMINE, METHYLENE BLUE, PHENYLSALICYLATE & BENZOIC ACID 158
Pro-Sof - See LAXATIVES, SOFTENER/ LUBRICANT 480
Pro-Sof Liquid Concentrate - See LAXATIVES, SOFTENER/LUBRICANT 480
Pro-Sof Plus - See
LAXATIVES, SOFTENER/LUBRICANT 480
LAXATIVES, STIMULANT 482
Prostaphlin - See PENICILLINS 646
ProStep - See NICOTINE 598
Prostigmin - See ANTIMYASTHENICS 128
Protease inhibitor - See PROTEASE INHIBITORS 688
PROTEASE INHIBITORS 688
Protectant (Ophthalmic) - See PROTECTANT (Ophthalmic) 690
PROTECTANT (Ophthalmic) 690
Prothazine - See ANTIHISTAMINES, PHENOTHIAZINE-DERIVATIVE 112
Prothazine Plain - See ANTIHISTAMINES, PHENOTHIAZINE-DERIVATIVE 112
Proton pump inhibitor - See PROTON PUMP INHIBITORS 692
PROTON PUMP INHIBITORS 692
Protonix - See PROTON PUMP INHIBITORS 692
Protonix Delayed-Release Oral Suspension - See PROTON PUMP INHIBITORS 692
Protophylline - See BRONCHODILATORS, XANTHINE 204
Protostat - See NITROIMIDAZOLES 606
Protrin - See
SULFONAMIDES 766
TRIMETHOPRIM 818
PROTRIPTYLINE - See ANTIDEPRESSANTS, TRICYCLIC 80
Protylol - See DICYCLOMINE 316
Proventil - See BRONCHODILATORS, ADRENERGIC 200
Proventil HFA - See BRONCHODILATORS, ADRENERGIC 200
Proventil Repetabs - See BRONCHODILATORS, ADRENERGIC 200
Provera - See PROGESTINS 680
ProveraPak - See PROGESTINS 680
Provigil - See STIMULANTS, AMPHETAMINE-RELATED 756
Prozac - See SELECTIVE SEROTONIN REUPTAKE INHIBITORS (SSRIs) 742
Prozac Weekly - See SELECTIVE SEROTONIN REUPTAKE INHIBITORS (SSRIs) 742
Prozine - See PHENOTHIAZINES 656
Prudoxin - See DOXEPIN (Topical) 346
Prulet - See LAXATIVES, STIMULANT 482
PSEUDOEPHEDRINE 694
PSORALENS 696
Psorcon - See ADRENOCORTICOIDS (Topical) 18
Psorent - See COAL TAR (Topical) 266
psoriGel - See COAL TAR (Topical) 266
PsoriNail - See COAL TAR (Topical) 266
PSYLLIUM - See LAXATIVES, BULK-FORMING 476
PT 105 - See APPETITE SUPPRESSANTS 146
Pulmicort Flexhaler - See ADRENOCORTICOIDS (Oral Inhalation) 14
Pulmicort Respules - See ADRENOCORTICOIDS (Oral Inhalation) 14

Pulmophylline - See BRONCHODILATORS, XANTHINE 204
Purge - See LAXATIVES, STIMULANT 482
Purinethol - See MERCAPTOPURINE 540
Purinol - See ANTIGOUT DRUGS 104
P.V. Carpine - See ANTIGLAUCOMA, CHOLINERGIC AGONISTS 100
P.V. Carpine Liquifilm - See ANTIGLAUCOMA, CHOLINERGIC AGONISTS 100
PVF - See PENICILLINS 646
PVF K - See PENICILLINS 646
P-V-Tussin - See
ANTIHISTAMINES 106
NARCOTIC ANALGESICS 584
PSEUDOEPHEDRINE 694
P-V-Tussin Tablets - See GUAIFENESIN 416
Pylera - See
BISMUTH SALTS 190
NITROIMIDAZOLES 606
TETRACYCLINES 782
PYRANTEL - See ANTHELMINTICS 50
Pyrazodine - See PHENAZOPYRIDINE 654
Pyregesic-C - See NARCOTIC ANALGESICS & ACETAMINOPHEN 586
PYRETHRINS & PIPERONYL BUTOXIDE - See PEDICULICIDES (Topical) 642
Pyribenzamine - See ANTIHISTAMINES 106
Pyridamole - See DIPYRIDAMOLE 326
Pyridiate - See PHENAZOPYRIDINE 654
Pyridium - See PHENAZOPYRIDINE 654
PYRIDOSTIGMINE - See ANTIMYASTHENICS 128
PYRIDOXINE (Vitamin B-6) 698
PYRILAMINE - See ANTIHISTAMINES 106
Pyrilamine Maleate Tablets - See ANTIHISTAMINES 106
Pyrinyl - See PEDICULICIDES (Topical) 642
PYRITHIONE - See ANTISEBORRHEICS (Topical) 132
Pyronium - See PHENAZOPYRIDINE 654
Pyroxine - See PYRIDOXINE (Vitamin B-6) 698
PYRVINIUM - See ANTHELMINTICS 50

Q

Qnasl - See ADRENOCORTICOIDS (Nasal Inhalation) 12
Qsymia - See
APPETITE SUPPRESSANTS 146
TOPIRAMATE 804
Qualaquin - See QUININE 706
Quarzan - See CLIDINIUM 256
Quasense - See CONTRACEPTIVES, ORAL & SKIN 278
QUAZEPAM - See BENZODIAZEPINES 176
Queltuss - See
DEXTROMETHORPHAN 312
GUAIFENESIN 416
Questran - See CHOLESTYRAMINE 248
Questran Light - See CHOLESTYRAMINE 248
QUETIAPINE 700
Quibron - See
BRONCHODILATORS, XANTHINE 204
GUAIFENESIN 416
Quibron 300 - See
BRONCHODILATORS, XANTHINE 204
GUAIFENESIN 416
Quibron-T - See BRONCHODILATORS, XANTHINE 204
Quibron-T Dividose - See BRONCHODILATORS, XANTHINE 204
Quibron-T/SR - See BRONCHODILATORS, XANTHINE 204
Quibron-T/SR Dividose - See BRONCHODILATORS, XANTHINE 204
Quick Pep - See CAFFEINE 216
QUINACRINE 702
Quinaglute Dura-Tabs - See QUINIDINE 704
Quinalan - See QUINIDINE 704
QUINAPRIL - See ANGIOTENSIN-CONVERTING ENZYME (ACE) INHIBITORS 44
QUINAPRIL & HYDROCHLOROTHIAZIDE - See ANGIOTENSIN-CONVERTING ENZYME (ACE) INHIBITORS & HYDROCHLOROTHIAZIDE 46
Quinate - See QUINIDINE 704
QUINESTROL - See ESTROGENS 372
QUINETHAZONE - See DIURETICS, THIAZIDE 338
Quinidex Extentabs - See QUINIDINE 704
QUINIDINE 704
QUININE 706
Quinora - See QUINIDINE 704
Quixin - See ANTIBACTERIALS (Ophthalmic) 66
Quixin Ophthalmic Solution - See ANTIBACTERIALS (Ophthalmic) 66
Qutenza - See CAPSAICIN 226
Qvar - See ADRENOCORTICOIDS (Oral-Inhalation) 14

R

R&C - See PEDICULICIDES (Topical) 642
R.A. - See KERATOLYTICS 470
RABEPRAZOLE - See PROTON PUMP INHIBITORS 692
RACEPINEPHRINE - See BRONCHODILATORS, ADRENERGIC 200
Radiostol - See VITAMIN D 840
Radiostol Forte - See VITAMIN D 840

RALOXIFENE 708
RALTEGRAVIR - See INTEGRASE INHIBITORS 450
RAMELTEON 710
RAMIPRIL - See ANGIOTENSIN-CONVERTING ENZYME (ACE) INHIBITORS 44
Ramses Contraceptive Foam - See CONTRACEPTIVES, VAGINAL 280
Ramses Contraceptive Vaginal Jelly - See CONTRACEPTIVES, VAGINAL 280
Ramses Crystal Clear Gel - See CONTRACEPTIVES, VAGINAL 280
Ranexa - See RANOLAZINE 712
Raniclor - See CEPHALOSPORINS 236
RANITIDINE - See HISTAMINE H_2 RECEPTOR ANTAGONISTS 422
RANOLAZINE 712
Rapaflo - See ALPHA ADRENERGIC RECEPTOR BLOCKERS 20
Rapinex Powder for Oral Suspension - See PROTON PUMP INHIBITORS 692
RASAGILINE - See MONOAMINE OXIDASE TYPE B (MAO-B) INHIBITORS 572
Raudixin - See RAUWOLFIA ALKALOIDS 714
Rauval - See RAUWOLFIA ALKALOIDS 714
Rauverid - See RAUWOLFIA ALKALOIDS 714
RAUWOLFIA ALKALOIDS 714
RAUWOLFIA SERPENTINA - See RAUWOLFIA ALKALOIDS 714
Rauzide - See
DIURETICS, THIAZIDE 338
RAUWOLFIA ALKALOIDS 714
Rayos - See ADRENOCORTICOIDS (Systemic) 16
Razadyne ER - See CHOLINESTERASE INHIBITORS 250
Reactine - See ANTIHISTAMINES, NONSEDATING 110
Reclast - See BISPHOSPHONATES 192
Reclomide - See METOCLOPRAMIDE 550
Recticare Anorectal - See ANESTHETICS (Rectal) 38
Rectiv - See NITRATES 602
Rectocort - See HYDROCORTISONE (Rectal) 430
Rederm - See ADRENOCORTICOIDS (Topical) 18
Redisol - See VITAMIN B-12 (Cyanocobalamin) 836
Redoxon - See VITAMIN C (Ascorbic Acid) 838
Redutemp - See ACETAMINOPHEN 8
Reese's Pinworm Medicine - See ANTHELMINTICS 50
Refenesen - See GUAIFENESIN 416
Refenesen Chest Congestion & Pain Relief PE - See
ACETAMINOPHEN 8
GUAIFENESIN 416
PHENYLEPHRINE 658
Refenesen PE - See
GUAIFENESIN 416
PHENYLEPHRINE 658
Refresh Eye Itch - See ANTIALLERGIC AGENTS (Ophthalmic) 56
Reglan - See METOCLOPRAMIDE 550
Regonol - See ANTIMYASTHENICS 128
Regranex - See BECAPLERMIN 172
Regroton - See RAUWOLFIA ALKALOIDS 714
Regulace - See
LAXATIVES, SOFTENER/LUBRICANT 480
LAXATIVES, STIMULANT 482
Regulax SS - See LAXATIVES, SOFTENER/LUBRICANT 480
Regulex - See LAXATIVES, SOFTENER/LUBRICANT 480
Regulex-D - See LAXATIVES, SOFTENER/LUBRICANT 480
Reguloid Natural - See LAXATIVES, BULK-FORMING 476
Reguloid Orange - See LAXATIVES, BULK-FORMING 476
Reguloid Orange Sugar Free - See LAXATIVES, BULK-FORMING 476
Regutol - See LAXATIVES, SOFTENER/LUBRICANT 480
Rela - See MUSCLE RELAXANTS, SKELETAL 576
Relaxadon - See BELLADONNA ALKALOIDS & BARBITURATES 174
Relenza - See ANTIVIRALS FOR INFLUENZA, NEURAMINIDASE INHIBITORS 140
Relief Eye Drops for Red Eyes - See PHENYLEPHRINE (Ophthalmic) 660
Relpax - See TRIPTANS 820
Remcol-C - See
ACETAMINOPHEN 8
ANTIHISTAMINES 106
DEXTROMETHORPHAN 312
Remeron - See MIRTAZAPINE 566
Remeron SolTab - See MIRTAZAPINE 566
Remicade - See TUMOR NECROSIS FACTOR BLOCKERS 822
Reminyl - See CHOLINESTERASE INHIBITORS 250
Renedil - See CALCIUM CHANNEL BLOCKERS 220
Renese - See DIURETICS, THIAZIDE 338
Renese-R - See RAUWOLFIA ALKALOIDS 714
Renin Inhibitor - See RENIN INHIBITORS 716

RENIN INHIBITORS 716
Renoquid - See SULFONAMIDES 766
Renova - See RETINOIDS (Topical) 722
REPAGLINIDE - See MEGLITINIDES 528
Repan - See
ACETAMINOPHEN 8
BARBITURATES 168
CAFFEINE 216
Repigmenting agent (Psoralen) - See PSORALENS 696
Reprexain CIII - See
ANTI-INFLAMMATORY DRUGS, NONSTEROIDAL (NSAIDs) 116
NARCOTIC ANALGESICS 584
Repreve - See DOPAMINE AGONISTS NONERGOT 344
Requip - See DOPAMINE AGONISTS NONERGOT 344
Requip XL - See DOPAMINE AGONISTS NONERGOT 344
Rescon-JR - See
ANTIHISTAMINES 106
PSEUDOEPHEDRINE 694
Rescon Mx - See
ANTICHOLINERGICS 72
ANTIHISTAMINES 106
PHENYLEPHRINE 658
Rescon Tablet - See
ANTICHOLINERGICS 72
ANTIHISTAMINES 106
PHENYLEPHRINE 658
Rescriptor - See NON-NUCLEOSIDE REVERSE TRANSCRIPTASE INHIBITORS 608
Rescula - See ANTIGLAUCOMA, PROSTAGLANDINS 102
Reserfia - See
DIURETICS, THIAZIDE 338
RAUWOLFIA ALKALOIDS 714
RESERPINE - See RAUWOLFIA ALKALOIDS 714
RESERPINE, HYDRALAZINE & HYDROCHLOROTHIAZIDE 718
RESORCINOL - See KERATOLYTICS 470
RESORCINOL & SULFUR - See KERATOLYTICS 470
Respaire-30 - See
GUAIFENESIN 416
PSEUDOEPHEDRINE 694
Respbid - See BRONCHODILATORS, XANTHINE 204
Restoril - See BENZODIAZEPINES 176
Resyl - See GUAIFENESIN 416
RETAPAMULIN - See ANTIBACTERIALS (Topical) 70
Retin-A Cream - See RETINOIDS (Topical) 722
Retin-A Cream Regimen Kit - See RETINOIDS (Topical) 722
Retin-A Gel - See RETINOIDS (Topical) 722
Retin-A Gel Regimen Kit - See RETINOIDS (Topical) 722
Retin-A Solution - See RETINOIDS (Topical) 722
Retinoic Acid - See RETINOIDS (Topical) 722
RETINOIDS (Oral) 720
RETINOIDS (Topical) 722
Retrovir - See NUCLEOSIDE REVERSE TRANSCRIPTASE INHIBITORS 610
Revatio - See ERECTILE DYSFUNCTION AGENTS 360
ReVia - See NALTREXONE 582
Reyataz - See PROTEASE INHIBITORS 688
Rezamid Lotion - See KERATOLYTICS 470
Rezira - See
NARCOTIC ANALGESICS 584
PSEUDOEPHENDRINE 694
Rheaban - See ATTAPULGITE 160
Rheumatrex - See METHOTREXATE 548
Rhinall - See PHENYLEPHRINE 658
Rhinall Children's Flavored Nose Drops - See PHENYLEPHRINE 658
Rhinatate - See
ANTIHISTAMINES 106
PHENYLEPHRINE 658
Rhinocort Aqua - See ADRENOCORTICOIDS (Nasal Inhalation) 12
Rhinocort Nasal Inhaler - See ADRENOCORTICOIDS (Nasal Inhalation) 12
Rhinocort Turbuhaler - See ADRENOCORTICOIDS (Nasal Inhalation) 12
Rhinosyn - See
ANTIHISTAMINES 106
PSEUDOEPHEDRINE 694
Rhinosyn-DM - See
ANTIHISTAMINES 106
DEXTROMETHORPHAN 312
PSEUDOEPHEDRINE 694
Rhinosyn-DMX Expectorant - See
DEXTROMETHORPHAN 312
GUAIFENESIN 416
Rhinosyn-PD - See
ANTIHISTAMINES 106
PSEUDOEPHEDRINE 694
Rhinosyn-X - See
DEXTROMETHORPHAN 312
GUAIFENESIN 416
PSEUDOEPHEDRINE 694
Rhodis - See ANTI-INFLAMMATORY DRUGS, NONSTEROIDAL (NSAIDs) 116

Rhodis-EC - See ANTI-INFLAMMATORY DRUGS, NONSTEROIDAL (NSAIDs) 116
Rhotrimine - See ANTIDEPRESSANTS, TRICYCLIC 80
Rhulicort - See ADRENOCORTICOIDS (Topical) 18
Rhythmol - See PROPAFENONE 684
RIBAVIRIN 724
RIBOFLAVIN (Vitamin B-2) 726
Rid-A-Pain - See ANESTHETICS (Mucosal-Local) 36
Rid-A-Pain Compound - See
ACETAMINOPHEN 8
SALICYLATES 736
Ridaura-Oral - See GOLD COMPOUNDS 412
Rifadin - See RIFAMYCINS 728
Rifamate - See
ISONIAZID 460
RIFAMYCINS 728
Rifampicin - See RIFAMYCINS 728
RIFAMPIN - See RIFAMYCINS 728
RIFAMYCINS 728
RIFAPENTINE - See RIFAMYCINS 728
RIFAXIMIN 730
RILPIVIRINE - See NON-NUCLEOSIDE REVERSE TRANSCRIPTASE INHIBITORS 608
Rilutek - See RILUZOLE 732
RILUZOLE 732
Rimactane - See RIFAMYCINS 728
RIMANTADINE - See ANTIVIRALS FOR INFLUENZA 138
RIMEXOLONE - See ANTI-INFLAMMATORY DRUGS, STEROIDAL (Ophthalmic) 122
Riomet - See METFORMIN 544
Riopan - See ANTACIDS 48
Riopan Extra Strength - See ANTACIDS 48
Riopan Plus - See
ANTACIDS 48
SIMETHICONE 748
Riopan Plus Double Strength - See ANTACIDS 48
Riopan Plus Extra Strength - See ANTACIDS 48
Riphen - See ASPIRIN 152
RISEDRONATE - See BISPHOSPHONATES 192
Risperdal - See SEROTONIN-DOPAMINE ANTAGONISTS 744
Risperdal Consta - See SEROTONIN-DOPAMINE ANTAGONISTS 744
Risperdal M-TAB - See SEROTONIN-DOPAMINE ANTAGONISTS 744
RISPERIDONE - See SEROTONIN-DOPAMINE ANTAGONISTS 744
Ritalin - See STIMULANT MEDICATIONS 754
Ritalin LA - See STIMULANT MEDICATIONS 754
Ritalin SR - See STIMULANT MEDICATIONS 754
RITONAVIR - See PROTEASE INHIBITORS 688
RIVAROXABAN - See FACTOR Xa INHIBITORS 382
RIVASTIGMINE - See CHOLINESTERASE INHIBITORS 250
Rivotril - See BENZODIAZEPINES 176
RIZATRIPTAN - See TRIPTANS 820
RMS Uniserts - See NARCOTIC ANALGESICS 584
Ro-Antoin - See NITROFURANTOIN 604
Robafen AC Cough - See
GUAIFENESIN 416
NARCOTIC ANALGESICS 584
Robafen DAC - See
GUAIFENESIN 416
NARCOTIC ANALGESICS 584
PSEUDOEPHEDRINE 694
Robafen DM - See
DEXTROMETHORPHAN 312
GUAIFENESIN 416
PSEUDOEPHEDRINE 694
Robafen Syrup - See GUAIFENESIN 416
Robamol - See MUSCLE RELAXANTS, SKELETAL 576
Robaxin - See MUSCLE RELAXANTS, SKELETAL 576
Robaxisal - See
ASPIRIN 152
MUSCLE RELAXANTS, SKELETAL 576
Robidex - See DEXTROMETHORPHAN 312
Robidone - See NARCOTIC ANALGESICS 584
Robigesic - See ACETAMINOPHEN 8
Robinul - See GLYCOPYRROLATE 410
Robinul Forte - See GLYCOPYRROLATE 410
Robitet - See TETRACYCLINES 782
Robitussin Chest Congestion - See GUAIFENESIN 416
Robitussin Children's Cough Long-Acting - See DEXTROMETHORPHAN 312
Robitussin Children's Cough & Cold Long-Acting - See
ANTIHISTAMINES 106
DEXTROMETHORPHAN 312
Robitussin Cough & Chest Congestion DM - See
DEXTROMETHORPHAN 312
GUAIFENESIN 416

Robitussin Cough & Chest Congestion DM Max - See
DEXTROMETHORPHAN 312
GUAIFENESIN 416
Robitussin Cough & Chest Congestion Sugar Free DM - See
DEXTROMETHORPHAN 312
GUAIFENESIN 416
Robitussin Cough & Cold CF - See
DEXTROMETHORPHAN 312
GUAIFENESIN 416
PHENYLEPHRINE 658
Robitussin Cough & Cold D - See
DEXTROMETHORPHAN 312
GUAIFENESIN 416
PSEUDOEPHEDRINE 694
Robitussin Cough & Cold Long-Acting - See
ANTIHISTAMINES 106
DEXTROMETHORPHAN 312
Robitussin Cough & Cold Nighttime - See
ANTIHISTAMINES 106
PHENYLEPHRINE 658
Robitussin Cough & Chest Congestion - See
DEXTROMETHORPHAN 312
GUAIFENESIN 416
Robitussin Cough Cold & Flu Nighttime - See
ACETAMINOPHEN 8
ANTIHISTAMINES 106
DEXTROMETHORPHAN 312
PHENYLEPHRINE 658
Robitussin Cough Gels Long Acting - See
DEXTROMETHORPHAN 312
Robitussin Cough Long-Acting - See
DEXTROMETHORPHAN 312
Robomol - See MUSCLE RELAXANTS, SKELETAL 576
Rocaltrol - See VITAMIN D 840
Rodex - See PYRIDOXINE (Vitamin B-6) 698
ROFECOXIB - See ANTI-INFLAMMATORY DRUGS, NONSTEROIDAL (NSAIDs) COX-2 INHIBITORS 118
ROFLUMILAST 734
Rogaine - See MINOXIDIL (Topical) 562
Rogaine Extra Strength for Men - See MINOXIDIL (Topical) 562
Rogaine for Men - See MINOXIDIL (Topical) 562
Rogaine for Women - See MINOXIDIL (Topical) 562
Rolaids - See ANTACIDS 48
Rolaids Antacid Cool - ANTACIDS 48
Rolaids Calcium Rich - See
ANTACIDS 48
CALCIUM SUPPLEMENTS 222
Rolaids Chewable - See ANTACIDS 48
Rolaids Extra Strength - See ANTACIDS 48
Rolaids Sodium Free - See ANTACIDS 48
Rolatuss Expectorant - See
ANTIHISTAMINES 106
NARCOTIC ANALGESICS 584
PHENYLEPHRINE 658
Rolatuss Plain - See
ANTIHISTAMINES 106
PHENYLEPHRINE 658
Roniacol - See NIACIN (Vitamin B-3, Nicotinic Acid, Nicotinamide) 596
Ronigen - See NIACIN (Vitamin B-3, Nicotinic Acid, Nicotinamide) 596
ROPINIROLE - See DOPAMINE AGONISTS NONERGOT 344
Ro-Profen - See ANTI-INFLAMMATORY DRUGS, NONSTEROIDAL (NSAIDs) 116
ROSIGLITAZONE - See THIAZOLIDINEDIONES 786
ROSUVASTATIN - See HMG-CoA REDUCTASE INHIBITORS 424
ROTIGOTINE - See DOPAMINE AGONISTS NONERGOT 344
Roubac - See
SULFONAMIDES 766
TRIMETHOPRIM 818
Rounox - See ACETAMINOPHEN 8
Rowasa - See MESALAMINE 542
Roxanol - See NARCOTIC ANALGESICS 584
Roxanol SR - See NARCOTIC ANALGESICS 584
Roxicet - See NARCOTIC ANALGESICS & ACETAMINOPHEN 586
Roxicodone - See NARCOTIC ANALGESICS 584
Roxilox - See NARCOTIC ANALGESICS & ACETAMINOPHEN 586
Roxiprin - See NARCOTIC ANALGESICS & ASPIRIN 588
Roychlor 10% - See POTASSIUM SUPPLEMENTS 666
Roychlor 20% - See POTASSIUM SUPPLEMENTS 666
Royonate - See POTASSIUM SUPPLEMENTS 666
Rozerem - See RAMELTEON 710
R-Tannamine - See
ANTIHISTAMINES 106
PHENYLEPHRINE 658
R-Tannamine Pediatric - See
ANTIHISTAMINES 106
PHENYLEPHRINE 658
R-Tannate - See
ANTIHISTAMINES 106
PHENYLEPHRINE 658
R-Tannate Pediatric - See
ANTIHISTAMINES 106
PHENYLEPHRINE 658

Rubion - See VITAMIN B-12 (Cyanocobalamin) 836
Rubramin - See VITAMIN B-12 (Cyanocobalamin) 836
Rubramin-PC - See VITAMIN B-12 (Cyanocobalamin) 836
Rufen - See ANTI-INFLAMMATORY DRUGS, NONSTEROIDAL (NSAIDs) 116
Rulox - See ANTACIDS 48
Rulox No. 1 - See ANTACIDS 48
Rulox No. 2 - See ANTACIDS 48
Rulox Plus - See ANTACIDS 48
Rum-K - See POTASSIUM SUPPLEMENTS 666
Ru-Tuss DE - See
GUAIFENESIN 416
PSEUDOEPHEDRINE 694
Ru-Tuss Expectorant - See
DEXTROMETHORPHAN 312
GUAIFENESIN 416
PSEUDOEPHEDRINE 694
Rycotin - See NIACIN (Vitamin B-3, Nicotinic Acid, Nicotinamide) 596
Ryna - See
ANTIHISTAMINES 106
PSEUDOEPHEDRINE 694
Ryna-C Liquid - See
ANTIHISTAMINES 106
NARCOTIC ANALGESICS 584
PSEUDOEPHEDRINE 694
Ryna-CX Liquid - See
GUAIFENESIN 416
NARCOTIC ANALGESICS 584
PSEUDOEPHEDRINE 694
Rynacrom - See CROMOLYN 282
Rynatan - See
ANTIHISTAMINES 106
PHENYLEPHRINE 658
Rynatan Pediatric - See
ANTIHISTAMINES 106
PHENYLEPHRINE 658
Rynatan-S Pediatric - See
ANTIHISTAMINES 106
PHENYLEPHRINE 658
Rynatuss - See
ANTIHISTAMINES 106
EPHEDRINE 356
PHENYLEPHRINE 658
Rynatuss Pediatric - See
ANTIHISTAMINES 106
EPHEDRINE 356
PHENYLEPHRINE 658
Rythmodan - See DISOPYRAMIDE 328
Rythmodan-LA - See DISOPYRAMIDE 328
Ryzolt - See TRAMADOL 808

S

SafeTussin 30 - See
DEXTROMETHORPHAN 312
GUAIFENESIN 416
Safyral - See
CONTRACEPTIVES, ORAL & SKIN 278
FOLIC ACID (Vitamin B-9) 396
Salac - See KERATOLYTICS 470
Salacid - See KERATOLYTICS 470
Sal-Acid Plaster - See KERATOLYTICS 470
Salactic Film Topical Solution - See KERATOLYTICS 470
Sal-Adult - See ASPIRIN 152
Salagen - See PILOCARPINE (Oral) 662
Salatin - See
ASPIRIN 152
CAFFEINE 216
Salazopyrin - See SULFASALAZINE 762
Salazosulfapyridine - See SULFASALAZINE 762
Sal-Clens Plus Shampoo - See KERATOLYTICS 470
Sal-Clens Shampoo - See KERATOLYTICS 470
Saleto-200 - See ANTI-INFLAMMATORY DRUGS, NONSTEROIDAL (NSAIDs) 116
Saleto-400 - See ANTI-INFLAMMATORY DRUGS, NONSTEROIDAL (NSAIDs) 116
Saleto-600 - See ANTI-INFLAMMATORY DRUGS, NONSTEROIDAL (NSAIDs) 116
Saleto-800 - See ANTI-INFLAMMATORY DRUGS, NONSTEROIDAL (NSAIDs) 116
Salflex - See SALICYLATES 736
Salgesic - See SALICYLATES 736
SALICYLAMIDE - See SALICYLATES 736
SALICYLATES 736
Salicylazosulfapyridine - See SULFASALAZINE 762
SALICYLIC ACID - See KERATOLYTICS 470
SALICYLIC ACID & SULFUR - See KERATOLYTICS 470
SALICYLIC ACID, SULFUR & COAL TAR - See ANTISEBORRHEICS (Topical) 132
Saligel - See KERATOLYTICS 470
Sal-Infant - See ASPIRIN 152
SALMETEROL - See BRONCHODILATORS, ADRENERGIC 200
Salocol - See
ASPIRIN 152
CAFFEINE 216
Salofalk - See MESALAMINE 542
Salonil - See KERATOLYTICS 470
Sal-Plant Gel Topical Solution - See KERATOLYTICS 470
SALSALATE - See SALICYLATES 736

Salsitab - See SALICYLATES 736
Saluron - See DIURETICS, THIAZIDE 338
Sanctura - See MUSCARINIC RECEPTOR ANTAGONISTS 574
Sanctura XR - See MUSCARINIC RECEPTOR ANTAGONISTS 574
Sandimmune - See CYCLOSPORINE 296
Sanorex - See APPETITE SUPPRESSANTS 146
Sans-Acne - See ANTIBACTERIALS FOR ACNE (Topical) 64
Saphris - See ASENAPINE 150
SAQUINAVIR - See PROTEASE INHIBITORS 688
Sarafem - See SELECTIVE SEROTONIN REUPTAKE INHIBITORS (SSRIs) 742
Sarisol No. 2 - See BARBITURATES 168
Sarna HC - See ADRENOCORTICOIDS (Topical) 18
Sarodant - See NITROFURANTOIN 604
S.A.S. Enteric-500 - See SULFASALAZINE 762
S.A.S.-500 - See SULFASALAZINE 762
Sastid (AL) Scrub - See KERATOLYTICS 470
Sastid Plain - See KERATOLYTICS 470
Sastid Plain Shampoo and Acne Wash - See KERATOLYTICS 470
Sastid Soap - See KERATOLYTICS 470
Satric - See NITROIMIDAZOLES 606
Savella - See SEROTONIN & NOREPINEPHRINE REUPTAKE INHIBITORS (SNRIs) 746
SAXAGLIPTIN - See DPP-4 INHIBITORS 348
Scabicide - See PEDICULICIDES (Topical) 642
SCE-A Vaginal Cream - See ESTROGENS 372
SCOPOLAMINE (Hyoscine) 738
Scot-Tussin - See
GUAIFENESIN 416
PHENYLEPHRINE 658
Scot-Tussin DM - See
ANTIHISTAMINES 106
DEXTROMETHORPHAN 312
Scot-Tussin Original 5-Action Cold Medicine - See
ANTIHISTAMINES 106
CAFFEINE 216
PHENYLEPHRINE 658
SALICYLATES 736
Scytera Foam - See COAL TAR (Topical) 266
Seasonale - See CONTRACEPTIVES, ORAL & SKIN 278
Seasonique - See CONTRACEPTIVES, ORAL & SKIN 278
Seba-Nil - See ANTIACNE, CLEANSING (Topical) 54
Sebasorb Liquid - See KERATOLYTICS 470
Sebex - See KERATOLYTICS 470
Sebex-T Tar Shampoo - See ANTISEBORRHEICS (Topical) 132
Sebucare - See KERATOLYTICS 470
Sebulex Antiseborrheic Treatment and Conditioning Shampoo - See KERATOLYTICS 470
Sebulex Antiseborrheic Treatment Shampoo - See KERATOLYTICS 470
Sebulex Conditioning Shampoo - See KERATOLYTICS 470
Sebulex Conditioning Suspension Shampoo - See ANTISEBORRHEICS (Topical) 132
Sebulex Cream Medicated Shampoo - See KERATOLYTICS 470
Sebulex Lotion Shampoo - See ANTISEBORRHEICS (Topical) 132
Sebulex Medicated Dandruff Shampoo with Conditioners - See KERATOLYTICS 470
Sebulex Medicated Shampoo - See KERATOLYTICS 470
Sebulex Regular Medicated Dandruff Shampoo - See KERATOLYTICS 470
Sebulex Shampoo - See KERATOLYTICS 470
Sebulon - See ANTISEBORRHEICS (Topical) 132
Sebutone - See ANTISEBORRHEICS (Topical) 132
SECOBARBITAL - See BARBITURATES 168
SECOBARBITAL & AMOBARBITAL - See BARBITURATES 168
Seconal - See BARBITURATES 168
Sectral - See BETA-ADRENERGIC BLOCKING AGENTS 182
Sedabamate - See MEPROBAMATE 538
Sedapap - See
ACETAMINOPHEN 8
BARBITURATES 168
Sedative - See
BARBITURATES 168
BELLADONNA ALKALOIDS & BARBITURATES 174
GUAIFENESIN 416
ZALEPLON 852
Sedative-hypnotic agent - See
BARBITURATES 168
ESZOPICLONE 374
TRIAZOLAM 812
ZOLPIDEM 858
Sedatuss - See DEXTROMETHORPHAN 312
Selective aldosterone blocker - See EPLERENONE 358
Selective norepinephrine reuptake inhibitor - See ATOMOXETINE 154
SELECTIVE PROGESTERONE RECEPTOR MODULATORS 740

SELECTIVE SEROTONIN REUPTAKE INHIBITORS (SSRIs) 742
SELEGILINE - See MONOAMINE OXIDASE TYPE B (MAO-B) INHIBITORS 572
SELENIUM SULFIDE - See ANTISEBORRHEICS (Topical) 132
Selexid - See PENICILLINS 646
Selpak - See MONOAMINE OXIDASE TYPE B (MAO-B) INHIBITORS 572
Selsun - See ANTISEBORRHEICS (Topical) 132
Selsun Blue - See ANTISEBORRHEICS (Topical) 132
Selsun Blue Dry Formula - See ANTISEBORRHEICS (Topical) 132
Selsun Blue Extra Conditioning Formula - See ANTISEBORRHEICS (Topical) 132
Selsun Blue Extra Medicated Formula - See ANTISEBORRHEICS (Topical) 132
Selsun Blue Oily Formula - See ANTISEBORRHEICS (Topical) 132
Selsun Blue Regular Formula - See ANTISEBORRHEICS (Topical) 132
Selzentry - See MARAVIROC 522
Semcet - See ACETAMINOPHEN 8
Semicid - See CONTRACEPTIVES, VAGINAL 280
Semprex-D - See
ANTIHISTAMINES 106
PSEUDOEPHEDRINE 694
Senexon - See LAXATIVES, STIMULANT 482
SENNA - See LAXATIVES, STIMULANT 482
SennaPrompt - See
LAXATIVES, BULK-FORMING 476
LAXATIVES, STIMULANT 482
SENNOSIDES - See LAXATIVES, STIMULANT 482
Senokot - See LAXATIVES, STIMULANT 482
Senokot-S - See
LAXATIVES, SOFTENER/LUBRICANT 480
LAXATIVES, STIMULANT 482
SenokotXTRA - See LAXATIVES, STIMULANT 482
Senolax - See LAXATIVES, STIMULANT 482
SensoGARD Canker Sore Relief - See ANESTHETICS (Mucosal-Local) 36
Sential - See ADRENOCORTICOIDS (Topical) 18
Septra - See
SULFONAMIDES 766
TRIMETHOPRIM 818
Septra DS - See
SULFONAMIDES 766
TRIMETHOPRIM 818
Ser-A-Gen - See RESERPINE, HYDRALAZINE & HYDROCHLOROTHIAZIDE 718
Seralazide - See RESERPINE, HYDRALAZINE & HYDROCHLOROTHIAZIDE 718
Serax - See BENZODIAZEPINES 176
Serentil - See PHENOTHIAZINES 656
Serentil Concentrate - See PHENOTHIAZINES 656
Serevent - See BRONCHODILATORS, ADRENERGIC 200
Serevent Diskus - See BRONCHODILATORS, ADRENERGIC 200
Seromycin - See CYCLOSERINE 294
Serophene - See CLOMIPHENE 260
Seroquel - See QUETIAPINE 700
Seroquel XR - See QUETIAPINE 700
SEROTONIN-DOPAMINE ANTAGONISTS 744
SEROTONIN & NOREPINEPHRINE REUPTAKE INHIBITORS (SNRIs) 746
Serpalan - See RAUWOLFIA ALKALOIDS 714
Serpasil - See RAUWOLFIA ALKALOIDS 714
Serpazide - See RESERPINE, HYDRALAZINE & HYDROCHLOROTHIAZIDE 718
SERTACONAZOLE - See ANTIFUNGALS (Topical) 88
Sertan - See PRIMIDONE 674
SERTRALINE - See SELECTIVE SEROTONIN REUPTAKE INHIBITORS (SSRIs) 742
Serutan - See LAXATIVES, BULK-FORMING 476
Serutan Toasted Granules - See LAXATIVES, BULK-FORMING 476
Serzone - See NEFAZODONE 590
sfRowasa - See MESALAMINE 542
Shogan - See ANTIHISTAMINES, PHENOTHIAZINE-DERIVATIVE 112
Shur-Seal - See CONTRACEPTIVES, VAGINAL 280
Sibelium - See CALCIUM CHANNEL BLOCKERS 220
Siblin - See LAXATIVES, BULK-FORMING 476
Siladryl - See ANTIHISTAMINES 106
Sildamac - See ANTIBACTERIALS, ANTIFUNGALS (Topical) 62
SILDENAFIL CITRATE - See ERECTILE DYSFUNCTION AGENTS 360
Silenor - See ANTIDEPRESSANTS, TRICYCLIC 80
Silexin Cough - See
DEXTROMETHORPHAN 312
GUAIFENESIN 416
SILODOSIN - See ALPHA ADRENERGIC RECEPTOR BLOCKERS 20
Silphen - See ANTIHISTAMINES 106

Silvadene - See ANTIBACTERIALS, ANTIFUNGALS (Topical) 62
Simaal 2 Gel - See ANTACIDS 48
Simaal Gel - See ANTACIDS 48
Simcor - See
HMG-CoA REDUCTASE INHIBITORS 424
NIACIN (Vitamin B-3, Nicotinic Acid, Nicotinamide) 596
SIMETHICONE 748
Simiron - See IRON SUPPLEMENTS 458
Simply Cough - See DEXTROMETHORPHAN 312
Simply Sleep - See ANTIHISTAMINES 106
Simply Stuffy - See PSEUDOEPHEDRINE 694
Simponi - See TUMOR NECROSIS FACTOR BLOCKERS 822
SIMVASTATIN - See HMG-CoA REDUCTASE INHIBITORS 424
Sinemet - See CARBIDOPA & LEVODOPA 230
Sinemet CR - See CARBIDOPA & LEVODOPA 230
Sinequan - See ANTIDEPRESSANTS, TRICYCLIC 80
Singulair - See LEUKOTRIENE MODIFIERS 488
Sinol Nasal Spray - See CAPSAICIN 226
Sinubid - See ACETAMINOPHEN 8
Sinumist-SR - See GUAIFENESIN 416
Sinupan - See
GUAIFENESIN 416
PHENYLEPHRINE 658
Sinus Buster - See CAPSAICIN 226
Sinus Relief - See
ACETAMINOPHEN 8
PSEUDOEPHEDRINE 694
Sinutab Maximum Strength Sinus Allergy Caplet - See
ACETAMINOPHEN 8
ANTIHISTAMINES 106
PSEUDOEPHEDRINE 694
Sinutab Non-Drying Liquid Caps - See
GUAIFENESIN 416
PSEUDOEPHEDRINE 694
Sinutab Sinus Caplets - See
ACETAMINOPHEN 8
PHENYLEPHRINE 658
SINUvent PE - See
GUAIFENESIN 416
PHENYLEPHRINE 658
SITAGLIPTIN - See DPP-4 INHIBITORS 348
Skelaxin - See MUSCLE RELAXANTS, SKELETAL 576
Skelex - See MUSCLE RELAXANTS, SKELETAL 576
Skelid - See BISPHOSPHONATES 192
Sklice Lotion - See PEDICULICIDES (Topical) 642
Sleep-Eze 3 - See ANTIHISTAMINES 106
Slo-Bid - See BRONCHODILATORS, XANTHINE 204
Slo-bid Gyrocaps - See BRONCHODILATORS, XANTHINE 204
Slo-Niacin - See NIACIN (Vitamin B-3, Nicotinic Acid, Nicotinamide) 596
Slo-Phyllin - See BRONCHODILATORS, XANTHINE 204
Slo-Phyllin GG - See
BRONCHODILATORS, XANTHINE 204
GUAIFENESIN 416
Slo-Phyllin Gyrocaps - See BRONCHODILATORS, XANTHINE 204
Slow Fe - See IRON SUPPLEMENTS 458
Slow-K - See POTASSIUM SUPPLEMENTS 666
Slow-Trasicor - See BETA-ADRENERGIC BLOCKING AGENTS 182
SMZ-TMP - See
SULFONAMIDES 766
TRIMETHOPRIM 818
Snap Back - See CAFFEINE 216
Snaplets-FR - See ACETAMINOPHEN 8
SODIUM BICARBONATE 750
SODIUM CITRATE & CITRIC ACID - See CITRATES 254
Sodium Cromoglycate - See CROMOLYN 282
SODIUM FLUORIDE 752
SODIUM PHOSPHATE - See LAXATIVES, OSMOTIC 478
SODIUM SALICYLATE - See SALICYLATES 736
Sodium Sulamyd - See ANTIBACTERIALS (Ophthalmic) 66
Sodol - See MUSCLE RELAXANTS, SKELETAL 576
Sofarin - See ANTICOAGULANTS (Oral) 74
Solage - See RETINOIDS (Topical) 722
Solatene - See BETA CAROTENE 180
Solazine - See PHENOTHIAZINES 656
Solfoton - See BARBITURATES 168
SOLIFENACIN - See MUSCARINIC RECEPTOR ANTAGONISTS 574
Solium - See BENZODIAZEPINES 176
Solodyn - See TETRACYCLINES 782
Soltamox - See TAMOXIFEN 772
Solu-Phyllin - See BRONCHODILATORS, XANTHINE 204
Solurex - See ADRENOCORTICOIDS (Systemic) 16
Solurex LA - See ADRENOCORTICOIDS (Systemic) 16

Soma - See MUSCLE RELAXANTS, SKELETAL 576
Soma Compound - See
ASPIRIN 152
NARCOTIC ANALGESICS 584
Soma Compound with Codeine - See MUSCLE RELAXANTS, SKELETAL 576
Sominex Formula 2 - See ANTIHISTAMINES 106
Somnol - See BENZODIAZEPINES 176
Somophyllin - See BRONCHODILATORS, XANTHINE 204
Somophyllin-12 - See BRONCHODILATORS, XANTHINE 204
Somophyllin-CRT - See BRONCHODILATORS, XANTHINE 204
Somophyllin-DF - See BRONCHODILATORS, XANTHINE 204
Somophyllin-T - See BRONCHODILATORS, XANTHINE 204
Sonata - See ZALEPLON 852
Sopamycetin Ophthalmic Ointment - See ANTIBACTERIALS (Ophthalmic) 66
Sopamycetin Ophthalmic Solution - See ANTIBACTERIALS (Ophthalmic) 66
Sopridol - See MUSCLE RELAXANTS, SKELETAL 576
Sorbitrate - See NITRATES 602
Sorbitrate SA - See NITRATES 602
Soriatane - See RETINOIDS (Oral) 720
Soridol - See MUSCLE RELAXANTS, SKELETAL 576
Sorilux - See VITAMIN D (Topical) 842
Sotacor - See BETA-ADRENERGIC BLOCKING AGENTS 182
SOTALOL - See BETA-ADRENERGIC BLOCKING AGENTS 182
Sotret - See ISOTRETINOIN 462
Spancap - See AMPHETAMINES 28
Span-FF - See IRON SUPPLEMENTS 458
Span-Niacin - See NIACIN (Vitamin B-3, Nicotinic Acid, Nicotinamide) 596
SPARFLOXACIN - See FLUOROQUINOLONES 392
Sparlon - See STIMULANTS, AMPHETAMINE RELATED 756
Spaslin - See BELLADONNA ALKALOIDS & BARBITURATES 174
Spasmoban - See DICYCLOMINE 316
Spasmoject - See DICYCLOMINE 316
Spasmolin - See BELLADONNA ALKALOIDS & BARBITURATES 174
Spasmophen - See BELLADONNA ALKALOIDS & BARBITURATES 174
Spasquid - See BELLADONNA ALKALOIDS & BARBITURATES 174
Spec-T Sore Throat Anesthetic - See ANESTHETICS (Mucosal-Local) 36
Spectazole - See ANTIFUNGALS (Topical) 88
Spectracef - See CEPHALOSPORINS 236
Spectrobid - See PENICILLINS 646
Spectro-Chlor Ophthalmic Ointment - See ANTIBACTERIALS (Ophthalmic) 66
Spectro-Chlor Ophthalmic Solution - See ANTIBACTERIALS (Ophthalmic) 66
Spectro-Genta - See ANTIBACTERIALS (Ophthalmic) 66
Spectro-Homatropine - See CYCLOPLEGIC, MYDRIATIC (Ophthalmic) 292
Spectro-Pentolate - See CYCLOPENTOLATE (Ophthalmic) 288
Spectro-Sporin - See ANTIBACTERIALS (Ophthalmic) 66
Spectro-Sulf - See ANTIBACTERIALS (Ophthalmic) 66
Spersadex - See ANTI-INFLAMMATORY DRUGS, STEROIDAL (Ophthalmic) 122
Spersaphrine - See PHENYLEPHRINE (Ophthalmic) 660
SPINOSAD - See PEDICULICIDES (Topical) 642
Spiriva - See BRONCHODILATORS, ANTICHOLINERGIC 202
SPIRONOLACTONE - See DIURETICS, POTASSIUM-SPARING 334
SPIRONOLACTONE & HYDROCHLOROTHIAZIDE - See DIURETICS, POTASSIUM-SPARING & HYDROCHLOROTHIAZIDE 336
Spirozide - See DIURETICS, POTASSIUM-SPARING & HYDROCHLOROTHIAZIDE 336
Sporanox - See ANTIFUNGALS, AZOLES 86
Sprix - See ANTI-INFLAMMATORY DRUGS, NONSTEROIDAL (NSAIDs) 116
SSD - See ANTIBACTERIALS, ANTIFUNGALS (Topical) 62
SSD AF - See ANTIBACTERIALS, ANTIFUNGALS (Topical) 62
SSKI - See POTASSIUM SUPPLEMENTS 666
S-T Cort - See ADRENOCORTICOIDS (Topical) 18
St. Joseph Adult Chewable Aspirin - See ASPIRIN 152
St. Joseph Antidiarrheal - See ATTAPULGITE 160
St. Joseph Aspirin Free Fever Reducer for Children - See ACETAMINOPHEN 8

INDEX

St. Joseph Companion Aspirin - See ASPIRIN 152
St. Joseph Cough Suppressant for Children - See DEXTROMETHORPHAN 312
Stadol NS - See BUTORPHANOL 214
Stagesic - See NARCOTIC ANALGESICS & ACETAMINOPHEN 586
Stalevo - See
COMT INHIBITORS 274
CARBIDOPA & LEVODOPA 230
Stamoist E - See
GUAIFENESIN 416
PSEUDOEPHEDRINE 694
STANOZOLOL - See ANDROGENS 34
Starlix - See MEGLITINIDES 528
Statex - See NARCOTIC ANALGESICS 584
Staticin - See ANTIBACTERIALS FOR ACNE (Topical) 64
Statobex - See APPETITE SUPPRESSANTS 146
Statuss Expectorant - See
NARCOTIC ANALGESICS 584
PHENYLEPHRINE 658
STAVUDINE - See NUCLEOSIDE REVERSE TRANSCRIPTASE INHIBITORS 610
Stavzor - See VALPROIC ACID 826
Staxyn - See ERECTILE DYSFUNCTION AGENTS 360
Stelara - See BIOLOGICS FOR PSORIASIS 188
Stelazine - See PHENOTHIAZINES 656
Stelazine Concentrate - See PHENOTHIAZINES 656
Stemetil - See PHENOTHIAZINES 656
Stemetil Liquid - See PHENOTHIAZINES 656
Stendra - See ERECTILE DYSFUNCTION AGENTS 360
Sterapred DS - See ADRENOCORTICOIDS (Systemic) 16
Steri-Units Sulfacetamide - See ANTIBACTERIALS (Ophthalmic) 66
Stieva-A Cream - See RETINOIDS (Topical) 722
Stieva-A Cream Forte - See RETINOIDS (Topical) 722
Stieva-A Gel - See RETINOIDS (Topical) 722
Stieva-A Solution - See RETINOIDS (Topical) 722
Stilphostrol - See ESTROGENS 372
Stimate - See DESMOPRESSIN 310
Stimulant - See ORPHENADRINE, ASPIRIN & CAFFEINE 626
Stimulant (Xanthine) - See CAFFEINE 216
STIMULANT MEDICATIONS 754
STIMULANTS, AMPHETAMINE-RELATED 756
Storz-Dexa - See ANTI-INFLAMMATORY DRUGS, STEROIDAL (Ophthalmic) 122
Storzolamide - See CARBONIC ANHYDRASE INHIBITORS 232
Stoxil Eye Ointment - See ANTIVIRALS (Ophthalmic) 142
Strattera - See ATOMOXETINE 154
Striant - See ANDROGENS 34
Stribild - See
COBICISTAT (not in book)
INTEGRASE INHIBITORS 450
NUCLEOSIDE REVERSE TRANSCRIPTASE INHIBITORS 610
NUCLEOTIDE REVERSE TRANSCRIPTASE INHIBITORS 612
Stri-Dex - See KERATOLYTICS 470
Stri-Dex Dual Textured Pads Maximum Strength - See KERATOLYTICS 470
Stri-Dex Dual Textured Pads Regular Strength - See KERATOLYTICS 470
Stri-Dex Dual Textured Pads Sensitive Skin - See KERATOLYTICS 470
Stri-Dex Maximum Strength Pads - See KERATOLYTICS 470
Stri-Dex Maximum Strength Treatment 10 Cream - See BENZOYL PEROXIDE 178
Stri-Dex Regular Strength Pads - See KERATOLYTICS 470
Stri-Dex Super Scrub Pads - See KERATOLYTICS 470
Stromectol - See ANTHELMINTICS 50
Stulex - See LAXATIVES, SOFTENER/ LUBRICANT 480
Suboxone Film - See BUPRENORPHINE & NALOXONE 206
Subsys - See NARCOTIC ANALGESICS 584
SUCRALFATE 758
Sucrets Cough Control - See DEXTROMETHORPHAN 312
Sucrets Maximum Strength - See ANESTHETICS (Mucosal-Local) 36
Sucrets Regular Strength - See ANESTHETICS (Mucosal-Local) 36
Sudafed 12 Hour - See PSEUDOEPHEDRINE 694
Sudafed 24-hour Tablets - See PSEUDOEPHEDRINE 694
Sudafed Multi-Symptom Cold & Cough - See
ACETAMINOPHEN 8
DEXTROMETHORPHAN 312
GUAIFENESIN 416
PSEUDOEPHEDRINE 694
Sudafed Nasal Decongestant Tablets - See PSEUDOEPHEDRINE 694

Sudafed Non-Drying Sinus Liquid Caps - See
GUAIFENESIN 416
PSEUDOEPHEDRINE 694
Sudafed PE Cold & Cough Caplets - See
ACETAMINOPHEN 8
DEXTROMETHORPHAN 312
GUAIFENESIN 416
PHENYLEPHRINE 658
Sudafed PE Maximum Strength Nasal Decongestant Tablets - See
PHENYLEPHRINE 658
Sudafed PE Quick Dissolve Strips Cherry Menthol - See PHENYLEPHRINE 658
Sudafed PE Severe Cold Caplets - See
ACETAMINOPHEN 8
ANTIHISTAMINES 106
PHENYLEPHRINE 658
Sudafed PE Sinus & Allergy Tablets - See
ANTIHISTAMINES 106
PHENYLEPHRINE 658
Sudafed PE Sinus Headache Caplets - See
ACETAMINOPHEN 8
PHENYLEPHRINE 658
Sufedrin - See PSEUDOEPHEDRINE 694
Sular - See CALCIUM CHANNEL BLOCKERS 220
Sul-Azo - See SULFONAMIDES & PHENAZOPYRIDINE 768
SULCONAZOLE - See ANTIFUNGALS (Topical) 88
Sulcrate - See SUCRALFATE 758
Sulcrate Suspension Plus - See
SUCRALFATE 758
Sulf-10 - See ANTIBACTERIALS (Ophthalmic) 66
SULFACETAMIDE (Ophthalmic) - See ANTIBACTERIALS (Ophthalmic) 66
Sulfa (Sulfonamide) - See
SULFASALAZINE 762
SULFONAMIDES 766
SULFACYTINE - See SULFONAMIDES 766
SULFADIAZINE - See
ANTIBACTERIALS, ANTIFUNGALS (Topical) 62
SULFONAMIDES 766
SULFADOXINE & PYRIMETHAMINE 760
Sulfair - See ANTIBACTERIALS (Ophthalmic) 66
Sulfair 10 - See ANTIBACTERIALS (Ophthalmic) 66
Sulfair 15 - See ANTIBACTERIALS (Ophthalmic) 66
Sulfair Forte - See ANTIBACTERIALS (Ophthalmic) 66
SULFAMETHIZOLE - See SULFONAMIDES 766
Sulfamethoprim - See
SULFONAMIDES 766
TRIMETHOPRIM 818
Sulfamethoprim DS - See
SULFONAMIDES 766
TRIMETHOPRIM 818
SULFAMETHOXAZOLE - See SULFONAMIDES 766
SULFAMETHOXAZOLE & PHENAZOPYRIDINE - See SULFONAMIDES & PHENAZOPYRIDINE 768
Sulfamide - See ANTIBACTERIALS (Ophthalmic) 66
Sulfaprim - See
SULFONAMIDES 766
TRIMETHOPRIM 818
Sulfaprim DS - See
SULFONAMIDES 766
TRIMETHOPRIM 818
SULFASALAZINE 762
Sulfatrim - See
SULFONAMIDES 766
TRIMETHOPRIM 818
Sulfatrim DS - See
SULFONAMIDES 766
TRIMETHOPRIM 818
Sulfex - See ANTIBACTERIALS (Ophthalmic) 66
Sulfimycin - See
ERYTHROMYCINS 368
SULFONAMIDES 766
SULFINPYRAZONE 764
SULFISOXAZOLE - See SULFONAMIDES 766
SULFISOXAZOLE & PHENAZOPYRIDINE - See SULFONAMIDES & PHENAZOPYRIDINE 768
SULFISOXAZOLE (Ophthalmic) - See ANTIBACTERIALS (Ophthalmic) 66
Sulfizole - See SULFONAMIDES 766
Sulfolax - See LAXATIVES, SOFTENER/LUBRICANT 480
Sulfonamide - See SULFONAMIDES & PHENAZOPYRIDINE 768
SULFONAMIDES 766
SULFONAMIDES & PHENAZOPYRIDINE 768
Sulfone - See DAPSONE 304
SULFONYLUREAS 770
Sulforcin - See KERATOLYTICS 470
Sulfoxaprim - See
SULFONAMIDES 766
TRIMETHOPRIM 818
Sulfoxaprim DS - See
SULFONAMIDES 766
TRIMETHOPRIM 818
SULFUR (Topical) - See KERATOLYTICS 470

INDEX

SULFURATED LIME - See ANTIACNE, CLEANSING (Topical) 54
SULINDAC - See ANTI-INFLAMMATORY DRUGS, NONSTEROIDAL (NSAIDs) 116
Sulmeprim - See
SULFONAMIDES 766
TRIMETHOPRIM 818
Sulsal Soap - See KERATOLYTICS 470
Sulten-10 - See ANTIBACTERIALS (Ophthalmic) 66
SUMATRIPTAN - See TRIPTANS 820
Sumavel DosePro - See TRIPTANS 820
Summit - See ACETAMINOPHEN 8
Sumycin - See TETRACYCLINES 782
Sunkist - See VITAMIN C (Ascorbic Acid) 838
Supac - See
ACETAMINOPHEN 8
ASPIRIN 152
CAFFEINE 216
Supasa - See ASPIRIN 152
SuperChar - See CHARCOAL, ACTIVATED 238
Supeudol - See NARCOTIC ANALGESICS 584
Suppap - See ACETAMINOPHEN 8
Suppress Cough with Dextromethorphan - See DEXTROMETHORPHAN 312
Supracaine - See ANESTHETICS (Mucosal-Local) 36
Suprax - See CEPHALOSPORINS 236
Suprazine - See PHENOTHIAZINES 656
Suprenza - See APPETITE SUPPRESSANTS 146
Supres - See
CENTRAL ALPHA AGONISTS 234
DIURETICS, THIAZIDE 338
SUPROFEN - See ANTI-INFLAMMATORY DRUGS, NONSTEROIDAL (NSAIDs) (Ophthalmic) 120
Surfak - See LAXATIVES, SOFTENER/ LUBRICANT 480
Surgam - See ANTI-INFLAMMATORY DRUGS, NONSTEROIDAL (NSAIDs) 116
Surgam SR - See ANTI-INFLAMMATORY DRUGS, NONSTEROIDAL (NSAIDs) 116
Surmontil - See ANTIDEPRESSANTS, TRICYCLIC 80
Susano - See BELLADONNA ALKALOIDS & BARBITURATES 174
Sust-A - See VITAMIN A 834
Sustaire - See BRONCHODILATORS, XANTHINE 204
Sustiva - See NON-NUCLEOSIDE REVERSE TRANSCRIPTASE INHIBITORS 608
Sutilan - See TIOPRONIN 798
Syllact - See LAXATIVES, BULK-FORMING 476
Syllamalt - See LAXATIVES, BULK-FORMING 476
Symadine - See ANTIVIRALS FOR INFLUENZA 138
Symbicort - See
ADRENOCORTICOIDS (Oral Inhalation) 14
BRONCHODILATORS, ADRENERGIC 200
Symbyax - See
OLANZAPINE 616
SELECTIVE SEROTONIN REUPTAKE INHIBITORS (SSRIs) 742
Symlin - See PRAMLINTIDE 668
SymlinPen - See PRAMLINTIDE 668
Symmetrel - See ANTIVIRALS FOR INFLUENZA 138
Sympathomimetic - See
BARBITURATES 168
BRONCHODILATORS, ADRENERGIC 200
EPHEDRINE 356
GUAIFENESIN 416
OXYMETAZOLINE (Nasal) 630
PHENYLEPHRINE 658
PSEUDOEPHEDRINE 694
STIMULANT MEDICATIONS 754
XYLOMETAZOLINE 850
Symphasic - See CONTRACEPTIVES, ORAL & SKIN 278
Synacort - See ADRENOCORTICOIDS (Topical) 18
Synalar - See ADRENOCORTICOIDS (Topical) 18
Synalar HP - See ADRENOCORTICOIDS (Topical) 18
Synalgos-DC - See
CAFFEINE 216
NARCOTIC ANALGESICS & ASPIRIN 588
Synamol - See ADRENOCORTICOIDS (Topical) 18
Synarel - See NAFARELIN 580
Syn-Captopril - See ANGIOTENSIN-CONVERTING ENZYME (ACE) INHIBITORS 44
Syn-Diltiazem - See CALCIUM CHANNEL BLOCKERS 220
Synemol - See ADRENOCORTICOIDS (Topical) 18
Synera - See ANESTHETICS (Topical) 40
Synflex - See ANTI-INFLAMMATORY DRUGS, NONSTEROIDAL (NSAIDs) 116
Synflex DS - See ANTI-INFLAMMATORY DRUGS, NONSTEROIDAL (NSAIDs) 116
Synkayvite - See VITAMIN K 846
Syn-Nadolol - See BETA-ADRENERGIC BLOCKING AGENTS 182

Synophylate - See BRONCHODILATORS, XANTHINE 204
Syn-Pindolol - See BETA-ADRENERGIC BLOCKING AGENTS 182
Synthroid - See THYROID HORMONES 792
Synvinolin - See HMG-CoA REDUCTASE INHIBITORS 424

T

Taclonex - See
ADRENOCORTICOIDS (Topical) 18
VITAMIN D (Topical) 842
TACROLIMUS - See IMMUNOSUPPRESSIVE AGENTS 442
TADALAFIL - See ERECTILE DYSFUNCTION AGENTS 360
TAFLUPROST - See ANTIGLAUCOMA, PROSTAGLANDINS 102
Tagamet - See HISTAMINE H_2 RECEPTOR ANTAGONISTS 422
Tagamet HB - See HISTAMINE H_2 RECEPTOR ANTAGONISTS 422
Talacen - See NARCOTIC ANALGESICS & ACETAMINOPHEN 586
TALBUTAL - See BARBITURATES 168
Talwin - See NARCOTIC ANALGESICS 584
Talwin Compound - See NARCOTIC ANALGESICS & ASPIRIN 588
Talwin Compound-50 - See NARCOTIC ANALGESICS & ASPIRIN 588
Talwin-NX - See NARCOTIC ANALGESICS 584
Tambocor - See FLECAINIDE ACETATE 390
Tamiflu - See ANTIVIRALS FOR INFLUENZA, NEURAMINIDASE INHIBITORS 140
Tamofen - See TAMOXIFEN 772
Tamone - See TAMOXIFEN 772
Tamoplex - See TAMOXIFEN 772
TAMOXIFEN 772
TAMSULOSIN - See ALPHA ADRENERGIC RECEPTOR BLOCKERS 20
Tanoral - See
ANTIHISTAMINES 106
PHENYLEPHRINE 658
Tapanol - See ACETAMINOPHEN 8
Tapanol Extra Strength - See ACETAMINOPHEN 8
Tapar - See ACETAMINOPHEN 8
Tapazole - See ANTITHYROID DRUGS 134
TAPENTADOL 774
Tar Doak - See COAL TAR (Topical) 266
Taraphilic - See COAL TAR (Topical) 266
Tarbonis - See COAL TAR (Topical) 266
Targretin - See RETINOIDS (Topical) 722
Tarka - See
ANGIOTENSIN-CONVERTING ENZYME (ACE) INHIBITORS 44
CALCIUM CHANNEL BLOCKERS 220
Taro-Carbamazepine - See CARBAMAZEPINE 228
Tarpaste - See COAL TAR (Topical) 266
Tarpaste Doak - See COAL TAR (Topical) 266
Tasmar - See COMT INHIBITORS 274
Tavist - See ANTIHISTAMINES 106
Tavist Allergy/Sinus/Headache - See
ACETAMINOPHEN 8
ANTIHISTAMINES 106
PSEUDOEPHEDRINE 694
Tavist-1 - See ANTIHISTAMINES 106
Taxol - See PACLITAXEL 632
TAZAROTENE - See RETINOIDS (Topical) 722
Tazorac - See RETINOIDS (Topical) 722
T-Cypionate - See ANDROGENS 34
T/Derm Tar Emollient - See COAL TAR (Topical) 266
T-Diet - See APPETITE SUPPRESSANTS 146
Tearisol - See PROTECTANT (Ophthalmic) 690
Tears Naturale - See PROTECTANT (Ophthalmic) 690
Tears Naturale Free - See PROTECTANT (Ophthalmic) 690
Tears Naturale II - See PROTECTANT (Ophthalmic) 690
Tears Renewed - See PROTECTANT (Ophthalmic) 690
Tecnal - See
ASPIRIN 152
BARBITURATES 168
Teczem - See
ANGIOTENSIN-CONVERTING ENZYME (ACE) INHIBITORS 44
CALCIUM CHANNEL BLOCKERS 220
Tega-Flex - See ORPHENADRINE 624
TEGASEROD 776
Tega-Span - See NIACIN (Vitamin B-3, Nicotinic Acid, Nicotinamide) 596
Tega-Vert - See ANTIHISTAMINES 106
Tegopen - See PENICILLINS 646
Tegretol - See CARBAMAZEPINE 228
Tegretol Chewtabs - See CARBAMAZEPINE 228
Tegretol CR - See CARBAMAZEPINE 228
Tegretol XR - See CARBAMAZEPINE 228
Tegrin Lotion for Psoriasis - See COAL TAR (Topical) 266
Tegrin Medicated Cream Shampoo - See COAL TAR (Topical) 266
Tegrin Medicated Shampoo Concentrated Gel - See COAL TAR (Topical) 266

Tegrin Medicated Shampoo Extra Conditioning Formula - See COAL TAR (Topical) 266
Tegrin Medicated Shampoo Herbal Formula - See COAL TAR (Topical) 266
Tegrin Medicated Shampoo Original Formula - See COAL TAR (Topical) 266
Tegrin Medicated Soap for Psoriasis - See COAL TAR (Topical) 266
Tegrin Skin Cream for Psoriasis - See COAL TAR (Topical) 266
Tekamlo - See
CALCIUM CHANNEL BLOCKERS 220
RENIN INHIBITORS 716
Tekturna - See RENIN INHIBITORS 716
Tekturna HCT - See
DIURETICS, THIAZIDE 338
RENIN INHIBITORS 716
Telachlor - See ANTIHISTAMINES 106
Teladar - See ADRENOCORTICOIDS (Topical) 18
Teldrin - See ANTIHISTAMINES 106
Telectin DS - See ANTI-INFLAMMATORY DRUGS, NONSTEROIDAL (NSAIDs) 116
TELITHROMYCIN 778
TELMISARTAN - See ANGIOTENSIN II RECEPTOR ANTAGONISTS 42
TEMAZEPAM - See BENZODIAZEPINES 176
Temgesic - See NARCOTIC ANALGESICS 584
Temovate - See ADRENOCORTICOIDS (Topical) 18
Temovate E - See ADRENOCORTICOIDS (Topical) 18
Temovate Emollient - See ADRENOCORTICOIDS (Topical) 18
Temovate Gel - See ADRENOCORTICOIDS (Topical) 18
Temovate Scalp Application - See ADRENOCORTICOIDS (Topical) 18
Tempo - See ANTACIDS 48
Tempra - See ACETAMINOPHEN 8
Tempra Caplets - See ACETAMINOPHEN 8
Tempra Chewable Tablets - See ACETAMINOPHEN 8
Tempra Double Strength - See ACETAMINOPHEN 8
Tempra Drops - See ACETAMINOPHEN 8
Tempra D.S. - See ACETAMINOPHEN 8
Tempra Infants - See ACETAMINOPHEN 8
Tempra Syrup - See ACETAMINOPHEN 8
Ten K - See POTASSIUM SUPPLEMENTS 666
Tencet - See
ACETAMINOPHEN 8
BARBITURATES 168
Tenex - CENTRAL ALPHA AGONISTS 234
TENOFOVIR - See NUCLEOTIDE REVERSE TRANSCRIPTASE INHIBITORS 612
Tenol - See ACETAMINOPHEN 8
Tenol Plus - See
ACETAMINOPHEN 8
ASPIRIN 152
Tenoretic - See BETA-ADRENERGIC BLOCKING AGENTS & THIAZIDE DIURETICS 184
Tenormin - See BETA-ADRENERGIC BLOCKING AGENTS 182
TENOXICAM - See ANTI-INFLAMMATORY DRUGS, NONSTEROIDAL (NSAIDs) 116
Tenuate - See APPETITE SUPPRESSANTS 146
Tenuate Dospan - See APPETITE SUPPRESSANTS 146
Tepanil - See APPETITE SUPPRESSANTS 146
Tepanil Ten-Tab - See APPETITE SUPPRESSANTS 146
Terazol 3 - See ANTIFUNGALS (Vaginal) 90
Terazol 7 - See ANTIFUNGALS (Vaginal) 90
TERAZOSIN - See ALPHA ADRENERGIC RECEPTOR BLOCKERS 20
TERBINAFINE - See ANTIFUNGALS (Topical) 88
TERBINAFINE (Oral) 780
TERBUTALINE - See BRONCHODILATORS, ADRENERGIC 200
TERCONAZOLE - See ANTIFUNGALS (Vaginal) 90
Terfluzine - See PHENOTHIAZINES 656
Terfluzine Concentrate - See PHENOTHIAZINES 656
TERIPARATIDE - See BONE FORMATION AGENTS 194
Terphan - See DEXTROMETHORPHAN 312
Terramycin - See TETRACYCLINES 782
Tersac Cleansing Gel - See KERATOLYTICS 470
Tersa-Tar Mild Therapeutic Shampoo with Protein and Conditioner - See COAL TAR (Topical) 266
Tersa-Tar Soapless Tar Shampoo - See COAL TAR (Topical) 266
Tersa-Tar Therapeutic Shampoo - See COAL TAR (Topical) 266
Tersi Foam - See ANTISEBORRHEICS (Topical) 132
Testa-C - See ANDROGENS 34
Testamone 100 - See ANDROGENS 34
Testaqua - See ANDROGENS 34
Testex - See ANDROGENS 34
Testim - See ANDROGENS 34
Testoderm with Adhesive - See ANDROGENS 34

Testoject-50 - See ANDROGENS 34
Testoject-LA - See ANDROGENS 34
Testone L.A. - See ANDROGENS 34
TESTOSTERONE - See ANDROGENS 34
Testred - See ANDROGENS 34
Testred-Cypionate 200 - See ANDROGENS 34
Testrin P.A. - See ANDROGENS 34
TETRACAINE - See
ANESTHETICS (Mucosal-Local) 36
ANESTHETICS (Rectal) 38
ANESTHETICS (Topical) 40
TETRACAINE & MENTHOL - See
ANESTHETICS (Rectal) 38
ANESTHETICS (Topical) 40
TETRACYCLINE - See TETRACYCLINES 782
TETRACYCLINE (Topical) - See ANTIBACTERIALS FOR ACNE (Topical) 64
TETRACYCLINES 782
Tetracyn - See TETRACYCLINES 782
TETRAHYDROZOLINE - See DECONGESTANTS (Ophthalmic) 306
Teveten - See ANGIOTENSIN II RECEPTOR ANTAGONISTS 42
Teveten HCT - See
ANGIOTENSIN II RECEPTOR ANTAGONISTS 42
DIURETICS, THIAZIDE 338
Texacort - See ADRENOCORTICOIDS (Topical) 18
T-Gel - See COAL TAR (Topical) 266
T/Gel Therapeutic Conditioner - See COAL TAR (Topical) 266
T/Gel Therapeutic Shampoo - See COAL TAR (Topical) 266
T-gesic - See NARCOTIC ANALGESICS & ACETAMINOPHEN 586
Thalitone - See DIURETICS, THIAZIDE 338
THC - See DRONABINOL (THC, Marijuana) 350
Theo-24 - See BRONCHODILATORS, XANTHINE 204
Theobid Duracaps - See BRONCHODILATORS, XANTHINE 204
Theobid Jr. Duracaps - See BRONCHODILATORS, XANTHINE 204
Theochron - See BRONCHODILATORS, XANTHINE 204
Theoclear L.A. 130 Cenules - See BRONCHODILATORS, XANTHINE 204
Theoclear L.A. 260 Cenules - See BRONCHODILATORS, XANTHINE 204
Theoclear-80 - See BRONCHODILATORS, XANTHINE 204
Theocot - See BRONCHODILATORS, XANTHINE 204
Theo-Dur - See BRONCHODILATORS, XANTHINE 204
Theo-Dur Sprinkle - See BRONCHODILATORS, XANTHINE 204
Theolair - See BRONCHODILATORS, XANTHINE 204
Theolair-SR - See BRONCHODILATORS, XANTHINE 204
Theolate - See
BRONCHODILATORS, XANTHINE 204
GUAIFENESIN 416
Theomar - See BRONCHODILATORS, XANTHINE 204
Theon - See BRONCHODILATORS, XANTHINE 204
Theophylline SR - See BRONCHODILATORS, XANTHINE 204
THEOPHYLLINE - See BRONCHODILATORS, XANTHINE 204
Theo-Sav - See BRONCHODILATORS, XANTHINE 204
Theospan SR - See BRONCHODILATORS, XANTHINE 204
Theo-SR - See BRONCHODILATORS, XANTHINE 204
Theostat - See BRONCHODILATORS, XANTHINE 204
Theostat 80 - See BRONCHODILATORS, XANTHINE 204
Theo-Time - See BRONCHODILATORS, XANTHINE 204
Theovent Long-acting - See BRONCHODILATORS, XANTHINE 204
Theox - See BRONCHODILATORS, XANTHINE 204
Therac Lotion - See KERATOLYTICS 470
Theracof Plus Multi-Symptom Cough and Cold Reliever - See
ACETAMINOPHEN 8
DEXTROMETHORPHAN 312
GUAIFENESIN 416
PHENYLEPHRINE 658
Theraflu Cold & Cough Hot Liquid - See
ANTIHISTAMINES 106
DEXTROMETHORPHAN 312
PHENYLEPHRINE 658
Theraflu Cold & Sore Throat Hot Liquid - See
ACETAMINOPHEN 8
ANTIHISTAMINES 106
PHENYLEPHRINE 658
Theraflu Daytime Severe Cold Caplets - See
ACETAMINOPHEN 8
DEXTROMETHORPHAN 312
PHENYLEPHRINE 658

Theraflu Daytime Severe Cold Hot Liquid - See
ACETAMINOPHEN 8
PHENYLEPHRINE 658
Theraflu Flu & Chest Congestion Hot Liquid - See
ACETAMINOPHEN 8
GUAIFENESIN 416
Theraflu Flu & Sore Throat Hot Liquid - See
ACETAMINOPHEN 8
ANTIHISTAMINES 106
PHENYLEPHRINE 658
Theraflu Nighttime Severe Cold Caplets - See
ACETAMINOPHEN 8
ANTIHISTAMINES 106
DEXTROMETHORPHAN 312
PHENYLEPHRINE 658
Theraflu Nighttime Severe Cold Hot Liquid - See
ACETAMINOPHEN 8
ANTIHISTAMINES 106
PHENYLEPHRINE 658
Theraflu Thin Strips Daytime Cold & Cough - See
DEXTROMETHORPHAN 312
PHENYLEPHRINE 658
Theraflu Thin Strips Multi-Symptom - See ANTIHISTAMINES 106
Theraflu Thin Strips Nighttime Severe Cold & Cough - See
ANTIHISTAMINES 106
PHENYLEPHRINE 658
Theraflu Warming Relief Daytime - See
ACETAMINOPHEN 8
DEXTROMETHORPHAN 312
PHENYLEPHRINE 658
Theraflu Warming Relief Nighttime - See
ACETAMINOPHEN 8
ANTIHISTAMINES 106
PHENYLEPHRINE 658
Theralax - See LAXATIVES, STIMULANT 482
Theramycin Z - See ANTIBACTERIALS FOR ACNE (Topical) 64
Theraplex T Shampoo - See COAL TAR (Topical) 266
Theraplex Z - See ANTISEBORRHEICS (Topical) 132
Therapy Bayer - See ASPIRIN 152
Therevac Plus - See LAXATIVES, SOFTENER/ LUBRICANT 480
Therevac-SB - See LAXATIVES, SOFTENER/ LUBRICANT 480
Thermazene - See ANTIBACTERIALS, ANTIFUNGALS (Topical) 62
Theroxide 5 Lotion - See BENZOYL PEROXIDE 178
Theroxide 10 Lotion - See BENZOYL PEROXIDE 178
Theroxide 10 Wash - See BENZOYL PEROXIDE 178
THIABENDAZOLE - See ANTHELMINTICS 50
Thiamazole - See ANTITHYROID DRUGS 134
<u>THIAMINE (Vitamin B-1)</u> 784
<u>THIAZOLIDINEDIONES</u> 786
<u>THIOGUANINE</u> 788
Thiola - See TIOPRONIN 798
THIOPROPAZATE - See PHENOTHIAZINES 656
THIOPROPERAZINE - See PHENOTHIAZINES 656
THIORIDAZINE - See PHENOTHIAZINES 656
Thiosol - See TIOPRONIN 798
Thiosulfil Forte - See SULFONAMIDES 766
<u>THIOTHIXENE</u> 790
Thiothixene HCl Intensol - See THIOTHIXENE 790
Thorazine - See PHENOTHIAZINES 656
Thorazine Concentrate - See PHENOTHIAZINES 656
Thorazine Spansule - See PHENOTHIAZINES 656
Thor-Prom - See PHENOTHIAZINES 656
Three Day Cream - See ANTIFUNGALS (Vaginal) 90
Thrive Gum - See NICOTINE 598
Thrive Lozenge - See NICOTINE 598
Thylline - See BRONCHODILATORS, XANTHINE 204
Thyrar - See THYROID HORMONES 792
Thyro-Block - See POTASSIUM SUPPLEMENTS 666
THYROGLOBULIN - See THYROID HORMONES 792
THYROID - See THYROID HORMONES 792
Thyroid hormone - See THYROID HORMONES 792
<u>THYROID HORMONES</u> 792
Thyroid Strong - See THYROID HORMONES 792
Thyrolar - See THYROID HORMONES 792
<u>TIAGABINE</u> 794
TIAPROFENIC ACID - See ANTI-INFLAMMATORY DRUGS, NONSTEROIDAL (NSAIDs) 116
Tiazac - See CALCIUM CHANNEL BLOCKERS 220
<u>TICAGRELOR</u> 796
Ticlid - See PLATELET INHIBITORS 664
TICLOPIDINE - See PLATELET INHIBITORS 664
Tigan - See TRIMETHOBENZAMIDE 816

Tija - See TETRACYCLINES 782
Tikosyn - See DOFETILIDE 342
TILUDRONATE - See BISPHOSPHONATES 192
Timodal - See ANTIGLAUCOMA, BETA BLOCKERS 96
Timolide - See BETA-ADRENERGIC BLOCKING AGENTS & THIAZIDE DIURETICS 184
TIMOLOL - See BETA-ADRENERGIC BLOCKING AGENTS 182
TIMOLOL & HYDROCHLOROTHIAZIDE - See BETA-ADRENERGIC BLOCKING AGENTS & THIAZIDE DIURETICS 184
TIMOLOL (Ophthalmic) - See ANTIGLAUCOMA, BETA BLOCKERS 96
Timoptic - See ANTIGLAUCOMA, BETA BLOCKERS 96
Timoptic in Ocudose - See ANTIGLAUCOMA, BETA BLOCKERS 96
Timoptic-XE - See ANTIGLAUCOMA, BETA BLOCKERS 96
Tinactin Aerosol Liquid - See ANTIFUNGALS (Topical) 88
Tinactin Aerosol Powder - See ANTIFUNGALS (Topical) 88
Tinactin Antifungal Deodorant Powder Aerosol - See ANTIFUNGALS (Topical) 88
Tinactin Cream - See ANTIFUNGALS (Topical) 88
Tinactin Jock Itch Aerosol Powder - See ANTIFUNGALS (Topical) 88
Tinactin Jock Itch Cream - See ANTIFUNGALS (Topical) 88
Tinactin Jock Itch Spray Powder - See ANTIFUNGALS (Topical) 88
Tinactin Plus Powder - See ANTIFUNGALS (Topical) 88
Tinactin Powder - See ANTIFUNGALS (Topical) 88
Tinactin Solution - See ANTIFUNGALS (Topical) 88
Tindal - See PHENOTHIAZINES 656
Tindamax - See NITROIMIDAZOLES 606
Ting Antifungal Cream - See ANTIFUNGALS (Topical) 88
Ting Antifungal Powder - See ANTIFUNGALS (Topical) 88
Ting Antifungal Spray Liquid - See ANTIFUNGALS (Topical) 88
Ting Antifungal Spray Powder - See ANTIFUNGALS (Topical) 88
TINIDAZOLE - See NITROIMIDAZOLES 606
TIOCONAZOLE - See ANTIFUNGALS (Vaginal) 90
Tioglis - See TIOPRONIN 798
TIOPRONIN 798
TIOTROPIUM - See BRONCHODILATORS, ANTICHOLINERGIC 202
Tipramine - See ANTIDEPRESSANTS, TRICYCLIC 80
TIPRANAVIR - See PROTEASE INHIBITORS 688
Tirend - See CAFFEINE 216
TISIT - See PEDICULICIDES (Topical) 642
TISIT Blue - See PEDICULICIDES (Topical) 642
Titralac - See
ANTACIDS 48
CALCIUM SUPPLEMENTS 222
Titralac Plus - See ANTACIDS 48
TIZANIDINE 800
Tobradex - See
ANTIBACTERIALS (Ophthalmic) 66
ANTI-INFLAMMATORY DRUGS, STEROIDAL (Ophthalmic) 122
Tobradex ST - See
ANTIBACTERIALS (Ophthalmic) 66
ANTI-INFLAMMATORY DRUGS, NON-STEROIDAL (NSAIDs) (Ophthalmic) 122
TOBRAMYCIN (Ophthalmic) - See ANTIBACTERIALS (Ophthalmic) 66
Tobrex - See ANTIBACTERIALS (Ophthalmic) 66
TOFACITINIB 802
Tofranil - See ANTIDEPRESSANTS, TRICYCLIC 80
Tofranil-PM - See ANTIDEPRESSANTS, TRICYCLIC 80
Tolamide - See SULFONYLUREAS 770
TOLAZAMIDE - See SULFONYLUREAS 770
TOLBUTAMIDE - See SULFONYLUREAS 770
TOLCAPONE - See COMT INHIBITORS 274
Tolinase - See SULFONYLUREAS 770
TOLMETIN - See ANTI-INFLAMMATORY DRUGS, NONSTEROIDAL (NSAIDs) 116
TOLNAFTATE - See ANTIFUNGALS (Topical) 88
TOLTERODINE - See MUSCARINIC RECEPTOR ANTAGONISTS 574
Tolu-Sed Cough - See
GUAIFENESIN 416
NARCOTIC ANALGESICS 584
Tolu-Sed DM Cough - See
DEXTROMETHORPHAN 312
GUAIFENESIN 416
Topamax - See TOPIRAMATE 804
Topamax Sprinkle Capsules - See TOPIRAMATE 804
Topex 5 Lotion - See BENZOYL PEROXIDE 178

Topex 10 Lotion - See BENZOYL PEROXIDE 178
Topicaine - See ANESTHETICS (Mucosal-Local) 36
Topicort - See ADRENOCORTICOIDS (Topical) 18
Topicort LP - See ADRENOCORTICOIDS (Topical) 18
Topicort Mild - See ADRENOCORTICOIDS (Topical) 18
Topicycline - See ANTIBACTERIALS FOR ACNE (Topical) 64
Topilene - See ADRENOCORTICOIDS (Topical) 18
TOPIRAMATE 804
Topisone - See ADRENOCORTICOIDS (Topical) 18
Topisporin - See ANTIBACTERIALS (Topical) 70
Toprol - See BETA-ADRENERGIC BLOCKING AGENTS 182
Toprol XL - See BETA-ADRENERGIC BLOCKING AGENTS 182
Topsyn - See ADRENOCORTICOIDS (Topical) 18
Toradol - See ANTI-INFLAMMATORY DRUGS, NONSTEROIDAL (NSAIDs) 116
TOREMIFENE 806
Tornalate - See BRONCHODILATORS, ADRENERGIC 200
TORSEMIDE - See DIURETICS, LOOP 332
Totacillin - See PENICILLINS 646
Touro A&H - See
ANTIHISTAMINES 106
PSEUDOEPHEDRINE 694
Touro DM - See
DEXTROMETHORPHAN 312
GUAIFENESIN 416
Touro Ex - See GUAIFENESIN 416
Touro LA Caplets - See
GUAIFENESIN 416
PSEUDOEPHEDRINE 694
Toviaz - See MUSCARINIC RECEPTOR ANTAGONISTS 574
T-Phyl - See BRONCHODILATORS, XANTHINE 204
T-Quil - See BENZODIAZEPINES 176
Trac Tabs 2X - See ATROPINE, HYOSCYAMINE, METHENAMINE, METHYLENE BLUE, PHENYLSALICYLATE & BENZOIC ACID 158
Tracleer - See ENDOTHELIN RECEPTOR ANTAGONISTS 354
Tradjenta - See DPP-4 INHIBITORS 348
TRAMADOL 808
Trancot - See MEPROBAMATE 538
Trandate - See BETA-ADRENERGIC BLOCKING AGENTS 182
Trandate HCT - See BETA-ADRENERGIC BLOCKING AGENTS & THIAZIDE DIURETICS 184
TRANDOLAPRIL - See ANGIOTENSIN-CONVERTING ENZYME (ACE) INHIBITORS 44
TRANEXAMIC ACID - See ANTIFIBRINOLYTIC AGENTS 84
Tranmep - See MEPROBAMATE 538
Tranquilizer - See
HYDROXYZINE 436
LOXAPINE 512
MEPROBAMATE 538
Tranquilizer (Benzodiazepine) - See BENZODIAZEPINES 176
Tranquilizer (Phenothiazine), antihistamine - See ANTIHISTAMINES, PHENOTHIAZINE-DERIVATIVE 112
Tranquilizer (Rauwolfia Alkaloid) - See RAUWOLFIA ALKALOIDS 714
Transderm-Nitro - See NITRATES 602
Transderm-Scop - See SCOPOLAMINE (Hyoscine) 738
Transderm-V - See SCOPOLAMINE (Hyoscine) 738
Trans-Plantar - See KERATOLYTICS 470
Trans-Ver-Sal - See KERATOLYTICS 470
Trantoin - See NITROFURANTOIN 604
Tranxene - See BENZODIAZEPINES 176
Tranxene T-Tab - See BENZODIAZEPINES 176
Tranxene-SD - See BENZODIAZEPINES 176
TRANYLCYPROMINE - See MONOAMINE OXIDASE (MAO) INHIBITORS 570
Trasicor - See BETA-ADRENERGIC BLOCKING AGENTS 182
Travamine - See ANTIHISTAMINES 106
Travatan - See ANTIGLAUCOMA, PROSTAGLANDINS 102
Travatan Z- See ANTIGLAUCOMA, PROSTAGLANDINS 102
TRAVOPROST - See ANTIGLAUCOMA, PROSTAGLANDINS 102
TRAZODONE 810
Trazon - See TRAZODONE 810
Trecator-SC - See ETHIONAMIDE 376
Trendar - See ANTI-INFLAMMATORY DRUGS, NONSTEROIDAL (NSAIDs) 116
Trental - See PENTOXIFYLLINE 652
TRETINOIN - See RETINOIDS (Topical) 722
Tretin-X - See RETINOIDS (Topical) 722
Trexall - See METHOTREXATE 548

Treximet - See
ANTI-INFLAMMATORY DRUGS, NONSTEROIDAL (NSAIDs) 116
TRIPTANS 820
Triacet - See ADRENOCORTICOIDS (Topical) 18
Triacin C Cough - See
ANTIHISTAMINES 106
NARCOTIC ANALGESICS 584
PSEUDOEPHEDRINE 694
Triad - See
ACETAMINOPHEN 8
BARBITURATES 168
Triadapin - See ANTIDEPRESSANTS, TRICYCLIC 80
Triaderm - See ADRENOCORTICOIDS (Topical) 18
Triafed - See
ANTIHISTAMINES 106
PSEUDOEPHEDRINE 694
Triafed with Codeine - See
ANTIHISTAMINES 106
NARCOTIC ANALGESICS 584
PSEUDOEPHEDRINE 694
Trialodine - See TRAZODONE 810
TRIAMCINOLONE - See ADRENOCORTICOIDS (Systemic) 16
TRIAMCINOLONE (Dental) - See ADRENOCORTICOIDS (Topical) 18
TRIAMCINOLONE (Nasal) - See ADRENOCORTICOIDS (Nasal Inhalation) 12
TRIAMCINOLONE (Oral Inhalation) - See ADRENOCORTICOIDS (Oral Inhalation) 14
TRIAMCINOLONE (Topical) - See ADRENOCORTICOIDS (Topical) 18
Triaminic Chest & Nasal Congestion - See
GUAIFENESIN 416
PHENYLEPHRINE 658
Triaminic Cold & Allergy - See
ANTIHISTAMINES 106
PHENYLEPHRINE 658
Triaminic Cough & Sore Throat - See
ACETAMINOPHEN 8
DEXTROMETHORPHAN 312
Triaminic-D Multi-Symptom Cold - See
ANTIHISTAMINES 106
DEXTROMETHORPHAN 312
PSEUDOEPHEDRINE 694
Triaminic Day Time Cold & Cough - See
DEXTROMETHORPHAN 312
PHENYLEPHRINE 658
Triaminic Decongestant Spray Nasal & Sinus Congestion - See XYLOMETAZOLINE 850
Triaminic Flu, Cough & Fever - See
ACETAMINOPHEN 8
ANTIHISTAMINES 106
DEXTROMETHORPHAN 312
Triaminic Long Acting Cough - See
DEXTROMETHORPHAN 312
Triaminic Night Time Cough & Cold - See
ANTIHISTAMINES 106
PHENYLEPHRINE 658
Triaminic Softchews Cough & Runny Nose - See
ANTIHISTAMINES 106
DEXTROMETHORPHAN 312
Triaminic Softchews Cough & Sore Throat - See
ACETAMINOPHEN 8
DEXTROMETHORPHAN 312
Triaminic Thin Strips Cold - See
PHENYLEPHRINE 658
Triaminic Thin Strips Daytime Cold & Cough - See
DEXTROMETHORPHAN 312
PHENYLEPHRINE 658
Triaminic Thin Strips Cough & Runny Nose - See ANTIHISTAMINES 106
Triaminic Thin Strips Long Acting Cough - See DEXTROMETHORPHAN 312
Triaminic Thin Strips Night Time Cold & Cough - See
ANTIHISTAMINES 106
PHENYLEPHRINE 658
TRIAMTERENE - See DIURETICS, POTASSIUM-SPARING 334
TRIAMTERENE & HYDROCHLOROTHIAZIDE - See DIURETICS, POTASSIUM-SPARING & HYDROCHLOROTHIAZIDE 336
Trianex - See ADRENOCORTICOIDS (Topical) 18
Trianide Mild - See ADRENOCORTICOIDS (Topical) 18
Trianide Regular - See ADRENOCORTICOIDS (Topical) 18
Triaphen - See ASPIRIN 152
Triaprin - See
ACETAMINOPHEN 8
BARBITURATES 168
Triasox - See ANTHELMINTICS 50
Triavil - See
ANTIDEPRESSANTS, TRICYCLIC 80
PHENOTHIAZINES 656
TRIAZOLAM 812
Triazole - See
SULFONAMIDES 766
TRIMETHOPRIM 818
Triazole DS - See
SULFONAMIDES 766
TRIMETHOPRIM 818
Tri-B3 - See NIACIN (Vitamin B-3, Nicotinic Acid, Nicotinamide) 596

TRIBASIC CALCIUM PHOSPHATE - See
CALCIUM SUPPLEMENTS 222
Tribavirin - See RIBAVIRIN 724
Tribenzor - See
ANGIOTENSIN II RECEPTOR
ANTAGONISTS 42
CALCIUM CHANNEL BLOCKERS 220
DIURETICS, THIAZIDE 338
Tribiotic - See ANTIBACTERIALS (Ophthalmic)
66
Trichlorex - See DIURETICS, THIAZIDE 338
TRICHLORMETHIAZIDE - See DIURETICS,
THIAZIDE 338
TRICITRATES - See CITRATES 254
Tricodene #1 - See NARCOTIC ANALGESICS
584
Tricodene Sugar Free - See
ANTIHISTAMINES 106
DEXTROMETHORPHAN 312
Tricom Caplets - See PSEUDOEPHEDRINE
694
Tricom Tablets - See
ACETAMINOPHEN 8
ANTIHISTAMINES 106
Triconsil - See ANTACIDS 48
Tricor - See FIBRATES 386
Tricosal - See SALICYLATES 736
Tri-Cyclen - See CONTRACEPTIVES, ORAL &
SKIN 278
Triderm - See ADRENOCORTICOIDS (Topical)
18
Tridesilon - See ADRENOCORTICOIDS
(Topical) 18
TRIDIHEXETHYL - See ANTICHOLINERGICS
72
Tridil - See NITRATES 602
Trifed - See
ANTIHISTAMINES 106
PSEUDOEPHEDRINE 694
Trifed-C Cough - See
ANTIHISTAMINES 106
NARCOTIC ANALGESICS 584
PSEUDOEPHEDRINE 694
TRIFLUOPERAZINE - See PHENOTHIAZINES
656
Trifluorothymidine - See ANTIVIRALS
(Ophthalmic) 142
TRIFLUPROMAZINE - See PHENOTHIAZINES
656
TRIFLURIDINE - See ANTIVIRALS (Ophthalmic)
142
Trigesic - See
ACETAMINOPHEN 8
ASPIRIN 152
CAFFEINE 216
Triglide - See FIBRATES 386
Trihexane - See ANTIDYSKINETICS 82
Trihexy - See ANTIDYSKINETICS 82
TRIHEXYPHENIDYL - See ANTIDYSKINETICS
82
Tri-Hydroserpine - See RESERPINE,
HYDRALAZINE &
HYDROCHLOROTHIAZIDE 718
Tri-K - See POTASSIUM SUPPLEMENTS 666
Trikacide - See NITROIMIDAZOLES 606
Trilafon - See PHENOTHIAZINES 656
Trilafon Concentrate - See PHENOTHIAZINES
656
Trilax - See
LAXATIVES, SOFTENER/LUBRICANT 480
LAXATIVES, STIMULANT 482
Trileptal - See OXCARBAZEPINE 628
Tri-Levlen - See CONTRACEPTIVES, ORAL &
SKIN 278
TriLipix - See FIBRATES 386
Trilisate - See SALICYLATES 736
Trilombrin - See ANTHELMINTICS 50
TRILOSTANE 814
Tri-Luma - See
ADRENOCORTICOIDS (Topical) 18
RETINOIDS (Topical) 722
Trimedine Liquid - See
ANTIHISTAMINES 106
DEXTROMETHORPHAN 312
PHENYLEPHRINE 658
TRIMEPRAZINE - See ANTIHISTAMINES,
PHENOTHIAZINE-DERIVATIVE 112
TRIMETHOBENZAMIDE 816
TRIMETHOPRIM 818
Trimeth-Sulfa - See
SULFONAMIDES 766
TRIMETHOPRIM 818
TRIMIPRAMINE - See ANTIDEPRESSANTS,
TRICYCLIC 80
Trimox - See PENICILLINS 646
Trimpex - See TRIMETHOPRIM 818
Trinalin Repetabs - See
ANTIHISTAMINES 106
PSEUDOEPHEDRINE 694
Tri-Nasal - See ADRENOCORTICOIDS (Nasal
Inhalation) 12
Tri-Norinyl - See CONTRACEPTIVES, ORAL &
SKIN 278
Tri-Ophthalmic - See ANTIBACTERIALS
(Ophthalmic) 66
Triotann - See
ANTIHISTAMINES 106
PHENYLEPHRINE 658

Triotann Pediatric - See
ANTIHISTAMINES 106
PHENYLEPHRINE 658
TRIOXSALEN - See PSORALENS 696
TRIPELENNAMINE - See ANTIHISTAMINES 106
Triphasil - See CONTRACEPTIVES, ORAL & SKIN 278
Triple Antibiotic - See ANTIBACTERIALS (Topical) 70
Triple X - See PEDICULICIDES (Topical) 642
Tri-Previfem - See CONTRACEPTIVES, ORAL & SKIN 278
TRIPROLIDINE - See ANTIHISTAMINES 106
TRIPTANS 820
Triptil - See ANTIDEPRESSANTS, TRICYCLIC 80
Trip-Tone - See ANTIHISTAMINES 106
Triquilar - See CONTRACEPTIVES, ORAL & SKIN 278
Trisoralen - See PSORALENS 696
Tri-Sprintec - See CONTRACEPTIVES, ORAL & SKIN 278
Tristatin II - See NYSTATIN 614
Trisulfam - See
SULFONAMIDES 766
TRIMETHOPRIM 818
Tritann Pediatric - See
ANTIHISTAMINES 106
PHENYLEPHRINE 658
Tri-Tannate - See
ANTIHISTAMINES 106
PHENYLEPHRINE 658
Tri-Tannate Plus Pediatric - See
ANTIHISTAMINES 106
PHENYLEPHRINE 658
Tri-Vi-Flor - See VITAMINS & FLUORIDE 848
Trivora - See CONTRACEPTIVES, ORAL & SKIN 278
Trizivir - See NUCLEOSIDE REVERSE TRANSCRIPTASE INHIBITORS 610
Trocal - See DEXTROMETHORPHAN 312
Trokendi XR - See TOPIRAMATE 804
Tronolane - See ANESTHETICS (Rectal) 38
Tronothane - See
ANESTHETICS (Rectal) 38
ANESTHETICS (Topical) 40
TROSPIUM - See MUSCARINIC RECEPTOR ANTAGONISTS 574
TROVAFLOXACIN - See FLUOROQUINOLONES 392
Trovan - See FLUOROQUINOLONES 392
Truphylline - See BRONCHODILATORS, XANTHINE 204
Trusopt - See ANTIGLAUCOMA, CARBONIC ANHYDRASE INHIBITORS 98
Truvada - See
NUCLEOSIDE REVERSE TRANSCRIPTASE INHIBITORS 610
NUCLEOTIDE REVERSE TRANSCRIPTASE INHIBITORS 612
Truxophyllin - See BRONCHODILATORS, XANTHINE 204
Trymegen - See ANTIHISTAMINES 106
Trymex - See ADRENOCORTICOIDS (Topical) 18
T-Stat - See ANTIBACTERIALS FOR ACNE (Topical) 64
Tubizid - See ISONIAZID 460
Tudorza Pressair - See BRONCHODILATORS, ANTICHOLINERGIC 202
Tuinal - See BARBITURATES 168
TUMOR NECROSIS FACTOR BLOCKERS 822
Tums - See
ANTACIDS 48
CALCIUM SUPPLEMENTS 222
Tums Dual Action - See
ANTACIDS 48
HISTAMINE H2 RECEPTOR ANTAGONISTS 422
Tums E-X - See
ANTACIDS 48
CALCIUM SUPPLEMENTS 222
Tums Extra Strength - See ANTACIDS 48
Tums Freshers - See ANTACIDS 48
Tums Kids - See ANTACIDS 48
Tums Lasting Effects - See ANTACIDS 48
Tums Liquid Extra Strength - See ANTACIDS 48
Tums Liquid Extra Strength with Simethicone - See ANTACIDS 48
Tums QuikPak - See ANTACIDS 48
Tums Smooth Dissolve - See ANTACIDS 48
Tussafed HCG Syrup - See
GUAIFENESIN 416
NARCOTIC ANALGESICS 584
PHENYLEPHRINE 658
Tussafin Expectorant - See
GUAIFENESIN 416
NARCOTIC ANALGESICS 584
PSEUDOEPHEDRINE 694
Tussar DM - See
ANTIHISTAMINES 106
DEXTROMETHORPHAN 312
PSEUDOEPHEDRINE 694
Tussar SF - See
GUAIFENESIN 416
NARCOTIC ANALGESICS 584

Tussar-2 - See
GUAIFENESIN 416
NARCOTIC ANALGESICS 584
PSEUDOEPHEDRINE 694
Tuss-DM - See
DEXTROMETHORPHAN 312
GUAIFENESIN 416
Tussend - See PSEUDOEPHEDRINE 694
Tussend Expectorant - See
PSEUDOEPHEDRINE 694
Tussend Liquid - See PSEUDOEPHEDRINE 694
Tussi-Bid - See
DEXTROMETHORPHAN 312
GUAIFENESIN 416
TussiCaps - See
ANTIHISTAMINES 106
NARCOTIC ANALGESICS 584
Tussigon - See
ANTICHOLINERGICS 72
NARCOTIC ANALGESICS 584
Tussionex - See
ANTIHISTAMINES 106
NARCOTIC ANALGESICS 584
Tussi-organidin - See GUAIFENESIN 416
Tussirex with Codeine Liquid - See
ANTIHISTAMINES 106
CITRATES 254
NARCOTIC ANALGESICS 584
PHENYLEPHRINE 658
SALICYLATES 736
Tussi-12 - See
ANTIHISTAMINES 106
PHENYLEPHRINE 658
Tusstat - See ANTIHISTAMINES 106
TV-Gan-25 - See ANTIHISTAMINES, PHENOTHIAZINE-DERIVATIVE 112
Twice-a-Day Nasal Spray - See
OXYMETAZOLINE (Nasal) 630
Twilite - See ANTIHISTAMINES 106
Twin-K - See POTASSIUM SUPPLEMENTS 666
Two-Dyne - See
ACETAMINOPHEN 8
BARBITURATES 168
CAFFEINE 216
Twynsta - See
ANGIOTENSIN II RECEPTOR ANTAGONISTS 42
CALCIUM CHANNEL BLOCKERS 220
Tylaprin with Codeine - See NARCOTIC ANALGESICS & ACETAMINOPHEN 586
Tylenol - See ACETAMINOPHEN 8
Tylenol 8 Hour - See ACETAMINOPHEN 8
Tylenol Allergy Multi-Symptom - See
ACETAMINOPHEN 8
ANTIHISTAMINES 106
PHENYLEPHRINE 658
Tylenol Allergy Multi-Symptom Nighttime - See
ACETAMINOPHEN 8
ANTIHISTAMINES 106
PHENYLEPHRINE 658
Tylenol Arthritis Pain - See
ACETAMINOPHEN 8
Tylenol Chest Congestion - See
ACETAMINOPHEN 8
GUAIFENESIN 416
Tylenol Cold Head Congestion Daytime - See
ACETAMINOPHEN 8
DEXTROMETHORPHAN 312
PHENYLEPHRINE 658
Tylenol Cold Head Congestion Nighttime - See
ACETAMINOPHEN 8
ANTIHISTAMINES 106
DEXTROMETHORPHAN 312
PHENYLEPHRINE 658
Tylenol Cold Head Congestion Severe - See
ACETAMINOPHEN 8
DEXTROMETHORPHAN 312
GUAIFENESIN 416
PHENYLEPHRINE 658
Tylenol Cold Multi Symptom Daytime - See
ACETAMINOPHEN 8
DEXTROMETHORPHAN 312
PHENYLEPHRINE 658
Tylenol Cold Multi Symptom Nighttime - See
ACETAMINOPHEN 8
ANTIHISTAMINES 106
DEXTROMETHORPHAN 312
PHENYLEPHRINE 658
Tylenol Cold Multi Symptom Severe - See
ACETAMINOPHEN 8
DEXTROMETHORPHAN 312
GUAIFENESIN 416
PHENYLEPHRINE 658
Tylenol Cold Severe Congestion Daytime - See
ACETAMINOPHEN 8
DEXTROMETHORPHAN 312
GUAIFENESIN 416
PSEUDOEPHEDRINE 694
Tylenol Concentrated Infants' Drops - See
ACETAMINOPHEN 8
Tylenol Cough & Severe Congestion Daytime - See
ACETAMINOPHEN 8
DEXTROMETHORPHAN 312
GUAIFENESIN 416
PHENYLEPHRINE 658

Tylenol Cough & Sore Throat Daytime - See
ACETAMINOPHEN 8
DEXTROMETHORPHAN 312
Tylenol Cough & Sore Throat Nighttime - See
ACETAMINOPHEN 8
ANTIHISTAMINES 106
DEXTROMETHORPHAN 312
Tylenol Extra Strength - See
ACETAMINOPHEN 8
Tylenol Extra Strength Rapid Release Gels - See ACETAMINOPHEN 8
Tylenol Junior Strength - See
ACETAMINOPHEN 8
Tylenol No.1 - See NARCOTIC ANALGESICS & ACETAMINOPHEN 586
Tylenol No.1 Forte - See NARCOTIC ANALGESICS & ACETAMINOPHEN 586
Tylenol PM - See
ACETAMINOPHEN 8
ANTIHISTAMINES 106
Tylenol Regular Strength - See
ACETAMINOPHEN 8
Tylenol Severe Allergy - See
ACETAMINOPHEN 8
ANTIHISTAMINES 106
Tylenol Sinus Congestion & Pain Daytime - See
ACETAMINOPHEN 8
PHENYLEPHRINE 658
Tylenol Sinus Congestion & Pain Nighttime - See
ACETAMINOPHEN 8
ANTIHISTAMINES 106
PHENYLEPHRINE 658
Tylenol Sinus Congestion & Pain Severe - See
ACETAMINOPHEN 8
GUAIFENESIN 416
PHENYLEPHRINE 658
Tylenol Sore Throat Daytime - See
ACETAMINOPHEN 8
Tylenol Sore Throat Nighttime - See
ACETAMINOPHEN 8
ANTIHISTAMINES 106
Tylenol with Codeine - See NARCOTIC ANALGESICS & ACETAMINOPHEN 586
Tylox - See NARCOTIC ANALGESICS & ACETAMINOPHEN 586
Ty-Pap - See ACETAMINOPHEN 8
Tyrodone - See
NARCOTIC ANALGESICS 584
PSEUDOEPHEDRINE 694

U

UAA - See ATROPINE, HYOSCYAMINE, METHENAMINE, METHYLENE BLUE, PHENYLSALICYLATE & BENZOIC ACID 158
Uceris - See ADRENOCORTICOIDS (Systemic) 16
Ugesic - See NARCOTIC ANALGESICS & ACETAMINOPHEN 586
Ulcidine - See HISTAMINE H_2 RECEPTOR ANTAGONISTS 422
Ulesfia - See PEDICULICIDES (Topical) 642
ULIPRISTAL - See SELECTIVE PROGESTERONE RECEPTOR MODULATORS 740
Uloric - See ANTIGOUT DRUGS 104
Ultra Pred - See ANTI-INFLAMMATORY DRUGS, STEROIDAL (Ophthalmic) 122
Ultra Tears - See PROTECTANT (Ophthalmic) 690
Ultracef - See CEPHALOSPORINS 236
Ultracet - See
ACETAMINOPHEN 8
TRAMADOL 808
Ultragesic - See NARCOTIC ANALGESICS & ACETAMINOPHEN 586
Ultralente - See INSULIN 446
Ultralente Iletin I - See INSULIN 446
Ultram - See TRAMADOL 808
Ultram ER - See TRAMADOL 808
Ultram ODT - See TRAMADOL 808
UltraMOP - See PSORALENS 696
Ultresa - See PANCRELIPASE 634
Ultravate - See ADRENOCORTICOIDS (Topical) 18
Ultrazine-10 - See PHENOTHIAZINES 656
UNDECYLENIC ACID - See ANTIFUNGALS (Topical) 88
Unguentine - See ANESTHETICS (Topical) 40
Unguentine Plus - See ANESTHETICS (Topical) 40
Unguentine Spray - See ANESTHETICS (Topical) 40
Uni-Bent Cough - See ANTIHISTAMINES 106
Unicort - See ADRENOCORTICOIDS (Topical) 18
Unilax - See
LAXATIVES, SOFTENER/LUBRICANT 480
LAXATIVES, STIMULANT 482
Unipen - See PENICILLINS 646
Uniphyl - See BRONCHODILATORS, XANTHINE 204
Unipres - See RESERPINE, HYDRALAZINE & HYDROCHLOROTHIAZIDE 718

INDEX

Uniretic - See
ANGIOTENSIN-CONVERTING ENZYME (ACE) INHIBITORS 44
DIURETICS, THIAZIDE 338
Unisom Nighttime Sleep Aid - See ANTIHISTAMINES 106
Unisom SleepGels Maximum Strength - See ANTIHISTAMINES 106
Uni-Tussin - See GUAIFENESIN 416
Uni-Tussin DM - See
DEXTROMETHORPHAN 312
GUAIFENESIN 416
Univasc - See ANGIOTENSIN-CONVERTING ENZYME (ACE) INHIBITORS 44
Univol - See ANTACIDS 48
Unproco - See
DEXTROMETHORPHAN 312
GUAIFENESIN 416
Urabeth - See BETHANECHOL 186
Urecholine - See BETHANECHOL 186
Urex - See METHENAMINE 546
Uribel - See ATROPINE, HYOSCYAMINE, METHENAMINE, METHYLENE BLUE, PHENYLSALICYLATE & BENZOIC ACID 158
Uridon - See DIURETICS, THIAZIDE 338
Uridon Modified - See ATROPINE, HYOSCYAMINE, METHENAMINE, METHYLENE BLUE, PHENYLSALICYLATE & BENZOIC ACID 158
Urimed - See ATROPINE, HYOSCYAMINE, METHENAMINE, METHYLENE BLUE, PHENYLSALICYLATE & BENZOIC ACID 158
Urinary alkalizer - See CITRATES 254
Urinary Antiseptic No. 2 - See ATROPINE, HYOSCYAMINE, METHENAMINE, METHYLENE BLUE, PHENYLSALICYLATE & BENZOIC ACID 158
Urised - See ATROPINE, HYOSCYAMINE, METHENAMINE, METHYLENE BLUE, PHENYLSALICYLATE & BENZOIC ACID 158
Uriseptic - See ATROPINE, HYOSCYAMINE, METHENAMINE, METHYLENE BLUE, PHENYLSALICYLATE & BENZOIC ACID 158
Urispas - See FLAVOXATE 388
Uritab - See ATROPINE, HYOSCYAMINE, METHENAMINE, METHYLENE BLUE, PHENYLSALICYLATE & BENZOIC ACID 158
Uritin - See ATROPINE, HYOSCYAMINE, METHENAMINE, METHYLENE BLUE, PHENYLSALICYLATE & BENZOIC ACID 158
Uritol - See DIURETICS, LOOP 332
Urobak - See SULFONAMIDES 766
Urocit-K - See CITRATES 254
Urodine - See PHENAZOPYRIDINE 654
Urogesic - See PHENAZOPYRIDINE 654
Urogesic-Blue - See ATROPINE, HYOSCYAMINE, METHENAMINE, METHYLENE BLUE, PHENYLSALICYLATE & BENZOIC ACID 158
Uro-KP-Neutral - See POTASSIUM SUPPLEMENTS 666
Uro-Mag - See ANTACIDS 48
Uroplus DS - See
SULFONAMIDES 766
TRIMETHOPRIM 818
Uroplus SS - See
SULFONAMIDES 766
TRIMETHOPRIM 818
Urotoin - See NITROFURANTOIN 604
Uro-Ves - See ATROPINE, HYOSCYAMINE, METHENAMINE, METHYLENE BLUE, PHENYLSALICYLATE & BENZOIC ACID 158
UroXatral - See ALPHA ADRENERGIC RECEPTOR BLOCKERS 20
Urozide - See DIURETICS, THIAZIDE 338
Urso - See URSODIOL 824
URSODIOL 824
Ursofalk - See URSODIOL 824
USTEKINUMAB - See BIOLOGICS FOR PSORIASIS 188
Uticort - See ADRENOCORTICOIDS (Topical) 18

V

Vagifem - See ESTROGENS 372
Vagistat - See ANTIFUNGALS (Vaginal) 90
Vagistat-1 - See ANTIFUNGALS (Vaginal) 90
VALACYCLOVIR - See ANTIVIRALS FOR HERPES VIRUS 136
Valadol - See ACETAMINOPHEN 8
Valadol Liquid - See ACETAMINOPHEN 8
VALDECOXIB - See ANTI-INFLAMMATORY DRUGS, NONSTEROIDAL (NSAIDs) COX-2 INHIBITORS 118
Valergen-10 - See ESTROGENS 372
Valergen-20 - See ESTROGENS 372
Valergen-40 - See ESTROGENS 372
Valisone - See ADRENOCORTICOIDS (Topical) 18
Valisone Reduced Strength - See ADRENOCORTICOIDS (Topical) 18
Valisone Scalp Lotion - See ADRENOCORTICOIDS (Topical) 18
Valium - See BENZODIAZEPINES 176

Valnac - See ADRENOCORTICOIDS (Topical) 18
Valorin - See ACETAMINOPHEN 8
Valorin Extra - See ACETAMINOPHEN 8
Valpin 50 - See ANTICHOLINERGICS 72
VALPROIC ACID 826
Valrelease - See BENZODIAZEPINES 176
VALSARTAN - See ANGIOTENSIN II RECEPTOR ANTAGONISTS 42
Valtrex - See ANTIVIRALS FOR HERPES VIRUS 136
Valturna - See
ANGIOTENSIN II RECEPTOR ANTAGONISTS 42
RENIN INHIBITORS 716
Vanacet - See NARCOTIC ANALGESICS & ACETAMINOPHEN 586
Vancenase - See ADRENOCORTICOIDS (Nasal Inhalation) 12
Vancenase AQ - See ADRENOCORTICOIDS (Nasal Inhalation) 12
Vanceril - See ADRENOCORTICOIDS (Oral Inhalation) 14
Vancocin - See VANCOMYCIN 828
VANCOMYCIN 828
Vandazole - See NITROIMIDAZOLES 606
Vanex Forte R - See ANTIHISTAMINES 106
Vanex-HD - See
ANTIHISTAMINES 106
NARCOTIC ANALGESICS 584
PHENYLEPHRINE 658
Vaniqa - See EFLORNITHINE (Topical) 352
Vanos - See ADRENOCORTICOIDS (Topical) 18
Vanoxide 5 Lotion - See BENZOYL PEROXIDE 178
Vanquin - See ANTHELMINTICS 50
Vanquis - See
ACETAMINOPHEN 8
ASPIRIN 152
Vanquish - See CAFFEINE 216
Vanseb Cream Dandruff Shampoo - See
ANTISEBORRHEICS (Topical) 132
KERATOLYTICS 470
Vanseb Lotion Dandruff Shampoo - See
ANTISEBORRHEICS (Topical) 132
KERATOLYTICS 470
Vanseb-T - See ANTISEBORRHEICS (Topical) 132
Vantin - See CEPHALOSPORINS 236
Vapocet - See NARCOTIC ANALGESICS & ACETAMINOPHEN 586
Vapo-Iso - See BRONCHODILATORS, ADRENERGIC 200
VARDENAFIL - See ERECTILE DYSFUNCTION AGENTS 360
VARENICLINE 830
Vascepa - See OMEGA-3 ACID ETHYL ESTERS 620
Vascor - See CALCIUM CHANNEL BLOCKERS 220
Vaseretic - See ANGIOTENSIN-CONVERTING ENZYME (ACE) INHIBITORS & HYDROCHLOROTHIAZIDE 46
Vasoclear - See DECONGESTANTS (Ophthalmic) 306
Vasoclear A - See DECONGESTANTS (Ophthalmic) 306
Vasocon - See DECONGESTANTS (Ophthalmic) 306
Vasocon Regular - See DECONGESTANTS (Ophthalmic) 306
Vasocon-A - See DECONGESTANTS (Ophthalmic) 306
Vasoconstrictor - See
CAFFEINE 216
ORPHENADRINE, ASPIRIN & CAFFEINE 626
Vasodilan - See ISOXSUPRINE 464
Vasodilator - See
CYCLANDELATE 284
INTERMITTENT CLAUDICATION AGENTS 452
ISOXSUPRINE 464
NIACIN (Vitamin B-3, Nicotinic Acid, Nicotinamide) 596
PAPAVERINE 638
Vasoprine - See ISOXSUPRINE 464
Vasotec - See ANGIOTENSIN-CONVERTING ENZYME (ACE) INHIBITORS 44
VCF - See CONTRACEPTIVES, VAGINAL 280
V-Cillin K - See PENICILLINS 646
Vectical - See VITAMIN D (Topical) 842
Veetids - See PENICILLINS 646
Veganin - See NARCOTIC ANALGESICS & ACETAMINOPHEN 586
Velosef - See CEPHALOSPORINS 236
Velosulin - See INSULIN 446
Velosulin Human - See INSULIN 446
Veltane - See ANTIHISTAMINES 106
Veltin Gel - See
ANTIBACTERIALS FOR ACNE (Topical) 64
RETINOIDS (Topical) 722
Vendone - See NARCOTIC ANALGESICS & ACETAMINOPHEN 586
VENLAFAXINE - See SEROTONIN & NOREPINEPHRINE REUPTAKE INHIBITORS (SNRIs) 746

INDEX

Ventolin - See BRONCHODILATORS, ADRENERGIC 200
Ventolin HFA - See BRONCHODILATORS, ADRENERGIC 200
Ventolin Rotocaps - See BRONCHODILATORS, ADRENERGIC 200
VePesid - See ETOPOSIDE 378
Veracolate - See LAXATIVES, STIMULANT 482
Veramyst - See ADRENOCORTICOIDS (Nasal Inhalation) 12
VERAPAMIL - See CALCIUM CHANNEL BLOCKERS 220
Verazinc - See ZINC SUPPLEMENTS 854
Verdeso Foam - See ADRENOCORTICOIDS (Topical) 18
Verelan - See CALCIUM CHANNEL BLOCKERS 220
Verelan PM - See CALCIUM CHANNEL BLOCKERS 220
Versabran - See LAXATIVES, BULK-FORMING 476
Versacaps - See
GUAIFENESIN 416
PSEUDOEPHEDRINE 694
Versacloz - See CLOZAPINE 264
Vertab - See ANTIHISTAMINES 106
Verukan Topical Solution - See KERATOLYTICS 470
Verukan-HP Topical Solution - See KERATOLYTICS 470
Vesicare - See MUSCARINIC RECEPTOR ANTAGONISTS 574
Vesprin - See PHENOTHIAZINES 656
Vexol - See ANTI-INFLAMMATORY DRUGS, STEROIDAL (Ophthalmic) 122
Vfend - See ANTIFUNGALS, AZOLES 86
V-Gan-50 - See ANTIHISTAMINES, PHENOTHIAZINE-DERIVATIVE 112
Viagra - See ERECTILE DYSFUNCTION AGENTS 360
Vibramycin - See TETRACYCLINES 782
Vibutal - See
ASPIRIN 152
BARBITURATES 168
Vicks Children's NyQuil - See
ANTIHISTAMINES 106
DEXTROMETHORPHAN 312
Vicks DayQuil Cold & Flu Symptom Relief Plus Vitamin C - See
ACETAMINOPHEN 8
DEXTROMETHORPHAN 312
PHENYLEPHRINE 658
Vicks DayQuil Cold/Flu Relief - See
ACETAMINOPHEN 8
DEXTROMETHORPHAN 312
PHENYLEPHRINE 658
Vicks DayQuil Cough - See DEXTROMETHORPHAN 312
Vicks DayQuil Mucus Control DM - See
DEXTROMETHORPHAN 312
GUAIFENESIN 416
Vicks DayQuil Mucus Control Liquid - See GUAIFENESIN 416
Vicks DayQuil Sinus LiquiCaps - See
ACETAMINOPHEN 8
PHENYLEPHRINE 658
Vicks Formula 44 Custom Care Body Aches - See ACETAMINOPHEN 8
Vicks Formula 44 Custom Care Chesty Cough - See
DEXTROMETHORPHAN 312
GUAIFENESIN 416
Vicks Formula 44 Custom Care Congestion - See
DEXTROMETHORPHAN 312
PHENYLEPHRINE 658
Vicks Formula 44 Custom Care Cough & Cold PM - See
ACETAMINOPHEN 8
ANTIHISTAMINES 106
DEXTROMETHORPHAN 312
Vicks Formula 44 Custom Care Dry Cough Suppressant - See DEXTROMETHORPHAN 312
Vicks NyQuil Cold & Flu Relief - See
ACETAMINOPHEN 8
ANTIHISTAMINES 106
DEXTROMETHORPHAN 312
Vicks NyQuil Cold & Flu Symptom Relief Plus Vitamin C - See
ACETAMINOPHEN 8
ANTIHISTAMINES 106
DEXTROMETHORPHAN 312
Vicks NyQuil Cough - See
ANTIHISTAMINES 106
DEXTROMETHORPHAN 312
Vicks NyQuil D - See
ACETAMINOPHEN 8
ANTIHISTAMINES 106
DEXTROMETHORPHAN 312
PSEUDOEPHEDRINE 694
Vicks NyQuil Less Drowsy Cold & Flu Relief Liquid - See
ACETAMINOPHEN 8
ANTIHISTAMINES 106
DEXTROMETHORPHAN 312
Vicks NyQuil Sinus LiquiCaps - See
ACETAMINOPHEN 8
ANTIHISTAMINES 106
PHENYLEPHRINE 658

Vicks Pediatric Formula 44e Cough & Chest Congestion Relief - See
DEXTROMETHORPHAN 312
GUAIFENESIN 416
Vicks Pediatric Formula 44m Cough & Cold Relief - See
ANTIHISTAMINES 106
DEXTROMETHORPHAN 312
Vicks Sinex - See PHENYLEPHRINE 658
Vicks Sinex 12-Hour Formula Decongestant Nasal Spray - See OXYMETAZOLINE (Nasal) 630
Vicks Sinex 12-Hour Ultra Fine Mist - See OXYMETAZOLINE (Nasal) 630
Vicks Sinex Nasal Spray - See PHENYLEPHRINE 658
Vicks VapoSyrup Severe Congestion Head & Chest Congestion Relief - See
GUAIFENESIN 416
PHENYLEPHRINE 658
Vicodin - See NARCOTIC ANALGESICS & ACETAMINOPHEN 586
Vicodin ES - See NARCOTIC ANALGESICS & ACETAMINOPHEN 586
Vicodin-Tuss - See
GUAIFENESIN 416
NARCOTIC ANALGESICS 584
Vicoprofen - See
ANTI-INFLAMMATORY DRUGS, NONSTEROIDAL (NSAIDs) 116
NARCOTIC ANALGESICS 584
Victoza - See GLP-1 RECEPTOR AGONISTS 406
Vi-Daylin/F - See VITAMINS & FLUORIDE 848
Videx - See NUCLEOSIDE REVERSE TRANSCRIPTASE INHIBITORS 610
Videx EC - See NUCLEOSIDE REVERSE TRANSCRIPTASE INHIBITORS 610
Vigamox - See ANTIBACTERIALS (Ophthalmic) 66
Viibryd - See VILAZODONE 832
VILAZODONE 832
Vimovo - See
ANTI-INFLAMMATORY DRUGS, NON-STEROIDAL (NSAIDs) 118
PROTON PUMP INHIBITORS 692
Vimpat - See LACOSAMIDE 472
Vincol - See TIOPRONIN 798
Viocase - See PANCRELIPASE 634
Vioform Hydrocortisone Cream - See ANTIBACTERIALS, ANTIFUNGALS (Topical) 62
Vioform Hydrocortisone Lotion - See
ADRENOCORTICOIDS (Topical) 18
ANTIBACTERIALS, ANTIFUNGALS (Topical) 62
Vioform Hydrocortisone Mild Cream - See ANTIBACTERIALS, ANTIFUNGALS (Topical) 62
Vioform Hydrocortisone Mild Ointment - See ANTIBACTERIALS, ANTIFUNGALS (Topical) 62
Vioform Hydrocortisone Ointment - See ANTIBACTERIALS, ANTIFUNGALS (Topical) 62
Vi-Penta F - See VITAMINS & FLUORIDE 848
Viprynium - See ANTHELMINTICS 50
Viracept - See PROTEASE INHIBITORS 688
Viramune - See NON-NUCLEOSIDE REVERSE TRANSCRIPTASE INHIBITORS 608
Viramune XR - See NON-NUCLEOSIDE REVERSE TRANSCRIPTASE INHIBITORS 608
Viranol - See KERATOLYTICS 470
Viranol Ultra - See KERATOLYTICS 470
Viravan DM - See
ANTIHISTAMINES 106
DEXTROMETHORPHAN 312
PHENYLEPHRINE 658
Virazid - See RIBAVIRIN 724
Virazole - See RIBAVIRIN 724
Viread - See NUCLEOTIDE REVERSE TRANSCRIPTASE INHIBITORS 612
Viridium - See PHENAZOPYRIDINE 654
Virilon - See ANDROGENS 34
Virolon IM - See ANDROGENS 34
Viroptic - See ANTIVIRALS (Ophthalmic) 142
Viscerol - See DICYCLOMINE 316
Visine - See DECONGESTANTS (Ophthalmic) 306
Visine L.R. - See DECONGESTANTS (Ophthalmic) 306
Viskazide - See BETA-ADRENERGIC BLOCKING AGENTS & THIAZIDE DIURETICS 184
Visken - See BETA-ADRENERGIC BLOCKING AGENTS 182
Vistacrom - See CROMOLYN 282
Vistaril - See HYDROXYZINE 436
Vitabec 6 - See PYRIDOXINE (Vitamin B-6) 698
VitaCarn - See LEVOCARNITINE 494
Vitalax Super Smooth Sugar Free Orange Flavor - See LAXATIVES, BULK-FORMING 476
Vitalax Unflavored - See LAXATIVES, BULK-FORMING 476
VITAMIN A 834
Vitamin A Acid Cream - See RETINOIDS (Topical) 722
Vitamin A Acid Gel - See RETINOIDS (Topical) 722

INDEX

VITAMIN B-3 - See NIACIN (Vitamin B-3, Nicotinic Acid, Nicotinamide) 596
VITAMIN B-12 (Cyanocobalamin) 836
VITAMIN C (Ascorbic Acid) 838
VITAMIN D 840
VITAMIN D (Topical) 842
VITAMIN E 844
VITAMIN K 846
Vitamin supplement - See
FOLIC ACID (Vitamin B-9) 396
NIACIN (Vitamin B-3, Nicotinic Acid, Nicotinamide) 596
PANTOTHENIC ACID (Vitamin B-5) 636
PYRIDOXINE (Vitamin B-6) 698
RIBOFLAVIN (Vitamin B-2) 726
THIAMINE (Vitamin B-1) 784
VITAMIN A 834
VITAMIN B-12 (Cyanocobalamin) 836
VITAMIN C (Ascorbic Acid) 838
VITAMIN D 840
VITAMIN E 844
VITAMIN K 846
Vitamins and minerals - See VITAMINS & FLUORIDE 848
VITAMINS & FLUORIDE 848
Viterra E - See VITAMIN E 844
Vituz - See
ANTIHISTAMINES 106
NARCOTIC ANALGESICS 584
Vivactil - See ANTIDEPRESSANTS, TRICYCLIC 80
Vivarin - See CAFFEINE 216
Vivelle - See ESTROGENS 372
Vivelle-Dot - See ESTROGENS 372
Vivitrol - See NALTREXONE 582
Vivol - See BENZODIAZEPINES 176
V-Lax - See LAXATIVES, BULK-FORMING 476
Vlemasque - See ANTIACNE, CLEANSING (Topical) 54
Vleminckx Solution - See ANTIACNE, CLEANSING (Topical) 54
Volmax - See BRONCHODILATORS, ADRENERGIC 200
Voltaren - See ANTI-INFLAMMATORY DRUGS, NONSTEROIDAL (NSAIDs) 116
Voltaren Gel - See DICLOFENAC (Topical) 314
Voltaren Ophtha - See ANTI-INFLAMMATORY DRUGS, NONSTEROIDAL (NSAIDs) (Ophthalmic) 120
Voltaren Ophthalmic - See ANTI-INFLAMMATORY DRUGS, NONSTEROIDAL (NSAIDs) (Ophthalmic) 120
Voltaren Rapide - See ANTI-INFLAMMATORY DRUGS, NONSTEROIDAL (NSAIDs) 116
Voltaren SR - See ANTI-INFLAMMATORY DRUGS, NONSTEROIDAL (NSAIDs) 116
Voltaren XR - See ANTI-INFLAMMATORY DRUGS, NONSTEROIDAL (NSAIDs) 116
Voltarol - See ANTI-INFLAMMATORY DRUGS, NONSTEROIDAL (NSAIDs) 116
Voltarol Retard - See ANTI-INFLAMMATORY DRUGS, NONSTEROIDAL (NSAIDs) 116
Vontrol - See DIPHENIDOL 322
VORICONAZOLE - See ANTIFUNGALS, AZOLES 86
VoSol - See ANTIBACTERIALS (Otic) 68
VoSol HC - See ANTIBACTERIALS (Otic) 68
VoSpire ER - See BRONCHODILATORS, ADRENERGIC 200
VP-16 - See ETOPOSIDE 378
Vusion - See ANTIFUNGALS (Topical) 88
Vytorin - See
EZETIMIBE 380
HMG-CoA REDUCTASE INHIBITORS 424
Vyvanse - See AMPHETAMINES 28

W

Wake-Up - See CAFFEINE 216
WARFARIN SODIUM - See ANTICOAGULANTS (Oral) 74
Warfilone - See ANTICOAGULANTS (Oral) 74
Wart-Off Topical Solution - See KERATOLYTICS 470
Wehamine - See ANTIHISTAMINES 106
Wehdryl - See ANTIHISTAMINES 106
Wehdryl-10 - See ANTIHISTAMINES 106
Wehdryl-50 - See ANTIHISTAMINES 106
Wehgen - See ESTROGENS 372
Welchol - See COLESEVELAM 270
Welchol Oral Suspension - See COLESEVELAM 270
Wellbutrin - See BUPROPION 208
Wellbutrin SR - See BUPROPION 208
Wellbutrin XL - See BUPROPION 208
Wellcovorin - See LEUCOVORIN 486
WellPatch Capsaicin Pain Patch - See CAPSAICIN 226
Westcort - See ADRENOCORTICOIDS (Topical) 18
Westhroid - See THYROID HORMONES 792
Wigraine - See
CAFFEINE 216
ERGOT DERIVATIVES 366
Winpred - See ADRENOCORTICOIDS (Systemic) 16
Winstrol - See ANDROGENS 34
Wintrocin - See ERYTHROMYCINS 368
Wolfina - See RAUWOLFIA ALKALOIDS 714

Women's Tylenol Menstrual Relief Caplets - See ACETAMINOPHEN 8
Wygesic - See NARCOTIC ANALGESICS & ACETAMINOPHEN 586
Wymox - See PENICILLINS 646
Wytensin - CENTRAL ALPHA AGONISTS 234

X

Xalatan - See ANTIGLAUCOMA, PROSTAGLANDINS 102
Xalcom - See
ANTIGLAUCOMA, BETA BLOCKERS 96
ANTIGLAUCOMA, PROSTAGLANDINS 102
Xanax - See BENZODIAZEPINES 176
Xanax XR - See BENZODIAZEPINES 176
Xarelto - See FACTOR Xa INHIBITORS 382
Xeljanz - See TOFACITINIB 802
Xeloda - See CAPECITABINE 224
Xenical - See ORLISTAT 622
Xerac BP 5 Gel - See BENZOYL PEROXIDE 178
Xeomin - See BOTULINUM TOXIN TYPE A 196
Xerac BP 10 Gel - See BENZOYL PEROXIDE 178
Xerese Cream - See
ADRENOCORTICOIDS (Topical) 18
ANTIVIRALS (Topical) 144
Xibrom - See ANTI-INFLAMMATORY DRUGS, NONSTEROIDAL (NSAIDs) (Ophthalmic) 120
Xifaxan - See RIFAXIMIN 730
Xodol - See NARCOTIC ANALGESICS & ACETAMINOPHEN 586
Xolegel Gel - See ANTIFUNGALS (Topical) 88
Xopenex - See BRONCHODILATORS, ADRENERGIC 200
Xopenex HFA - See BRONCHODILATORS, ADRENERGIC 200
X-Prep Liquid - See LAXATIVES, STIMULANT 482
X-Seb - See KERATOLYTICS 470
Xylocaine - See
ANESTHETICS (Mucosal-Local) 36
ANESTHETICS (Topical) 40
Xylocaine Viscous - See ANESTHETICS (Mucosal-Local) 36
XYLOMETAZOLINE 850
Xyralid Cream - See
ADRENOCORTICOIDS (Topical) 18
ANESTHETICS (Topical) 40
Xyralid LP Lotion - See
ADRENOCORTICOIDS (Topical) 18
ANESTHETICS (Topical) 40
Xyralid RC - See
ANESTHETICS (Rectal) 38
HYDROCORTISONE (Rectal) 430
Xyzal - See ANTIHISTAMINES, NON-SEDATING 110

Y

Yasmin - See CONTRACEPTIVES, ORAL & SKIN 278
Yaz - See CONTRACEPTIVES, ORAL & SKIN 278
Yodoquinol - See IODOQUINOL 454
Yodoxin - See IODOQUINOL 454

Z

Zaditor - See ANTIALLERGIC AGENTS (Ophthalmic) 56
Zagam - See FLUOROQUINOLONES 392
ZAFIRLUKAST - See LEUKOTRIENE MODIFIERS 488
ZALEPLON 852
Zanaflex - See TIZANIDINE 800
ZANAMIVIR - See ANTIVIRALS FOR INFLUENZA, NEURAMINIDASE INHIBITORS 140
Zantac - See HISTAMINE H_2 RECEPTOR ANTAGONISTS 422
Zantac 75 - See HISTAMINE H_2 RECEPTOR ANTAGONISTS 422
Zantac-C - See HISTAMINE H_2 RECEPTOR ANTAGONISTS 422
Zantac Efferdose - See HISTAMINE H_2 RECEPTOR ANTAGONISTS 422
Zantac Geldose - See HISTAMINE H_2 RECEPTOR ANTAGONISTS 422
Zantryl - See APPETITE SUPPRESSANTS 146
Zapex - See BENZODIAZEPINES 176
Zarontin - See ANTICONVULSANTS, SUCCINIMIDE 78
Zaroxolyn - See DIURETICS, THIAZIDE 338
Zeasorb-AF Powder - See ANTIFUNGALS (Topical) 88
Zebeta - See BETA-ADRENERGIC BLOCKING AGENTS 182
Zebrax - See
BENZODIAZEPINES 176
CLIDINIUM 256
Zecuity - See TRIPTANS 820
Zegerid Capsule - See
PROTON PUMP INHIBITORS 692
SODIUM BICARBONATE 750
Zegerid Chewable Tablets - See
ANTACIDS 48
PROTON PUMP INHIBITORS 692
SODIUM BICARBONATE 750

Zegerid OTC - See
PROTON PUMP INHIBITORS 692
SODIUM BICARBONATE 750
Zegerid Powder - See
PROTON PUMP INHIBITORS 692
SODIUM BICARBONATE 750
Zelepar - See MONOAMINE OXIDASE TYPE B (MAO-B) INHIBITORS 572
Zelnorm - See TEGASEROD 776
Zenpep - See PANCRELIPASE 634
Zentrip - See ANTIHISTAMINES, PIPERAZINE 114
Zephrex-D - See PSEUDOEPHEDRINE 694
Zerit - See NUCLEOSIDE REVERSE TRANSCRIPTASE INHIBITORS 610
Zeroxin-5 Gel - See BENZOYL PEROXIDE 178
Zeroxin-10 Gel - See BENZOYL PEROXIDE 178
Zestoretic - See ANGIOTENSIN-CONVERTING ENZYME (ACE) INHIBITORS & HYDROCHLOROTHIAZIDE 46
Zestril - See ANGIOTENSIN-CONVERTING ENZYME (ACE) INHIBITORS 44
Zetar - See COAL TAR (Topical) 266
Zetar Emulsion - See COAL TAR (Topical) 266
Zetar Medicated Antiseborrheic Shampoo - See COAL TAR (Topical) 266
Zetia - See EZETIMIBE 380
Zetonna - See ADRENOCORTICOIDS (Nasal Inhalation) 12
Zetran - See BENZODIAZEPINES 176
Ziac - See BETA-ADRENERGIC BLOCKING AGENTS & THIAZIDE DIURETICS 184
Ziagen - See NUCLEOSIDE REVERSE TRANSCRIPTASE INHIBITORS 610
Ziana Gel - See
ANTIBACTERIALS FOR ACNE (Topical) 64
RETINOIDS (Topical) 722
ZIDOVUDINE - See NUCLEOSIDE REVERSE TRANSCRIPTASE INHIBITORS 610
Zilactin-L - See ANESTHETICS (Mucosal-Local) 36
ZILEUTON - See LEUKOTRIENE MODIFIERS 488
ZINC ACETATE - See ZINC SUPPLEMENTS 854
ZINC GLUCONATE - See ZINC SUPPLEMENTS 854
ZINC SULFATE - See ZINC SUPPLEMENTS 854
<u>ZINC SUPPLEMENTS</u> 854
Zinc-220 - See ZINC SUPPLEMENTS 854
Zincate - See ZINC SUPPLEMENTS 854
Zincon - See ANTISEBORRHEICS (Topical) 132
Zioptan - See ANTIGLAUCOMA, PROSTAGLANDINS 102
<u>ZIPRASIDONE</u> 856
Zipsor - See ANTI-INFLAMMATORY DRUGS, NONSTEROIDAL (NSAIDs) 116
Zirgan - See ANTIVIRALS (Ophthalmic) 142
Zithromax - See MACROLIDE ANTIBIOTICS 518
Zmax - See MACROLIDE ANTIBIOTICS 518
ZNP - See ANTISEBORRHEICS (Topical) 132
Zocor - See HMG-CoA REDUCTASE INHIBITORS 424
Zoderm - See BENZOYL PEROXIDE 178
Zoderm Ready Pads - See BENZOYL PEROXIDE 178
ZOLEDRONIC ACID - See BISPHOSPHONATES 192
ZOLMITRIPTAN - See TRIPTANS 820
Zoloft - See SELECTIVE SEROTONIN REUPTAKE INHIBITORS (SSRIs) 742
<u>ZOLPIDEM</u> 858
ZolpiMist - See ZOLPIDEM 858
Zometa - See BISPHOSPHONATES 192
Zomig - See TRIPTANS 820
Zomig Nasal Spray - See TRIPTANS 820
Zomig-ZMT - See TRIPTANS 820
Zonalon - See DOXEPIN (Topical) 346
Zonegran - See ZONISAMIDE 860
<u>ZONISAMIDE</u> 860
Zorprin - See ASPIRIN 152
Zostrix - See CAPSAICIN 226
Zostrix-HP - See CAPSAICIN 226
Zostrix Neuropathy Cream - See
ANESTHETICS (Topical) 40
CAPSAICIN 226
Zovia 1/35E - See CONTRACEPTIVES, ORAL & SKIN 278
Zovia 1/50E - See CONTRACEPTIVES, ORAL & SKIN 278
Zovirax - See ANTIVIRALS FOR HERPES VIRUS 136
Zovirax Cream - See ANTIVIRALS (Topical) 144
Zutripro - See
ANTIHISTAMINES 106
NARCOTIC ANALGESICS 584
PSEUDOEPHEDRINE 694
Zyban - See BUPROPION 208
Zyclara - See CONDYLOMA ACUMINATUM AGENTS 276
Zydone - See NARCOTIC ANALGESICS & ACETAMINOPHEN 586
Zyflo CR - See LEUKOTRIENE MODIFIERS 488

Zylet - See
ANTIBACTERIALS (Ophthalmic) 66
ANTI-INFLAMMATORY DRUGS, STEROIDAL (Ophthalmic) 122
Zyloprim - See ANTIGOUT DRUGS 104
Zymar - See ANTIBACTERIALS (Ophthalmic) 66
Zymenol - See LAXATIVES, SOFTENER/ LUBRICANT 480
Zyprexa - See OLANZAPINE 616
Zyprexa Relprevv - See OLANZAPINE 616
Zyprexa Zydis - See OLANZAPINE 616
Zyrtec - See ANTIHISTAMINES, NONSEDATING 110
Zyrtec Allergy - See ANTIHISTAMINES, NONSEDATING 110
Zyrtec Children's Allergy Syrup - See ANTIHISTAMINES, NONSEDATING 110
Zyrtec Children's Chewable - See ANTIHISTAMINES, NONSEDATING 110
Zyrtec Children's Hives Relief Syrup - See ANTIHISTAMINES, NONSEDATING 110
Zyrtec D - See
ANTIHISTAMINES, NONSEDATING 110
PSEUDOEPHEDRINE 694
Zyrtec Eye Drops - See ANTIALLERGIC AGENTS (Ophthalmic) 56
Zytopic Cream - See ADRENOCORTICOIDS (Topical) 18
Zyvox - See LINEZOLID 502

Emergency Guide for Overdose Victims

These are basic steps in recognizing and treating immediate effects of drug overdose.

Take just 5 to 10 seconds to check for a response from the victim. In an adult, check for *normal* breathing. In a child, check for the *presence* or *absence* of breathing (a child may be breathing in a pattern that is not normal, but is adequate).

IF VICTIM IS NOT BREATHING:

Adults and children over age 1:

1. Call 911. The emergency dispatcher can help coach you through CPR (cardiopulmonary resuscitation) until experienced help arrives. If there are other persons available, have one call 911 and one or more persons perform CPR.
2. Begin CPR. Open the victim's airway—tilt the head back and lift chin. Pinch the victim's nose and prepare to give two rescue breaths. Give the first rescue breath (last one second) into his or her mouth. The chest should rise. If it does, give the second breath. If the chest does not rise after the first breath, reopen the airway.
3. Then place your hands on the breastbone in the middle of the chest. Use the heel of both hands (stacked) and push down on the chest 1½ to 2 inches 30 times right between the nipples. Pump hard and fast at the rate of 100/minute (faster than once per second). Let the chest rebound between pumps. For a child ages 1 to 8, use 1 hand or 2 hands as needed to compress the chest one third to one half its depth.
4. Continue with 2 breaths and 30 pumps until victim is breathing or medical help arrives. This ratio is the same for one-person and two-person CPR. In two-person CPR the person pumping the chest stops while the other gives mouth-to-mouth breathing.

Infants under age 1 (excluding newborns):

1. If there are other persons present, have one call 911 and one or more persons begin CPR. If you are alone, perform about 5 cycles or 2 minutes of CPR and then call 911.
2. Begin CPR. Place infant on his or her back. Open the airway—tilt head back and lift chin. Do not tilt the head too far back. Cover the infant's mouth and nose with your mouth. Give 2 small gentle breaths. Each breath should be 1 second long. The infant's chest should rise with each breath.
3. Then place two fingers in the center of the chest just below the nipples. Give 30 gentle chest compressions at the rate of 100 per minute. Press down about one-third the depth of the chest.
4. Continue with 2 breaths and 30 pumps until victim is breathing or medical help arrives. This ratio is the same for one-person and two-person CPR. In two-person CPR the person pumping the chest stops while the other gives mouth-to-mouth breathing.

Note: For all victims, don't try to make the victim vomit. If vomiting does occur, turn the victim's head to the side and try to sweep out or wipe off the vomit. Continue with CPR. Save vomit to take to emergency room for analysis. Take medicine or empty pill bottles with you to emergency room.

IF VICTIM IS UNCONSCIOUS AND BREATHING:

1. Call 911 for medical help.
2. If you are in a location where you can't get emergency help immediately, take victim to the nearest emergency room. Monitor the victim's breathing.
3. Don't try to make victim vomit. If vomiting occurs, save vomit to take to emergency room for analysis.
4. Take medicine or empty pill bottles with you to emergency room.

IF VICTIM IS DROWSY:

1. Call 911 for medical help.
2. If you are in a location where you can't get emergency help immediately, take victim to the nearest emergency room. Monitor the victim's breathing.
3. Don't try to make victim vomit. If vomiting occurs, save vomit to take to emergency room for analysis.
4. Take medicine or empty pill bottles with you to emergency room.

IF VICTIM IS ALERT:

1. Call 911 for medical help or call Poison Control Center–1-800-222-1222 (in the United States) for instructions.
2. If you can't get medical help quickly, take victim to nearest emergency room.
3. Take medicine or empty pill bottles with you to emergency room.

IF VICTIM HAS NO SYMPTOMS, BUT YOU SUSPECT AN OVERDOSE:

1. Call Poison Control Center 1-800-222-1222 (in the United States).
2. Describe the suspect drug with as much information as you can quickly gather. The center will give emergency instructions.
3. Consider calling the victim's doctor or your doctor for instructions.
4. If you have no telephone, take victim to the nearest emergency room.
5. Take medicine or empty pill bottles with you to emergency room.

A note about CPR training: Just about everyone can benefit by taking a certified course in first aid and learn to perform cardiopulmonary resuscitation (CPR). Courses taught by certified instructors are the best way to learn CPR. To find a course in your area, contact:

American Heart Association: 800-242-8721 or check website at www.americanheart.org.

American Red Cross: call the local office or check website at www.redcross.org.

Also, classes are offered in almost every city and town, at YMCAs, civic centers, schools, doctors' offices, and elsewhere.

Emergency Guide for Anaphylaxis Victims

The following are basic steps in recognizing and treating immediate effects of a severe allergic reaction, which is called *anaphylaxis*.

Some people may be highly sensitive to drugs. An anaphylactic reaction to a drug can be life-threatening! Persons suffering these allergic symptoms need immediate emergency treatment!

Symptoms of anaphylaxis:

- **Itching**
- **Rash**
- **Hives**
- **Runny nose**
- **Wheezing**
- **Paleness**
- **Cold sweats**
- **Low blood pressure**
- **Coma**
- **Cardiac arrest**

IF VICTIM IS UNCONSCIOUS AND NOT BREATHING:

1. Call 911. The emergency dispatcher may be able to coach you through CPR until experienced help arrives. If there are other persons available, have one call 911 and one or more persons perform CPR (cardiopulmonary resuscitation).
2. Check to see if the person is carrying special medication (e.g., Epi-Pen or allergy kit) to inject to counter the effects of the allergic attack. If so, inject it if you know how to do so. Avoid oral medication if the person is not breathing.
3. Begin CPR. See instructions 2 through 4 under Emergency Guide for Overdose Victims on page 1088 (2nd previous page).

IF VICTIM IS UNCONSCIOUS AND BREATHING:

1. Call 911 for medical help.
2. Check to see if the person is carrying special medication to inject to counter the effects of the allergic attack. If so, inject it if you know how to do so.
3. Take medicine or empty bottles with you to emergency room for analysis.

IF VICTIM IS CONSCIOUS:

1. Ask the person if he or she is carrying special medication to inhale, swallow or inject to counter the effects of the allergic attack. Help the person use the medication.
2. Give the person an antihistamine pill, if it is available.
3. Encourage the person to breathe slowly and deeply. Stay calm and be reassuring.

DISCLAIMER: The information provided in Emergency Guide for Overdose Victims and Emergency Guide for Anaphylaxis Victims is of a general nature and should not be used as a substitute for professional medical advice, emergency treatment instructions, or formal first aid training. If you think you or a family member may suffer from an allergic or other disease that requires attention, you should discuss it with your health care provider.